Clinical Immunology and Serology

A Laboratory Perspective

FIFTH EDITION

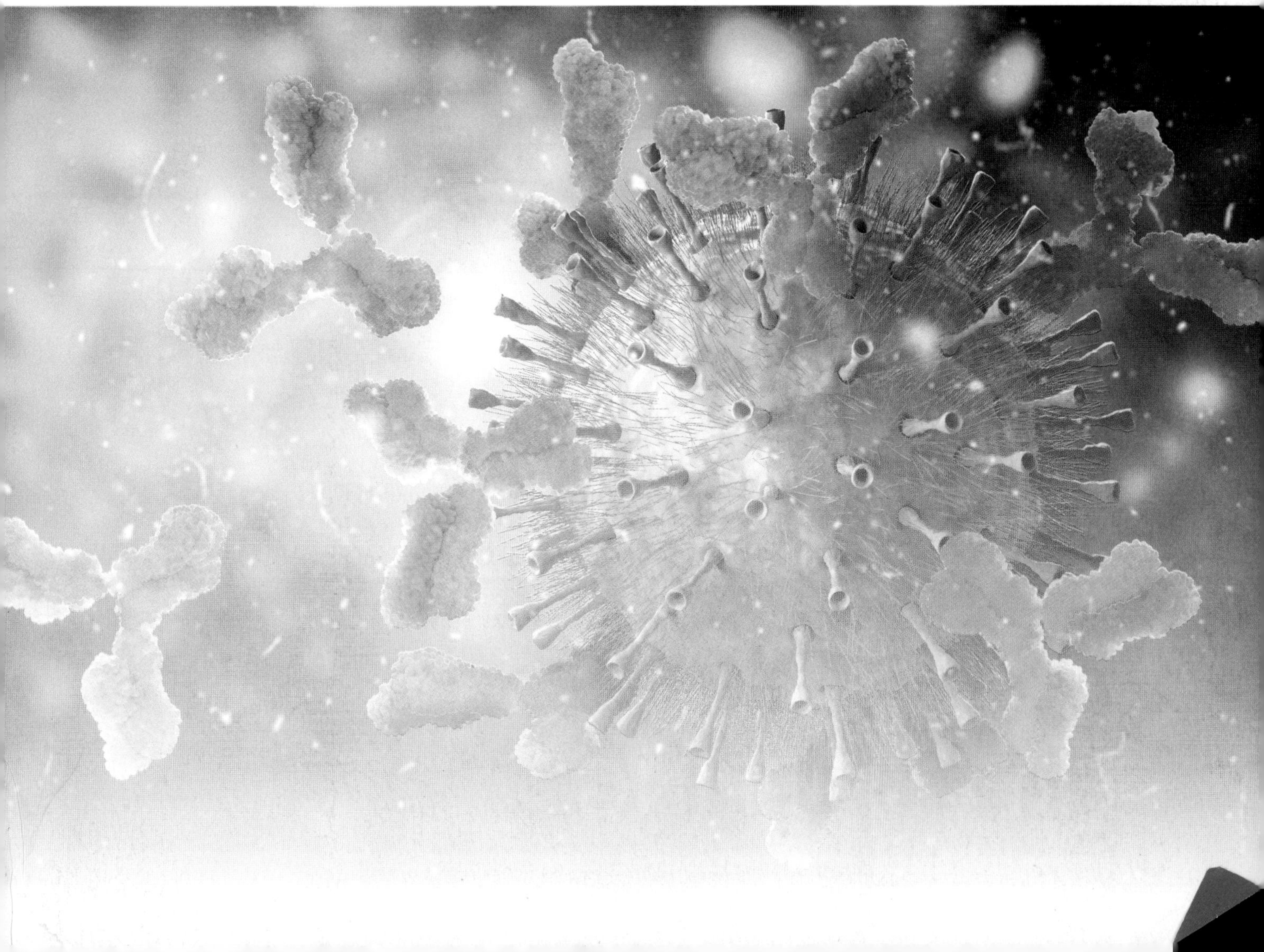

Clinical Immunology and Serology

A Laboratory Perspective

FIFTH EDITION

Linda E. Miller, PhD, I, MB^{CM}(ASCP)SI
Professor of Clinical Laboratory Science
SUNY Upstate Medical University
Syracuse, New York

Christine Dorresteyn Stevens, EdD, MT(ASCP)
Professor Emeritus of Clinical Laboratory Science
Western Carolina University
Cullowhee, North Carolina

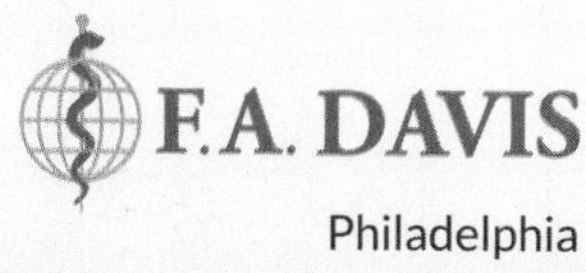

Philadelphia

F.A. Davis Company
1915 Arch Street
Philadelphia, PA 19103
www.fadavis.com

Printed in the United States of America.

Last digit indicates print number: 10 9 8 7 6 5 4 3 2 1

Publisher: Christa Fratantoro
Director of Content Development: George W. Lang
Senior Developmental Editor: Dean W. DeChambeau
Content Project Manager: Julie Chase
Art and Design Manager: Carolyn O'Brien

As new scientific information becomes available through basic and clinical research, recommended treatments and drug therapies undergo changes. The author(s) and publisher have done everything possible to make this book accurate, up-to-date, and in accord with accepted standards at the time of publication. The author(s), editors, and publisher are not responsible for errors or omissions or for consequences from application of the book, and make no warranty, expressed or implied, in regard to the contents of the book. Any practice described in this book should be applied by the reader in accordance with professional standards of care used in regard to the unique circumstances that may apply in each situation. The reader is advised always to check product information (package inserts) for changes and new information regarding dose and contraindications before administering any drug. Caution is especially urged when using new or infrequently ordered drugs.

Library of Congress Cataloging-in-Publication Data

Names: Stevens, Christine Dorresteyn, author. | Miller, Linda E., author.
Title: Clinical immunology and serology : a laboratory perspective / Linda E. Miller, Christine Dorresteyn Stevens.
Description: Fifth edition. | Philadelphia : F.A. Davis Company, [2021] | Christine Dorresteyn Stevens' name appears first in previous editions. | Includes bibliographical references and index.
Identifiers: LCCN 2020046540 (print) | LCCN 2020046541 (ebook) | ISBN 9780803694408 (paperback) | ISBN 9780803694415 (ebook)
Subjects: MESH: Immunity--physiology | Immune System Diseases--diagnosis | Immunologic Techniques | Immunologic Tests | Serologic Tests
Classification: LCC RB46.5 (print) | LCC RB46.5 (ebook) | NLM QW 540 | DDC 616.07/56--dc23
LC record available at https://lccn.loc.gov/2020046540
LC ebook record available at https://lccn.loc.gov/2020046541MILLE

To my wonderful family, for their love and support; to the Clinical Laboratory Science faculty at SUNY Upstate Medical University, in appreciation of their expertise and collegiality; and especially to my students, who have inspired me to share my passion for immunology over the years.

— L.E.M.

To my wonderful family: Eric, Kathy, Hannah, and Matthew, and Kevin, Melissa, Turner, and Avery for their love and encouragement and to Bayard for his love and faith in me.

— C.D.S.

Preface

Clinical Immunology and Serology: A Laboratory Perspective is designed to meet the needs of medical laboratory science students on both the 2- and 4-year levels. It uniquely combines practical information about laboratory testing with a discussion of the theory behind the testing and the diseases for which the tests are used. For practicing laboratorians and other health professionals, the book may serve as a valuable reference about new developments in the field of immunology.

The fifth edition of *Clinical Immunology and Serology: A Laboratory Perspective* is built on the success of the first four editions. The organization of the chapters is based on the experience of many years of teaching immunology to medical laboratory science students. The book is divided into four major sections: I. Nature of the Immune System; II. Basic Immunologic Procedures; III. Immune Disorders; and IV. Serological and Molecular Diagnosis of Infectious Disease. The sections build upon one another, and the chapters relate previous material to new material by means of boxes titled Connections and Clinical Correlations. These features help the students recall information from previous chapters and bridge theory with actual clinical diagnosis and testing. Information in the chapters is related to real-world events to make it more interesting for the student and to show the important role that immunology plays in people's daily lives. The Study Guide Tables at the end of most of the chapters can be used as study tools by the students.

Section I of this edition has been revised to provide a more in-depth discussion on basic immune mechanisms, building a strong foundation for understanding the pathogenesis of diseases related to abnormalities of the immune system. All the chapters in Sections II, III, and IV have been updated to include new information about laboratory testing and treatments for immunologic diseases. For example, information on the Globally Harmonized System and root cause analysis has been added to Chapter 8—Safety and Quality Management. Chapter 9—Principles of Serological Testing—has been revised to include additional examples to help students perform the types of dilutions commonly used in serology. The chapters on Labeled Immunoassays (Chapter 11) and Molecular Diagnostic Techniques (Chapter 12) have been revised to include principles and illustrations for newer technologies that have been incorporated into the clinical laboratory. Additional autoimmune diseases have been added to the chapter on Autoimmunity (Chapter 15). Chapter 18—Immunoproliferative Diseases—has been revised to include updated information on the immunophenotype and cytogenetic abnormalities associated with selected hematologic malignancies. New information on testing for Lyme disease and leptospirosis is presented in Chapter 21—Spirochete Diseases.

The book remains a practical introduction to the field of clinical immunology that combines essential theoretical principles with serological and molecular techniques commonly used in the clinical laboratory. The theory is comprehensive but concise, and the emphasis is on direct application to the clinical laboratory. The text is readable and user-friendly, with learning outcomes, chapter outlines, and a glossary of all key terms. Each chapter is a complete learning module that contains theoretical principles, illustrations, definitions of relevant terminology, and review questions and case studies that help to evaluate learning.

For the instructor, there are many online resources at FADavis.com to assist in course development. Part of this edition was written in the early phases of the COVID-19 pandemic, when many course instructors were forced to convert teaching materials that would normally be presented in the classroom to an online or remote-learning format. The resources provided with this edition can serve as valuable tools to the instructor in developing course materials that can be used not only in in-person teaching but also in online or hybrid learning environments. They include updated PowerPoint slides, suggested learning activities and laboratory exercises, additional case studies, and an expanded bank of test questions that can be used for review or test preparation.

Because the field of immunology continues to grow so rapidly, the challenge in writing this book has been to ensure adequate coverage but to keep it on an introductory level. Every chapter has been revised to include current practices as of the time of writing. It is hoped that this book will kindle an interest in both students and laboratory professionals in this exciting and dynamic field.

Contributors

ART CONSULTANT

Joseph G. Cannon, PhD

Professor and Kellett Chair of Allied Health Sciences
Clinical Laboratory Sciences Program
Augusta University
Augusta, Georgia

CONTRIBUTORS

Thomas S. Alexander, PhD, D(ABMLI)

Immunologist
Summa Health System
Akron, Ohio
Professor of Pathology
Northeast Ohio Medical University
Rootstown, Ohio

Lela Buckingham, PhD, MB(ASCP), DLM(ASCP)

Director, Medical Oncology
Rush Medical Laboratories
Rush University Medical Center
Chicago, Illinois

Marjorie Schaub Di Lorenzo, MT(ASCP)SH

Program Coordinator
Phlebotomy Technician Program
Nebraska Methodist College
Omaha, Nebraska

Bradley Dixon, MD, FASN

Associate Professor of Pediatrics and Medicine
School of Medicine
University of Colorado
Denver, Colorado

Ashley Frazer-Able, PhD, D(ABMLI)

Director, Exsera BioLabs
Assistant Professor
School of Medicine
University of Colorado
Denver, Colorado

Aaron Glass, PhD

Assistant Professor
Department of Clinical Laboratory Science
SUNY Upstate Medical University
Syracuse, New York

Jeannie Guglielmo, MS, MAT, MLS(ASCP)CM

Clinical Assistant Professor
Department of Clinical Laboratory Sciences
Stony Brook University
Stony Brook, New York

Songkai Hu, MA, MLS(ASCP)CM

Dry Reagent Specialist, Flow Cytometry
Beckman Coulter Life Sciences
Los Angeles, California
Clinical Instructor of Flow Cytometry
Stony Brook University
Stony Brook, New York

Paul R. Johnson, PhD, MBA, MT(ASCP), DABCC

Associate Professor
Department of Clinical Laboratory Science
Upstate Medical University
State University of New York
Syracuse, New York

Deborah Josko, PhD, MLT(ASCP)M,SM

Associate Professor and Director
Medical Laboratory Science Program
Clinical Laboratory and Medical Imaging Sciences
Rutgers University–School of Health Professions
Newark, New Jersey

Nadine M. Lerret, PhD, MLS(ASCP)CM

Assistant Professor
Medical Laboratory Science Rush University
Chicago, Illinois

Hamida Nusrat, PhD, PHM(CDPH) SM(ASCP)CM

Faculty, Clinical Laboratory Science Internship Program
San Francisco State University
San Francisco, California
Adjunct Professor
University of California Berkeley
Berkeley, California

John L. Schmitz, PhD, D(ABMLI, ABHI)
Professor
Department of Pathology and Laboratory Medicine
University of North Carolina at Chapel Hill
Chapel Hill, North Carolina

James L. Vossler, MS, MLS^{CM}(ASCP)SM^{CM}
Assistant Professor
Department of Clinical Laboratory Science
SUNY Upstate Medical University
Syracuse, New York

Reviewers

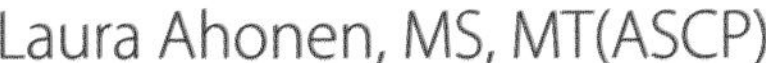

Laura Ahonen, MS, MT(ASCP)
MLT Program Director
School of Health Sciences
Northcentral Technical College
Wausau, Wisconsin

Beverly J. Barham, PhD, MPH, MT(ASCP)
Professor
Health Sciences
Illinois State University
Normal, Illinois

Roger Beckering, MEd, BA, MLT(ASCP)
Faculty MLT/MLS
Brookline College
Phoenix, Arizona

Lisa Ann Blankinship, PhD
Associate Professor
Biology
University of North Alabama
Florence, Alabama

Jimmy L. Boyd, MLS(ASCP), MS/MHS
Department Chair/Program Director
Medical Laboratory Sciences
Arkansas State University–Beebe
Beebe, Arkansas

Lee Ellen Brunson-Sicilia, MHS, MLS(ASCP)^{CM}
Instructor
Clinical Laboratory Science
LSU Health
Shreveport, Louisiana

Grace Leu Burke, MSCLS, MT(ASCP)
Assistant Professor
Medical Laboratory Science
University of Alaska Anchorage
Anchorage, Alaska

Jason Costenbader, MLS(ASCP)
Instructor
Medical Laboratory Technician Program
McCann School of Business and Technology
Allentown, Pennsylvania

Rosemary Duda, MT(ASCP) MS, SM, I
Program Director
Medical Laboratory Science
Franciscan Health Hammond
Hammond, Indiana

Karen Escolas, EdD, MT(ASCP)
Chair/Program Director
Medical Laboratory Technology
Farmingdale State College
Farmingdale, New York

Jackie Frank, MT(ASCP)
Program Director
MLT Program
Pima Medical Institute
Colorado Springs, Colorado

Michele G. Harms, MS, MLS(ASCP)
Program Director
Medical Laboratory Science Program
UPMC Chautauqua WCA Hospital
Jamestown, New York

Virginia Haynes, MS, MLS(ASCP)^{CM}
Program Director
Medical Laboratory Technician
Lake Superior College
Duluth, Minnesota

Lisa Hochstein, MS, MLS(ASCP)
Associate Professor/Program Director
Clinical Health Professions
St. John's University
Queens, New York

Robin M. Hughes, MT(ASCP)
Adjunct Faculty
Clinical Laboratory Technology
St. Louis Community College–Forest Park
St. Louis, Missouri

Marnie Imhoff, MBA, MLS(ASCP)
Assistant Professor
Medical Laboratory Science
University of Nebraska Medical Center
Omaha, Nebraska

Melissa Jamerson, PhD, MLS(ASCP)

Assistant Professor
Clinical Laboratory Sciences
Virginia Commonwealth University
Richmond, Virginia

Ali Jazirehi, CLS, PhD

Associate Professor
Biological Sciences
California State University Los Angeles
Los Angeles, California

Steve Johnson, MS, MT(ASCP)

Program Director
School of Medical Technology
Saint Vincent Hospital
Erie, Pennsylvania

Jennifer Jones, MAEd, MLS(ASCP)

Program Director
Medical Laboratory Technology
Davidson County Community College
Thomasville, North Carolina

Deborah Josko, PhD, MLT(ASCP)M, SM

Associate Professor and Director
Medical Laboratory Science Program
Clinical Laboratory and Medical Imaging Sciences
Rutgers University–School of Health Professions
Newark, New Jersey

Cecelia W. Landin, EdD, MLS(ASCP)^CM^

Clinical Associate Professor
Clinical Laboratory Science
Marquette University
Milwaukee, Wisconsin

Nadine M. Lerret, PhD, MLS(ASCP)^CM^

Assistant Professor
Medical Laboratory Science
Rush University
Chicago, Illinois

Brigitte Morin, MS

Senior Lecturer Biological Sciences
Michigan Technological University
Houghton, Michigan

Hamida Nusrat, PhD, PHM(CDPH), SM(ASCP)^CM^

Faculty, Clinical Laboratory Science Internship Program
San Francisco State University
San Francisco, California
Adjunct Professor, University of California Berkeley
Berkeley, California

Kristen Pesavento, MA, MLS(ASCP)

Manager, MS in Medical Laboratory Science Program
Pathology and Laboratory Medicine
Loyola University Chicago
Maywood, Illinois

Kristina B. Pierce, MS, MLS

Coordinator, Teaching Laboratory
MLS Division, Pathology
University of Utah
Salt Lake City, Utah

Joan Polancic, MSEd, MLS(ASCP)^CM^

Program Director
Denver Health
School of Medical Laboratory Science
Denver, Colorado

Amy L. Raugh, MS, MT(ASCP)

Assistant Professor
Health and Public Service
Harrisburg Area Community College
Harrisburg, Pennsylvania

Karen A. Reiner, PhD, MT(ASCP)

Department Chair
Medical Laboratory Sciences
Andrews University
Berrien Springs, Michigan

Teri J. Ross, MS, MT(ASCP)SBB

Program Director, Phlebotomy; Instructor, Clinical Laboratory Science
School of Allied Health Professions
Loma Linda University
Loma Linda, California

Jo Ellen Russell, MBA, MT(ASCP), RHIT, RMA(AMT)

Director of Medical Technologies (MLT, HIT)
Health Sciences
Panola College
Carthage, Texas

Paul K. Small, PhD

Professor of Biology
Eureka College
Eureka, Illinois

Debra St. George, MS(ASCP)

Department Chair
Clinical Laboratory Science
Bristol Community College
Fall River, Massachusetts

Terri A. Talbot, MHSA, MT(ASCP)
SETH Laboratory Coordinator
Simulation Education
Franciscan Missionaries of Our Lady University
Baton Rouge, Louisiana

Lorraine Torres, EdD, MT(ASCP)
Program Director
Clinical Laboratory Science
The University of Texas at El Paso
El Paso, Texas

Amanda Voelker, MT(ASCP), MPH
Clinical Coordinator, Instructor
Medical Laboratory Sciences
Northern Illinois University
Dekalb, Illinois

Mary Warren, RHIT
Instructor
Medical Billing and Coding
Erwin Technical College
Tampa, Florida

Melissa White, MA, BS
Assistant Professor; MLT Program Director
School of Health Careers
Pierpont Community & Technical College
Fairmont, West Virginia

Stephen M. Wiesner, PhD, MT(ASCP), FACSc
Associate Professor
Center for Allied Health Programs
University of Minnesota
Minneapolis, Minnesota

Reannon Wilkerson, MS, MLS(ASCP)
Medical Laboratory Technician Instructor
Calhoun Community College
Huntsville, Alabama

Robin L. Woodard, PhD, MT(ASCP)
Associate Professor
Natural Sciences
University of Virginia–Wise
Wise, Virginia

Joan M. Young, MT(ASCP), MHA
MLT Program Director
Health Occupations
Southwest Wisconsin Technical College
Fennimore, Wisconsin

Acknowledgments

We are grateful for the assistance we received from many individuals during the preparation of this fifth edition. We would like to express a special appreciation to our chapter contributors, whose expertise enriched this book: Thomas Alexander, Lela Buckingham, Marjorie Di Lorenzo, Bradley Dixon, Ashley Frazer-Able, Aaron Glass, Jeannie Guglielmo, Songkai Hu, Paul Johnson, Deborah Josko, Nadine Lerret, Hamida Nusrat, John Schmitz, and James Vossler.

We would like to acknowledge everyone at F.A. Davis for their hard work in making this book a reality. A special thank-you goes to Christa Fratantoro, publisher for Health Professions, for her innovative ideas for the fifth edition, as well as her patience and encouragement during periods of unanticipated delays in the process. We also appreciate the efforts of Dean DeChambeau, our developmental editor, whose eye for detail was invaluable, and to our content project manager, Julie Chase, for her role in the review process. We extend thanks to Joe Cannon, who changed our ideas into workable full-color illustrations that began with the fourth edition, and to Daniel Domzalski, the illustration coordinator who worked on the figures for this edition. We would also like to thank Kimberly Whiter for her hard work and innovative ideas in revising the online Instructor's Guide and expanding the online test bank that accompany this book. A special thanks goes to Roxanne Klaas, project manager with S4Carlisle Publishing Services, for her efficient coordination of the production of this book. Thanks to George Lang and everyone else behind the scenes at F.A. Davis who helped this book come to life.

Our immunology students—past, present, and future—are the reason for writing this book. We hope that this text will inspire interest in the field of immunology and help to make a very complex subject easier to understand.

Finally, a big thank-you goes to our families, whose support, encouragement, and patience made it possible for us to engage in this labor of love.

Contents

SECTION IV

Nature of the Immune System

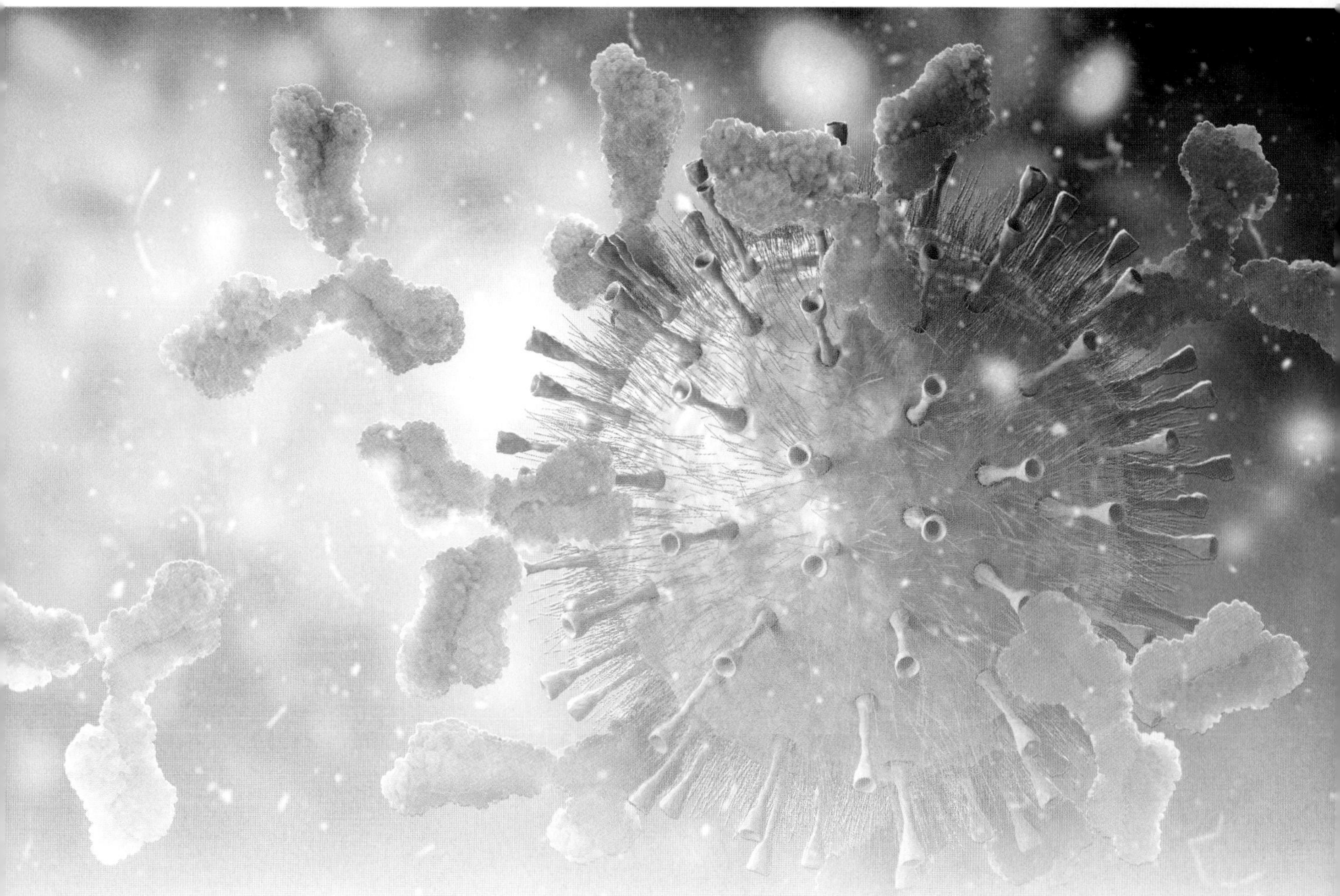

1 Introduction to Immunity and the Immune System

Christine Dorresteyn Stevens, EdD, MT(ASCP)

LEARNING OUTCOMES

After finishing this chapter, you should be able to:

1. Discuss how immunology as a science began with the study of immunity.
2. Describe what is meant by an attenuated vaccine.
3. Explain how the controversy over humoral versus cellular immunity contributed to expanding knowledge in the field of immunology.
4. Contrast innate and adaptive immunity.
5. Describe the types of white blood cells (WBCs) capable of phagocytosis.
6. Discuss the roles of macrophages, mast cells, and dendritic cells in the immune system.
7. Identify the two primary lymphoid organs and discuss the main functions of each.
8. List four secondary lymphoid organs and discuss their overall importance to immunity.
9. Describe the function and architecture of a lymph node.
10. Compare a primary and a secondary follicle.
11. Define "cluster of differentiation" (CD).
12. Differentiate the roles of T cells and B cells in the immune response.
13. Discuss how natural killer (NK) cells differ from T lymphocytes.

CHAPTER OUTLINE

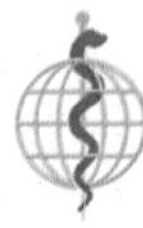

Go to FADavis.com for the laboratory exercises that accompany this text.

KEY TERMS

Adaptive immunity
Antibodies
Antigens
Attenuation
B lymphocytes
Basophils
Bone marrow
Cell-mediated immunity
Chemotaxins
Clusters of differentiation (CD)
Cytokines
Dendritic cells
Diapedesis
Eosinophils
Germinal center
Hematopoiesis
Humoral immunity
Immunity
Immunology
Innate (natural) immunity
Leukocytes
Lymph nodes
Lymphocyte
Macrophages
Mast cells
Memory cells
Monocytes
Natural killer (NK) cells
Neutrophil
Periarteriolar lymphoid sheath (PALS)
Phagocytosis
Plasma cells
Primary follicles
Primary lymphoid organs
Secondary follicles
Secondary lymphoid organs
Spleen
T lymphocytes
Thymocytes
Thymus

Although humans have been trying for centuries to unravel the secrets of preventing disease, the field of immunology is a relatively new science. **Immunology** can be defined as the study of a host's reactions to foreign substances that are introduced into the body. Such foreign substances that induce a host response are called **antigens.** Antigens are all around us in nature. They vary from substances, such as pollen, that may make us sneeze to serious bacterial pathogens, such as *Staphylococcus aureus* or Group A *Streptococcus,* that can cause life-threatening illnesses. The study of immunology has given us the ability to prevent diseases such as smallpox, polio, diphtheria, and measles through the development of vaccines. In addition, understanding how the immune system works has made successful organ transplantation possible and has given us new tools to treat diseases such as cancer and autoimmune diseases. Immunological techniques have affected testing in many areas of the clinical laboratory and allowed for such testing to be more precise and automated. Thus, the study of immunology is important to many areas of medicine. We begin this chapter by providing a brief look at the history of immunology. An introduction to the cells and tissues of the immune system follows to help the student form a basis for understanding how the immune response works. In later chapters, we will apply this knowledge to principles of testing for specific diseases.

Immunity and Immunization

Immunology as a science has its roots in the study of **immunity:** the condition of being resistant to infection. The first recorded attempts to deliberately induce immunity date back to the 15th century when people living in China and Turkey inhaled powder made from smallpox scabs in order to produce protection against this dreaded disease. The hypothesis was that if a healthy individual was exposed as a child or a young adult, the effects of the disease would be minimized. However, rather than providing protection, the early exposure had a fatality rate of 30%. Further refinements did not occur until the late 1700s when an English country doctor by the name of Edward Jenner was able to successfully prevent infection with smallpox by injecting a less harmful substance—cowpox—from a disease affecting cows. Details of the development of this first vaccine can be found in Chapter 25.

The next major development in disease prevention did not occur until almost a hundred years later when Louis Pasteur, often called the "father of immunology," observed by chance that older bacterial cultures accidentally left out on a laboratory bench for the summer would not cause disease when injected into chickens **(Fig. 1–1).** Subsequent injections of more virulent organisms had no effect on the birds that had been previously exposed to the older cultures. In contrast, chickens that were not exposed to the older cultures died after being injected with the new fresh cultures. In this manner, the first attenuated vaccine was discovered; this event can be considered the birth of immunology. **Attenuation,** or change, means to make a pathogen less virulent; it takes place through heat, aging, or chemical means. Attenuation remains the basis for many of the immunizations that are used today. Pasteur applied this same principle of attenuation to the prevention of rabies in exposed individuals. He was thus the first scientist to introduce the concept that vaccination could be applied to any microbial disease.

Innate Versus Adaptive Immunity

In the late 1800s, scientists began to identify the actual mechanisms that produce immunity in a host. Élie Metchnikoff, a Russian scientist, observed under a microscope that foreign objects introduced into transparent starfish larvae became surrounded by motile amoeboid-like cells that attempted to destroy the penetrating objects. This process was later termed **phagocytosis,** meaning "cells that eat cells." He hypothesized that immunity to disease was based on the action of these

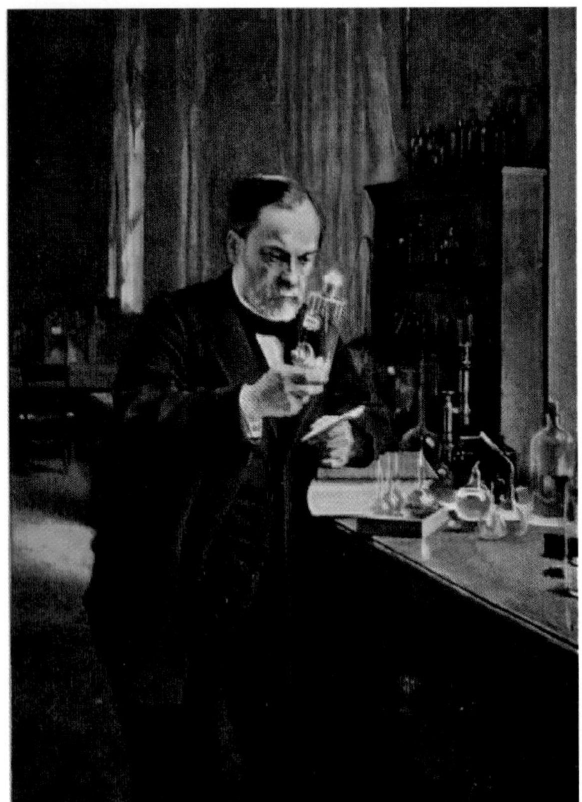

FIGURE 1–1 Louis Pasteur. *(Courtesy of the National Library of Medicine.)*

scavenger cells and was a natural, or innate, host defense. He was eventually awarded a Nobel Prize for his pioneering work.

Other researchers contended that noncellular elements in the blood were responsible for protection from microorganisms. Emil von Behring demonstrated that diphtheria and tetanus toxins, which are produced by specific microorganisms as they grow, could be neutralized by the noncellular portion of the blood, or serum, of animals previously exposed to the microorganisms. Von Behring was awarded the first Nobel Prize in Physiology for his work with serum therapy. The theory of **humoral immunity** was thus born and sparked a long-lasting dispute over the relative importance of cellular immunity versus humoral immunity.

In 1903, an English physician named Almroth Wright linked the two theories by showing that the immune response involved both cellular and humoral elements. He observed that certain humoral, or circulating, factors called *opsonins* acted to coat bacteria so that they became more susceptible to ingestion by phagocytic cells. These serum factors include specific proteins known as *antibodies,* as well as other factors called *acute-phase reactants* that increase nonspecifically in any infection. **Antibodies** are serum proteins produced by certain lymphocytes when exposed to a foreign substance, and they react specifically with that foreign substance (see Chapter 5).

These discoveries showed that there were two major branches of immunity, currently referred to as innate immunity and adaptive immunity. **Innate,** or **natural immunity,** is the individual's ability to resist infection by means of normally present body functions. Innate defenses are considered nonadaptive or nonspecific and are the same for all pathogens or foreign substances to which one is exposed. No prior exposure is required and the response lacks memory and specificity, but the effect is immediate. Many of these mechanisms are subject to influence by such factors as nutrition, age, fatigue, stress, and genetic determinants.

Adaptive immunity, in contrast, is a type of resistance that is characterized by specificity for each individual pathogen, or microbial agent, and the ability to remember a prior exposure. Memory and specificity result in an increased response to that pathogen upon repeated exposure, something that does not occur in innate immunity. Both systems are necessary to maintain good health. In fact, they operate in combination and depend on one another for maximal effectiveness. Certain key cells are considered essential to both systems, and they will be discussed next.

Cells of the Innate Immune System

Leukocytes in Peripheral Blood

White blood cells (WBCs), or **leukocytes,** in the peripheral blood play a key role in both innate and adaptive immunity. Leukocytes defend against invasion by bacteria, viruses, fungi, and other foreign substances. There are five principal types of leukocytes in peripheral blood: neutrophils, eosinophils, basophils, monocytes, and lymphocytes. The first four types are all part of innate immunity. Because lymphocytes are considered part of adaptive immunity, they will be considered in a separate section. Several cell lines that are found in the tissues, namely, mast cells, macrophages, and dendritic cells, will also be discussed in this chapter because they all contribute to the process of immunity.

All blood cells arise from a type of cell called a *hematopoietic stem cell* (HSC). Approximately one and one-half billion WBCs are produced in the bone marrow daily. To form WBCs, the HSC gives rise to two distinct types of precursor cells: common myeloid precursors (CMPs) and common lymphoid precursors (CLPs). CMPs give rise to the WBCs that participate in phagocytosis, which are known as the *myeloid line.* Phagocytic cells are key to innate immunity, but they are also important in processing antigens for the adaptive response. Lymphocytes arise from CLPs and form the basis of the adaptive immune response. Mature lymphocytes are found in the tissues as well as in peripheral blood. Refer to **Figure 1–2** for a simplified scheme of blood cell development, known as **hematopoiesis.**

Neutrophils

The **neutrophil,** or polymorphonuclear neutrophilic (PMN) leukocyte, represents approximately 50% to 70% of the total peripheral WBCs in adults. These cells are around 10 to 15 µm in diameter with a nucleus that has between two and five lobes, which are connected by thin, threadlike filaments **(Fig. 1–3).** Hence, they are often called *segmented neutrophils,* or "segs." They contain a large number of neutral staining granules when stained with Wright stain, two-thirds of which are specific granules; the remaining one-third are called

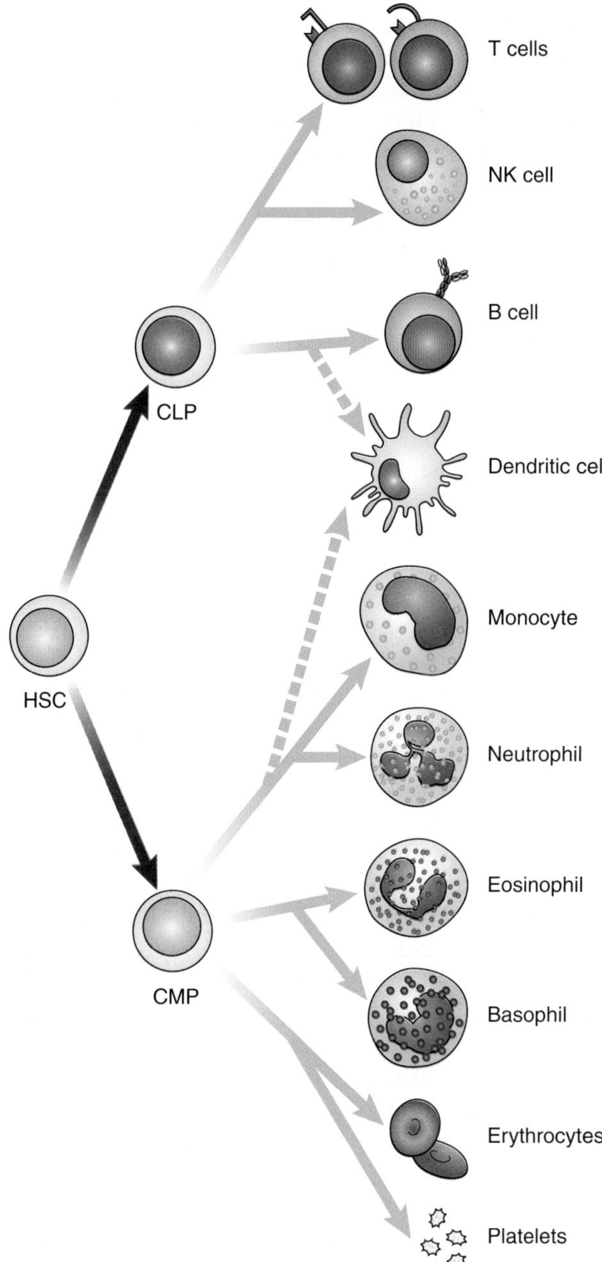

FIGURE 1–2 Simplified scheme of hematopoiesis. In the marrow, HSCs give rise to two different lines—a CLP and a CMP. CLPs give rise to T/NK progenitors, which differentiate into T and NK cells, and to B-cell progenitors, which become B cells and dendritic cells. The CMP differentiates into another type of dendritic cell, monocytes/macrophages, neutrophils, eosinophils, basophils, erythrocytes, and platelets.

azurophilic granules. Azurophilic or primary granules contain antimicrobial products such as myeloperoxidase, lysozyme, elastase, proteinase-3, cathepsin G, and defensins, which are small proteins that have antibacterial activity. Specific granules, also known as *secondary granules*, contain lysozyme, lactoferrin, collagenase, gelatinase, and components essential for the oxidative burst. See Chapter 2 for a discussion of the oxidative burst, which takes place during phagocytosis. The main function of neutrophils is phagocytosis, resulting in the destruction of foreign particles.

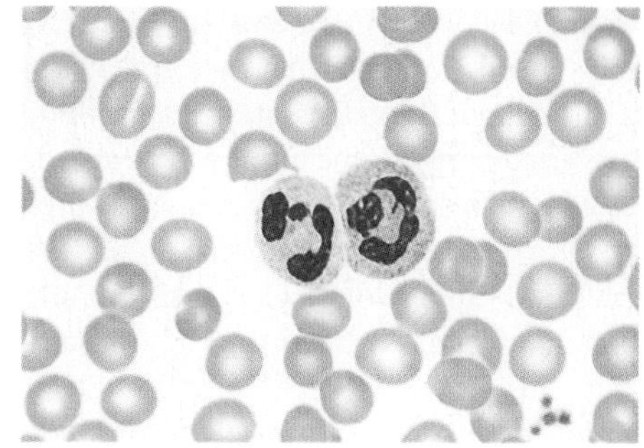

FIGURE 1–3 Neutrophils. (*From Harmening D.* Clinical Hematology and Fundamentals of Hemostasis. *5th ed. Philadelphia, PA: F.A. Davis; 2009: Fig. 1–4.*)

Normally, half of the total neutrophil population in peripheral blood is found in a marginating pool adhering to blood vessel walls, whereas the rest of the neutrophils circulate freely for approximately 6 to 8 hours. There is a continuous interchange, however, between the marginating and the circulating pools. Margination occurs to allow neutrophils to move from the circulating blood to the tissues through a process known as **diapedesis,** or movement through blood vessel walls. They are attracted to a specific area by chemotactic factors. **Chemotaxins** are chemical messengers that cause cells to migrate in a particular direction. Once in the tissues, neutrophils have a life span of up to several days. Normally, the influx of neutrophils from the bone marrow equals the output from the blood to the tissues to maintain a steady state. However, in the case of acute infection, an increase of neutrophils in the circulating blood can occur almost immediately. These cells are then driven rapidly to the site of an infection.

Eosinophils

Eosinophils are approximately 10 to 15 μm in diameter and normally make up between 1% and 4% of the circulating WBCs in a nonallergic person. Their number increases in an allergic reaction or in response to certain parasitic infections. The nucleus is usually bilobed or ellipsoidal and is often eccentrically located **(Fig. 1–4).** Eosinophils take up the acid eosin dye, and

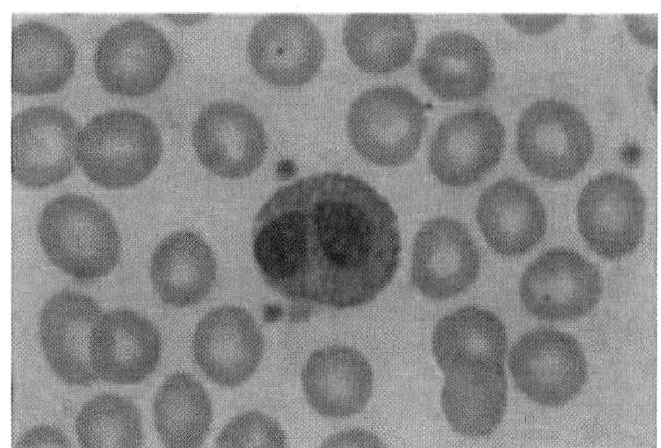

FIGURE 1–4 Eosinophil. (*From Harmening D.* Clinical Hematology and Fundamentals of Hemostasis. *5th ed. Philadelphia, PA: F.A. Davis; 2009: Fig. 1–6.*)

the cytoplasm is filled with large orange to reddish-orange granules. Granules in eosinophils, which are spherical and evenly distributed throughout the cell, contain a large number of previously synthesized proteins, including eosinophil-derived neurotoxin, peroxidase, histamine, proteases, **cytokines** (chemical messengers), growth factors, and cationic proteins.

Eosinophils are capable of phagocytosis but are much less efficient than neutrophils because they are present in smaller numbers and they lack digestive enzymes. Eosinophils are able to neutralize basophil and mast cell products. In addition, they can use cationic proteins released during degranulation to damage cell membranes and kill larger parasites, such as helminth worms, that cannot be phagocytized. (See Chapter 22 for details.) However, the most important role of eosinophils is regulation of the adaptive immune response through cytokine release.

Basophils

Basophils are the least numerous of the WBCs found in peripheral blood, representing less than 1% of all circulating WBCs. The smallest of the granulocytes, basophils are slightly larger than red blood cells (RBCs) (between 10 to 15 μm in diameter) and contain coarse, densely staining deep-bluish-purple granules that often obscure the bilobed nucleus **(Fig. 1–5).** Constituents of these granules include histamine, cytokines, growth factors, and a small amount of heparin, all of which have an important function in inducing and maintaining allergic reactions. Histamine contracts smooth muscle, and heparin is an anticoagulant. In addition, basophils regulate some T-helper (Th) cell responses and stimulate B cells to produce the antibody immunoglobulin E (IgE). Basophils have a short life span of only a few hours in the bloodstream; they are then removed and destroyed by macrophages in the spleen.

Monocytes

Monocytes are the largest cells in the peripheral blood, with a diameter that can vary from 12 to 20 μm (the average is 18 μm). One distinguishing feature of monocytes is an irregularly folded or horseshoe-shaped nucleus that occupies almost one-half of the entire cell's volume **(Fig. 1–6).** The abundant cytoplasm stains a dull grayish blue and has a ground-glass appearance because of the presence of fine, dustlike granules. These granules are actually of two types. The first type contains peroxidase, acid phosphatase, and arylsulfatase, indicating that these granules are similar to the lysosomes of neutrophils. The second type of granule may contain β-glucuronidase, lysozyme, and lipase, but no alkaline phosphatase. Digestive vacuoles may also be observed in the cytoplasm. Monocytes make up between 2% and 10% of total circulating WBCs; however, they do not remain in the circulation for long. They stay in peripheral blood for up to 30 hours; then, they migrate to the tissues and become known as **macrophages**.

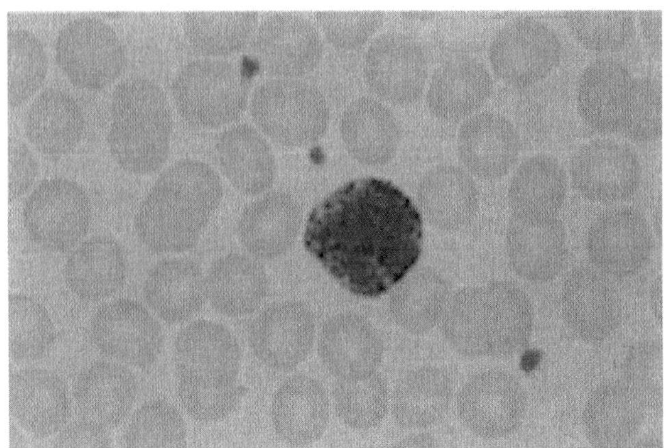

FIGURE 1–5 Basophil. (*From Harmening D.* Clinical Hematology and Fundamentals of Hemostasis. *5th ed. Philadelphia, PA: F.A. Davis; 2009: Fig. 1–7.*)

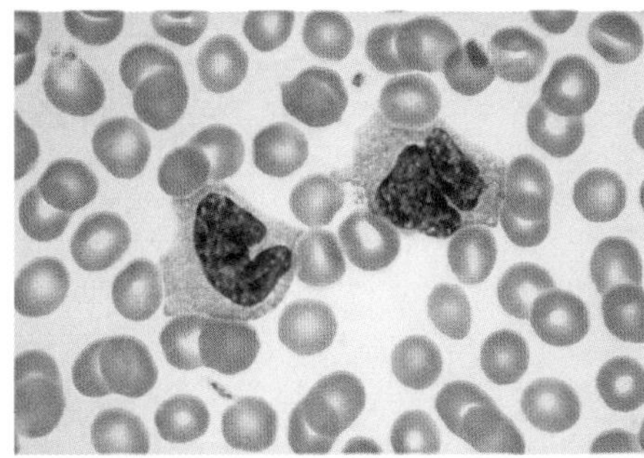

FIGURE 1–6 Two monocytes. (*From Harmening D.* Clinical Hematology and Fundamentals of Hemostasis. *5th ed. Philadelphia, PA: F.A. Davis; 2009: Fig. 1–13.*)

Tissue Cells

Macrophages

All macrophages arise from monocytes, which can be thought of as macrophage precursors, because additional differentiation and cell division take place in the tissues. The transition from monocyte to macrophage in the tissues is characterized by progressive cellular enlargement to between 25 and 80 μm. Unlike monocytes, macrophages contain no peroxidase. Tissue distribution appears to be a random phenomenon.

Macrophages have specific names according to their particular tissue location. Macrophages in the lungs are called *alveolar macrophages*; in the liver, *Kupffer cells*; in the brain, *microglial cells*; in the bone, *osteoclasts*; and in connective tissue, *histiocytes*. Macrophages may not be as efficient as neutrophils in phagocytosis because their motility is slow compared with that of the neutrophils. Some macrophages progress through the tissues by means of amoeboid action, whereas others are immobile. However, their life span appears to be in the range of months rather than days.

Macrophages play an important role in initiating and regulating both innate and adaptive immune responses. Their innate immune functions include phagocytosis, microbial killing, anti-tumor activity, intracellular parasite eradication, and secretion of cell mediators. Killing activity is enhanced when macrophages become "activated" by contact with microorganisms or cytokines that are released by certain lymphocytes during the immune response. (See Chapter 6 for a complete discussion of cytokines.) Macrophages play a major role in the adaptive immune response by presenting phagocytosed antigens to T lymphocytes.

Mast Cells

Tissue **mast cells** resemble basophils, but they come from a different lineage. Mast cells are distributed throughout the body in a wide variety of tissues, such as skin, connective tissue, and the mucosal epithelial tissue of the respiratory, genitourinary, and digestive tracts. Mast cells are larger than basophils, with a diameter of up to 20 μm, and have a small ovoid nucleus with many granules **(Fig. 1–7)**. Unlike basophils, they have a long life span of between 9 and 18 months. The enzyme content of the granules in mast cells helps to distinguish them from basophils because they contain serine proteases, heparin, and neutrophil chemotactic factor, as well as histamine. Mast cells act to increase vascular permeability and increase blood flow to the affected area. Mast cells also play a role in allergic reactions, as well as functioning as antigen-presenting cells (APCs). Because of their versatility, mast cells function as a major conduit between the innate and adaptive immune systems.

Dendritic Cells

Dendritic cells are so named because they are covered with long, membranous extensions that resemble nerve cell dendrites. They were discovered by Steinman and Cohn in 1973. Progenitors in the bone marrow give rise to dendritic cell precursors that travel to lymphoid as well as nonlymphoid tissue. They are classified according to their tissue location in a similar manner to macrophages. After capturing an antigen in the tissue by phagocytosis or endocytosis, dendritic cells travel to the nearest lymph node and present the antigen to T lymphocytes to initiate the adaptive immune response in a similar way as macrophages. Dendritic cells, however, are considered the most effective APC in the body, as well as the most potent phagocytic cell.

Cells of the Adaptive Immune System

The key cell involved in the adaptive immune response is the **lymphocyte.** Lymphocytes represent between 20% and 40% of the circulating WBCs. The typical small lymphocyte is similar in size to RBCs (7 to 10 μm in diameter) and has a large rounded nucleus that may be somewhat indented. The nuclear chromatin is dense and tends to stain a deep blue **(Fig. 1–8)**. Cytoplasm is sparse, containing few organelles and no specific granules, and consists of a narrow ring surrounding the nucleus. The cytoplasm stains a lighter blue. These cells are unique because they arise from an HSC and then are further differentiated in the primary lymphoid organs, namely, the bone marrow and the thymus. Lymphocytes can be divided into three major populations—T cells, B cells, and innate lymphoid cells (of which natural killer [NK] cells are the most prominent type)—based on specific functions and the proteins on their cell surfaces. In the peripheral blood of adults, approximately 10% to 20% of lymphocytes are B cells, 61% to 80% are T cells, and 10% to 15% are NK cells.

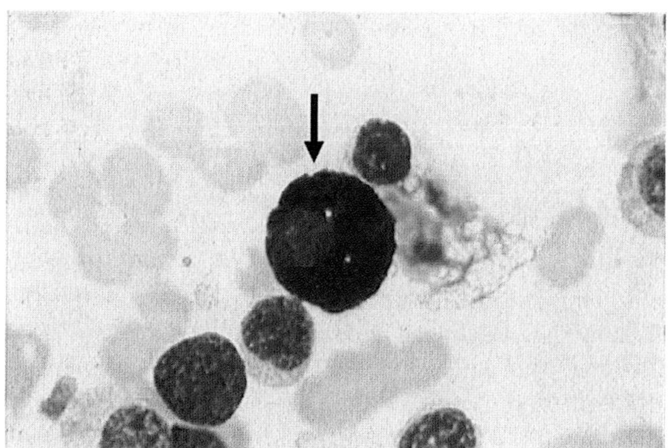

FIGURE 1–7 Mast cell. *(From Harmening D.* Clinical Hematology and Fundamentals of Hemostasis. *5th ed. Philadelphia, PA: F.A. Davis; 2009: Fig. 1–13.)*

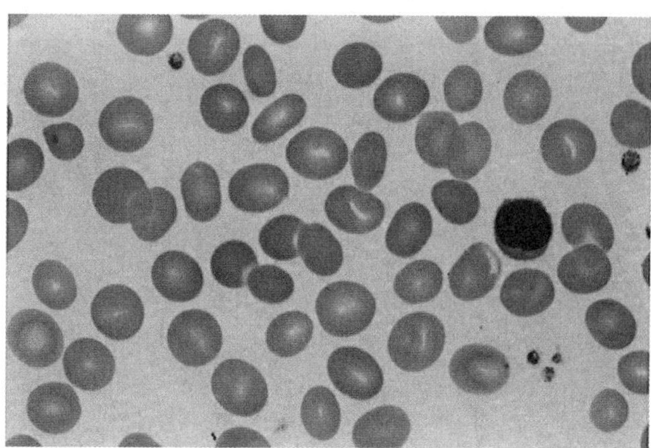

FIGURE 1–8 Typical lymphocyte found in peripheral blood. *(From Harr R.* Clinical Laboratory Science Review. *4th ed. Philadelphia, PA: F.A. Davis; 2013: Color Plate 31.)*

The three types of cells are difficult to distinguish visually. In the laboratory, proteins, or antigens, on cell surfaces can be used to identify each lymphocyte subpopulation. In order to standardize the nomenclature, scientists set up the Human Leukocyte Differentiation Antigens Workshops to relate research findings. Panels of antibodies from different laboratories were used for analysis, and antibodies reacting similarly with standard cell lines were said to define **clusters of differentiation (CD)**. As each antigen, or CD, was found, it was assigned a number. The list of CD designations currently numbers more than 400. **Table 1–1** lists some of the most important CD numbers used to identify lymphocytes.

B Cells and Plasma Cells

B cells are derived from a lymphoid precursor that differentiates to become either a T cell, B cell, or NK cell depending on exposure to different cytokines. B cells remain in the environment provided by bone marrow stromal cells. B-cell precursors go through a developmental process that prepares them for their role in antibody production and, at the same time, restricts the types of antigens to which any one cell can respond. They are able to generate highly specific cell surface receptors through genetic recombination of their immunoglobulin genes (see Chapter 5 for details). The end result

Table 1–1 Surface Markers on T, B, and NK Cells

ANTIGEN	CELL TYPE	FUNCTION
CD3	Thymocytes, T cells	Found on all T cells; associated with T-cell antigen receptor
CD4	Th cells, monocytes, macrophages	Identifies Th cells; also found on most Treg cells
CD8	Thymocyte subsets, Tc cells	Identifies Tc cells
CD16	NK cells, macrophages, neutrophils	Low affinity Fc receptor for antibody; mediates phagocytosis
CD19	B cells, follicular dendritic cells	Part of B-cell coreceptor; regulates B-cell development and activation
CD20	B cells	B-cell activation and proliferation
CD21	B cells, follicular dendritic cells	Receptor for complement component C3d; part of B-cell coreceptor with CD19
CD56	NK cells, subsets of T cells	Cell adhesion

is a **B lymphocyte** programmed to produce a unique antibody molecule. B cells can be recognized by the presence of membrane-bound antibodies of two types, namely, immunoglobulin M (IgM) and immunoglobulin D (IgD). Other surface proteins that appear on the B cell include CD19, CD20, CD21, and class II major histocompatibility complex (MHC) molecules (see Chapter 3).

Plasma cells represent the most fully differentiated B lymphocyte, and their main function is antibody production. They are not normally found in the blood; rather, they are located in germinal centers in the peripheral lymphoid organs or they reside in the bone marrow. Plasma cells are spherical or ellipsoidal cells between 10 and 20 µm in size that are characterized by the presence of abundant cytoplasmic immunoglobulin and little to no surface immunoglobulin (**Fig. 1–9**). The nucleus is eccentric or oval with heavily clumped chromatin that stains darkly. An abundant endoplasmic reticulum and a clear, well-defined Golgi zone are present in the cytoplasm. Plasma cells can be long-lived in lymphoid organs and continually produce antibodies. Antibodies are the major contributor to humoral immunity.

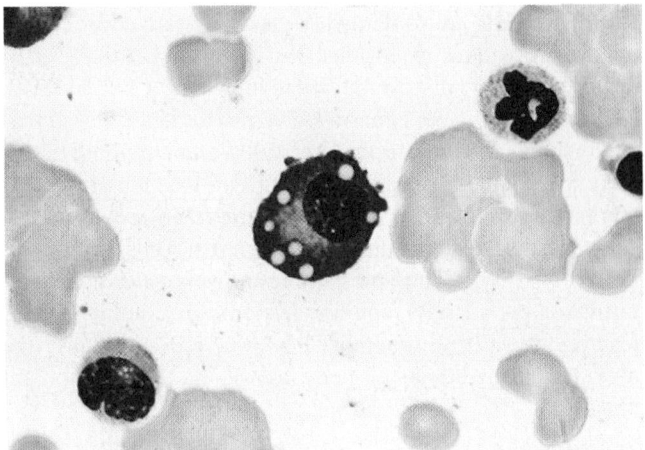

FIGURE 1–9 A typical plasma cell. (*From Harmening D.* Clinical Hematology and Fundamentals of Hemostasis. *5th ed. Philadelphia, PA: F.A. Davis; 2009: Fig. 1–47.*)

T Cells

T lymphocytes are so named because they differentiate in the thymus. Lymphocyte precursors called **thymocytes** enter the thymus from the bone marrow through the bloodstream. As they mature, the T cells express unique surface markers that allow them to recognize foreign antigens bound to cell membrane proteins called *MHC molecules*. T cells have multiple roles in the immune system. They produce cytokines that stimulate B cells to make antibodies, they kill tumor cells and virus-infected cells, and they regulate innate and adaptive immune responses. The processes in which T cells have a primary role are collectively known as **cell-mediated immunity.**

Three main subtypes of T cells can be distinguished according to their unique functions: helper T cells (Th), cytotoxic T cells (Tc), and regulatory T cells (Treg). All T cells possess the CD3 marker on their cell surface, and the T-cell subtypes can be identified by the presence of either CD4 or CD8 as well. T cells bearing the CD4 receptor are mainly either Th or Treg cells, whereas the CD8-positive (CD8+) population consists of Tc cells. The ratio of CD4+ to CD8+ cells is approximately 2:1 in peripheral blood. Th cells help B cells to make antibody, Tc cells kill virally infected cells and tumor cells, and Treg cells help to control the actions of other T cells.

Innate Lymphoid Cells and Natural Killer Cells

The innate lymphoid cells are a family of related cells that have important roles in innate immunity and tissue remodeling. These cells share three main properties: (1) They have a lymphoid morphology, (2) they do not possess antigen-specific receptors, and (3) they do not have myeloid and dendritic cell markers. A principal type of innate lymphoid cell is the **natural killer (NK) cell.** NK cells are so named because they have the ability to kill target cells without prior exposure to them. NK cells do not require the thymus for development but appear to mature in the bone marrow itself. NK cells are generally larger than T cells and B cells, at approximately 15 μm in diameter, and contain kidney-shaped nuclei with condensed chromatin and prominent nucleoli. Described as large granular lymphocytes, NK cells make up 10% to 15% of the circulating lymphoid pool and are found mainly in the liver, spleen, and peripheral blood.

There are no surface markers that are unique to NK cells, but they express a specific combination of antigens that can be used for identification. Two such antigens are CD16 and CD56. CD16 is a receptor for the antigen-nonspecific part of antibody molecules. (See Chapter 5 for more details.) Because of the presence of CD16, NK cells are able to make contact with and then lyse any cell coated with antibodies (see Chapter 2). NK cells continuously scan for protein irregularities on host cells, and they represent the first line of defense against virally infected cells and tumor cells. NK cells are also capable of recognizing foreign cells and destroying them. Granules found in NK cells contain serine proteases called *granzymes*, and release of these enzymes causes target cell death.

Although NK cells have traditionally been considered part of the innate immune system because they can respond to a variety of antigens, they are thought to play an important role as a transitional cell that bridges the innate and the adaptive immune responses against pathogens.

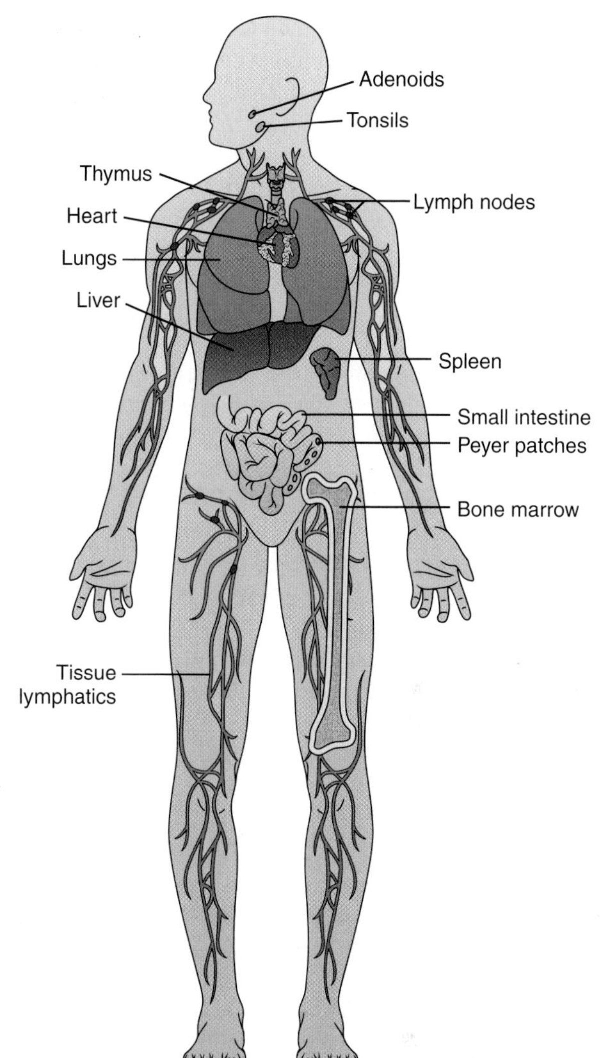

FIGURE 1–10 Sites of lymphoreticular tissue. Primary organs include the bone marrow and the thymus. Secondary organs are distributed throughout the body and include the spleen, lymph nodes, and MALT. The spleen filters antigens in the blood, whereas the lymphatic system filters fluid from the tissues.

Organs of the Immune System

Just as the cells of the immune system have diverse functions, so, too, do key organs that are involved in the development of the immune response. The bone marrow and thymus are considered the **primary lymphoid organs** where maturation of B lymphocytes and T lymphocytes takes place, respectively. The secondary lymphoid organs provide a location where contact with foreign antigens can occur **(Fig. 1–10). Secondary lymphoid organs** include the spleen, lymph nodes, and various types of mucosal-associated lymphoid tissues (MALT). The primary and secondary organs are differentiated according to their function in both adaptive and innate immunity.

Primary Lymphoid Organs

Bone Marrow

Bone marrow is considered one of the largest tissues in the body, and it fills the core of all long flat bones. It is the main source of HSCs, which develop into erythrocytes, granulocytes, monocytes, platelets, and lymphocytes. Each of these lines has specific precursors that originate from the pluripotent stem cells.

Some lymphocyte precursors remain in the marrow to mature and become NK cells or B cells. B cells received their name because they were originally found to mature in birds in an organ called the *bursa of Fabricius,* which is similar to the appendix in humans. After searching for such an organ in humans, it was discovered that B-cell maturation takes place within the bone marrow itself. Thus, the naming of these cells was appropriate. Other lymphocyte precursors go to the thymus and develop into T cells, so named because of where they mature. Immature T cells appear in the fetus as early as 8 weeks in the gestational period. Thus, differentiation of lymphocytes appears to take place very early in fetal development and is essential to acquisition of immunocompetence by the time the infant is born.

Thymus

T cells develop their identifying characteristics in the **thymus,** which is a small, flat, bilobed organ found in the thorax, or chest cavity, right below the thyroid gland and overlying the heart. In humans, the thymus reaches a weight of 30 to 40 g by puberty and then gradually shrinks in size. It was first thought that the thymus produces enough virgin T lymphocytes early in life to seed the entire immune system, making the organ unnecessary later on. However, it now appears that although the thymus diminishes in size as humans age, it is still capable of producing T lymphocytes, although at a reduced rate.

Each lobe of the thymus is divided into smaller lobules filled with epithelial cells that play a central role in the differentiation process. Maturation of T cells takes place during a 3-week period as cells filter through the thymic cortex to the medulla. Different surface antigens are expressed as T cells mature. In this manner, a repertoire of T cells is created to protect the body from foreign invaders. Mature T lymphocytes are then released from the medulla.

Secondary Lymphoid Organs

Once lymphocytes mature in the primary organs, they are released and make their way to secondary lymphoid organs, which include the spleen, lymph nodes, cutaneous-associated lymphoid tissue (CALT), and MALT in the respiratory, gastrointestinal, and urogenital tracts. It is within these secondary organs that the main contact with foreign antigens takes place. Lymphocyte circulation between the secondary organs is complex and is regulated by different cell surface adhesion molecules and by cytokines.

Each lymphocyte spends most of its life span in solid tissue, entering the circulation only periodically to go from one secondary lymphoid organ to another. Lymphocytes in these organs travel through the tissue and then return to the bloodstream by way of the thoracic duct. The thoracic duct is the largest lymphatic vessel in the body. It collects most of the body's lymph fluid and empties it into the left subclavian vein. The majority of circulating lymphocytes are T cells. Continuous recirculation increases the likelihood of a T lymphocyte coming into contact with the specific antigen with which it can react.

Lymphocytes are segregated within the secondary lymphoid organs according to their particular functions. T lymphocytes are effector cells that serve a regulatory role, whereas B lymphocytes produce antibodies. It is in the secondary lymphoid organs that contact of the B and T lymphocytes with foreign antigens is most likely to take place.

Lymphopoiesis, or multiplication of lymphocytes, occurs in the secondary lymphoid tissues and is strictly dependent on antigenic stimulation. Formation of lymphocytes in the bone marrow, however, is antigen-independent, meaning that lymphocytes are constantly being produced without the presence of specific antigens. Most naïve or resting lymphocytes die within a few days after leaving the primary lymphoid organs unless activated by the presence of a specific foreign antigen. Antigen activation gives rise to long-lived memory cells and shorter-lived effector cells that are responsible for the generation of the immune response.

Spleen

The **spleen,** the largest secondary lymphoid organ, has a length of approximately 12 cm and weighs 150 g in the adult. It is located in the upper-left quadrant of the abdomen just below the diaphragm and is surrounded by a thin capsule of connective tissue. The organ can be characterized as a large discriminating filter, as it removes old and damaged cells and foreign antigens from the blood.

Splenic tissue can be divided into two main types: red pulp and white pulp. The red pulp makes up more than one-half of the total volume, and it is rich in macrophages. The major function of the red pulp is to destroy old RBCs, platelets, and some pathogens. Blood flows from the arterioles into the red pulp and then exits by way of the splenic vein. The white pulp comprises approximately 20% of the total weight of the spleen and contains the lymphoid tissue, which is arranged around arterioles in a **periarteriolar lymphoid sheath (PALS) (Fig. 1–11).** This sheath contains mainly T cells. Attached to the sheath are **primary follicles,** which contain B cells that are not yet stimulated by antigens. Surrounding the PALS is a marginal zone containing dendritic cells that trap antigens. Lymphocytes enter and leave this area by means of the many capillary branches that connect to the arterioles. The spleen receives a blood volume of approximately 350 mL/minute, which allows lymphocytes and macrophages to constantly survey for infectious agents or other foreign matter.

Lymph Nodes

Lymph nodes serve as central collecting points for lymph fluid from adjacent tissues. Lymph fluid is a filtrate of the blood and arises from the passage of water and low-molecular-weight

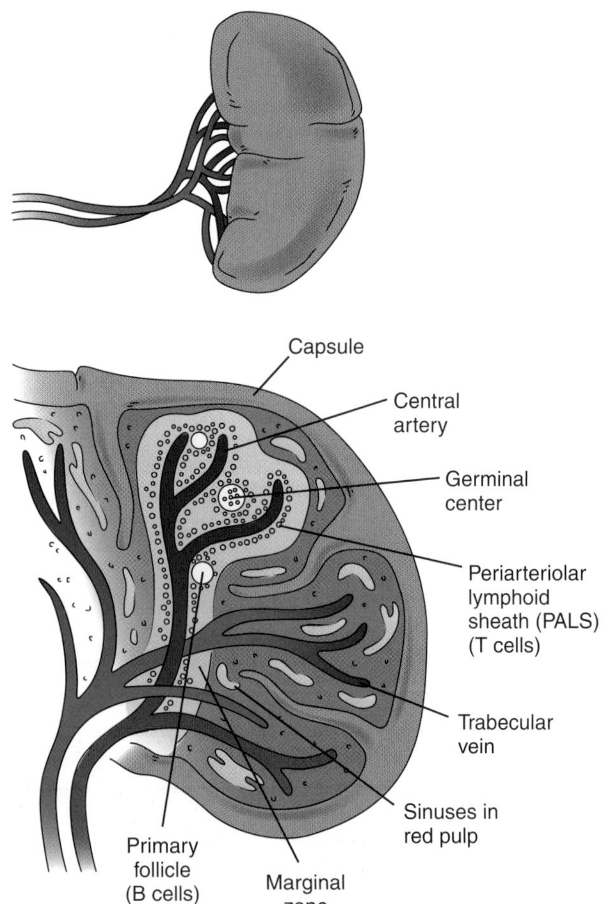

FIGURE 1–11 Cross-section of the spleen showing organization of the lymphoid tissue. T cells surround arterioles in the PALS. B cells are just beyond in follicles. When stimulated by antigens, the B cells form germinal centers. All the lymphoid tissue is referred to as the *white pulp*.

solutes out of blood vessel walls and into the interstitial spaces between cells. Some of this interstitial fluid returns to the bloodstream through venules, but a portion flows through the tissues and is eventually collected in thin-walled vessels known as *lymphatic vessels*. Lymph nodes are located along lymphatic ducts and are especially numerous near the joints and where the arms and legs join the body (see Fig. 1–10).

Filtration of interstitial fluid from around cells in the tissues is an important function of these organs because it allows contact between lymphocytes and foreign antigens from the tissues to take place. Whereas the spleen helps to protect us from foreign antigens in the blood, the lymph nodes provide the ideal environment for contact with foreign antigens that have penetrated into the tissues. The lymph fluid flows slowly through spaces called *sinuses*, which are lined with macrophages, creating an ideal location where phagocytosis can take place. The node tissue is organized into an outer cortex, a paracortex, and an inner medulla **(Fig. 1–12).**

Lymphocytes and any foreign antigens present enter nodes via afferent lymphatic vessels. Numerous lymphocytes also enter the nodes from the bloodstream by means of specialized venules called *high endothelial venules*, which are located in the paracortical areas of the node tissues. The outermost layer, the cortex, contains macrophages and aggregations of B cells in primary follicles similar to those found in the spleen. These are the mature, resting B cells that have not yet been exposed to antigens. Specialized cells called *follicular dendritic cells* are also located here. These cells exhibit a large number of receptors for antibodies and help to capture antigens to present to T cells and B cells.

Secondary follicles consist of antigen-stimulated proliferating B cells. The interior of a secondary follicle is known as the **germinal center** because it is here that transformation of the B cells takes place. When exposed to an antigen, plasma cells (see Fig. 1–9), which actively secrete antibodies, and **memory cells**, which can quickly develop into plasma cells, are formed. Thus, the lymph nodes provide an ideal environment for the generation of B-cell memory, or the ability of the immune system to react more quickly to a foreign substance it has already encountered in the past.

T lymphocytes are mainly localized in the paracortex, the region between the follicles and the medulla. T lymphocytes are in close proximity to APCs called *interdigitating cells*. The medulla is less densely populated than the cortex but contains some T cells (in addition to B cells), macrophages, and numerous plasma cells.

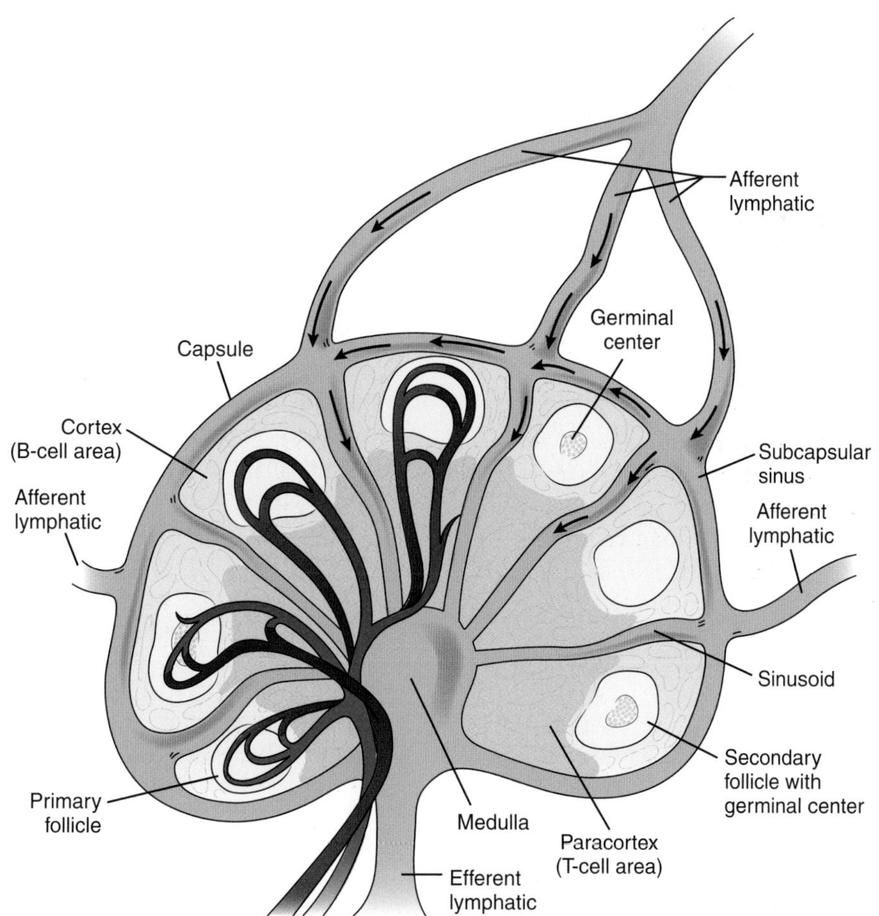

FIGURE 1–12 Structure of a lymph node. A lymph node is surrounded by a fibrous outer capsule. Right underneath is the subcapsular sinus, where lymph fluid drains from afferent lymphatic vessels. The outer cortex contains collections of B cells in primary follicles. When stimulated by antigens, secondary follicles are formed. T cells are found in the paracortical area. Fluid drains slowly through sinusoids to the medullary region and out the efferent lymphatic vessel to the thoracic duct.

Particulate antigens are removed from the fluid as it travels across the node from cortex to medulla. Fluid and lymphocytes exit by way of the efferent lymphatic vessels. Such vessels form a larger duct that eventually connects with the thoracic duct and the venous system. Therefore, lymphocytes are able to recirculate continuously between lymph nodes and the peripheral blood.

If contact with an antigen takes place, lymphocyte traffic shuts down. Lymphocytes able to respond to a particular antigen proliferate in the node. Accumulation of lymphocytes and other cells causes the lymph nodes to become enlarged, a condition known as *lymphadenopathy.* As lymphocyte traffic resumes, recirculation of expanded numbers of lymphocytes occurs.

Other Secondary Organs

Additional areas of lymphoid tissue include the mucosal-associated tissue known as *MALT*. MALT is found in the gastrointestinal, respiratory, and urogenital tracts. Some examples include the tonsils; appendix; and Peyer's patches, a specialized type of MALT located at the lower ileum of the intestinal tract. These mucosal surfaces represent some of the main ports of entry for foreign antigens, and thus, numerous macrophages and lymphocytes are localized here.

The skin is considered the largest organ in the body, and the epidermis contains several intraepidermal lymphocytes. Most of these are T cells, which are uniquely positioned to combat any antigens that enter through the skin. In addition, monocytes, macrophages, and dendritic cells are found here. The collective term for these cells is the *CALT* (cutaneous-associated lymphoid tissue).

All these secondary organs function as potential sites for contact with foreign antigens, and they increase the probability of an immune response. Within each of these secondary organs, T and B cells are segregated and perform specialized functions. B cells differentiate into memory cells and plasma cells and are responsible for humoral immunity or antibody formation. T cells play a role in cell-mediated immunity; as such, they produce sensitized lymphocytes that secrete cytokines. As we discussed, both cell-mediated immunity and humoral immunity are key components of the adaptive immune response.

SUMMARY

- Immunology has its roots in the study of immunity—the condition of being resistant to disease.
- Edward Jenner performed the first vaccination against smallpox by using material from cowpox lesions.
- Louis Pasteur is considered the father of immunology for his use of attenuated vaccines.
- Élie Metchnikoff was the first to observe phagocytosis, the process by which cells eat other cells.
- Immunity has two branches: innate and adaptive. Innate immunity is the ability of the body to resist infection through means of preexisting barriers or nonspecific mechanisms that can be activated quickly. Adaptive immunity is characterized by specificity for antigen, memory, and dependence upon lymphocytes.
- There are two main types of adaptive immune responses: (1) humoral immunity, which involves production of antibodies by B lymphocytes and plasma cells, and (2) cell-mediated immunity, which is carried out by T lymphocytes to destroy internal pathogens.
- All blood cells arise from multipotent HSCs in the bone marrow during a process called *hematopoiesis*.
- The five principal types of leukocytes are neutrophils, eosinophils, basophils, monocytes, and lymphocytes.
- Tissue cells involved in immunity include mast cells, dendritic cells, and macrophages that arise from monocytes.
- Cells that are involved in the innate immune response and are actively phagocytic include neutrophils, monocytes, macrophages, and dendritic cells.
- Lymphocytes are the key cells involved in the adaptive immune response because they have antigen-specific receptors.
- *CD* stands for "clusters of differentiation," which are proteins found on cell surfaces that can be used for identification of specific cell types and stages of differentiation.
- B cells are a type of lymphocyte that develop in the bone marrow and are capable of secreting antibody when they mature into plasma cells. They can be identified by the presence of CD19, CD20, and surface antibody.
- T cells acquire their specificity in the thymus and consist of two subtypes: CD4+, which are mainly Th or Treg cells, and CD8+, which are Tc cells. The CD3 marker is present on all T-cell subtypes.
- NK cells are lymphocytes that arise from a lymphocyte precursor but do not develop in the thymus. NK cells can kill virally infected or cancerous target cells without previous exposure to them.
- In humans, the bone marrow and the thymus are considered the primary lymphoid organs where lymphocytes mature. B cells remain in the bone marrow to mature, whereas T cells develop their specific characteristics in the thymus.
- The secondary lymphoid organs are the sites in which lymphocytes come into contact with foreign antigens and become activated in the adaptive immune response. Secondary lymphoid organs include the spleen, lymph nodes, MALT, and CALT.

Study Guide: Cells of the Immune System

CELL TYPE	WHERE FOUND	FUNCTION
Neutrophils	50%–70% of circulating WBCs, also in tissue	First responders to infection, phagocytosis
Eosinophils	1%–4% of circulating WBCs	Kill parasites, neutralize basophil and mast cell products, regulate mast cells
Basophils	Less than 1% of circulating WBCs	Produce inflammatory mediators that induce and maintain allergic reactions
Mast cells	Skin, connective tissue, mucosal epithelium	Produce inflammatory mediators that induce and maintain allergic reactions
Monocytes	2%–10% of circulating WBCs	Phagocytosis; migrate to tissues to become macrophages
Macrophages	Lungs, liver, brain, bone, connective tissue, other tissues	Phagocytosis; kill intracellular parasites; tumoricidal activity; antigen presentation to T cells
Dendritic cells	Skin, mucous membranes, heart, lungs, liver, kidney, other tissues	Most potent type of phagocytic cell; most effective at antigen presentation
Lymphocytes	20%–40% of circulating WBCs; also found in lymph nodes, spleen, other secondary lymphoid organs	Key cells in adaptive immune responses. Major types are T cells, B cells, and NK cells.

(continued)

Study Guide: Cells of the Immune System—cont'd

CELL TYPE	WHERE FOUND	FUNCTION
B lymphocytes	Develop in bone marrow and migrate to secondary lymphoid organs. Found in peripheral blood and follicles in lymph nodes and spleen	Key role in humoral immune response. Possess antibody receptors that bind to specific antigen. Mature into plasma cells.
Plasma cell	Bone marrow; germinal centers in secondary lymphoid organs	Secrete antibodies into blood and other body fluids
T lymphocytes	Mature in thymus. Also found in peripheral blood and secondary lymphoid organs. Located in paracortex in lymph nodes and PALS in spleen.	Key role in cell-mediated immunity. Different subtypes produce cytokines that help or suppress adaptive and innate immune responses.
NK cells	Develop in bone marrow. Found in peripheral blood, liver, and spleen.	Kill target cells such as tumors or virus-infected host cells without prior exposure

Comparison of T Cells, B Cells, and NK Cells

T CELLS	B CELLS	NK CELLS
Develop in the thymus	Develop in the bone marrow	Develop in the bone marrow
Found in lymph nodes, thoracic duct fluid 60%–80% of circulating lymphocytes in blood	Found in bone marrow, spleen, lymph nodes; 10%–20% of circulating lymphocytes in blood	Found in spleen, liver; 10%–15% of circulating lymphoid cells in blood
Adaptive immunity: end products of activation are cytokines	Adaptive immunity: end product of activation is antibody	Bridge innate and adaptive immunity: lysis of virally infected cells and tumor cells
Antigens include CD2, CD3, CD4, and CD8	Antigens include CD19, CD20, CD21, surface antibody	Antigens include CD16, CD56

Primary and Secondary Lymphoid Organs

LYMPHOID ORGAN CATEGORY	ORGANS INVOLVED	FUNCTION
Primary	Bone marrow	Produces HSCs; maturation of B cells and NK cells
	Thymus	Maturation of T cells
Secondary		Places where contact between T cells, B cells, and antigens occur
	Spleen	Filters blood
	Lymph nodes	Filter lymphatic fluid
	MALT CALT	Protects mucosal surfaces Prevents antigens from penetrating the skin

CASE STUDIES

1. A 13-year-old girl had her ears pierced at a small jewelry store in a mall. Although she was instructed to clean the area around the earrings with alcohol, she forgot to do so for the first 2 days. On the third day, she noticed that the area around one earlobe was red and slightly swollen.

Questions

a. Are the girl's symptoms most likely caused by innate immunity or adaptive immunity?
b. What types of cells would you expect to see in the affected earlobe tissue?

2. You and a friend are discussing the relative merits of immunizations. Your friend says that he doesn't want to get a tetanus booster shot because he has a good immune system and his natural defenses will take care of any possible infection. You have just been studying this subject in your immunology class.

Questions

a. What argument could you make to convince him that a tetanus booster is a good idea?
b. What would you tell him about the types of cells involved in the response to a vaccine?

REVIEW QUESTIONS

1. Pasteur's discovery of attenuated vaccines is based on which of the following principles?
   a. Attenuated vaccines mainly stimulate the innate immune system.
   b. Attenuated vaccines usually cause severe disease.
   c. Attenuated pathogens are changed to become less virulent.
   d. Attenuated pathogens are stronger than unchanged ones.

2. Which WBC is capable of further differentiation in tissues?
   a. Neutrophil
   b. Eosinophil
   c. Basophil
   d. Monocyte

3. The cells that Metchnikoff first observed are associated with which phenomenon?
   a. Innate immunity
   b. Adaptive immunity
   c. Humoral immunity
   d. Specific immunity

4. Where are all undifferentiated lymphocytes made?
   a. Bone marrow
   b. Spleen
   c. Thymus
   d. Lymph nodes

5. How do NK cells differ from T cells?
   a. NK cells are better at phagocytosis than T cells.
   b. NK cells require the thymus for development, and T cells do not.
   c. Only NK cells are found in lymph nodes.
   d. Only NK cells are able to kill target cells without prior exposure to them.

6. Which cell is the most potent phagocytic cell in the tissue?
   a. Neutrophil
   b. Dendritic cell
   c. Eosinophil
   d. Basophil

7. The ability of an individual to resist infection by means of normally present body functions is called
   a. innate immunity.
   b. humoral immunity.
   c. adaptive immunity.
   d. cross-immunity.

8. A cell characterized by a nucleus with two to five lobes, a diameter of 10 to 15 µm, and a large number of neutral-staining granules is identified as a(n)
   a. eosinophil.
   b. monocyte.
   c. basophil.
   d. neutrophil.

9. Which of the following is a primary lymphoid organ?
   a. Lymph node
   b. Spleen
   c. Thymus
   d. MALT

10. What type of cells would be found in a primary follicle?
    a. Unstimulated B cells
    b. Germinal centers
    c. Plasma cells
    d. Memory cells

11. Which of the following is a distinguishing feature of B cells?
    a. Act as helper cells
    b. Presence of surface antibody
    c. Able to kill target cells without prior exposure
    d. Active in phagocytosis

12. Where do lymphocytes mainly come in contact with antigens?
    a. Secondary lymphoid organs
    b. Bloodstream
    c. Bone marrow
    d. Thymus

13. Which of the following is found on the T-cell subset known as *helpers*?
    a. CD19
    b. CD4
    c. CD8
    d. CD56

14. Which of the following statements best characterizes adaptive immunity?
    a. Relies on normally present body functions
    b. Response is similar for each exposure
    c. Specificity for each individual pathogen
    d. Involves only cellular immunity

15. The main function of T cells in the immune response is to
    a. produce cytokines that regulate both innate and adaptive immunity.
    b. produce antibodies.
    c. participate actively in phagocytosis.
    d. respond to target cells without prior exposure.

16. Which of the following is a function of antibodies?
    a. Phagocytosis
    b. Neutralization of bacterial toxins
    c. Recruitment of macrophages
    d. Activation of T cells

17. Immunity can be defined as
    a. the study of medicines used to treat diseases.
    b. a specific population at risk for a disease.
    c. the condition of being resistant to disease.
    d. the study of the noncellular portion of the blood.

18. A blood cell that has reddish-staining granules and is able to kill large parasites describes
    a. basophils.
    b. monocytes.
    c. neutrophils.
    d. eosinophils.

19. Which of the following statements best describes a lymph node?
    a. It is considered a primary lymphoid organ.
    b. It removes old RBCs.
    c. It collects fluid from the tissues.
    d. It is where B cells mature.

20. Antigenic groups identified by different sets of antibodies reacting in a similar manner to certain standard cell lines best describes
    a. cytokines.
    b. clusters of differentiation (CD).
    c. neutrophilic granules.
    d. opsonins.

Innate Immunity

2

Christine Dorresteyn Stevens, EdD, MT(ASCP)
and Nadine Lerret, PhD, MLS^{CM}(ASCP)

LEARNING OUTCOMES

After finishing this chapter, you should be able to:

1. Differentiate between the external and internal defense systems.
2. Give examples of several external defense mechanisms.
3. Describe how normal flora act as a defense against pathogens.
4. Define "pathogen-associated molecular pattern" (PAMP) and provide some examples.
5. Discuss the role of pattern recognition receptors (PRRs) in both the innate and adaptive immune responses.
6. Describe the function of Toll-like receptors (TLRs) in the immune system.
7. Discuss the role of acute-phase reactants in the innate immune response.
8. Explain how each of the following acute-phase reactants contributes to innate immunity: C-reactive protein (CRP), serum amyloid A (SAA), complement, alpha$_1$-antitrypsin (AAT), haptoglobin, fibrinogen, and ceruloplasmin.
9. Determine the significance of abnormal levels of acute-phase reactants.
10. Describe the process of inflammation.
11. List the steps in the process of phagocytosis.
12. Discuss the intracellular mechanism for destruction of foreign particles during the process of phagocytosis.
13. Explain the importance of phagocytosis in both innate and adaptive immunity.
14. Explain how natural killer (NK) cells recognize target cells.
15. Describe two methods that NK cells use to kill target cells.
16. Discuss the defining characteristics and functions of innate lymphoid cells (ILCs).

CHAPTER OUTLINE

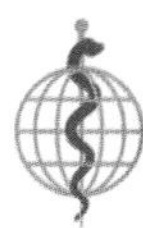

Go to FADavis.com for the laboratory exercises that accompany this text.

KEY TERMS

Acute-phase reactants
Alpha$_1$-antitrypsin (AAT)
Antibody-dependent cellular cytotoxicity (ADCC)
Ceruloplasmin
Chemotaxis
Complement
C-reactive protein (CRP)
Defensins
Diapedesis
External defense system
Fibrinogen
Haptoglobin
Inflammation
Innate immunity
Innate lymphoid cell (ILC)
Internal defense system
Microbiota
Opsonins
Oxidative burst
Pathogen-associated molecular patterns (PAMPs)
Pattern recognition receptors (PRRs)
Phagocytosis
Phagolysosome
Phagosome
Serum amyloid A (SAA)
Toll-like receptor (TLR)

Humans are protected by two systems of immunity—innate and adaptive—as we discussed in Chapter 1. **Innate immunity** consists of the defenses against infection that are ready for immediate action when a host is attacked by a pathogen. If a pathogen manages to evade these defenses, there is a coordinated series of interactions between various cells and molecules to destroy any invading pathogens before disease can occur. These defenses are considered nonadaptive or nonspecific; regardless of the infectious agent to which the body is exposed, innate immunity produces the same response. Components of innate immunity can be thought of as the first responders because they react immediately to infectious agents. Adaptive immunity, in contrast, is a more tailored response. It takes a longer time to be activated, but it is more specific and longer lasting. The two systems, however, are highly interactive and interdependent; innate immunity actually sets the stage for the more specific and longer-lasting adaptive immune response.

The innate immune system is composed of two parts: the external defense system and the internal defense system. The external defense system consists of anatomical barriers designed to keep microorganisms from entering the body. If these defenses are overcome, then the internal defense system is triggered within minutes and clears invaders as quickly as possible. Internal defenses include cellular responses that recognize specific molecular components of pathogens. Both of these systems work together to promote phagocytosis. The process of **phagocytosis,** as defined in Chapter 1, is the engulfment and destruction of foreign cells or particles by leukocytes, macrophages, and other cells. Importantly, phagocytosis and resulting inflammation bring cells and humoral factors to the injured area, orchestrating the healing process. If healing begins and inflammation is resolved as quickly as possible, the tissues are less likely to be damaged. The innate immune system is so efficient that most pathogens are destroyed before they ever encounter cells of the adaptive immune response.

External Defense System

The **external defense system** is composed of physical, chemical, and biological barriers that function together to prevent most infectious agents from entering the body **(Fig. 2–1).** First and foremost are the unbroken skin and the mucosal membrane surfaces. The outer layer of the skin, the epidermis, contains several layers of tightly packed epithelial cells. These cells are coated with a protein called *keratin*, making the skin impermeable to most infectious agents. The outer skin layer is renewed every few days to keep it intact. The dermis is a thicker layer just underneath the epidermis that is composed of connective tissue with blood vessels, hair follicles, sebaceous glands, sweat glands, and white blood cells (WBCs), including macrophages, dendritic cells, and mast cells. To understand how important a role the skin plays, one has only to consider how vulnerable victims of severe burns are to infection.

Not only does the skin serve as a major structural barrier, but the presence of several secretions on the skin discourages the growth of microorganisms. Lactic acid in sweat, for instance, and fatty acids from sebaceous glands maintain the skin at a pH of approximately 5.6. This acidic pH keeps most microorganisms from growing. In addition, human skin cells produce psoriasin, a small protein that has antibacterial effects, especially against gram-negative organisms such as *Escherichia coli.*

Additionally, each of the various organ systems in the body has its own unique defense mechanisms. In the respiratory tract, mucous secretions block the adherence of bacteria to epithelial cells. These secretions contain small proteins called *surfactants* that are produced by the epithelial cells and bind to microorganisms to help move pathogens out. The motion of the cilia that line the nasopharyngeal passages clears away almost 90% of the deposited material. The simple acts of coughing and sneezing also help to move pathogens out of the respiratory tract. The flushing action of urine, plus its slight acidity, helps to remove many potential pathogens from the genitourinary tract. Lactic acid production in the female genital tract keeps the vagina at a pH of about 5, which is another means of preventing the invasion of pathogens. In the digestive tract, the stomach's hydrochloric acid keeps the pH as low as 1. We take in many microorganisms with food and drink, and the low pH serves to halt microbial growth. Lysozyme—an enzyme found in many bodily secretions, such as tears and

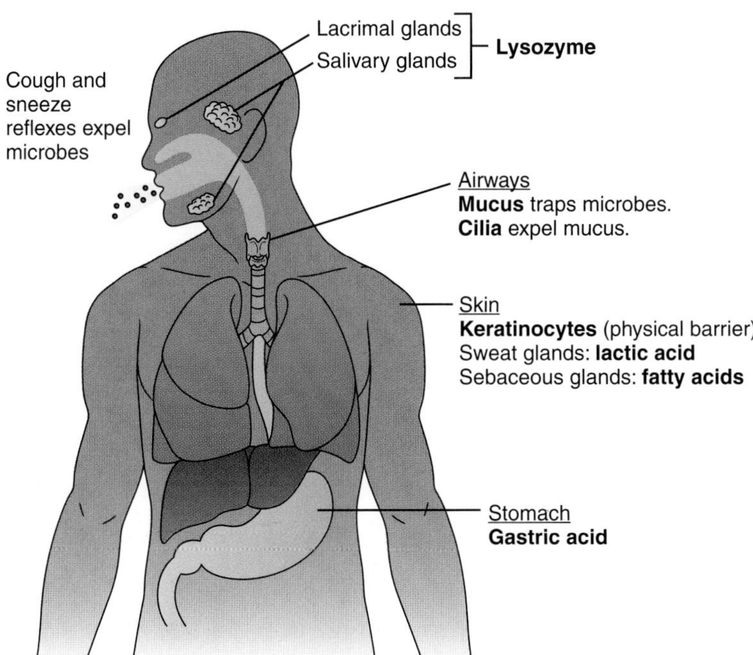

FIGURE 2–1 The external defense system.

saliva—attacks the cell walls of microorganisms, especially those that are gram-positive.

In many locations of the human body, the presence of microbiota (formerly known as *normal flora*) helps to keep pathogens from establishing themselves in these areas. **Microbiota** consist of a mix of bacteria that are normally found at specific body sites and do not typically cause disease. The significance of microbiota is readily demonstrated by looking at the side effects of antimicrobial therapy. For example, women who take an antibiotic for a urinary tract infection (UTI) frequently develop a yeast infection because of the presence of *Candida albicans*. In this case, antimicrobial therapy depletes not only the pathogenic bacteria but also the microorganisms that ordinarily compete with such opportunists that are normally present in very small numbers. Interestingly, the dynamic and bilateral interaction between resident microbes of the digestive tract (the gut microbiome) and the innate immune system is now a focus of investigation with regard to therapies for systemic diseases such as inflammatory bowel disease and metabolic syndrome.

Internal Defense System

If microorganisms do penetrate the barriers of the external defense system, the innate immune system has additional mechanisms to destroy foreign invaders. The **internal defense system** is composed of both cells and soluble factors that have specific and essential functions. Cells that are capable of phagocytosis play a major role in the internal defenses (see Chapter 1). Phagocytic cells engulf and destroy most of the foreign cells or particles that enter the body; this is the most important function of the internal defense system. Phagocytosis is enhanced by specific receptors on cells that capture invaders through identification of unique microbial substances. In addition, soluble factors called *acute-phase reactants* act by several different mechanisms to facilitate contact between microbes and phagocytic cells and to bind to and recycle important proteins after the process of phagocytosis has taken place. Both cellular receptors and soluble factors are described in more detail here.

Pattern Recognition Receptors

The internal defense system is designed to recognize molecules that are unique to infectious organisms. Macrophages and dendritic cells constituting between 10% and 15% of the total cellular population in the tissues are the most important cells involved in pathogen recognition. They are able to distinguish pathogens from normally present molecules in the body by means of receptors known as **pattern recognition receptors (PRRs)**, which are also found on neutrophils, eosinophils, monocytes, mast cells, and epithelial cells. These receptors are encoded by the host's genomic DNA and act as sensors for extracellular infection. PRRs thus play a pivotal role as a second line of defense if microorganisms penetrate the external barriers. Once these receptors bind to a pathogen, phagocytic cells become activated and are better able to engulf and eliminate microorganisms. Activated cells then secrete proinflammatory cytokines and chemokines, chemical messengers that make capillaries more permeable and recruit additional phagocytic cell types to the area of infection. Cytokines and chemokines also trigger the adaptive immune response.

PRRs are able to distinguish self from nonself by recognizing substances, known as **pathogen-associated molecular patterns (PAMPs)**, which are only found in microorganisms. Some examples of PAMPs include peptidoglycan in gram-positive bacteria, lipopolysaccharide in gram-negative bacteria, zymosan in yeast, and flagellin in bacteria with flagellae.

Charles Janeway's discovery of the first receptor in humans, the **Toll-like receptor (TLR),** had a major impact on the understanding of innate immunity. Toll is a protein originally discovered in the fruit fly *Drosophila,* where it plays an important role in innate immunity in the adult fly. Very similar molecules were found on human leukocytes and some other cell types. The highest concentration of TLRs occurs on monocytes, macrophages, and dendritic cells **(Fig. 2–2)**.

TLRs make up a large family of receptors strategically located in various cellular compartments; some are found in the cytoplasm, whereas others are found on cell surfaces **(Table 2–1)**. TLR1, TLR2, TLR4, TLR5, and TLR6 are found on cell surfaces, whereas TLR3, TLR7, TLR8, and TLR9 are found in the endosomal compartment of a cell. Each of these receptors recognizes a different microbial product. For example, TLR2 recognizes teichoic acid and peptidoglycan found in gram-positive bacteria; TLR4 recognizes lipopolysaccharide, which is found in gram-negative bacteria; and TLR5 recognizes bacterial flagellin **(Fig. 2–3)**. The function of TLR10 is thought to be anti-inflammatory.

TLRs are membrane-spanning glycoproteins that share a common structural element called *leucine-rich repeats* (LRRs). Once TLRs bind to their particular substances, host immune responses are rapidly activated by the production of cytokines and chemokines. Neutrophils are recruited to the area because of increased capillary permeability; in addition, macrophages and dendritic cells become more efficient because of increased expression of adhesion molecules on their cell surfaces. These processes enhance phagocytosis and, importantly, provide a vital link between the innate and adaptive immune systems, which work together to destroy most pathogens that humans are exposed to before disease sets in. In addition to TLRs, there are several other families of receptors that activate innate immune responses. One such family is the C-type lectin receptor (CLR). CLRs are plasma membrane receptors found on monocytes, macrophages, dendritic cells, neutrophils, B cells, and T-cell subsets. These receptors bind to mannan and β-glucans found in fungal cell walls (see Chapter 22). Although the initial signaling pathway differs from TLRs, the end result is the same—the production of cytokines and chemokines to eliminate microbes.

Other families of receptors that recognize pathogens include retinoic acid–inducible gene-I-like receptors (RLRs) and nucleotide-binding oligomerization domain (NOD)-like

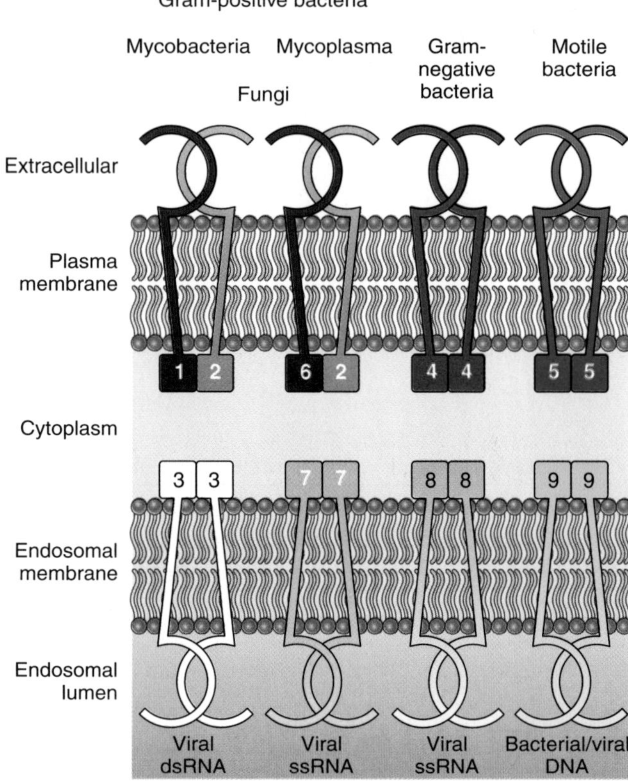

FIGURE 2–2 Toll-like receptors on a WBC membrane. Each of the 10 different TLRs recognizes a different pathogenic product. TLRs found on the cell surface tend to form dimers to increase chances of binding to a foreign substance.

Table 2–1 The 10 Human Toll-Like Receptors

RECEPTOR	SUBSTANCE RECOGNIZED	TARGET MICROORGANISM
TLR Receptors Found on Cell Surfaces		
TLR1	Lipopeptides	Mycobacteria
TLR2	Peptidoglycan, lipoproteins, zymosan	Gram-positive bacteria, mycobacteria, yeasts
TLR4	Lipopolysaccharide, fusion proteins, mannan	Gram-negative bacteria, respiratory syncytial virus, fungi
TLR5	Flagellin	Bacteria with flagellae
TLR6	Lipopeptides, lipoteichoic acid, zymosan	Mycobacteria, gram-positive bacteria, yeasts
TLR Receptors Found in Endosomal Compartments		
TLR3	Double-stranded RNA	RNA viruses
TLR7	Single-stranded RNA	RNA viruses
TLR8	Single-stranded RNA	RNA viruses
TLR9	Double-stranded DNA	DNA viruses, bacterial DNA
TLR10	Unknown	Unknown

A

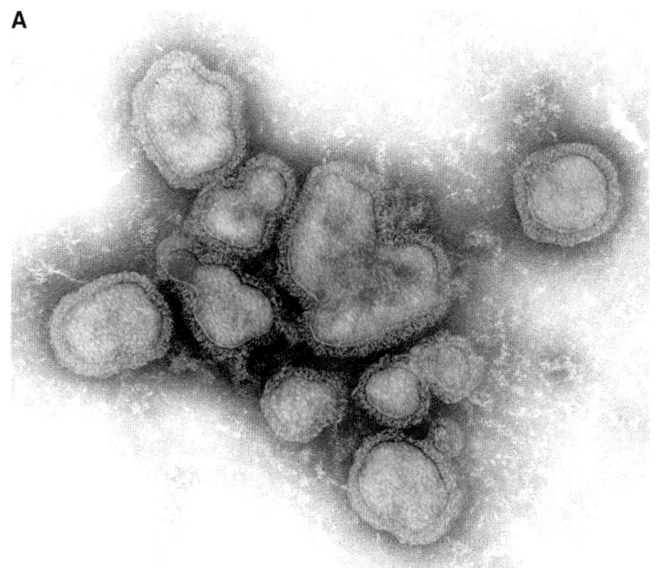

B

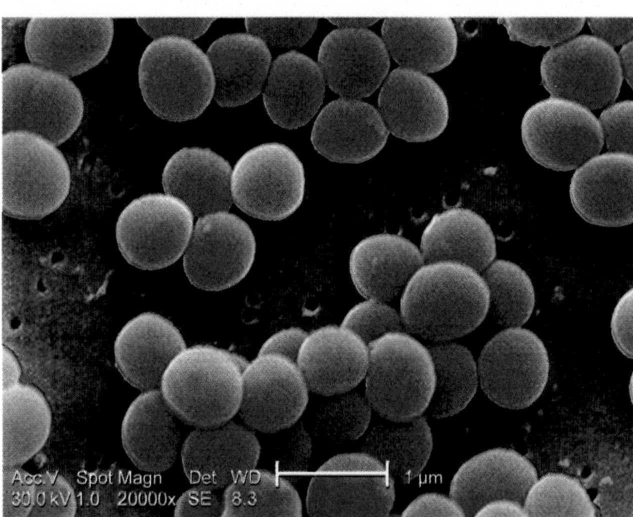

FIGURE 2–3 (A) Digitally colored and negative stained transmission electron micrograph of the influenza A virus, an RNA virus that TLR3, TLR7, and TLR8 recognize as foreign. (B) Scanning electron micrograph of *Staphylococcus aureus;* gram-positive bacteria that are recognized by the TLR2 receptor. *(A. Courtesy of the CDC/FA Murphy, Public Health Image Library. B. Courtesy of the CDC/Matthew Arduino, Public Health Image Library, DRPH.)*

receptors (NLRs). The RLR family recognizes RNA from RNA viruses in the cytoplasm of infected cells and induces inflammatory cytokines and type I interferons. Type I interferons inhibit viral replication and induce apoptosis (cell death) in infected cells. NLRs provide immune surveillance in the cytoplasm, where they bind ligands from microbial pathogens, such as peptidoglycan, flagellin, viral RNA, and fungal hyphae. NLRs also have the ability to form an *inflammasome*, a multiprotein unit that can activate apoptotic (controlled-cell-death) proteins and proinflammatory cytokines.

Pattern Recognition Receptors and Disease

Although PRRs are essential for protection against pathogens, inappropriate PRR responses have been found to contribute to acute and chronic inflammation as well as to systemic autoimmune diseases. For example, mutations in NLRs may result in Crohn's disease, a painful inflammatory disease of the bowel. Additionally, in systemic lupus erythematosus, there is a higher concentration of antibodies to self–nucleic acids, which activate dendritic cells through TLR9. Therefore, a tight regulatory network of PRR signaling is critical to ensure the elimination of invading pathogens while avoiding harmful immune reactions that can cause pathology.

Acute-Phase Reactants

In addition to the cells and receptors that enhance the destruction of pathogens, the internal defense system also consists of soluble factors called acute-phase reactants that contribute to the innate immune response. **Acute-phase reactants** are normal serum constituents that rapidly increase or decrease in concentration because of infection, injury, or trauma to the tissues. Those that increase are termed *positive acute-phase reactants*, whereas those that decrease, such as albumin and transferrin, are known as *negative acute-phase reactants*. In this chapter, we will discuss positive acute-phase reactants. Many of these proteins act by binding to microorganisms and promoting adherence, the first step in phagocytosis. Others help to limit destruction caused by the release of proteolytic enzymes from WBCs as the process of phagocytosis takes place. Some of the most important positive acute-phase reactants are C-reactive protein (CRP), serum amyloid A (SAA), complement components, alpha$_1$-antitrypsin (AAT), haptoglobin, fibrinogen, and ceruloplasmin. They are produced primarily by hepatocytes (liver parenchymal cells) within 12 to 24 hours in response to an increase in cytokines (see Chapter 6 for a complete discussion of cytokines). The major cytokines involved in inflammation are interleukin-1 (IL-1), interleukin-6 (IL-6), and tumor necrosis factor-α (TNF-α), all of which are produced by monocytes and macrophages. **Table 2–2** summarizes characteristics of the main positive acute-phase reactants.

C-Reactive Protein

C-reactive protein (CRP) is a trace constituent of serum originally thought to be an antibody to the C-polysaccharide of pneumococci. It was discovered by Tillet and Francis in 1930 when they observed that serum from patients with *Streptococcus pneumoniae* infection precipitated with a soluble extract of the bacteria. Now CRP is known to have a more generalized role in innate immunity.

CRP has a molecular weight of between 118,000 and 144,000 daltons and has a structure that consists of five identical subunits held together by noncovalent bonds. It is a member of the family known as the *pentraxins*, all of which are proteins with five subunits. CRP acts somewhat similar to an antibody because it is capable of *opsonization* (the coating of foreign particles), agglutination, precipitation, and activation of complement by the classical pathway. However, binding is

Table 2-2 Characteristics of Acute-Phase Reactants

PROTEIN	RESPONSE TIME (HR)	NORMAL CONCENTRATION (MG/DL)	INCREASE	FUNCTION
C-reactive protein	4–6	0.5	1,000X	Opsonization, complement activation
Serum amyloid A	24	5	1,000X	Activates monocytes and macrophages
Alpha$_1$-antitrypsin	24	200–400	2–5X	Protease inhibitor
Fibrinogen	24	200–400	2–5X	Clot formation
Haptoglobin	24	40–290	2–10X	Binds hemoglobin
Ceruloplasmin	48–72	20–40	2X	Binds copper and oxidizes iron
Complement C3	48–72	60–140	2X	Opsonization, lysis

calcium-dependent and nonspecific. The main substrate is phosphocholine, a common constituent of microbial membranes. CRP also binds to small ribonuclear proteins; phospholipids; peptidoglycan; and other constituents of bacteria, fungi, and parasites. In addition, CRP promotes phagocytosis by binding to specific receptors found on monocytes, macrophages, and neutrophils. Thus, CRP can be thought of as a primitive, nonspecific form of an antibody molecule that is able to act as a defense against microorganisms or foreign cells until specific antibodies can be produced.

CRP is a relatively stable serum protein, with a half-life of about 18 hours. It increases rapidly, within 4 to 6 hours following infection, surgery, or other trauma to the body. Levels increase dramatically, as much as a hundredfold to a thousand-fold, reaching a peak value within 48 hours. CRP also declines rapidly with cessation of the stimuli. Elevated levels are found in conditions such as bacterial infections, rheumatic fever, viral infections, malignant diseases, tuberculosis, and after a heart attack. Additionally, the median CRP value for an individual increases with age, reflecting an increase in subclinical inflammatory conditions.

Because the levels rise and then decline so rapidly, CRP is the most widely used indicator of acute inflammation. Although CRP is a nonspecific indicator of disease or trauma, monitoring of its levels can be useful clinically to follow a disease process and observe the response to treatment of inflammation and infection. It is a nonsurgical means of following the course of malignancy and organ transplantation because a rise in the level may mean a return of the malignancy or, in the case of transplantation, the beginning of organ rejection. CRP levels can also be used to monitor the progression or remission of autoimmune diseases. Laboratory assays for CRP are sensitive, reproducible, and relatively inexpensive.

Clinical Correlations

CRP and Rheumatoid Arthritis

Rheumatoid arthritis (RA) is an autoimmune disease characterized by inflammation of the joints. CRP is often used to monitor patients with RA because the CRP concentration reflects the intensity of the inflammatory response. CRP levels decrease when therapy is successful in reducing inflammation.

CRP has also received attention as a risk marker for cardiovascular disease. In accord with the finding that atherosclerosis (coronary artery disease) may be the result of a chronic inflammatory process, an increased level of CRP has been shown to be a significant risk factor for myocardial infarction, ischemic stroke, and peripheral vascular disease in men and women who are at an intermediate risk for cardiovascular disease. When inflammation is chronic, increased amounts of CRP react with endothelial cells that line blood vessel walls, predisposing them to vasoconstriction, platelet activation, thrombosis (clot formation), and vascular inflammation.

The ability to monitor CRP is significant because cardiovascular disease is the number-one cause of mortality in the United States and the world today. The Centers for Disease Control and Prevention (CDC) has recommended that a serum CRP concentration of lower than 1 mg/L is associated with a low risk for cardiovascular disease, 1 to 3 mg/L is associated with an average risk, and greater than 3 mg/L is associated with a high risk. Normal levels in adults range from approximately 0.47 to 1.34 mg/L. The mean CRP level for people with no coronary artery disease is 0.87 mg/L. Thus, monitoring of CRP is now an established clinical tool to evaluate subtle chronic systemic inflammation, and when used in conjunction with traditional clinical laboratory methods, it may be an important preventative measure in determining the potential risk of heart attack or stroke. High-sensitivity CRP testing has the necessary lower level of detection of 0.01 mg/L, which enables measurement of much smaller increases than the traditional latex agglutination screening test.

One clinically relevant property of CRP is that it is easily destroyed by heating serum to 56°C for 30 minutes. The destruction of CRP is often necessary in the laboratory because it may interfere with certain tests for the presence of antibodies.

Serum Amyloid A

Serum amyloid A (SAA) is the other major protein besides CRP whose concentration can increase almost a thousand-fold in response to infection or injury. It is an apolipoprotein that is synthesized in the liver and has a molecular weight of 11,685 daltons. Normal circulating levels are approximately 5 to 8 ug/mL. In plasma, SAA has a high affinity for high-density lipoprotein

(HDL) cholesterol and is transported by HDL to the site of infection. SAA appears to act as a chemical messenger, similar to a cytokine, and it activates monocytes and macrophages to produce products that increase inflammation. It has been found to increase significantly more in bacterial infections than in viral infections. Levels reach a peak between 24 and 48 hours after an acute infection. SAA can also be increased because of chronic inflammation, atherosclerosis, and cancer. Because SAA has been found in atherosclerotic lesions, it is thought to contribute to localized inflammation in coronary artery disease. Elevated levels may predict a worse outcome for the patient.

Complement

Complement refers to a series of serum proteins that are normally present and contribute to inflammation. Nine complement proteins are activated by bound antibodies in a sequence known as the *classical pathway;* additional numbers are involved in the alternative pathway that is triggered by the presence of microorganisms. The major functions of complement are opsonization, chemotaxis, and lysis of cells. Complement is discussed in detail in Chapter 7.

> **Connections**
>
> **Complement**
>
> The complement protein C5a is a potent anaphylatoxin and chemotaxin. As such, C5a functions to increase vascular permeability and to attract WBCs to the site of inflammation.

Alpha$_1$-Antitrypsin

Alpha$_1$-antitrypsin (AAT) is a 52-kD protein that is primarily synthesized in the liver. It is the major component of the alpha band when serum is electrophoresed. Although the name implies that it acts against trypsin, it is a general plasma inhibitor of proteases released from leukocytes. Elastase, one such protease, is an enzyme secreted by neutrophils during inflammation that can degrade elastin and collagen. In chronic pulmonary inflammation, elastase activity damages lung tissue. Thus, AAT acts to counteract the effects of neutrophil invasion during an inflammatory response. It also regulates the expression of proinflammatory cytokines such as TNF-α, interleukin-1β, and interleukin-6, mentioned previously. Therefore, activation of monocytes and neutrophils is inhibited, limiting the harmful side effects of inflammation.

AAT deficiency can result in premature emphysema, especially in individuals who smoke or who have frequent exposure to noxious chemicals. In such a deficiency, uninhibited proteases remain in the lower respiratory tract, leading to destruction of parenchymal cells in the lungs and to the development of emphysema or idiopathic pulmonary fibrosis. It has been estimated that as many as 100,000 Americans suffer from this deficiency, although many of them are undiagnosed. There are at least 75 alleles of the gene coding for AAT, and 17 of these are associated with low production of the enzyme. One variant gene for AAT is responsible for a complete lack of production of the enzyme; individuals who inherit this gene are at risk of developing liver disease and emphysema. Homozygous inheritance of this particular gene may lead to the development of cirrhosis, hepatitis, or hepatoma in early childhood. The only treatment is a liver transplant.

AAT can also react with any serine protease, such as proteases generated by the triggering of the complement cascade or fibrinolysis. Once bound to AAT, the protease is completely inactivated and is subsequently removed from the area of tissue damage.

Haptoglobin

Haptoglobin is an alpha$_2$-globulin with a molecular weight of 100,000 daltons. It binds irreversibly to free hemoglobin released by intravascular hemolysis. Haptoglobin thus acts as an antioxidant to provide protection against oxidative damage mediated by free hemoglobin. Once bound, the complex is cleared rapidly by macrophages in the liver. A two- to tenfold increase in haptoglobin can be seen following inflammation, stress, or tissue necrosis. Early in the inflammatory response, however, haptoglobin levels may drop because of intravascular hemolysis, consequently masking the protein's behavior as an acute-phase reactant. Thus, plasma levels must be interpreted in light of other acute-phase reactants. Normal plasma concentrations range from 40 to 290 mg/dL.

Fibrinogen

Fibrinogen is an acute-phase protein involved in the coagulation pathway. A small portion is cleaved by thrombin to form fibrils that make up a fibrin clot. The molecule is a dimer with a molecular weight of 340,000 daltons. Normal levels range from 200 to 400 mg/dL. The clot increases the strength of a wound and stimulates endothelial cell adhesion and proliferation, which are critical to the healing process. Formation of a clot creates a barrier that helps prevent the spread of microorganisms further into the body. Fibrinogen makes blood more viscous and serves to promote aggregation of red blood cells (RBCs) and platelets. Increased levels may contribute to an increased risk for developing coronary artery disease.

Ceruloplasmin

Ceruloplasmin consists of a single polypeptide chain with a molecular weight of 132,000 daltons. It is the principal copper-transporting protein in human plasma, binding more than 70% of the copper found in plasma by attaching six cupric ions per molecule. Additionally, ceruloplasmin acts as an enzyme, converting the toxic ferrous ion (Fe^{2+}) to the nontoxic ferric form (Fe^{3+}). The normal plasma concentration for adults is 20 to 40 mg/dL.

A depletion of ceruloplasmin is found in Wilson's disease, an autosomal recessive genetic disorder characterized by a massive increase of copper in the tissues. Normally, circulating copper is absorbed out of the circulation by the liver and either combined with ceruloplasmin and returned to the plasma or excreted into the bile duct. In Wilson's disease, copper accumulates in the liver and subsequently in other tissues, such as the brain, corneas, kidneys, and bones. Treatment involves long-term chelation therapy to remove the copper or a liver transplant.

Inflammation

When pathogens breach the outer barriers of innate immunity, both cellular and humoral mechanisms are involved in a complex, highly orchestrated process known as *inflammation*. **Inflammation** can be defined as the body's overall reaction to injury or invasion by an infectious agent. Each individual reactant plays a role in initiating, amplifying, or sustaining the reaction, and a delicate balance must be maintained for the process to be quickly and efficiently resolved. The four cardinal signs or clinical symptoms of inflammation are redness (erythema), swelling (edema), heat, and pain. Major events that occur rapidly after tissue injury are as follows:

1. Release of chemical mediators such as histamine from injured mast cells, which causes dilation of the blood vessels. This results in increased blood flow to the affected area, producing redness and heat.
2. Increased capillary permeability caused by contraction of the endothelial cells lining the vessels. The increased permeability of the vessels allows fluids in the plasma to leak into the tissues, resulting in the swelling and pain associated with inflammation.
3. Migration of WBCs, mainly neutrophils, from the capillaries to the surrounding tissue in a process called **diapedesis.** As the endothelial cells of the vessels contract, neutrophils move through the endothelial cells of the vessel and out into the tissues. Soluble mediators, which include acute-phase reactants, chemokines, and cytokines, act as chemoattractants to initiate and control the response. Neutrophils are mobilized within 30 to 60 minutes after the injury, and their emigration may last 24 to 48 hours.
4. Migration of macrophages to the injured area. Migration of macrophages and dendritic cells from surrounding tissue occurs several hours later and peaks at 16 to 48 hours.
5. Acute-phase reactants stimulate phagocytosis of microorganisms. Macrophages, neutrophils, and dendritic cells all attempt to clear the area through phagocytosis; in most cases, the healing process is completed with a return to normal tissue structure **(Fig. 2–4).**

The *acute* inflammatory response acts to combat the early stages of infection and also begins a process that repairs tissue damage. However, when the inflammatory process becomes prolonged, it is said to be *chronic*. The failure to remove microorganisms or injured tissue may result in continued tissue damage and loss of function.

Connections

Inflammation and Disease

Although inflammation is essential to the body's defense against pathogens, prolonged inflammation can cause harm to the host. The tissue damage resulting from chronic inflammation is the basis for the pathogenesis of many autoimmune diseases, in which the body mounts an immune response against self-antigens.

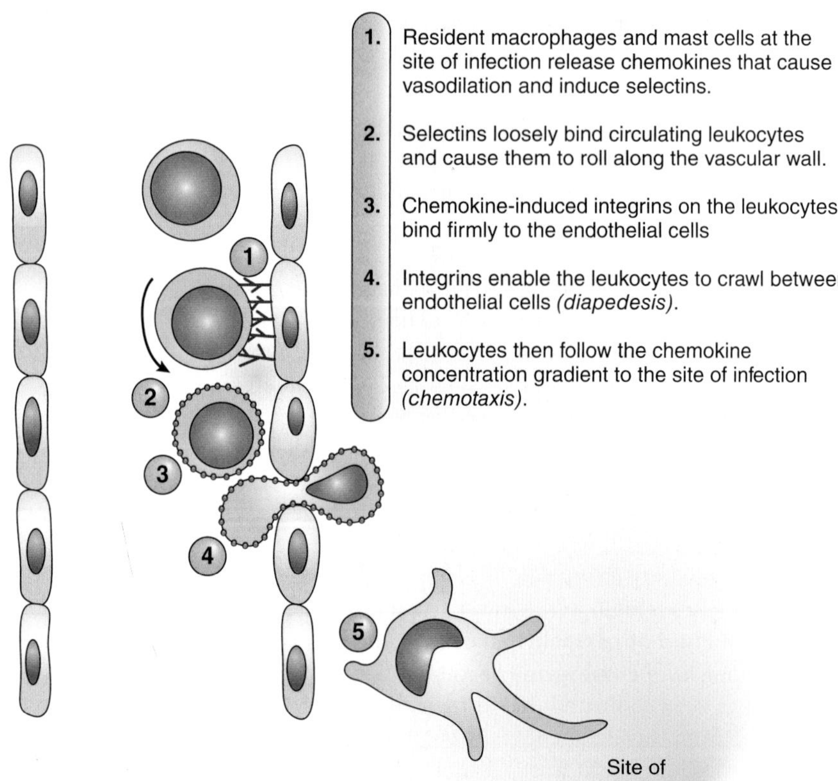

1. Resident macrophages and mast cells at the site of infection release chemokines that cause vasodilation and induce selectins.
2. Selectins loosely bind circulating leukocytes and cause them to roll along the vascular wall.
3. Chemokine-induced integrins on the leukocytes bind firmly to the endothelial cells
4. Integrins enable the leukocytes to crawl between endothelial cells (diapedesis).
5. Leukocytes then follow the chemokine concentration gradient to the site of infection (chemotaxis).
1
2
3
4
5
Site of infection

FIGURE 2–4 Local inflammatory events.

Phagocytosis

The main purpose of the inflammatory response is to attract cells to the site of infection and remove foreign cells or pathogens by means of phagocytosis. Although the acute-phase reactants enhance the process of phagocytosis, it is the cellular elements of the internal defense system that play the major role. The cells that are most active in phagocytosis are neutrophils, monocytes, macrophages, and dendritic cells, as discussed in Chapter 1.

Once the WBCs are attracted to the area, the actual process of phagocytosis consists of seven main steps **(Fig. 2–5)**:

1. Physical contact between the WBC and the foreign cell
2. Outflowing of the cytoplasm to surround the microorganism
3. Formation of a phagosome
4. Fusion of lysosomal granules with the phagosome
5. Formation of the phagolysosome with release of lysosomal contents
6. Digestion of microorganisms by hydrolytic enzymes
7. Release of debris to the outside of the cell by exocytosis

Physical contact occurs as neutrophils bind loosely to adhesion molecules called *selectins* on the endothelial cells lining the blood vessels. This causes the neutrophils to roll along the vascular wall in a random pattern until they encounter the site of injury or infection. They adhere firmly to adhesion molecules on the endothelial cell wall called *integrins* and penetrate through to the tissue by means of diapedesis. This adhering process is aided by **chemotaxis,** whereby cells are attracted to the site of inflammation by chemical substances such as soluble bacterial factors or acute-phase reactants, including complement components and CRP. Macrophages and dendritic cells already reside in the tissues. Receptors on neutrophils, macrophages, and dendritic cells bind to certain molecular patterns on a foreign particle surface, as discussed previously. This binding process is enhanced by *opsonins*, a term derived from the Greek word meaning "to prepare for eating." **Opsonins** are serum proteins that attach to a foreign cell or pathogen and help prepare it for phagocytosis. CRP, complement components, and antibodies are all important opsonins. Opsonins may act by neutralizing the surface charge on the foreign particle, making it easier for the cells to approach one another. In addition to receptors for pathogens themselves, phagocytic cells also have receptors for immunoglobulins and complement components, which aid in contact and in initiating ingestion (see Chapters 5 and 7).

Once contact with surface receptors occurs, phagocytic cells secrete chemoattractants such as cytokines and chemokines that recruit additional cells to the site of infection. Neutrophils are followed by monocytes, after which macrophages and dendritic cells arrive at the site. Macrophages and dendritic cells are not only able to ingest whole microorganisms, but they can also remove injured or dead host cells.

After attachment to a foreign cell or pathogen has occurred, the cell membrane invaginates, and pseudopodia (outflowing of cytoplasm) surround the pathogen. The pseudopodia fuse to completely enclose the pathogen, forming a structure known as a **phagosome.** The phagosome is moved toward the center of the cell. Lysosomal granules quickly migrate to the phagosome, and fusion between granules and the phagosome occurs. At this point, the fused elements are known as a **phagolysosome.** The granules contain lysozyme, myeloperoxidase, and other proteolytic enzymes. The contents of the granules are released into the phagolysosome, and digestion

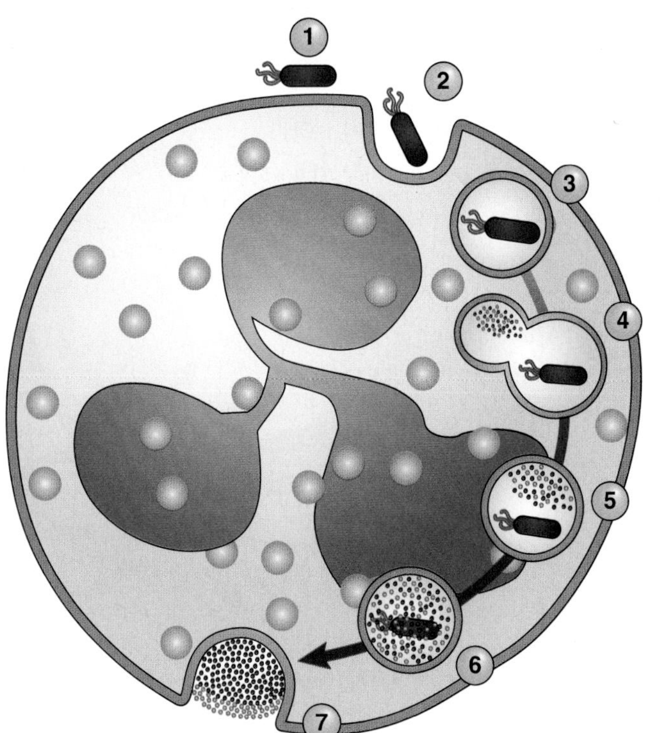

1. Adherence: physical contact between the phagocytic cell and the microorganism occurs, aided by opsonins.
2. Engulfment: outflowing of cytoplasm to surround the microorganism.
3. Formation of phagosome: microorganism is completely surrounded by a part of the cell membrane.
4. Granule contact: lysosomal granules contact and fuse with the phagosome.
5. Formation of the phagolysosome: contents of the lysosome are emptied into this membrane-bound space.
6. Digestion of the microorganism by hydrolytic enzymes.
7. Excretion: contents of phagolysosome are expelled to the outside by exocytosis.

FIGURE 2–5 Steps involved in phagocytosis.

occurs. Any undigested material is excreted from the cells by exocytosis. Heavily opsonized particles are taken up in as little as 20 seconds, and killing is almost immediate.

The elimination of pathogens actually occurs by two different processes: an oxygen-dependent pathway and an oxygen-independent pathway. In the oxygen-dependent process, an increase in oxygen consumption, known as the **oxidative burst,** occurs within the cell as the pseudopodia enclose the particle within a vacuole. This mechanism generates considerable energy through oxidative metabolism. The hexose monophosphate shunt is used to change nicotinamide adenine dinucleotide phosphate (NADP) to its reduced form by adding a hydrogen atom. Electrons then pass from NADPH to oxygen in the presence of NADPH oxidase, a membrane-bound enzyme that is only activated through conformational change triggered by microbes themselves. A radical known as superoxide (O_2^-) is then formed. Superoxide is highly toxic but can be rapidly converted to even more lethal products. By adding hydrogen ions, the enzyme superoxide dismutase (SD) converts superoxide to hydrogen peroxide or the hydroxyl radical •OH.

Hydrogen peroxide has long been considered an important bactericidal agent and is more stable than any of the free radicals. Its antimicrobial effect is further enhanced by the formation of hypochlorite ions through the action of the enzyme myeloperoxidase in the presence of chloride ions. Hypochlorite is a powerful oxidizing agent and is highly toxic for microorganisms. It is the main component of household bleach used to disinfect surfaces **(Fig. 2–6).**

NADPH oxidase also plays a major role in the oxygen-independent pathway. NADPH oxidase depolarizes the membrane when fusion with the phagosome occurs, allowing hydrogen and potassium ions to enter the vacuole. This alters the pH, which in turn activates proteases that contribute to microbial elimination. Some of these lytic enzymes include small cationic proteins called **defensins.** When defensins are released from lysosomal granules, they are able to cleave segments of bacterial cell walls without the benefit of oxygen. Defensins kill a wide spectrum of organisms, including both gram-positive and gram-negative bacteria, many fungi, and some viruses. Cathepsin G is another example of a protein that is able to damage bacterial cell membranes. Chapter 1 lists some of the contents of neutrophil granules.

The importance of NADPH oxidase in the elimination of microbes is demonstrated by the fact that a lack of it may lead to an increased susceptibility to infection. Patients with chronic granulomatous disease have a genetic mutation that causes a defect in NADPH oxidase, resulting in an inability to kill bacteria during the process of phagocytosis. Individuals with this disease suffer from recurring, severe bacterial infections (see Chapter 19).

Following phagocytosis, macrophages and dendritic cells mature and are able to process peptides from pathogens for presentation to T cells. T cells then interact with B cells to

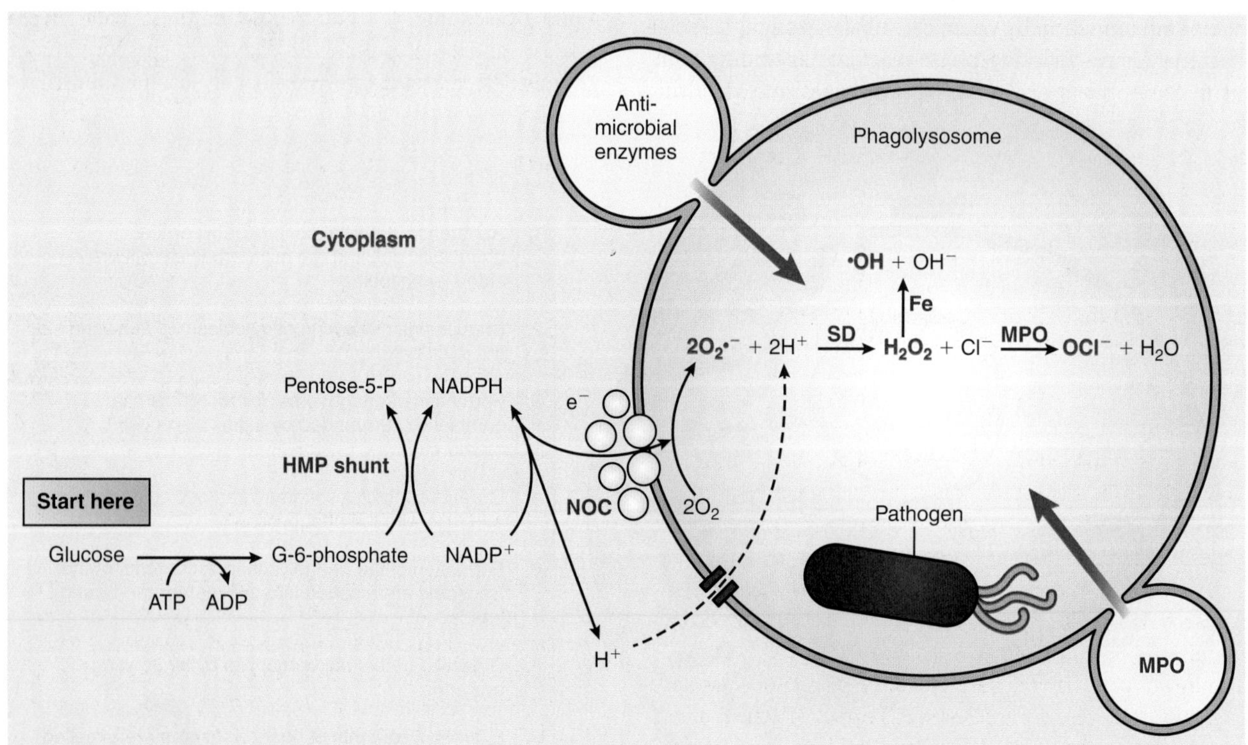

FIGURE 2–6 Creation of oxygen radicals in the phagocytic cell. The hexose monophosphate (HMP) shunt reduces NADP+ to NADPH. NADPH reduces oxygen to superoxide ($2O_2^-$) when the NADPH oxidase complex (NOC) is assembled in the membrane of the phagolysosome. Superoxide dismutase (SD) catalyzes the conversion of superoxide to hydrogen peroxide (H_2O_2). Myeloperoxidase (MPO) catalyzes the formation of hypochlorite (OCl^-), a very powerful oxidizing agent. Hydroxyl radicals (•OH), which are also powerful oxidizing agents, may also be formed if iron ions are present.

produce antibodies (see Chapter 4 for details). Because T cells are not able to respond to intact pathogens, phagocytosis is a crucial link between the innate and the adaptive immune systems.

Action of Natural Killer Cells

Another important cellular defense that is part of innate immunity is the action of natural killer (NK) cells. Although phagocytosis is important in eliminating infectious agents, NK cells represent the first line of defense against virally infected cells, tumor cells, and cells infected with other intracellular pathogens. NK cells have the ability to recognize damaged cells and to eliminate such target cells without prior exposure to them. The fact that they lack specificity in their response is essential to their function as early defenders against pathogens. By quickly engaging infected target cells, NK cells give the immune system time to activate the adaptive response of specific T and B cells.

Connections

NK Cells and Defense Against Tumors

NK cells are thought to play a key role in immunosurveillance by continually patrolling the body for cancerous cells and eliminating them before they become clinically apparent.

NK cell activity is enhanced by exposure to cytokines such as interleukin-12, interferon-α, and interferon-β. Because these cytokines rise rapidly during a viral infection, NK cells are able to respond early during an infection, and their activity peaks in about 3 days, well before antibody production or a naïve cytotoxic T-cell response. They localize in the tissues in areas where inflammation is occurring and where dendritic cells are found. Once activated, NK cells themselves become major producers of cytokines such as interferon-gamma (IFN-γ) and TNF-α that help to recruit T cells. In addition, NK cells release various colony-stimulating factors that act on developing granulocytes and macrophages. Thus, the actions of NK cells have a major influence on both innate and adaptive immunity.

Mechanism of Cytotoxicity

NK cells constantly monitor the body for potential target cells by contacting them through two main classes of binding receptors on their surface: inhibitory receptors, which deliver inhibitory signals, and activating receptors, which deliver signals to activate the cytotoxic mechanisms. The balance between activating and inhibitory signals enables NK cells to distinguish healthy cells from infected or cancerous ones.

The inhibitory signal is based on recognition of class I major histocompatibility complex (MHC) proteins, which are expressed on all healthy cells (see Chapter 3 for details). If NK cells react with class I MHC proteins, then the natural killing process is inhibited. Examples of this type of inhibitory receptor include killer cell immunoglobulin-like receptors (KIRs) and CD94/NKG2A receptors, both of which bind class I MHC molecules.

Diseased and cancerous cells may lose their ability to produce MHC proteins. NK cells are thus triggered by a lack of MHC antigens, sometimes referred to as recognition of "missing self." This lack of inhibition appears to be combined with an activating signal switched on by the presence of proteins produced by cells under stress, namely, those cells that are cancerous or infected with a pathogen.

Examples of activating receptors that bind stress proteins are CD16 and NKG2D. If an inhibitory signal is not received when binding to activating receptors occurs, then NK cells release substances called *perforins* and *granzymes* **(Fig. 2–7).** These substances are released into the space between the NK cell and the target cell. Perforins are proteins that form channels (pores) in the target cell membrane. Granzymes are packets of enzymes that may enter through the channels and mediate cell lysis. The elimination of target cells can occur in as little as 30 to 60 minutes. Thus, depending on the signals,

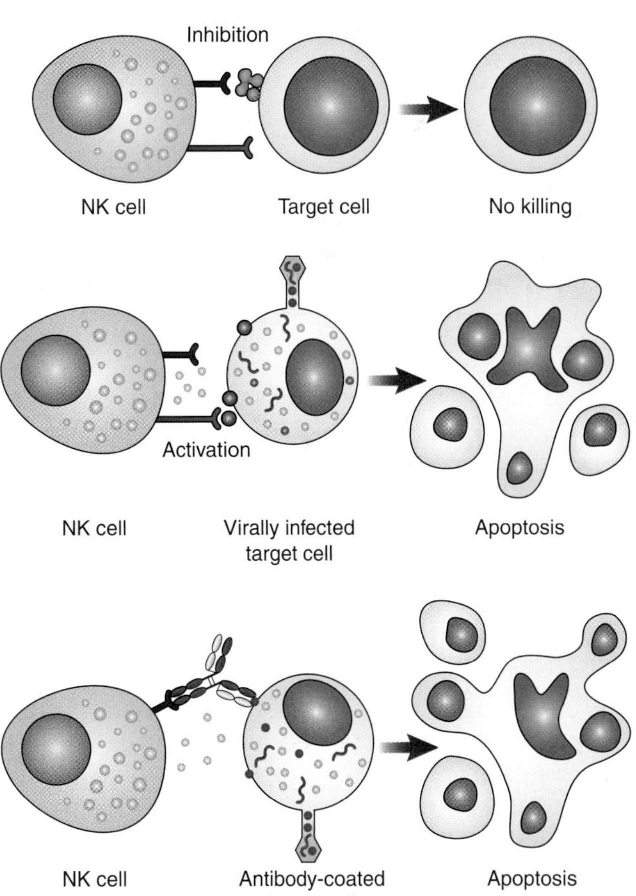

FIGURE 2–7 Actions of NK cells. NK cells are constantly surveying cells in the body. (A) If class I MHC protein is present and there are no foreign or stress proteins, then an inhibitory signal is sent to the NK cell, no killing occurs, and the normal cell is released. (B) If an activating receptor is engaged by a foreign or stress protein and class I MHC is altered or missing ("missing self"), then no inhibitory signal is given, granzymes and perforins are released, and the infected or diseased cell is eliminated by apoptosis. (C) Alternatively, infected cells may express foreign proteins on their surface that are recognized by antibody. NK cells express CD16 receptors that bind the immobilized antibody and activate the release of perforins and granzymes *(antibody-dependent cellular cytotoxicity).*

the NK cell either proceeds to activate cell destruction or detaches and moves on to search for another target cell.

Antibody-Dependent Cellular Cytotoxicity

A second method of destroying target cells is also available to NK cells. NK cells recognize and lyse antibody-coated target cells through a process called **antibody-dependent cellular cytotoxicity (ADCC)** (see Fig. 2–7). Binding occurs through the surface receptors, CD16 (FcγIII) and CD32 (FcγRIIC), which bind to the Fc portion of human immunoglobulins. Lysis of the target cell requires contact with the NK cell, followed by release of cytotoxic granules. Target cell destruction occurs outside of the NK cell and does not involve phagocytosis or complement fixation. ADCC is recognized as an important contributor to the anti-tumor activity of many monoclonal antibodies used as tumor immunotherapy (see Chapter 17). However, this method is not unique to NK cells, as monocytes, macrophages, and neutrophils also exhibit such receptors and act in a similar manner. Nonetheless, the overall importance of NK cells as a defense mechanism is demonstrated by the fact that patients who lack these cells have recurring, serious viral infections and an increased incidence of tumors.

Innate Lymphoid Cells

Innate lymphoid cells (ILCs) are a growing family of immune cells that develop from the common lymphoid progenitor but do not express markers of the lymphocyte lineage. ILCs are found predominantly at mucosal sites and contribute to the innate response to infectious agents at these sites through the rapid release of immunoregulatory cytokines. One key example of the role of ILCs in the innate immune response is through their secretion of IFN-γ. This cytokine activates the production of reactive oxygen species, such as superoxide and hydrogen peroxide, in phagocytic cells to be used in the oxidative burst.

SUMMARY

- Innate immunity encompasses all the body's normally present defense mechanisms for resisting disease. It is characterized by lack of antigen specificity, no need for a prior exposure to antigen, and a similar response with each exposure.
- External defenses include structural barriers such as skin, mucous membranes, cilia, and secretions such as lactic acid and lysozyme, that keep microorganisms from entering the body.
- Internal defenses include both cells capable of phagocytosis and acute-phase reactants that enhance the process of phagocytosis. Cells that are most active in phagocytosis include neutrophils, monocytes, macrophages, and dendritic cells.
- PRRs are molecules on host cells that recognize substances found only on pathogens. They are found on neutrophils, monocytes, eosinophils, mast cells, and dendritic cells. Once receptors bind a pathogen, phagocytosis can take place.
- Importantly, all PRRs play a critical role in not just the innate immune response, but also in the establishment of an adaptive immune response, acting as a bridge between the two arms of the immune system.
- PAMPs are molecules found only on pathogens but not on host cells, allowing the host cells to distinguish them from self. They are recognized by the PRRs.
- Positive acute-phase reactants are serum proteins that increase rapidly in response to infection or injury. They include CRP, SAA, complement components, AAT, haptoglobin, fibrinogen, and ceruloplasmin.
- CRP is the acute-phase reactant that is most widely monitored by the laboratory; it increases 100 to 1,000 times in response to infection or trauma, acts as an opsonin, and is able to fix complement.
- Acute-phase reactants increase the likelihood of phagocytosis of pathogens and help healing occur.
- The first step in phagocytosis is physical contact between the phagocytic cell and the foreign particle.
- Cytoplasm flows around the foreign particle to form a phagosome. Fusion of the phagosome with lysosomal granules creates a phagolysosome. Inside this structure, enzymes such as lysozyme and myeloperoxidase are released and the foreign particle is digested.
- Creation of hypochlorite and hydroxyl ions, which damage protein irreversibly, occurs in the oxygen-dependent phase of phagocytosis.
- Phagocytosis must occur before the specific immune response can be initiated, so this process is essential to both innate and adaptive immunity.
- Inflammation is the body's response to injury or invasion by a pathogen. It is characterized by increased blood supply to the affected area, increased capillary permeability, migration of neutrophils to the surrounding tissue, and migration of macrophages to the injured area.
- The process by which cells are attracted to the area of infection is called *chemotaxis*.
- NK cells are able to kill target cells that are infected with a virus or other intracellular pathogen. They also recognize and destroy malignant cells.
- The action of NK cells does not require prior exposure and is nonspecific. NK cells recognize a lack of class I MHC protein found on normal cells. This capability is called *recognition of missing self*.
- NK cells bind to and kill any antibody-coated target cells, such as cancer cells and virus-infected cells.
- NK cells represent an important link between the innate and adaptive immune systems.
- ILCs rapidly secrete cytokines that can activate other innate cells, specifically phagocytic cells.

Study Guide: Mechanisms of Innate Immunity

TYPE OF DEFENSE	EXAMPLE	FUNCTION
External	Skin and mucous membranes	Biological barriers
	Lactic acid	Reduces growth of microorganisms
	Cilia	Move pathogens out of respiratory tract
	Stomach acid	Low pH keeps pathogens from growing
	Urine	Flushes out pathogens from the body
	Lysozyme	Attacks cell walls of pathogens
	Microbiota (normal flora)	Compete with pathogens Produce antimicrobial peptides
Internal	WBCs	Produce cytokines and chemokines Neutrophils, macrophages, and dendritic cells participate in phagocytosis and inflammation NK cells destroy target cells using granzymes and perforins
	Pattern recognition receptors (e.g., TLRs)	Help phagocytic cells recognize pathogens
	Acute-phase reactants	Recruit WBCs for phagocytosis Coat pathogens to enhance phagocytosis Remove debris

CASE STUDIES

1. A 45-year-old male named Rick went to his physician for an annual checkup. Although he was slightly overweight, his laboratory results indicated that both his total cholesterol and his HDL cholesterol were within normal limits. His fibrinogen level was 450 mg/dL, and his CRP level was 3.5 mg/dL. His physical examination was perfectly normal. The physician cautioned Rick that he might be at risk for a future heart attack, and he counseled him to be sure to exercise and eat a healthy, low-fat diet. Rick's wife told him that as long as his cholesterol level was normal, he didn't have anything to worry about.

   Question

   a. Who is correct? Explain your answer.

2. A 20-year-old female college student went to the infirmary with symptoms of malaise, fatigue, sore throat, and a slight fever. A complete blood count (CBC) was performed, and both the RBC and WBC count were within normal limits. A normal WBC count ruled out the possibility of a bacterial infection. A rapid strep test was performed, which was negative. A rapid screening test for infectious mononucleosis was indeterminate (neither positive nor negative), whereas a slide agglutination test for CRP was positive. Results of a semiquantitative CRP determination indicated an increased level of approximately 20 mg/dL. The student was advised to return in a few days for a repeat mono test.

   Questions

   a. What conditions might cause a rise in CRP?
   b. Would an increase in CRP be consistent with the possibility of infectious mononucleosis?

REVIEW QUESTIONS

1. The enhancement of phagocytosis by coating of foreign particles with serum proteins is called
   a. opsonization.
   b. agglutination.
   c. extravasation.
   d. chemotaxis.

2. Which of the following plays an important role as an external defense mechanism?
   a. Phagocytosis
   b. C-reactive protein
   c. Lysozyme
   d. Complement

3. The process of inflammation is characterized by all of the following *except*
   a. increased blood supply to the area.
   b. migration of WBCs.
   c. decreased capillary permeability.
   d. increase of acute-phase reactants.

4. Skin, lactic acid secretions, stomach acidity, and the motion of cilia represent which type of immunity?
   a. Innate
   b. Cross
   c. Adaptive
   d. Auto

5. The structure formed by the fusion of engulfed material and enzymatic granules within the phagocytic cell is called a
   a. phagosome.
   b. lysosome.
   c. vacuole.
   d. phagolysosome.

6. The presence of human microbiota (normal flora) acts as a defense mechanism by which of the following methods?
   a. Maintaining an acid environment
   b. Competing with potential pathogens
   c. Keeping phagocytes in the area
   d. Coating mucosal surfaces

7. Measurement of CRP levels can be used for all of the following *except*
   a. monitoring drug therapy with anti-inflammatory agents.
   b. tracking the progress of an organ transplant.
   c. diagnosis of a specific bacterial infection.
   d. determining active phases of rheumatoid arthritis.

8. Pattern recognition receptors act by
   a. recognizing molecules common to both host cells and pathogens.
   b. recognizing molecules that are unique to pathogens.
   c. helping to spread infection because they are found on pathogens.
   d. all recognizing the same pathogens.

9. Which of the following are characteristics of acute-phase reactants?
   a. Rapid increase following infection
   b. Enhancement of phagocytosis
   c. Nonspecific indicators of inflammation
   d. All of the above

10. Which is the most potent agent formed in the phagolysosome for the elimination of microorganisms?
    a. Proteolytic enzymes
    b. Hydrogen ions
    c. Hypochlorite ions
    d. Superoxide

11. Which acute-phase reactant helps to prevent the formation of peroxides and free radicals that may damage tissues?
    a. Haptoglobin
    b. Fibrinogen
    c. Ceruloplasmin
    d. Serum amyloid A

12. Which statement best describes TLRs?
    a. They protect adult flies from infection.
    b. They are found on all host cells.
    c. They only play a role in adaptive immunity.
    d. They enhance phagocytosis.

13. The action of CRP can be distinguished from that of an antibody because
    a. CRP acts before the antibody appears.
    b. only the antibody triggers the complement cascade.
    c. binding of the antibody is calcium-dependent.
    d. only CRP acts as an opsonin.

14. How does innate immunity differ from adaptive immunity?
    a. Innate immunity requires prior exposure to a pathogen.
    b. Innate immunity depends upon normally present body functions.
    c. Innate immunity develops later than adaptive immunity.
    d. Innate immunity is more specific than adaptive immunity.

15. A 40-year-old male who is a smoker develops symptoms of premature emphysema. The symptoms may be caused by a deficiency of which of the following acute-phase reactants?
    a. Haptoglobin
    b. Alpha$_1$-antitrypsin
    c. Fibrinogen
    d. Ceruloplasmin

16. Which statement best describes NK cells?
    a. Their response against pathogens is very specific.
    b. They only react when an abundance of MHC antigens is present.
    c. They react when both an inhibitory and activating signal is triggered.
    d. They are able to kill target cells without previous exposure to them.

Nature of Antigens and the Major Histocompatibility Complex

3

Aaron Glass, PhD, MB^{CM}(ASCP)

LEARNING OUTCOMES

After finishing this chapter, you should be able to:

1. Define and characterize the nature of immunogens.
2. Differentiate an immunogen from an antigen.
3. Discuss several biological properties of individuals that influence the nature of the immune response.
4. Describe four important traits of immunogens that affect their ability to stimulate a host response.
5. Define *haptens* and describe some of their characteristics.
6. Describe the relationship between an epitope and an antigen.
7. Discuss the functions of adjuvants.
8. Differentiate heterophile antigens from alloantigens and autoantigens.
9. Explain what a haplotype is in regard to inheritance of major histocompatibility complex (MHC) antigens.
10. Describe the differences in the structure of class I and class II MHC molecules.
11. Contrast the transport of antigen to cell surfaces by class I and class II MHC molecules.
12. Describe the role of transporters associated with antigen processing (TAPs) in selecting peptides for binding to class I MHC molecules.
13. Discuss the differences in the sources and types of antigens processed by class I and class II MHC molecules.
14. Explain the clinical significance of the class I and class II MHC molecules.

CHAPTER OUTLINE

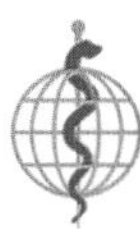

Go to FADavis.com for the laboratory exercises that accompany this text.

KEY TERMS

Adjuvant
Alleles
Alloantigens
Antigen
Antigen presentation
Autoantigens
Class I MHC (HLA) molecules
Class II MHC (HLA) molecules
Conformational epitope
Epitope
Haplotype
Haptens
Heteroantigens
Heterophile antigens
Immunogenicity
Immunogens
Invariant chain (Ii)
Linear epitopes
Major histocompatibility complex (MHC)
Transporters associated with antigen processing (TAP1 and TAP2)

A hallmark of innate immunity is the body's ability to respond nonspecifically to infection by recognizing broad classes of molecular patterns found on the surface and inside of pathogens. In contrast, the adaptive immune system recognizes very specific molecular regions from individual pathogens. The key cells responsible for the specificity, diversity, and memory associated with adaptive immunity are the lymphocytes, which can be further subdivided into T and B cells. Two key terms used to define substances that are targeted by adaptive immune responses are *antigen* and *immunogen*. An **antigen** is a substance that is specifically recognized by the adaptive immune system, whereas an **immunogen** is a substance capable of causing an adaptive response. The chief distinction between antigens and immunogens is the ability of the latter to successfully stimulate an immune response. To achieve this, certain conditions must be met, meaning that some antigens in and of themselves are not immunogenic. Thus, all immunogens are antigens, but not all antigens are necessarily immunogens. Despite this distinction, immunologists generally use these terms interchangeably.

One of the most exciting areas of immunological research focuses on how and why we respond to certain antigens. It is currently understood that multiple factors influence our response to antigens: unique biological properties of the individual, the nature of the antigen itself, antigen processing in conjunction with inherited **major histocompatibility complex (MHC)** molecules, and antigen presentation to T cells. This chapter focuses on all these areas and discusses potential clinical implications of some recent findings.

Factors Influencing the Immune Response

Many factors are known to influence whether an antigen is actually immunogenic. These factors can arise from the biology of the host, the way in which the host encounters the antigen, and the nature of the antigen itself. Outbred populations such as humans exhibit diverse biological properties, meaning that each person has unique traits—and certain traits can strongly influence the nature of the immune response. Factors including age, health status, and genetics are all important in determining whether an immune response is mounted against a particular antigen. Similarly, the dosage and route of exposure to an antigen also influence the promotion of an immune response. Finally, and fundamentally, not all antigens are equivalent in their ability to stimulate an immune response.

In general, elderly individuals are more likely to have a decreased response to antigenic stimulation. At the other end of the age scale, neonates do not fully respond to immunogens because their immune systems are not completely developed. Overall health plays a role because individuals who are malnourished, fatigued, or stressed are less likely to mount a successful immune response.

An individual's genetic composition plays a major role in determining the immune response, or lack thereof, to an antigen. Although many genes influence both innate and adaptive immunity, the MHC genes exert perhaps the most profound overall influence. The MHC is a system of genes that code for cell surface molecules that play an important role in antigen recognition. Further details are found in a later section in this chapter.

To stimulate an adaptive immune response, a certain amount of antigen must be introduced into the body. Small quantities of antigen, as would be found in very minor infections, simply do not meet the lower threshold required for activation of an adaptive immune response. Throughout the human life span, such minor infections occur continuously and are quickly and efficiently cleared by innate immune mechanisms, reserving adaptive immunity for persistent infections that involve relatively greater quantities of antigen. However, very large quantities of antigen can be detrimental to the development of an immune response by encouraging lymphocyte *tolerance*, or a state of ignorance, toward a particular antigen.

There are many ways that we come in contact with antigens in nature. How and where antigens enter our bodies can impact the amount of antigen required to generate an immune response. Possible routes of exposure include intravenous (into a vein), intradermal (into the skin), subcutaneous (beneath the skin), intramuscular, and oral. One mechanism explaining the differential response to antigens is that each of these routes ultimately shuttles antigens to different secondary lymphoid tissues, where antigens encounter distinct populations of immune cells. For example, a deep puncture wound may allow antigens to be introduced intravenously and carried by the blood to the spleen, where an immune response will be mounted. On the other hand, superficial cuts and scratches may lead antigens to enter subcutaneously, in which case they are delivered to local lymph nodes. Oral introduction of antigen can be counterproductive to immunity, as this route of entry is associated with the development of *oral tolerance,* a phenomenon where antigens delivered via the gastrointestinal tract are ignored by the cells of the adaptive immune system. This mechanism is believed to have evolved so that we do not mount an immune response against the foods we eat.

Traits of Antigens and Immunogens

In general, **immunogenicity**—the ability of an antigen to stimulate a host response—depends on the following characteristics: (1) macromolecular size, (2) foreignness, (3) chemical composition and molecular complexity, and (4) the ability to be processed and presented within MHC molecules. Usually, an immunogen must have a molecular weight of at least 10,000 daltons (Da) to be recognized by the immune system, and the most effective immunogens typically have a molecular weight of more than 100,000 Da. However, there are exceptions, because a few substances with a molecular weight of lower than 1,000 Da have been known to induce an immune response. For the most part, the greater the molecular weight, the more potent the molecule is as an immunogen.

Another characteristic shared by strong immunogens is *foreignness*, or un-relatedness to the host. To prevent the immune system from attacking the body's own cells and tissues, lymphocytes are carefully selected during their development to ensure that the pool of mature lymphocytes responds only to antigens *not* recognized as self. Typically, the more taxonomically distant an antigen's source is from the host, the greater the likelihood that host lymphocytes will react to it, dramatically increasing the probability that the antigen will be a successful immunogen. For example, plant protein is a better immunogen for an animal than is material from a related animal. Occasionally, however, autoantibodies, or antibodies to self-antigens, exist. This is the exception rather than the rule; this phenomenon is discussed in Chapter 15.

Immunogenicity is also determined by a substance's chemical composition and molecular complexity. Proteins and polysaccharides are the most effective immunogens. In contrast, synthetic polymers such as nylon or Teflon are made up of a few simple repeating units with no bending or folding within the molecule, and these materials are nonimmunogenic. For this reason, they are used in making artificial heart valves, elbow replacements, and other medical devices.

The immunogenicity of a substance is also strongly influenced by the type of molecules it is composed of. Proteins are highly immunogenic when compared with other biomolecules, such as polysaccharides, nucleic acids, and lipids. The mechanisms underlying the strong immunogenicity of proteins is related to (1) differences in how the T and B lymphocytes detect antigens and (2) a requirement for interactions between B cells and T cells for an effective antibody response to occur. These concepts will be discussed in Chapter 4.

Proteins are composed of a variety of subunits known as *amino acids,* which are covalently linked together in polypeptide chains of varying length. The linear sequence of amino acids comprises the *primary* structure of a protein. Each type of amino acid incorporated into a protein possesses distinct chemical properties, and interactions between the amino acids within a protein's primary structure cause the chain to bend, kink, and loop, forming basic three-dimensional shapes, or *secondary* structures. Two common secondary structures found in proteins are known as *alpha helices*, which have peptide chains that twist to form a spiral, and beta pleated sheets, in which chains form undulating zig zags that coalesce into a planar shape. In the third, or *tertiary,* level of protein structure, these basic secondary structures fold upon themselves once again, bringing distant regions of the primary amino acid chain together and embodying the spatial or three-dimensional orientation of the entire molecule. At the final level of protein structure, known as *quaternary,* two or more polypeptide chains come together, forming a multimeric unit **(Fig. 3–1).** The interactions between amino acids that dictate the overall three-dimensional shape of a protein are very complex but can

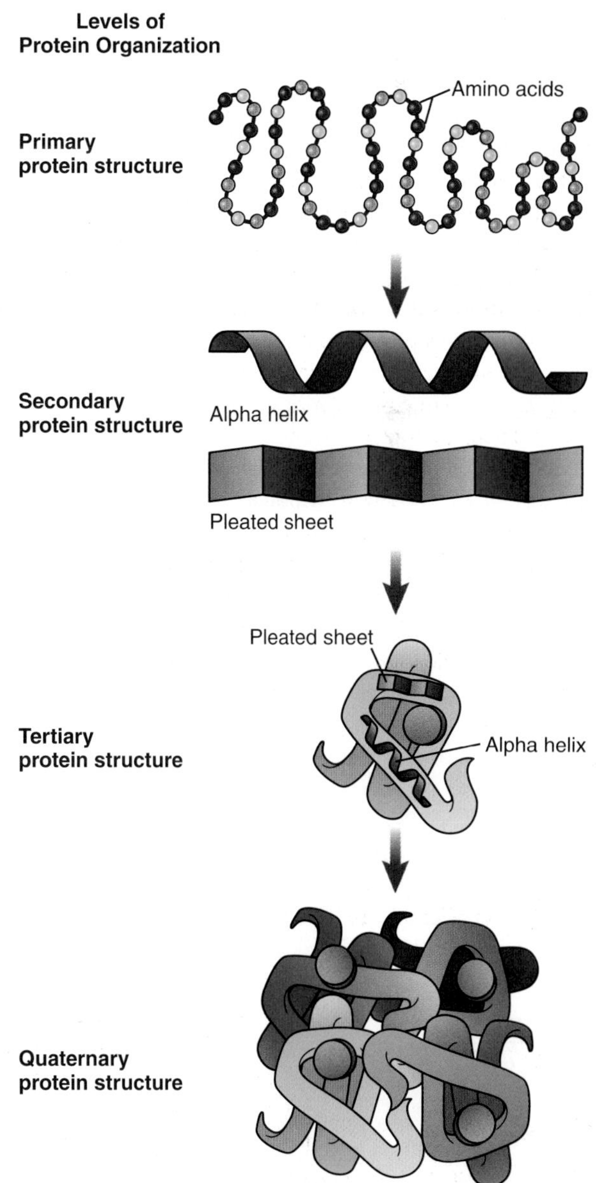

FIGURE 3–1 Levels of protein organization.

ultimately be traced back to the sequence of peptides found in the primary structure.

The activating receptors of both T and B lymphocytes are capable of reacting to specific proteins, but the levels of protein structure at which this detection occurs are very different. T cells, as you will learn later in this chapter, detect small fragments of a protein, known as *peptides*, and rely on MHC molecules to cradle these peptides for antigen recognition to occur. Thus, T cells "see" the primary structures, or amino acid sequences, of small pieces of a protein. The receptors on B cells, on the other hand, are activated by binding to amino acids on a protein's exterior. Therefore, B cells "see" the exposed tertiary or quaternary structures of a protein.

An effective B-cell response to most antigens (one that involves the production of high-affinity antibodies and results in immunological memory) requires "help" from T cells. In other words, to mount an appropriate B-cell response, T cells must also be activated so that they can provide necessary physical and chemical signals to the B cell.

Polysaccharides are less immunogenic than proteins because of their smaller relative size and because T cells do not recognize carbohydrates. Therefore, exposure to pure polysaccharide does not result in T-cell activation, and B cells that respond to a particular polysaccharide antigen will not receive crucial T-cell help. As immunogens, carbohydrates most often occur in the form of glycolipids or glycoproteins. Many of the blood group antigens are composed of such carbohydrate complexes. For example, the A, B, and H blood group antigens are glycolipids, and the Rh and Lewis antigens are glycoproteins. Other carbohydrates that are important immunogens are the capsular polysaccharides of bacteria such as *Streptococcus pneumoniae*. Pure nucleic acids and lipids are not immunogenic by themselves, although a response can be generated when they are attached to a suitable carrier molecule. This is the case for autoantibodies to DNA that are formed in systemic lupus erythematosus (SLE). These autoantibodies are actually stimulated by a DNA–protein complex rather than by DNA itself.

Finally, for a substance to elicit an immune response, it must be subject to antigen processing, which involves enzymatic digestion to create small peptides or pieces that can be complexed to MHC molecules for presentation to responsive T lymphocytes. The particular MHC molecules expressed by an individual also govern responsiveness to specific antigens. Each person only inherits genes encoding a limited repertoire of MHC molecules, as we will discuss in the section on the genes coding for MHC molecules.

Epitopes

Although an immunogen must have a molecular weight of at least 10,000 Da, only a small portion of the total molecule is actually recognized by each individual lymphocyte. This key portion of the immunogen is known as the *antigenic determinant* or *epitope*. **Epitopes** are the precise molecular shapes or configurations recognized by B cells, or the peptide sequences detected by T cells. Large molecules may contain numerous epitopes, and each one is capable of triggering the production of a specific antibody or activating a T cell. B cells may recognize two types of epitopes: (1) **linear epitopes** that consist of sequential amino acids on a single polypeptide chain or (2) **conformational epitopes** that result from the folding of one or more polypeptide chains, bringing together amino acids that may be distant from each other so that they are recognized together **(Fig. 3–2).** Triggering of a B-lymphocyte response requires that epitopes be found on the surface of a molecule, accessible to the B-cell receptor, and that these sites contain more than one copy of the epitope so that cross-linking of the B-cell receptors may occur. This can be accomplished by as few as 6 to 15 amino acids. In contrast, T cells detect only linear epitopes that are liberated once a protein has been degraded. This means that many T cells are able to respond to cryptic epitopes found hidden within the interiors of large proteins that are not available for B-cell recognition. As mentioned previously, T-cell recognition also requires that these peptide antigens are presented by MHC molecules.

Haptens

Many substances are too small to be recognized by B cells but can stimulate a response if combined with a larger molecule. A **hapten** is a substance that is nonimmunogenic by itself but is able to form new antigenic determinants when combined with a larger carrier molecule. Thus, a hapten is an antigen but not an immunogen. Bound to its carrier, the hapten is able to initiate the production of antibodies that can react with the hapten even in the absence of the carrier. Small size and the presence of a solitary determinant site renders haptens incapable of antibody-mediated precipitation or agglutination because cross-linking with more than one antibody molecule is not possible **(Fig. 3–3).**

Examples of haptens found in nature are the *catechols* contained within the poison ivy plant *(Rhus radicans)*. Once in contact with the skin, these catechols join with tissue proteins to form the immunogens that give rise to contact dermatitis. Another example of haptens coupling with normal proteins in the body to provoke an immune response occurs with certain drug–protein conjugates. The best-known example occurs with penicillin, which can result in a life-threatening allergic response.

Karl Landsteiner, an Austrian scientist perhaps best known for his discovery of the ABO blood groups, conducted the most famous study of haptens. In his book *The Specificity of Serological Reactions*, published in 1917, he detailed the results of an exhaustive study of haptens that has contributed greatly to our knowledge of antigen–antibody reactions. Landsteiner immunized rabbits with haptens attached to a carrier molecule, then tested the serum to measure how the antibodies produced reacted with different haptens. He discovered that antibodies not only recognize chemical features such as polarity, hydrophobicity, and ionic charge, but the

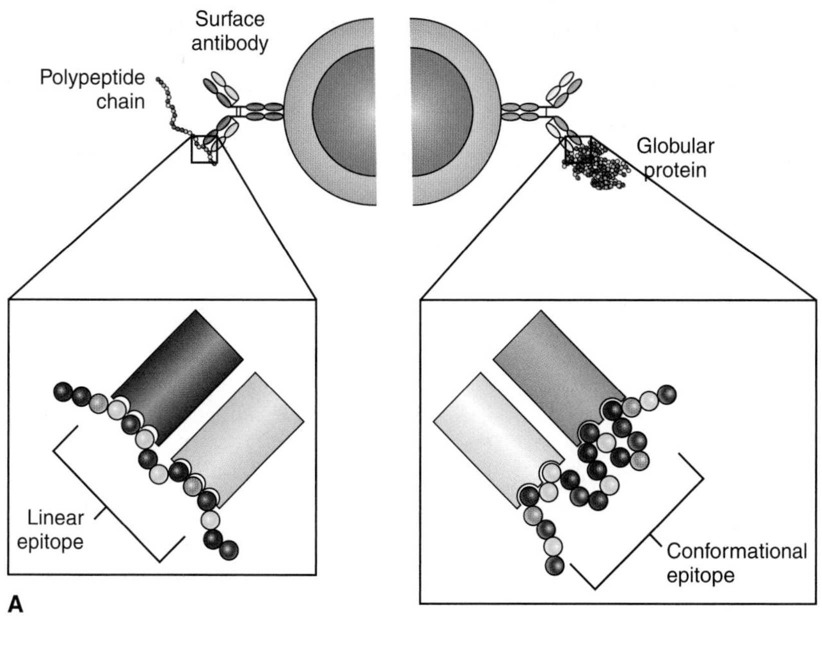

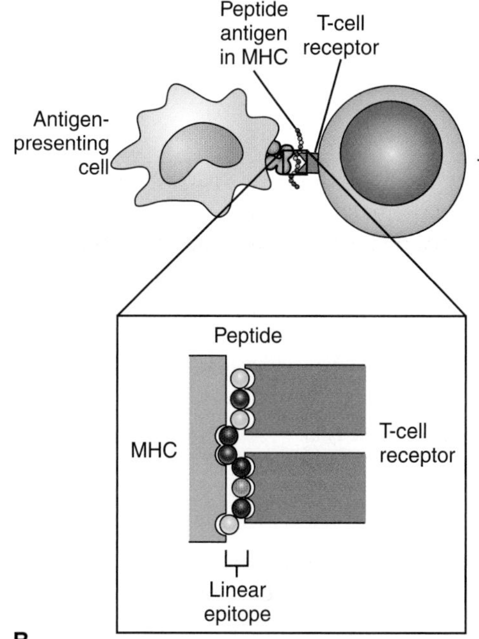

FIGURE 3–2 Linear versus conformational epitopes. (A) Linear epitopes consist of sequential amino acids on a single polypeptide chain, whereas conformational epitopes result from the folding of a polypeptide chain or chains, placing nonsequential amino acids in close proximity. B cells are capable of responding to antigens containing both linear and conformational epitopes. (B) T cells are only able to respond to linear epitopes that are displayed in MHC molecules. Unlike B cells, these linear epitopes need not be found at the surface of a protein; they may be buried within the molecule.

overall three-dimensional configuration is also important. The spatial orientation and the chemical complementarity are responsible for the lock-and-key relationship that allows for tight binding between antibody and epitope **(Fig. 3–4)**. Today, it is known that many therapeutic drugs and hormones can function as haptens.

Adjuvants

Proteins and glycoproteins are not necessarily highly immunogenic when administered by themselves. The generation of a robust immune response against proteins and related biomolecules often requires stimulation of innate immunity, especially antigen-presenting cells (APCs), such as dendritic cells. Substances delivered simultaneously with antigen for the purpose of potentiating, or enhancing, the immune response are known as **adjuvants.**

Adjuvants are able to increase the immunogenicity of an antigen by stimulating innate immune receptors, such as Toll-like receptors, that detect the presence of infection or danger. Adjuvants are also thought to work by preventing antigen from diffusing away from a site of inoculation, which allows innate immune cells to accumulate in the site. In this way, adjuvants *trick* the immune system into acting as if an infection is under way, even if the antigen inoculum given to a patient is essentially harmless.

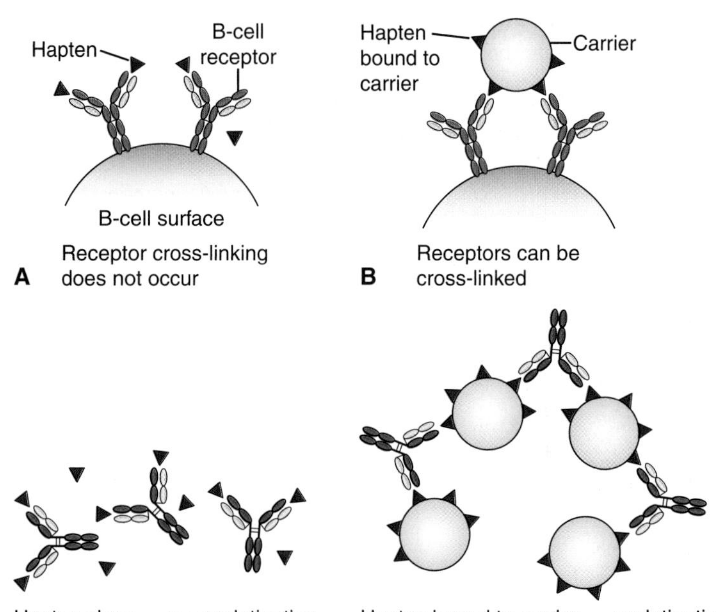

FIGURE 3–3 Characteristics of haptens. (A) Haptens bind B-cell receptors, but the receptors are not cross-linked; therefore, no activation occurs (not immunogenic). (B) Hapten or carrier complexes cross-link receptors, leading to B-cell activation and antibody production (immunogenic). (C) Although haptens can bind to the antibody-binding sites (antigenic), no agglutination can occur. Hence, the reaction cannot be visualized. (D) When bound to carriers, the haptens contribute to the formation of an interconnected lattice, which is the basis for precipitation and agglutination reactions.

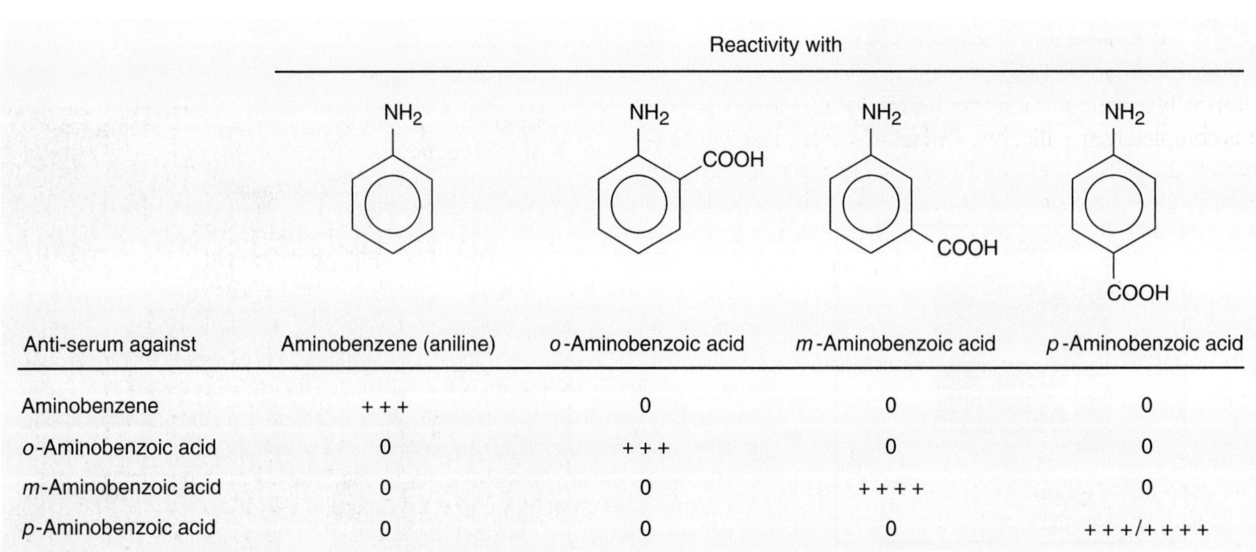

Anti-serum against	Reactivity with: Aminobenzene (aniline)	o-Aminobenzoic acid	m-Aminobenzoic acid	p-Aminobenzoic acid
Aminobenzene	+ + +	0	0	0
o-Aminobenzoic acid	0	+ + +	0	0
m-Aminobenzoic acid	0	0	+ + + +	0
p-Aminobenzoic acid	0	0	0	+ + +/+ + + +

FIGURE 3–4 Landsteiner's study of the specificity of haptens. Spatial orientation of small groups is recognized, because antibodies made against aminobenzene coupled with a carrier will not react with other similar haptens. The same is true for anti-serum to *o*-aminobenzoic acid, *m*-aminobenzoic acid, and *p*-aminobenzoic acid. Antibody to a carboxyl group in one location would not react with a hapten, which has the carboxyl group in a different location. *(From Landsteiner K.* The Specificity of Serological Reactions. *Revised Edition. New York, NY: Dover Press; 1962.)*

Many vaccines use adjuvants to achieve protective immunity against the target antigen (see Chapter 25). Those vaccines that do not require adjuvants are usually composed of whole pathogens or substances derived from pathogens that have been killed or weakened. Some vaccines consist of microbes that have been altered so that they are capable of limited replication within a human host but cannot establish a productive infection. In vaccines composed of such live or killed pathogens, no adjuvant is required, because the pathogen itself supplies the immune danger signals necessary to stimulate an immune response.

Most newer vaccines, however, consist of recombinant protein antigens that have been manufactured in a sterile laboratory setting. Such protein antigens alone are not ideal immunogens, requiring vaccines containing them to be formulated with adjuvants to trigger an immune response. The improvement of existing adjuvants and the design of new adjuvants is a rapidly developing field in immunology.

Relationship of Antigens to the Host

Antigens can be placed in broad categories according to their relationship to the host. **Autoantigens** are those antigens that belong to the host. These do not evoke an immune response under normal circumstances. However, if an immune response does occur to autoantigens, it may result in an autoimmune disease. Refer to Chapter 15 for a discussion of some of the most well-known autoimmune diseases. **Alloantigens** are from other members of the host's species and are capable of eliciting an immune response. They are important to consider in tissue transplantation and in blood transfusions. **Heteroantigens** are from other species, such as other animals, plants, or microorganisms.

Heterophile antigens are heteroantigens that exist in unrelated plants or animals but are either identical or closely related in structure so that an antibody against either antigen will cross-react with the other. An example of this is the human blood Group A and B antigens, which are related to bacterial polysaccharides. It is believed that anti-A antibody, which is normally found in individuals with blood types other than A (e.g., type B and type O), is originally formed after exposure to pneumococci or other similar bacteria. Naturally occurring anti-B antibody is formed after exposure to a similar bacterial cell wall product. The presence of naturally occurring antibodies is an important consideration in selecting the correct blood type for transfusion purposes.

Normally in serological reactions, it is ideal to use a reaction that is completely specific, but the fact that cross-reactivity exists can be helpful for certain diagnostic purposes. Indeed, the first laboratory assay for infectious mononucleosis (IM) was based on a heterophile antibody reaction. During the early stages of IM, a heterophile antibody is formed, stimulated by an unknown antigen. This antibody was found to react with sheep red blood cells (RBCs), which formed the basis of the Paul–Bunnell test for mononucleosis (see Chapter 23). This procedure was a useful screening test when the causative agent of IM, Epstein–Barr virus, had not yet been identified. Current rapid screening tests for IM detect heterophile antibodies present in the sera of infected patients that cross-react with horse or bovine RBC antigens.

The cross-reactivity between patient antibodies against Epstein–Barr virus, the causative agent of IM, and sheep, horse, or bovine RBC antigens is fortuitous in that it can aid in the detection of the disease. The presence of certain heterophile antibodies in patient sera can also confound clinical immunoassays. In many assays for specific analytes, animal antibodies are used as reagents. Such antibody reagents may be bound to a surface and used to capture an analyte from a patient sample, or they may be covalently bound to reporter molecules, such as enzymes or fluorescent dyes, and used to detect the presence and quantity of an analyte. In rare cases, patient-produced heterophile antibodies can link together the reagent antibodies used for antigen capture and the reagent antibodies used for detection of the analyte, falsely elevating its apparent level. This concept is discussed in more detail in Chapter 11. In these situations, the presence of heterophile antibodies is detrimental to the work of the clinical laboratory scientist.

Major Histocompatibility Complex

For years, scientists searched to identify possible immune response genes that would account for differences in how individuals respond to particular antigens. Today we know that the genetic capability to mount an immune response is linked to a group of molecules originally referred to as *human leukocyte antigens* (HLAs). The French scientist Dausset gave them this name because they were first defined by discovering an antibody response to circulating white blood cells (WBCs). These molecules are now known as *MHC molecules* because they determine whether transplanted tissue is histocompatible and accepted by the recipient or if it is recognized as foreign and rejected. MHC molecules are actually found on all nucleated cells in the body, and they play a pivotal role in the development of both humoral and cell-mediated immunity. Although MHC molecules were initially identified by their antigenicity in the context of organ transplantation, their main immune function is to serve as carriers of peptide antigens for recognition by T cells. Unlike B cells, whose surface receptors bind to antigen directly, T cells require antigens to be cradled within MHC molecules for recognition to occur.

Connections

The Florida Panther

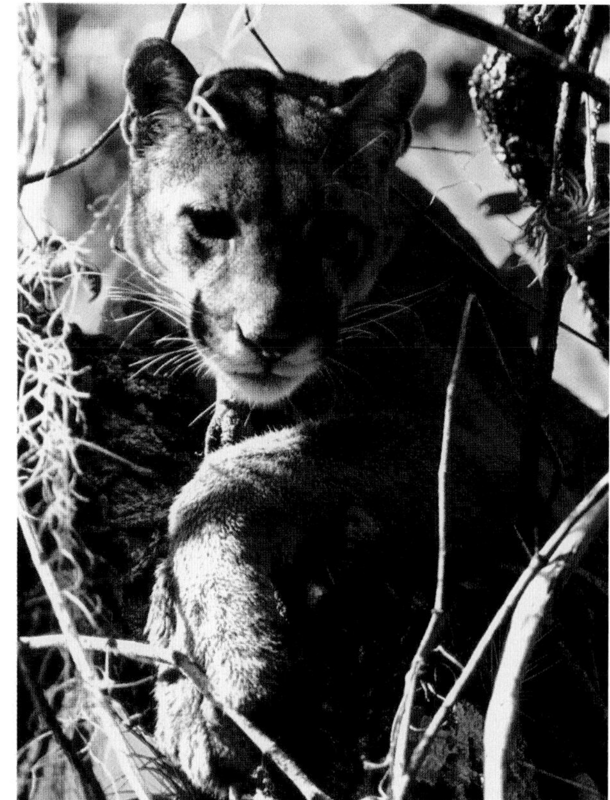

FIGURE 3–5 The Florida panther. *(John Hollingsworth/U.S. Fish and Wildlife Service.)*

Polymorphism of the MHC genes in a species is thought to serve as a protection against infectious diseases because diverse genes allow for a response to a wide variety of antigens. The fate of the Florida panther is a good example of what happens when there is a lack of genetic diversity in a particular population **(Fig. 3–5)**. In the early 1990s, only about 20 to 25 adult panthers remained in Florida because of a combination of factors, including destruction of their habitat and inbreeding. The latter severely decreased the genetic pool of the population. It has been postulated that the panthers became increasingly susceptible to viral diseases because of the limited polymorphism of the MHC antigens. Conservationists decided to increase the strength of the gene pool by moving eight females from the Texas population to Florida.

Now, more than two decades after introducing new females into the population, the Florida panthers have exhibited a marked improvement in health and fitness. The increased diversity of the MHC genes allowed for a response to diverse pathogens. The Florida panthers are able to withstand disease better because of the introduction of these new genes into the population.

Genes Coding for MHC Molecules (HLA Antigens)

MHC molecules are encoded by the most polymorphic gene system found in humans, meaning that each allele in this region of the human genome varies greatly among different individuals. Because the role of MHC genes is so essential for immunity, this high degree of polymorphism is thought to improve our chances of survival as a species, because it allows for an immune response to diverse pathogens (also see Connections box). Genes coding for the MHC molecules in humans are found on the short arm of chromosome 6 and are divided into three categories or classes. Class I genes are found at three different locations or loci, termed *A*, *B*, and *C*. Class II genes are situated in the D region, and there are several different loci, known as *DR*, *DQ*, and *DP*. For class I molecules, there is only one gene coding for each particular molecule. Class II molecules, in contrast, have one gene that codes for the α chain of the molecule and one or more genes that code for the β chain. The area of class III genes lies between the class I and class II regions on chromosome 6. Class III genes code for the complement proteins, C4a, C4b, C2, and B, as well as cytokines such as tumor necrosis factor (TNF) **(Fig. 3–6)**.

The class I and class II molecules are involved in antigen recognition by T cells; in this role, they influence the repertoire of antigens to which lymphocytes can respond. In contrast, class III molecules are secreted proteins that have an immune function, but they are not expressed on cell surfaces, as are class I and II. Class III molecules also have a completely different structure compared with the other two classes.

When the human population is considered as a whole, many alternate forms, or alleles, of each MHC gene are found. Different **alleles** of a gene code for slightly different varieties of the same product. The MHC system is described as highly polymorphic because there are so many possible alleles at each location. At the time this chapter was written, 6,082 different HLA-A alleles, 7,256 HLA-B alleles, and 5,842 HLA-C alleles had been identified within the human population.

The probability that any two individuals will express the same MHC molecules is very low. Each person inherits two copies of chromosome 6; thus, there is a possibility of two different alleles for each gene on the chromosome unless that person is homozygous (has the same alleles) at a given location. These genes are described as *codominant,* meaning that all alleles that an individual inherits code for products that are expressed on cells. Because the MHC genes are closely linked, they are inherited together as a package called a **haplotype.** Thus, each inherited chromosomal region consists of a specific combination of genes for HLA-A, -B, -C, -DR, -DP, and -DQ. The full genotype would consist of two genes of each type at a particular locus (see Chapter 16).

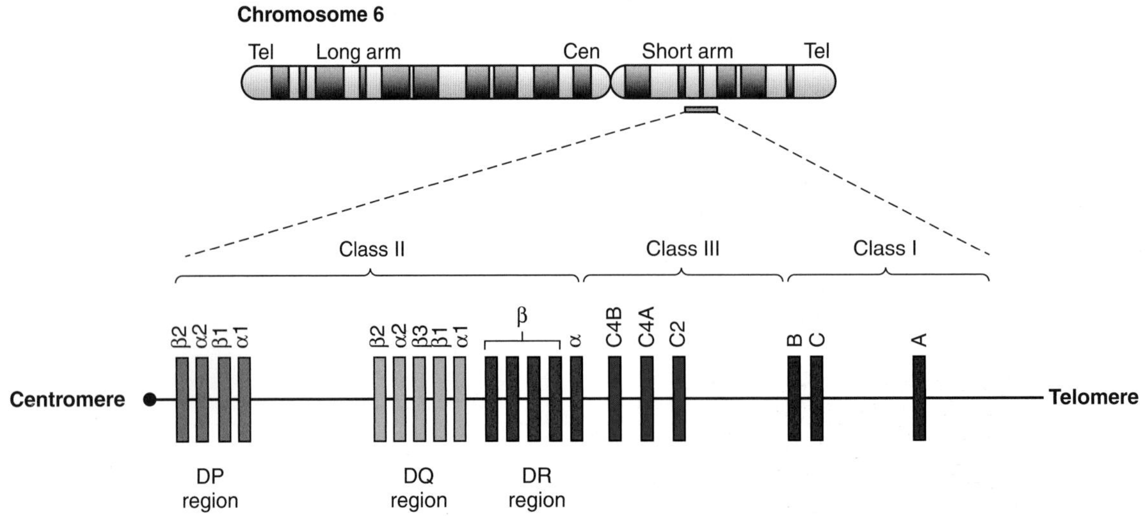

FIGURE 3–6 The major histocompatibility complex. Location of the class I, II, and III genes on chromosome 6. Class I consists of loci A, B, and C, whereas class II has at least three loci: DR, DQ, and DP.

One haplotype is inherited from each parent. Because there are numerous alleles or variant forms at each locus, an individual's MHC type is about as unique as a fingerprint. Because of the tremendous diversity of alleles, more than 1.7 billion different class I haplotypes alone are possible in the human population. The frequency of particular HLA alleles differs significantly among different ethnic populations and can sometimes be used to trace an individual's ancestry or ethnic origins. The uniqueness of the HLA antigens creates a major problem in matching organ donors to recipients because these antigens are highly immunogenic. However, in cases of disputed paternity, polymorphisms can be used as a helpful identification tool.

Clinical Correlations

HLA Nomenclature

Traditionally, HLA nomenclature had been defined serologically through the use of a battery of antibodies. Advances in DNA sequencing have made the identification of actual genes possible. The nomenclature has become correspondingly more complex. For instance, the notation HLA DRB1*1301 indicates that the actual gene involved in coding for the β chain of an HLA DR1 antigen is the number 13, and the 01 is a specific subtype.

Expression of Class I and II MHC Molecules

Each of the class I and II MHC genes codes for a protein that appears on cell surfaces. All the proteins of a particular class share structural similarities and are found on the same types of cells. Whereas **class I MHC (HLA) molecules** are expressed on all nucleated cells, **class II MHC (HLA) molecules** are found primarily on APCs. Their differing structures, as explained in the text that follows, are tailored to their specific functions in the adaptive immune response.

Structure of Class I MHC Molecules

Although class I MHC molecules are expressed on all nucleated cells, levels of expression can vary among various cell types. Class I expression is highest on lymphocytes and myeloid cells and low or undetectable on liver hepatocytes, neural cells, muscle cells, and sperm. This may explain why engraftment of HLA-mismatched livers can be quite successful, whereas other solid-organ transplants require a much closer MHC match between donor and recipient. Additionally, HLA-C antigens are expressed at a much lower level than HLA-A and HLA-B antigens, so the latter two are the most important class I MHC antigens to match for transplantation.

Each class I antigen is a glycoprotein dimer made up of two noncovalently linked polypeptide chains **(Fig. 3–7).** The α chain has a molecular weight of 44,000 Da. A lighter chain associated with it, called a β_2-*microglobulin*, has a molecular weight of 12,000 Da and is encoded by a single gene on chromosome 15 that is not polymorphic. This means that within an individual and across the human population, all class I molecules contain identical β_2-*microglobulin*. The class I α chain is folded into three domains—α1, α2, and α3—and it is inserted into the cell membrane via a hydrophobic transmembrane segment. The three external domains consist of about 90 amino acids each; the transmembrane domain has about 25 hydrophobic amino acids, along with a short stretch of about 5 hydrophilic amino acids, as well as an anchor of 30 amino acids. β_2-microglobulin does not penetrate the cell membrane, but it is essential for proper folding of the α chain.

X-ray crystallographic studies indicate that the α1 and α2 domains of class I MHC molecules each contain an alpha helix. In the tertiary structure of the molecule, these alpha helices are brought together to form the walls of a deep groove. This furrow is found at the top of the MHC molecule (facing away from the cell membrane) and functions as the peptide-binding site. This binding site is able to hold peptides between 8 and 11 amino acids long. Most of the polymorphism found in class

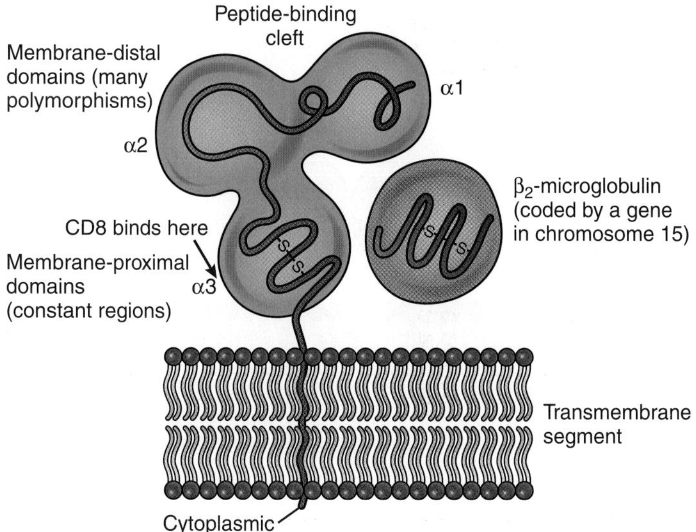

FIGURE 3–7 General structure of a class I MHC molecule. Class I MHC molecules consist of an α chain with three domains and a shorter chain, β_2–microglobulin, common to all class I molecules.

I molecules resides in the $\alpha 1$ and $\alpha 2$ regions, whereas the $\alpha 3$ region and β_2-microglobulin are relatively constant. The $\alpha 3$ region reacts with CD8 molecules on cytotoxic T cells.

HLA-E, -F, and -G are considered *nonclassical* class I MHC molecules. HLA-E and -F are generally not expressed on the surfaces of cells and don't present peptide antigen to cytotoxic T cells. Instead, HLA-E and -F play other important roles in immunity. HLA-G plays a role unique among the MHC-related proteins: HLA-G is primarily expressed on fetal trophoblast cells during the first trimester of pregnancy. Placental trophoblast cells represent points of direct contact between maternal and fetal tissue—a potential source of alloantigens. HLA-G molecules are thought to contribute to maternal immune tolerance of the fetus by protecting placental tissue from the action of natural killer (NK) cells. HLA-G binds to NK inhibitory receptors, preventing an NK-cell-driven cytotoxic response. (See Chapter 2 for the action of NK cells.)

Structure of Class II MHC Molecules

Class II MHC molecules are found on APCs, including B lymphocytes, monocytes, macrophages, dendritic cells, and thymic epithelial cells. Because dendritic cells are considered the most effective APCs, they express high levels of class II MHC on their surface.

The major class II molecules—HLA-DP, -DQ, and –DR—consist of two noncovalently bound polypeptide chains that are encoded by separate genes in the MHC gene complex. This type of quaternary protein structure is often referred to as a *heterodimer* because it comprises two ("dimer") dissimilar polypeptide chains ("hetero"). HLA-DR is expressed at the highest level because it accounts for about one-half of all the class II molecules found on a particular cell. Among the class II MHC genes, the DRβ gene is the most highly polymorphic; over 3,300 different alleles are known at this time. DP molecules are found in the shortest supply.

Both the class II MHC α chain, with a molecular weight of 34,000 Da, and the β chain, with a molecular weight of 29,000 Da, are anchored to the cell membrane **(Fig. 3–8).** The α chain and the β chain each contain two domains, numbered 1 and 2. In the heterodimeric quaternary structure of class II MHC molecules, the $\alpha 1$ and $\beta 1$ domains each contribute an alpha helix, forming the peptide-binding site, which is analogous to the groove found on class I molecules (see Fig. 3–7). However, in class II MHC molecules, both ends of the peptide-binding cleft are open, allowing the capture of longer peptides, as compared with class I molecules. The $\alpha 2$ domains and the $\beta 2$ domains are evolutionarily conserved in a similar manner to the $\alpha 3$ and β_2-microglobulin components found in class I molecules.

As with class I MHC molecules, three *nonclassical* class II genes have been identified—HLA-DM, -DN, and -DO. The products of these genes have been shown to play a regulatory role in antigen processing. DM helps to load peptides onto class II molecules, whereas DO modulates antigen binding. The function of DN is not known at this time.

Role of Class I and II Molecules in the Immune Response

The main role of the class I and II MHC molecules is **antigen presentation,** the process by which peptide fragments derived from degraded proteins are transported to the plasma membrane, allowing recognition by T lymphocytes. As mentioned previously, T cells can only "see" and respond to peptide antigens when the antigens are combined with MHC molecules.

Whereas one individual expresses (at most) only six different class I molecules (two copies each of HLA-A, -B, and

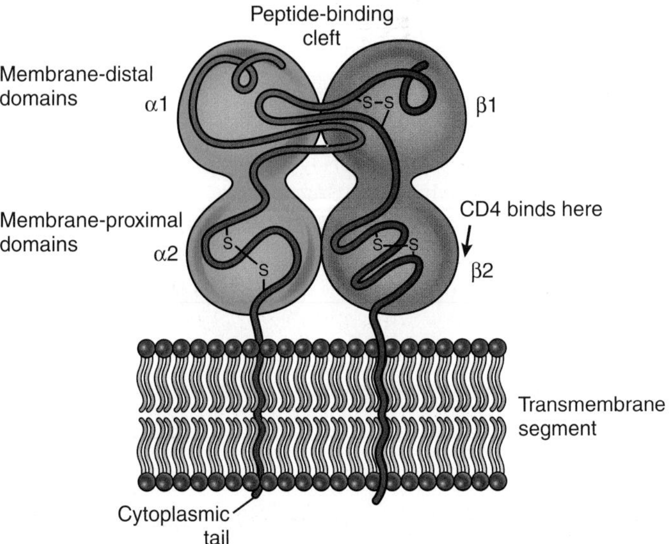

FIGURE 3–8 General structure of class II MHC molecule. Class II MHC molecules consist of an α chain and a β chain, each of which has two domains.

–C) and six class II molecules (two each of HLA-DR, -DP, and –DQ), each of these MHC molecules is capable of presenting a large number of diverse antigenic peptides to T cells. This is possible because the binding of peptides to MHC molecules is promiscuous and not highly specific. This allows humans to respond to many different antigens, which is important for the survival of the species.

It is thought that these two main classes of MHC have evolved to deal with two distinct types of infections: those that attack cells from the outside (such as bacteria) and those that attack from the inside (viruses and other intracellular pathogens). Class I molecules mainly present cytoplasmic peptide antigens to CD8 (cytotoxic) T cells, whereas class II molecules present extracellular antigens to CD4 (helper) T cells. Extracellular proteins presented by class II molecules are those taken into the cell from the outside by processes such as phagocytosis and degraded within intracellular vacuoles. Class I molecules are thus the watchdogs of viral, tumor, and intracellular parasitic antigens that are synthesized within the cell, whereas class II molecules help to mount an immune response to bacterial infections or other pathogens usually found outside of cells. In either case, for a T-cell response to be triggered, peptides must be available in adequate supply for MHC molecules to bind, they must be able to bind to MHC effectively, and they must be recognized by a T-cell receptor. Some viruses, such as herpes simplex and adenovirus, have managed to block the immune response by interfering with one or more processes involved in antigen presentation. These viruses are able to maintain a lifelong presence in the host.

The dramatic functional differences between class I and II MHC can largely be attributed to the mechanisms responsible for the processing and delivery of peptide antigen to the MHC molecules themselves. The following sections highlight the differences in the intracellular pathways that feed antigen into each type of MHC.

The Class I MHC–Peptide Presentation Pathway

The class I MHC presentation pathway is sometimes referred to as the *endogenous* pathway of antigen presentation, because both the peptides and MHC molecules arise from within the same cell. The endogenous peptide antigens presented by class I MHC represent a sampling of the many polypeptide chains that compose the proteins found within the cell's cytosol. In a healthy cell, these peptides derive from host proteins; however, tumor cells or those infected with a virus or parasitic bacterium also contain aberrant proteins that are unique to the tumor or are produced by the invading pathogen. The class I MHC presentation pathway provides cytotoxic T lymphocytes a means of surveilling the interiors of cells throughout the body, allowing T cells to search for peptides associated with infection or malignancy.

Cytoplasmic proteins enter the class I pathway by undergoing proteolysis in an enzyme complex known as the *proteasome* **(Fig. 3–9)**. This macromolecular structure contains dozens of enzymatic subunits arranged cylindrically to form a proteolytic tunnel. To generate peptide fragments, whole proteins are unfolded and threaded into the core of the proteasome, which cleaves the proteins into peptide chains. The resultant peptides are released from the proteasome into the cytosol.

Class I MHC molecules are synthesized by ribosomes associated with the rough endoplasmic reticulum. As the α chain is being manufactured, several important *chaperone* proteins associate with it to ensure that the nascent MHC molecule folds into the appropriate three-dimensional tertiary shape. One important chaperone, known as *calnexin*, stabilizes the α chain until it binds to β_2-microglobulin. When β_2-microglobulin binds, calnexin is released, and two additional chaperone molecules—calreticulin and tapasin—associate with the complex and help to stabilize it for peptide binding.

When synthesis of MHC molecules is complete, their antigen-binding sites are oriented toward the interior of the endoplasmic reticulum, whereas the peptide antigens generated by proteasomal degradation are located within the cytoplasm. Two **transporters associated with antigen processing, TAP1** and **TAP2,** are essential for shuttling antigenic peptides into the lumen of the endoplasmic reticulum, allowing the peptides to interact with newly formed class I MHC molecules. TAP-driven translocation is dependent on adenosine triphosphate (ATP) and is most efficient for peptides of 8 to 16 amino acids in length. The TAP transporters are brought into close proximity with class I molecules by tapasin, a protein that bridges transporter and MHC, so that peptides can be directly loaded. Once the α chain has bound the peptide, the class I MHC peptide complex is rapidly transported to the cell surface (see Fig. 3–9).

The class I pathway is capable of generating thousands of peptides from proteins that have undergone proteasomal digestion, but only a small fraction of these will actually become antigens. The binding of peptides to class I MHC is dictated by several variables, all of which must be met for successful presentation to occur. The first consideration in the binding of peptides to the MHC groove is the length of the peptide chain. As the class I MHC binding groove is closed at its ends, it can accommodate peptides of no longer than 11 amino acids. Peptide binding itself is determined by complementary noncovalent interactions between the peptide and the amino acids comprising the alpha helices that form the binding groove. In most cases, the interactions between peptide and MHC molecule are dictated by fewer than a handful of individual intermolecular interactions. Different class I molecules have slightly different binding affinities, and these small differences determine the particular antigens to which an individual will respond.

It is estimated that a single cell may express between 100,000 and 200,000 copies of each class I molecule at its surface, meaning that many different peptides are simultaneously displayed in this manner. As few as 10 to 100 class I MHC complexes bearing the same peptide antigen may be sufficient to induce a CD8 cytotoxic T-cell response. In healthy cells, all class I MHC molecules contain self-peptides that are

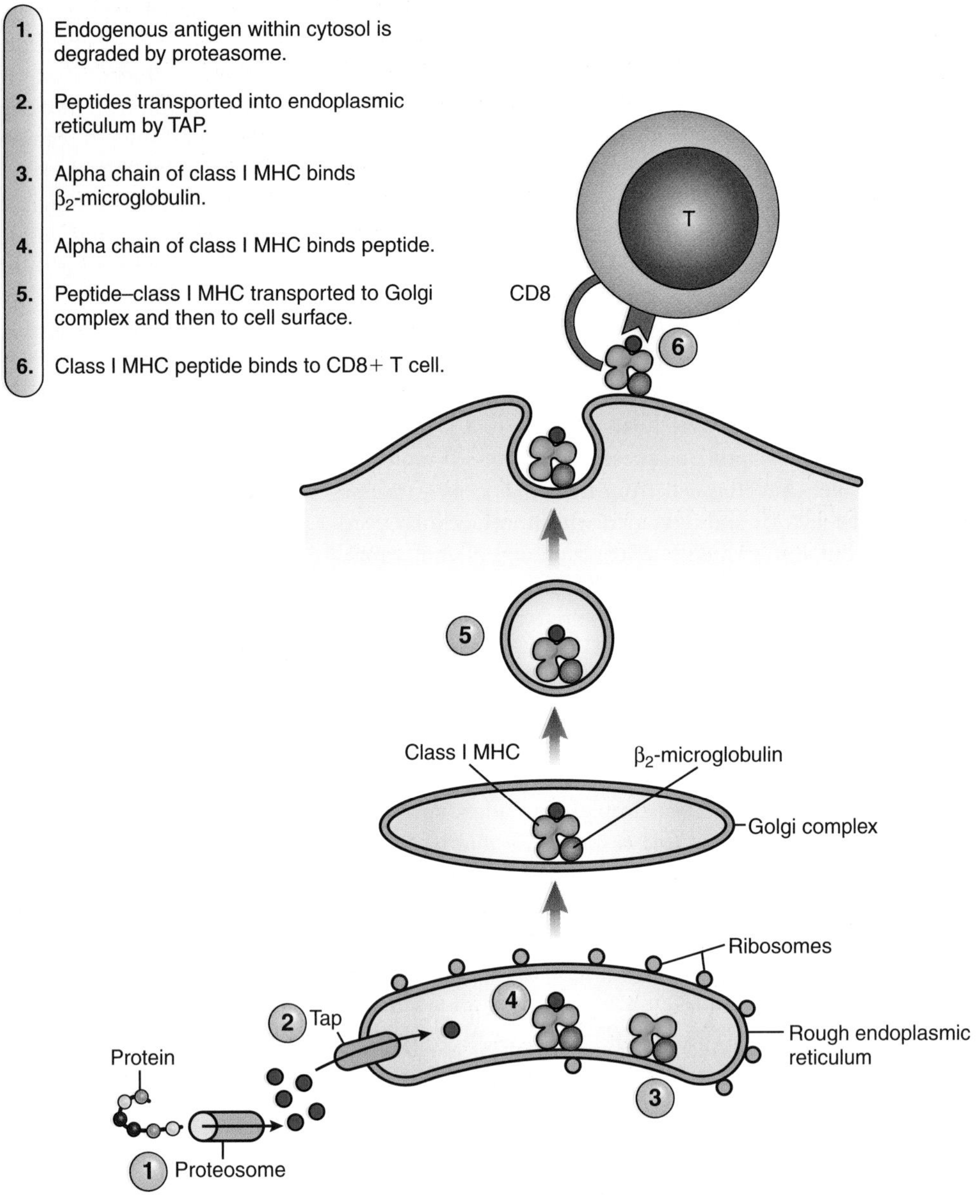

1. Endogenous antigen within cytosol is degraded by proteasome.
2. Peptides transported into endoplasmic reticulum by TAP.
3. Alpha chain of class I MHC binds β_2-microglobulin.
4. Alpha chain of class I MHC binds peptide.
5. Peptide–class I MHC transported to Golgi complex and then to cell surface.
6. Class I MHC peptide binds to CD8+ T cell.

T
CD8
6
5
Class I MHC
β_2-microglobulin
Golgi complex
Ribosomes
2 Tap
4
Rough endoplasmic reticulum
Protein
3
1 Proteosome

FIGURE 3–9 Antigen-processing pathway for endogenous antigens. Cytoplasmic proteins are degraded and fed into the MHC class I pathway for presentation to CD8+ cytotoxic T cells.

ignored by patrolling T cells. In diseased cells, some of the peptides displayed originate from microbial proteins or proteins associated with cancer. The display of thousands of class I molecules complexed to antigen allows CD8+ T cells to continuously check the body's cells for the presence of nonself antigen. If a T cell that recognizes a particular foreign peptide antigen in class I MHC makes contact with a cell presenting that antigen, the T cell may be triggered to lyse the infected cell **(Fig. 3–10)**.

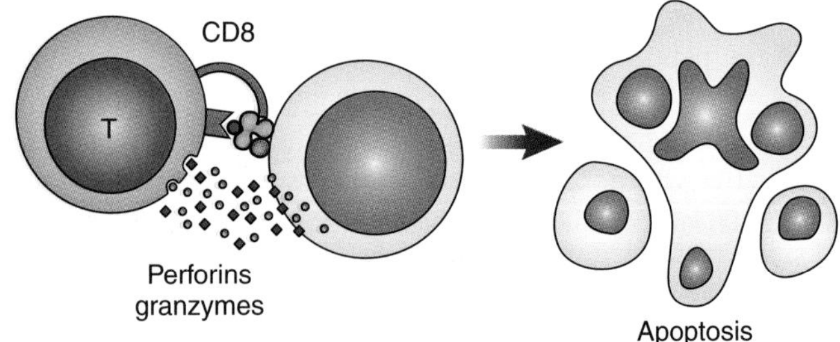

FIGURE 3–10 CD8 T cells recognize antigen in association with class I MHC. If endogenous antigens are recognized as being foreign by the T cell, cytotoxic molecules are released, resulting in destruction of the target cell.

The Class II MHC–Peptide Presentation Pathway

Class II MHC molecules function in the presentation of *exogenous* antigens to T cells, that is, peptide antigens that are derived from proteins found outside of the presenting cell. For presentation of exogenous antigens to occur, extracellular proteins must be taken up by means of either phagocytosis or endocytosis, processes by which cells ingest materials by enclosing them in a small portion of the plasma membrane. Proteins that are captured in this way are digested by hydrolytic enzymes that accumulate within the lumen of the vesicle, resulting in peptide chains of 13 to 18 amino acids in size. Dendritic cells, the immune cells considered to be the most potent activators of T cells, are excellent at capturing and digesting exogenous antigens from bacteria and other microbes in this way.

Similar to class I MHC molecules, class II molecules are synthesized in the rough endoplasmic reticulum **(Fig. 3–11).** Immediately after synthesis, class II molecules associate with a protein known as the **invariant chain (Ii),** a 31-kDa protein present in great excess of the actual number of class II molecules being synthesized. Ii is required during the production of class II MHC molecules to prevent endogenous peptides within the endoplasmic reticulum from binding to the class II peptide-binding groove. Thus, Ii serves as a placeholder, ensuring that only exogenous peptide antigens will be bound to MHC II molecules. Ii may also aid in bringing α and β chains together, a signal required for newly translated class II molecules to move from the endoplasmic reticulum into the Golgi complex, and then to enter endocytic or phagocytic vesicles where digested exogenous antigens are located.

Within endosomal compartments, class II molecules encounter peptides derived from exogenous proteins previously ingested by the presenting cell. In order for peptide antigens to bind to MHC II, Ii must first be degraded by a protease, leaving just a small fragment called *class II invariant chain peptide* (CLIP) attached to the peptide-binding cleft. CLIP is then exchanged for an exogenous peptide whose selective binding to the cleft is favored by the low pH of the endosomal compartment. Nonclassical class II MHC molecules such as HLA-DM assist with CLIP removal and guide exogenous peptides into the binding groove. Because the MHC II binding groove is open at both ends, the length of peptides that can be accommodated within it extends from 10 to nearly 30 amino acids (although the optimal size is between 12 and 16 amino acids). This is in contrast to class I MHC molecules, which have closed ends, constraining the length of peptides that can bind.

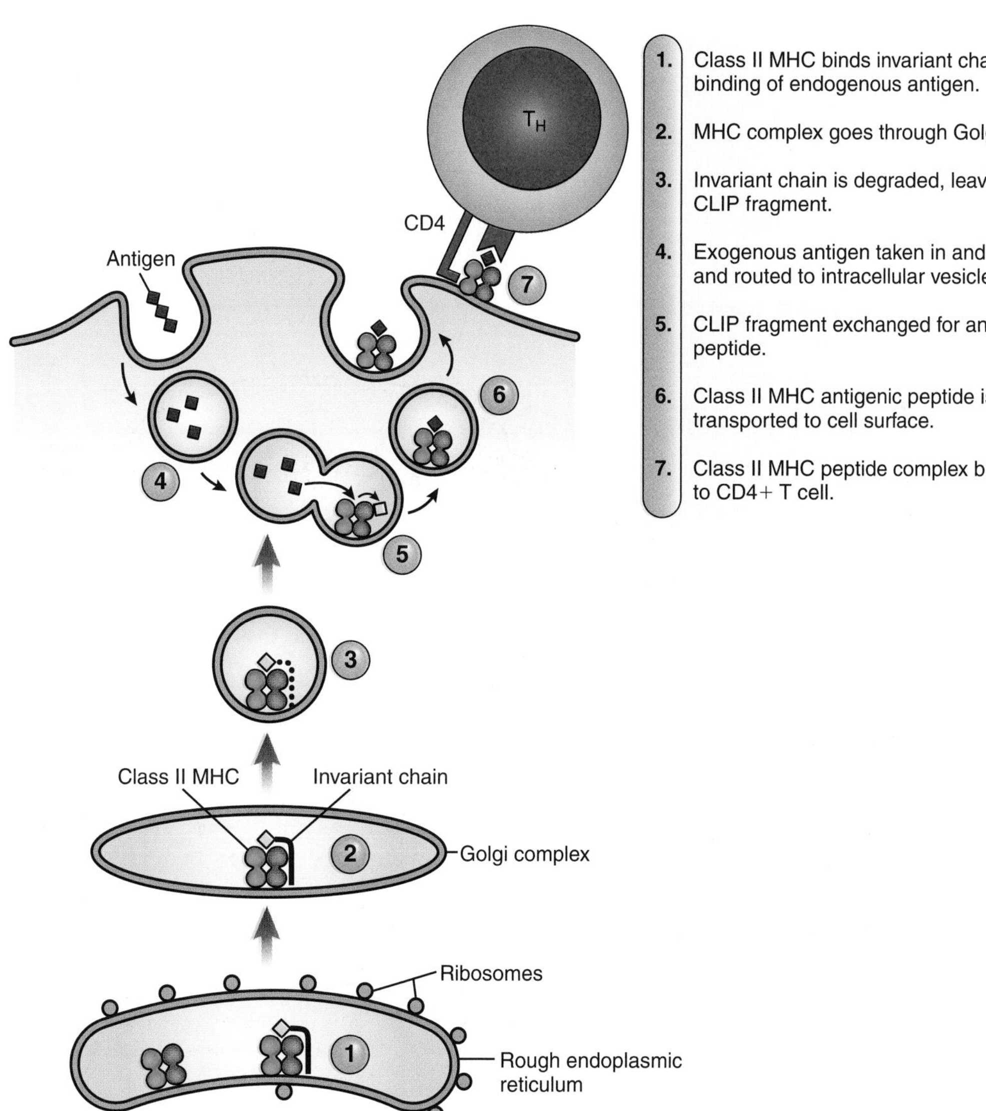
T$_H$
CD4
Antigen
7
6
4
5
3
Class II MHC
Invariant chain
2
Golgi complex
Ribosomes
1
Rough endoplasmic reticulum
1. Class II MHC binds invariant chain to block binding of endogenous antigen.
2. MHC complex goes through Golgi complex.
3. Invariant chain is degraded, leaving CLIP fragment.
4. Exogenous antigen taken in and degraded and routed to intracellular vesicle.
5. CLIP fragment exchanged for antigenic peptide.
6. Class II MHC antigenic peptide is transported to cell surface.
7. Class II MHC peptide complex binds to CD4+ T cell.

FIGURE 3–11 Antigen-processing pathway for exogenous antigen. The binding site of class II MHC molecules is first occupied by an invariant chain (Ii). This is degraded and exchanged for short exogenous peptides in an endosomal compartment. The exogenous peptide class II MHC complex is then transported to the cell surface.

With MHC class II molecules (as with class I molecules), only some of the amino acid residues within the peptide antigen, perhaps 7 to 10, mediate binding to the groove. For class II MHC, however, hydrogen bonding occurs along the length of the captured peptide, whereas binding of peptide to class I molecules occurs mostly at the amino and carboxy-terminal ends. The class II binding groove also features several pockets that can accommodate amino acids with large side chains, giving the class II molecule greater flexibility in the variety of peptides that can be bound.

Once peptide antigen has bound to an MHC II molecule, the class II protein–peptide complex is stabilized and transported to the cell surface (see Fig. 3–11). Once there, class II molecules bearing nonself antigen serve as essential signals for the activation of CD4 helper T cells. Helper T cells orchestrate the adaptive immune response, influencing the activities of other immune cells, including macrophages, cytotoxic T cells, and antibody-secreting B cells **(Fig. 3–12)**.

Clinical Significance of MHC

Given the near-ubiquitous expression of MHC molecules in tissues throughout the body and their critical importance in immunity, identifying an individual's MHC genotype and understanding the implications for health is of considerable clinical importance. Laboratory MHC testing is typically carried out before tissue transplantation because an immune response against either class I or class II molecules can induce graft rejection. Modern transplant HLA testing involves the use of molecular techniques to determine the MHC types of both donor and recipient, as well as serological testing to detect the presence of antibodies in the recipient targeting the MHC molecules of a potential donor. The role of the laboratory in transplantation is presented in Chapter 16.

Inheritance of certain HLA types may predispose individuals to the development of autoimmunity. The closest association between MHC expression and autoimmunity is between

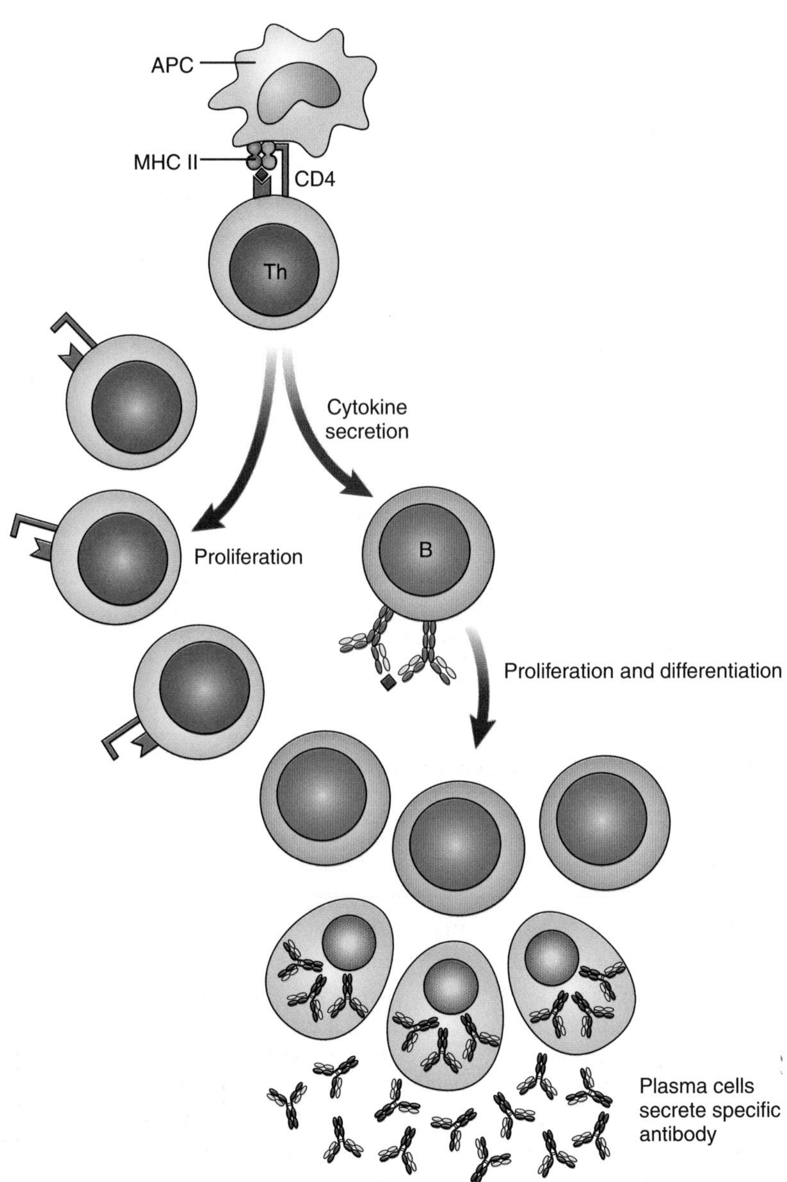

FIGURE 3–12 CD4+ T cells recognize exogenous antigen on phagocytic APCs along with class II MHC. CD4+ helper T cells are stimulated by contact when antigen and clonal expansion takes place. These cells secrete cytokines that cause an antigen-activated B cell to proliferate and differentiate into plasma cells, which make antibodies.

Table 3–1 Association of HLA Alleles and Disease

DISEASE	SYMPTOMS	HLA ALLELE	STRENGTH OF ASSOCIATION
Ankylosing spondylitis	Inflammation of the vertebrae of the spine	B27	+++
Celiac disease	Diarrhea, weight loss, intolerance to gluten	DQ2 DQ8	+++ +
Rheumatoid arthritis	Inflammation of multiple joints	DR4	+
Type 1 diabetes	Increase in blood glucose because of destruction of insulin-producing cells	DQ8 DQ2	++ +

+++ = very strong association, ++ = strong association, + = clear association. (From Margulies DH, Natarajan K, Rossjohn J, and McCluskey J. Major histocompatibility complex (MHC) molecules: structure, function, and genetics. In: Paul WE, ed. Fundamental Immunology. *6th ed. Philadelphia, PA: Wolters Kluwer, Lippincott Williams & Wilkins; 2012; Ch 21:487–523.)*

the inheritance of the class I molecule HLA-B27 and a disease called *ankylosing spondylitis*—a progressive chronic inflammatory disorder affecting the vertebrae of the spine. See **Table 3–1** for other links between HLA antigens and autoimmune diseases. This topic is discussed more fully in Chapter 15.

However, the centrality of antigen presentation by both class I and class II molecules in immunity is much more consequential than their roles in transplantation and autoimmunity. MHC molecules determine the types of peptide antigen to which an individual can mount an adaptive immune response, potentially defining a person's ability to overcome an infection. Although MHC molecules typically can bind a broad variety of peptides, small biochemical differences in the molecules can amount to large differences in the immune system's ability to react to a specific antigen. For instance, it is possible that nonresponders to a particular vaccine do not have the genetic capacity to respond to the vaccine antigen. On the other hand, the presence of a particular MHC protein may confer additional protection against an infection, as seen in the example of HLA B8 and increased resistance to HIV infection. It is therefore foreseeable that, in the future, determination of an individual's HLA type may be routinely performed on all patients and considered a standard laboratory technique.

Much of the recent research in this area has focused on the types of peptides that can be bound by particular MHC molecules. Future developments may include tailoring vaccines to certain groups of such molecules. As more is learned about antigen processing and presentation, researchers can specifically develop vaccines containing certain amino acid sequences that serve as immunodominant epitopes. These vaccines may avoid the risk associated with using live organisms. Additionally, if an individual suffers from allergies, knowing a person's MHC type may also help predict the types of allergens to which he or she may respond. Certain drug hypersensitivities have also been linked to particular HLA alleles, and knowledge of one's HLA genes might prevent severe reactions to these drugs. Another area for future research is the development of possible tumor vaccines based on an individual's MHC type. It is likely that knowledge of the MHC molecules will affect many areas of patient care in the future.

SUMMARY

- Immunogens are substances that are capable of stimulating an adaptive immune response—either in the form of antibody production by B cells or the activation of T cells.
- The term *antigen* describes a substance recognized by the adaptive immune system but that may not necessarily elicit an adaptive response by itself (as in the case of haptens).
- The immunogenicity, or ability of a substance to stimulate an immune response, is influenced by factors such as age, health, route of inoculation, and genetic capacity.
- Most immunogens are high-molecular-weight proteins (at least 100,000 Da) or polysaccharides that are foreign to the host.
- Although immunogens are fairly large molecules, the response of each B and T cell is directed against a small portion of the entire molecule, or epitope.
- B cells recognize epitopes found on the exterior of a protein—those regions that antibodies can reach. B cells can target linear epitopes, which are made of sequential amino acids in the peptide chain, or conformational epitopes produced by twisting and folding of the primary chain to bring distant amino acid residues together in the same epitope.
- In contrast, T cells only recognize linear epitopes bound to MHC molecules, but these epitopes can come from any region of the protein—even parts of the peptide chain that are buried deeply inside and hidden from antibodies.
- Haptens are substances that are too small to provoke an adaptive immune response alone but stimulate such a response when combined with a carrier.
- Once an antibody response is generated, haptens are capable of reacting with that antibody, but precipitation or agglutination reactions will not occur because the complexes formed are too small.
- Adjuvants are substances that can be mixed with antigen to enhance the immune response. Adjuvants usually contain

inert materials that simulate infection or prevent antigen from diffusing away from the site of inoculation.
- Antigens can be characterized by their relationship to the host. Autoantigens are those that belong to the host; alloantigens are from the same species as the host but are not identical to the host; heteroantigens are from other species.
- Heterophile antigens exist in unrelated species, but their structure is so similar that antibody formed to one antigen will cross-react with antigen from a different species.
- The MHC encodes class I and class II molecules, which play a major role in antigen presentation to T cells.
- So many different alleles are found in the human population for each MHC gene that the MHC system is considered the most polymorphic in the genome of our species.
- Class I and class II molecules bind peptides within cells and transport them to the plasma membrane, where the peptides can be recognized by T cells.
- Class I MHC molecules are found on all nucleated cells; these molecules associate with foreign antigens, such as viral proteins, synthesized within a host cell. This is known as the *endogenous pathway* for antigen presentation.
- Class II molecules are only found on APCs (B cells, monocytes, macrophages, dendritic cells, and thymic epithelium). These molecules associate with foreign antigens taken into the cell from the outside, in the pathway known as *exogenous antigen presentation*.
- Class I MHC molecules consist of an α chain encoded by the MHC complex, as well as a second lighter chain called *β_2-microglobulin* encoded by a gene on chromosome 15.
- Class II MHC molecules have an α and a β chain, both of which are encoded by genes in the MHC complex.
- Class I molecules present endogenous antigen to CD8+ T cells, triggering a cytotoxic reaction.
- Class II molecules present exogenous antigen to CD4+ T cells, which are helper cells involved in antibody production.

Study Guide: A Comparison of Class I and Class II MHC Molecules

	CLASS I MHC MOLECULES	CLASS II MHC MOLECULES
Cellular distribution	All nucleated cells	B cells, monocytes, macrophages, dendritic cells, thymic epithelial cells
Structure	One α chain and β_2-microglobulin	An α chain and a β chain
Classes	A, B, C	DP, DQ, DR
Size of peptides bound	8 to 11 amino acids	10 to 30 amino acids (12 to 16 optimally)
Nature of peptide binding cleft	Closed at both ends	Open at both ends
Interaction with T cells	Presents endogenous antigen to CD8+ T cells	Presents exogenous antigen to CD4+ T cells

CASE STUDIES

1. A 15-year-old boy needs to have a kidney transplant because of the effects of severe diabetes. His family members consist of his father, mother, and two sisters. All of them are willing to donate a kidney so that he can discontinue dialysis. He is also on a list for a cadaver kidney. His physician suggests that the family be tested first for the best HLA match.

Questions

a. How many alleles are shared by mother and son? Father and son?
b. What are the chances that one of the sisters would be an exact match?
c. Is there a possibility that a cadaver kidney might be a better match than any of the family members'?

2. A zombie plague is ravaging the world and decimating the human population. You are one of a few hundred million survivors. Chaos reigns. Although you haven't yet completed your training in immunology, you are visited by government agents and conscripted into designing a vaccine to protect against the plague. When you arrive at a secret military laboratory, you are told that the zombie pathogen has been identified and isolated. It's your mission to design an effective vaccine.

Questions

a. Other researchers have purified several different antigens from the plague virus: a lipid, a nucleic acid fragment, a polysaccharide, and a protein. Which of these plague antigens would make the most effective vaccine, and why?
b. Now that you have selected an antigen to use in the vaccine, what additional component might be required to make an effective zombie plague vaccine? What purpose does this additional component serve?

REVIEW QUESTIONS

1. All of the following are characteristics of an effective immunogen *except*
   a. internal complexity.
   b. large molecular weight.
   c. the presence of numerous epitopes.
   d. found on host cells.

2. Which of the following best describes a hapten?
   a. Cannot react with antibody
   b. Immunogenic only when coupled to a carrier
   c. Has multiple determinant sites that can cross-link B-cell receptors
   d. A large chemically complex molecule

3. Which would be the most effective immunogen?
   a. Protein with a molecular weight of 200,000
   b. Lipid with a molecular weight of 250,000
   c. Polysaccharide with a molecular weight of 220,000
   d. DNA with a molecular weight of 175,000

4. Which of the following individuals would likely respond most strongly to a bacterial infection?
   a. An adult who is 75 years of age
   b. A malnourished 40-year-old
   c. A weightlifter who is 35 years old
   d. A newborn baby

5. Which best describes an epitope?
   a. A peptide that must be at least 10,000 MW
   b. An area of an antigen recognized only by T cells
   c. A segment of sequential amino acids only
   d. A key portion of the antigen

6. Adjuvants act by which of the following methods?
   a. Activate innate immune cells
   b. Facilitate rapid diffusion of antigen from the tissues
   c. Inhibit presentation of peptide antigens to T cells
   d. Decrease recruitment of APCs

7. A heterophile antigen is one that
   a. is a self-antigen.
   b. exists in unrelated plants or animals.
   c. has been used previously to stimulate an antibody response.
   d. is from the same species but is different from the host.

8. Which of the following is true of class II MHC (HLA) antigens?
   a. They are found on B cells and macrophages.
   b. They are found on all nucleated cells.
   c. They are also known as *HLA-A*, *-B*, and *-C*.
   d. They are coded for on chromosome 9.

9. Class II MHC molecules are recognized by which of the following?
   a. CD4+ T cells
   b. CD8+ T cells
   c. NK cells
   d. Neutrophils

10. Which of the following best describes the role of TAP?
    a. Binds to class II molecules to help block the antigen-binding site
    b. Binds to class I proteins in proteasomes
    c. Transports peptides into the lumen of the endoplasmic reticulum
    d. Helps cleave peptides for transport to endosomes

11. What is the purpose of the invariant chain in antigen processing associated with class II MHC molecules?
    a. Helps transport peptides into the endoplasmic reticulum
    b. Blocks binding of endogenous peptides
    c. Binds to CD8+ T cells
    d. Cleaves peptides into the proper size for binding

12. An individual is recovering from a bacterial infection and tests positive for antibodies to a protein normally found in the cytoplasm of this bacterium. Which of the following statements is true of this situation?
    a. Class I molecules have presented bacterial antigen to CD8+ T cells.
    b. Class I molecules have presented bacterial antigen to CD4+ T cells.
    c. Class II molecules have presented bacterial antigen to CD4+ T cells.
    d. B cells have recognized bacterial antigen without help from T cells.

13. In relation to a human, alloantigens would need to be considered in which of the following events?
    a. Transplantation of a kidney from one individual to another
    b. Vaccination with the polysaccharide coat of a bacterial cell
    c. Oral administration of a live but heat-killed virus particle
    d. Grafting skin from one area of the body to another

14. Which is characteristic of class I MHC molecules?
    a. Consist of one α and one β chain
    b. Bind peptides made within the cell
    c. Able to bind whole protein antigens
    d. Coded for by HLA-DR, -DP, and -DQ genes

15. Which best explains the difference between immunogens and antigens?
    a. Only antigens are large enough to be recognized by T cells.
    b. Only immunogens can react with antibody.
    c. Only immunogens can trigger an immune response.
    d. Only antigens are recognized as foreign.

16. When a child inherits one set of six HLA genes together from one parent, this is called a(n)
    a. genotype.
    b. haplotype.
    c. phenotype.
    d. allotype.

17. HLA molecules A, B, and C belong to which MHC class?
    a. Class I
    b. Class II
    c. Class III
    d. Class IV

Adaptive Immunity

4

Aaron Glass, PhD, MB^{CM}(ASCP)

LEARNING OUTCOMES

After finishing this chapter, you should be able to:

1. Compare and contrast adaptive immunity and innate immunity.
2. Discuss the role of the thymus in T-cell maturation.
3. Describe the T-cell receptor (TCR) for antigen.
4. Explain how positive and negative selection contribute to T-cell development.
5. List and describe five different subsets of CD4 T helper (Th) cells.
6. Describe the maturation of a B cell from the pro–B-cell stage to the plasma cell stage.
7. Contrast the antigen-independent and antigen-dependent phases of B-cell development.
8. Explain how cytotoxic T cells recognize and kill target cells.
9. Discuss the role of class I major histocompatibility complex (MHC) and class II MHC molecules in the presentation of antigens to T cells.
10. Compare and contrast the immune response to T-dependent antigens with the response to T-independent antigens.
11. Discuss how Th cells influence the B-cell antibody response.
12. Explain the importance of T cells and B memory cells to the adaptive immune response.
13. Indicate surface markers characteristic of T and B lymphocytes in various stages of development.

CHAPTER OUTLINE

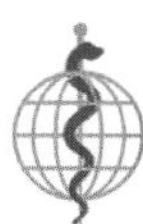

Go to FADavis.com for the laboratory exercises that accompany this text.

KEY TERMS

Adaptive immunity
Allelic exclusion
Antigen-dependent phase
Antigen-independent phase
B-cell receptor (BCR)
Cell-mediated immunity
Central tolerance
Chemokines
Clonal expansion
Cytotoxic T cells
Double-negative (DN) thymocytes
Double-positive (DP) thymocytes
Effector cells
Humoral immunity
Immature B cells
Isotype switching
Memory cells
MHC restriction
Negative selection
Plasma cell
Positive selection
Pre-B cells
Pro-B cells
Single-positive (SP) stage
Surrogate light chain
T-cell receptor (TCR)
T-dependent antigens
T follicular helper (Tfh) cells
Th1 cells
Th2 cells
T helper (Th) cells
T-independent antigens
T regulatory (Treg) cells
Thymocytes

As you learned in Chapter 2, the concept of innate immunity encompasses the body's barrier defenses, such as the skin; phagocytic cells, such as macrophages and neutrophils; and preformed soluble factors, including complement proteins. Innate immunity is general in nature—entire classes of pathogens elicit nearly identical innate responses, and these responses are unchanging through time. In contrast, **adaptive immunity** is characterized by:

- Specificity for individual microbes and pathogens
- Memory of prior exposures to antigen
- Enhancement of responses upon repeated exposures to the same threat

When compared with innate immunity, adaptive immunity represents a more *tailored,* or pathogen-specific, response. One tradeoff for this high degree of specificity is the time required after an initial exposure to a pathogen for an adaptive response to be mounted (often several days). Once under way, the adaptive response is highly effective and can often provide lifelong immunity against reinfection.

Adaptive immunity is traditionally divided into two main branches: (1) ***cell-mediated* immunity,** which is carried out by cells of the immune system, and (2) ***humoral* immunity,** which is mediated by soluble factors (antibodies) found in the liquid portions of body fluids. T lymphocytes, or T cells, are responsible for the cell-mediated arm of adaptive immunity, whereas B lymphocytes, or B cells, produce the antibodies that enable humoral immunity.

T lymphocytes can be divided into two broad categories, cytotoxic T cells and helper (Th) T cells **(Fig. 4–1).** The immune function of **cytotoxic T cells** is to kill target cells infected with intracellular pathogens, such as viruses and certain bacteria. Cytotoxic T cells are also capable of killing cancerous cells. In contrast, Th cells don't directly kill cells but instead control the immune response through the secretion of *cytokines,* or signaling molecules that allow communication between immune cells. Th cells can be further divided into several subpopulations based on the types of cytokines they secrete.

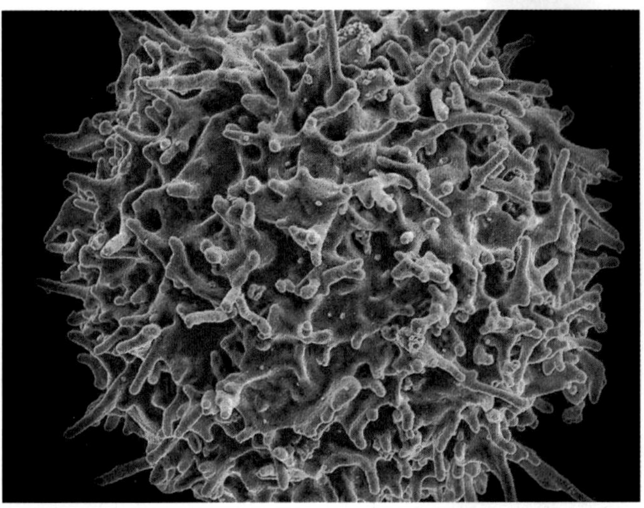

FIGURE 4–1 Scanning electron micrograph of a typical T cell. *(Courtesy of National Institute of Allergy and Infectious Diseases [NIAID].)*

B cells are responsible for producing antibodies (or immunoglobulins). Antibodies carry out many different roles in immunity, such as (1) labeling targets for ingestion by phagocytes, (2) rendering viruses and toxins inert through neutralization, and (3) blocking the adhesion of microbes to body tissues (see Chapter 5).

One key difference between the lymphocytes of adaptive immunity and the various cells of innate immunity is that the genes coding for the primary receptors that activate lymphocytes undergo rearrangement during the early stages of T-cell or B-cell development. In theory, following gene rearrangement, each individual lymphocyte is equipped to respond to a unique epitope associated with a specific pathogen (see Chapter 5). By virtue of each lymphocyte possessing a slightly different receptor specificity, the adaptive immune system, as a whole, represents an immune army that is theoretically capable of combating any conceivable infectious threat. When infection occurs, only the lymphocytes responsive to epitopes found on or in the invading pathogen(s) are activated and proliferate, a process known as **clonal expansion.** Clonal expansion is so named because proliferating lymphocytes give rise to populations of cells with genetically identical receptors that are specific for the same epitope, and these populations therefore represent *clones* of each other.

The characteristic delay between an initial infection and an effective adaptive response arises because a handful of pathogen-responsive lymphocytes must undergo a massive clonal expansion before reaching the large number of effector cells needed to alter the course of an infection. Most of the progeny generated during clonal expansion are **effector cells:** T cells that secrete cytokines or are cytotoxic, or B cells that produce antibodies. However, a small proportion of the clones become **memory cells;** that is, they enter a quiescent state and become long-lived. Memory cells lie in wait for reinfection with the same microbe. When memory cells encounter their specific epitope, they activate rapidly, resulting in a swifter response of greater magnitude than the primary response.

The production of lymphocytes by the body, also known as *lymphocyte differentiation*, begins very early in fetal development—a necessity because the rudiments of adaptive immunity must be in place at birth. Progenitors of T and B cells appear in the fetal liver as early as 8 weeks of pregnancy. Later in fetal development, the bone marrow becomes the source of new lymphocytes and remains the primary producer of hematopoietic cells at birth and throughout adult life. The earliest precursors of T and B lymphocytes are generated by asymmetric division of lymphoid progenitor cells. *Asymmetry* in this context refers to the concept that when a progenitor cell divides into two, one of the resulting daughter cells begins to take on the characteristics of a lymphocyte, whereas the other daughter cell retains the stem cell–like plasticity of a lymphoid progenitor.

The following sections provide a more detailed description of lymphocyte differentiation and how these maturation processes relate to the function of T and B cells in the adaptive immune response.

T-Cell Differentiation

Soon after their formation, T-cell precursors leave the bone marrow and are transported by circulating blood to the thymus, a primary lymphoid organ located in the upper thorax, roughly between the sternum and heart (the "T" in *T cell* derives from "thymus"). Thymic tissue can be divided into two histologically distinct regions: an outer cortex and inner medulla (**Fig. 4–2**).

Once in the thymus, T-cell precursors become known as **thymocytes.** Newly arriving thymocytes enter at the cortico-medullary junction—the border between the medulla and cortex. Entering thymocytes immediately begin to migrate toward the thymic cortex under the direction of **chemokines,** or cytokines that control the movement of cells. During a 3-week period, thymocytes slowly move from the thymic cortex into the medulla. During this time, various differentiation processes occur, such as rearrangement of the **T-cell receptor (TCR)** genes, changes in the expression of thymocyte cell surface markers, the selection of thymocytes with functional receptors, and the deletion of thymocytes with self-reactive potential. Interactions with *stromal,* or supporting, cells within the thymus are critical for each of these differentiation processes. These essential thymic stromal cells include macrophages, dendritic cells, and fibroblasts, in addition to thymic epithelial cells. The major stages of T-cell development—the double-negative (DN) stage, double-positive (DP) stage, and mature T cells—are discussed in the sections that follow. Key markers found on T cells in the various stages are listed in **Table 4–1.**

Connections

CD Markers

Recall from Chapter 1 that key cluster of differentiation (CD) markers are found on the surface of immune cells, including lymphocytes. CD markers provide a sort of *fingerprint*, allowing the classification of T and B cells and their developmental stage. These markers are bound by fluorescent-tagged antibody reagents, which allow the number of lymphocytes positive for each marker to be determined using a technique called *flow cytometry* (see Chapter 13). This type of analysis is routinely used in the diagnosis of leukemias, lymphomas, and immunodeficiency diseases such as AIDS. See Chapters 18 and 19 for details.

Double-Negative Stage

The two major subdivisions of T cells, cytotoxic T cells (Tc) and Th cells, can be identified by their differential expression of two important cell surface markers, CD4 and CD8. CD4 is commonly used to identify Th cells, whereas CD8 is a very reliable marker of cytotoxic T cells. Because their ultimate fate has yet to be decided, early thymocytes lack both CD4 and CD8 and are therefore known as **double-negative (DN) thymocytes.** DN thymocytes aggregate in the outer cortex of

Table 4–1 Stages of T-Cell Development

	DEVELOPMENTAL STAGE		
	DOUBLE NEGATIVE (DN)	**DOUBLE POSITIVE (DP)**	**SINGLE POSITIVE (SP)**
Key CD Markers	CD3	CD3 CD4 CD8	CD3 *Either* CD4 or CD8
T-Cell Receptor	—	TCR α/β	TCR α/β

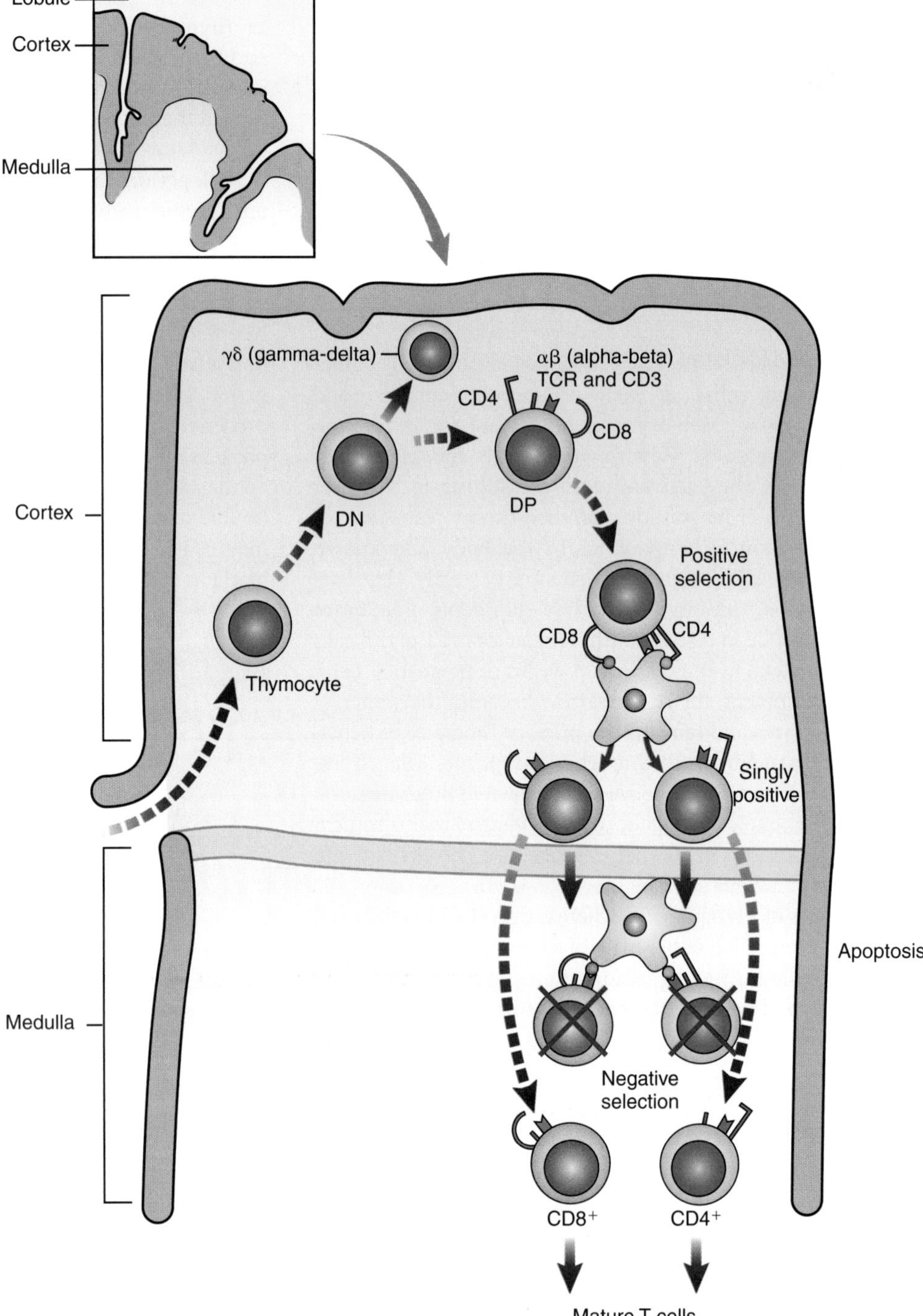

FIGURE 4–2 T-cell maturation in the thymus. T-lymphocyte precursors (thymocytes) enter the thymus at the corticomedullary junction and migrate into the cortex as DN (lacking both CD4 and CD8) thymocytes. It is at this point that TCR rearrangement begins. A small percentage of DN thymocytes express gamma-delta (γδ) chains, whereas the majority develop alpha-beta (αβ) chains and become DP thymocytes. Positive selection occurs as DP thymocytes encounter thymic stromal cells, allowing interactions between major histocompatibility complex (MHC) molecules and newly formed TCRs. Thymocytes that are successfully positively selected proceed to the single-positive (SP) stage and express either CD4 or CD8, depending on the type of MHC their TCR interacts with. Further interactions with thymic macrophages or dendritic cells allow negative selection, where potentially autoreactive thymocytes die by apoptosis before they can escape to the periphery. Thymocytes that successfully navigate these developmental hurdles exit the thymus as mature CD4 and CD8 T cells.

the thymus, where they actively proliferate under the influence of the cytokines, such as interleukin-7 (IL-7).

It is during the DN stage of T-cell development that rearrangement of the genes coding for the TCR begins **(Fig. 4–3).** Occurring at random, this shuffling and altering of the TCR genes results in the expression of a unique antigen receptor by each individual thymocyte—the underlying basis for a highly diverse population of T cells capable of responding to the myriad of antigens a person might encounter during a lifetime. The TCR is composed of two transmembrane proteins, the alpha (α) and beta (β) chains, each of which possesses an intracellular signaling domain, a membrane-spanning domain, and an extracellular domain tipped with a variable region. The variable regions of the α and β chains are responsible for recognition of antigen and are therefore the only portions of the TCR genes that undergo rearrangement.

Before rearrangement, the genes encoding the variable region of the TCR β chain (found on chromosome 7) are divided

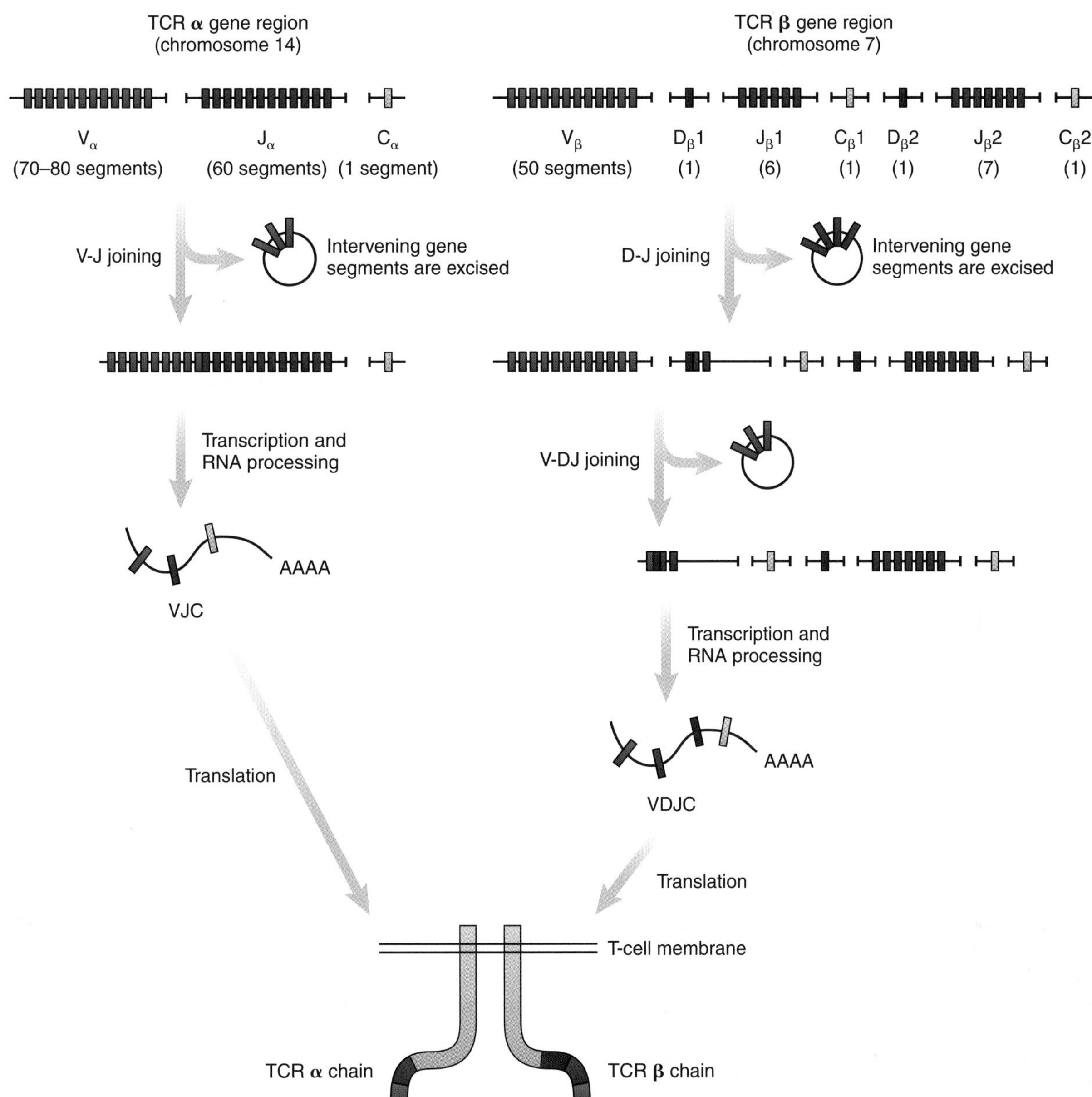

FIGURE 4–3 TCR gene organization and rearrangement. The TCR consists of two chains, α and β. The TCR α chain genes are located on chromosome 14 and consist of a series of variable (Vα) gene segments, a series of joining (Jα) gene segments, and a single constant (Cα) gene segment. In contrast, the TCR β chain genes are found on chromosome 7 and have a similar genetic structure to the TCR α genes except for the addition of diversity gene segments (Dβ) and duplicate regions of D (Dβ1 and Dβ2), J (Jβ1 and Jβ2), and C (Cβ1 and Cβ2) gene segments. During thymic development, the TCR genes undergo rearrangement, during which stepwise cleavage and joining events occur. Therefore, VJ and C are brought together in the TCR α chain, and VDJ and C are brought together in the TCR β chain. The variable region of each TCR chain, which interacts with MHCs and associated antigen peptides, is encoded by rearranged VD and J gene segments, whereas the C gene segments encode transmembrane and intercellular signaling domains.

into three large sections named *V*, *D*, and *J*, each containing multiple segments. During rearrangement, enzymes activated in DN thymocytes clip genomic DNA and begin stitching it back together in a way that randomly aligns one V segment, one D segment, one J segment, and a segment encoding the constant region. These enzymes are imprecise in the nucleotide positions at which DNA cleavage and ligation occur, a property that enhances TCR diversity but also introduces the possibility that some rearrangements will shift the translational frame of the gene in such a way as to result in a nonfunctional TCR. In cases where rearrangement leads to a faulty TCR β chain, developing T cells employ two strategies aimed at generating a functional protein. First, because T cells are diploid, the β chain genes on both copies of chromosome 7 simultaneously undergo rearrangement, doubling the probability of a functional β chain being produced. Second, the enzymes that mediate TCR gene rearrangement continue clipping and stitching variable-region DNA until a functional TCR is generated.

To test the functionality of the TCR β chains produced by gene rearrangement, a surrogate α chain with no variable region is temporarily expressed and forms a *pre-TCR* with the newly rearranged beta chain. If the DN thymocyte expresses a functional β chain, the pre-TCR provides survival signals to the T cell, ushering it into the next phase of T-cell differentiation, known as the *DP stage*.

Early on, some thymocytes, representing 10% or less of the total number, rearrange and express two other TCR chains—gamma (γ) and delta (δ)—when there is not a productive rearrangement of DNA coding for a β chain. Referred to as *gamma-delta (γδ) T cells*, this unique population of T lymphocytes proceeds down an alternate developmental pathway, typically remaining negative for both CD4 and CD8. Interestingly, γδ T cells represent the dominant T-cell population in the skin, intestinal epithelium, and pulmonary epithelium. Their tasks include wound healing and protection of the epithelium. In contrast to Th cells and cytotoxic T cells, γδ T cells do not require antigen presentation by major histocompatibility complex (MHC) proteins, suggesting that γδ T cells represent an important bridge between innate and adaptive immunity.

Double-Positive Stage

Successful pre-TCR signaling because of the presence of a functioning TCR β chain allows developing thymocytes to cross a developmental threshold, initiating rearrangement of the TCR α chain. In contrast to the TCR β chain, α chain gene variable regions are divided into only two sections, V and J (see Fig. 4–3). Despite this fact, the process of α chain rearrangement is mechanistically identical to that of the β chain and similarly results in segments from the V and J regions being connected to a constant region. The appearance of a functional α chain on the cell surface sends a signal to suppress any further TCR gene rearrangements. Concurrently with α chain rearrangement, thymocytes become both CD4-positive (CD4+) and CD8-positive (CD8+); in this stage of T-cell development, thymocytes are referred to as **double-positive (DP) thymocytes.**

As mentioned in the previous section, thymocytes are diploid cells with the potential to express two different α and β chains, should successful rearrangement of all four TCR genes occur. In this unlikely event, either of the β chains could pair with either α chain, resulting in a single T cell with four different TCR specificities (α1+β1, α1+β2, α2+β1, α2+β2). However, abundant experimental evidence has shown that each T cell recognizes only one antigenic peptide. This specificity for a single epitope arises because once a functional version of the β and α chains is produced, expression of the corresponding TCR gene on the opposite chromosome is permanently shut off—a process known as **allelic exclusion.**

The TCR α and β chains occur in a complex with six other molecules common to all T cells, known collectively as the *CD3/TCR complex*. The six chains of the nonspecific CD3 portion of the complex assist in intracellular signaling when an antigen binds to the TCR. These chains occur in three pairs:

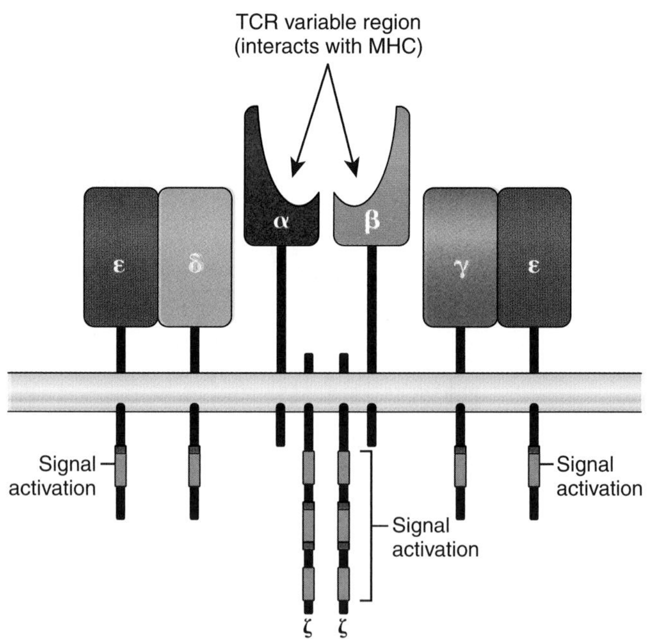

FIGURE 4–4 The CD3/TCR complex. The main structures are the TCR and the α and β chains, which are responsible for binding to MHCs. Four other types of chains that associate with the α and β chains in the TCR complex are collectively known as *CD3*. These are the ε, γ, δ, and ζ molecules that are essential for transmitting a signal to the T cell's interior when antigen binding occurs. Note that the γ and δ chains found here are different from the γδ chains of the γδ TCR.

delta-epsilon (δ-ε), gamma-epsilon (γ-ε), and a tau-tau (ζ-ζ) chain that is in the cytoplasm of the cell **(Fig. 4–4).**

T-cell receptors do not recognize peptide antigen alone (see Chapter 3). Instead, peptide antigen must be held in an MHC molecule, or "presented" to T cells, a requirement known as **MHC restriction.** This property of T cells is established during the DP stage of thymocyte development. Because gene rearrangement produces TCRs with nearly unlimited specificities, each newly formed receptor must be tested for its ability to interact with MHC through the process of **positive selection (Fig. 4–5).** During positive selection, thymocytes encounter stromal cells in the thymic cortex that express MHC class I and II proteins. These initial interactions between the DP thymocyte's TCR and stromal MHC determine the thymocyte's fate: Thymocytes that have TCRs that bind with very high affinity to MHC, or those that fail to bind to MHC at all, are induced to die by apoptosis. Only those DP thymocytes with receptors that bind moderately to MHC survive and proceed to the next step of maturation. This is important because T cells with receptors that bind to MHC too strongly have a high potential to react with self-antigens, and those with TCRs that don't bind to MHC can't function as mature T cells.

Two important molecules for establishing the MHC restriction of T cells are CD4 and CD8, which bind to MHC class I and class II molecules, respectively. During the DP stage, thymocytes express both CD4 and CD8. Depending on which class of MHC molecule a positively selected thymocyte

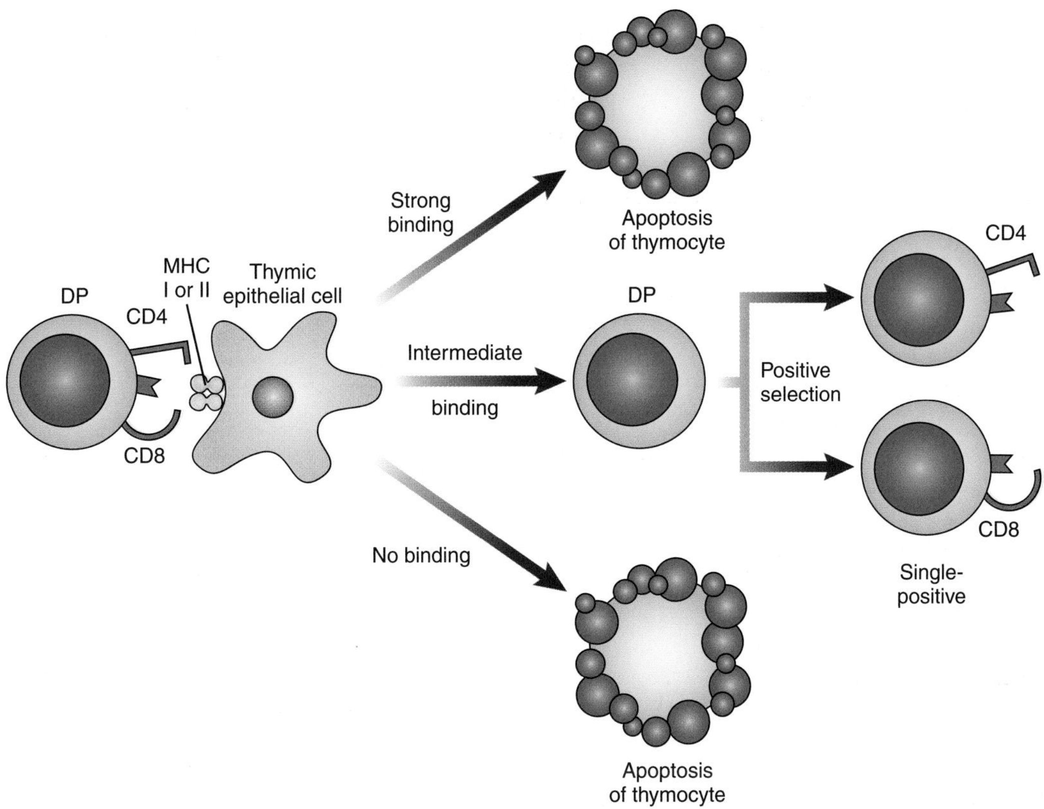

FIGURE 4–5 Positive selection of thymocytes in the thymic cortex. DP thymocytes (expressing both CD4 and CD8) interact with thymic epithelial cells. If very strong bonding occurs, those thymocytes are eliminated by apoptosis. If very weak or no bonding occurs, those thymocytes are also eliminated. Therefore, SP thymocytes (CD4 or CD8) that can interact with MHC, but don't interact *too strongly,* could signify future reactivity with self-antigens.

recognizes, the expression of the opposite marker begins to decrease substantially. Ultimately, thymocytes possessing TCRs that recognize MHC-II express CD4, whereas those that bind to MHC-I express CD8. Stable expression of either CD4 or CD8 and loss of expression of the opposite marker signify the entrance of the thymocyte into the next phase of differentiation, the "**single-positive**" **(SP) stage.**

Single-Positive Stage

Thymocytes that survive positive selection must overcome one final developmental hurdle before exiting the thymus as mature T cells. A second selection process, known as **negative selection,** takes place in the corticomedullary and medulla regions of the thymus. In negative selection, thymic stromal cells express a variety of self-antigens and present peptide fragments of these antigens to positively selected thymocytes **(Fig. 4–6).** A strong reaction between a thymocyte's TCR and any of the self-peptides presented by the thymic stroma indicates a high potential for autoreactivity. To prevent such self-reactive T cells from leaving the thymus and subsequently attacking the body's own cells and tissues, thymocytes with strongly binding TCRs are negatively selected and undergo apoptosis.

Mature T Cells

Once a T cell exits the thymus, it is considered *mature*. Mature T cells that have not yet encountered the specific peptide epitope recognized by their TCR are referred to as "naïve." To enhance the probability of a mature naïve T cell encountering its specific antigen, these cells spend their lives circulating and recirculating between the bloodstream and lymphatics. During this time, each naïve T cell forms many contacts with MHC molecules on antigen-presenting cells (APCs) throughout the body. The journey to activation may last several years for an individual naïve T cell. Most will recirculate in vain, never uniting with an APC bearing the peptide antigen recognized by their TCR.

When antigen recognition occurs, T lymphocytes are activated and differentiate into functionally active cells. Activated CD4+ Th cells immediately begin to proliferate and secrete cytokines. Signals found within the environment where Th- cell activation occurs, such as cytokines secreted by nearby APCs, influence which cytokines are produced by the Th cells. CD8+ cytotoxic T cells are also activated by antigen recognition. Responsive to stimulation by APCs as well as cytokines produced by Th cells, cytotoxic T cells proliferate and begin to seek and destroy cells displaying their specific antigen.

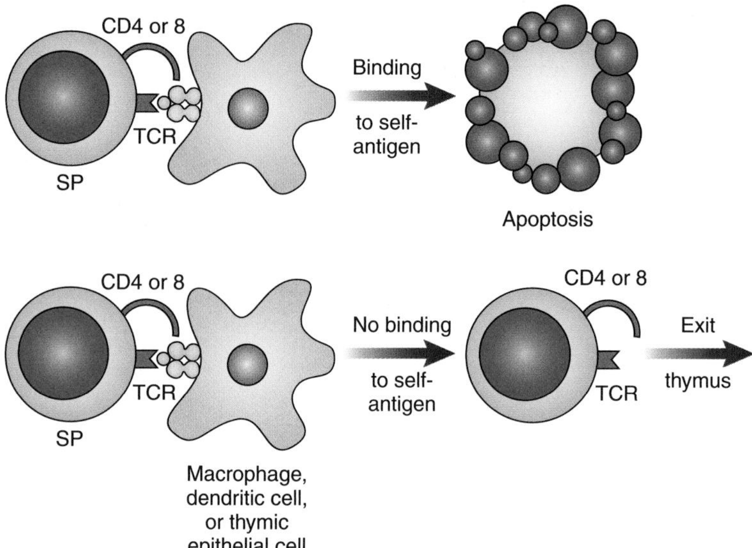

FIGURE 4–6 Negative selection of thymocytes in the thymic medulla. When self-antigen is presented by a macrophage, dendritic cell, or thymic epithelial cell to a TCR on a thymocyte, the thymocyte is eliminated by apoptosis.

Stages in B-Cell Differentiation

Similar to T cells, B cells are derived from a hematopoietic stem cell that develops into an early lymphocyte progenitor in the bone marrow. Unlike T cells, which leave the bone marrow and travel to the thymus to mature, B cells mature within the bone marrow itself. There, stromal cells form special niches, promoting the maturation of B-cell precursors. Similar to T cells, B-cell precursors go through an ordered developmental process that prepares them for their role in antibody production and, at the same time, restricts the specific antigen to which any one B cell can respond.

The first phase of B-cell development in the bone marrow, which results in mature B cells that have not yet been exposed to antigen, is known as the **antigen-independent phase.** This phase can be divided according to formation of several distinct subpopulations: **pro-B cells** (progenitor B cells), **pre-B cells** (precursor B cells), **immature B cells,** and mature B cells. For B cells that reach maturity and encounter their specific antigen, an **antigen-dependent phase** of development begins. The antigen-dependent phase typically involves the generation of plasma cells and, in many cases, long-lived memory B cells. **Figure 4–7** depicts the changes that occur as B cells mature from the pro-B stage to become memory cells or plasma cells. Key markers found on B cells in different developmental stages are listed in **Table 4–2.**

Pro-B Cells

At the earliest developmental stage, B-cell progenitors receive signals from bone marrow stromal cells through cell-to-cell contact as well as soluble cytokines, such as IL-7. This signaling induces the expression of several *transcription factors,* or proteins that control the expression of genes. Some important transcription factors expressed within pro-B cells are E2A, early B-cell factor (EBF), interferon regulatory factor 8 (IFR8), and paired box protein 5 (PAX5). Working in concert, these factors drive the expression of genes that distinguish pro-B cells from progenitor cells. Such gene expression is required for continued survival and development of the pro-B cell.

One of the most important events of the pro-B cell phase is rearrangement of the **B-cell–receptor (BCR)** genes. The BCR is simply a cell surface version of an immunoglobulin, or antibody molecule. Although structurally and functionally very different, BCRs share many similarities with T-cell receptors. For instance, both BCRs and TCRs:

- Are composed of two different chains (TCRs consist of α and β chains, whereas BCRs contain *heavy* and *light* chains)
- Have variable regions, which determine their epitope specificity
- Contain constant regions, which allow for intracellular signaling and activation of the lymphocyte expressing them
- Have similar gene regions (i.e., V, D, and J)
- Use similar mechanisms for gene rearrangement

Similar to T-cell development, the BCR genes undergo rearrangement in a stepwise manner, beginning with the heavy-chain genes. As with the TCR β chain, the heavy-chain genes contain multiple V, D, and J segments. Enzymes bring together one V, one D, and one J segment by looping out intervening DNA. The enzyme terminal deoxynucleotidyl transferase incorporates random nucleotides into the joints between V-D and D-J. Because of this targeted gene rearrangement, pro-B cells generate unique BCR genes not found in the genome, and (theoretically) not shared with any other B cell (see Chapter 5).

Because of the random nature of the process, the possibility exists that certain BCR heavy-chain rearrangements may shift the gene out of frame or result in a stop codon in the middle of the gene, leading to a nonfunctional heavy chain. In such instances, rearrangement continues until a functional

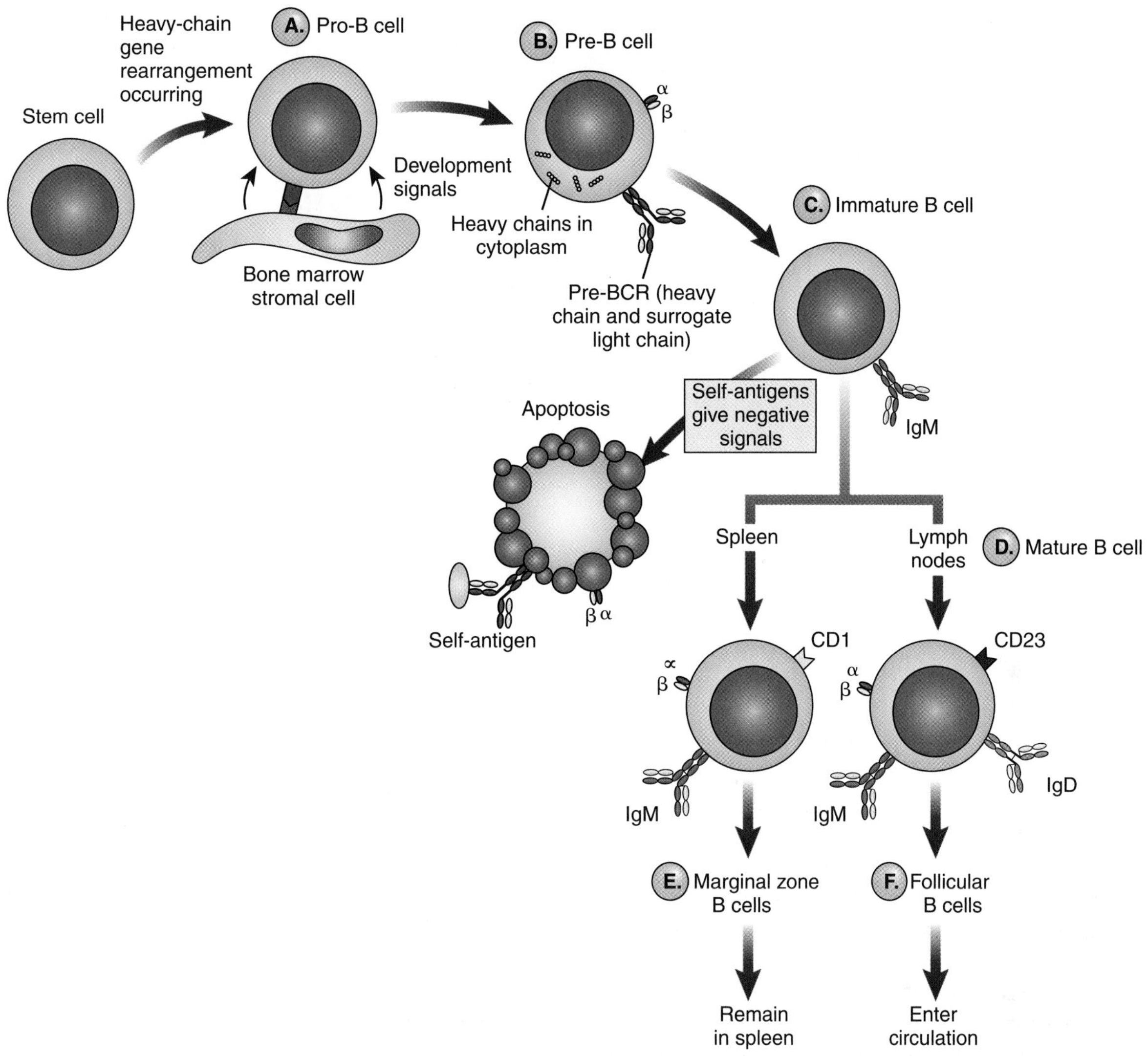

FIGURE 4–7 B-cell development. Selected markers are shown for the various stages in the differentiation of B cells. (A) Pro-B cell. (B) Pre-B cell. (C) Immature B cell. (D) Mature B cell. (E) Marginal-zone B cell. (F) Follicular B cell. Stages A through C occur within the bone marrow, whereas stages E and F occur in the spleen and lymph nodes, respectively.

Table 4–2 Stages of B-Cell Development

	DEVELOPMENTAL STAGE				
	PRO-B CELL	**PRE-B CELL**	**IMMATURE B CELL**	**MATURE B CELL**	**PLASMA CELL**
Key CD Markers	CD10 CD19	CD10 CD19 CD20	CD10 CD19 CD20 CD21 CD40	CD19 CD20 CD21 CD40	CD138
B-Cell Receptor	—	Pre-BCR: Immunoglobulin (Ig) heavy chain Surrogate light chain	Functional BCR: Immunoglobulin M (IgM) heavy chains and κ or λ light chains	Functional BCR: Immunoglobulin D (IgD) or IgM heavy chains and κ or λ light chains	—
MHC II	+	+	++	++	-

Connections

Epitope

Recall from Chapter 3 that an epitope is a part of the antigen that binds to the BCR and triggers activation of the B cell. The variable portion of the BCR, which is coded for by selected V, D, and J genes, is unique to each BCR and determines the specificity of the BCR for a particular epitope.

heavy chain can be produced using the gene templates for either heavy-chain allele. As with the TCR, once heavy-chain rearrangement is completed successfully on one chromosome, allelic exclusion silences expression of the heavy-chain gene on the opposite chromosome. For a pro-B cell to progress to the next phase of differentiation, at least one heavy-chain gene must undergo successful rearrangement.

Pre-B Cells

Once production of successfully rearranged heavy chains begins, developing B cells enter the pre–B-cell stage of differentiation. During the pre–B-cell stage, heavy chains accumulate in the cytoplasm. However, some heavy chains travel to the cell surface and combine with an unusual light-chain molecule called a **surrogate light chain,** as well as two shorter chains, Ig-α and Ig-β, which are signal-transducing subunits, to form a structure known as the pre–B-cell receptor (pre-BCR). Pre-B cells that assemble the pre-BCR undergo several rounds of cell division, resulting in many clones of the original cell, all of which express an identical heavy chain.

Simultaneously with the appearance of the pre-BCR at the surface of the cell, light-chain gene rearrangement begins. Humans, similar to most mammals, possess two different types of light-chain genes: κ and λ. Similar to the TCR α genes, the κ and λ light-chain loci are composed of multiple V and J segments. During rearrangement, a V segment, J segment, and light-chain constant region are stitched together.

Once successfully rearranged light chains are expressed, macromolecular complexes comprised of two light chains and two heavy chains are formed. These *immunoglobulins* are fastened together by disulfide bonds and journey to the cell surface to replace the pre-BCR. Because the heavy chains synthesized during the pre–B-cell stage incorporate the μ constant region, the first class of immunoglobulin produced is immunoglobulin M (IgM). The appearance of a functional BCR on the B-cell surface signifies entry of the cell into the next phase of development, the *immature B cell.*

Connections

Immunoglobulins

As you will learn in Chapter 5, immunoglobulins consist of two heavy chains and two light chains connected together by disulfide bonds. The immunoglobulins are grouped into five major classes based on the type of heavy chain they contain: IgM, immunoglobulin G (IgG), immunoglobulin A (IgA), immunoglobulin D (IgD), and immunoglobulin E (IgE). Each immunoglobulin molecule, regardless of class, contains two identical light chains, which are either both κ or both λ.

Immature B Cells

The appearance of a functional IgM BCR on the cell surface indicates that rearrangement of the genes encoding the receptor is now complete, and that a new B cell exists with the potential to produce antibody for a specific and unique epitope. Similar to T-cell receptors, the immunoglobulin variable regions, found on both the light and heavy chains, determine the antigen specificity of the immature B cell and its IgM BCR.

Because gene rearrangement produces BCRs with random specificities, the likelihood is high that some newly formed BCRs may respond to self-antigen. Therefore, B cells (similar to T cells) require a process of negative selection. When they reach maturity, B cells respond to binding of antigen to the BCR by activation, proliferation, and antibody production. In contrast, immature B cells respond to the same signals by halting their development and undergoing apoptosis. Thus, the majority of B cells capable of producing antibody to self-antigens are deleted before even exiting the bone marrow. The elimination of B cells that bear self-reactive receptors is known as **central tolerance,** and it is estimated that more than 90% of B cells die in this manner (see Chapter 15).

In addition to the appearance of IgM BCRs at the cell surface, numerous other surface markers begin to appear during the immature B-cell phase. CD21, CD40, and class II MHC molecules are just some of the proteins and glycoproteins that decorate the external membrane of the immature B cell. These markers are not only useful for laboratory identification of B cells, but they are also essential to the function of B cells—especially their role in antigen presentation to CD4+ Th cells. For instance, CD21 acts as a receptor for a breakdown product of the complement component C3, known as *C3d* (see Chapter 7 for details on complement). The presence of the CD21 receptor enhances the likelihood of contact between B cells and antigens because antigens frequently become coated with complement fragments during the immune response. CD40 and class II MHC are important for the interaction of B cells with Th cells.

A B cell that expresses a functional IgM BCR, survives selection by not reacting to self-antigens, and begins to display certain B-cell markers (CD21, CD40, and MHC) is considered a mature B cell. B cells that have achieved these milestones exit the bone marrow and are carried in the blood to the spleen for the next stage in their development.

Mature B Cells

In the spleen, immature B cells develop into one of two types of mature B cells, known as *follicular B cells* and *marginal-zone B cells.* Follicular B cells constantly recirculate between the blood and secondary lymphoid organs in search of their specific antigens, whereas marginal-zone B cells remain in the

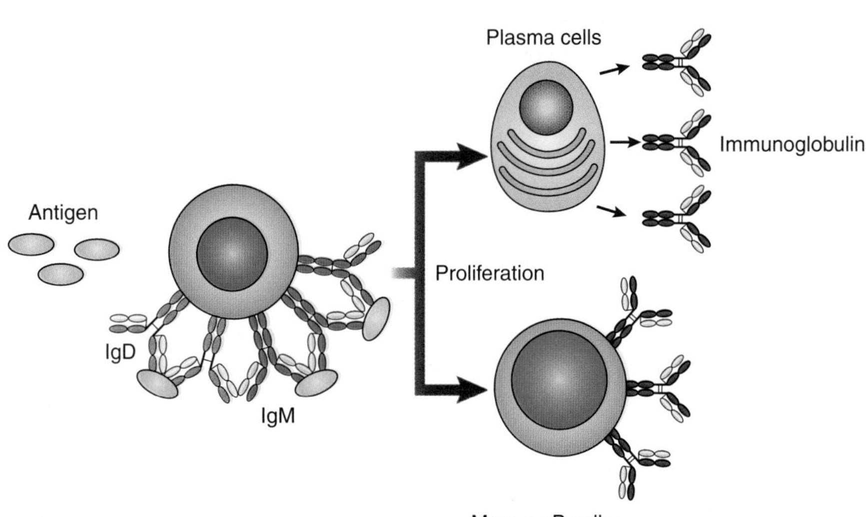

FIGURE 4–8 B-cell activation. B cells bind to antigen by means of immunoglobulin receptors (IgM and IgD). B cells activated by encountering antigen proliferate and may, upon receiving help from T cells, become antibody-secreting plasma cells or memory B cells capable of responding rapidly upon re-exposure to the same antigen.

spleen to respond quickly to blood-borne pathogens. Both marginal-zone and follicular B cells produce antibody, but the circumstances that trigger antibody production, the types of antibody produced, and the duration of the response are very different between these two populations.

The majority of mature B cells are destined to become follicular B cells. The term *follicular* refers to the region of the lymph node where this type of mature B cell tends to localize during its movements throughout the body (see Chapter 1). Lymphoid follicles represent dense clusters of naïve B cells awaiting exposure to their specific antigens. When antigen recognition occurs, follicular B cells make contact with CD4+ follicular helper (Tfh) cells. Cooperation between antigen-activated B cells and Tfh cells is critical for many B-cell processes, including the formation of immunologic memory.

Marginal-zone B cells receive their name from the anatomical site in which they are most concentrated, the marginal sinus of the spleen. Experimental evidence suggests that BCR specificity plays a role in determining which mature B cells come to reside in the spleen, because most marginal-zone B cells recognize polysaccharide antigens found on common bacterial pathogens. When marginal-zone B cells contact their specific antigens, they don't receive help from Tfh cells. Instead, they differentiate into IgM-secreting plasma cells, each producing vast quantities of anti-microbial IgM, and only stopping once the invading microbes have been eliminated. Because Tfh cell help is essential for the formation of immunologic memory, the marginal-zone response must begin anew upon each exposure to a particular polysaccharide antigen.

In addition to an IgM BCR, most mature B cells also express an IgD form of the BCR. The IgM and IgD BCRs expressed on a particular B cell have the same antigenic specificity, although it is not clear how much of a role IgD actually plays in sensing antigen or activation of the B cell. Nevertheless, the presence of both IgM and IgD on the cell membrane signifies a mature B cell.

When a BCR binds its specific antigen, multiple BCR molecules are brought together, initiating an intracellular signaling cascade. These signals drive the B cell to enter a proliferative stage where it divides rapidly to produce both antibody-secreting plasma cells and, for follicular B cells, memory B cells **(Fig. 4–8).**

Plasma Cells

The histological appearance of **plasma cells** reflects their role as fully differentiated antibody-production factories (see Fig. 1–9). Plasma cells express very little immunoglobulin on their surface membranes but have abundant cytoplasmic immunoglobulin. As gene transcription is dominated by that of the antibody-coding genes, the oval-shaped nuclei of plasma cells often contain heavily clumped, dark-staining chromatin. To accommodate translation and post-translational processing of the large quantities of antibody being manufactured, plasma cells possess ample endoplasmic reticulum and a well-defined Golgi. Resident plasma cells are a common feature of the bone marrow and the germinal centers found in peripheral lymphoid organs. Similar to lymphoid progenitor cells, plasma cells survive in bone marrow niches surrounded by stromal cells, which provide stimulation to plasma cells via cytokines. Stromal cell support allows plasma cells to be long-lived and fosters their continual production of antibodies. In contrast, plasma cells located in tissues other than the bone marrow produce antibody for only a short time before dying. A key surface marker found on plasma cells is CD138.

The Role of T Cells in the Adaptive Immune Response

When infection occurs in the body's tissues, APCs such as macrophages and dendritic cells are among the first immune cells to respond. Sensing the presence of danger via innate receptors, such as Toll-like receptors (see Chapter 2), APCs engulf pathogens at these distal sites of infection and carry associated antigens to local lymph nodes. Upon arrival at lymph nodes near the site of infection, antigen-laden APCs encounter naïve T cells in the process of patrolling for antigen. Because gene rearrangement imbues each T cell with a TCR of a different specificity, very few circulating naïve T cells (only about 1 in 10^5) are specific for any given antigen. Therefore, the continuous recirculation of naïve T cells between the blood and lymph nodes greatly increases the likelihood of an APC connecting with one or more of the few T cells whose TCRs recognize the antigens carried by the APC.

Antigen Presentation

The primary mode of communication between T cells and APCs involves direct cell-to-cell contact (discussed in more detail in Chapter 3). Using an immunologic process known as *antigen presentation,* APCs display peptide antigens to T cells via major histocompatibility molecules (MHC, also called *human leukocyte antigen* [HLA]). MHC molecules cradle antigenic peptides in a manner similar to a bun holding a hot dog and allow the TCR to bind along the entire length of the peptide. Humans and related mammals express two different forms of MHC protein, MHC class I and MHC class II. The overall structures and functions of MHC class I and class II are similar. However, the source of the peptides presented by each type of MHC and the type of T cell each MHC class interacts with are quite different.

As we discussed in Chapter 3, class I MHC molecules present peptide antigens derived from cytoplasmic sources, such as endogenous peptides manufactured by healthy cells. In diseased cells, the antigens presented by class I MHC might include peptides associated with intercellular bacteria, viruses, or even proteins associated with cancer. Class I MHC molecules present antigen to cytotoxic T cells—the T-cell population most useful for destroying malignant cells or cells infected with intracellular pathogens. The interaction between the cytotoxic TCR and class I MHC is stabilized by CD8, a reliable marker for cytotoxic T cells.

In contrast, class II MHC molecules present peptides captured from the extracellular space, such as those derived from extracellular microbes. Class II MHC molecules allow APCs to present such extracellular-derived peptide antigens to Th cells. Similar to cytotoxic T cells, an additional protein is required to stabilize the interaction between class II MHC and the Th TCR, and this role is filled by CD4. Thus, CD4 is commonly used as a marker to identify Th cells in the laboratory.

When a naïve T cell enters secondary lymphoid tissues and encounters APCs, multiple contacts occur between the T cells' TCR and peptides presented in MHC molecules on the surfaces of the APCs. If the TCR recognizes one of the many antigens being presented by an APC, an intracellular signaling cascade is initiated within the T cell. Importantly, TCR signaling alone is not sufficient to activate a naïve T cell. For activation to occur, the APC must also provide costimulation to the T cell by expressing CD80 or CD86, molecules that ligate the T-cell surface protein CD28. The combination of signals that arises when the TCR recognizes its specific peptide and CD28 is ligated transforms a naïve T cell into an activated T cell.

Actions of T Helper and T Regulatory Cells

T helper (Th) cells are not phagocytic, cannot kill infected cells, and are incapable of the production and secretion of antibodies. Nonetheless, Th cells are arguably the most important cells of the adaptive response. The importance of Th cells derives from their role in driving the activities of other immune cells that act directly to fight infection (macrophages, cytotoxic T cells, and B cells). When activated by APCs, Th cells travel to infected tissues to orchestrate the immune response via the secretion of cytokines.

Several subsets of activated Th cells exist, of which the most prominent are termed *Th1*, *Th2*, and *Th17* cells, each of which has a different role in immune responses **(Fig. 4–9).** The ability of newly activated Th cells to *differentiate* into these various subsets is influenced by the cytokines present during activation. Each Th subset, in turn, produces a unique set of cytokines capable of driving the immune response to target a particular type of infection.

Th1 cells produce interferon-gamma (IFN-γ), interleukin-2 (IL-2), and tumor necrosis factor-α (TNF-α), cytokines that activate CD8+ cytotoxic lymphocytes and macrophages to fight intracellular parasites. **Th2 cells** produce a variety of cytokines, including interleukins (IL) IL-4, IL-5, IL-6, IL-9, IL-10, and IL-13. The essential role of Th2 cells is to control the clearance of extracellular parasites, such as intestinal worms. Th2 cells are also thought to play a role in allergy. Th17 cells produce the cytokines IL-17 and IL-22, which lead to the recruitment of granulocytes in response to an extracellular bacterial infection. Granulocyte activity can sometimes cause immune-mediated damage. Because of this, the Th17 response is often associated with pathology.

An additional Th subpopulation, called **T regulatory (Treg) cells,** possess the CD4 antigen as well as CD25. These cells comprise approximately 5% of all CD4+ T cells. Tregs play an important role in suppressing the immune response to self-antigens and harmless antigens, such as those in common foods. They inhibit the proliferation of other T-cell populations by secreting inhibitory cytokines. Because they possess TCRs that recognize antigenic peptide in MHC class II, the response of Tregs is antigen-specific.

To assist B cells in antibody production, a special subpopulation of Th cells, known as **T follicular helper (Tfh) cells,** remains in the lymph nodes and interacts with B cells and plasma cells there. Tfh cells provide essential signaling to B cells as they undergo processes such as activation, immunoglobulin class switching, affinity maturation, and the formation of B-cell memory. These processes will be discussed in more detail in a later section of this chapter.

During the many rounds of cell division that follow Th-cell activation, two distinct populations of cells are formed. Most

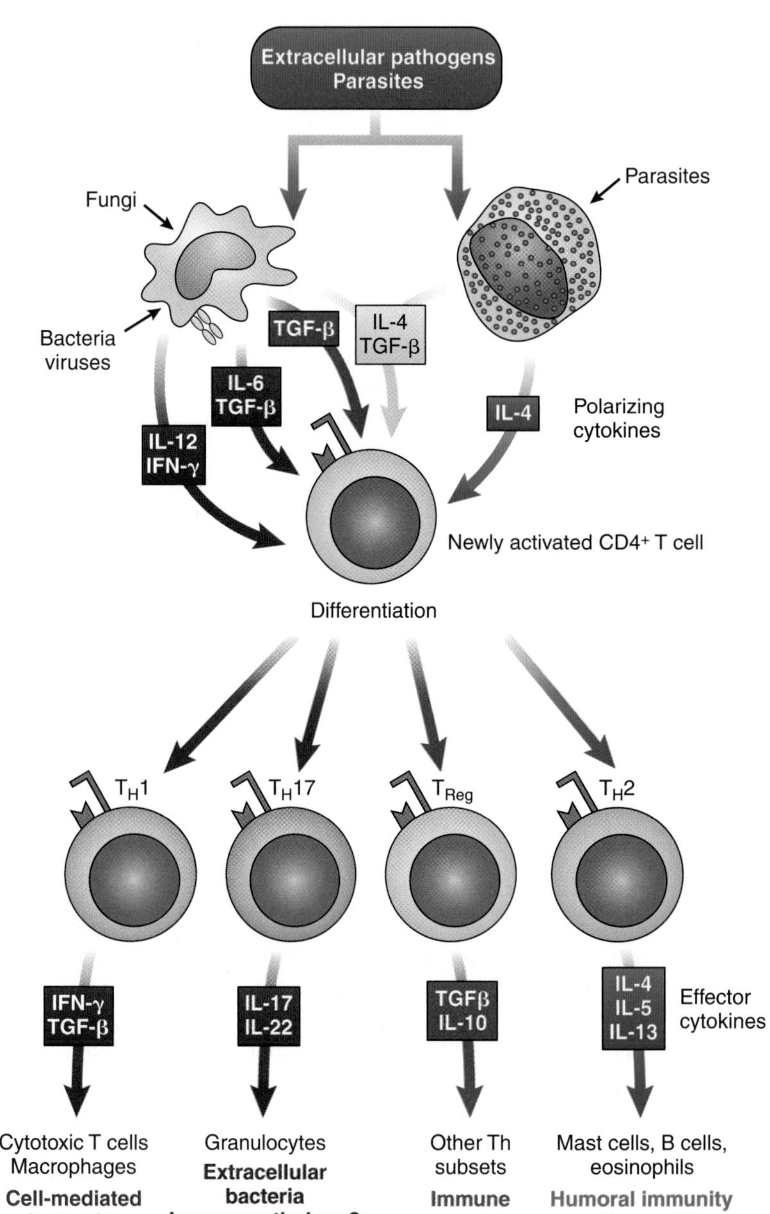

FIGURE 4–9 T helper (Th) subsets. Depending on the type of pathogen encountered, APCs secrete a specific combination of polarizing cytokines that direct newly activated CD4+ Th cells to further differentiate into one of four subsets: Th1, Th2, Treg, or Th17. These specialized T cells release different types of cytokines to coordinate an appropriate immune response against the pathogen.

Th cells begin to secrete cytokines and may travel to infected tissues where their activities are most needed. A small percentage of the Th cells generated after activation will differentiate into memory cells. Memory Th cells enter a quiescent state and await re-exposure to their specific antigen. If and when contact with antigen occurs again, memory cells respond rapidly by re-entering cell division and immediately secreting appropriate cytokines.

Action of Cytotoxic T Cells

CD8-expressing cytotoxic T cells (Tc), also known as *cytotoxic T lymphocytes* (CTLs), play a different role than Th cells. Activated cytotoxic T cells migrate to sites of infection and initiate apoptosis in cells infected with intracellular parasites and viruses. Unlike NK cells, which fulfill a similar role but recognize infection through germline-encoded receptors, the activity of cytotoxic T cells is driven by TCR recognition and is therefore antigen-specific.

Upon recognition of peptide antigen in class I MHC on the surface of a target cell, cytotoxic T cells kill their targets using two primary strategies: (1) the release of cytotoxic granules from the T-cell cytoplasm or (2) ligation of death receptors on a target cell's surface. In either case, the target cell rapidly undergoes apoptosis **(Fig. 4–10).**

Cytotoxic T-cell granules contain two toxic substances: perforins and granzymes. Perforins are proteins that insert into target-cell membranes and polymerize to form pores. Granzymes are *serine proteases,* a class of enzymes that can initiate the fragmentation of DNA in the target cell. TCR recognition of antigen by a cytotoxic T cell causes accumulation of granules in the T-cell cytoplasm adjacent to the

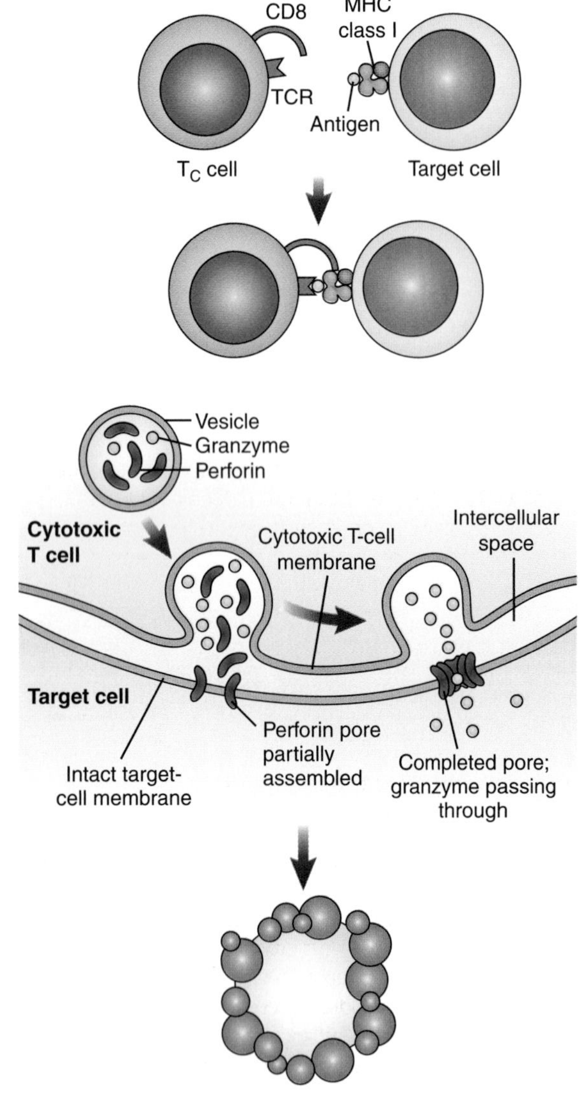

FIGURE 4–10 Activation of cytotoxic T cells. The CD8+ T cell recognizes foreign peptide antigen presented in class I MHC. When binding occurs, vesicles containing perforin and granzymes move toward the point of contact with the target cell. Granules fuse with the membrane and release their lytic contents into the space between the T cell and target cell. Perforin inserts itself into the target-cell membrane and polymerizes to form a pore. Granzymes enter the target cell and induce apoptosis.

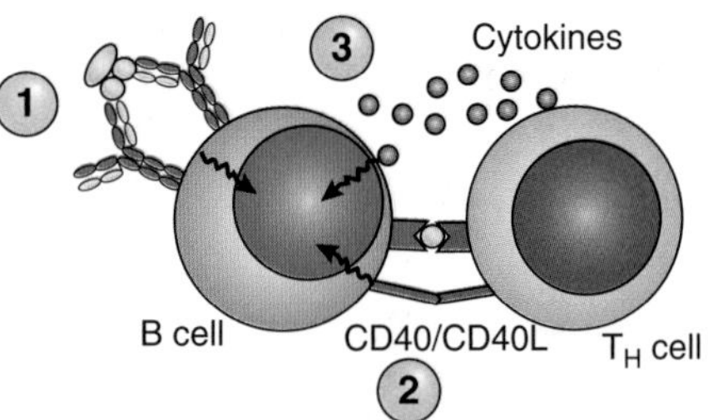

FIGURE 4–11 Activating signals for T-dependent antigens. (1) T-dependent antigens bind to immunoglobulin receptors on B cells. The antigen is processed and delivered to CD4+ T cells. The Th cell binds by means of its CD3-TCR complex and (2) delivers further activating signals through binding of CD40 on the B cell to the CD40L receptor on the Th cell. (3) Cytokines are released from the T cell and enhance B-cell transformation to plasma cells.

target cell. Subsequently, the granules are released by the T cell in the direction of the target cell. Almost immediately, perforin begins forming holes in the target-cell membrane, through which granzymes can enter. Once in the target cell, granzymes activate nuclease enzymes that cleave DNA and disrupt mitochondria. With its genetic material shredded and energy levels dropping, the target cell quietly dies by apoptosis.

Cytotoxic T cells are also capable of inducing apoptosis in target cells by ligation of death receptors. In this situation, TCR recognition of antigen complexed with target-cell MHC leads to expression of the death-inducing protein Fas-ligand (FasL) by the T cell. When FasL binds to Fas on the target-cell membrane, apoptotic pathways similar to those activated by the granzymes are set in motion.

The Role of B Cells in the Adaptive Immune Response

As mentioned previously, the essential first step in the activation of a mature B cell is exposure of the IgM BCR to its specific antigenic epitope. Antigen recognition by the different types of mature B cells (follicular and marginal zone) occurs in different anatomical regions—the lymph nodes and the spleen, respectively. Because the follicular B-cell response depends heavily on the activity of Tfh cells to promote an effective antibody response, antigens that provoke this type of response are often referred to as **T-dependent antigens (Fig. 4–11).** Correspondingly, as marginal-zone B cells don't require the help of Tfh cells, the antigens recognized by marginal-zone B cells are referred to as **T-independent antigens (Fig. 4–12).**

Immune Response to T-Dependent Antigens

Because of the requirement for T-cell help, T-dependent antigens are almost always proteins, because proteins are the only type of antigen that can stimulate a T-cell response. To reach the lymph nodes, where mature naïve follicular B cells reside, protein antigens may travel suspended or dissolved within lymphatic fluid, or they may be carried by macrophages or dendritic cells. Regardless of the means by which protein antigens are brought to lymph nodes from areas of infection or inoculation, they arrive at the B-cell–rich follicles in their *native* state (that is, not processed or denatured). This fact is central to the concept that BCRs

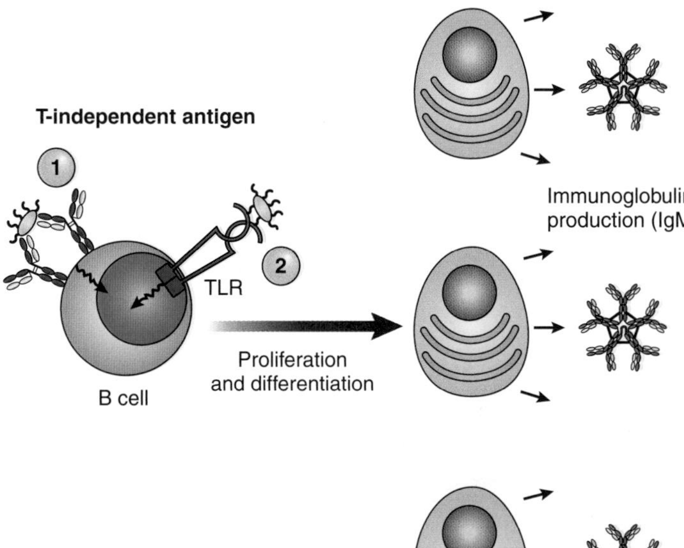

FIGURE 4–12 Activating signals for T-independent antigens. (1) T-independent antigens can bind to B cells through immunoglobulin receptors and trigger B-cell transformation directly. Several antigen receptors must be cross-linked in order to activate a B cell directly. (2) Antigens can also be bound to B cells' innate immune receptors, such as TLRs.

bind to antigenic epitopes exposed on an antigen's surface **(Fig. 4–13)**.

When a follicular B cell and its specific antigen are united, the BCR locates its epitope and binds the antigen securely via surface immunoglobulin. BCR antigen recognition initiates a cascade of intracellular signaling within the B cell, driving the cell into an activated state. In response to BCR signaling, the B-cell cytoskeleton is mobilized to internalize the bound antigen using a process known as *endocytosis*. Antigen uptake allows for digestion of the antigen and presentation of its constituent peptides on class II MHC molecules on the B-cell surface.

Following activation, B cells migrate to the edges of follicles, where they begin to interact with Tfh cells. In this context, B cells act as APCs, presenting peptide fragments derived from internalized antigen to Tfh cells. If TCR binding to one of these antigenic peptides occurs, a T cell–B cell pair is formed, and the T-dependent phase of the B-cell response begins.

To complement BCR signaling, Tfh cells provide activated B cells with two additional signals that contribute to the B-cell response. The first signal provided by the T cell requires physical contact between T cells and B cells. TCR recognition of peptide antigen causes Tfh cells to express CD40 ligand (CD40L), which binds to CD40 on B cells.

T cells also signal to B cells through the secretion of cytokines. For instance, T cells secrete IL-2, which binds to CD25 expressed on B cells and spurs them to enter a phase of rapid cell division. Each daughter cell produced during this replicative explosion will inherit an identical BCR to that of the parent B cell and will therefore recognize the same antigen. Daughter B cells produced during the proliferative phase of the T-dependent response have two potential fates: Some remain in contact with T cells and differentiate into IgM-secreting plasma cells, whereas others form *germinal centers* within follicles and participate in a series of processes that enhance the antibody response through time.

The germinal center reaction involves three overlapping processes: immunoglobulin isotype switching, affinity maturation, and memory-cell generation. Germinal center formation requires interaction with T cells, specifically the affiliation of CD40 with CD40L and the secretion of cytokines.

IgM is the most common class of immunoglobulin molecule incorporated into the BCRs of marginal-zone B cells and follicular B cells before and at very early times after antigen recognition. However, B cells can express other classes of immunoglobulin through precisely controlled rearrangement of the heavy-chain genes. Other types of immunoglobulin include IgG, which is the predominant form of antibody found in the blood; IgA, which is found in the intestines and the body's secretions; and IgE, which is associated with allergy. Each of these antibody classes has a different function in immunity and plays a different role in protecting the body from infection.

Connections

Mutation of CD40L Gene Causes Immunodeficiency

When the delicate balance between T- and B-cell interaction is disrupted, immune deficiencies may result. An X-linked mutation causing a CD40L deficiency on Th cells is linked to disruption of immunoglobulin class switching. In patients with this mutation, normal or increased levels of IgM are present, but B cells are unable to produce other antibody classes. IgG and IgA levels are decreased, leading to an increased susceptibility to infections. See Chapter 17 for further discussion on immunodeficiency diseases.

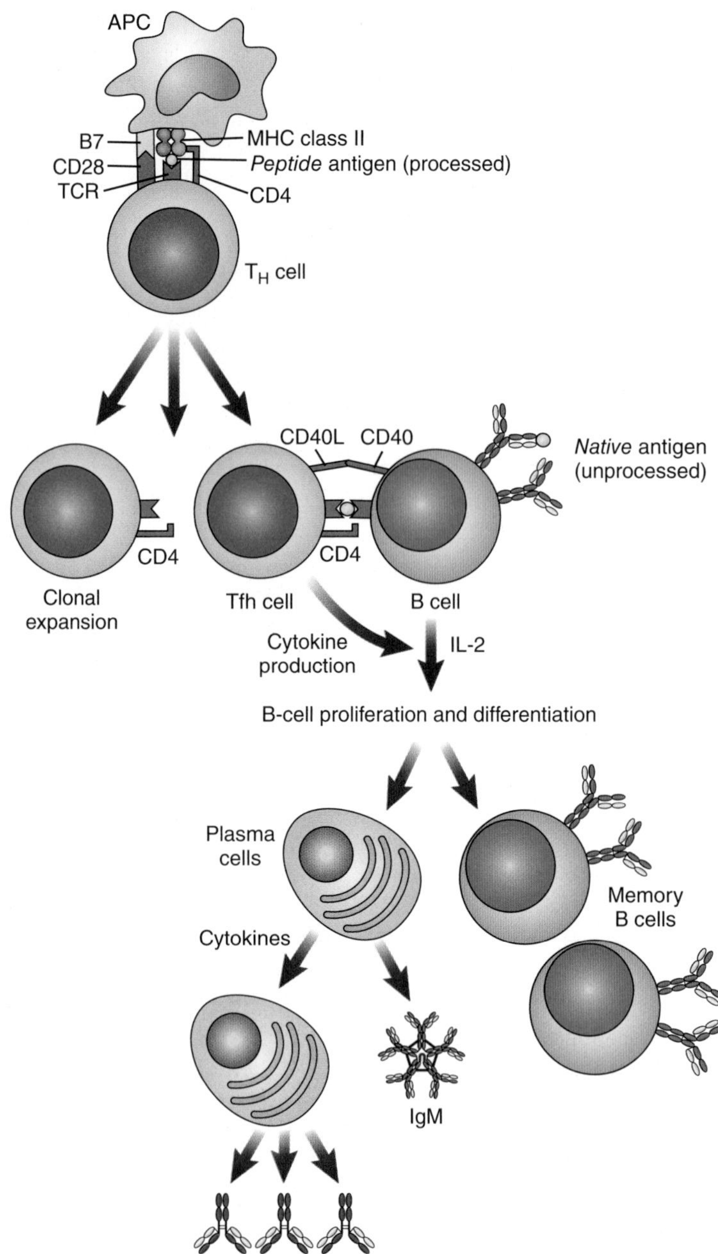

FIGURE 4–13 T- and B-cell cooperation in the immune response. CD4+ T cells recognize exogenous antigen on a macrophage, along with class II MHC. Binding between CD28 and B7 enhances interaction between the cells. Th cells go through clonal expansion and produce cytokines, including IL-2. B cells capable of responding to the same antigen present antigen to Th cells through the class II MHC receptor. The TCR binds antigen, and CD4 binds to class II MHC. CD40L binds to the costimulatory molecule CD40, enhancing the reaction. Cytokine production by the T cell causes B cells to proliferate and produce plasma cells, which secrete antibody.

Under the direction of T cells, germinal center B cells can change which class of antibody they express, a process referred to as **isotype switching.** Isotype switching not only changes the type of immunoglobulin comprising the BCR, but it also determines the class of antibody secreted once the B cell differentiates into a plasma cell. The gene recombination that occurs during isotype switching is specific to the constant region of the heavy chains, meaning that the target epitope recognized by the immunoglobulin does not change; only the general structure of the antibody is altered.

Affinity maturation refers to a process by which immunoglobulins bind antigen with increasing strength (affinity) through the course of an immune response, resulting in the production of even more effective antibodies. This feat is accomplished through *somatic hypermutation,* or the appearance of mutations in immunoglobulin gene variable regions. Because of somatic hypermutation, daughter cells are produced with slightly different antigen-binding abilities. Daughter cells whose BCRs have a greater affinity for antigen receive survival signals, whereas those with lesser antigen affinity die by apoptosis. In this way, affinity maturation represents an *evolution* of the antibody response throughout the battle against an infection.

For each generation of daughter cells produced within the germinal center, three basic populations of cells are formed: plasma cells, memory cells, and B cells that remain in the germinal center to continue the process of affinity maturation. Plasma cells exit lymph nodes and secrete large quantities of antibody of the isotype and affinity achieved during that replicative generation. Memory cells may remain in the lymph nodes or travel to the tissues. Memory cells do not require antigen stimulation for survival, allowing them to lie in wait for re-exposure to antigen. When a memory B cell is re-exposed to antigen, it can rapidly respond with the production of high-affinity, class-switched antibody.

Immune Response to T-Independent Antigens

Some populations of B cells, including marginal-zone B cells, don't interact with T cells during their response to antigen. The T-independent antigens recognized by these B cells are often polymers, such as polysaccharides. The presence of many repeating elements on these antigens causes cross-linking of multiple BCRs on a single B cell, inducing proliferation and antibody production (see Fig. 4–12). Examples of T-independent antigens include plant lectins, polymerized proteins with repeating molecular patterns, and lipopolysaccharides found in bacterial cell walls. Because T cells don't participate in this type of B-cell response, processes such as isotype switching, affinity maturation, and memory formation do not occur. Consequently, these antigens elicit IgM production only, and the induction of memory does not occur to any great extent.

SUMMARY

- Adaptive immunity is characterized by specificity, memory, and enhancement upon repeated exposure to the same antigen.
- The immune cells responsible for mediating adaptive immunity are the lymphocytes, which can be subdivided into T and B lymphocytes (T cells and B cells).
- Adaptive immunity can be broadly divided into two branches: *cell-mediated* immunity (T cells) and *humoral* immunity (antibodies produced by B cells).
- All lymphocytes arise in the bone marrow from hematopoietic stem cells (lymphoid progenitor cells), but T cells and B cells undergo very different maturation processes.
- B lymphocytes remain in the bone marrow for the majority of their maturation, whereas T cells exit the bone marrow to undergo a thymic phase of development.
- The primary antigen receptors of the lymphocytes undergo genetic rearrangement so that each naïve lymphocyte expresses a unique receptor with a different specificity than other lymphocytes.
- After gene rearrangement, each lymphocyte expresses a different primary receptor and therefore recognizes a very specific target. Taken as a whole, the body's lymphocyte population can respond to an almost unlimited variety of pathogens.
- The T-cell receptor (TCR) is composed of two protein chains called α and β. TCRs allow T cells to recognize peptide antigen, but the peptide must be presented by an MHC molecule on the surface of an APC.
- The BCR is composed primarily of an immunoglobulin molecule on the surface of the B cell. BCRs allow B cells to detect their antigen, which is usually exposed on the surface of an antigenic substance.
- In the thymus, T cells undergo several stages of differentiation before becoming naïve T cells capable of patrolling the body and responding to antigen. These stages are characterized by the expression of the surface molecules CD4 and CD8: double-negative (DN), double-positive (DP), and single-positive (SP).
- B-cell development can be divided into a series of *antigen independent* stages, consisting of pro-, pre-, and mature B cells. B cells that survive antigen-independent development and encounter their specific antigens enter an *antigen-dependent* phase where they can become antibody-secreting plasma cells or memory cells.
- When a lymphocyte detects its specific antigen, it proliferates substantially, a phase known as *clonal expansion,* resulting in a large population of cells that respond to a particular target.
- The CD4 molecule helps stabilize the interaction between the TCR and class II MHC molecules and is used as a marker to identify helper T cells (Th cells). CD8 does the same between the TCR and class I MHC and serves as a marker of cytotoxic T cells.
- Cytotoxic (CD 8+) T cells can induce apoptosis in cells infected with intracellular pathogens or malignant cells, whereas Th cells (CD4+) secrete cytokines to direct the immune response.
- When they reach maturity, B cells become one of two populations, follicular B cells or marginal-zone B cells. Follicular B cells patrol and occupy B-cell follicles found in lymph nodes, whereas marginal-zone B cells spend their lives in the marginal sinus of the spleen.

Study Guide: Comparison of T and B Cells

T CELLS	B CELLS
Develop in the thymus	Develop in the bone marrow
Found in blood (60%–80% of circulating lymphocytes), thoracic duct fluid, lymph nodes	Found in bone marrow, spleen, lymph nodes
End products of T helper or cytotoxic T-cell activation are cytokines	End product of B-cell activation is antibody
Surface markers include CD2 (all T cells), CD3 (all T cells), CD4 (T helper and regulatory T cells), CD8 (cytotoxic T cells)	Surface markers include CD19, CD20, CD21, CD40, class II MHC

CASE STUDIES

1. A 2-year-old boy is sent for immunologic testing because of recurring respiratory infections, including several bouts of pneumonia. The results show decreased immunoglobulin levels, especially of IgG. Although his white blood cell (WBC) count was within the normal range, his lymphocyte count was low. Flow cytometry was performed to determine the levels of different classes of lymphocytes. The result showed a decrease in CD4+ cells. The CD19+ lymphocyte population was normal.

Questions

a. How can these findings be interpreted?
b. How can this account for his recurring infections?

2. You and a friend in your immunology class are discussing how the body is able to fight infection. Your friend states that as long as you have a good innate immune system and you can make antibodies, then a decrease in CD8+ T cells is not really important.

Question

a. How do you respond to your friend?

REVIEW QUESTIONS

1. Which MHC molecule is necessary for antigen recognition by CD4+ T cells?
   a. Class I
   b. Class II
   c. Class III
   d. No MHC molecule is necessary.

2. Which would be characteristic of an immune response to a T-independent antigen?
   a. The IgG antibody is produced exclusively.
   b. Large numbers of memory cells are produced.
   c. Antigens bind only one receptor on B cells.
   d. Antigens are often polysaccharides.

3. *Humoral immunity* refers to which of the following?
   a. Production of antibody by plasma cells
   b. Production of cytokines by T cells
   c. Elimination of virally infected cells by cytotoxic cells
   d. Downregulation of the immune response

4. Where does antigen-independent maturation of B lymphocytes take place?
   a. Bone marrow
   b. Thymus
   c. Spleen
   d. Lymph nodes

5. In the thymus, positive selection of immature T cells is based upon recognition of which of the following?
   a. Self-antigens
   b. Stress proteins
   c. MHC antigens
   d. μ chains

6. Which of these is/are found on a mature B cell?
   a. IgG and IgD
   b. IgM and IgD
   c. α and β chains
   d. CD3

7. How do cytotoxic T cells kill target cells?
   a. They produce antibodies that bind to the cell.
   b. They engulf the cell by phagocytosis.
   c. They stop protein synthesis in the target cell.
   d. They produce granzymes that stimulate apoptosis.

8. Which of the following can be directly attributed to antigen-stimulated T cells?
   a. Humoral response
   b. Plasma cells
   c. Cytokines
   d. Antibody

9. Which is a distinguishing feature of a pre-B cell?
   a. μ chains in the cytoplasm
   b. Complete IgM on the surface
   c. Presence of CD21 antigen
   d. Presence of CD25 antigen

10. When does genetic rearrangement for coding of antibody light chains take place during B-cell development?
   a. Before the pre-B cell stage
   b. As the cell becomes an immature B cell
   c. Not until the cell becomes a mature B cell
   d. When the B cell becomes a plasma cell

11. Which of the following antigens is found on "helper" T cells?
   a. CD4
   b. CD8
   c. CD11
   d. CD21

12. Which of the following would represent a DN thymocyte?
   a. CD3+CD4–CD8+
   b. CD3–CD4+CD8–
   c. CD3+CD4–CD8–
   d. CD2–CD3–CD4+CD8–

13. Which of the following best describes the TCR for antigen?
   a. It consists of IgM and IgD molecules.
   b. It is the same for all T cells.
   c. It is present in the DN stage.
   d. α and β chains are unique for each antigen.

14. Laboratory results belonging to a 3-year-old patient showed the following: normal CD4+ T-cell count, normal CD19+ B-cell count, low CD8+ T-cell count. Which aspect of immunity would be affected?
   a. Production of antibody
   b. Formation of plasma cells
   c. Elimination of virally infected cells
   d. Downregulation of the immune response

15. Which of the following is a unique characteristic of adaptive immunity?
   a. Ability to fight infection
   b. Ability to remember a prior exposure to a pathogen
   c. A similar response to all pathogens encountered
   d. Process of phagocytosis to destroy a pathogen

16. Clonal deletion of T cells as they mature is important in which of the following processes?
   a. Elimination of autoimmune responses
   b. Positive selection of CD3/TCR receptors
   c. Allelic exclusion of chromosomes
   d. Elimination of cells unable to bind to MHC antigens

17. Where are germinal centers found?
   a. In the thymus
   b. In the bone marrow
   c. In peripheral blood
   d. In lymph nodes

5 Antibody Structure and Function

Linda E. Miller, PhD, MB^{CM}(ASCP)SI

LEARNING OUTCOMES

After finishing this chapter, you should be able to:

1. Diagram the general structure of an immunoglobulin and recognize its major components.
2. Identify the electrophoretic fraction of serum that contains the majority of immunoglobulins.
3. Differentiate between isotypes, allotypes, and idiotypes.
4. Differentiate between the light chains and heavy chains of immunoglobulins and indicate the Greek letters that denote each type.
5. Discuss the effects of treating an immunoglobulin molecule with papain, pepsin, or mercaptoethanol.
6. Describe the major characteristics of the five immunoglobulin classes found in humans.
7. Relate the differences in the structures of the five immunoglobulin classes to their functions.
8. Discuss how the immunoglobulin G (IgG) subclasses differ in functional capability.
9. Describe the functions of the J chain and the secretory component (SC) and indicate in which immunoglobulin classes they are found.
10. Discuss how immunoglobulin D (IgD) differs from other immunoglobulin types.
11. Identify the types of cells that immunoglobulin E (IgE) binds to in allergic reactions.
12. Compare and contrast the primary and secondary antibody responses to antigen.
13. Describe the genes that code for the immunoglobulin proteins, and explain how they combine to code for a unique antibody molecule.
14. Explain how immunoglobulin class switching occurs on a genetic level.
15. Explain how the clonal selection hypothesis contributes to antibody specificity.
16. Outline the traditional process of mouse monoclonal antibody production.
17. Discuss some clinical and research applications of monoclonal antibodies.

CHAPTER OUTLINE

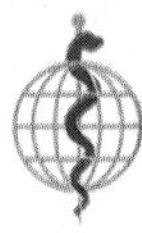

Go to FADavis.com for the laboratory exercises that accompany this text.

KEY TERMS

Affinity maturation
Allelic exclusion
Allotype
Anamnestic response
Antibody
Antibody-dependent cellular cytotoxicity (ADCC)
Class switching
Clonal selection hypothesis
Constant region
Domains
Fab fragments
F(ab')$_2$ fragment
Fc fragment
Heavy (H) chains
Hinge region
Hybridoma
Idiotype
Immunoglobulin
Isotype
Joining (J) chain
Kappa (κ) chains
Lambda (λ) chains
Light (L) chains
Monoclonal antibody
Opsonization
Paratope
Primary antibody response
Secondary antibody response
Secretory component (SC)
Tetrapeptide
Variable region

In 1890, the scientists Emil von Behring and Shibasaburo Kitasato described a substance in the blood that could neutralize the toxin produced by the bacteria that cause diphtheria. The substance that was responsible for this and similar activities was later termed *antibody.* As we discussed in Chapter 4, antibodies are the main element of the humoral arm of the adaptive immune response. They are found on the surface of B cells, where they serve as receptors that specifically recognize foreign antigens to initiate the immune response. When B lymphocytes are stimulated by antigen, they undergo differentiation into plasma cells, which secrete antibodies into the blood and other body fluids. There, antibodies perform biological activities that inactivate antigens such as toxins and help to eliminate harmful microorganisms from the body.

Another term for **antibody** is **immunoglobulin,** based on the fact that these molecules are globular proteins that play a role in immunity. Immunoglobulins are glycoproteins that are composed of 86% to 98% polypeptide and 2% to 14% carbohydrate. They constitute approximately 20% of plasma proteins in healthy individuals and can be detected by performing serum protein electrophoresis. In this process, serum is placed on an agarose gel, and an electrical current is applied to separate the proteins. If electrophoresis is carried out at a pH of 8.6, most serum proteins can be separated on the basis of size and charge. Five distinct bands are obtained in this manner. Immunoglobulins are the slowest-moving proteins and appear primarily in the gamma (γ) band **(Fig. 5–1).** Because the gamma band contains most of the antibody activity, antibodies have also been referred to as *gamma globulins.*

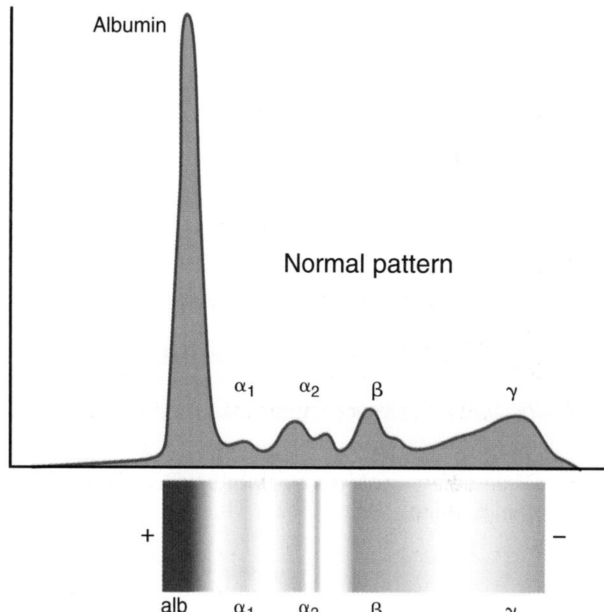

FIGURE 5–1 Serum electrophoresis. Serum is subjected to an electrical charge, and proteins are separated on the basis of size and charge. Antibodies are found in the gamma region because they are the slowest-migrating proteins and have a charge that is close to neutral. Hence, they do not move far from the origin.

Detection of immunoglobulins by electrophoresis and testing for specific antibodies by other laboratory methods are very helpful in the diagnosis of many types of diseases. Knowledge of the type of immunoglobulin produced is important in blood banking as well as in the interpretation of laboratory tests that are based on a patient's immune response to a specific antigen. Detection of specific antibodies is very helpful in the diagnosis of a variety of diseases, including infections, allergies, autoimmune diseases, and immunoproliferative diseases. Laboratory tests to detect antibodies for the purpose of diagnosing these diseases will be discussed in more detail in later chapters of this book.

Immunoglobulins are divided into five major classes based on a part of the molecule called the heavy chain. These classes are designated as IgG, IgM, IgA, IgD, and IgE (with *Ig* being the abbreviation for *immunoglobulin*). The heavy chains within these classes are denoted by the Greek letters γ (gamma), μ (mu), α (alpha), δ (delta), and ε (epsilon), respectively. Some of the Ig classes also contain subclasses, which have slight differences in their heavy chains. Although each class has distinct properties, all immunoglobulin molecules share many common features, and their basic structure is similar.

In this chapter, we present the nature of this generalized structure and discusses the characteristics of each immunoglobulin type. Specific functions for each of the classes are examined in relation to their structural differences. We will then proceed to discuss the cellular and genetic basis by which the specificity and diversity of antibodies arise. Finally, we will describe how highly specific antibodies, known as *monoclonal antibodies*, can be produced in the laboratory and used in a variety of clinical and research situations.

General Structure of Immunoglobulins

The basic structure of immunoglobulins was first discovered in the 1950s and 1960s because of biochemical analyses performed by two scientists—Gerald Edelman, of the Rockefeller Institute in the United States, and Rodney Porter, at Oxford University in England. They chose to work with immunoglobulin G (IgG), the most abundant of all the antibodies. For their contributions, these men shared the Nobel Prize in Physiology and Medicine in 1972. The key findings of these scientists and others are summarized in **Table 5–1.**

Two-Dimensional Structure

Because of this research, scientists developed an understanding of the basic structure of the IgG molecule. In its two-dimensional form, IgG can be visualized as a symmetrical molecule consisting of two larger peptide chains, known as **heavy (H) chains,** bound to two smaller peptide chains, called **light (L) chains (Fig. 5–2).** The heavy chains of IgG are denoted by the Greek letter for G (gamma or γ); they have a molecular weight of approximately 50,000 and are unique to the IgG molecule. The light chains have a molecular weight of about 22,000 and can be one of two types: **kappa (κ) chains** or **lambda (λ) chains**. The κ and λ chains differ by just a few amino acid substitutions along their length, and there are no functional differences between the two types. Both κ and λ light chains are found in all five classes of immunoglobulins, but only one type is present in a given molecule.

The heavy and light chains are held together by disulfide (S–S) bonds and other forces, including hydrogen bonds, hydrophobic forces, and electrostatic attractions. The sulfhydryl bonds can be broken by treatment of the molecule with a reducing agent, such as mercaptoethanol. The exact number of disulfide bonds differs among antibody classes and subclasses. The **tetrapeptide** structure of an antibody, indicated by the formula H_2L_2, serves as the basic structural unit of all the immunoglobulin classes, although the type of heavy chain is unique to each class and the number of units may vary, depending on the class.

Sequencing of the amino acids in the heavy and light chains revealed that each chain has a single variable region and one or more constant regions. The **variable region** is located in the first 110 amino acids of the molecule at the amino terminal. It is unique to each antibody molecule and allows the molecule to bind specifically to a particular antigen. The **constant regions** of the molecule, from amino acid 111 to the carboxyl terminal, are the same in each immunoglobulin class or subclass and are responsible for the biological functions that play a role in immune defense against an antigen. The IgG molecule has three constant regions, CH1, CH2, and CH3. CH2 and CH3 are responsible for binding to complement and Fc receptors on phagocytic cells, respectively. The importance of these functions will be discussed in the later section on immunoglobulin G.

Treatment With Proteolytic Enzymes

Porter and another scientist, Alfred Nisonoff, used the proteolytic enzymes papain and pepsin, respectively, to elucidate the structure of IgG. As you can see in Figure 5–2, papain

Table 5–1 Scientific Discoveries: Understanding the Structure and Function of Immunoglobulins

SCIENTIST(S)	DISCOVERY
Von Behring and Kitasato	Discovered that a substance in blood could neutralize activity of diphtheria toxin
Henry Bence Jones	Discovered monoclonal light chains in the urine of patients with multiple myeloma, facilitating the characterization of the Ig light chains
Arne Tiselius and Elvin Kabat	Separated serum into protein fractions by electrophoresis and identified the gamma globulin fraction as the main source of immunoglobulins
Rodney Porter	Used the enzyme papain to cleave IgG into the fragments Fab and Fc
Gerald Edelman	Performed analytic ultracentrifugation to separate immunoglobulins on the basis of molecular weight; unfolded the IgG molecule with urea and disrupted the disulfide bonds with mercaptoethanol
Alfred Nisonoff	Used the enzyme pepsin to cleave IgG to produce the fragment $F(ab')_2$

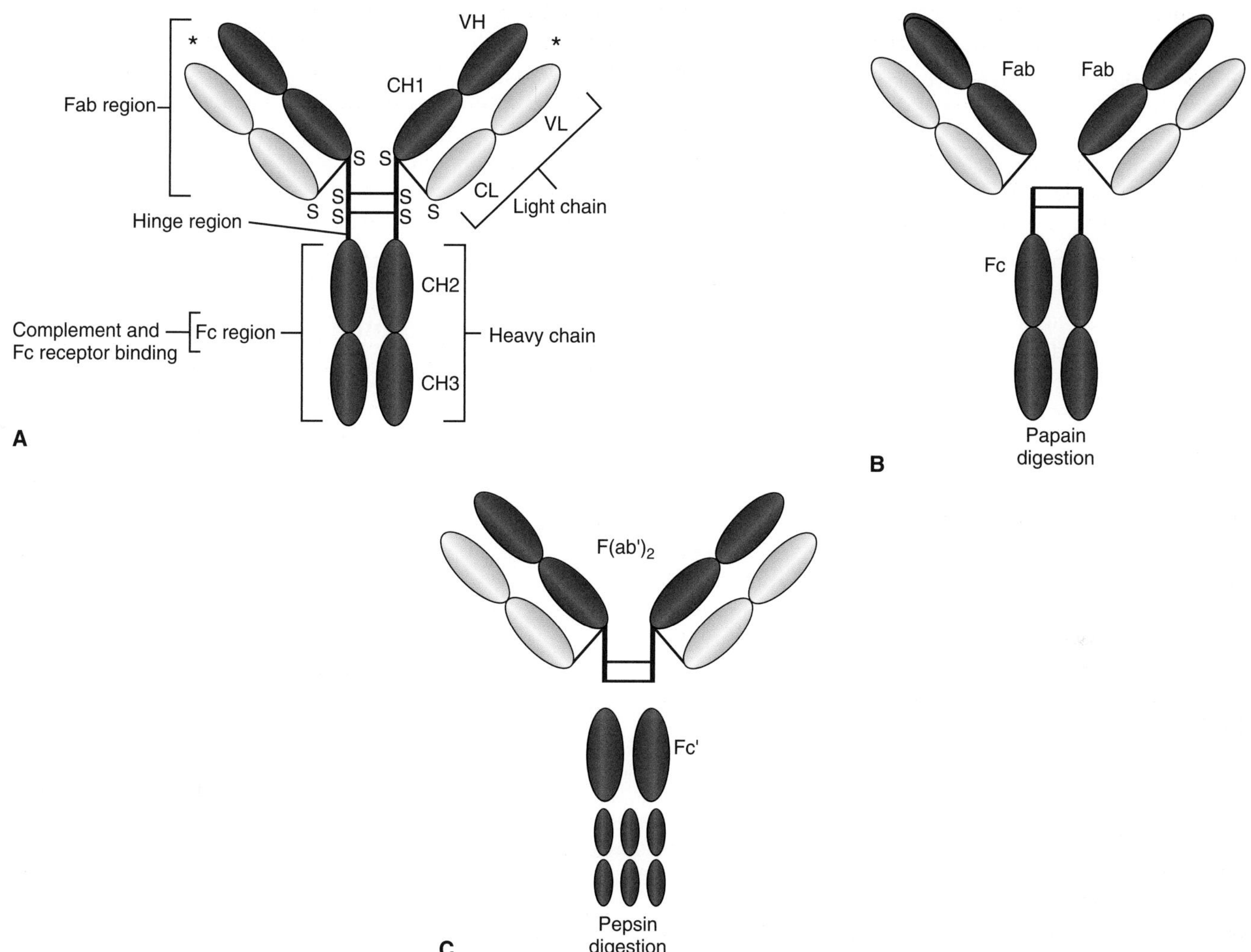

FIGURE 5–2 Basic structure of an immunoglobulin molecule. (A) Immunoglobulin G is made up of two heavy chains (50,000 MW each) and two light chains (22,000 MW each), held together by disulfide bonds. Intrachain disulfide bonds create looped regions or domains. The amino-terminal end of each chain is a variable region, whereas the carboxy-terminal end consists of one or more constant regions. (B) Papain digestion yields two Fab fragments and an Fc portion. (C) Pepsin digestion yields an $F(ab')_2$ fragment with all the antibody activity, as well as an Fc′ portion.

cleaves the IgG molecule below the set of disulfide bonds that holds the two heavy chains together, resulting in the formation of three fragments. Two of these fragments, located at the amino-terminal end of the molecule, are identical and have antigen-binding capability; hence, they are known as the **Fab fragments** (fragment antigen binding). Each Fab fragment thus consists of one light chain and one-half of a heavy chain held together by disulfide bonding. The third fragment, consisting of the carboxy-terminal halves of two heavy chains held together by S–S bonds, was designated as the **Fc fragment** because it spontaneously crystallized at 4°C. The Fc portion of the molecule does not bind antigen and contains the constant regions CH2 and CH3, which are responsible for important biological activities.

In contrast to papain, the enzyme pepsin cleaves IgG at the carboxy-terminal side of the interchain disulfide bonds, yielding a single fragment with a molecular weight of 100,000 daltons that contains all the antigen-binding ability, known as a **$F(ab')_2$ fragment.** An additional fragment called *Fc′* is created in the carboxy-terminal portion of the molecule, which is disintegrated into several smaller pieces and has no biological activity. The enzymes papain and pepsin are still used today to obtain immunoglobulin fragments with the desired activities, and the terms *Fab, Fc,* and *$F(ab')_2$* are commonly used to describe various portions of the antibody molecule.

Hinge Region

The segment of heavy chain located between the CH1 and CH2 regions is known as the **hinge region.** It is rich in hydrophobic residues and has a high proline content that allows for flexibility of the molecule. The ability to bend lets the two antigen-binding sites operate independently and engage in an angular motion relative to each other and to the Fc stem. Thus, two Fab arms can cover a good bit of territory. Such flexibility also assists in effector functions, including initiation of the complement cascade (see Chapter 7) and binding to cells with specific receptors for the Fc portion of the molecule. Gamma, delta, and alpha chains all have a hinge region, but mu and epsilon chains do not. However, the CH2 domains of these latter two chains are paired in such a way as to confer flexibility to the Fab arms.

In addition to the four polypeptide chains, all types of immunoglobulins contain a carbohydrate portion, which is localized between the CH2 domains of the two heavy chains. The carbohydrate has several important functions, including (1) increasing the solubility of immunoglobulin, (2) providing protection against degradation of the molecule, and (3) enhancing functional activity of the Fc domains. The latter function may be the most important because glycosylation appears to be critical for recognition by Fc receptors that are found on phagocytic cells.

Isotypes, Allotypes, and Idiotypes

Amino acid sequencing of the immunoglobulin peptide chains revealed the presence of antigenic determinants that can react with other antibodies produced by immunization of heterologous species. These antigenic determinants can be classified into one of three groups: isotypes, allotypes, and idiotypes **(Fig. 5–3).**

Isotypes are unique amino acid sequences that are common to all immunoglobulin molecules of a given class or subclass. They are identical in all individuals of a given species and differ from one species to another. Isotypes comprise constant regions of the heavy chains that are unique to each immunoglobulin class and give each type its name. Hence, the isotypes of the classes are known as γ for IgG, μ for IgM, α for IgA, δ for IgD, and ϵ for IgE. Antibodies to human isotypes can be prepared by immunizing animals with human serum. For example, goat antibodies directed against human IgG can be prepared after immunizing goats with human serum, and these antibodies can be used as reagents in immunoassays.

Minor variations of amino acid sequences that are present in some individuals of the same species but not others are known as **allotypes.** Allotypes occur in the four IgG subclasses, in one IgA subclass, and in the λ light chain. These genetic markers are found in the constant region and are inherited in a simple Mendelian fashion. Some of the best-known examples of allotypes are variations of the γ chain known as G1m3 and G1m17. Individuals can produce antibodies against allotypes they do not have if they are exposed through pregnancy or transfusion.

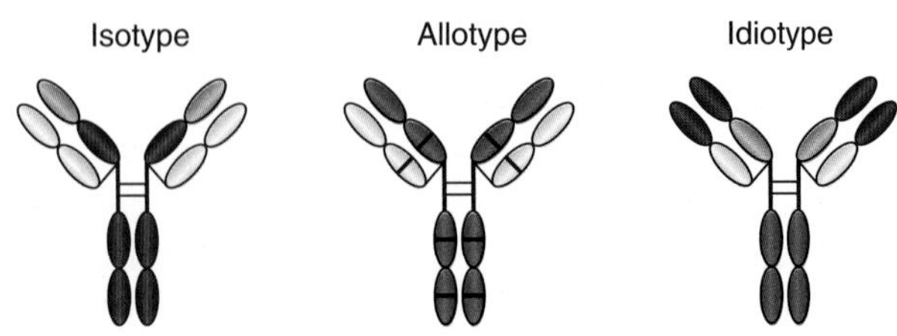

FIGURE 5–3 Antibody variations (shown in black). (A) Isotype—the heavy chain that is unique to each immunoglobulin class. (B) Allotype—genetic variations in the constant regions. (C) Idiotype—variations in variable regions that give individual antibody molecules specificity.

The variable portions of each immunoglobulin chain are unique to a specific antibody molecule, and they constitute what is known as the **idiotype** of the molecule. The amino-terminal ends of both heavy chains and light chains contain these regions, which are essential to the formation of the antigen-binding site. Together, they serve as the antigen-recognition unit.

Three-Dimensional Structure of Antibodies

The immunoglobulin structure is similar to other molecules belonging to the immunoglobulin superfamily, a group of glycoproteins that share a common ancestral gene. This gene originally coded for 110 amino acids, but it has been duplicated and mutated through time. Each type of immunoglobulin is made up of several regions called **domains,** which consist of approximately 110 amino acids. Although the different immunoglobulin classes may have differing numbers of domains, the three-dimensional structure of each is essentially the same.

The basic four-chain structure of all immunoglobulin molecules does not actually exist as a straight Y shape but is in fact folded into compact globular subunits based on the formation of balloon-shaped loops at each of the domains. Intrachain disulfide bonds stabilize these globular regions. Within each of these regions or domains, the polypeptide chain is folded back and forth on itself to form what is called a *β-pleated sheet*. The folded domains of the heavy chains line up with those of the light chains to produce a cylindrical structure called an *immunoglobulin fold* **(Fig. 5–4).** Antigen is captured within the fold by binding to a small number of amino acids at strategic locations on each chain known as *hypervariable regions.*

Three small hypervariable regions consisting of approximately 30 amino acid residues are found within the variable regions of both heavy and light chains. Each of these regions, called *complementarity-determining regions* (CDRs), is between 9 and 12 residues long. They occur as loops in the folds of the variable regions of both light and heavy chains. The antigen-binding site, or **paratope,** is actually determined by the apposition of the six hypervariable loops, three from each chain (see Fig. 5–4). Antigen binds in the middle of the CDRs, with at least four of the CDRs involved in the binding. Thus, a small number of amino acids can create an immense diversity of antigen-binding sites.

Antibody Classes

As we mentioned previously, there are five major classes of immunoglobulins—IgG, IgM, IgA, IgD, and IgE—and some of these can be further divided into subclasses. The structural and functional properties of the individual antibody classes are summarized in **Table 5–2** and are discussed in the following sections.

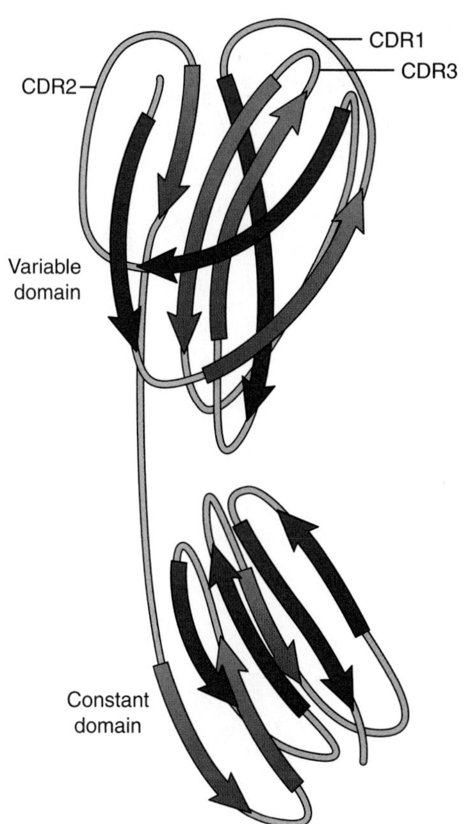

FIGURE 5–4 Three-dimensional structure of a light chain. In this ribbon diagram tracing the polypeptide backbone, β strands (polypeptide chains) are shown as wide ribbons, with other regions as narrow strings. Each of the two globular domains consists of a barrel-shaped assembly of seven to nine antiparallel β strands (polypeptide chains). The three hypervariable regions (CDR1, CDR2, and CDR3) are flexible loops that project outward from the amino-terminal end of the V_L domain.

Immunoglobulin G (IgG)

IgG is the predominant immunoglobulin in humans, comprising approximately 70% to 75% of the total serum immunoglobulins. In adults, the normal serum concentration of IgG ranges from 800 to 1,600 mg/dL. As you can see in Table 5–2, IgG has the longest half-life of any immunoglobulin class, approximately 23 days, which may help to account for its predominance in human serum.

IgG is a monomer, consisting of one tetrapeptide unit, with a molecular weight of 150,000 and a sedimentation coefficient of 7S. The sedimentation coefficient, or number of Svedberg units, is a measure of the rate by which the molecule sediments in a high-speed ultracentrifuge, and the S-value reflects the molecular weight of the molecule. There are four major IgG subclasses with the following distribution: IgG1, 66%; IgG2, 23%; IgG3, 7%; and IgG4, 4%. The γ heavy chains of these subclasses have slight variations in their constant-region amino acid sequences and differ in the number and position of disulfide bridges, as seen in **Figure 5–5.** Variability in the hinge region affects the ability to reach for antigen and the ability to initiate important biological functions, as you will learn in the following discussion. In general, IgG1 and IgG3 are produced in response to protein antigens, whereas IgG2 and IgG4 are associated with polysaccharide antigens.

All subclasses have the ability to cross the placenta except IgG2.

IgG has many important functions in the humoral immune response. The major functions of IgG include the following:

1. The CH2 region of IgG is able to bind to complement, a series of proteins that interact with antibodies to combat foreign antigens (see Chapter 7 for details). Activation

Table 5–2 Properties of Immunoglobulins

	IgG	IgM	IgA	IgD	IgE
Molecular weight	150,000	900,000	160,000 for the monomer	180,000	190,000
Sedimentation coefficient	7 S	19 S	7 S	7 S	8 S
Serum half-life (days)	23	6	5	1–3	2–3
Serum concentration (mg/dL)	800–1,600	120–150	70–350	1–3	0.005
Percent of total immunoglobulin	70–75	10	10–15	≤1	0.02
Heavy chain	γ	μ	α	δ	ϵ
Heavy-chain subclasses	γ1, γ2, γ3, γ4	None	α1, α2	None	None
Heavy-chain molecular weight	50,000–60,000	70,000	55,000–60,000	62,000	70,000–75,000
Number of constant domains in heavy chain	3	4	3	3	4
Carbohydrate content (percent)	2–3	12	7–11	9–14	12
Electrophoretic migration	γ2–α1	γ1–β2	γ2–β1,2	γ1	γ1
Complement fixation	Yes	Yes	No	No	No
Crosses placenta	Yes	No	No	No	No

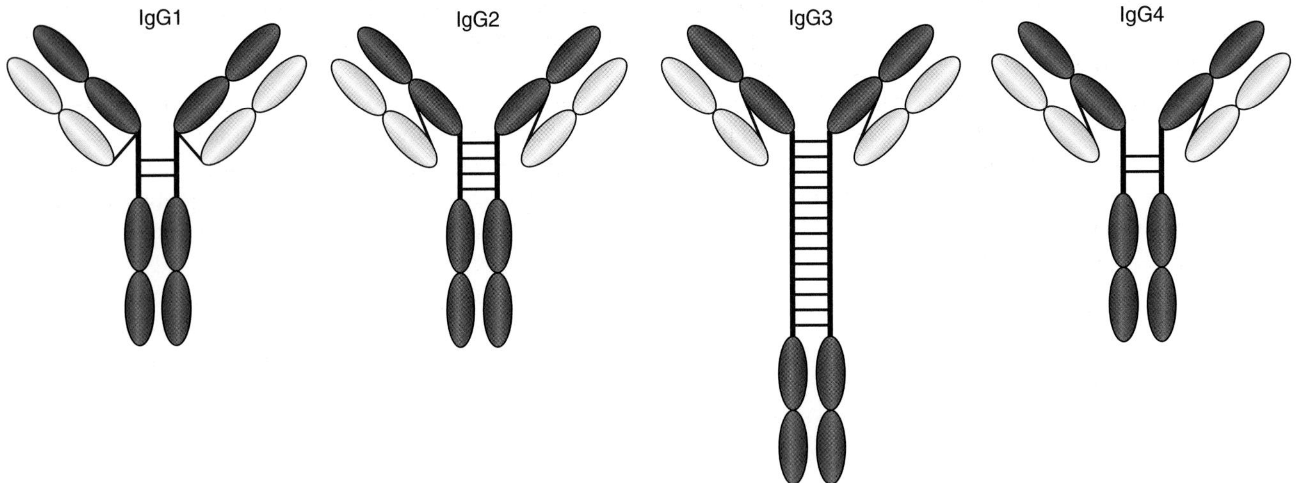

FIGURE 5–5 The four IgG subclasses are IgG1, IgG2, IgG3, and IgG4. These differ in the number and linkages of the disulfide bonds.

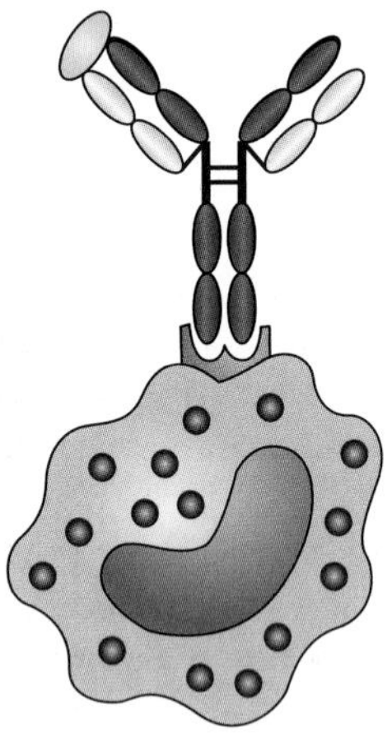

FIGURE 5–6 Opsonization. IgG coats the antigen and binds to Fc receptors on phagocytic cells.

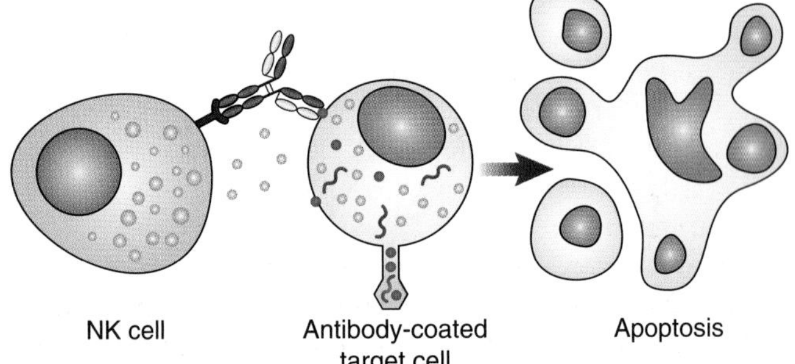

FIGURE 5–7 Antibody-dependent cellular cytotoxicity (ADCC). The Fab portion of IgG antibody binds to an antigen, whereas the Fc portion binds to receptors on macrophages, neutrophils, or NK cells, triggering the release of enzymes that destroy cells expressing the antigen. The figure shows an NK cell destroying an antibody-coated virus-infected host cell by ADCC.

of complement results in an enhanced inflammatory response and destruction of foreign cells such as bacteria. IgG3 is the most efficient subclass to bind complement because it has the largest hinge region and the largest number of interchain disulfide bonds. IgG1 is the second most efficient subclass to perform this function. In contrast, IgG2 and IgG4 have shorter hinge segments, which tend to make them poor mediators of complement activation.

2. IgG is an important mediator of **opsonization,** or the coating of a foreign antigen that leads to enhanced phagocytosis. This process occurs because macrophages, monocytes, and neutrophils have receptors on their surfaces that are specific for the Fc region of IgG. Binding of the CH3 region of IgG to the Fc receptor enhances contact between antigen and phagocytic cells and increases the efficiency of phagocytosis **(Fig. 5–6).** IgG1 and IgG3 are particularly good opsonins because they bind most strongly to Fc receptors.
3. A similar process in which IgG participates is **antibody-dependent cellular cytotoxicity (ADCC)**. In this process, IgG binds to Fc receptors on the surface of macrophages, monocytes, neutrophils, and natural killer (NK) cells. In this case, however, the antigen is not engulfed; instead, binding triggers the release of enzymes by the cells, which destroy the antigen extracellularly **(Fig. 5–7).**
4. Another important function of IgG is its ability to bind to bacterial toxins and viruses and neutralize their activity. IgG is effective in this process because it has a high diffusion coefficient that allows it to enter extravascular spaces more readily than the other immunoglobulin types.
5. IgG is the only type of antibody that can cross the placenta. This ability is present because the placenta possesses receptors for the Fc region of IgG molecules, which take up the antibodies by receptor-mediated endocytosis and transport them to the fetal blood. This function is mediated by IgG1, IgG3, and IgG4. Passive transfer of maternal IgG to the fetus is especially important in providing immunity to the newborn during its first few months of life, when its immune system is immature. The level of maternal IgG declines steadily according to its half-life, so by about 6 months of age, its levels are negligible; however, the infant will have started to make its own IgG by that time. Adult levels of IgG are reached at about 6 or 7 years of age.

6. IgG also participates in agglutination reactions (clumping of large particles) and precipitation (immune complexes falling out of a solution); see Chapter 10. Agglutination and precipitation reactions take place *in vitro*, although it is not known how significant a role these reactions play in vivo. IgG is better at precipitation reactions than at agglutination because precipitation involves small soluble particles, which are brought together more easily by the relatively small IgG molecule.

Immunoglobulin M (IgM)

IgM is known as a *macroglobulin* because it is the largest of all the immunoglobulin classes, having a sedimentation rate of 19 S, which represents a molecular weight of approximately 900,000 d. In the serum, IgM exists as a pentamer of five monomeric units held together by a glycoprotein known as the **J** or **joining chain,** whose cysteine residues form disulfide bonds that link the carboxy-terminal ends of adjacent monomers together to form a star-like shape **(Fig. 5–8).** Each monomer contains μ heavy chains and either κ or λ light chains. The μ heavy chains possess one more constant domain, CH4, adding to the large size of the molecule. Treatment of the pentamer with mercaptoethanol dissociates the molecule into its monomeric units. The monomer form of the μ heavy chain can also be found on the surface of B cells, and its expression is important to the process of B-cell maturation.

The half-life of IgM is about 6 days, and it accounts for between 5% and 10% of all serum immunoglobulins. In healthy adults, serum concentrations range from 120 to 150 mg/dL. IgM shares some of the same functions as IgG but performs them more effectively because of its multiple binding sites. For example, IgM is the most efficient of all the immunoglobulins at triggering the classical pathway of complement because a single molecule can initiate the reaction when complement binds to two adjacent CH2 regions (see Chapter 7). This probably represents the most important function of IgM. The larger number of binding sites also makes IgM more efficient at agglutination reactions than IgG. Because IgM is a pentamer, it can bind up to 10 separate antigens or bind to multivalent antigens. The high valency of IgM antibodies helps to overcome the fact that they tend to have a low affinity for antigen.

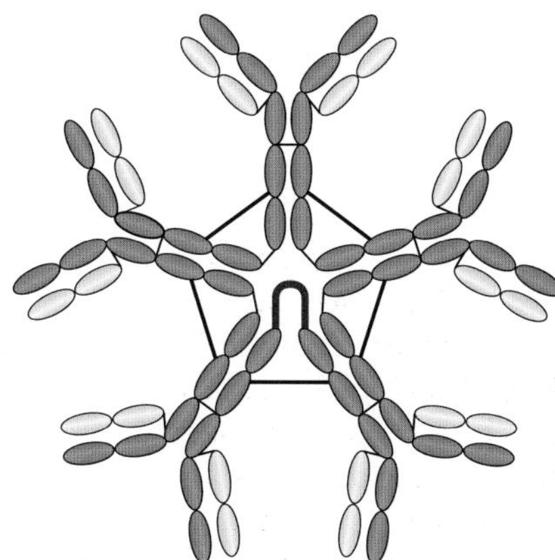

FIGURE 5–8 The pentameric structure of IgM is linked by a J chain (shown in red). Each arm can bend out of the plane to capture antigen.

Because of its large size, IgM is found mainly in the intravascular pool and not in other body fluids or tissues. It can neutralize bacterial toxins and viruses, but it cannot cross the placenta. IgM is known as the *primary response antibody* because it is the first to appear after antigenic stimulation and the first to appear in the maturing infant. It is synthesized only as long as antigen remains present because there are no memory cells for IgM. As we will see in later chapters, IgM can be used to diagnose an acute infection because its presence indicates a primary exposure to antigen.

Immunoglobulin A (IgA)

In the serum, IgA represents 10% to 15% of all circulating immunoglobulin, with a normal adult serum concentration of 70 to 350 mg/dL. It is a monomer with a molecular weight of approximately 160,000 and a sedimentation coefficient of 7 S. Upon electrophoresis, IgA migrates between the β and γ regions. The heavy chain of IgA is called α, and it contains one variable and three constant regions. There are two subclasses of IgA, designated *IgA1* and IgA2. They differ in content by 22 amino acids, 13 of which are located in the hinge region and are deleted in IgA2. The lack of this region appears to make IgA2 more resistant to some bacterial proteinases that are able to cleave IgA1. Hence, IgA2 is the predominant form in secretions at mucosal surfaces, whereas IgA1 is mainly found in serum. The major role of serum IgA is as an anti-inflammatory agent. Serum IgA appears to downregulate IgG-mediated phagocytosis, chemotaxis, bactericidal activity, and cytokine release.

IgA2 is found as a dimer along the respiratory, urogenital, and intestinal mucosa; it also appears in breast milk, colostrum, saliva, tears, and sweat. The dimer consists of two monomers held together by a J chain, as seen in IgM. The J chain is essential for the polymerization and secretion of IgA. Secretory IgA is synthesized in plasma cells found mainly in mucosal-associated lymphoid tissue and is released in dimeric form. IgA is synthesized at a much greater rate than that of IgG—approximately 3 grams per day in the average adult—but because it is mainly in secretory form, the serum concentration is much lower.

Another protein, called the **secretory component (SC)**, is later attached to the Fc region around the hinge portion of the α chains. This protein is derived from epithelial cells found in close proximity to the plasma cells. As **Figure 5–9** indicates, an SC precursor is present on the surface of epithelial cells and serves as a specific receptor for IgA. Plasma cells are attracted to subepithelial tissue, where they secrete IgA, which binds to the precursor. Once binding takes place, the IgA and SC precursor are taken inside the cell and released at the opposite surface by a process known as *transcytosis*. The vesicle carrying IgA and the SC receptor fuses with the membrane on the cell's opposite side; a small fragment of SC is then cleaved to liberate the IgA dimer with the remaining SC. The SC may

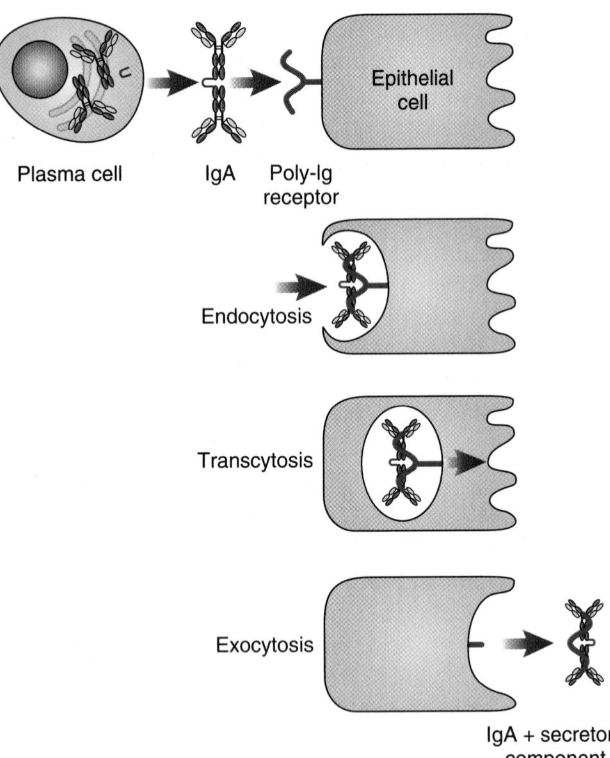

FIGURE 5–9 Formation of secretory IgA. IgA is secreted as a dimer from plasma cells and is captured by specific receptors on epithelial cells. The receptor is actually an SC, which binds to IgA and exits the cell along with it.

thus act to facilitate transport of IgA to mucosal surfaces. It also makes the dimer more resistant to enzymatic digestion by masking sites that would be susceptible to protease cleavage.

The main function of secretory IgA is to patrol mucosal surfaces and act as a first line of defense by preventing antigens from penetrating farther into the body. IgA plays an important role in neutralizing toxins produced by microorganisms and helps to prevent bacterial and viral adherence to mucosal surfaces. Complexes of IgA and antigen are easily trapped in mucus and then eliminated by the ciliated epithelial cells of the respiratory or intestinal tract. This prevents pathogens from colonizing the mucosal epithelium.

Furthermore, because IgA is found in breast milk, breastfeeding helps to maintain the health of newborns by passively transferring antibodies and greatly decreasing infant death from both respiratory and gastrointestinal infections. Additionally, neutrophils, monocytes, and macrophages possess specific receptors for IgA. Binding to these sites triggers a respiratory burst and degranulation, indicating that IgA is capable of acting as an opsonin.

It appears that IgA is not capable of fixing complement by the classical pathway, although aggregation of immune complexes may trigger the alternate complement pathway (see Chapter 7). Lack of complement activation may actually assist in clearing antigen without triggering an inflammatory response, thus minimizing tissue damage.

Immunoglobulin D (IgD)

IgD was not discovered until 1965, when it was found in a patient with multiple myeloma, a cancer of the plasma cells. It is extremely scarce in the serum, representing less than 0.001% of total immunoglobulins. It is synthesized at a low level and has a half-life of only 1 to 3 days. The molecule has a molecular weight of approximately 180,000 and migrates as a fast γ protein. The delta (δ) heavy chain has a molecular weight of 62,000 and appears to have an extended hinge region consisting of 58 amino acids.

Because of its unusually long hinge region, IgD is more susceptible to proteolysis than other immunoglobulins. This may be the main reason for its short half-life. In the secreted form in the serum, IgD does not appear to serve a protective function because it does not bind complement, it does not bind to neutrophils or macrophages, and it does not cross the placenta.

Most of the IgD is found on the surface of immunocompetent but unstimulated B lymphocytes. It is the second type of immunoglobulin to appear (IgM being the first), and it may play a role in B-cell activation, although its function is not completely understood. The high level of surface expression and its intrinsic flexibility make IgD an ideal early responder to antigen. Unlike B cells bearing only IgM receptors, those with both IgM and IgD receptors are capable of responding to T-cell help and switching to synthesis of IgG, IgA, or IgE. Thus, IgD may play a role in regulating B-cell maturation and differentiation.

Immunoglobulin E (IgE)

IgE is best known for its very low concentration in serum and the fact that it has the ability to activate mast cells and basophils. It is the least abundant immunoglobulin in the serum, accounting for only 0.0005% of total serum immunoglobulins, with a normal adult serum concentration of about 0.005 mg/dL. The molecular weight of IgE is approximately 190,000, making it an 8S molecule, and it has a carbohydrate content of 12%. The epsilon (ϵ) heavy chain is composed of one variable and four constant domains. A single disulfide bond joins each ϵ chain to a light chain, and two disulfide bonds link the heavy chains to one another.

IgE is the most heat-labile of all immunoglobulins; heating to 56°C for between 30 minutes and 3 hours results in conformational changes and loss of ability to bind to target cells. IgE does not participate in typical immunoglobulin reactions such as complement fixation, agglutination, or opsonization. Additionally, it is incapable of crossing the placenta. Instead, shortly after synthesis, it attaches to basophils, Langerhans cells, eosinophils, and tissue mast cells through high-affinity receptors for the Fc portion of the ϵ chain (Fc ϵ RI), which are found exclusively on the surface of these cells. The molecule binds at the CH3 domain, leaving the antigen-binding sites free to interact with specific antigen **(Fig. 5–10).** Plasma cells that produce IgE are located primarily in the lungs and in the skin.

Mast cells are also found mainly in the skin and in the lining of the respiratory and alimentary tracts. One such cell may have several hundred thousand receptors, each capable of binding to an IgE molecule. When two adjacent IgE molecules on a mast cell bind specific antigen, a cascade of cellular events is initiated that results in degranulation of the mast cells with the release of vasoactive amines such as histamine and heparin. The release of these mediators induces what is known as a *type I* immediate hypersensitivity or allergic reaction (see Chapter 14). Typical reactions include hay fever, asthma, vomiting and diarrhea, hives, and life-threatening anaphylactic shock.

IgE appears to be a nuisance antibody; however, it may serve a protective role by triggering an acute inflammatory reaction that recruits neutrophils and eosinophils to the area to help destroy invading antigens that have penetrated IgA defenses. Eosinophils, in particular, play a major part in the destruction of large antigens, such as parasitic worms, that cannot be easily phagocytized (see Chapter 22 for details).

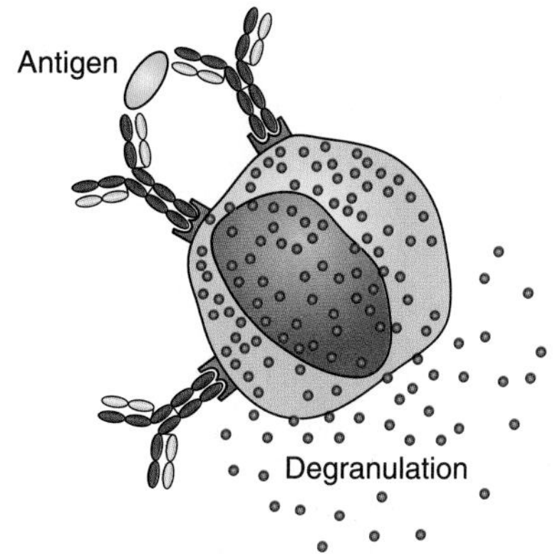

FIGURE 5–10 IgE binds to specific Fc ϵ receptors on mast cells. When antigen bridges two nearby IgE molecules, the membrane is disturbed, degranulation results, and chemical mediators are released.

Immunologic Memory: Primary and Secondary Antibody Responses

As we discussed in earlier chapters, one of the key features of the adaptive immune response is immunologic memory, or the ability of the immune system to respond more rapidly and effectively to an antigen upon repeated exposure. The first time an individual is exposed to an antigen, he or she mounts what is called a **primary antibody response.** This response is characterized by a long time period, or lag phase, between the encounter with the antigen and the production of detectable antibody. During the lag phase, which typically lasts between 4 and 7 days, T and B lymphocytes are being activated to respond to the antigen by the T-dependent mechanism of antibody production that was discussed in Chapter 4. This process results in the generation of antibody-secreting plasma cells. Antigen-specific IgM antibody is produced first, followed by specific IgG antibody **(Fig. 5–11).** The amounts of antibody produced are relatively low and decline during the span of a few weeks.

Some of the activated B cells from the primary response will not develop into plasma cells but, rather, expand into clones of long-lived memory cells. These memory cells have undergone

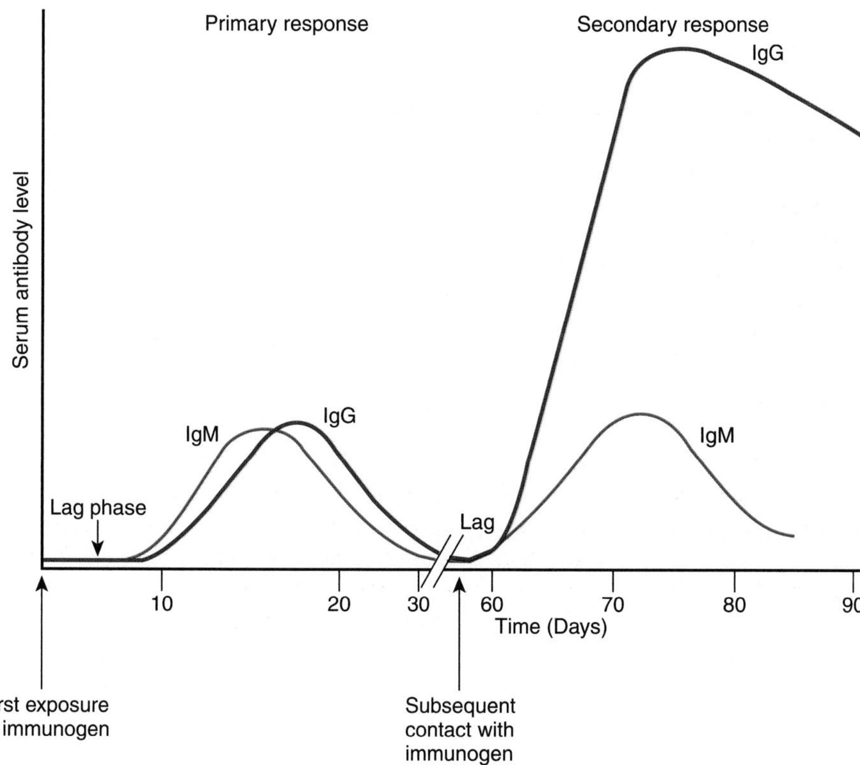

FIGURE 5–11 Primary and secondary antibody responses. Memory lymphocytes are generated during the primary response, and these cells can respond more effectively upon subsequent exposure to the same antigen. As compared with the primary response, the secondary or anamnestic response has a shorter lag phase; a much more rapid increase in antibody titer, mainly IgG; and greater persistence of IgG over time.

Clinical Correlations

Serologic Testing

The antibody responses shown in Figure 5-11 are the basis for serology testing for infectious diseases. The antibody classes can be used to differentiate an acute immune response, characterized by IgM only, from the response occurring later in the course of infection (IgM plus IgG) and a past infection (IgG only). See Chapters 20 to 23.

genetic changes that allow them to resist apoptosis; express high-affinity antigen receptors; and switch their production from IgM to another isotype, predominantly IgG. Therefore, if the memory B cells are exposed to the same antigen weeks, months, or even years later, they can rapidly differentiate into plasma cells, and larger amounts of antibody are produced. The memory response is also referred to as the **secondary antibody response,** or **anamnestic response.** As you can see in Figure 5–10, this response has a shorter lag phase (~1 to 2 days) and results in the production of low levels of IgM that rapidly decline, as in the primary response. More importantly, it results in higher levels of another immunoglobulin isotype (usually IgG). IgG levels decline slowly and persist in the body for longer periods, sometimes providing life-long immunity to the antigen. The key differences between the primary and secondary antibody responses are summarized in **Table 5–3**. The memory response serves as the basis for the booster injections that are given in routine vaccination schedules to optimize the immunity of the recipient to potentially harmful pathogens (see Chapter 25).

Antibody Specificity and Diversity

Other important features of adaptive immunity are its specificity for a particular antigen and its ability to respond to a diverse array of antigens in our environment. It is estimated that humans have the potential to respond to between 10^7 and 10^9 different antigens. Yet, when an individual is exposed to a particular antigen, the immune system produces antibodies that are specific for that antigen and not for unrelated antigens. For example, a person infected with Group A *Streptococcus* bacteria will make antibodies to antigens possessed by those bacteria and not to *Staphylococcus* bacteria. You may be wondering how this is possible. In this section, we will explore the genetic basis for antigen specificity and diversity and discuss how these characteristics are achieved on a cellular level.

Clonal Selection

As we previously discussed, in addition to their presence in the blood and other body fluids, immunoglobulins are found on the surface membrane of B cells, where they serve as receptors for antigens. Through the years, scientists discovered that the body has numerous clones of lymphocytes, each possessing surface receptors with a unique antigen specificity. When the body is exposed to an antigen, the antigen selectively binds to receptors on the cells capable of responding to it, causing only those cells to proliferate and mount the antibody responses we discussed in Chapter 4. This process, first hypothesized by the scientist Paul Ehrlich in the early 1900s and confirmed independently by Niels Jerne and Macfarlane Burnet in the 1950s, is called the **clonal selection hypothesis.** Today, clonal selection is considered to be a fundamental concept of the immune response **(Fig. 5–12).**

Furthermore, as you will learn in the next section, individual lymphocytes are genetically preprogrammed to produce an immunoglobulin receptor with a single antigen specificity. This process occurs before contact with antigen, during maturation of the B cells in the bone marrow. In a similar fashion, antigen-specific T-cell receptors are generated during maturation of the T cells in the thymus (see Chapter 4). Because of this remarkable process, mature lymphocytes that have seeded the lymphoid tissues are prepared to respond to a diverse array of potentially harmful antigens long before the body actually encounters them.

Immunoglobulin Genes

Before the concept of clonal selection became established, scientists wondered how this hypothesis could be reconciled with the genetic basis for antibody diversity. The central dogma of molecular genetics is that one gene codes for one polypeptide. However, if there were separate genes to code for all the antibody molecules to every possible antigen, an overwhelming amount of DNA would be needed, much more than could be packaged into a cell nucleus. In 1965, Dreyer and Bennett proposed a solution to this dilemma by suggesting that the constant and variable portions of immunoglobulin chains are actually coded for by separate genes. They hypothesized that there was a small number of genes coding for the constant region and a larger number coding for the variable region. This notion implied that although all lymphocytes originate with identical genetic germline DNA, diversity is created by a series of events whereby separate gene segments

Table 5-3 Comparison of Primary and Secondary Antibody Responses

	PRIMARY RESPONSE	SECONDARY RESPONSE
Time to antibody production	Longer lag phase	Shorter lag phase; faster appearance of antibody
Antibody classes	IgM, followed by IgG	IgM, followed by a greater predominance of IgG
Antibody titer	Relatively low; declines in a few weeks	High IgG titer, which declines slowly and persists for a long time
Antibody affinity for antigen	Low affinity	High affinity

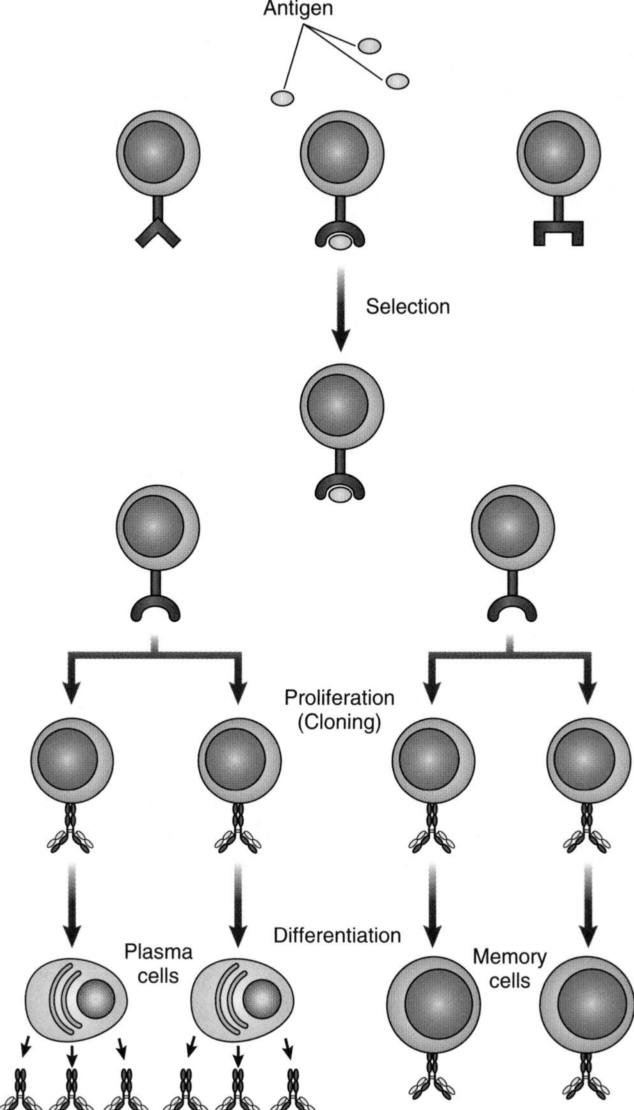

FIGURE 5–12 Clonal selection. Antigen binds only to B lymphocytes expressing receptors specific for the antigen. Those B cells are stimulated to divide and differentiate into plasma cells that secrete antibody specific for the antigen (in this example, the B cell in the middle).

are selected and joined together as the B cell matures. Susumu Tonegawa's pioneering work provided scientific evidence for this hypothesis, and he was awarded the Nobel Prize in 1987 for his monumental discovery.

Tonegawa's experiments with DNA revealed that chromosomes do not contain intact immunoglobulin genes but, rather, building blocks from which genes can be assembled. Human immunoglobulin genes are found in three unlinked clusters: Heavy-chain genes are located on chromosome 14, κ light-chain genes are on chromosome 2, and λ light-chain genes are on chromosome 22. Within each of these clusters, a selection process occurs. The genes cannot be transcribed and translated into functional antibody molecules until this rearrangement, assisted by special recombinase enzymes, takes place. Gene rearrangement involves a cutting-and-splicing process that removes much of the intervening DNA, resulting in a functional gene that codes for a specific antibody. Once this rearrangement occurs in a B lymphocyte, it permanently changes its DNA.

Rearrangement of Heavy-Chain Genes

The selection process begins with rearrangement of the genes for the heavy chains. All heavy chains are derived from a single region on the long arm of chromosome 14. The genes that code for the variable region of the heavy chain are divided into three groups—V_H, D, and J. There are approximately 45 functional V_H (variable) genes, 23 D (diversity) genes, and six J (joining) genes. All the V, D, and J genes are present in the germline DNA of a bone marrow stem cell. In addition, there is a set of genes that codes for the constant region (C). This set includes one gene for each heavy-chain isotype. They are located in the following order: Cμ, Cδ, Cγ3, Cγ1, Cα1, Cγ2, Cγ4, Cε, and Cα2, as shown in **Figure 5–13.** Only one of these constant regions is selected at any one time.

As the B cell matures and the heavy chain is constructed, a random choice is made from each of the sections so as to include one V_H gene, one D gene, one J gene, and one constant-region gene. Joining of these segments occurs in two steps: First, in pro-B cells, one D gene and one J gene are randomly chosen and are joined by means of a recombinase enzyme after the intervening DNA is deleted (see Fig. 5–13). Next, in the pre–B-cell stage, a V gene is joined to the DJ complex, resulting in a rearranged VDJ gene. The VDJ gene combination codes for the entire variable region of the heavy chain. Thus, during the process of B-cell maturation, the pieces are spliced together to commit that B lymphocyte to making antibody of a single specificity.

If a successful rearrangement of DNA on one chromosome 14 occurs, then the genes on the second chromosome are not rearranged; this phenomenon is known as **allelic exclusion.** If the first rearrangement is nonproductive, then rearrangement of the second set of genes on the other chromosome 14 occurs. This mechanism maintains clonal specificity by ensuring that each B cell only expresses a single antigen receptor.

Next, the variable-and constant-region genes are joined. This process occurs at the ribonucleic acid (RNA) level, thus conserving the DNA of the constant regions. During transcription and synthesis of messenger ribonucleic acid (mRNA), a constant region is spliced to the VDJ complex. Because Cμ is the region closest to the J region, μ heavy chains are the first to be synthesized; these are the markers of the pre-B lymphocytes. The Cδ region, which lies closest to the Cμ region, is often transcribed along with Cμ. The presence of DNA for both the Cμ and Cδ regions allows for mRNA for IgD and IgM to be transcribed at the same time. Thus, a B cell could express IgD and IgM with the same variable domain on its surface at the same time.

Light-Chain Rearrangement

Because light-chain rearrangement occurs only after μ chains appear, μ-chain synthesis represents a pivotal step in the process. Light chains exhibit a similar genetic rearrangement, except they lack a D region. Recombination of segments on

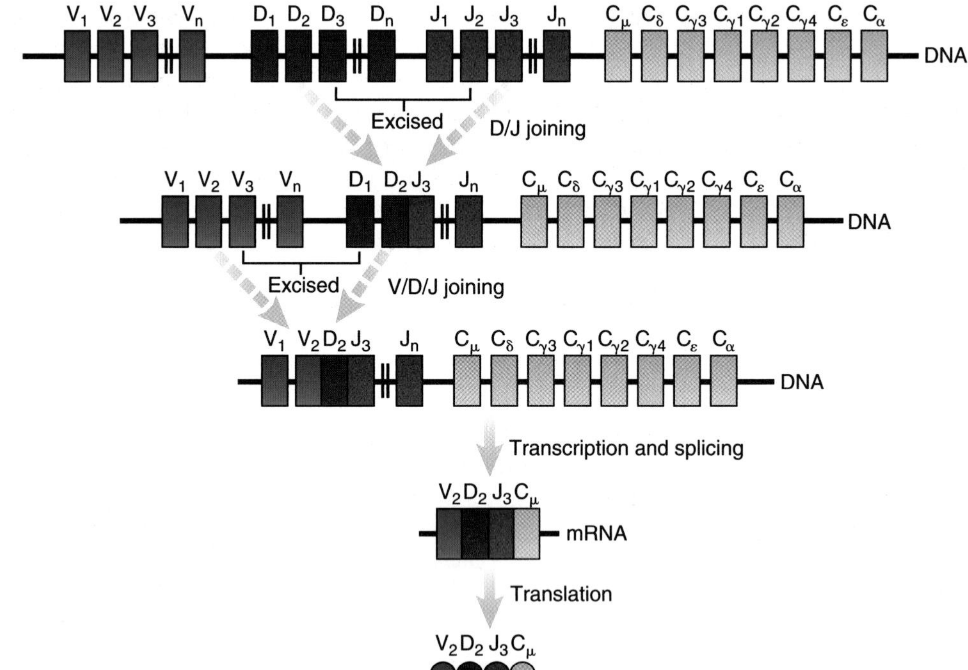

FIGURE 5–13 Genes Coding for immunoglobulin heavy chains. Four separate regions on chromosome 14 code for heavy chains. DJ regions are spliced first, and then this segment is joined to a variable region. When RNA synthesis occurs, one constant region is attached to the VDJ combination; μ heavy chains are made first, but the cell retains its capacity to produce immunoglobulin of another class.

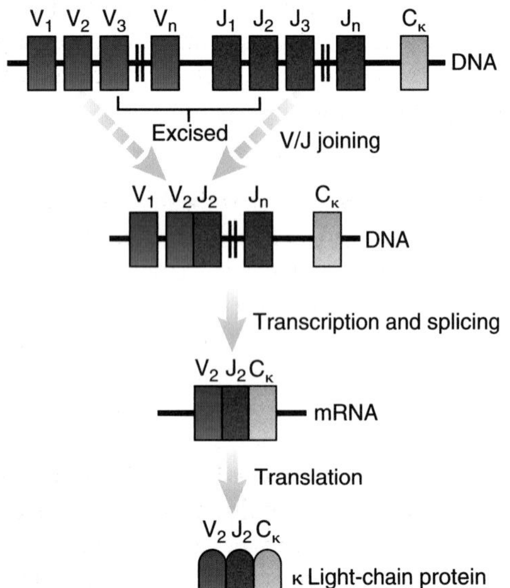

FIGURE 5–14 Assembly and expression of the λ-light-chain locus. A DNA rearrangement fuses one V segment to one J segment. The VJ segment is then transcribed along with a unique C region to form mature λ mRNA. Unarranged J segments are removed during RNA splicing.

chromosome 2, coding for κ chains, occurs before that on chromosome 22, which codes for λ chains.

The κ locus contains approximately 35 V_κ, five J_κ, and one functional C_κ segment. The process of VJ joining is accomplished by cutting out intervening DNA. This results in the V_κ and J_κ segments becoming permanently joined to one another on the rearranged chromosome. Transcription begins at one end of the V_κ segment and proceeds through the J_κ and C_κ segments. J segments that have not been rearranged are removed by RNA splicing, which occurs during translation **(Fig. 5–14)**.

A productive rearrangement of the κ genes with subsequent protein production keeps the other chromosome 2 from rearranging and shuts down any recombination of the λ-chain locus on chromosome 22. Only if a nonfunctioning gene product arises from κ rearrangement does λ-chain synthesis occur. The λ locus contains approximately 30 V_λ, 4 J_λ, and 4 functional C_λ segments. If functional heavy and light chains are not produced in a B lymphocyte by these rearrangements, then that cell dies by apoptosis.

Light chains are then joined with μ chains to form a complete IgM antibody, which first appears in immature B cells. Once IgM and IgD are present on the surface membrane, the B lymphocyte is fully mature and capable of responding to antigen (see Chapter 4).

Additional Sources of Diversity

The process of VDJ recombination is just one way in which diversity is generated in the creation of B-cell antigen receptors. The recombinase enzymes, RAG-1 and RAG-2, are essential for initiating VDJ recombination during B-cell maturation. These enzymes recognize specific recombination signal sequences in the DNA that flank all immunoglobulin gene segments. However, joining of the V, J, and D segments doesn't always occur at a fixed position, so each sequence can vary by a small number of nucleotides. This variation, called *junctional diversity,* is a major contributor to diversity in the variable-region genes. Furthermore, additional nucleotides may be added at the junctions.

Another source of variation occurs at the protein level. Once the immunoglobulin chains are synthesized, different heavy chains can combine with different light chains to produce functional antibody molecules.

A final source of variation, called *somatic hypermutation*, can occur after the B cell has had contact with the antigen. During the T-cell–dependent antibody response, cytokines are produced that stimulate the B cells to divide so that the response to the antigen is enhanced. Genetic mutations occur at a very high rate in the variable regions of the immunoglobulin genes during this period of rapid B-cell proliferation. Mutations in some of these B cells result in immunoglobulin receptors that can bind the antigen more strongly, and these B cells become the dominant clones as the immune response evolves. This process, called **affinity maturation,** results in a more effective response to the antigen.

Thus, there are several sources of immunoglobulin diversity: the large variety of V, J, D, and C combinations for each type of chain; junctional diversity; different possibilities for light-and heavy-chain combinations; and somatic hypermutation. All these processes, taken together, result in more than enough antibody configurations to allow us to respond to any antigen in our environment.

Immunoglobulin Class Switching

As we discussed earlier, the first immunoglobulin to be synthesized during the immune response is IgM. This occurs because the Cμ gene is the constant-region gene that is closest to the VDJ genes. As the immune response progresses, B cells may become capable of producing antibody of another class, a phenomenon called **class switching.**

Production of other immunoglobulin isotypes occurs because of a process called *switch recombination,* whereby a portion of the constant-region DNA is deleted and the remaining C_H genes are placed adjacent to the variable-region genes. This allows the same VDJ region to be coupled with a different C region to produce antibody of a different class (i.e., IgA, IgG, or IgE) but having identical specificity for antigen. Contact with T cells and cytokines determines where switching takes place and which C_H gene will be transcribed. For example, the cytokine IL-4 provides the signal for transcription of the Cε gene and deletion of the intervening sequences. The resulting production of IgE antibody might be helpful in defense against parasitic infections. Thus, class switching allows the B cells to change their production to a different antibody isotype, which would be most effective in defending against a particular type of pathogen encountered by the host.

Monoclonal Antibodies

The normal response to an antigen results in the production of polyclonal antibodies because even a purified antigen has multiple epitopes that stimulate a variety of B cells. In contrast, **monoclonal antibodies** are derived from a single parent antibody-producing cell that has reproduced many times to form a clone. All the cells in the clone are identical, and the antibody produced by each of these cells is exactly the same as that produced by every other cell in the clone. Monoclonal antibodies are directed against a specific epitope on an antigen.

The knowledge that B cells are genetically preprogrammed to synthesize a very specific antibody has been used to develop monoclonal antibodies for diagnostic testing. In 1975, Georges Kohler and Cesar Milstein developed a technique to produce antibody arising from a single B cell, and this method has revolutionized serological testing. They were awarded the Nobel Prize in 1984 for their pioneering research.

Hybridomas

A normal B cell can only survive for a short time in culture. To develop a cell line that produces antibody but can live for a long period of time, Kohler and Milstein combined an activated B cell with a myeloma cell, a cancerous plasma cell that can be grown indefinitely in the laboratory. The fusion product of these two cell types is called a **hybridoma.** The particular myeloma cell line that was chosen to make the hybridoma was not capable of producing its own antibody. In addition, this cell line was deficient in the enzyme hypoxanthine-guanine phosphoribosyltransferase (HGPRT), making it incapable of synthesizing nucleotides from hypoxanthine and thymidine, substances needed for DNA synthesis. The fact that these myeloma cells could not make their own DNA meant that they would die unless they were fused to a B cell that had the enzymes necessary to synthesize DNA. This deficiency kept the myeloma cells from reproducing on their own.

Hybridoma Production

The production of hybridomas begins by immunizing a mouse with the desired antigen. After a time, the mouse's spleen cells are harvested because the spleen is a rich source of B lymphocytes. The spleen cells are combined with myeloma cells in the presence of polyethylene glycol (PEG), a surfactant that brings about fusion of the cells to produce a hybridoma. Only a small percentage of the cells actually fuse, and some of these are not hybridomas but, rather, two myeloma cells or two spleen cells combined together. After fusion, all cells are placed in culture using a selective medium called *HAT,* which contains hypoxanthine, aminopterin, and thymidine. The culture medium allows the hybridoma cells to grow but does not allow the fused myeloma cells or fused spleen cells to survive. The myeloma cells die because the two pathways of nucleotide synthesis (the salvage pathway and the de novo pathway) are blocked under these conditions. The salvage pathway, which builds DNA from degradation of old nucleic acids, is blocked because the myeloma cell line is deficient in the required enzymes HGPRT and thymidine kinase. The de novo pathway, which makes DNA from new nucleotides, is blocked by the presence of aminopterin. Consequently, the myeloma cells die. Normal B cells cannot be maintained continuously in cell culture, so these die as well. This leaves only the fused hybridoma cells, which have the ability to reproduce indefinitely in culture (acquired from the myeloma cell) and the ability to synthesize nucleotides by the HGPRT and thymidine kinase pathway (acquired from the normal B cell) **(Fig. 5–15).**

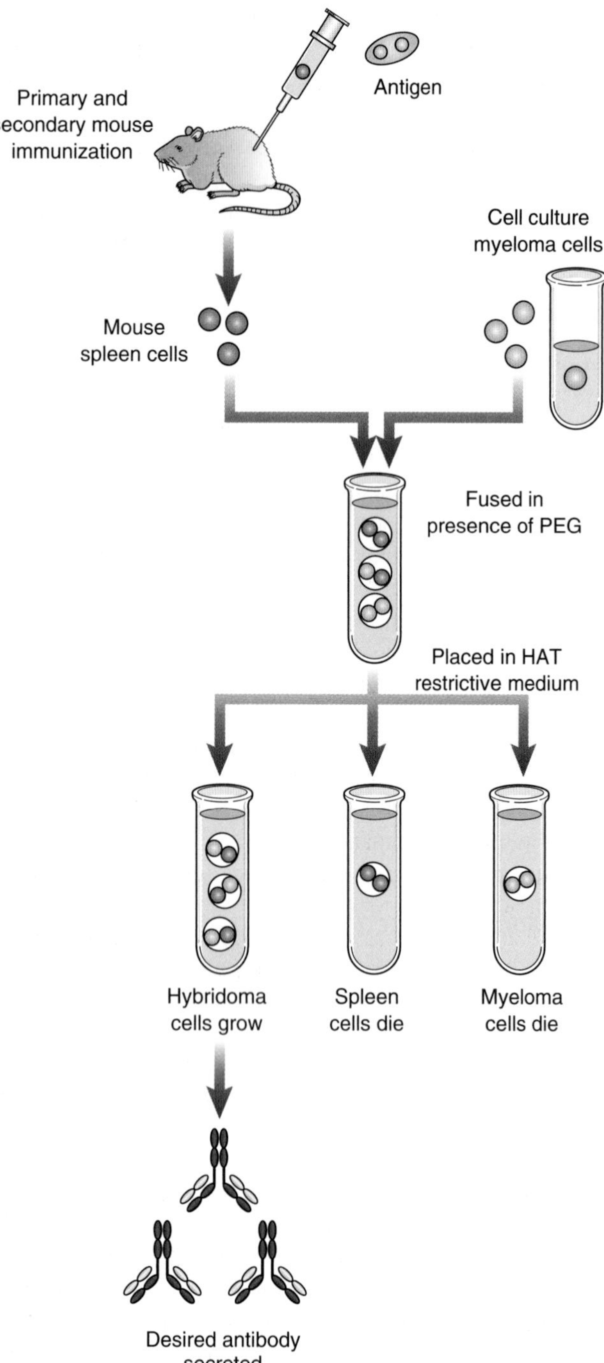

FIGURE 5–15 Formation of a hybridoma in monoclonal antibody production. A mouse is immunized, and spleen cells are removed. These cells are fused with nonsecreting myeloma cells and then plated in a restrictive culture medium. Only the hybridoma cells will grow in this medium, where they synthesize and secrete a monoclonal immunoglobulin specific for a single determinant on an antigen.

Selection of Specific Antibody-Producing Clones

The hybridoma cells are then diluted and placed in microtiter wells, where they are allowed to grow. Each well contains a single clone and is screened for the presence of the desired antibody in the culture supernatant. Once the desired clones are identified, they are cultured in larger quantities. These hybridomas can be maintained in cell culture indefinitely and produce an abundant supply of monoclonal antibody that reacts with a single antigen epitope.

Clinical and Research Applications

Monoclonal antibodies were initially used *in vitro*, as reagents in laboratory tests. A familiar example is pregnancy testing, which uses antibody specific for the β chain of human chorionic gonadotropin, thereby eliminating many false-positive reactions. Other examples include tests that detect tumor antigens or measure hormone levels. Before the development of monoclonal antibodies, antibody reagents could only be produced by immunizing animals such as horses or goats with the desired antigen and isolating polyclonal antibodies from the animal serum. The primary advantages of monoclonal antibody reagents are that they provide decreased lot-to-lot variation and increased specificity toward a single epitope, rather than multiple epitopes of an antigen. These advantages have led to the widespread use of monoclonal antibodies in laboratory tests that identify various types of lymphocytes and other white blood cells on the basis of their cell surface markers.

Connections

CD4 T-Cell Quantitation

An example of a laboratory test that uses monoclonal antibodies to detect lymphocytes is CD4 T-cell quantitation. CD4 T cells (i.e., T helper cells) are the main target of the HIV virus, and a decrease in the number of CD4 T cells in the peripheral blood is a hallmark characteristic of HIV infection and its end stage, AIDS. The CD4 T cells are detected by fluorescent-labeled antibodies to the T-cell antigen, CD3, and the helper-T-cell marker, CD4. The amount of fluorescence emitted by the cells is recorded by an instrument called a *flow cytometer* (see Chapters 13 and 25).

Monoclonal antibodies have subsequently been used as therapeutic agents to treat a variety of diseases, especially cancer and autoimmune disorders. Some examples include the antibody trastuzumab (Herceptin), directed against the HER-2 protein, which is amplified in some breast cancer patients; rituximab (Rituxan), which targets the B-cell marker CD20 and is used to treat patients with non-Hodgkin lymphoma and other B-cell malignancies; and adalimumab (Humira), a monoclonal antibody that blocks the action of tumor necrosis factor-α (TNF-α), a cytokine that plays a pathogenic role in rheumatoid arthritis.

A major limitation of using mouse monoclonal antibodies as therapeutic agents is that they are highly immunogenic for humans, inducing the development of human-anti-mouse antibodies (HAMAs) that can cause severe hypersensitivity reactions (see Chapter 25). Therefore, several techniques have been developed to reduce such reactions by constructing monoclonal antibodies that are made of more human protein and less mouse protein. Chimeric and humanized monoclonal antibodies have been generated by using molecular techniques to graft the entire antibody-combining site or CDRs from mouse antibodies onto the rest of a human immunoglobulin. More recently, fully human monoclonal antibodies have been produced by transgenic mice in which the mouse immunoglobulin genes have been replaced by human immunoglobulin genes. The spleen cells from the transgenic mice immunized with a specific antigen can be used to generate hybridoma cell lines, as described previously. Libraries of genetically engineered bacteriophages (viruses that infect bacteria), yeast, or mammalian cells can be used to clone the antibody genes of interest, and along with next-generation sequencing (see Chapter 12), select for antibodies that have a high binding affinity for antigen.

The use of monoclonal antibodies as therapeutic agents continues to grow. This represents a rapidly developing area in pharmacology that is impacting several fields of medicine by changing treatment options for numerous diseases. (See Chapter 25 for additional information about the use of monoclonal antibodies.)

SUMMARY

- The basic structural unit for all immunoglobulins is a tetrapeptide composed of two light chains and two heavy chains joined together by disulfide bonds.
- The five classes of antibodies are IgM, IgG, IgA, IgD, and IgE. IgG, IgD, and IgE exist as monomers. IgA has a dimeric form in the secretions, whereas IgM is a pentamer whose subunits are held together by a J chain.
- Kappa and lambda light chains are found in all types of immunoglobulins, but the heavy chains differ for each immunoglobulin class.
- Each immunoglobulin molecule has constant and variable regions. The variable region is at the amino-terminal end, called the Fab fragment; this determines the specificity of that molecule for a particular antigen.
- The constant region, located at the carboxy-terminal end of the molecule, contains the Fc fragment and is responsible for binding to complement and to effector cells such as neutrophils, basophils, eosinophils, and mast cells.
- *Opsonization* refers to the coating of a foreign antigen by antibody to enhance phagocytosis through binding of the Fc portion of the antibody to receptors on neutrophils and macrophages.
- ADCC is a process by which IgG binds to Fc receptors on macrophages, monocytes, neutrophils, and NK cells, triggering the release of enzymes that cause extracellular destruction of antigen.
- The five different types of heavy chains are called *isotypes*. Isotypes are unique to each Ig class or subclass within a species.
- Minor variations in a particular type of heavy chain are called *allotypes*. Allotypes are genetically determined markers that are shared by some individuals of the same species.
- The variable portion of the heavy and light chains unique to a particular immunoglobulin molecule is known as the *idiotype*. Idiotypes are essential to the formation of unique antigen-binding sites.
- IgG is relatively small and easily penetrates into tissues. IgG is a monomer that is capable of binding to complement, mediating opsonization, participating in ADCC, and neutralizing bacterial toxins. It is the only immunoglobulin that can cross the placenta.
- IgM is a large pentamer whose subunits are held together by a protein known as the *J chain*. IgM is more efficient at complement fixation than IgG because of its more numerous binding sites for complement. IgM is also very efficient in agglutinating antigens. IgM is known as the *primary response antibody* because it is the first Ig to appear in the maturing infant and the first to be produced by the host during an immune response.
- IgA is a dimer that is the main Ig in the body's secretions. Secretory IgA contains a J chain and an secretory component that protects it from enzymatic digestion while it patrols mucosal surfaces. IgA is also found in breast milk and thus is involved in the passive transfer of immunity from mother to infant.
- An extended hinge region gives IgD an advantage as a surface receptor for antigen.
- IgE binds to mast cells to initiate an inflammatory response that plays a role in allergic reactions.
- The primary antibody response is mounted after the first time an individual is exposed to an antigen. The primary response has a relatively long lag phase (usually 5 to 7 days before antibody can be detected) and results in low levels of IgM and IgG, which decline during a period of a few weeks.
- The secondary response to antigen, also known as the *memory* or *anamnestic response*, occurs after a second or subsequent exposure of the host to the same antigen. The secondary response occurs more rapidly than the primary response because of the activation of memory lymphocytes. The amount of IgM is similar to that of the primary response, whereas IgG may be up to 100 times greater than that of the primary response. The IgG levels decline slowly and provide long-term immunity to the antigen.
- Clonal selection is a fundamental concept of the immune response. In this process, when antigen is introduced into the body, it binds to unique receptors on selected B cells, stimulating only those B cells to divide and differentiate into plasma cells that produce antibody specific for that antigen.
- Several genes code for the variable and constant regions of a particular immunoglobulin: The V_H, D, and J genes code for the variable portion of the Ig heavy chains, and there is one constant-region gene for each Ig class; a similar set of genes code for the Ig light chains, except they do not include the D genes. Through a random-selection

process, the individual gene segments are joined to make antibody of a single specificity. The antibody appears on the surface of B lymphocytes, where it serves as a receptor for antigen.

- Antibody diversity results from several different mechanisms: VDJ gene recombination, junctional diversity, various combinations of heavy and light chains, and somatic hypermutation.
- During the course of the immune response, Ig production switches from IgM to another Ig class because of genetic recombination between the constant-region genes for the different heavy chains.
- Monoclonal antibodies are made by hybridoma cells, which are created by fusing an antibody-producing B cell with a malignant myeloma cell line that contributes the property of immortality. The fused cells are isolated in a selective medium called *HAT*. Those hybridomas secreting the desired antibody are then grown in larger quantities.
- Monoclonal antibodies are used as reagents in laboratory tests and as therapies for the treatment of various diseases.

Study Guide: The Five Classes of Immunoglobulins

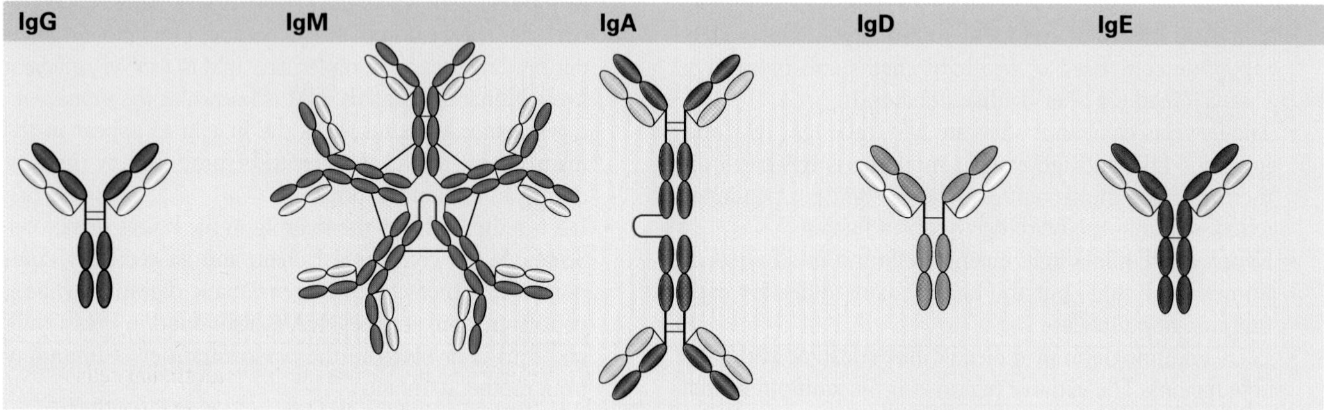

IgG	IgM	IgA	IgD	IgE
Most abundant in serum Binds complement Binds to receptors on phagocytic cells Able to cross placenta Increases with second exposure to antigen	Primary response antibody Pentamer with 10 antibody-binding sites Binds efficiently to complement Causes efficient agglutination of antigens Indicates acute infection	Monomer in serum and dimer in secretions Protects mucosal surfaces Present in breast milk Has secretory component	Present as an antigen receptor on B-cell membrane Role in B-cell activation Identifies mature B cells	Binds to mast cells and basophils Triggers allergic response Role in response to parasites

CASE STUDIES

1. A 15-year-old male exhibited symptoms of fever, fatigue, nausea, and sore throat. He went to his primary care physician, who ordered a rapid strep test and a test for infectious mononucleosis to be performed in the office. The rapid strep test result was negative, but the test result for infectious mononucleosis was faintly positive. The patient mentioned that he thought he had mononucleosis about 2 years earlier, but it was never officially diagnosed. His serum was sent to a reference laboratory to test with specific Epstein-Barr viral antigens. The results indicated the presence of IgM only.

Questions

a. Is this a new or reactivated case of mononucleosis? Explain your answer.
b. How do the results relate to the difference between a primary and a secondary response to exposure to the same antigen?

2. A 10-year-old female experienced one cold after another in the springtime. She had missed several days of school, and her mother was greatly concerned. The mother took her daughter to the pediatrician, worried that her daughter might be immunocompromised because she couldn't seem to fight off infections. A blood sample was obtained and sent to a reference laboratory for a determination of antibody levels, including an IgE level. The patient's IgM, IgG, and IgA levels were all normal for her age, but her IgE level was greatly increased.

Questions

a. What does the increase in IgE signify?
b. Should there be a concern about the patient being immunocompromised?

REVIEW QUESTIONS

1. Which of the following is characteristic of variable domains of immunoglobulins?
   a. They occur on both the heavy and light chains.
   b. They represent the complement-binding site.
   c. They are at the carboxy-terminal ends of the molecules.
   d. They are found only on heavy chains.

2. All of the following are true of IgM *except* that it
   a. can cross the placenta.
   b. fixes complement.
   c. has a J chain.
   d. is a primary response antibody.

3. How does the structure of IgE differ from that of IgG?
   a. IgG has an SC, and IgE does not.
   b. IgE has one more constant region than IgG.
   c. IgG has more antigen-binding sites than IgE.
   d. IgG has more light chains than IgE.

4. How many antigen-binding sites does a typical IgM molecule have?
   a. 2
   b. 4
   c. 6
   d. 10

5. An Fab fragment consists of
   a. two heavy chains.
   b. two light chains.
   c. one light chain and one-half of a heavy chain.
   d. one light chain and an entire heavy chain.

6. Which antibody best protects mucosal surfaces?
   a. IgA
   b. IgG
   c. IgD
   d. IgM

7. Which of the following pairs represents two different immunoglobulin allotypes?
   a. IgM and IgG
   b. IgM1 and IgM2
   c. Anti-human IgM and anti-human IgG
   d. IgG1m3 and IgG1m17

8. The structure of a typical immunoglobulin consists of which of the following?
   a. Two light chains and two heavy chains
   b. Four light chains and two heavy chains
   c. Four light chains and four heavy chains
   d. Two light chains and four heavy chains

9. Which of the following are light chains of antibody molecules?
   a. Kappa
   b. Gamma
   c. Mu
   d. Alpha

10. If the results of serum protein electrophoresis show a significant decrease in the gamma band, which of the following is a likely possibility?
    a. Normal response to active infection
    b. Multiple myeloma
    c. Immunodeficiency disorder
    d. Monoclonal gammopathy

11. The subclasses of IgG differ mainly in
    a. the type of light chain.
    b. the arrangement of disulfide bonds.
    c. the ability to act as opsonins.
    d. molecular weight.

12. Which best describes the role of the SC of IgA?
    a. A transport mechanism across endothelial cells
    b. A means of joining two IgA monomers together
    c. An aid to trapping antigen
    d. Enhancement of complement fixation by the classical pathway

13. Which is thought to be the main function of IgD?
    a. Protection of the mucous membranes
    b. Removal of antigens by complement fixation
    c. Activation of B cells
    d. Destruction of parasitic worms

14. Which antibody is best at agglutination and complement fixation?
    a. IgA
    b. IgG
    c. IgD
    d. IgM

15. Which of the following can be attributed to the clonal selection hypothesis of antibody formation?
    a. Plasma cells make generalized antibody.
    b. B cells are preprogrammed for specific antibody synthesis.
    c. Proteins can alter their shape to conform to antigen.
    d. Cell receptors break off and become circulating antibody.

16. All of the following are true of IgE *except* that it
   a. fails to fix complement.
   b. is heat stable.
   c. attaches to tissue mast cells.
   d. is increased in the serum of allergic persons.

17. Which best describes coding for immunoglobulin molecules?
   a. All genes are located on the same chromosome.
   b. Light-chain gene rearrangement occurs before heavy-chain gene rearrangement.
   c. Four different regions are involved in coding for heavy chains.
   d. Lambda gene rearrangement occurs before kappa gene rearrangement.

18. What is the purpose of HAT medium in the preparation of monoclonal antibody?
   a. Fusion of the two cell types
   b. Restricting the growth of myeloma cells
   c. Restricting the growth of spleen cells
   d. Restricting antibody production to the IgM class

19. Papain digestion of an IgG molecule results in which of the following?
   a. Two Fab′ fragments and one Fc′ fragment
   b. One $F(ab')_2$ fragment and one Fc′ fragment
   c. Two Fab fragments and two Fc fragments
   d. Two Fab fragments and one Fc fragment

20. Which antibody provides protection to the growing fetus because it is able to cross the placenta?
   a. IgG
   b. IgA
   c. IgM
   d. IgD

21. Which best characterizes the secondary response?
   a. Equal amounts of IgM and IgG are produced.
   b. There is an increase in IgM only.
   c. There is a large increase in IgG but not IgM.
   d. The lag phase is the same as in the primary response.

Cytokines 6

Aaron Glass, PhD, MB(ASCP)[CM]

LEARNING OUTCOMES

After finishing this chapter, you should be able to:

1. Define *cytokine.*
2. Define and describe the term *cytokine storm* and relate its medical importance.
3. Distinguish between autocrine, paracrine, and endocrine effects of cytokines.
4. Define *pleiotropy* as it relates to cytokine activities.
5. Explain the functions of interleukin-1 (IL-1) in mediating the immune response.
6. Explain the effects of tumor necrosis factors (TNFs).
7. Discuss how interleukin-6 (IL-6) affects inflammation and other activities of the immune system.
8. Determine the role of chemokines in the chemotaxis of white blood cells (WBCs).
9. Compare the functions of type 1 and type 2 interferons (IFNs).
10. Describe the actions of interleukin-2 (IL-2) on its target cells.
11. Discuss the biological roles of the hematopoietic growth factors.
12. Discuss cytokines involved in differentiation of T helper (Th) cell subpopulations: Th1, Th2, Th17, and T regulatory (Treg).
13. Explain the biological role of colony-stimulating factors (CSFs).
14. Describe current types of anti-cytokine therapies.
15. Describe clinical assays for cytokines.

CHAPTER OUTLINE

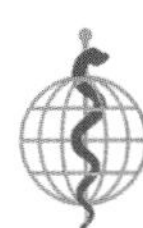

Go to FADavis.com for the laboratory exercises that accompany this text.

KEY TERMS

Antagonism
Autocrine
Cascade
Chemokines
Colony-stimulating factor (CSF)
Cytokines
ELISpot
Endocrine
Endogenous pyrogen
Erythropoietin (EPO)
Granulocyte colony-stimulating factor (G-CSF)
Granulocyte–macrophage colony-stimulating factor (GM-CSF)
Hypercytokinemia
Interferons (IFNs)
Interleukin
Macrophage colony-stimulating factor (M-CSF)
Paracrine
Pleiotropy
Proinflammatory
Redundancy
Synergistic
T helper 1 cells (Th1)
T helper 2 cells (Th2)
T helper 17 cells (Th17)
T regulatory (Treg) cells
Transforming growth factor-beta (TGF-β)
Tumor necrosis factor (TNF)

Introduction to Cytokines

Successful immunity requires coordination between immune cells, which may be widely dispersed throughout the body. Therefore, a form of intercellular communication between immune cells is necessary to orchestrate a successful immune response. **Cytokines** are chemical messengers that regulate immunity, influencing both the innate and adaptive responses to infection.

Produced by many immune and nonimmune cells, all cytokines are small proteins that bind to and activate receptors located on target cells. Many cytokines are produced in response to infectious stimuli; for example, bacterial lipopolysaccharides (LPSs), flagellin, and other bacterial products cause innate immune cells to release a host of *proinflammatory* cytokines. The effects of cytokines include regulation of growth, differentiation, and gene expression by many different cell types. After release, most cytokines are rapidly degraded in the extracellular environment, limiting their activity.

Many cytokines exhibit the properties of pleiotropy and redundancy. **Pleiotropy** means that a single cytokine can have many different actions. **Redundancy** occurs when different cytokines activate some of the same pathways and genes. Redundancy may be explained by the fact that many cytokines share receptor subunits. Thus, some cytokines may have overlapping effects and may alter the activity of many of the same genes.

Cytokine activity can be classified according to the distance traveled between the producing cell and its target cell(s). Some cytokines act locally, impacting only the producing cell or a few nearby cells, whereas other cytokines transmit their messages throughout the entire body. Cytokines that bind to receptors on the same cell from which they were secreted are said to signal in an **autocrine** manner. Cytokines that act on cells within the tissue region surrounding their cellular source transmit **paracrine** signals. Some cytokines diffuse into the bloodstream, allowing them to influence cells far from the cell or cells that produce them. In these cases, the cytokines are behaving as hormones, acting in an **endocrine** fashion **(Fig. 6–1)**.

Understanding the roles of individual cytokines in immunity is complicated by the fact that many do not act alone but, rather, in conjunction with other cytokines. Even an innocuous infection may result in the production of many different cytokines, some of which exert opposing activities. Successful immune responses often involve the expression of a *network* of cytokines, each influencing a different aspect of leukocyte activity and resulting in elimination of the infection.

In these networks, cytokines can interact in several ways. If the effects of two different cytokines complement and enhance each other, the interaction is called **synergistic (Fig. 6–2)**. In contrast, if one cytokine counteracts the action of another, **antagonism** occurs (see Fig. 6–2). Many cytokines induce the production of additional cytokines by target cells, resulting in a cytokine **cascade.** Each of these forms of network interaction can be observed in the example of the cytokine interferon-γ (IFN-γ). IFN-γ causes certain T lymphocytes to secrete additional IFN-γ as well as an **interleukin (IL)** called *interleukin-2*. IFN-γ synergizes with the cytokine tumor necrosis factor-α (TNF-α) to activate macrophages and antagonizes the cytokine interleukin-4 (IL-4) by preventing IL-4 from influencing T lymphocytes.

Cytokine interactions are powerful determinants of immunity, and the pattern of cytokines produced in response to a particular infection can spell the difference between an effective or inappropriate immune response. In extreme circumstances, massive overproduction and dysregulation of cytokines can result in hyperstimulation of the immune response or **hypercytokinemia,** a condition commonly referred to as *cytokine storm.* Instead of orchestrating an effective immune response against a pathogen, cytokine storms may lead to shock, multiorgan failure, or even death. Several human pathogens induce cytokine storms, including pathogenic viruses (e.g., influenza A) and bacteria (e.g., *Francisella tularensis*). Cytokine storms have been implicated in the lethality of the 1918 influenza pandemic among young adults. Historical

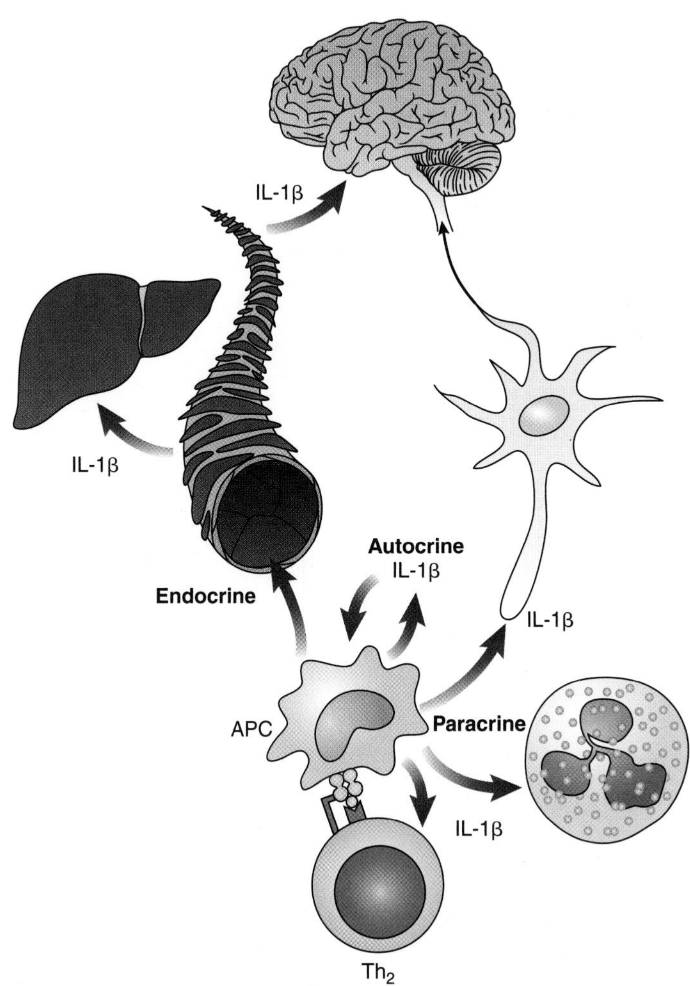

FIGURE 6–1 Range of cytokine actions. Autocrine: Cytokine acts on the cell that secreted it (e.g., IL-1β increases activation of antigen-presenting cell [APC)]. Paracrine: Cytokine acts on nearby cells (e.g., IL-1β stimulates Th cells, activates neutrophils, and depolarizes neurons). Endocrine: Cytokine travels through blood vessels to distant cells (e.g., IL-1β stimulates acute-phase protein synthesis in the liver, as well as fever induction in the hypothalamus).

documents suggest that many 1918 influenza deaths resulted not from the virus itself but because of the production of extremely high levels of **proinflammatory** cytokines, such as TNF-α and interleukin-1β (IL-1β), which promote inflammation. When present in the blood at high concentrations, these cytokines cause hypotension, fever, and edema and can precipitate organ failure and death.

Given the destructive effects of cytokine storms, it is clear that the inflammatory response must be closely regulated to prevent damaging systemic inflammation. Anti-inflammatory cytokines antagonize the effects of TNF-α and IL-1β, thus resolving inflammation and limiting collateral damage to host cells. **Table 6–1** displays major proinflammatory and anti-inflammatory cytokines.

Initially, immunologists named cytokines based on either their activities or the immune cell population that produced them. Using this system, a cytokine that was observed to kill cancer cells was named "tumor necrosis factor," cytokines released from lymphocytes were called *lymphokines*, monocytes produced monokines, and leukocytes secreted interleukins that influenced other leukocytes. At times, the same cytokine was referred to by different names, leading to confusion.

More recently, cytokines have been grouped into families, which include TNF, IFN, chemokine, transforming growth factor (TGF), and **colony-stimulating factor (CSF).** Instead of reclassifying the interleukins into structurally or functionally similar families, they have been numbered IL-1 to IL-40. Selected cytokines from each of these groups will be discussed in this chapter.

The growth in clinical applications for cytokines, cytokine antagonists, and cytokine receptor antagonists in conditions such as rheumatoid arthritis (RA), asthma, and Crohn's disease have increased the demand for cytokine assays in the clinical laboratory. In addition, the clinical laboratory plays an important role in assessing treatment modalities, effectiveness, and potential gene-replacement therapies for numerous immunodeficiency syndromes and leukemias caused by defects in cytokines, their receptors, or their signal transduction circuits.

The following sections will discuss cytokines according to their participation in either the innate immune response or the adaptive immune response. The major cytokines and their functions are summarized in the Study Guides at the end of this chapter.

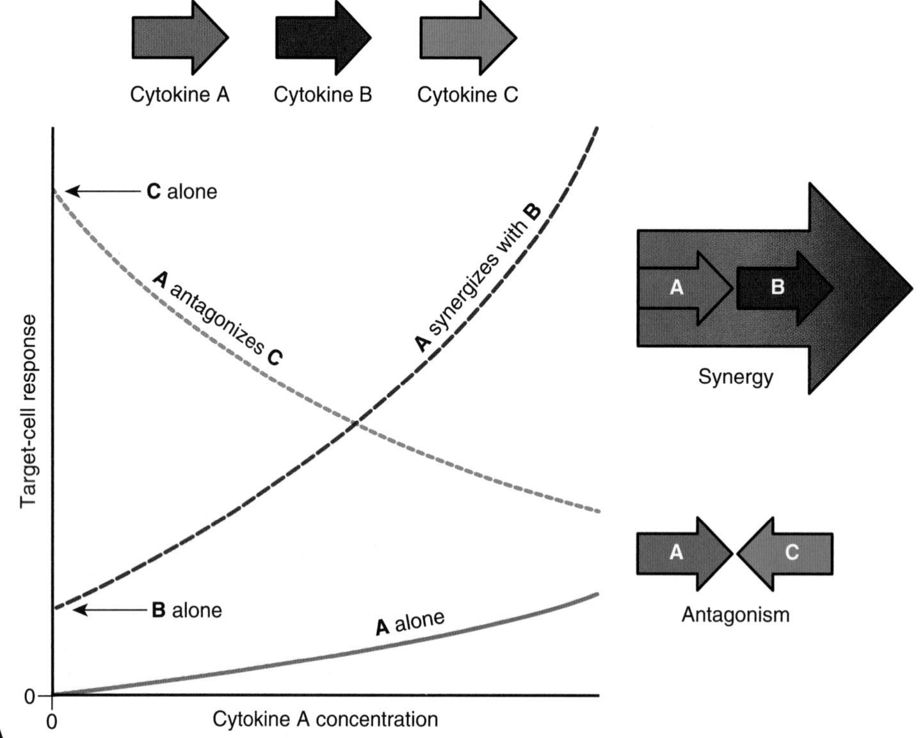

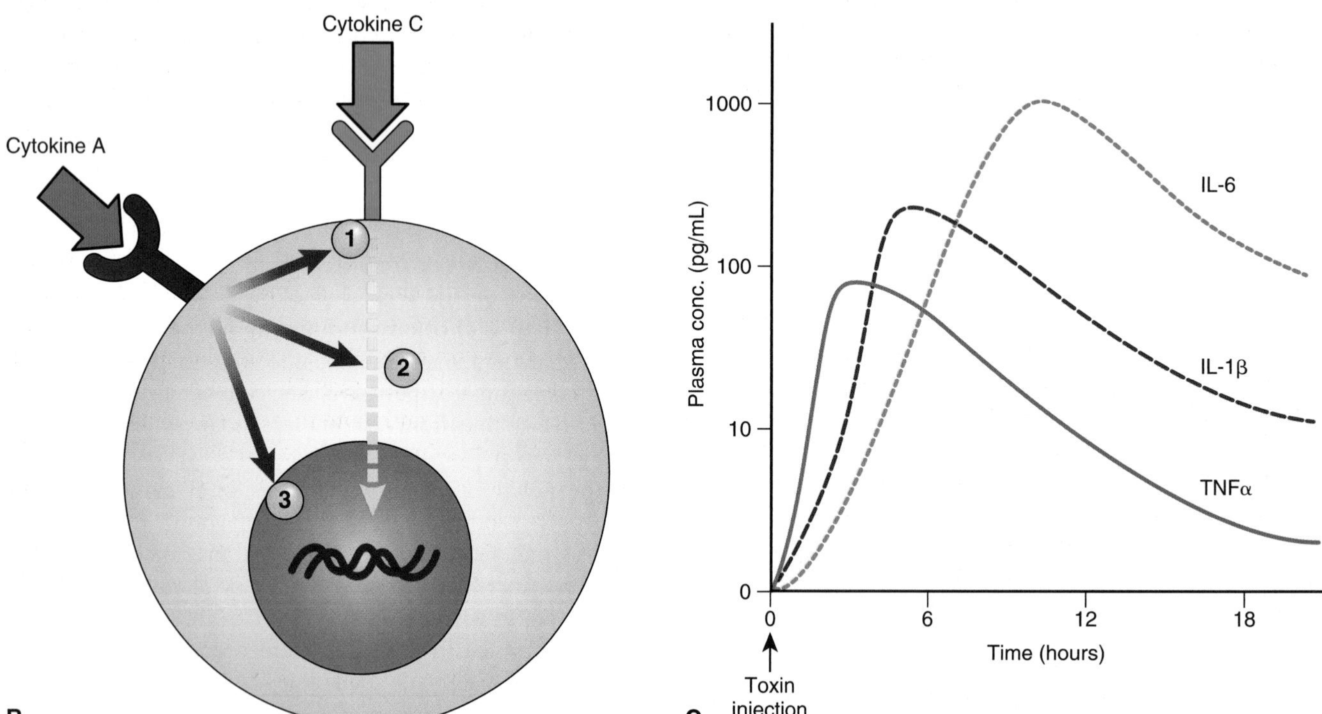

FIGURE 6–2 (A) Cytokine characteristics of synergy, antagonism, and cascade induction. Synergy: Neither cytokine A nor B induces a strong response individually; however, when combined, the net response is much greater than the sum of the individual responses. Antagonism: Individually, cytokine C induces a strong response, and cytokine A induces a weak (but positive) response. When combined, cytokine A diminishes the action of cytokine C. In this illustration, the concentrations of cytokines B and C are held constant, whereas cytokine A increases along the horizontal axis. (B) Synergistic and antagonistic interactions may be the result of cytokine A (1) altering the expression or function of the receptor for cytokine C, (2) altering the activity of a key enzyme in the signaling pathway for cytokine C, or (3) altering the stability or translation of the mRNA induced by cytokine C. (C) Cytokines can induce the release of other cytokines in an amplifying cascade. For example, following intravenous injection of a bacterial toxin, TNF-α is first released by monocytes and macrophages. Both the toxin and TNF-α induce the subsequent release of IL-1β. Then all three induce interleukin 6 (IL-6) release from a wide variety of cell types.

Table 6–1 Examples of Major Proinflammatory and Anti-Inflammatory Cytokines

MAJOR PROINFLAMMATORY CYTOKINES	MAJOR ANTI-INFLAMMATORY CYTOKINES
TNF-α	TGF-β
IL-1	IL-10
IL-6	IL-13
IFN-γ	IL-35

Cytokines in the Innate Immune Response

Cytokines and the Innate Response to Extracellular Microbes

For most species of pathogenic bacteria and fungi, infections begin once the body's epithelial barriers, such as the skin, have been breached. The first immune cells to encounter invading microorganisms are tissue-resident phagocytes, such as macrophages and dendritic cells (DCs). These sentinel immune cells detect infection using innate receptors (Toll-like receptors and similar pattern recognition receptors) that recognize molecular patterns (pathogen-associated molecular patterns [PAMPs]) found on diverse types of microbes. Binding of macrophage and DC receptors to their corresponding PAMPs induces the production and secretion of inflammatory cytokines (see Chapter 2).

The primary cytokines provoked by infection with extracellular microbes are interleukin-1 (IL-1), interleukin-6 (IL-6), and TNF-α. Once produced, these cytokines diffuse away from their sources to mediate a handful of local (paracrine) effects, including (1) increased capillary permeability, which allows soluble anti-microbial proteins (complement, C-reactive protein, etc.) to enter the tissues from blood plasma; (2) increased platelet aggregation, which helps to seal off local blood vessels, preventing dissemination of the infection into the blood; and (3) alteration of adhesion molecule expression on capillary endothelial cells, which enhances entry of leukocytes from the blood into inflamed tissues.

Severe infections can stimulate the production of larger quantities of inflammatory cytokines, causing systemic (endocrine) effects, including (1) an increase in body temperature, which may make the body less hospitable to invading microbes; (2) an increase in the production of immune cells by the bone marrow and acute-phase reactants by the liver; and (3) the subjective feeling of being ill. These effects are responsible for many of the physical symptoms of inflammation, including fever, swelling, pain, and infiltration of immune cells into damaged tissues. Perhaps the most important role of these inflammatory cytokines is the recruitment of effector cells, such as neutrophils and monocytes, into inflamed tissues.

The Interleukin-1 (IL-1) Cytokine Family

IL-1 is a family of 11 structurally and functionally related cytokines. The best characterized of the IL-1 cytokines are IL-1α, IL-1β, and IL-1RA (IL-1 receptor antagonist). IL-1β and IL-1RA are expressed in monocytes, macrophages, and DCs. In contrast, IL-1α is expressed in innate phagocytic cells and can also be detected in epithelial cells from the skin, lungs, and gastrointestinal tract.

Many microbial components induce the production of IL-1, such as LPS, lipoteichoic acid, bacterial or viral nucleic acids, and even other cytokines. Although the genes encoding IL-1α and IL-1β have lower than 30% sequence homology, experimental studies have demonstrated that both have very similar biological effects. One substantial difference between these two forms of IL-1 is that IL-1α is retained within the cell cytoplasm and is only released after cell death. The presence of free IL-1α helps to attract inflammatory cells to areas where cells and tissues are being damaged or killed.

In contrast to IL-1α, IL-1β is released from macrophages and monocytes. IL-1β mediates most of the local (paracrine) and systemic (hormonal) activity attributed to IL-1, including activation of phagocytes, fever, and production of acute-phase proteins. Before secretion, IL-1β must be cleaved intracellularly to an active form (see Clinical Correlation "Inflammasomes Link Gout and Alum to Inflammation").

One of the most important paracrine effects of IL-1β is the recruitment of immune cells into inflamed tissues. Binding of IL-1β to IL-1 receptors on blood vessel endothelial cells alters adhesion molecule expression and stimulates the production of chemokines. These changes cause immune cells such as granulocytes and monocytes to stop moving through the blood and begin *diapedesis,* a process where blood leukocytes pass through vessel walls and enter inflamed tissues (see Chapter 2).

IL-1β is sometimes referred to as **endogenous pyrogen** because of its ability to induce fever. IL-1 receptors on neurons of the hypothalamus allow this brain organ to respond to the presence of systemic IL-1β by increasing body temperature. Fever serves several purposes during infection. For instance, higher body temperatures (1) inhibit the growth of many bacteria and fungi; (2) increase the microbicidal activities of macrophages and neutrophils; and (3) contribute to feelings of discomfort and fatigue, compelling sick individuals to reduce activity and conserve energy to combat the infection. In addition to causing fever, IL-1β also induces the production of specific CSFs in the bone marrow, spurring the production and release of additional immune cells into the circulation that can be recruited to serve as reinforcements in responding to infection or tissue damage.

In contrast to proinflammatory IL-1α and IL-1β, IL-1RA has an anti-inflammatory effect. This cytokine is so named because it *antagonizes*, or *works against*, the activity of other IL-1 cytokines. IL-1RA accomplishes this antagonism by binding to only one of the two transmembrane proteins that compose the IL-1 receptor. When ligated by proinflammatory IL-1α or IL-1β, these two receptor subunits are brought together, initiating an intracellular signaling cascade that alerts the target cell to the presence of IL-1. Because IL-1RA binds to only one IL-1 receptor subunit and repels the other, IL-1RA prevents receptor subunits from coming together to initiate signaling, even in the presence of IL-1α or IL-1β. In this way, IL-1RA helps to regulate the physiological response to IL-1 and turn off the response when no longer needed.

Clinical Correlation

Inflammasomes Link Gout and Alum to Inflammation

Secretion of the biologically active form of IL-1β requires processing of the cytokine from an inactive pro-IL-1β form to an active form. This processing is accomplished by multiprotein complexes known as *inflammasomes,* which assemble within the cytoplasm of innate immune cells in response to danger associated molecular patterns (DAMPs). Central to the activity of inflammasomes is the enzyme caspase-1, which cleaves pro-IL-1β into active IL-1β. Following catalytic processing, active IL-1β is released from the cell, transmitting a powerful inflammatory signal.

Inflammasome activation and IL-1β release occur in response to infection but can also occur in "sterile" inflammatory diseases such as gout. In gout, a surplus of uric acid leads to crystal deposition in the body's tissues. One specific type of uric acid crystal, monosodium urate, has been shown to act as a DAMP, causing inflammasome assembly. Drugs that block IL-1β signaling dramatically reduce the pain and inflammation associated with gout.

Interestingly, the adjuvant alum has also been shown to cause inflammasome activation. Adjuvants are substances that enhance immune responses, and adjuvants such as alum are often incorporated into vaccines to help stimulate immunity for the purposes of protection (see Chapter 25). In this case, the release of active IL-1β and the inflammatory signaling driven by the cytokine cause the immune system to associate the harmless molecules found in the vaccine with *danger,* leading to an immune response and providing protection against the harmful substances or pathogens that the vaccine is intended to mimic.

Tumor Necrosis Factors

The cytokines that comprise the **tumor necrosis factor (TNF)** superfamily were first identified in the laboratory as products of macrophages and lymphocytes. The name *tumor necrosis factor* emerged from the observation that these cytokines induce lysis of mouse tumor cells. In all, the TNF superfamily encompasses 19 proteins that exhibit diverse immunologic functions. Structurally, the TNF superfamily members are manufactured as transmembrane proteins. Functionally, some TNFs remain cell-attached, transmitting messages only when the producing cell and target cell are in contact. An example of a surface-bound TNF we discussed in Chapter 4 is CD40 ligand, which is essential for signaling between T and B lymphocytes. Other TNFs are released from the cell surface by enzymatic cleavage, after which they diffuse into the extracellular space, allowing signaling across a distance. In regard to inflammation, the most important TNF is TNF-α.

Microbial substances such as LPS, a component of the cell walls of gram-negative bacteria, are major inducers of TNF-α production. Innate immune receptor signaling in macrophages leads to the production of a TNF-α precursor protein. Similar to other TNF superfamily members, this TNF-α precursor is translated directly into membranes of the endoplasmic reticulum and is then sorted into vesicles destined for the cell surface. As TNF-α precursor proteins arrive at the macrophage plasma membrane, the transmembrane domains are enzymatically removed, and the resultant soluble polypeptide fragments reassemble in groups of three (called *homotrimers*), representing the active form of TNF-α.

TNF-α is a ligand for two receptors, TNF receptors 1 and 2 (TNFR1 and TNFR2). TNFR1 is constitutively expressed on many cells and tissues throughout the body, whereas the expression of TNFR2 is limited to cells of hematopoietic origin and endothelial cells. Compared with the interaction between other cytokines and their receptors, TNFR1 and TNFR2 bind soluble TNF-α with a comparatively low affinity, evidenced by the TNF-α trimer binding and falling off of TNFR repeatedly. If levels of TNF-α near the membrane of the target cell reach a critical concentration, the TNF-α trimer draws together three TNFR molecules. As with IL-1, this close approximation of TNFR cytoplasmic domains leads to the initiation of downstream intracellular signaling. This signaling is responsible for the TNF-driven effects on target cells, such as alteration of adhesion molecule expression by endothelial cells.

In addition to TNF-α, another soluble TNF, known as *TNFβ* (or "lymphotoxin"), was identified by immunologists. As its pseudonym suggests, TNFβ is produced by lymphocytes and causes cell death, or *cytotoxicity,* in many different types of cells. A closer look at the biology of TNFβ using animals with a deletion of the TNFβ gene revealed that this cytokine also acts as an important signal during the development of lymphoid tissues in the gastrointestinal immune system. Recent studies have indicated that TNFβ is produced by a unique class of lymphocytes known as *lymphoid-tissue inducer cells.* Without these cells, or the TNFβ they produce, secondary lymphoid tissues, such as the mesenteric lymph nodes and Peyer's patches, fail to form.

Interleukin-6

(IL-6)

The third cytokine most prominently associated with the inflammatory response is IL-6. Structurally, IL-6 is related to

Clinical Correlation

The Role of Cytokine Storm in Ebola Virus Infection

The Ebola virus causes one of the most serious and fatal diseases known to humans **(Fig. 6–3)**. Ebola is a single-stranded RNA virus capable of infecting many different cell types throughout the body, including immune cells such as macrophages and DCs. Within a few days of exposure, symptoms become apparent. Infected individuals exhibit severe headache, fever, muscle pain, fatigue, diarrhea, vomiting, abdominal pain, and unexplained bruising or hemorrhaging. Ebola is extremely infectious and spreads quickly through a population, as evidenced by a major outbreak across West Africa in 2014.

In response to Ebola virus infection, immune cells release a massive amount of proinflammatory cytokines, including IL-1β, TNF-α, and IL-6. The cytokines produced and the magnitude of their concentrations in the blood have led immunologists to refer to this phenomenon as a "cytokine storm." Although infection with Ebola virus causes widespread cell death, many scientists have hypothesized that this aggressive cytokine response is the primary driver of Ebola pathogenesis. TNF-α, in particular, causes the blood vessels to become more permeable, resulting in dangerously low blood pressure. As the platelet count drops, excessive bleeding occurs from every orifice in the body. Death typically results in 1 to 2 weeks after infection. Interestingly, the virus inhibits the production of anti-viral cytokines known as *IFNs* (IFN-α and IFN-β) by infected cells.

The cytokine storm associated with Ebola infection exemplifies the essential (but complicated) role of cytokines in the immune response. If regulation of these powerful immune mediators is lost, their benefits can be easily transformed into harmful and potentially lethal effects.

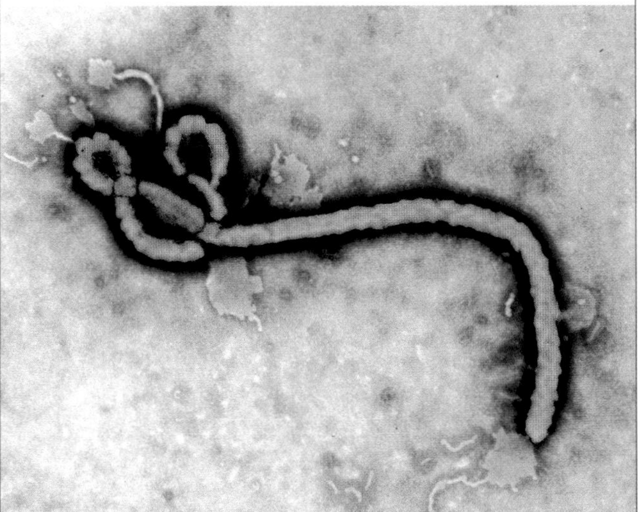

FIGURE 6–3 False-colored micrograph of the Ebola virus virion. *(Courtesy of the CDC/Frederick A. Murphy, Public Health Image Library.)*

many other cytokines, including the type I IFNs and several hematopoietic growth factors (discussed later in this chapter), consisting of a single polypeptide chain that winds into four helices that then fold upon themselves in a complicated tertiary structure. Two identical IL-6 polypeptide chains come together to form a homodimer, which represents the active form of the cytokine. Macrophages and monocytes are a common source of IL-6, but many other cell types are known to produce this cytokine, including endothelial cells, fibroblasts, some varieties of lymphocytes, and even skeletal muscle cells.

The activity of IL-6 is highly pleiotropic, influencing many biological systems. Functioning as an innate cytokine, IL-6 stimulates the production of acute-phase proteins by liver hepatocytes and increases the production and release of granulocytes by the bone marrow. In adaptive immunity, IL-6 increases the activation of B and T lymphocytes and modulates immunoglobulin synthesis by causing B cells to proliferate and differentiate into plasma cells. Interestingly, adipose tissue can serve as a source of IL-6, forming a potential mechanistic link between obesity and inflammation.

Similar to many cytokine receptors, the IL-6 receptor is composed of multiple subunits: one subunit specific to IL-6, known as the *IL-6 receptor* (IL-6R), and a signal-transducing subunit shared by many type I cytokines and growth factors, called *glycoprotein 130* (gp130). With IL-6 bound, the IL-6R subunit assembles with gp130, prompting a conformational change in the latter. This structural change in gp130 allows its cytoplasmic domains to initiate intracellular signaling cascades, driving the expression of IL-6-mediated genes that code for products such as C-reactive protein, complement proteins, and fibrinogen.

Chemokines

Not all cytokines result in changes in gene expression in their target cells. **Chemokines** are a subgroup of cytokines that influence the motility and migration of their target cells. *Chemokine* is derived from the words *cytokine* and *chemotaxis,* the latter term meaning "movement of a cell toward a stimulus." Most immune cell movement arises from the activities of chemokines, including recruitment to and movement through areas of infection and inflammation and the continual migration of lymphocytes between the blood and lymphoid tissues.

Chemokines are classified into four families based on the sequence of amino acids found in their N-termini, specifically, the positioning of cysteine residues. The CXC group of chemokines contains a single amino acid, "X," between the first and second cysteines. In the CC group, the cysteines are found together, with no intervening amino acid. Another group—the C chemokines—has only a single cysteine. Finally, the CX3C chemokines have three amino acids between the cysteines. Since their discovery, the number of chemokines has grown. Currently, more than 40 chemokines and 20 chemokine receptors have been identified; select chemokines and receptors are displayed in **Table 6–2.**

Many proinflammatory cytokines, including TNF-α and IL-6, induce the production of chemokines. In an inflammatory context, one of the most important effects of chemokines is the recruitment of leukocytes from the blood into infected or damaged tissues. Chemokines accomplish this recruitment

Table 6–2 Select Chemokines and Their Receptors

CHEMOKINE GROUP	CHEMOKINE NAMES	CHEMOKINE RECEPTORS
CC Chemokines	CCL2	CCR2
	CCL3	CCR1 CCR5
	CCL4	CCR5
	CCL5	CCR1 CCR3 CCR5
	CCL11	CCR3
	CCL19	CCR7
	CCL20	CCR6
	CCL25	CCR9
CXC Chemokines	CXCL1 CXCL2 CXCL3 CXCL5 CXCL7	CXCR2
	CXCL8	CXCR1 CXCR2
	CXCL9 CXCL10 CXCL11	CXCR3-A CXCR3-B
	CXCL12	CXCR4

by modulating the adhesion between leukocytes and the endothelial cells that line blood vessels. These interactions cause the leukocytes to *roll* along capillary walls, similar to a tennis ball rolling over a sheet of Velcro, and to subsequently exit the blood vessel and enter into the tissues (see Chapter 2).

Another important role of chemokines comes into play after leukocytes, such as neutrophils and monocytes, have entered inflamed tissues. Chemokine receptors allow these immune cells to detect chemokine gradients that exist within inflamed tissues. Engagement of these receptors causes a reorganization of the immune cell cytoskeleton, increasing actin polymerization near the cell surface that faces the higher concentration of chemokine. Therefore, responding immune cells migrate in the direction of the chemokine source, allowing them to pinpoint the exact location of damaged or infected cells.

In many cases, the expression of chemokine receptors changes throughout the life span of an immune cell. For example, DCs are responsible for initiating an adaptive immune response by presenting antigens to T- and B-lymphocytes (see Chapter 4). The activation of DCs by exposure to microbial substances causes them to express specific chemokine receptors, sensitizing them to chemokines produced by lymphatic endothelial cells. Following the gradient of these chemokines, DCs carrying microbial antigens journey into and through lymphatic capillaries. Eventually, the activated DCs arrive at local lymph nodes, where they interact with naïve T and B lymphocytes.

Transforming Growth Factor-β

Three isoforms of **transforming growth factor-β (TGF-β)**, named TGF-β1, TGF-β2, and TGF-β3, encompass the main constituents of the cytokine and growth factor superfamily of the same name. TGF-β was originally characterized as a factor that induced growth arrest in tumor cells. Later, it was identified as a factor that induces anti-proliferative activity in a wide variety of cell types. Active TGF-β is primarily a regulator of cell growth, differentiation, apoptosis, migration, and the inflammatory response. Thus, it acts as a control to help downregulate the inflammatory response when it is no longer needed.

In the immune response, TGF-β functions as both an activator and an inhibitor of proliferation, depending on the developmental stage of the affected cells. TGF-β regulates the expression of CD8 in CD4–CD8 thymocytes and acts as an autocrine inhibitory factor for immature thymocytes. It inhibits the activation of macrophages and the growth of many different somatic cell types and functions as an anti-inflammatory factor for mature T cells. TGF-β blocks the production of IL-12 and strongly inhibits the induction of IFN-gamma (IFN-γ). In addition, the production of TGF-β by **T helper 2 (Th2)** cells is now recognized as an important factor in the establishment of oral tolerance to bacteria normally found in the mouth. In activated B cells, TGF-β typically inhibits proliferation and may function as an autocrine regulator to limit the expansion of activated cells.

Interferon-α and Interferon-β (Type I Interferons)

The **interferons (IFNs)** were first identified as soluble substances produced by virally infected cells that *interfere* with the ability of viruses to replicate by making host cells less hospitable to viral takeover. IFNs are grouped as type I, type II, and type III, according to the IFN receptor that they interact with. The type I IFNs, consisting of IFN-α and IFN-β, are perhaps the most important cytokines in the response to viral infection. Because type II IFN production is associated with one particular form of adaptive immune response, known as a *Th1 response*, this form of IFN will be discussed in a later section of this chapter.

Type I IFNs are produced by many cell types. IFN-α is mainly the product of DCs and macrophages, whereas IFN-β can be produced by a wide variety of infected cells. The effects of IFN signaling in target cells are manifold and include halting protein translation and inducing production of RNases that target viral RNAs. These changes inhibit viral replication, slowing viral spread by preventing productive cellular infection. For most viral infections, this helps limit the infection to one relatively small area of the body. Type I IFNs also function to recruit innate lymphocytes, such as natural killer (NK) cells, to sites of viral infection. When ligated by IFN-α or IFN-β, type I IFN receptors cause NK cells to become activated, traffic to virally infected tissues, and rapidly expand in number. The combination of IFN-α and IFN-β activity and NK cell killing constitutes the most important innate defense mechanism against viral infection.

To augment the activity of NK cells, type I IFNs also enhance the expression of class I major histocompatibility complex (MHC) proteins on target cells. As discussed in more detail in Chapters 3 and 4 of this text, class I MHC molecules are important for the presentation of foreign (viral) peptide antigens to cytotoxic T cells. Increased expression of MHC I improves the likelihood that virus-specific T cells will recognize the presence of infection and induce apoptosis of the infected cell.

In addition to their role in combating viral infections, evidence is mounting that IFN-α and IFN-β also help protect against certain malignancies. Experiments in mice have shown that animals lacking type I IFN receptors are prone to the development of cancer. Human studies indicate that IFN is required for some cancer chemotherapies to work effectively, and that cancer patients expressing high levels of IFN-regulated genes have a greater probability of survival. A final piece of evidence in support of the anti-cancer role of type I IFNs is that recombinant IFN-α, which is manufactured in genetically modified cultured cells, can be used to augment other therapies in certain malignancies.

Type I IFNs have also found important roles as treatments for certain inflammatory and autoimmune diseases. For example, recombinant IFN-β is used as a treatment for multiple sclerosis (MS). The anti-inflammatory effect of IFN-β is most likely attributable to its tremendous pleiotropy. Decreased expression of MHC class II molecules on DCs, increased production of IL-10, and induction of apoptosis in B lymphocytes have all been noted in subjects receiving IFN-β therapy. Isolating the precise mechanism(s) underlying the anti-inflammatory effect of IFN-β treatment is difficult, however, because more than 500 different genes are influenced by type I IFNs.

Cytokines in the Adaptive Immune Response

Innate immunity is able to eradicate, or successfully control, most bacterial, fungal, and viral infections. Cytokines perform essential roles in these innate defenses, allowing the coordination and cooperation of many different cells and molecules. While these early battles are under way, the adaptive arm of immunity becomes sensitized to the infection and begins to scale up a specific response. Although the majority of human infections are terminated before an adaptive response is required, overcoming infections with the most dangerous pathogens usually requires that an adaptive response be mounted.

The cytokines involved in the innate immune response are produced by many different cell types. In contrast, the cytokines associated with adaptive immunity are mainly secreted by T lymphocytes, especially CD4-positive T helper (Th) cells. Th cells can be divided into several subpopulations, based upon the profile of cytokines they produce. Currently, immunologists have characterized at least four types of Th cells: **T helper 1 (Th1)**, Th2, **T helper 17 (Th17)**, and **T regulatory (Treg) cells.** Each of these different Th-cell subpopulations has a different immune function and produces a different array of cytokines.

As described earlier in this chapter, the initiation of an adaptive T-lymphocyte response begins when DCs arrive in lymph nodes, carrying antigens gathered from an area of infection. DCs present fragments of pathogen-derived antigens to hundreds or thousands of lymph node Th cells, but T-cell activation only occurs upon ligation of a T-cell receptor specific for one of the presented fragments. This activation event initiates an expansion of CD4+ Th cells specific to antigens associated with the ongoing infection (see Chapter 4).

Following activation, Th cells undertake a process known as *differentiation,* during which they are transformed into Th1, Th2, Th17, or Treg cells. The particular subset into which a Th cell differentiates is strongly influenced by the cytokines found in the lymph node during T-cell activation and early differentiation **(Fig. 6–4).** DC production of the cytokine IL-12 causes differentiation to the Th1 lineage, a change often observed in infections requiring a cell-mediated adaptive response, whereas the presence of IL-4 drives antibody-mediated immunity. Th17 cells arise in the presence of IL-23, whereas Tregs are produced in response to TGF-β.

Cytokines Produced by Th1 Cells

As we previously mentioned, the differentiation of naïve Th cells to the Th1 lineage is strongly influenced by the presence of the cytokine IL-12, which is secreted by DCs in response to infections with viruses and intracellular bacteria (such as

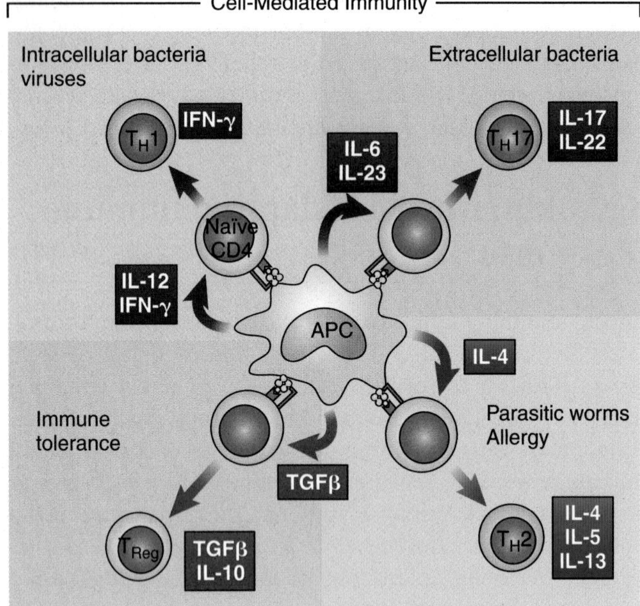

FIGURE 6–4 Subpopulations of T cells. Depending on the pathogen encountered, antigen-presenting cells (APCs) secrete a specific combination of polarizing cytokines that direct naïve Th cells to differentiate into specialized subsets (Th1, Th2, Th17, or Treg). Each T-cell subpopulation exerts different types of immune functions. The release of effector cytokines coordinates an appropriate immune response against the pathogen. *(Figure courtesy of Dr. Aaron Glass.)*

Mycobacterium tuberculosis or *Listeria monocytogenes*). The hallmark of Th1 cells is high-level expression of the proliferative cytokine IL-2 and the type II IFN, IFN-γ. As pathogen-specific Th1 cells expand to combat infection, these cytokines promote cell-mediated immunity in the form of CD8-positive cytotoxic T cells that kill infected host cells and activated macrophages that are more effective at killing intracellular bacteria. In addition to stimulating cell-mediated immunity, Th1 cells secrete cytokines that cause antigen-activated B cells to produce IgG1 and IgG3 antibodies capable of opsonizing pathogens (coating with antibodies to make phagocytosis more effective) and fixing complement. The Th1-driven antibody response augments cell-mediated immunity.

Interleukin-2 (IL-2)

The alternate name for IL-2, *T-cell growth factor,* is not fully indicative of the high degree of pleiotropy exhibited by this essential cytokine. IL-2 drives the growth and differentiation of both T and B cells and enhances the lytic activity of NK cells. In cooperation with IFN-γ, IL-2 causes naïve helper T cells to differentiate into Th1 cells, creating a feed-forward mechanism that can skew the adaptive immune response toward Th1.

The IL-2 receptor (IL-2R) is composed of three protein subunits, called α, β, and γ. Before activation, naïve T cells express a low-affinity form of the IL-2R, which is composed of only the β and γ subunits. Activation spurs the T cell to produce both IL-2 and the α subunit of IL-2R. When all three receptor subunits are present, a high-affinity IL-2R is formed, imbuing the T cell with an exquisite sensitivity to IL-2.

Clinical Correlation

The Common Gamma Chain (γc) and Severe Combined Immunodeficiency

The IL-2R shares its γ subunit with the receptors for several other cytokines, including IL-4, IL-7, IL-9, IL-15, and IL-21. Given the structural similarities of these receptors and their incorporation of the γc, these cytokines comprise a family known as the *common γ-chain cytokines.*

Individuals who develop or inherit mutations in the γc gene exhibit severe impairment of immunity. Because the γc gene is carried on the X chromosome, the resultant immunodeficiency is referred to as *X-linked severe combined immunodeficiency disease*, or XSCID (see Chapter 19). The effects of XSCID on the immune system are so pronounced that without treatment, males who inherit a defective γc gene succumb to infection before their first birthday. In one famous case of XSCID, David Vetter (known as the "Bubble Boy") was raised in a germ-free environment to protect him from the normally harmless microorganisms that can be lethal to an XSCID patient. Today, hematopoietic stem cell transfer and bone marrow transplantation can be used to successfully treat XSCID if a compatible donor is found and the patient is treated in the first year of life.

The severity of XSCID is attributable to the fact that so many cytokine receptors incorporate the γc subunit. Among other immune irregularities, XSCID results in disrupted NK cell development and a lack of functional T and B lymphocytes. Both innate and adaptive immunity are impacted.

Some strains of laboratory mice also harbor mutations in the γc gene, making them important immunologic tools. Although susceptible to infection, these animals are unable to reject foreign tissues because of their lack of functional adaptive immunity. If housed in a germ-free environment, these animals can be engrafted with cells and tissues from other animal species, including humans. SCID mice are important experimental models for understanding human immunity and testing new therapies.

Interferon-γ (IFN-γ)

The primary cytokine of the Th1 response, IFN-γ, influences the expression of more than 200 target-cell genes. Because Th1 cytokines are associated with cell-mediated immunity, IFN-γ tends to increase the expression of genes that shape the responses of T cells and macrophages. For example, a major function of IFN-γ is the enhancement of antigen presentation by class I and class II MHC molecules. Increased expression of class I and II MHC molecules on antigen-presenting cells (APCs) increase the probability that peptide antigens will be presented to T lymphocytes capable of responding to the infection. IFN-γ is also a potent activator of macrophages, dramatically increasing their ability to kill ingested microbes. The resulting "super" macrophages possess enhanced phagocytic and cytotoxic abilities. IFN-γ is involved in the regulation and activation of CD4+ Th1 cells, CD8+ cytotoxic T lymphocytes, and NK cells. Thus, IFN-γ influences the immune response in several key ways.

Cytokines Produced by Th2 Cells

As mentioned previously, the cytokines produced by Th2 cells propel the adaptive response in the direction of antibody-mediated immunity. Perhaps the most influential of the Th2 cytokines are IL-4 and IL-10. Both of these cytokines are important regulators of the immune response but have opposite effects.

Interleukin-4 (IL-4)

IL-4 is one of the key cytokines regulating Th2 immune activities and helps drive antibody responses in a variety of diseases. The IL-4 receptor is expressed on lymphocytes and on numerous nonhematopoietic cell types. IL-4 activity on naïve T cells turns on the genes that generate Th2 cells and turns off the genes that promote Th1 cells.

Th2 cells are responsible for regulating many aspects of the immune response, including those related to allergies, autoimmune diseases, and parasites. IL-4 induces the production of MHC-I, IL-4, IL-5, IL-13, and the costimulatory molecules CD80 and CD86. IL-4 also stimulates the production of IgG2a and IgE and, along with IL-5, drives the differentiation and activation of eosinophils in both allergic immune responses and responses to parasitic infections. IL-13 is a cytokine with many of the same properties as IL-4; both cytokines induce worm expulsion and favor IgE-class switching. IL-13, however, differs from IL-4 because it also plays an anti-inflammatory role by inhibiting activation and cytokine secretion by monocytes.

Interleukin-10 (IL-10)

In contrast to the cytokines previously discussed, IL-10 primarily has inhibitory effects on the immune system. It is produced by monocytes, macrophages, CD8+ T cells, and CD4+ Th2 cells and has anti-inflammatory and suppressive effects on Th1 cells. It also inhibits antigen presentation by macrophages and DCs. In addition, one of the major effects of IL-10 is inhibition of IFN-γ production by suppressing IL-12 synthesis by accessory cells and promoting a Th2 cytokine pattern. Thus, IL-10 serves as an antagonist of IFN-γ —it is a downregulator of the immune response.

Cytokines Associated With T-Regulatory Cells

Tregs comprise the third major subclass of CD4-positive T cells. Tregs can be identified by the expression of CD4, CD25 (the IL-2R α subunit), and the transcription factor FoxP3. Some Tregs are formed during thymic development, whereas others differentiate from naïve T cells in the periphery. Tregs formed outside of the thymus are sometimes referred to as *induced Tregs (iTregs)*.

Tregs are essential for establishing peripheral tolerance to a wide variety of self-antigens as well as harmless antigens, such as those found in foods and the environment (see Chapter 15). Clinically, Tregs may be found in transplanted tissue and help to establish tolerance to the graft. In some cases, Treg-mediated tolerance to certain antigens can be harmful. For example, Tregs can protect tumor cells from an immune attack by dampening the activity of cancer-fighting T cells.

Although Tregs have been studied intensely by immunologists for many years, the mechanisms underpinning their immune suppression remain incompletely understood. Some hypotheses for how Tregs suppress immunity include (1) the production of suppressive cytokines, such as IL-10 and TGF-β; (2) disruption of T-cell metabolism; (3) direct cytotoxic killing of T cells and APCs; and (4) modulation of signaling between APC and T cells. All these mechanisms, and others not yet considered, likely contribute to the activity of this essential cell population.

Th17 Cytokines in Innate and Adaptive Immune Responses

The Th17 subset secretes the IL-17 family of cytokines and plays critical roles in both innate and adaptive immune responses. Key cytokines that differentiate T cells to maintain them as Th17 cells are TGF-β and IL-6. Interleukin-23, produced by macrophages and DCs, also plays a role in finalizing the commitment to Th17 cells.

IL-17A, the first IL-17 identified, is the most studied IL-17 cytokine. Other IL-17 family members include IL-17B, IL-17C, IL-17D, IL-17E, and IL-17F. Most of the IL-17 cytokine family members are potent proinflammatory cytokines and induce expression of TNF-α, IL-1β, and IL-6 in epithelial cells, endothelial cells, keratinocytes, fibroblasts, and macrophages.

Th17 cells play an important role in host defense against bacterial and fungal infections at mucosal surfaces. Upon an encounter with bacteria or fungi, APCs secrete cytokines, which differentiate Th17 subsets of cells. Th17 cells invade the infected area and secrete IL-17 cytokines necessary for the continuous recruitment of neutrophils. Th17 cells in the local tissue may be important for long-term maintenance of the anti-microbial response during chronic bacterial infections. Mucosal surfaces, in response to IL-17 cytokine stimulation, secrete anti-microbial peptides. IL-17A and IL-17F induce epithelial cells, endothelial cells, and fibroblasts to produce CXC ligand 8 (CXCL-8), which is crucial for the recruitment of neutrophils to the site of inflammation. IL-17A and IL-17F also act together with granulocyte–macrophage CSF to produce CXCL-8 in macrophages, which also signals neutrophils to the site.

The fine regulation of APC cytokines (IL-23 or IL-12) and Th17 development may also be important for anti-microbial defense. Dysregulation of Th17 cell subsets and secreted cytokines has been implicated in the pathogenesis of multiple inflammatory diseases and several autoimmune conditions, including RA, MS, inflammatory bowel disease (IBD), and psoriasis.

IL-17 can produce proinflammatory mediators from myeloid and synovial fibroblasts and perpetuate the inflammatory process in RA. Increased numbers of Th17 cells and IL-17A have also been observed in asthmatic and allergic patients. IL-17A directly induces IgE production by B cells; higher amounts of IL-17A and IL-17F in patient lungs have been associated with more severe asthma. Interestingly, removal of Th17 cells from the peripheral blood mononuclear cells (PBMCs) of allergic asthma patients has led to decreased levels of IgE.

Hematopoietic Growth Factors

Several cytokines produced during innate and adaptive immune responses stimulate the proliferation and differentiation of bone marrow progenitor cells. Thus, the responses that require a supply of leukocytes produce mediators to provide those cells. The primary mediators of hematopoiesis are called CSFs because they stimulate the formation of colonies of cells in the bone marrow. The CSFs include IL-3, **erythropoietin (EPO)**, **granulocyte colony-stimulating factor (G-CSF)**, **macrophage colony-stimulating factor (M-CSF)**, and **granulocyte–macrophage colony-stimulating factor (GM-CSF).** In response to inflammatory cytokines such as IL-1, the different CSFs act on bone marrow cells at different developmental stages and promote specific colony formation for the various cell lineages. IL-3 is a multi-lineage CSF that induces bone marrow stem cells to form T and B cells. In conjunction with IL-3, the CSFs direct immature bone marrow stem cells to develop into red blood cells (RBCs), platelets, and the various types of white blood cells (WBCs) **(Fig. 6–5).** IL-3 acts on bone marrow stem cells to begin the differentiation cycle; the activity of IL-3 alone drives the stem cells into the lymphocyte differentiation pathway.

GM-CSF acts to drive differentiation toward other WBC types. If M-CSF is activated, the cells become macrophages. M-CSF also increases phagocytosis, chemotaxis, and additional cytokine production in monocytes and macrophages. If G-CSF is activated, the cells become neutrophils. G-CSF enhances the function of mature neutrophils and affects the survival, proliferation, and differentiation of all cell types in the neutrophil lineage. It decreases IFN-γ production, increases IL-4 production in T cells, and mobilizes multipotent stem cells from the bone marrow. These stem cells are used to repair damaged tissues and create new vasculature to reconstruct the tissues following an infection. However, IL-3, in conjunction with GM-CSF, drives the development of basophils and mast cells, whereas the addition of IL-5 to IL-3 and GM-CSF drives the cells to develop into eosinophils. The net effect is an increase in WBCs to respond to the ongoing inflammatory processes.

EPO regulates RBC production in the bone marrow, but it is primarily produced in the kidneys. Recombinant EPO is licensed for clinical use and is administered to improve RBC counts for individuals with anemia and for those with cancer who have undergone radiation therapy or chemotherapy. RBC proliferation induced by EPO improves oxygenation of

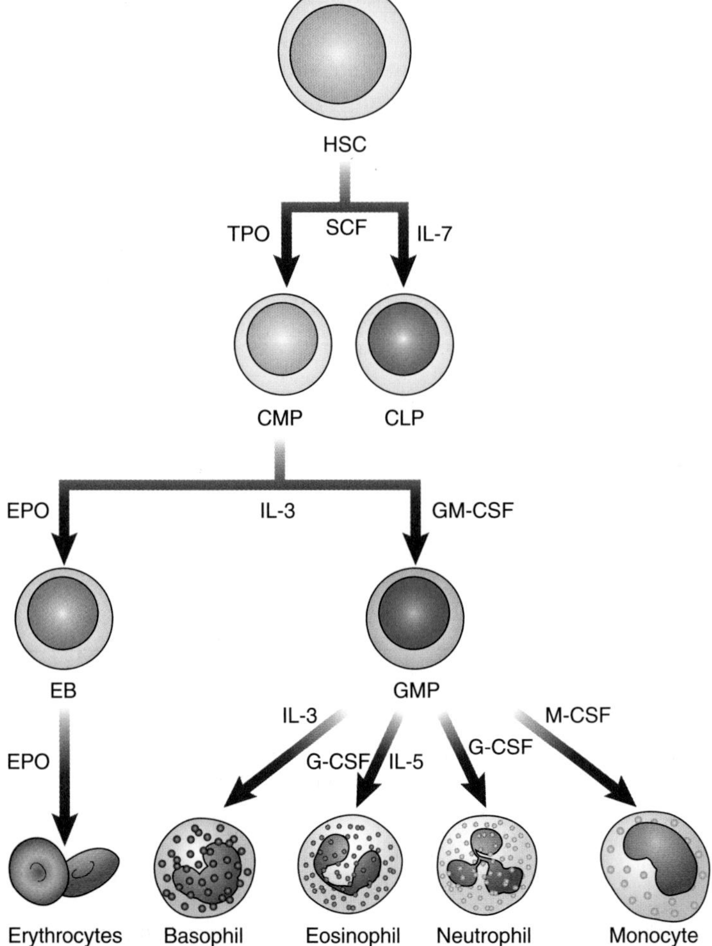

FIGURE 6–5 Influence of CSFs on growth and differentiation of blood cells. Growth of hematopoietic stem cells (HSCs) requires stem cell factor (SCF) with differentiation determined by IL-7 or thrombopoietin (TPO). Growth of common myeloid progenitors (CMPs) depends upon IL-3. Differentiation is driven by GM-CSF or EPO. Common granulocyte/monocyte precursors (GMPs) differentiate into granulocytes in response to G-CSF. Further specificity is provided by IL-3 or IL-5. M-CSF promotes the development of monocytes. CLP = common lymphoid progenitor; EB = erythroblast.

the tissues and eventually switches off EPO production. The normal serum EPO values range from 5 to 28 U/L but must be interpreted in relation to the hematocrit because levels can increase up to a thousand-fold during anemia.

Cytokine and Anti-Cytokine Therapies

In addition to being produced in response to infection, cytokines may also contribute to the pathology of many autoimmune and other inflammatory diseases. Anti-cytokine therapy is a rapidly growing field that aims to break the vicious cycle of chronic inflammation by targeting the interaction between specific cytokines and their cognate receptors. A few examples of such therapies will be discussed here.

The first anti-cytokine therapeutics used in humans were mostly murine monoclonal antibodies. However, structural differences between mouse and human immunoglobulins often resulted in immune responses against the drugs, rendering the treatment noneffective. Newer anti-cytokine agents have been greatly improved using recombinant DNA techniques to generate humanized monoclonal antibodies that are much less immunogenic **(Fig. 6–6)**. An example is infliximab (e.g., Remicade), a chimeric antibody containing human constant regions and murine variable regions that bind specifically to human TNF-α. Infliximab is a valuable treatment option for patients with Crohn's disease, RA, ulcerative colitis, and other autoimmune diseases because it blocks TNF-α activity very rapidly, dramatically reducing inflammation.

Another approach to anti-cytokine therapy is the development of a class of hybrid proteins containing cytokine receptor binding sites attached to immunoglobulin constant regions. Etanercept (e.g., Enbrel), for example, is a member of this class that has been approved for use in humans. Etanercept consists of the extracellular domains of the type 2 TNF receptor fused to the heavy-chain constant region of IgG1. The fusion protein can bind TNF-α and block its activity. It has a 4.8-day half-life in serum. Etanercept remains an important, cost-effective treatment option in patients with RA, ankylosing spondylitis, psoriatic arthritis or psoriasis, and pediatric arthritis and psoriasis. Etanercept effectively reduces signs and symptoms, disease activity, and disability and improves health-related quality of life, and these benefits are sustained during long-term treatment.

The blockade of IL-17 function has also been a therapeutic target. An IL-17 blocking antibody to prevent IL-17 mediated pathogenesis, known as *ixekizumab*, has been approved for the treatment of plaque psoriasis, psoriatic arthritis, and ankylosing spondylitis. Monoclonal antibodies that block IL-17 receptors or IL-23, which enhances the differentiation of Th17 lymphocytes, have also been approved for the treatment of psoriasis.

Clinical Assays for Cytokines

Clinical evaluation of the cytokine profile in a patient could be of prognostic and diagnostic value to the physician when treating autoimmune diseases, infections, allergic conditions, or other inflammatory disorders. Several cytokine assay formats are available for basic and clinical research, including multiplexed enzyme-linked immunosorbent assays (ELISAs), microbead assays, and **ELISpot** assays.

Multiplexed ELISAs use several detector antibodies bound to individual microwells or antibody microarrays and allow for simultaneous detection of several cytokines from serum or plasma in a single test run. In the microarray format, each well on the slide contains a microarray of spotted antibodies, with "spots" for each of the cytokines plus additional "spots" for positive and negative controls. The replicate spots allow for the acquisition of reliable quantitative data from a single sample.

Microbead assays allow for the simultaneous detection of multiple cytokines in a single tube (see Chapter 11). Each bead type has its own fluorescent wavelength, which, when combined with the fluorescent secondary antibody bound to a specific cytokine, allows for the detection of up to 100 different analytes in one tube. The use of a multiplexed bead array enables simultaneous measurement of a multitude of biomarkers; these include acute-phase reactants such as CRP; proinflammatory cytokines; Thl and Th2 distinguishing cytokines such as IFN-γ, IL-2, IL-4, IL-5, and IL-10; CSFs; and others.

ELISA and microbead assays allow the quantitation of cytokine levels in a sample of plasma or cell culture supernatant but reveal no information about the cytokine source. In contrast, ELISpot assays allow the detection and enumeration of individual cytokine-secreting cells. ELISpot assays accomplish this feat by employing a modified ELISA technique on immune cells stimulated in vitro.

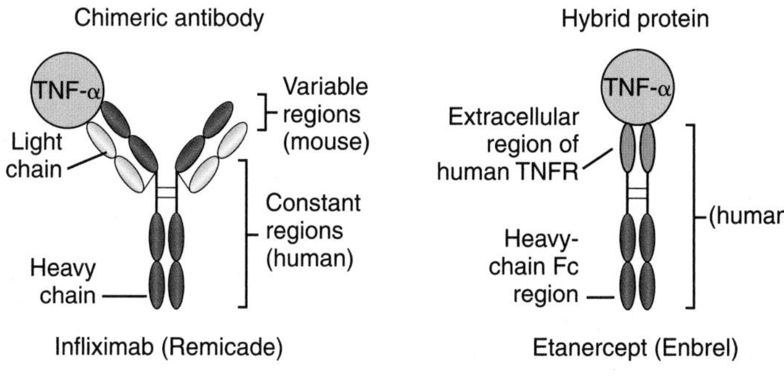

FIGURE 6–6 Anti-cytokine antagonists of TNF-α. Infliximab is a chimeric monoclonal antibody composed of human constant regions fused to mouse variable regions. The mouse variable regions bind to TNF-α, preventing it from interacting with the TNF receptor (TNFR). Etanercept is a hybrid protein consisting of the extracellular (ligand binding) domains of the human TNFR (green), coupled with a human immunoglobulin constant region. Etanercept acts as a decoy, sequestering bound TNF-α so that it cannot interact with TNF receptors on target cells. *(Figure courtesy of Dr. Aaron Glass.)*

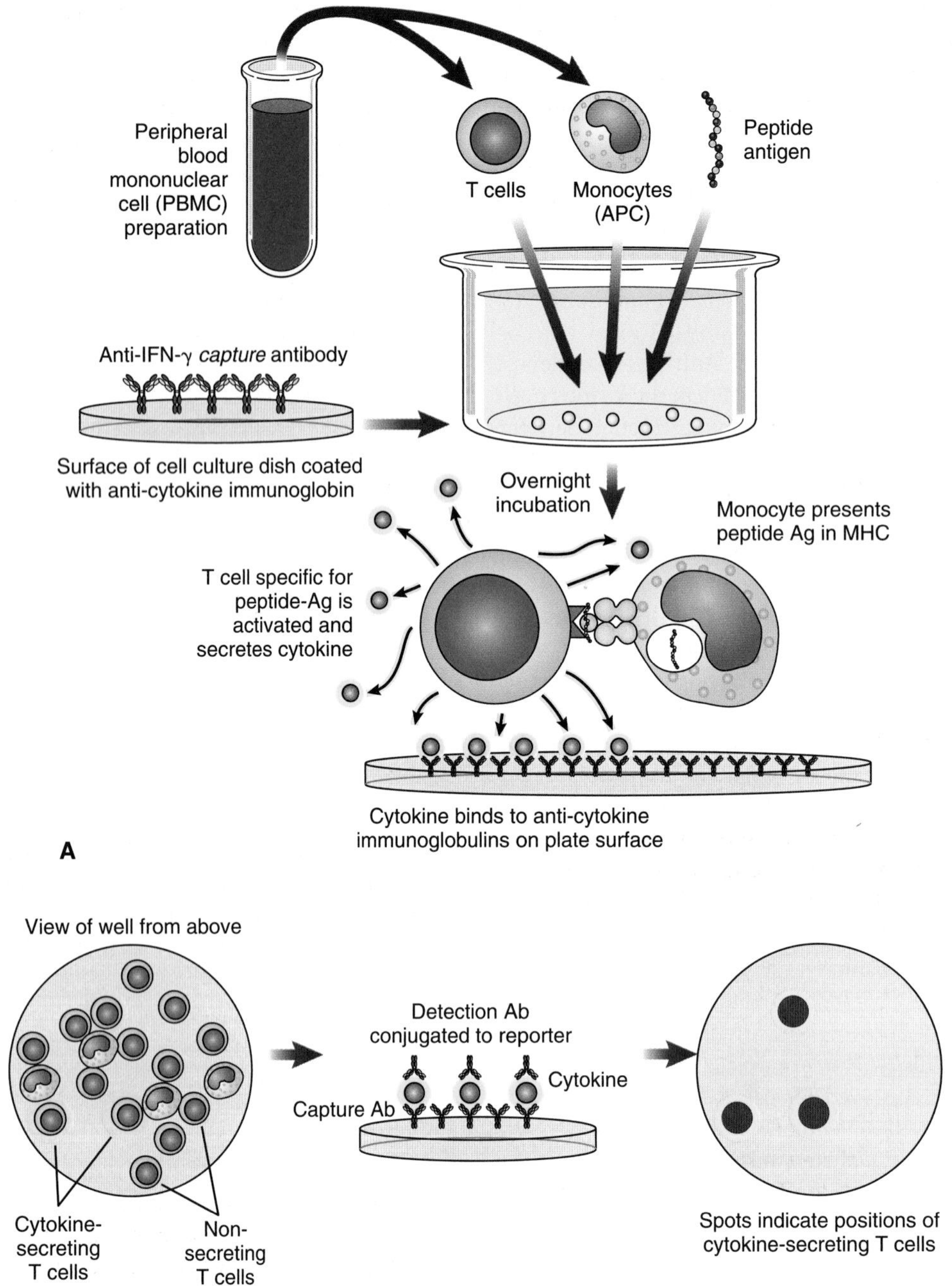

FIGURE 6–7 The ELISpot assay. (A) PBMCs are loaded into a plate precoated with capture antibody specific to the target cytokine (IFN-γ in this example). The PBMCs are incubated overnight in the presence of a synthetic peptide antigen, which is processed by monocytes and presented to T cells. T cells responsive to the peptide antigen are stimulated to secrete cytokines, including IFN-γ. (B) Target cytokine binds to the capture antibody and remains fixed to the plate even after the cells are washed away. A labeled detection antibody is added to the plate and binds to the target cytokine (IFN-γ), if present. After excess detection antibody is removed, "spots" indicate the positions where responsive T cells formerly rested on the microplate bottom. These spots can be quantified to assess the number of T cells in a given volume of sample that produce IFN-γ in response to the peptide antigen. *(Figure courtesy of Dr. Aaron Glass.)*

One clinical application that exemplifies ELISpot is the detection of circulating Th1 cells that secrete IFN-γ in response to an antigen **(Fig. 6–7).** Th1 cells, similar to all T lymphocytes, are highly specific in their responses—each Th1 cell possesses a unique T-cell receptor and recognizes a discrete polypeptide antigen. Adding a synthetic protein antigen to T cells co-cultured with APCs will elicit the production of cytokines, including IFN-γ, by Th1 cells reactive to peptide fragments derived from the larger protein.

ELISpot assays are performed using cell culture microplates coated with cytokine-specific *capture* antibodies. For example, IFN-γ ELISpot assays use capture antibodies that bind to an epitope found on IFN-γ. Samples of PBMCs are prepared from venous blood by gradient centrifugation. Because the granulocyte fraction is discarded, PBMCs represent only circulating lymphocytes and monocytes.

In the first step of an ELISpot protocol, PBMCs are added to the wells of the antibody-coated microplate and treated with a synthetic protein antigen. An incubation period allows for uptake and presentation of the antigen by monocytes, which serve as APCs. In culture, some T cells recognize peptide fragments derived from the protein antigen and begin producing cytokines. Most T cells in a given sample, however, have receptor specificities that do not match epitopes found within the protein antigen and will not respond.

During the incubation period, antigen-responsive Th1 cells secrete cytokines as they rest at the bottom of the microplate well. Because the T cells are in close contact with the plate-bound capture antibodies, molecules of the target cytokine (IFN-γ in this example) are rapidly immobilized, forming a halo of antibody-bound cytokine directly beneath each IFN-γ –secreting T cell.

Following the incubation period, PBMCs and any soluble substances, such as cytokines, are washed from the microplate wells, leaving only the target cytokine bound to capture antibodies. Next, a *detection* antibody, specific to the target cytokine, is added to the wells. In our example, the detection antibody binds to IFN-γ at an epitope different from that bound by the capture antibody, allowing molecules of IFN-γ to be *sandwiched* between the plate-bound capture antibody and the detection antibody. Depending on the ELISpot protocol, detection antibodies may feature a biotin-streptavidin labeling system or may be covalently conjugated to an enzyme or fluorophore (see Chapter 11).

Regardless of the specifics of individual protocols, the role of the ELISpot detection antibody is to produce a visual signal indicating where target cytokine is bound to capture antibody. The "spots" represent tiny, elliptical silhouettes of captured IFN-γ speckling the plate bottom where antigen-responsive Th1 cells once resided. The spots can be counted with a microscope or with an automated ELISpot instrument.

Clinical Correlation

T-SPOT.TB Test

The T-SPOT.TB Test is an ELISpot method used to evaluate the cell-mediated immune response to *Mycobacterium tuberculosis*. In this test, PBMCs from a patient are incubated in microtiter wells that have been coated with *M. tuberculosis*–specific antigens. Cells from patients who have been exposed to *M. tuberculosis* are stimulated to release IFN-γ, and dark blue spots are produced in the locations of the IFN-γ–secreting cells following addition of the detection antibody. Clinical significance is determined by the number of spots produced, in comparison with controls (see Chapter 14).

One drawback of protein-based technologies is the short half-life of certain cytokines. This can be overcome by looking at RNA expression in cells using reverse-transcription polymerase chain reaction (PCR). The PCR product is made using a fluorescent-labeled primer and can be hybridized to either solid-phase or liquid microarrays. Solid-phase arrays have up to 40,000 spots containing specific single-stranded DNA (ssDNA) oligonucleotides representing individual genes. Clinically useful arrays generally have substantially fewer genes represented. Fluorescence of a spot indicates that the gene was expressed in the cell and that the cell was producing the cytokine.

The liquid arrays use the same beads as the antibody microbead arrays discussed earlier. However, instead of antibodies, these beads have oligonucleotides on their surfaces and allow up to 100 different complementary DNAs (cDNAs) to be identified. The combination of the bead fluorescence and the fluorescence of the labeled cDNA produces an emission spectrum that identifies the cytokine gene that was expressed in the cells.

Real-time PCR has emerged as a means of detecting cytokine responses at the level of gene expression. This type of testing is much faster than traditional PCR. See Chapter 12 for a discussion of molecular techniques.

SUMMARY

- Cytokines are small, soluble proteins secreted by immune cells and a variety of other cells. They act as chemical messengers to regulate the immune system.
- Cytokine production is induced in response to specific, stimuli such as bacterial LPS, flagellin, or other bacterial products.
- The effects of cytokines in vivo include regulation of growth, differentiation, and gene expression by many different cell types.
- If a cytokine has an autocrine effect, it affects the same cell that secreted it.
- A cytokine can have a paracrine effect when it affects a target cell in close proximity. Occasionally, cytokines will exert systemic or endocrine activities.
- Individual cytokines do not act alone but in conjunction with many other cytokines that are induced during the process of immune activation. The combined cytokines produce a spectrum of activities that lead to the rapid generation of innate and adaptive immune responses.
- Massive overproduction of cytokines is called a "cytokine storm" that leads to shock, multiorgan failure, or even death, thus contributing to pathogenesis.
- The pleiotropic nature of cytokine activity relates to the ability of a cytokine to affect many different types of cells.
- *Redundancy* refers to the ability of several different cytokines to activate some of the same cells.
- The major cytokines involved in the initial stages of the inflammatory response are IL-1, IL-6, TNF-α, and the chemokines. These cytokines are responsible for many of the physical symptoms attributed to inflammation, such as fever, swelling and pain, as well as cellular infiltrates moving into damaged tissues.

- Naïve T cells can differentiate into Th1, Th2, Treg, or Th17 cell lineages, with the help of cytokines involved in the adaptive immune response.
- The Th1 lineage is driven by the expression of IL-12 by DCs and is primarily responsible for cell-mediated immunity.
- Th2 cells drive antibody-mediated immunity and are regulated by IL-4.
- Treg cells are derived from naïve T cells in response to IL-10 and TGF-β and help to regulate the activities of other T cells.
- Th17 cells produce IL-17, a proinflammatory cytokine that induces expression of TNF-α, IL-1β, and IL-6. IL-17 also recruits neutrophils to an infected area.
- CSFs are responsible for inducing differentiation and growth of all WBC types.
- Anti-cytokine therapies are aimed at disrupting the interaction between cytokines and their specific receptors in autoimmune inflammatory diseases such as RA, Crohn's disease, and plaque psoriasis.
- Cytokine assay formats available for basic and clinical research include ELISpot assays, multiplexed ELISAs, and microbead assays.
- ELISpot assays are ELISAs on in vitro stimulated T cells that allow quantitation of the number of T cells that secrete specific cytokines in response to a protein antigen.
- Multiplexed ELISAs and microbead assays can simultaneously detect several cytokines in a sample.

Study Guide: Cytokines Associated With Innate Immunity

CYTOKINE	SECRETED BY	ACTIONS
Interleukin-1 β (IL-1β)	Monocytes, macrophages, DCs	Inflammation, fever, initiation of the acute-phase response
Tumor necrosis factor-alpha (TNF-α)	Monocytes, macrophages, neutrophils, NK cells, activated T cells	Inflammation, initiation of the acute-phase response, death of tumor cells
Interleukin-6 (IL-6)	Monocytes, macrophages, endothelial cells, Th2 cells	Initiation of the acute-phase response, activation of B and T cells
Transforming growth factor-beta (TGF-β)	T cells, macrophages, other cell types	Inhibition of both T- and B-cell proliferation, induction of IgA, inhibition of macrophages
Interferon-alpha (IFN-α), Interferon-beta (IFN-β)	Macrophages, DCs, virally infected cells	Protects cells against viruses, increases class I MHC expression, activates NK cells

Study Guide: Cytokines Associated With Adaptive Immunity

CYTOKINE	SECRETED BY	ACTIONS
Interleukin-2 (IL-2)	T cells	Growth and proliferation of T and B cells, NK activation and proliferation
Interleukin-4 (IL-4)	Th2 cells, mast cells	Promotion of Th2 differentiation, stimulation of B cells to switch to IgE production
Interleukin-5 (IL-5)	Th2 cells	Eosinophil generation and activation, B-cell differentiation
Interleukin-10 (IL-10)	Th2 cells, monocytes, macrophages	Suppression of Th2 cells, inhibition of antigen presentation, inhibition of IFN-γ
Interferon-gamma (IFN-γ)	Th1 cells, CD8+ T cells, NK cells	Activation of macrophages, increased expression of class I and II MHC molecules, increased antigen presentation

CASE STUDY

A 55-year-old woman being treated for acute lymphocytic leukemia (ALL) was not responding well to chemotherapy. Her physicians felt that increasing the dosage of her chemotherapy drugs was necessary to eliminate the cancer. However, laboratory results showed the patient was severely neutropenic (477 neutrophils/mL) because of the drugs. The medical team could not risk further lowering of the neutrophil count because of the increased risk of infection. Therefore, it was necessary to treat the patient for neutropenia in order to continue with chemotherapy. The patient was also enrolled in a research study designed to look at cytokine expression in ALL patients with neutropenia. The study used a liquid bead array to detect the CSFs and the cytokines typically seen in the innate immune response and in Th1 and Th2 responses.

Questions

a. What CSF should the physicians prescribe to overcome the neutropenia?
b. What are some of the cytokines that might be detected in a Th1-type response?
c. What are some of the cytokines that might be detected in a Th2-type response?

REVIEW QUESTIONS

1. The ability of a single cytokine to alter the expression of several genes is called
   a. redundancy.
   b. pleiotropy.
   c. autocrine stimulation.
   d. the endocrine effect.

2. Which of the following effects can be attributed to IL-1?
   a. Mediation of the innate immune response
   b. Differentiation of stem cells
   c. Halted growth of virally infected cells
   d. Stimulation of mast cells

3. Which of the following precursors is a target cell for IL-3?
   a. Myeloid precursors
   b. Lymphoid precursors
   c. Erythroid precursors
   d. All of the above

4. A lack of IL-4 may result in which of the following effects?
   a. Inability to fight off viral infections
   b. Increased risk of tumors
   c. Lack of IgM
   d. Decreased eosinophil count

5. Which of the following cytokines is also known as the *T-cell growth factor*?
   a. IFN-γ
   b. IL-12
   c. IL-2
   d. IL-10

6. Which of the following represents an autocrine effect of IL-2?
   a. Increased IL-2 receptor expression by the Th cell producing it
   b. Macrophages signaled to the area of antigen stimulation
   c. Proliferation of antigen-stimulated B cells
   d. Increased synthesis of acute-phase proteins throughout the body

7. IFN-α and IFN-β differ in which way from IFN-γ?
   a. IFN-α and IFN-β are called *immune IFNs*, and IFN-γ is not.
   b. IFN-α and IFN-β primarily activate macrophages, whereas IFN-γ halts viral activity.
   c. IFN-α and IFN-β are made primarily by activated T cells, whereas IFN-γ is made by fibroblasts.
   d. IFN-α and IFN-β inhibit viral replication, whereas IFN-γ stimulates antigen presentation by class II MHC molecules.

8. A patient in septic shock caused by a gram-negative bacterial infection exhibits the following symptoms: high fever, very low blood pressure, and disseminated intravascular coagulation. Which cytokine is the most likely contributor to these symptoms?
   a. IL-2
   b. TNF
   c. IL-12
   d. IL-7

9. IL-10 acts as an antagonist to what cytokine?
   a. IL-4
   b. TNF-α
   c. IFN-γ
   d. TGF-β

10. Which would be the best assay to measure a specific cytokine?
   a. Blast formation
   b. T-cell proliferation
   c. Measurement of leukocyte chemotaxis
   d. ELISA testing

11. Selective destruction of Th cells by the HIV virus contributes to immune suppression by which means?
   a. Decrease in IL-1
   b. Decrease in IL-2
   c. Decrease in IL-8
   d. Decrease in IL-10

12. Why might a CSF be given to a cancer patient?
    a. Stimulate activity of NK cells
    b. Increase the production of certain types of leukocytes
    c. Decrease the production of TNF
    d. Increase the production of mast cells

13. Which of the following would result from a lack of TNF?
    a. Decreased ability to fight gram-negative bacterial infections
    b. Increased expression of class II MHC molecules
    c. Decreased survival of cancer cells
    d. Increased risk of septic shock

14. Which cytokine acts to promote differentiation of T cells to the Th1 subclass?
    a. IL-4
    b. IFN-γ
    c. IL-12
    d. IL-10

15. What is the major function of Treg cells?
    a. Suppression of the immune response by producing TNF
    b. Suppression of the immune response by inducing IL-10
    c. Proliferation of the immune response by producing IL-2
    d. Proliferation of the immune response by inducing IL-4

16. Th17 cells affect the innate immune response by inducing production of which cytokines?
    a. IFN-γ and IL-2
    b. IL-4 and IL-10
    c. IL-2 and IL-4
    d. TNF-α and IL-6

The Complement System

7

Bradley Dixon, MD, and Ashley Frazer-Abel, PhD, D(ABMLI)

LEARNING OUTCOMES

After finishing this chapter, you should be able to:

1. Describe the roles of the complement system.
2. Differentiate between the classical, alternative, and lectin pathways and indicate the proteins and activators involved in each.
3. Discuss the formation of the three principal units of the classical pathway: recognition, activation, and membrane attack units.
4. Explain how C3 plays a key role in all three pathways of complement activation.
5. Discuss regulators of the complement system and their roles in inhibiting the complement pathways.
6. Describe deficiencies of complement components and the diseases they cause.
7. Describe potential disease manifestations of improper complement regulation.
8. Differentiate tests for functional activity of complement from measurement of individual complement components.
9. Analyze laboratory findings to indicate disease implications in relation to complement abnormalities.
10. Discuss clinical applications of complement therapeutics and their effects on laboratory tests for complement.

CHAPTER OUTLINE

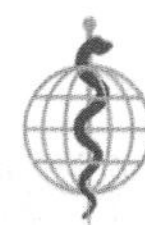

Go to FADavis.com for the laboratory exercises that accompany this text.

KEY TERMS

Activation unit
Alternative pathway
Anaphylatoxin
Atypical hemolytic uremic syndrome (aHUS)
Bystander lysis
C1 inhibitor (C1-INH)
C3 glomerulopathies (C3G)
C4-binding protein (C4BP)
Chemotaxin
Classical pathway
Complement receptor type 1 (CR1)
Decay-accelerating factor (DAF)
Factor H
Factor I
Hemolytic titration (CH50) assay
Hemolytic uremic syndrome (HUS)
Hereditary angioedema (HAE)
Immune adherence
Lectin pathway
Mannose-binding lectin (MBL)
Membrane attack complex (MAC)
Membrane cofactor protein (MCP)
Opsonins
Paroxysmal nocturnal hemoglobinuria (PNH)
Properdin
Recognition unit
S protein

As we described in Chapter 2, complement is a complex series of more than 50 proteins of the innate immune system. These soluble and cell-bound proteins have an important role in responding to infection, but they are also important for their strong proinflammatory properties. Complement can lyse foreign cells, opsonize and tag foreign invaders for clearance, and direct the adaptive immune system to the site of infection. Complement activation can also have proinflammatory effects because of its ability to increase vascular permeability, recruit monocytes and neutrophils to the area of antigen concentration, and trigger secretion of immunoregulatory molecules that amplify the immune response. In their proinflammatory role, complement proteins serve as an important link between innate and adaptive immunity, but these properties are increasingly recognized for their role in a growing list of disease pathologies. In such circumstances, complement activates the host's immune system, often through a lack of proper control, leading to several potential outcomes that stretch far beyond infection.

The interplay of complement with disease is also seen when the important "housekeeping" roles of complement are lost. Complement recognizes cellular debris, such as apoptotic cells and immune complexes, tagging it for removal by innate immune cells. The loss of these functions is part of the link between complement and rheumatological diseases. Because of its potential for far-reaching effects, complement activation needs to be carefully regulated. The need for tight control has been recognized by the medical field, as exemplified by the advent of therapeutics directed at regulating various components of the complement system.

Pathways of the Complement System

The complement system can be activated in three different ways. The first pathway described, the **classical pathway,** involves nine proteins that are triggered primarily by antigen–antibody complexes. In the 1950s, Pillemer and colleagues discovered an antibody-independent pathway that plays a major role as a natural defense system. This second pathway is called the **alternative pathway.** The third pathway, likely the most ancient of the three, is the **lectin pathway,** and it is another antibody-independent means of activating complement proteins. In this pathway, **mannose-** (or mannan-) **binding lectin (MBL)** in the serum adheres to mannose sugar in the cell walls or outer coating of bacteria, viruses, yeast, and protozoa. Similarly, the ficolins and collectins can bind to pathogen-associated molecular patterns to activate the lectin pathway. Although each of these pathways will be considered separately, activation typically involves more than one pathway.

Most plasma complement proteins are synthesized in the liver, with the exception of C1 components, which are mainly produced by intestinal epithelial cells, and Factor D, which is made in adipose tissue. Other cells, such as monocytes and macrophages, are additional sources of early complement components, including C1, C2, C3, and C4. Most of these proteins are inactive precursors, or zymogens, which are converted to active enzymes in a very precise order. **Table 7–1** lists the characteristics of the main complement proteins.

The Classical Pathway

The classical pathway, the first activation cascade described, is the main antibody-directed mechanism for triggering complement activation. However, not all immunoglobulins are able to activate this pathway. The immunoglobulin (Ig) classes that can activate the classical pathway are IgM, IgG1, IgG2, and IgG3, but not IgG4, IgA, or IgE. IgM is the most efficient of the activating immunoglobulins because it has multiple binding sites for complement; thus, it takes only one molecule attached to two adjacent antigenic determinants to initiate the cascade **(Fig. 7–1).** Two IgG molecules must attach to antigen within 30 to 40 nm of each other before complement can bind; it may take at least 1,000 IgG molecules to ensure that there are two close enough to initiate such binding. Research has demonstrated that a raft of six IgG molecules is ideal for interacting with C1q to initiate the classical pathway. Some epitopes, notably the Rh group, are too far apart on the cell for this to occur; therefore, they are unable to fix complement.

Table 7–1 Proteins of the Complement System

SERUM PROTEIN (molecular weight)	CONCENTRATION (μg/mL)	FUNCTION	DISEASE ASSOCIATION
Classical Pathway			
C1q (410 kDa)	150	Binds to Fc region of IgM and IgG, synaptic pruning	SLE; recurrent infections
C1r (85 kDa)	50	Activates C1s	
C1s (85 kDa)	50	Cleaves C4 and C2	
C4 (205 kDa)	300–600	Part of C3 convertase (C4b)	Often asymptomatic; RA, SLE, or infection
C2 (102 kDa)	25	Binds to C4b—forms C3 convertase	SLE, recurrent infection, may be asymptomatic
Lectin Pathway			
MBL (200–600 kDa)	0.0002–10	Binds to mannose	Mostly asymptomatic, bacterial infection, some autoimmunity
MASP-1 (93 kDa)	1.5–12	Unknown	3MC syndrome
MASP-2 (76 kDa)	Unknown	Cleaves C4 and C2	Mostly asymptomatic, respiratory infections
Alternative Pathway			
Factor B (93 kDa)	200	Binds to C3b to form C3 convertase	*Neisseria* and pneumococcal infections; aHUS with gain of function
Factor D (24 kDa)	2	Cleaves Factor B	Bacterial infection
Properdin (55 kDa)	15–25	Stabilizes C3bBb–C3 convertase	Severe recurrent infection
Terminal Pathway			
C3 (190 kDa)	1, 200	Key intermediate in all pathways	Severe recurrent infection; aHUS, C3G, AMD with gain of function
C5 (190 kDa)	80	Initiates MAC	*Neisseria* infection
C6 (110 kDa)	45	Binds to C5b in MAC	
C7 (100 kDa)	90	Binds to C5bC6 in MAC	
C8 (150 kDa)	55	Starts pore formation on membrane	
C9 (70 kDa)	60	Polymerizes to cause cell lysis	No known disease association

aHUS = atypical hemolytic uremic syndrome; AMD = age-related macular degeneration; C1-INH = C1 inhibitor; C3G = C3 glomerulopathy; DAF = decay-accelerating factor; Fc = fragment crystallizable; Ig = immunoglobulin; MAC = membrane attack complex; MASP-1 and -2 = MBL-associated serine proteases; MBL = mannose-binding lectin; RA = rheumatoid arthritis; SLE = systemic lupus erythematosus.

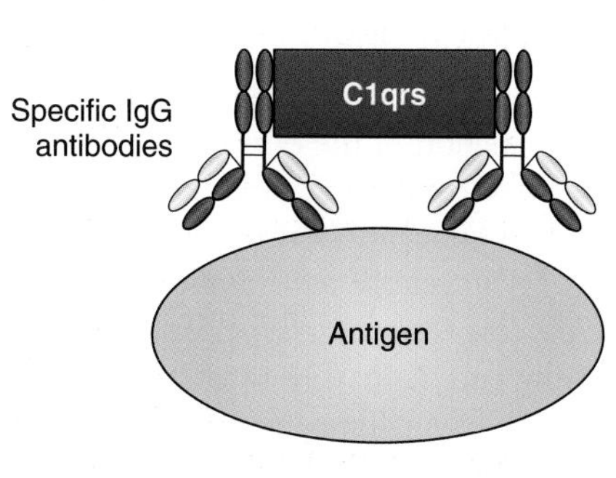

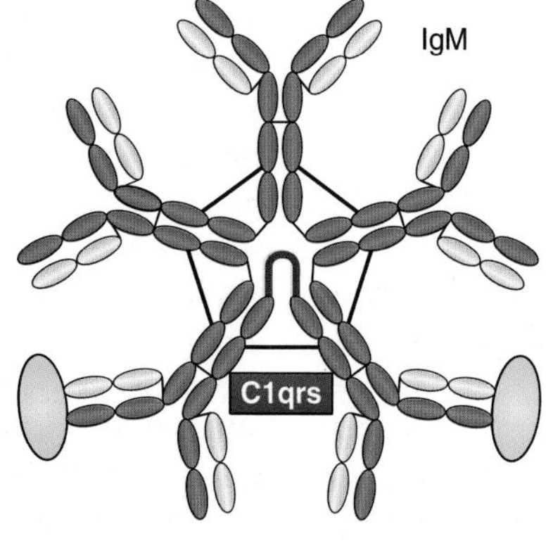

FIGURE 7–1 Binding of C1q to IgG (2 molecules required) and IgM (1 molecule required).

Connections

Discovery of Complement and Its Properties

Jules Bordet was awarded the Nobel Prize in 1919 for his role in elucidating the nature of complement. Complement was originally recognized in the 1890s; Paul Ehrlich coined the term *complement* because the proteins complement the action of antibody in destroying microorganisms. Present as a substance in normal nonimmune serum, complement is part of the innate immune system. Complement is considered an acute-phase reactant because levels rise during an infection. It also has a unique property of being easily inactivated (i.e., heat-labile) by heating serum to 56°C for 30 minutes. Refer to Chapter 2 for a further description of the innate immune system.

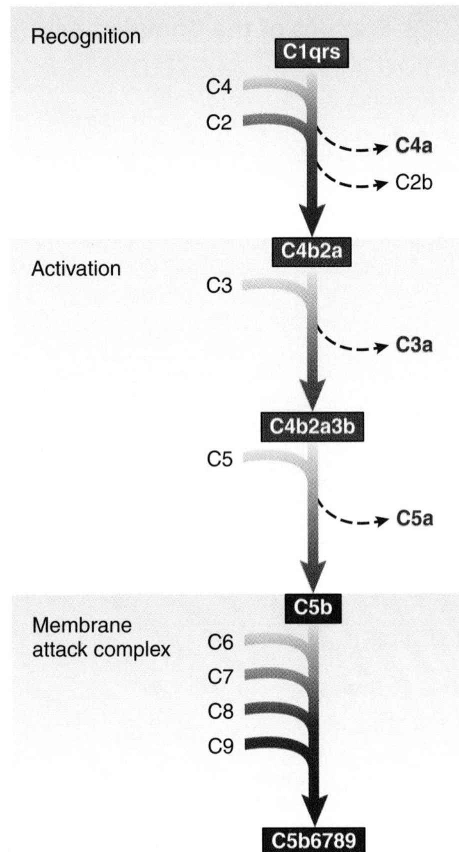

FIGURE 7–2 The classical complement cascade. C1qrs is the recognition unit that binds to the Fc portion of two antibody molecules. C1s is activated and cleaves C4 and C2 to form C4bC2a, also known as *C3 convertase.* C3 convertase cleaves C3 to form C4b2a3b, known as *C5 convertase.* The combination of C4bC2aC3b is the activation unit. C5 convertase cleaves C5. C5b attracts C6, C7, C8, and C9, which bind together, forming the MAC. C9 polymerizes to cause lysis of the target cell.

Within the IgG group, IgG3 is the most effective, followed by IgG1 and then IgG2.

In addition to antibodies, a few substances can bind complement directly to initiate the classical cascade. These include C-reactive protein (CRP), several viruses, mycoplasmas, some protozoa, and certain gram-negative bacteria such as *Escherichia coli.* However, most infectious agents can directly activate only the alternative or lectin pathways.

Complement activation can be divided into three main stages, each involving a combination of specific complement components to form a functional complex. The first stage involves the formation of the **recognition unit,** which, in the case of the classical pathway, is C1. Once C1 is bound, the next components activated are C4, C2, and C3, known collectively as the **activation unit** of the classical pathway (and the lectin pathway). C5 through C9 comprise the **membrane attack complex (MAC)**; this last unit completes the lysis of foreign particles. Each of these is discussed in detail in the following sections. **Figure 7–2** depicts a simplified scheme of the entire pathway. Note that the complement proteins were named as they were discovered, before the sequence of activation was known—hence the irregularity in the numbering system.

The first complement component of the classical pathway to bind is C1, a molecular complex of 740 kDa. It consists of three subunits—C1q, C1r, and C1s—which require the presence of calcium to maintain structure. The complex is made up of one C1q subunit, two C1r subunits, and two C1s subunits **(Fig. 7–3).** Although the C1q unit is the part that binds to antibody molecules, the C1r and C1s subunits generate enzyme activity to begin the cascade.

Formation of the Recognition Unit

C1q has a molecular weight of 410 kDa and is composed of six globular heads with a collagen-like tail portion. This structure has been likened to a bouquet of tulips with six blossoms extending outward (see Fig. 7–3). As long as calcium is present in the serum, C1r and C1s remain associated with C1q.

C1q binds to the Fc regions from two (or ideally six) adjacent antibody molecules, and at least two of the globular heads of C1q must be bound to initiate the classical pathway. C1r and C1s are serine protease proenzymes, or zymogens. As binding of C1q occurs, both are converted into active enzymes. Autoactivation of C1r results from a conformational change that takes place as C1q is bound. Once activated, C1r cleaves a thioester bond on C1s, which, in turn, activates it. Activated C1r is extremely specific because its only known substrate is C1s. Likewise, C1s has a limited specificity, with its only substrates being C4 and C2. Once C1s is activated, the recognition stage ends.

Formation of the Activation Unit

Phase two, the activation phase, begins when C1s cleaves C4 and ends with the production of the enzyme C3 convertase **(Fig. 7–4).** C4 is the second most abundant complement protein, with a serum concentration of approximately 600 µg/mL. C1s cleaves C4 to release a 77-amino acid fragment called *C4a.* In the process, it opens a thioester-containing active site on the remaining part, C4b. C4b must bind to protein or carbohydrate within a few seconds, or it will react with water molecules to form iC4b, which is rapidly degraded.

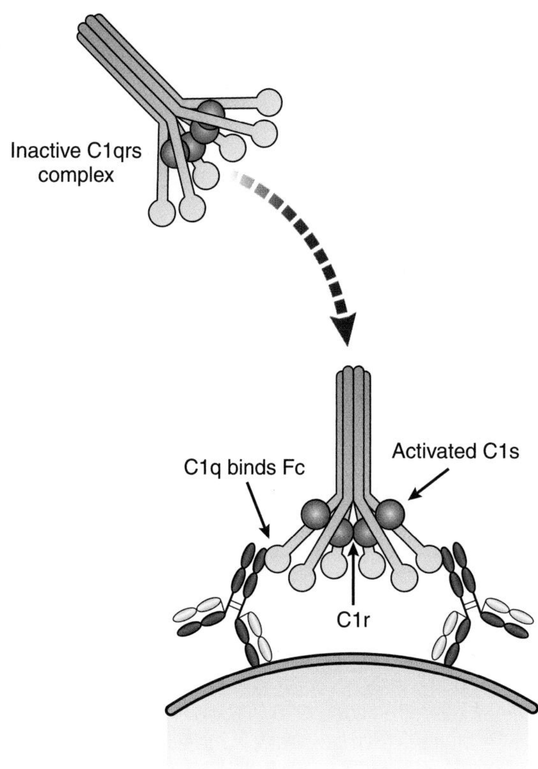

FIGURE 7–3 Structure of C1qrs. When two or more globular heads of C1q attach to bound immunoglobulin molecules, the collagen-like stalks change their configuration. The resulting shape change causes C1r to become a serine protease, which cleaves a small fragment of C1s, uncovering the C1s protease, whose only targets are C4 and C2.

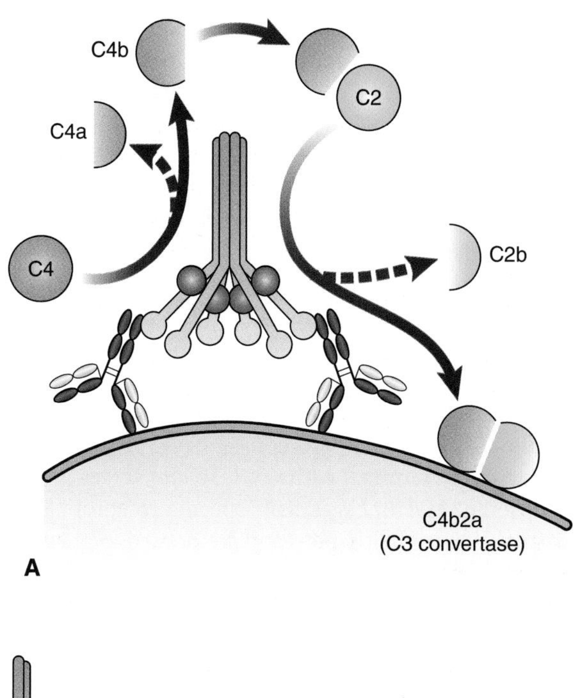

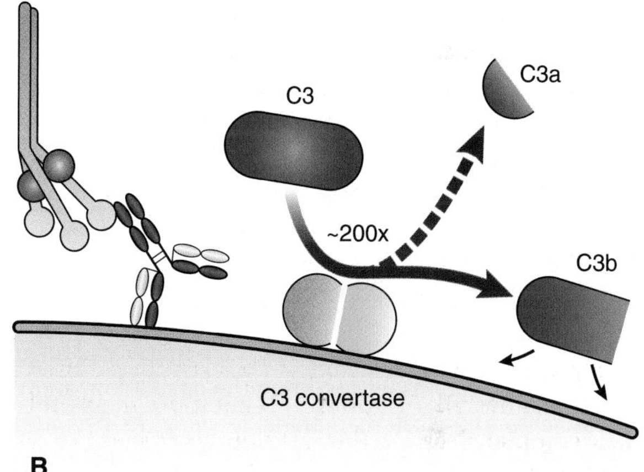

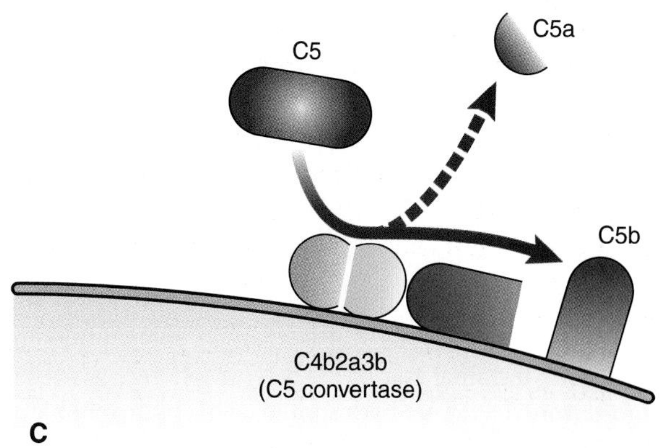

FIGURE 7–4 Formation of the activation unit. (A) Activated C1qrs cleaves C4 and C2, with the larger pieces, C4b and C2a, binding to the target-cell surface and forming the enzyme C3 convertase. (B) Each C3 convertase cleaves ~200 C3 molecules into C3a and C3b. C3b is a powerful opsonin that binds to the target in many places. (C) Some C3b associates with C4bC2a, forming C4bC2aC3b, also known as *C5 convertase*. This convertase cleaves C5 into the anaphylatoxin, C5a, and C5b, which binds to the target cell.

Thus, C4b binds mainly to antigen in clusters that are within a 40-nm radius of C1. This represents the first amplification step in the cascade because for every C1 molecule attached, approximately 30 molecules of C4 are split and attached.

C2 is the next component to be activated. When combined with C4b in the presence of magnesium ions, C2 is cleaved by C1s to form the fragments, C2a (which has a molecular weight of 70 kDa) and C2b (which has a molecular weight of 34 kDa) (see Fig. 7–4A). This is the only case in which the letter "a" has been designated for the larger cleavage piece with enzyme activity. The short life of these reactive species serves as a mechanism of control, keeping the reaction localized.

The combination of C4b and C2a is known as *C3 convertase* (see Fig. 7–4B). The C4bC2a complex is an active enzyme. This complex is not very stable. The half-life is estimated to be between 15 seconds and 3 minutes, so C3 must be bound quickly. If binding does occur, C3 is cleaved into two fragments, C3a and C3b.

C3, the major and central constituent of the complement system, is present in the plasma in a concentration of 1 mg/mL to 1.5 mg/mL. It serves as the pivotal point of convergence of all three complement pathways. The cleavage of C3 to C3b represents the most significant step in the entire process of complement activation. The C3 molecule has a molecular weight of 190 kDa and consists of two polypeptide chains, alpha (α) and beta (β). The α chain contains a highly reactive thioester group. When C3a is removed by cleavage of a single bond in the α chain, the thioester is exposed; the remaining piece, C3b, is then capable of binding to hydroxyl groups on carbohydrates and proteins in the immediate vicinity. C3b is estimated to have a half-life of 60 microseconds if not bound to antigen. Therefore, only a small percentage of cleaved C3 molecules bind to adjacent surfaces; most are hydrolyzed by water molecules and decay in the fluid phase.

The cleavage of C3 represents a second and major amplification process because about 200 molecules are split for every molecule of C4bC2a. In addition to being required for the activation of the terminal pathway, C3b also serves as a powerful opsonin. Macrophages have specific receptors for C3b (discussed later in the chapter) and are primed to phagocytize antigen that has bound C3b. Large numbers of molecules are needed for this to occur, hence the need for amplification.

If C3b is bound within 40 nm of the C4bC2a, a new enzyme known as *C5 convertase* (C4bC2aC3b) is created. Figure 7–4C depicts this last step in the formation of the activation unit. The cleaving of C5 with deposition of C5b at another site on the cell membrane constitutes the beginning of the MAC.

The Membrane Attack Complex (MAC)

C5 consists of two polypeptide chains, α and β, which are linked by disulfide bonds to form a molecule with a molecular weight of about 190 kDa. C5 convertase, consisting of C4bC2aC3b, splits C5 into two fragments, a 74-amino acid fragment known as *C5a*, which is released into the circulation, and C5b, which attaches to the cell membrane, forming the beginning of the MAC. The splitting of C5 and the cleavage of C3 represent the most significant biological consequences of the complement system, as explained in the section on biological manifestations of complement activation. However, C5b is extremely labile and is rapidly inactivated unless binding to C6 occurs.

Once C6 is bound to C5b, subsequent binding of C7, C8, and multiple molecules of C9 occurs. The complex of C5b-C6-C7-C8 and C9 is known as *C5b-9* or the *MAC*. None of these proteins has enzymatic activity; they are all present in much smaller amounts in serum than the preceding components. C6 and C7 have similar physical and chemical properties. C8 is made up of three dissimilar chains, α, β, and γ, joined by disulfide bonds. C9 is a single polypeptide chain. The carboxy-terminal end of C9 is hydrophobic, whereas the amino-terminal end is hydrophilic. The hydrophobic part serves to anchor the MAC within the target membrane. Formation of the membrane attack unit is pictured in **Figure 7–5.** If the complex is soluble in circulation, it is known as *sC5b-9*. Measurement of the level of *sC5b-9* is an indicator of the amount of terminal pathway activation that is occurring. When formed, the MAC produces a pore of 70 to 100Å that allows ions to pass in and out of the membrane. Destruction of target cells actually occurs through an influx of water and a corresponding loss of electrolytes. The presence of C9 greatly accelerates lysis. However, sufficient perturbation of the membrane can occur in the absence of C9 so that deficiencies in C9 appear largely benign.

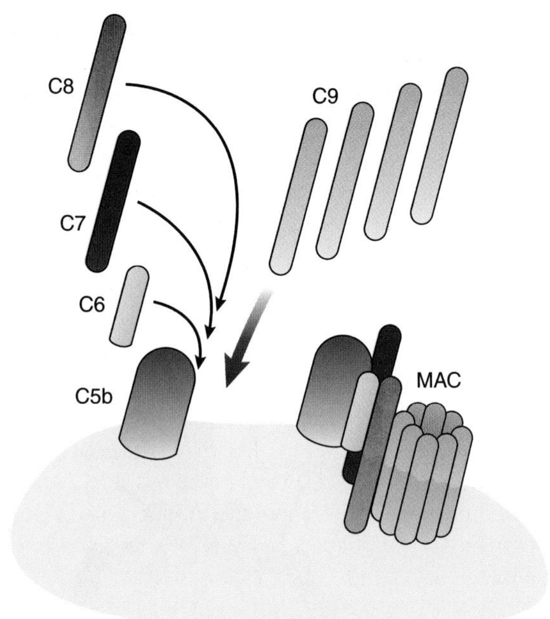

FIGURE 7–5 Formation of the MAC. C5b binds to the target cell, and C6 and C7 attach to C5b. C8 binds to these associated molecules and begins (along with C7) to penetrate the cell membrane. Multiple C9 molecules bind to C5bC6C7C8 and polymerize to form a transmembrane channel, the MAC, which causes lysis of the cell.

The Lectin Pathway

The lectin pathway represents another means of activating complement. Instead of activation through antibody binding, the lectin pathway is activated by direct recognition of surface moieties that are found on pathogens. This pathway provides an additional link between the innate and acquired immune response because it involves nonspecific recognition of carbohydrates that are common constituents of microbial cell walls and that are distinct from those found on human cell surfaces. The lectin pathway also plays an important role as a defense mechanism in infancy, during the interval between the loss of maternal antibody and the acquisition of a full-fledged antibody response to pathogens. Although this pathway is the most recently described of the three activation pathways of complement, it is probably the most ancient.

The early lectin pathway molecules are structurally similar to those of the classical pathway; the classical and lectin pathways even share the components C4 and C2. Once C4 and C2 are cleaved, the rest of the pathway is identical to the classical pathway. The role C1q serves in the classical pathway is filled by three classes of recognition molecules in the lectin pathway: lectins, ficolins, and collectins. The structure of all three classes of recognition molecules is similar to that of C1q. One key protein, called *mannose-binding lectin* (MBL), binds to mannose or related sugars in a calcium-dependent manner to initiate this pathway. These sugars are found in glycoproteins or carbohydrates of a wide variety of microorganisms, such as bacteria, yeasts, viruses, and some parasites. MBL is considered an acute-phase protein because it is produced in the liver and is normally present in the serum but increases during an initial inflammatory response.

After MBL binds to mannose on the surface of microorganisms, serine proteases called *MBL-associated serine proteases* (MASPs) associate with the complex. The enzymatic function of the MASPs is triggered, resembling the roles of C1r and C1s in the classical pathway. There are currently three MASPs identified: MASP-1, MASP-2, and MASP-3. Although the recognition molecules are different for the lectin pathway, activation soon converges on the same C4 and C2 molecules that are involved in the classical pathway. From this point, activation of the lectin and classical pathways is indistinguishable. One difference is that there is mounting evidence for a possible bypass for the lectin pathway, where C3 is activated in the absence of C4 and C2 activation.

The Alternative Pathway

First described by Pillemer and his associates in the early 1950s, the alternative pathway was originally named for the protein **properdin,** a protein in normal serum with a concentration of approximately 5 to 15 µg/mL. Although the alternative pathway can be activated on its own, it appears that it functions largely as an amplification loop for activation started from the classical or lectin pathways. In addition to properdin, two other serum proteins, Factor B and Factor D, are unique to the alternative pathway. The alternative pathway is summarized in **Figure 7–6.**

Activation of the pathway begins with C3. Triggering substances for the alternative pathway include bacterial cell walls, especially those containing lipopolysaccharide; fungal cell walls; yeast; viruses; virally infected cells; tumor cell lines; and some parasites, especially trypanosomes. All these can serve as sites for binding the complex C3bBb, one of the key products of this pathway.

The alternative pathway also acts as a monitoring system, with a continual baseline level of activation, which must be kept in check. This continual low-level activation occurs through the fact that native C3 is not stable in plasma. Water is able to hydrolyze the C3 thioester bond, thus spontaneously activating a small number of these molecules. A C3b-like molecule, often referred to as $C3_{H2O}$, is formed by this spontaneous hydrolysis and can start activation of the alternative pathway,

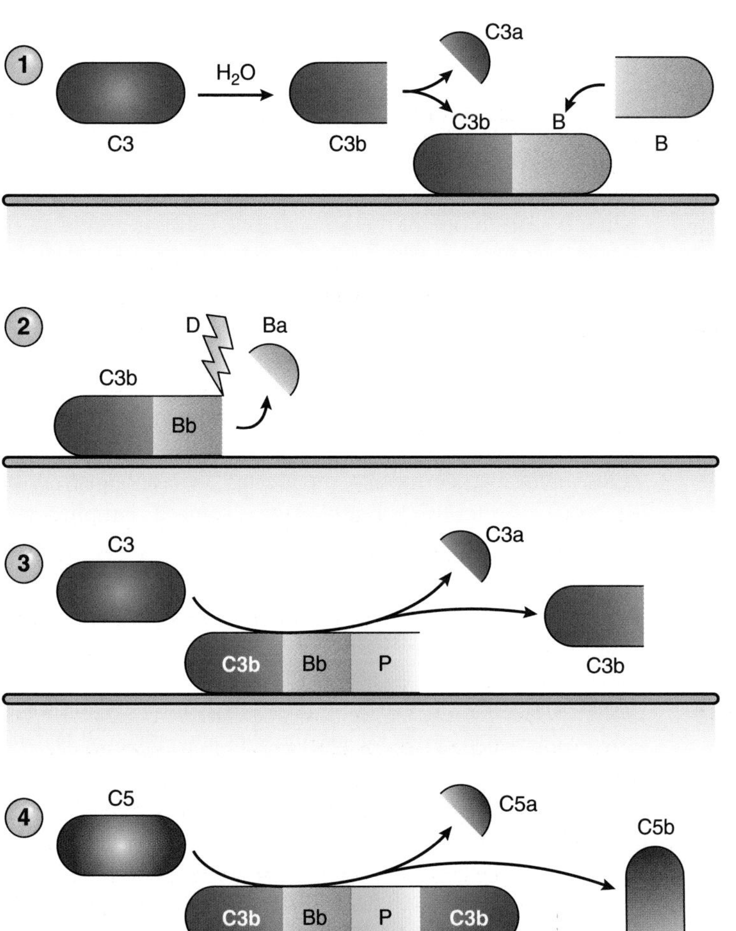

1. C3 is hydrolyzed by water to produce C3b, which binds Factor B, and together they attach to target cell surface.
2. B is cleaved by Factor D into the fragments Ba and Bb. Bb combines with C3b to form C3bBb, an enzyme with C3 convertase activity.
3. More C3 is cleaved, forming more C3bBb. This enzyme is stabilized by properdin, and it continues to cleave additional C3.
4. If a molecule of C3 remains attached to the C3bBbP enzyme, the convertase now has the capability to cleave C5. The C5 convertase thus consists of C3bBbP3b. After C5 is cleaved, the pathway is identical to the classical pathway.

FIGURE 7–6 The alternative pathway.

similar to the crossover activation initiated in the classical or lectin pathways. Once formed, the C3b or $C3_{H2O}$ acts as the seed of activation of the alternative pathway. C3b binds to Factor B, which has a molecular weight of 93 kDa and is fairly abundant in the serum, at a level of around 200 µg/ mL. Once bound to C3b, Factor B can be cleaved by Factor D. The role of Factor B is thus analogous to that of C2 in the classical pathway because it forms an integral part of a C3 convertase.

Factor D is a plasma protein that goes through a conformational change when it binds to Factor B. The concentration of Factor D in the plasma is the lowest of all the complement proteins, approximately 2 µg/mL. Factor D is a serine protease that cleaves Factor B into two pieces: Ba (with a molecular weight of 33 kDa) and Bb (with a molecular weight of approximately 60 kDa). Bb remains attached to C3b, forming the initial *C3 convertase* of the alternative pathway. Bb is rapidly inactivated unless it becomes bound to a site on one of the triggering cellular antigens.

As the alternative pathway convertase, C3bBb is then capable of cleaving additional C3 into C3a and C3b. Some C3b attaches to cellular surfaces and acts as a binding site for more Factor B, resulting in an amplification loop; activation initiated by the classical or lectin pathways is amplified to levels of biological consequence. All C3 present in plasma would be rapidly converted by this method were it not for the fact that the enzyme C3bBb is extremely unstable unless properdin binds to the complex. Binding of properdin increases the half-life of C3bBb from 90 seconds to several minutes. In this manner, optimal rates of alternative pathway activation are achieved.

C3bBb can also cleave C5, but it is much more efficient at cleaving C3. If, however, some of the C3b produced remains bound to the C3 convertase in combination with properdin, the complex is stabilized. The resulting enzyme, C3bBbC3bP, has a high affinity for C5 and exhibits C5 convertase activity. Thus, C5 is cleaved to produce C5b, the first part of the MAC. From this point on, the alternative, lectin, and classical pathways are identical. **Figure 7–7** shows the convergence of all three pathways.

System Controls

Activation of complement could cause tissue damage and have devastating systemic effects if it were allowed to proceed uncontrolled. To ensure that infectious agents and not self-antigens are destroyed and that the reaction remains localized, several plasma proteins act as system regulators. In addition, there are specific receptors on certain cells that also exert a controlling influence on the activation process. In fact, approximately one-half of the complement components serve as controls for critical steps in the activation process. Because activation of C3 is the pivotal step in all pathways, the majority of the control proteins are aimed at halting accumulation of C3b. However, there are controls at all crucial steps along the way. Regulators will be discussed according to their order of appearance in each of the three pathways. A brief summary of these is found in **Table 7–2.**

Regulation of the Classical and Lectin Pathways

C1 inhibitor (C1-INH) inhibits activation at the first stages of both the classical and lectin pathways. Its main role is to inactivate C1 by binding to the active sites of C1r and C1s. Therefore, Clr and Cls become instantly and irreversibly dissociated from C1q. C1q remains bound to antibody, but all enzymatic activity ceases. C1-INH also inactivates MASP-2, binding to the MBL-MASP complex, thus halting the lectin pathway. Similar to most of the other complement proteins, it is mainly synthesized in the liver; however, monocytes also may be involved to some extent in its production. As a suicide inhibitor, one C1-INH can only inhibit one serine protease. Importantly for hereditary angioedema (HAE), as will be described later, C1-INH is also responsible for the control of several serine proteases of the contact system, a plasma protease cascade that activates inflammation and coagulation.

A rare regulator for just the lectin pathway, called *MAp19*, has been described. Also referred to as *MAp44*, there is still some work to be done to fully elucidate the importance of this splice variant of MASP-2. However, genetic polymorphisms in MAp19 have been associated with changes in mortality in patients receiving kidney transplants, largely because of infection.

Further formation of C3 convertase in the classical and lectin pathways is inhibited by four main regulators: soluble **C4-binding protein (C4BP)** and three cell-bound receptors, **complement receptor type 1 (CR1), membrane cofactor protein** (**MCP**, also known as *CD46*), and **decay-accelerating factor** (**DAF**, **also known as** *CD55*). All these act in concert with **Factor I,** a serine protease that inactivates C3b and C4b when bound to one of these regulators. C4BP is abundant in the plasma and is capable of combining with either fluid-phase or cell-bound C4b. Thus, C4BP blocks C4b from binding to C2 and directs degradation by Factor I. If C4BP attaches to cell-bound C4b, it can dissociate it from C4bC2a complexes, controlling further classical pathway activation.

CR1, also known as *CD35*, is a large polymorphic glycoprotein found mainly on the cell surface of peripheral blood cells, including neutrophils, monocytes, macrophages, erythrocytes, eosinophils, B lymphocytes, some T lymphocytes, and follicular dendritic cells. It binds C3b and C4b but has the greatest affinity for C3b. Once bound to CR1, both C4b and C3b can then be degraded by Factor I.

Importantly, CR1 also plays a key role in the clearance of immune complexes. CR1 is a key receptor on platelets and red blood cells (RBCs), which bind C3b-coated immune complexes, and facilitate their trafficking to the liver and spleen. It is there that fixed tissue macrophages strip the immune complexes from the RBCs, process the complexes, and return the RBCs intact to the circulation. The ability of cells to bind complement-coated particles is referred to as **immune adherence.**

MCP, or CD46, has a molecular weight of between 50 kDa and 70 kDa and is found on the cell membrane of virtually all epithelial and endothelial cells except erythrocytes. MCP is the most efficient cofactor for Factor I–mediated cleavage of C3b. It can serve as a cofactor for cleavage of C4b, but it is not

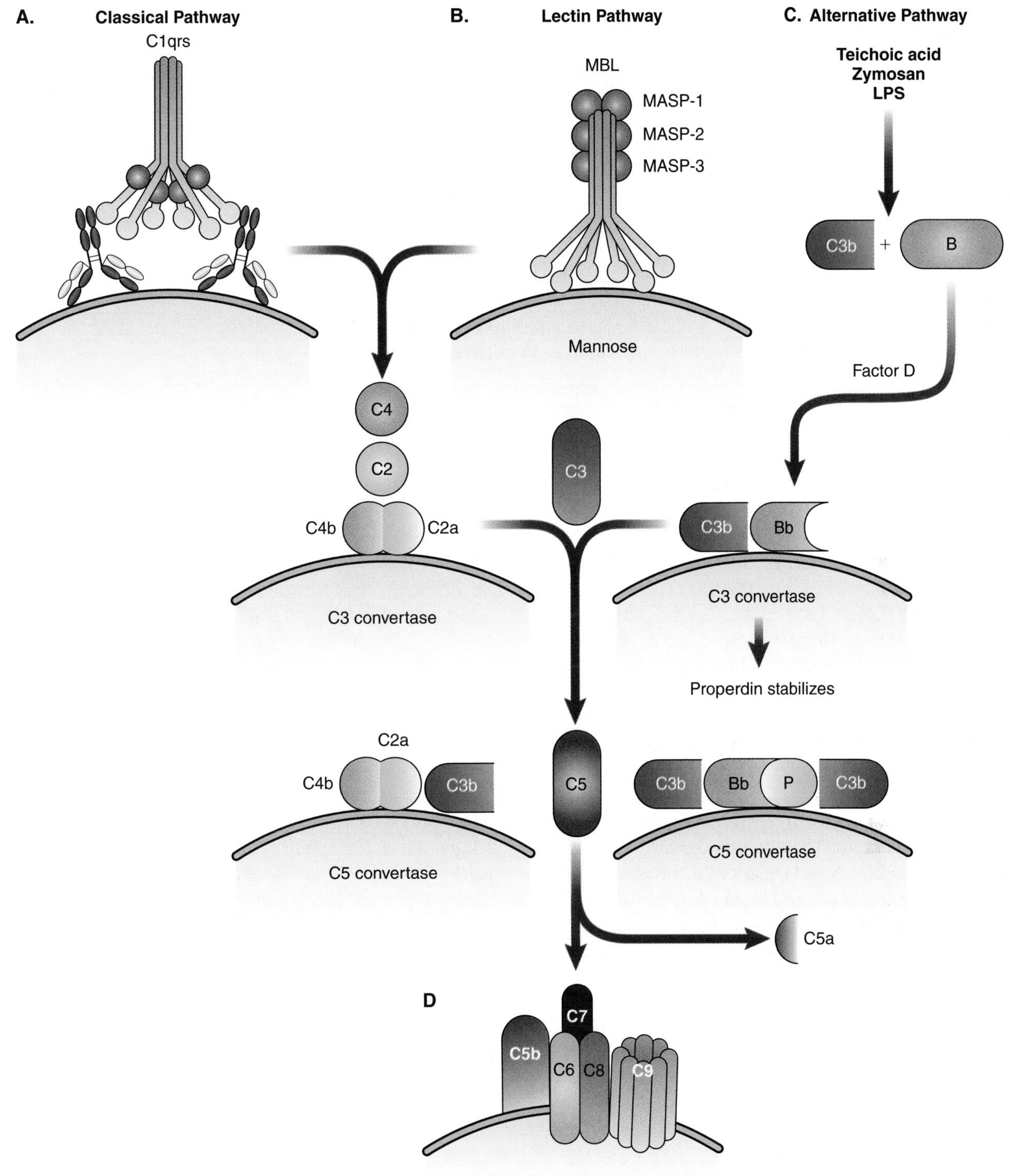

FIGURE 7–7 Convergence of the classical, alternative, and lectin pathways. Note that C3 is a key component in each pathway. (A) The binding of C1qrs to two IgG antibody molecules activates the classical pathway. Activation of C1s leads to the production of C4b2a, a C3 convertase that cleaves C3 into C3a and C3b. C3b combines with C4b2a to produce a C5 convertase, which cleaves C5 into C5a and C5b. (B) The lectin pathway is triggered by binding of MBP to mannose on bacterial cell walls. MASP-1, MASP-2, and MASP-3 bind to form an activated C1-like complex. MASP-2 cleaves C2 and C4 then the lectin pathway proceeds similar to the classical pathway. (C) The alternative pathway is started by hydrolysis of C3 to produce C3b in the presence of activating substances from microorganisms, such as lipopolysaccharides (LPS). C3b reacts with Factor B and Factor D to produce a C3 convertase, C3bBb. Properdin stabilizes the complex, producing a C5 convertase that consists of C3bBbC3bP. (D) After C5 is cleaved, the remaining steps are common to all three pathways, resulting in formation of the MAC (C5b6789).

Table 7–2 Plasma Complement Regulators

SERUM PROTEIN	CONCENTRATION (mg/mL)	FUNCTION	DISEASE ASSOCIATION
C1 inhibitor (C1-INH)	240	Dissociates C1r and C1s from C1q	Hereditary angioedema
Factor I	35	Cleaves C3b and C4b	aHUS or C3G; AMD with gain of function
Factor H	300–450	Cofactor with I to inactivate C3b; prevents binding of B to C3b	
C4-binding protein (C4BP)	250	Acts as a cofactor with I to inactivate C4b	Atypical morbus, Behcet's disease, angioedema, protein S deficit
S protein (vitronectin)	500	Prevents attachment of the C5b67 complex to cell membranes	

aHUS = atypical hemolytic uremic syndrome; AMD = age-related macular degeneration; C3G = C3 glomerulopathy.

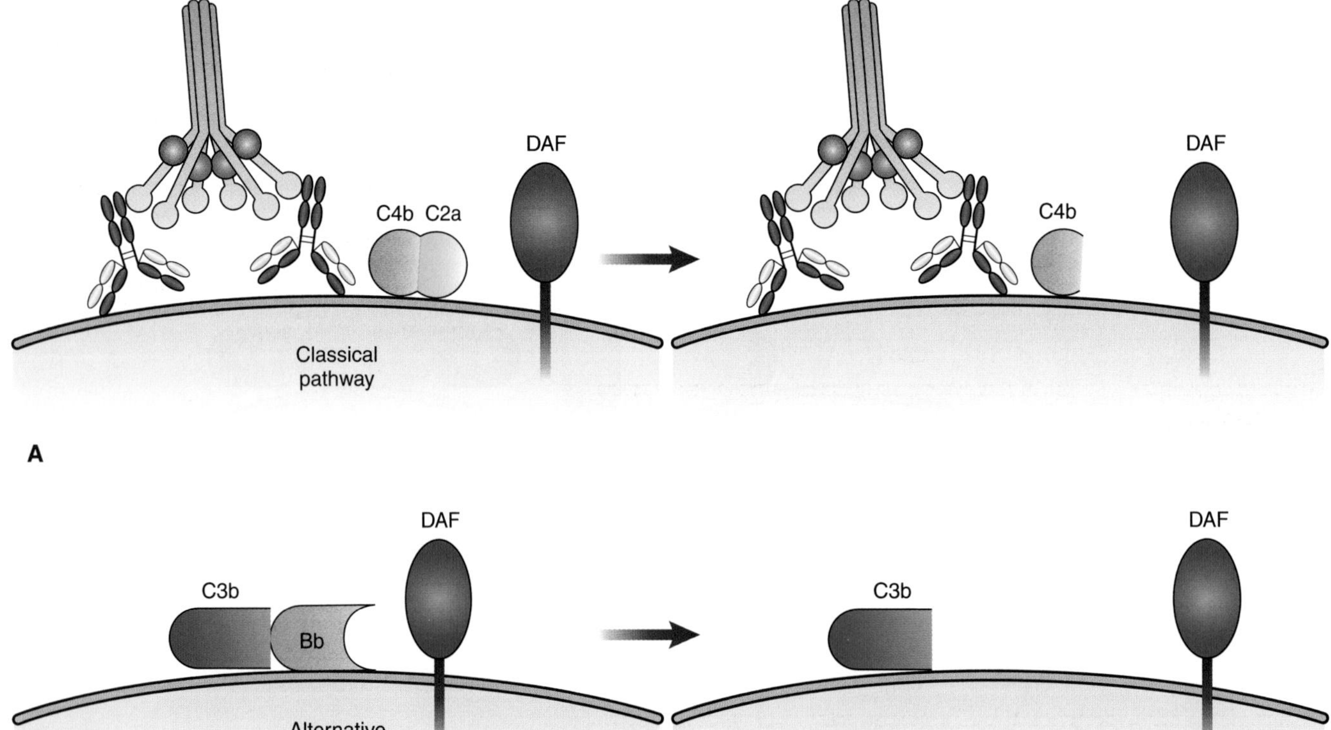

FIGURE 7–8 Inhibitory effects of DAF. (A) In the classical pathway, DAF dissociates C2a from C4b. (B) In the alternative pathway, when C3b binds to cell surfaces that have DAF present, DAF helps dissociate Bb from binding to C3b.

as effective as C4BP. MCP also helps to control the alternative pathway because binding of Factor B to C3b is inhibited.

A third complement receptor, called *DAF* or *CD55*, is a membrane glycoprotein that has a wide tissue distribution. It is found on peripheral blood cells, endothelial cells, fibroblasts, and numerous types of epithelial cells. DAF is capable of dissociating the C3 convertases of both the classical and alternative pathways. It can bind to both C3b and C4b in a manner similar to CR1. It does not prevent initial binding of either C2 or Factor B to the cell but can rapidly dissociate both from their binding sites, thus preventing the assembly of an active C3 convertase.

The carboxy-terminal portion of DAF is covalently attached to a glycophospholipid anchor that is inserted into the outer layer of the membrane lipid bilayer. This arrangement allows DAF mobility within the membrane so that it can reach C3 convertase sites that are not immediately adjacent to it **(Fig. 7–8).**

The presence of DAF on host cells protects them from **bystander lysis.** It is one of the main mechanisms used in discrimination of self from nonself because foreign cells do not possess this substance. However, it does not permanently modify C3b or C4b; they are capable of re-forming elsewhere as active convertases.

Regulation of the Alternative Pathway

The principal soluble regulator of the alternative pathway is **Factor H,** which acts by binding to C3b to prevent the binding of Factor B. C3b in the fluid phase has a hundredfold-greater affinity for Factor H than for Factor B, but on cell surfaces, C3b preferentially binds to Factor B. Factor H also accelerates the dissociation of the C3bBb complex on cell surfaces. When Factor H binds to C3bBb, Bb becomes displaced. In this manner, C3 convertase activity is curtailed in plasma and on cell surfaces.

Additionally, Factor H acts as a cofactor that facilitates the degradation of C3b by Factor I. It appears that only those molecules with tightly bound Factor H acquire high-affinity binding sites for Factor I. When Factor I binds, a conformational change takes place that allows it to cleave C3b. On cellular surfaces, C3b is cleaved into C3f, which is released into the plasma, and iC3b, which remains attached but is no longer an active enzyme. iC3b is further broken down to C3c and C3dg by Factor I in conjunction with another cofactor, the CR1 receptor **(Fig. 7–9).** With this key role in complement regulation, it should not be surprising that Factor H has been shown to play a role in a variety of disorders (discussed in the text that follows).

Regulation of Terminal Components

S protein is a soluble control protein that acts at a deeper level of complement activation. Also known as *vitronectin,*

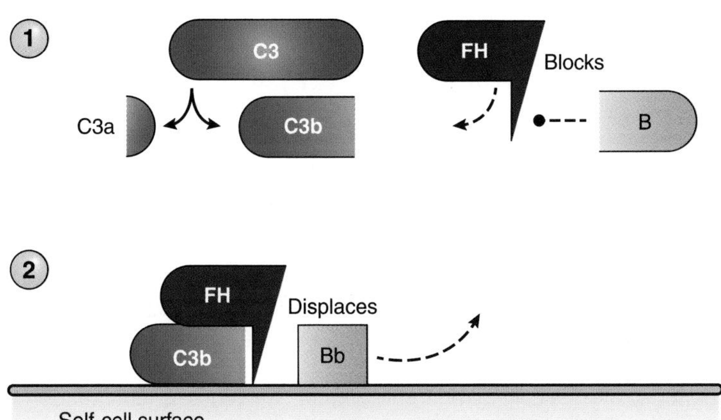

1. Factor H (FH) competes with Factor B (B) for binding to spontaneously (hydrolytically) activated C3b.
2. Factor H dissociates any C3bBb complexes that form on self-cell surfaces.
3. Factor H is a cofactor with Factor I (FI), enabling cleavage of C3b. The resulting iC3b loses enzymatic activity but is still an opsonin.
4. CR1 is a cofactor with FI, enabling cleavage of iC3b. The resulting C3dg is an opsonin and a cofactor in B-cell stimulation.

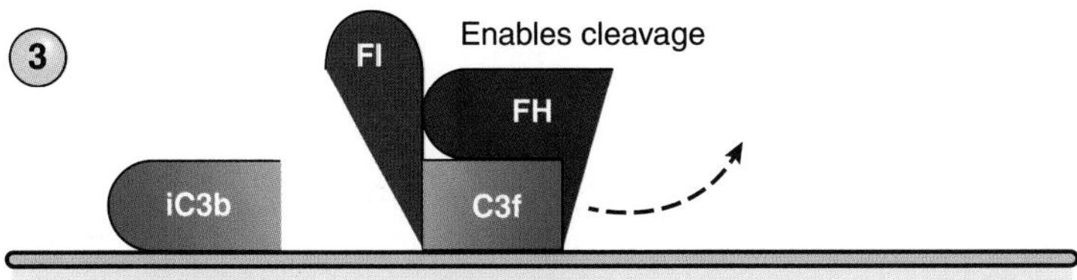

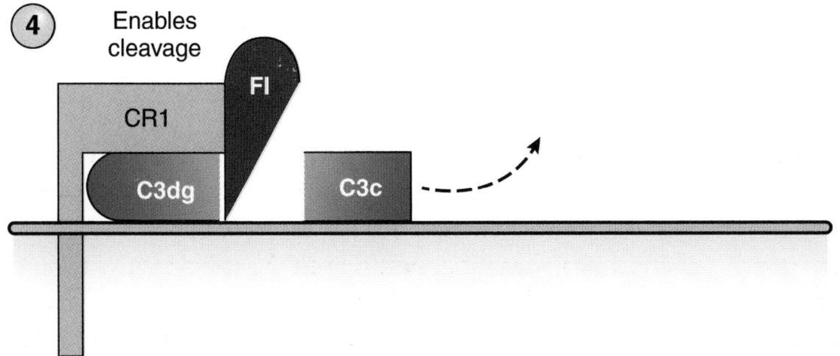

FIGURE 7–9 Complement controls. CR1 receptor acts as a cofactor in the inactivation of C3b. Factor I cleaves C3b to form C3dg and C3c. C3dg is not an effective opsonin and is not capable of further participation in the complement cascade.

S protein interacts with the C5b-7 complex as it forms in the fluid phase and prevents it from binding to cell membranes. Binding of C8 and C9 still proceeds, but polymerization of C9 does not occur; therefore, the complex is unable to insert itself into the cell membrane or to produce lysis.

A receptor, known by various terms, including *membrane inhibitor of reactive lysis* (MIRL) or *CD59*, also acts to block formation of the MAC. CD59 is widely distributed on the cell membranes of all circulating blood cells, including RBCs, and on endothelial, epithelial, and many other types of cells. **Table 7–3** lists the complement receptors and indicates the types of cells on which they are found.

Complement Receptors and Their Biological Roles

Some complement receptors found on host cells amplify and enhance the immune response by augmenting phagocytosis and stimulating accessory cells rather than acting as regulators (see Table 7–3). CR1 has been discussed in the previous section. A second receptor, CR2 (or CD21), is found mainly on B lymphocytes and follicular dendritic cells. Ligands for CR2 include degradation products of C3b, such as C3dg, C3d, and iC3b. In addition, the Epstein-Barr virus gains entry to B cells by binding to this receptor. CR2 is present only on mature B cells and is lost when differentiation to plasma cells occurs. CR2 plays an important role as part of the B-cell co-receptor for antigen. Acting in concert with CD19, it binds complement-coated antigen and cross-links it to membrane immunoglobulin to activate B cells. In this manner, immune complexes are more effective at enhancing B-cell differentiation and producing memory cells than is antigen by itself.

Another receptor, CR3 (CD11b/CD18), found on monocytes, macrophages, neutrophils, and natural killer (NK) cells, specifically binds particles opsonized with iC3b, a C3b degradation product. It does this in a calcium-dependent manner. The CR3 receptor plays a key role in mediating phagocytosis of particles coated with these complement fragments **(Fig. 7–10)**. These proteins trigger surface adhesion and increased activity of phagocytic cells. Patients whose white blood cells (WBCs) lack these receptors fail to exhibit functions such as chemotaxis, surface adherence, and aggregation.

Table 7-3 Receptors on Cell Membranes for Complement Components

RECEPTOR	LIGAND	CELL TYPE	FUNCTION	DISEASE ASSOCIATION
CR1 (CD35)	C3b, iC3b, C4b	RBCs, neutrophils, monocytes, macrophages, eosinophils, B and T cells, follicular dendritic cells	Cofactor for Factor I; mediates transport of immune complexes	SLE
CR2 (CD21)	C3dg, C3d, iC3b	B cells, follicular dendritic cells, epithelial cells	B-cell co-receptor for antigen with CD19	Infections, connected to CVID
CR3 (CD11b/CD18)	iC3b, C3d, C3b	Monocytes, macrophages, neutrophils, NK cells	Adhesion and increased activity of phagocytic cells	LAD
CR4 (CD11c/CD18)	iC3b, C3b	Monocytes, macrophages, neutrophils, NK cells, activated T and B cells, dendritic cells	Adhesion and increased activity of phagocytic cells	
DAF (CD55)	C3b, C4b	RBCs, neutrophils, platelets, monocytes, endothelial cells, fibroblasts, T cells, B cells, epithelial cells	Dissociates C2b or Bb from binding sites, thus preventing formation of C3 convertase	PNH; protein-losing enteropathy
MIRL (CD59)	C8	RBCs, neutrophils, platelets, monocytes, endothelial cells, epithelial cells	Prevents insertion of C9 into cell membrane	PNH; polyneuropathy
MCP (CD46)	C3b, C4b	Neutrophils, monocytes, macrophages, platelets, T cells, B cells, endothelial cells	Cofactor for Factor I cleavage of C3b and C4b	aHUS

aHUS = atypical hemolytic uremic syndrome; C1-INH = C1 inhibitor; CVID = common variable immune deficiency; DAF = decay-accelerating factor; LAD = leukocyte adhesion deficiency; MASP-2 = mannose-associated serine protease; MBL = mannose-binding lectin; MIRL = membrane inhibitor of reactive lysis; NK = natural killer; PNH = paroxysmal nocturnal hemoglobinuria; RBC = red blood cell; SLE = systemic lupus erythematosus.

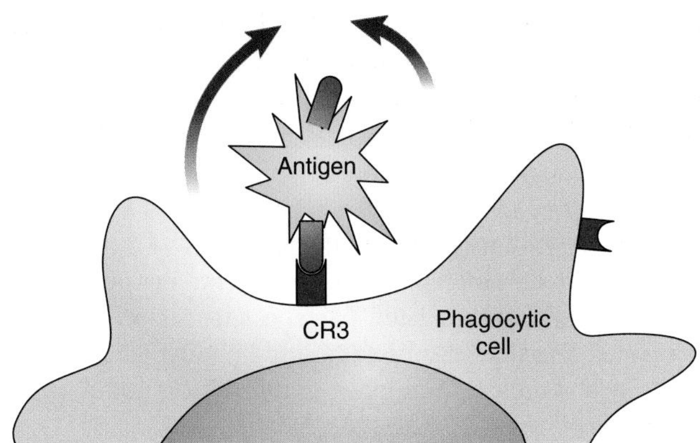

FIGURE 7–10 Role of C3b in opsonization. C3b is an important opsonin that coats antigens to enhance phagocytosis. Receptors for C3b (CR3) on the membrane of a phagocytic cell, such as a neutrophil or macrophage, bind C3b and pull the membrane around to envelop the antigen.

Deficiencies in phagocytosis are also noted. These individuals have an impaired capacity to bind iC3b-coated particles and are subject to recurrent infections.

The CR4 (CD11c/CD18) receptor is very similar to CR3 in that it also binds iC3b fragments in a calcium-dependent fashion. CR4 proteins are found on neutrophils, monocytes, tissue macrophages, activated T cells, dendritic cells, NK cells, and activated B cells. Neutrophils and monocytes, however, possess smaller amounts of CR4 than of CR3. Their function appears to be similar to that of CR3, and they may assist neutrophil adhesion to the endothelium during inflammation.

Receptors specific for C1q are found on neutrophils, monocytes, macrophages, B cells, platelets, and endothelial cells. These receptors, known as *collectin receptors*, bind the collagen portion of C1q and generally enhance the binding of C1q to Fc receptors. Interacting only with bound C1q, the receptors appear to increase uptake of immune complexes opsonized with C1q by phagocytic cells. C1q may also act to enhance the respiratory burst triggered by IgG binding to Fc receptors on neutrophils.

Biological Manifestations of Complement Activation

Activation of complement is a very effective means of amplifying the inflammatory response to destroy and clear foreign antigens. The cycle does not always have to proceed to lysis for this to be accomplished; hence, some of the initiating proteins are much more plentiful than proteins that form the MAC. Complement proteins also serve as a means of linking innate and adaptive immunity. They act as opsonins to facilitate recognition and subsequent destruction by phagocytic cells; in addition, they play a major role in the uptake and presentation of antigens so that a specific immune response can occur. Research has demonstrated that complement can facilitate B-cell activation and is necessary for maintaining immunologic memory. Effector molecules generated earlier in the cascade play a major role in all these areas. Such molecules can be classified into three main categories: anaphylatoxins, chemotaxins, and opsonins.

An **anaphylatoxin** is a small proinflammatory peptide that causes increased vascular permeability, contraction of smooth muscle, and release of histamine from basophils and mast cells. The activation products C3a and C5a are anaphylatoxins. Both of these have molecular weights between 9 and 11 kDa and are formed as cleavage products from larger complement components. Of these molecules, C5a is the most potent; it is at least 200 times more powerful than C3a. This increased potency of C5a is illustrated by the fact that C5a retains much of its proinflammatory capabilities after the terminal arginine is removed by carboxypeptidase, forming C5adesArg. In contrast, removal of the terminal arginine of C3a to form the C3adesArg reduces its proinflammatory properties.

C3a and C5a attach to specific receptors on neutrophils, basophils, mast cells, eosinophils, smooth muscle cells, and vascular endothelium. C3a attaches to the C3a receptor (C3aR), whereas C5a attaches to the C5a receptor (C5aR). When binding occurs on basophils and mast cells, histamine is released, increasing vascular permeability and causing contraction of smooth muscles. C5a causes neutrophils to release proteolytic enzymes, oxygen radicals, and prostaglandins, which aid in the destruction of foreign antigens.

C5a also serves as a **chemotaxin** for neutrophils, basophils, eosinophils, mast cells, monocytes, and dendritic cells. In this manner, these cells are directed to the source of antigen concentration. Because of increased vascular permeability, neutrophils migrate from blood vessels to the tissues and tend to aggregate.

Binding of C5a to monocytes causes them to undergo an oxidative burst that includes increased production of proteolytic enzymes, neutrophil chemotactic factor, platelet-activating factors, interleukin-1 (IL-1), and toxic oxygen metabolites. IL-1 is a member of the proinflammatory cytokine family that enhances T-cell activation. The activation may produce fever and lead to an increase in acute-phase reactants, both of which are characteristic of an inflammatory response.

An important function of complement is opsonization. As complement activation proceeds, the peptides C4b, C3b, iC3b, and C3dg are generated and accumulate on cell membranes. These peptides serve as **opsonins** by binding to specific receptors on erythrocytes, neutrophils, monocytes, and macrophages to facilitate phagocytosis and clearance of foreign substances or cellular debris. In addition, attachment of C3 products to an antigen has been found to enhance the B-cell response to the antigen.

Complement has historically been considered only as a cascade of circulating proteins important in innate immunity. However, there is growing evidence of important roles for complement outside this narrow perspective, particularly in neural development (synaptic pruning) and in intercellular regulation. It remains to be seen how intercellular complement, or its deficiencies, manifest in human disease. These roles of complement point to the potential need to test for intracellular complement activation and to consider the effects of release of intracellular complement on plasma testing in the future.

Complement and Disease States

Although complement acts as a powerful weapon to combat infection by amplifying phagocytosis, in some cases it can actually contribute to tissue damage or death. Complement can be harmful if

- It is activated systemically on a large scale, as in gram-negative septicemia.
- It is activated by tissue necrosis, such as myocardial infarction.
- Lysis of RBCs occurs.

In the case of septicemia caused by a gram-negative organism, large quantities of C3a and C5a are generated, leading to neutrophil aggregation and clotting. Damage to the tiny pulmonary capillaries and interstitial pulmonary edema may result.

Tissue injury following obstruction of the blood supply, such as occurs in a myocardial infarction or heart attack, can cause complement activation and deposition of MACs on cell surfaces. Receptors for C3a and C5a have been found in coronary plaques, indicating that complement components may increase the damage to heart tissue.

Cell lysis may be another end result of complement activation. Hemolytic diseases such as cold agglutinin hemolytic anemia are characterized by the presence of an autoantibody that binds at low temperatures. When these cells warm up, complement fixation results in lysis. (See Chapter 15 for a more complete discussion of complement-mediated autoimmune diseases.)

Abnormalities of Major Pathway Complement Components

Although excess activation of the complement system can result in disease states, as is discussed in a later section, the lack of individual components also has a deleterious effect. Hereditary deficiency of any complement protein, with the exception of C9, usually manifests itself in increased susceptibility to infection and delayed clearance of immune complexes. Most of these conditions are inherited with an autosomal recessive inheritance pattern and are quite rare, occurring in much less than 1% of the general population. A lack of C2 is the most common deficiency. C2-deficient individuals are more prone to recurrent streptococcal and staphylococcal infections. Because the Factor B locus is near the C2 gene, C2-deficient persons are often reported to have decreases in Factor B also. Although rare, deficiencies of early components of the classical pathway, including C1q, C4, and C2, may also cause a lupus-like syndrome because of failure to clear immune complexes from the circulation.

A second deficiency that occurs with some frequency is that of MBL. Deficiencies and polymorphisms in MBL occur in about 30% of the population. The health consequences of such variation in MBL levels remain unclear. Lack of MBL has been associated with pneumonia, sepsis, and meningococcal disease in infants; however, the majority of individuals deficient in MBL appear to have no deleterious effects.

The most serious deficiency is that of C3 because it is the key mediator in all three activation pathways. C3 deficiencies are, however, extremely rare. Individuals with a C3 deficiency are prone to developing severe, recurrent, life-threatening infections with encapsulated bacteria such as *Streptococcus pneumoniae* and may also be subject to immune complex diseases. Such complexes can lodge in the kidneys and result in glomerulonephritis.

It appears that a deficiency of any of the terminal components of the complement cascade (C5–C8) causes increased susceptibility to systemic *Neisseria* infections, including meningococcal meningitis and disseminated gonorrheal disease.

Abnormalities of Regulatory Complement Components

A prime example of a disease caused by a missing or defective regulatory component is **paroxysmal nocturnal hemoglobinuria (PNH).** Individuals with this disease have RBCs that are deficient in DAF. Hence, the RBCs are subject to lysis by means of the bystander effect once the complement system has been triggered. These individuals have a deficiency in linking DAF to its glycophospholipid anchor, preventing its insertion into the cell membrane. When C3b is deposited on erythrocytes through activation of any of the pathways, the result is complement-mediated intravascular and extravascular hemolysis, resulting in a chronic hemolytic anemia.

DAF deficiency has been associated with a lack of CD59 (MIRL), and both are implicated in PNH. CD59 has the same glycophospholipid anchor found in DAF; therefore, the gene deficiency affects both molecules. As mentioned previously, CD59 prevents insertion of C9 into the cell membrane by binding to the C5b-8 complex, inhibiting formation of transmembrane channels. Both DAF and CD59 are important in protecting RBCs against bystander lysis.

Another complement deficiency disorder that involves a regulatory protein is **hereditary angioedema (HAE).** HAE is characterized by recurrent attacks of swelling that affect the extremities, the skin, the gastrointestinal tract, and other mucosal surfaces. This disease is caused by a deficiency or lack of C1-INH. Although C1-INH was named for its role in controlling complement, it is the function of C1-INH in controlling the contact pathway of the coagulation system that is critical in this disease. C1-INH is a serpin (serine protease inhibitor) that controls many of the serine proteases on contact. The lack of C1-INH causes an increase in C1s activity and creation of C2b, resulting in localized swelling that can be either subcutaneous or found within the gastrointestinal or upper respiratory tract. Normally, this spontaneously subsides in 48 to 72 hours, but if the edema occurs in the area of the oropharynx, life-threatening upper-airway obstruction may develop. These attacks can be quite debilitating, even when they are not life threatening, so there is a need for proper diagnosis for these patients.

HAE is classified into two types: type I and type II. Type I is characterized by a decrease in the C1-INH protein; type II has normal levels of C1-INH, but the function is decreased. The genetic cause of either type is a heterozygous mutation in the *SERPING1* gene that codes for either a dysfunctional or an inactive C1-INH protein and is inherited in an autosomal dominant pattern. In addition to the hereditary forms of the disorder, there are acquired forms that result from either consumption of C1-INH or from autoantibodies blocking the function of C1-INH. To differentiate the acquired and hereditary forms, measurement of C1q can be helpful; C1q will be low in the acquired forms but not in the hereditary forms. Measurement of C4 can also be a very helpful screen for HAE, particularly during an attack, because patients usually exhibit a drop in C4 at that time. C2 can also be low, but measurement of C4 is more accessible.

In addition to these well-described diseases of failed control of the complement system, there is a growing number of disorders that are found to be associated with deficiencies, polymorphisms, or autoantibodies involving one or multiple complement components. Key among these is a group of rare kidney disorders associated with complement, referred to as **hemolytic uremic syndrome (HUS).** HUS is one of the most common causes of acute renal failure in children worldwide and is characterized by hemolytic anemia, low platelet count, and acute renal failure. The primary cause of HUS in the majority of cases is exposure to a Shiga toxin from an acute diarrheal illness, most commonly caused by Shiga-toxin–producing strains of *Escherichia coli*. In approximately 5% of cases, HUS occurs in the absence of Shiga-toxin exposure and is caused by mutations in complement regulatory proteins. This condition is known as **atypical hemolytic uremic syndrome (aHUS).** The genetic mutations associated with aHUS include those of Factor H, MCP, Factor I, Factor B, C3, and thrombomodulin, as well as inactivating autoantibodies against Factor H. aHUS may have an acute or gradual onset; otherwise, the clinical presentation is similar to HUS.

Dysregulation of complement has also been implicated in **C3 glomerulopathy (C3G),** a disease that causes inflammation of the glomeruli of the kidneys, leading to hematuria, proteinuria, hypertension, and gradual decline of kidney function. The two forms of C3 glomerulopathy, called *dense deposit disease* (DDD) and C3 *glomerulonephritis* (C3GN), have recently been reclassified from an older description of these diseases known as *membranoproliferative glomerulonephritis* (MPGN) on the basis of isolated or dominant presence of C3 by immunofluorescence through a kidney biopsy. Analysis of these patients has shown that a minority of patients (10%–15%) with C3G have mutations or polymorphisms in complement proteins, specifically C3, Factor B, Factor H, or Factor I. Most patients (up to 60% of patients with C3GN and up to 80% of patients with DDD) have acquired autoantibodies that cause complement dysregulation, known as *C3 nephritic factors* (C3NeFs).

A C3NeF is an antibody that binds the C3-convertase from the alternative pathway, C3bBb, holding it together and making it impervious to the normal control mechanisms. In this way, a C3NeF leads to uncontrolled cleavage of C3 with concomitant uncontrolled deposition of C3 in the glomeruli of the kidneys. C3 glomerulopathy (C3G) caused by C3NeF is clinically indistinguishable from the hereditary form of the disorder. It is only with laboratory measurement of the presence or absence of a C3NeF that the nature of the disorder can be differentiated. In addition, an investigation of a possible complement deficiency can be complicated by depletion of complement components caused by consumption through activation. Laboratory testing is the key way to differentiate the acquired forms from the hereditary forms of complement disorders.

Laboratory Detection of Complement Abnormalities

Determining the levels of complement components can be useful in diagnosing disease. Hereditary deficiencies can be identified, and much can be learned about inflammatory or autoimmune states by monitoring the consumption of complement proteins because of activation of complement by antigen–antibody complexes. Techniques to determine complement abnormalities generally fall into two categories: (1) measurement of components as antigens in serum and (2) measurement of functional activity. Many assays that are unavailable in routine clinical laboratories are available in specialized laboratories. Some of the more common assays will be discussed in the text that follows.

Immunologic Assays of Individual Components

Some of the most common methods of complement-level measurement are based on the principle of antigen–antibody equivalence. For this testing, the level of antibody to the component is kept constant; when the antibody and antigen are in equilibrium, immune complexes will form that can be detected. The most common methods for measuring individual complement proteins are nephelometry and immunoturbidimetry. Historically, radial immunodiffusion (RID) was also utilized (see Fig. 10–5), but this technique has become less common in favor of the more automated methods. C3 and C4 levels are routinely measured in most clinical laboratories by automated nephelometry or immunoturbidimetry. Measurement of these and other complement proteins relies on the precipitation of immune complexes produced when the patient sample (i.e., the source of complement) is incubated with a reagent antibody directed against the corresponding complement component. Nephelometry measures the concentration of an individual complement protein according to the amount of light scattered by the antigen–antibody mixture, whereas immunoturbidimetry is based on the reduction in light transmission resulting from immune complex formation (refer to Chapter 10 for more details).

None of the previously discussed assays is able to distinguish whether the molecules are functionally active. Thus, although the preceding techniques give quantitative results and are relatively easy to perform, test results must be interpreted carefully. Therefore, it may be important to use other methods, such as enzyme-linked immunosorbent assay (ELISA), for measurement of the activation fragments, particularly in relation to testing for the diseases of improper complement control.

Assays for the Classical Pathway

Assays that measure lysis, the endpoint of complement activation, are functional tests that are frequently run in conjunction with testing of individual components and have become more important with the advent of complement-blocking therapies. The **hemolytic titration (CH50) assay** was the original assay used for this purpose. This assay measures the amount of patient serum required to lyse 50% of a standardized concentration of antibody-sensitized sheep erythrocytes. Because all proteins from C1 to C9 are necessary for this to occur, functional or quantitative absence of any one component will result in an abnormal CH50, essentially reducing this number to zero.

The titer is expressed in CH50 units, which is the reciprocal of the dilution that is able to lyse 50% of the sensitized RBCs. The 50% point is used because this is when the maximum change in lytic activity per unit change in complement occurs **(Fig. 7–11).** Most laboratories need to establish their own normal values.

The newer and more common version of this test is based on the ability of complement in the patient sample to lyse antibody-coated liposomes that release an enzyme (glucose-6-phosphate dehydrogenase). The enzyme reacts with a substrate solution (NAD plus glucose-6-phosphate) to produce NADH. The resulting absorbance, which can be measured by most laboratory analyzers, is proportional to the complement activity in the sample. The test is simpler to perform than traditional CH50 testing and is more reproducible for the standard laboratory. However, this form of classical pathway function testing, although well suited for immunodeficiency diagnosis, may not be ideal for following the efficacy of complement inhibition. One reason for the discrepancy is that the liposomal assays involve testing at acidic pH, whereas the ELISA and hemolytic methods involve physiological pH. Regardless of which assay is used, individual laboratories must establish their own normal values.

More recently, 96-well ELISA assays have been developed to test complement function. These assays rely on activation of complement at the surface of the plate, followed by detection of neo-epitopes on C9 that are only present when the component is part of the terminal complement complex (TCC, also known as the *MAC*). These assays can be easily adapted by the general immunology laboratory. The ability to accurately follow the effectiveness of therapeutic complement blockade requires a method such as ELISA to provide the high sensitivity required to detect low levels of specific complement products.

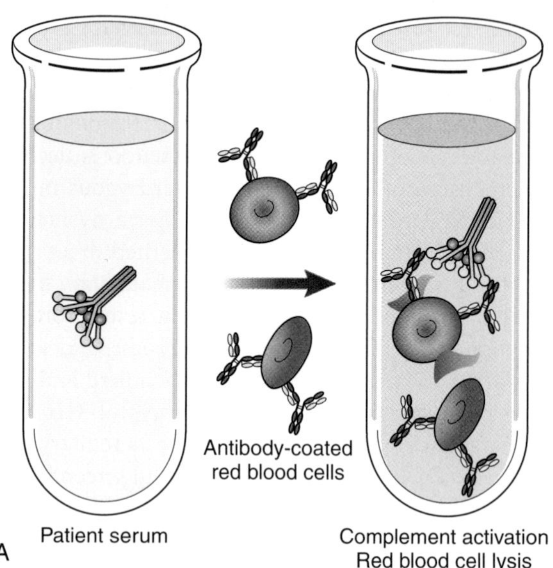

Serum to be tested is diluted serially and added to sensitized sheep red blood cells. The tubes are incubated at 37°C and then centrifuged to pellet the unlysed cells.

The CH50 is defined as the reciprocal of the dilution that causes lysis of 50% of the cells used in the assay.

In the example shown, the CH50 would be about 80 U/mL.

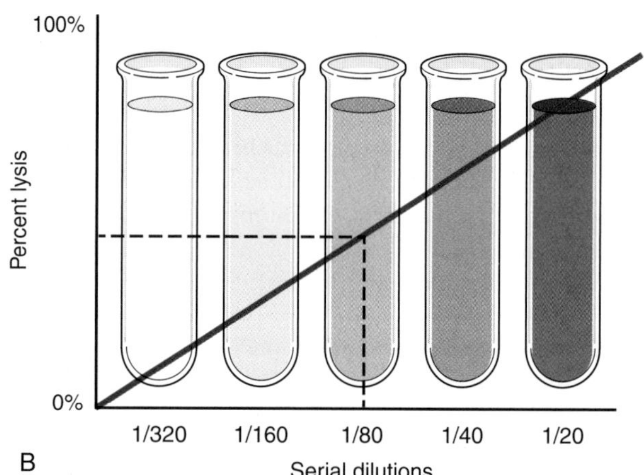

FIGURE 7–11 CH50 testing. (A) Antibody-coated RBCs are added to patient serum. This activates the complement in the sample, and the RBCs are lysed. Although only C1qrs is shown for simplicity, this test requires C1 through C9 to be present in order for lysis to occur. The degree of lysis indicates the functional capacity of the complete classical pathway. (B) CH50 methodology.

Alternative and Lectin Pathway Assays

Alternative pathway activation can be measured by several different means. An AH50 can be performed in the same manner as the CH50, except magnesium chloride and ethylene glycol tetraacetic acid (EGTA) are added to the buffer, and calcium is left out. This buffer chelates calcium, blocking classical pathway activation. Rabbit RBCs are used as the indicator because they provide an ideal surface for alternative pathway activation.

An additional means of testing for alternative pathway function is by ELISA. One such test can detect C3bBbP or C3bP complexes in very small quantities. Microtiter wells are typically coated with bacterial lipopolysaccharide to trigger activation of the alternative pathway.

One test system has been developed that can determine the activity of all three pathways. Strips used for the classical pathway are coated with IgM, strips for the alternative pathway are coated with lipopolysaccharide, and strips for the MBL pathway are coated with mannose. Such testing is easy to perform as it does not depend on the use of animal erythrocytes, which may be hard to obtain. Deficiencies can be detected using the combined test results.

Testing Levels of Complement Activation

With increased recognition of the role improper complement control plays in a growing list of diseases, there is increased interest in being able to monitor the balance of complement activation and control. Measurement of C3 and C4 levels has been used for monitoring in autoimmune-mediated diseases, but tests for intact complement components are not as sensitive as those that measure the fragments formed upon activation. Assays that test for complement activation are generally ELISA or multiplex versions of immunoassays (see Chapter 11 for more explanation of ELISAs). Measuring complement fragments has several potential benefits. First, these tests are more sensitive to any complement activation, so they can more easily separate a change from baseline. Second, measuring anaphylatoxin (C3a, and C5a) levels directly can be informative about the degree of inflammation that is being driven by complement. Third, by measuring individual fragments, it is possible to determine which pathway or pathways are activated and where any control is achieved in the cascade of complement activation. Specifically, measuring C4a will reflect classical/lectin pathway activation, and Bb or Ba will demonstrate the level of alternative pathway activation. There is also much interest in measuring the soluble version of the MAC, sC5b-9 (also known as *sMAC* or *TCC*). The sC5b-9 level is a measure of the level of activation reaching the terminal pathway, the pathway with the greatest biological effects.

Unfortunately, there are also problems with measuring the fragments. As many of these fragments are strongly proinflammatory, the body has developed mechanisms to control their action; therefore, most have very short half-lives in the circulation. C5a has the shortest half-life, at less than 1 minute. Another complication of tests measuring activation fragments of complement is that they are also very susceptible to *ex vivo* increases associated with blood collection. The use of ethylenediaminetetraacetic acid (EDTA) plasma is therefore necessary to chelate the calcium necessary for classical and lectin pathway activation and also to avoid the cross-pathway cleavage of complement during the clotting process. Even in EDTA tubes, a delay in processing or storage at –20°C can lead to dramatic increases in measured levels. Therefore, it is best to process complement specimens quickly and store them at –80°C within 2 hours of draw. This is also important for the functional assays but far less critical for the measurements of intact parent components such as C3 and C4.

Interpretation of Laboratory Findings

Interpretation of complement laboratory testing can be complicated by the effects of post-draw handling, as well as by the use of complement therapeutics. In complement-function tests, decreased levels of complement components or activity may be caused by decreased production by the patient, consumption of components because of certain diseases, or *in vitro* consumption from post-draw handling. The third condition must be ruled out before either of the other two is considered. Specimen handling is extremely important. The tube should be spun down, and the serum should be frozen at –80°C or placed on dry ice if it is not tested within 2 hours. If a sample is left at room temperature, stored at –20°C, or subjected to multiple freeze-and-thaw cycles, artificially low complement function will be measured. In such situations, results may be invalid, and the test needs to be repeated with a fresh specimen. It is important to keep in mind that improper post-draw handling of a sample would cause the test to return an abnormally low value; it is very unlikely for improper preanalytical handling to lead to a false-normal result.

Specimen handling is also critical when testing for activation markers, such as C3a or sC5b-9. These tests require an EDTA plasma tube to chelate calcium and help control post-draw complement activation. If a serum tube is used by mistake, the clotting process will produce a large increase in these fragments post-draw that may obscure any activation occurring in the patient. It is important to centrifuge the specimen, remove the plasma from the cells, and freeze the sample at –80°C within 2 hours of draw. Failure to freeze the sample promptly will lead to an artificially elevated result. Assays for standard measurements of C3 and C4 have been developed so as not to be as sensitive to specimen handling; however, they cannot distinguish between intact C3 or C4 and their activation fragments.

If a complement deficiency is suspected, it is possible to narrow down the possible candidate components with CH50 and AH50 assays. If the CH50 is low but the AH50 is normal, the components unique to the classical pathway should be investigated. If the CH50 is normal but the AH50 is low, the alternative pathway components need to be investigated. If both the CH50 and AH50 are low, suspicion should be on the components of the terminal pathway (as well as C3) because those components are shared by both the classical and alternative pathways. Although this analysis will be true for most patients, it is also possible, if there is sufficient activation of complement through any one pathway, that enough components could be consumed to lower the function of the other pathways. As previously stated, complement activation is rarely limited to just one pathway. Such consumption can result from the loss of a control protein, the presence of an autoantibody, an ongoing infection, or other activation circumstances.

Once the CH50 and AH50 hemolytic assays have been performed, it is appropriate to test the levels or function of individual complement components as directed by the relative results of the CH50 and AH50. For many of the components, an antigen level is sufficient to determine where the deficiency lies; however, there are a few instances in which measurement of the function would be more informative. For example, it is necessary to measure the function of C1 because it is a three-subunit protein. The loss of one of the three subunits would not put the level of C1 out of normal range, but it would render the remaining two subunits nonfunctional. In addition, C2 type II deficiency results from a genetic mutation in C2 that renders the protein nonfunctional but does not decrease the level of expression. In type II HAE, C1-INH may be present in normal levels but be nonfunctional.

A typical screening test for complement abnormalities usually includes determination of the following: C3 and C4, as well as hemolytic capacity through CH50. Testing for products of complement activation such as C3a, C4a, C5a, Bb, and Ba (as well as breakdown products, including iC3b and C4d) can also be performed as a means of monitoring inflammatory processes such as rheumatoid arthritis and SLE. **Table 7–4** presents some of the possible screening results from ELISA testing and correlates these with deficiencies of individual factors. An understanding of these patterns may be helpful in differentiating hereditary deficiencies from activation states that consume available complement components. Additional testing would be necessary, however, to actually pinpoint hereditary deficiencies.

With the advent of complement-targeted therapeutics, there is not only more demand to measure complement but also a need to appreciate the effect of complement-inhibiting drugs on the complement assays. If given in sufficient dose, a complement inhibitor, such as eculizumab (a monoclonal antibody directed against C5), will inhibit complement activity. This would be reflected in a low CH50 or AH50 measurement. This is also expected to lead to lower levels of activation markers, but only those downstream of the point of inhibition. For example, eculizumab would reduce levels of sC5b-9 but not C3a.

Complement Therapeutics

With increased recognition of the role of the complement system in the pathogenesis of many different diseases, several complement-targeted therapeutic agents have received approval for clinical use or are under investigation through human clinical trials. These agents are specifically targeted at key points in the complement pathways, thus determining the specific laboratory testing that is best suited for monitoring the treatment response and disease activity in patients receiving these agents.

Agents targeting the classical pathway are currently limited to the treatment of HAE, restoring C1-INH function by providing recombinant protein. Such treatment during an HAE crisis would be expected to restore classical pathway activity to normal, which would be evident by both an increase in C4 and C2 levels and normalization of low classical pathway function (CH50). A monoclonal antibody targeting C1s is also under development for cold agglutinin autoimmune hemolytic anemia and would be expected to cause a low CH50 by blocking classical pathway activation. The lectin pathway is also a target for therapeutic agents in clinical development, specifically a monoclonal antibody targeting MASP-2 under development for IgA nephropathy, a kidney disease in which the lectin pathway has been implicated in the pathogenesis.

Complement therapeutics targeting the alternative pathway are currently in advanced stages of clinical development for diseases in which the activation of this pathway is dysregulated, such as aHUS, C3G, and PNH. These agents, which include monoclonal antibodies, small molecules, and peptides targeting proteins such as Factor B, C3, and Factor D, would be expected to cause decreased functional hemolytic activity

Table 7–4 Diagnosis of Complement Abnormalities

IMPAIRED FUNCTION OR DEFICIENCY	CLASSICAL PATHWAY	LECTIN PATHWAY	ALTERNATIVE PATHWAY
C1q, C1r, C1s	Low	Normal	Normal
C4, C2	Low	Low	Normal
MBL, MASP-2, MASP-3	Normal	Low	Normal
Factor B, Factor D, and properdin	Normal	Normal	Low
C3, C5, C6, C7, C8, C9	Low	Low	Low
C1-INH	Low	Low	Normal
Factor H and Factor I	Low	Low	Low
Improperly handled sera	Low	Low	Low

Adapted from Seelen MA, et al. An enzyme-linked immunosorbent assay-based method for functional analysis of the three pathways of the complement system. In: Detrick B, Hamilton RG, and Folds JD, eds. Manual of Molecular and Clinical Laboratory Immunology. *7th ed. Washington, DC: ASM Press; 2006:124.*

of the alternative pathway (AH50). In addition, by halting activation, levels of C3 would be expected to rise to normal, and activation fragments such as Bb, Ba, and C3a would be expected to decrease to within the normal range.

Formation of C5a and the MAC through the terminal complement pathway has been the subject of much clinical investigation for therapeutic development, leading to successful approval of the first complement inhibitor targeting this pathway. Eculizumab, a monoclonal antibody targeting the C5 protein, has been clinically approved for use in patients with aHUS or PNH. Eculizumab reduces disease symptoms by inhibiting C5, leading to a decrease in sC5b-9 levels and decreased activity of both the classical and alternative pathways (CH50 and AH50). Several other agents targeting C5 through inhibition with peptides or monoclonal antibodies, knockdown of gene expression with silencing RNA (siRNA), and blocking the C5aR are under development.

SUMMARY

- The complement system is a series of more than 50 soluble and cell-bound proteins that interact with the innate and adaptive immune systems to enhance host defenses against infection.
- Activities of complement include lysis of foreign or damaged cells, opsonization, increase in vascular permeability, and attraction of monocytes and macrophages to areas where they are needed. Thus, complement can influence the inflammatory state of the host.
- The classical complement pathway is triggered by IgG or IgM binding to the surface of pathogens. Nine major proteins (C1–C9) are involved in this pathway.
- Three distinct units are involved in the classical pathway. They are the recognition unit consisting of C1qrs; the activation unit consisting of C2, C4, and C3; and the MAC, consisting of C5, C6, C7, C8, and C9.
- The lectin pathway is activated by carbohydrates present in microbial cell walls and serves as an important link between the innate and adaptive immune responses. Proteins distinct to the lectin pathway include MBL, MASP-1, MASP-2, and MASP-3.
- The alternative pathway can be triggered by bacterial and fungal cell walls, yeast, viruses, tumor cells, and certain parasites. Factors unique to the alternative pathway include Factor B, Factor D, and properdin.
- The alternative pathway has an important role in amplifying activation that starts with the classical or lectin pathway.
- Complement activation that is clinically important usually involves more than one pathway.
- All three pathways terminate with formation of the MAC.
- Plasma protein regulators of the complement system play a very important role because, if uncontrolled, complement activation could have devastating systemic effects.
- Soluble regulators include C1-INH, C4BP, Factor H, Factor I, and S protein.
- Examples of cell-bound regulators are CR1, MCP, and DAF.
- Specific complement receptors found on host cells amplify the immune response by enhancing phagocytosis and stimulating other accessory cells. Some of these receptors include CR1, CR2, CR3, CR4, and collectin receptors.
- Effector molecules generated during complement activation play a major role in the inflammation, recognition and presentation of antigens, activation of B cells, and maintenance of immunologic memory. They are classified as anaphylatoxins, chemotaxins, and opsonins.
- Anaphylatoxins (C3a, C5a) increase vascular permeability, whereas chemotaxins (C5a) attract phagocytic cells to a specific area, and opsonins (C3b, C4b, iC3b, C3dg) coat damaged or foreign cells to enhance phagocytosis.
- Deficiencies of complement components can place an individual at risk for certain infections.
- Missing or deficient regulators are the cause of diseases such as PNH and HAE.
- Improper control of complement can lead to several diseases related to inflammation, such as aHUS, C3G, and age-related macular degeneration.
- The aHUS is a thrombotic microvascular disease that is rooted in improper control of the alternative pathway of complement caused by genetic mutations in the complement system.
- There are three main methods for testing classical pathway function: hemolytic CH50, automated liposomal CH50, and ELISA assays. The results of these assays may not agree when very low levels of complement are present.
- Complement proteins such as C3 and C4 are quantitated routinely using automated nephelometry or immunoturbidimetry assays.
- Complement levels may vary between different assays and laboratories, so it is important to compare results to the laboratory reference range.
- The hemolytic titration or CH50 assay is a measure of RBC lysis, the endpoint of complement activation in the classical pathway. The AH50 assay is a similar test for measuring the activity of the alternative pathway.

Study Guide: Biologic Functions of Selected Complement Activation Products

FUNCTION	DEFINITION	COMPLEMENT PRODUCTS INVOLVED
Membrane attack complex	Product generated in the terminal steps of complement activation that creates a pore in the membrane of the target cell, leading to cell lysis	C5b6789
Anaphylatoxin activity	Release of histamine from mast cells and basophils, producing increased vascular permeability and contraction of smooth muscle	C5a, C3a
Chemotaxis	Migration of WBCs toward the site of antigen concentration	C5a
Opsonization	Coating of an antigen to facilitate phagocytosis	C3b, C4b, iC3b, C3dg

CASE STUDIES

1. A 3-year-old child has a history of serious infections and is currently hospitalized with meningitis. The doctor suspects that he may have a complement deficiency and orders testing. The following results are obtained: decreased CH50, decreased AH50, and normal C4 and C3 levels.

Questions

a. What do the results indicate about the possible pathway(s) affected?
b. Which component(s) are likely to be lacking?
c. What follow-up testing would be recommended?

2. A 25-year-old female appeared at the local hospital's emergency department with symptoms of abdominal pain as well as severe vomiting and swelling of the legs and hands. She stated that she has had these symptoms on several previous occasions. After ruling out appendicitis, the physician ordered a battery of tests, including some for abnormalities of complement components. The following results were obtained: RBC and WBC count normal, total serum protein normal, CH50 decreased, alternative pathway function normal, C3 and C1q levels normal, and C4 and C2 levels decreased.

Questions

a. What symptoms led physicians to consider a possible complement abnormality?
b. What are possible reasons for a decrease in both C4 and C2? What information does the normal C1q add?
c. What other testing would confirm your suspicions?

REVIEW QUESTIONS

1. The classical complement pathway is activated primarily by
   a. most viruses.
   b. antigen–antibody complexes.
   c. fungal cell walls.
   d. mannose in bacterial cell walls.

2. Which of the following is characteristic of complement components?
   a. Normally present in serum
   b. Mainly synthesized by B cells
   c. Present as active enzymes
   d. Heat stable

3. All of the following are true of the recognition unit *except*
   a. it consists of C1q, C1r, and C1s.
   b. the subunits require calcium for binding together.
   c. binding occurs at the Fc region of antibody molecules.
   d. C1q becomes an active esterase.

4. Which of the following is referred to as *C3 convertase*?
   a. C1qrs
   b. C4bC2a
   c. C3bBb
   d. All of the above
   e. Only b and c

5. Mannose-binding protein in the lectin pathway is most similar to which classical pathway component?
   a. C3
   b. C1rs
   c. C1q
   d. C4

6. Which of the following describes the role of properdin in the alternative pathway?
   a. Stabilization of C3 convertase
   b. Conversion of B to Bb
   c. Inhibition of C3 convertase formation
   d. Binding and cleavage of Factor B

7. Which best characterizes the MAC?
   a. Each pathway uses different factors to form it.
   b. C5 through C9 are not added in any particular order.
   c. One MAC unit is sufficient to lyse any type of cell.
   d. C9 polymerizes to form the transmembrane channel.

8. All of the following represent functions of the complement system *except*
   a. decreased clearance of antigen–antibody complexes.
   b. lysis of foreign cells.
   c. increase in vascular permeability.
   d. migration of neutrophils to the tissues.

9. Which of the following are diseases associated with complement deficiencies or improper control?
   a. Age-related macular degeneration (AMD)
   b. Paroxysmal nocturnal hemoglobinuria (PNH)
   c. Atypical hemolytic uremic syndrome
   d. C3 glomerulopathy
   e. All of the above
   f. Only c and d

10. Which of the following is *not* true of the amplification loop in complement activation?
    a. Improper control can lead to disease.
    b. It can amplify activation that is initiated by the classical pathway.
    c. C3b is the product that is increased.
    d. Increasing amounts of C1qrs are produced.

11. Factor H acts by competing with which of the following for the same binding site?
    a. Factor B
    b. Factor D
    c. C3b
    d. Factor I

12. Which best describes the role of CR2 on cell membranes?
    a. Binds C1qrs to inactivate it
    b. Acts as co-receptor on B cells for antigen
    c. Increases clearance of immune complexes
    d. Binds particles opsonized with C3b

13. Which of the following would be expected to be true for the testing of a patient who is on a complement C5 inhibitor?
    a. Low CH50
    b. Low AH50
    c. High sC5b-9
    d. All of the above
    e. Only a and b

14. Which of the following best characterizes HUS?
    a. It is a common cause of renal failure in children.
    b. It never has neurological manifestations.
    c. It is associated with a high platelet count.
    d. It is associated with antibody to C3 convertase.

15. The CH50 test measures which of the following?
    a. Patient serum required to lyse 50% of sensitized sheep RBCs
    b. Functioning of both the classical and alternative pathways
    c. Genetic deficiencies of any of the complement components
    d. Functioning of the lectin pathway only

16. A decreased CH50 level and a normal AH50 level indicate which deficiency?
    a. Decrease in components in the lectin pathway only
    b. Decrease in components in the alternative pathway only
    c. Decrease in components of both classical and alternative pathways
    d. Decrease in components of the classical pathway only

17. Which best describes the role of an anaphylatoxin?
    a. Coats cells to increase phagocytosis
    b. Attracts WBCs to the area of antigen concentration
    c. Increases production of interleukin-1
    d. Increases permeability of blood vessels

18. Which of the following is *not* a cofactor for Factor I?
    a. Factor H
    b. C4-binding protein
    c. Membrane cofactor protein (MCP, CD46)
    d. C3bBbC3b

19. A lack of C1-INH has been associated with which of the following conditions?
    a. Paroxysmal nocturnal hemoglobinuria
    b. Hemolytic uremic syndrome
    c. Hereditary angioedema
    d. Increased bacterial infections

20. If a specimen for complement testing was left on a laboratory bench overnight and not properly frozen, which of the following would be true?
    a. A CH50 level would be falsely low.
    b. An AH50 level would be falsely high.
    c. A measure of C3a would be falsely low.
    d. A C3 level by nephelometry would be changed.

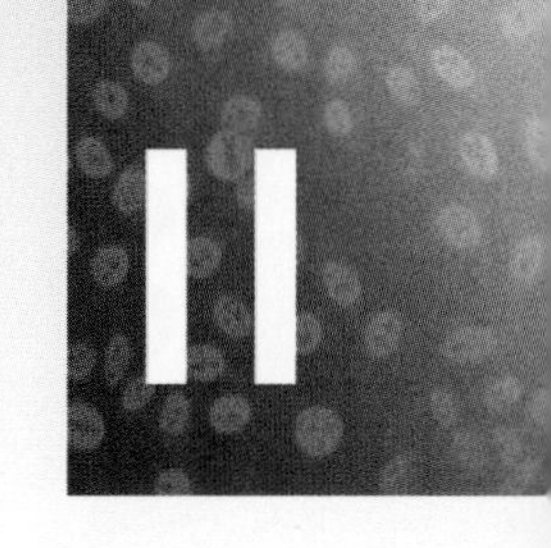

Basic Immunologic Procedures

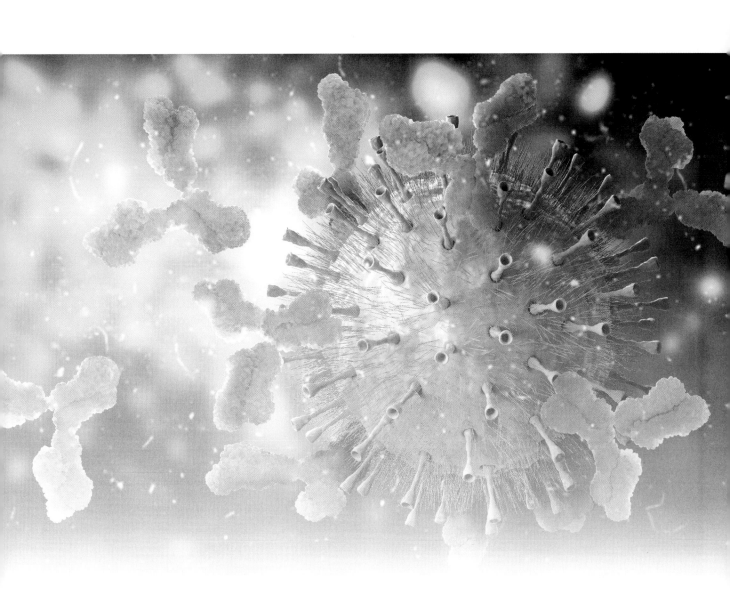

8 Safety and Quality Management

Marjorie Schaub Di Lorenzo, MT(ASCP)SH

LEARNING OUTCOMES

After finishing this chapter, you should be able to:

1. Define and give an example of the types of safety hazards encountered in the laboratory.
2. Describe the six components of the chain of infection and the safety precautions that will break the chain.
3. Correctly perform hand hygiene procedures following Centers for Disease Control and Prevention (CDC) guidelines.
4. Describe the types of personal protective equipment (PPE) used by laboratory personnel.
5. Define Standard Precautions (SPs) and state their purpose.
6. State the acceptable procedures for disposal, decontamination, and spill control of biological waste in the laboratory.
7. Discuss the federal regulations and guidelines for preparing and shipping patient samples from the laboratory.
8. Explain the requirements mandated by the Occupational Exposure to Bloodborne Pathogens compliance directive.
9. Discuss the purpose of a Chemical Hygiene Plan, the information contained in a Safety Data Sheet (SDS), and the use of the Globally Harmonized System (GHS).
10. Describe precautions that laboratory personnel should take when radioactive, electrical, fire, and physical hazards are encountered.
11. Explain the RACE (Rescue, Alarm, Contain, Extinguish or Evacuate) and PASS (Pull, Aim, Squeeze, Sweep) actions to be taken when a fire is discovered.
12. State and interpret the components of the National Fire Protection Association (NFPA) hazardous material labeling system.
13. Define the preexamination (preanalytical), examination (analytical), and postexamination (postanalytical) components of quality management (QM).
14. Distinguish between the components of internal, external, and electronic quality control (QC), and external quality assessment (EQA; proficiency testing).

CHAPTER OUTLINE

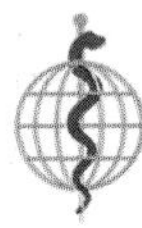

Go to FADavis.com for the laboratory exercises that accompany this text.

15. Discuss the roles of the Clinical Laboratory Improvement Amendments (CLIA), Clinical and Laboratory Standards Institute (CLSI), The Joint Commission (TJC), and the College of American Pathologists (CAP) in the regulation of health care.
16. State and describe the 12 quality system essentials (QSEs) used in a quality management system (QMS).
17. Describe the purpose of quality indicators.
18. List the six areas of the Lean system and describe how it can benefit the laboratory.
19. State the purpose of the Six Sigma methodology in a QMS.
20. Demonstrate knowledge of root cause analysis (RCA) as it relates to laboratory testing.

KEY TERMS

Accuracy
Biohazard
Biohazardous materials
Bloodborne pathogens (BBPs)
Chain of infection
Chemical Hygiene Plan
Clinical and Laboratory Standards Institute (CLSI)
Clinical Laboratory Improvement Amendments (CLIA)
Coefficient of variation (CV)
Control mean
Delta check
Examination variables
External quality assessment (EQA)
Fomite
Globally Harmonized System (GHS)
Infection control
The Joint Commission (TJC)
Lean system
Occupational Safety and Health Administration (OSHA)
Personal protective equipment (PPE)
Postexamination variables
Postexposure prophylaxis (PEP)
Precision
Preexamination variables
Proficiency testing
Quality control (QC)
Quality indicators
Quality management (QM)
Quality management system (QMS)
Quality system essentials (QSEs)
Reliability
Root cause analysis (RCA)
Safety Data Sheet (SDS)
Shift
Six Sigma
Standard of care
Standard deviation (SD)
Standard Precautions (SPs)
Trend
Turnaround time (TAT)
Variable

Laboratory Hazards

The clinical laboratory contains a wide variety of safety hazards, many capable of producing serious injury or life-threatening disease. To work safely in this environment, clinical laboratorians must learn what hazards exist and the basic safety precautions associated with them. They must apply the basic rules of common sense required for everyday safety. Some hazards are unique to the health-care environment, and others are encountered routinely throughout life **(Table 8–1)**. It is essential that laboratory personnel know where all safety equipment is located and be trained in all aspects of its use on a yearly basis.

Biological Hazards

In the immunology laboratory, the most significant hazard exists in obtaining and testing patient specimens. Understanding how microorganisms are transmitted **(chain of infection)** is necessary to prevent infection. The chain of infection requires a continuous link between six elements: an infectious agent, a reservoir, a portal of exit, a means of transmission, a portal of entry, and a susceptible host.

Chain of Infection Elements

Infectious Agents (Pathogens). Infectious agents consist of bacteria, fungi, parasites, and viruses. The chain can be broken by early detection and treatment of infections to reduce the opportunity for growth of pathogens.
Reservoir. A reservoir is a place where the infectious agent can live and multiply, such as a contaminated clinical specimen or an infected patient. Humans and animals (hosts) or contaminated inanimate objects **(fomites)** that contain blood, urine, or other body fluids make ideal reservoirs. Disinfecting the work area kills the infectious agent and eliminates the reservoir, thereby breaking the chain.

Table 8–1 Types of Safety Hazards

TYPE	SOURCE	POSSIBLE INJURY
Biological	Infectious agents	Bacterial, fungal, viral, or parasitic infections
Sharp	Needles, lancets, and broken glass	Cuts, punctures, or bloodborne pathogen (BBP) exposure
Chemical	Preservatives and reagents	Exposure to toxic, carcinogenic, or caustic agents
Radioactive	Equipment and radioisotopes	Damage to a fetus or generalized overexposure to radiation
Electrical	Ungrounded or wet equipment and frayed cords	Burns or shock
Fire or explosive	Open flames and organic chemicals	Burns or dismemberment
Physical	Wet floors, heavy boxes, and patients	Falls, sprains, or strains

Portal of Exit. The infectious agent leaves the reservoir through a portal of exit, such as through the nose, mouth, and mucous membranes, as well as in the blood or other body fluids, and is transmitted to a susceptible source to continue the chain of infection. The chain is broken when contaminated materials are placed in biohazard containers and by keeping tubes and specimen containers sealed. When contaminated materials are in the appropriate containers that remain sealed, the infectious agent still has a reservoir but no means of exit.

Means of Transmission. An infectious agent that has left the reservoir must have a way to reach a susceptible host. Means of transmission include:

- Direct contact (the unprotected host touches the patient, specimen, or a contaminated object)
- Droplet (the host inhales infected aerosol droplets from a patient or specimen)
- Airborne (the host inhales dried aerosol particles circulating on the air currents or dust particles)
- Vehicle (the host ingests contaminated food or water)
- Vector (from an animal or mosquito bite)

Hand sanitizing and adhering to **Standard Precautions (SPs)** are methods to break the chain.

Portal of Entry. The infectious agent now must enter a new reservoir through a portal of entry, which can be the same as the portal of exit. Reservoirs include mucous membranes of the nose, mouth, and eyes; breaks in the skin; and open wounds to complete the chain of infection. Disinfection, sterilization, and strict adherence to SPs block the portal of entry, thus breaking the chain.

Susceptible Host. Possible sources of infection include other patients, health-care personnel, or visitors. Patients receiving chemotherapy, the elderly, and immunocompromised patients are susceptible hosts. The immune system is still developing in newborns and infants and begins to weaken as people age, making these groups of patients more susceptible to infection. The immune system also is depressed by stress, fatigue, and lack of proper nutrition, which contribute to the susceptibility of patients and health-care personnel. Once the chain of infection is complete, the infected host then becomes another source able to transmit the microorganisms to others. To break the chain, health-care personnel must stay current with required immunizations, be tested for immunity, and maintain a healthy lifestyle.

The most likely source of infection in serological testing is through contact with patient specimens; the main concern is exposure to viruses such as the hepatitis viruses and HIV. Therefore, safety precautions are designed to protect health-care workers from exposure to potentially harmful infectious agents. The ultimate goal of biological safety is to prevent completion of the chain by preventing transmission. The **infection control** team develops procedures to control and monitor infections occurring within health-care facilities. **Figure 8–1** contains the universal symbol for **biohazardous material** and illustrates the chain of infection and how it can be broken by following safety practices.

Preventing transmission of microorganisms from infected sources to susceptible hosts is critical in controlling the spread of infection. Procedures used to prevent microorganism transmission include hand hygiene, wearing **personal protective equipment (PPE)**, isolating highly infective or highly susceptible patients, and properly disposing of contaminated materials. Strict adherence to guidelines published by the Centers for Disease Control and Prevention (CDC) and the **Occupational Safety and Health Administration (OSHA)** is essential.

Hand Hygiene

Hand contact represents the number-one method of infection transmission. Hands should always be sanitized before patient contact; after gloves are removed; before leaving the work area; whenever the hands have been knowingly contaminated; before going to designated break areas; before and after using bathroom facilities; and after blowing your nose, coughing, or sneezing. Hand hygiene includes both hand washing and using alcohol-based antiseptic cleansers. Alcohol-based cleansers are not recommended after contact with spore-forming bacteria, including *Clostridium difficile* and *Bacillus* sp.

The CDC's guidelines for the correct hand-washing technique are pictured in **Figure 8–2.** If using alcohol-based cleansers, apply the cleanser to the palm of one hand. Rub your hands together and over the entire cleansing area,

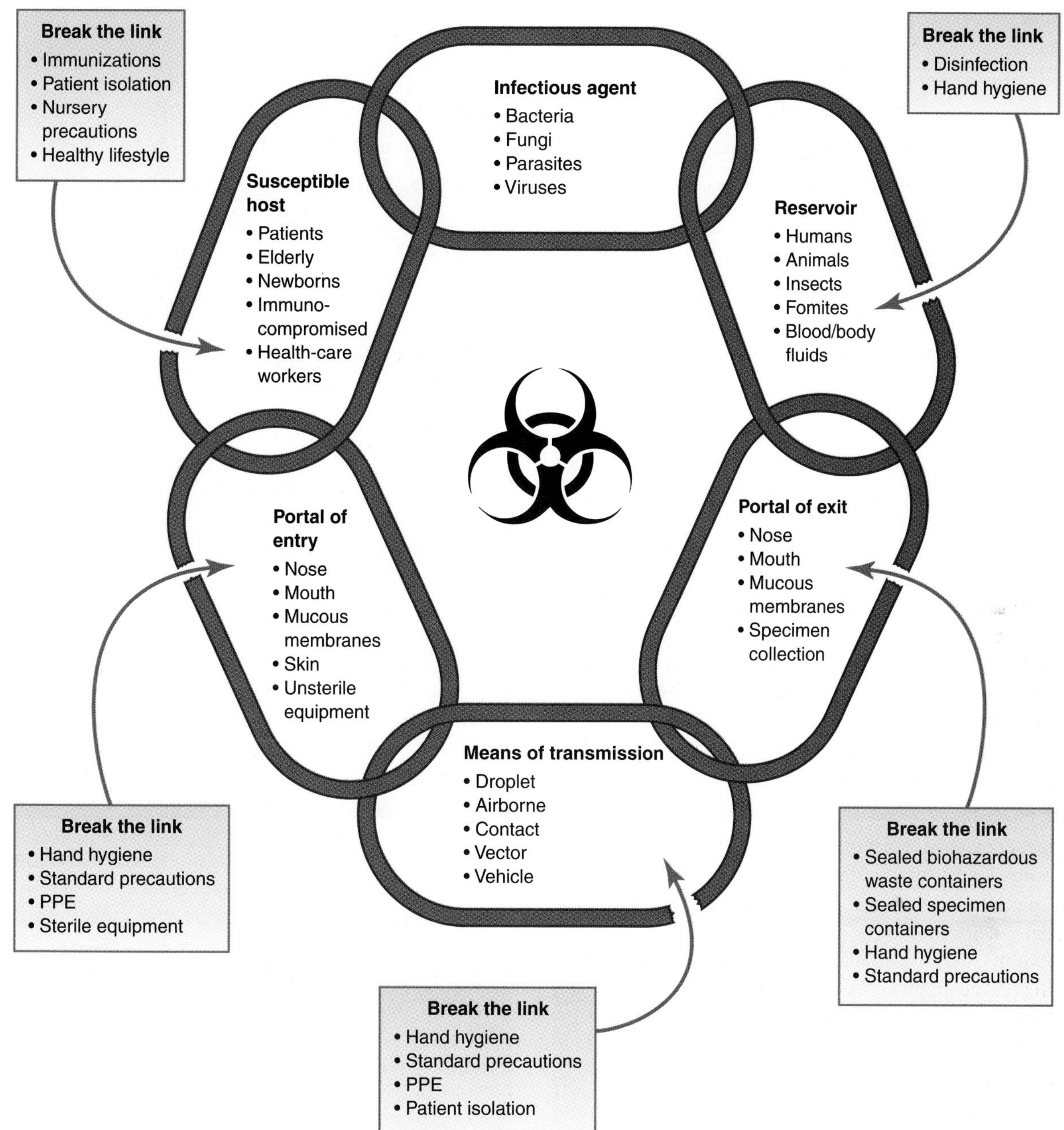

FIGURE 8–1 Chain of infection and safety practices related to the biohazard symbol. *(From Strasinger SK, DiLorenzo MS.* The Phlebotomy Textbook. *4th ed. Philadelphia, PA: F.A. Davis, Philadelphia; 2018, with permission.)*

including between the fingers and thumbs. Continue rubbing until the alcohol dries.

Personal Protective Equipment (PPE)

PPE used by laboratorians includes gloves, gowns or laboratory coats, masks, goggles, face shields, and Plexiglas countertop shields.

Gloves. Gloves are worn to protect the health-care worker's hands from contamination by patient body substances and to protect the patient from possible microorganisms on the health-care worker's hands. Gloves must be worn when working with patients, when processing specimens and performing testing procedures, and when cleaning equipment and work areas. However, wearing gloves is not a substitute for hand sanitizing. Hands must always be sanitized when gloves are removed. Gloves used in the laboratory should be removed when noticeably contaminated or damaged and before leaving the laboratory. A variety of gloves are available, including sterile and nonsterile, powdered and unpowdered, and latex and nonlatex.

In the immunology laboratory, fluid-resistant laboratory coats with wrist cuffs are worn at all times to protect skin and clothing from contamination by patient specimens. They must be completely buttoned, with the gloves pulled over the cuffs. Both gloves and laboratory coats should be changed as soon as possible if they become visibly soiled and must be removed when leaving the laboratory.

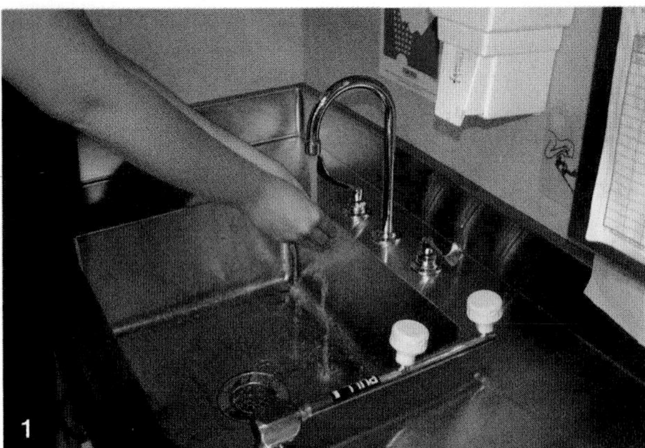
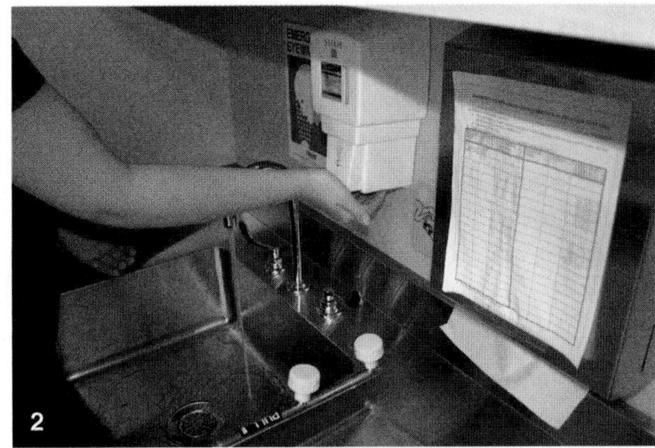
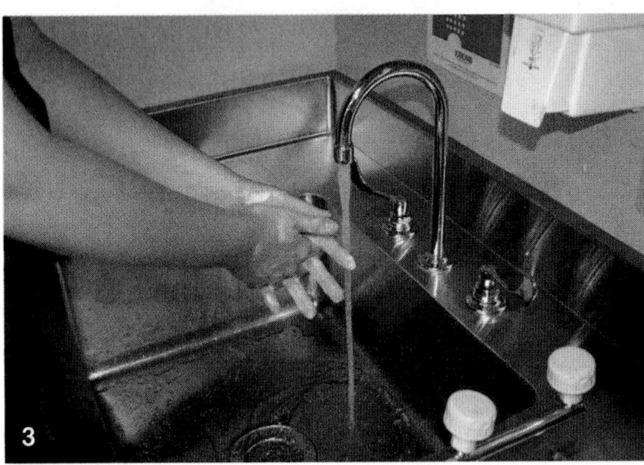
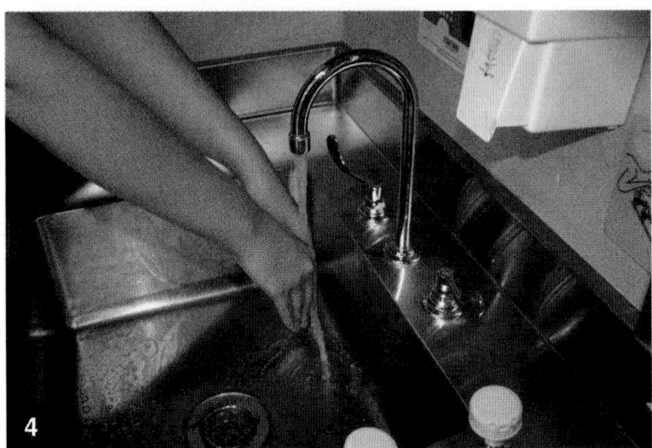
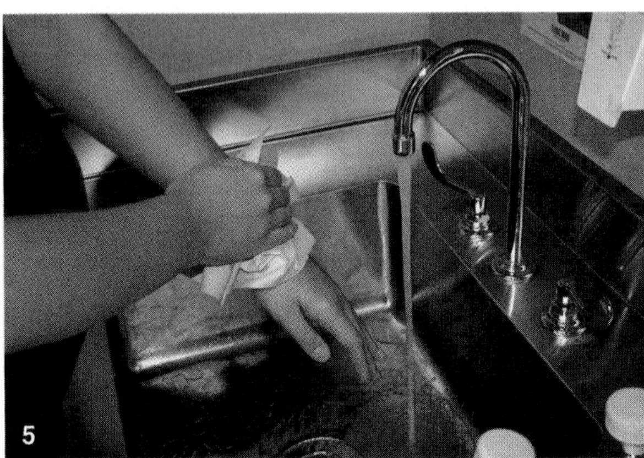
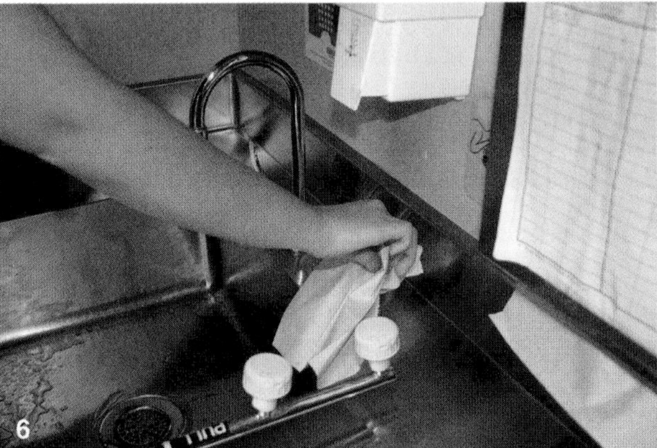

FIGURE 8–2 Hand hygiene. *(From Strasinger SK, DiLorenzo MS.* Urinalysis and Body Fluids. *6th ed. Philadelphia, PA: F.A. Davis; 2014, with permission.)*

1. Remove jewelry. Wet hands with warm water. Do not allow any part of the body to touch the sink.
2. Apply soap, preferably antimicrobial.
3. Rub to form a lather, create friction, and loosen debris. Thoroughly clean between the fingers and under the fingernails for at least 20 seconds; include thumbs and wrists in the cleaning.
4. Rinse hands in a downward position to prevent recontamination of hands and wrists.
5. Dry hands with a paper towel.
6. Turn off the faucets with a clean paper towel to prevent contamination.

Connections

Latex Allergy
Laboratory Coats

Allergy to latex is decreasing among health-care workers because of the availability of other types of gloves. However, laboratorians should be alert for symptoms of reactions associated with latex contact, including irritant contact dermatitis that produces patches of dry, itchy irritation on the hands; delayed hypersensitivity reactions resembling poison ivy that appear 24 to 48 hours following exposure; and true immediate hypersensitivity reactions often characterized by facial flushing and respiratory difficulty (see Chapter 14). Hand sanitizing immediately after removal of gloves and avoiding powdered gloves may aid in preventing the development of latex allergy. Any signs of a latex reaction should be reported to a supervisor because a true latex allergy can be life-threatening.

Masks, Goggles, and Face Shields. The mucous membranes of the eyes, nose, and mouth must be protected from specimen splashes and aerosols. A variety of protective equipment is available, including goggles, full-face plastic shields, and Plexiglas countertop shields **(Fig. 8–3)**. To avoid splashes and aerosols, remove specimen caps under a Plexiglas shield or with gauze. Transfer pipettes should be used when aliquoting samples from a specimen container. Never centrifuge specimens in uncapped tubes or in uncovered centrifuges. When specimens are received in containers with contaminated exteriors, the exterior of the container must be disinfected; if necessary, a new specimen may be requested.

Standard Precautions

The CDC developed SPs by combining recommendations of Universal Precautions (UPs) and Body Substance Isolation (BSI) procedures. Under UPs, all patients were assumed to be potential carriers of **bloodborne pathogens (BBPs)**. The BSI modified UPs by requiring that gloves be worn when encountering blood or any other body substance. The CDC continually modifies SPs as changes occur in the health-care environment. SPs assume every person in the health-care setting is potentially infected or colonized by an organism that could be transmitted. SPs apply to blood, all body fluids, mucous membranes, and nonintact skin and emphasize hand washing.

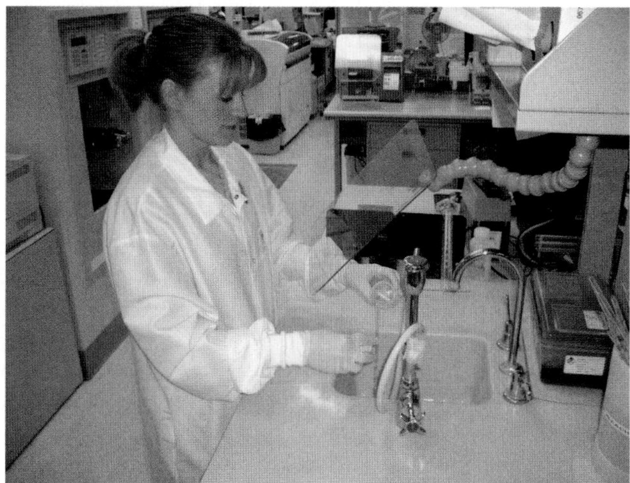

FIGURE 8–3 PPE using a plastic shield. *(From Strasinger SK, DiLorenzo MS. Urinalysis and Body Fluids. 6th ed. Philadelphia, PA: F.A. Davis; 2014, with permission.)*

SPs that apply directly to the laboratory are as follows:

- *Hand hygiene*—Hand hygiene includes both hand washing and the use of alcohol-based antiseptic cleansers. Sanitize hands after touching blood, body fluids, secretions, excretions, and contaminated items, whether or not gloves are worn. Sanitize hands immediately after gloves are removed, between patient contacts, and when otherwise indicated to avoid transfer of microorganisms to other environments.
- *Gloves*—Wear gloves (clean, nonsterile gloves are adequate) when touching blood, body fluids, secretions, excretions, and contaminated items. Remove gloves promptly after use, before touching noncontaminated items and environmental surfaces, and before going to another patient. Sanitize hands immediately to avoid transfer of microorganisms to other patients or environments.
- *Mask, nose, and eye protection*—Wear a mask and eye protection or a face shield to protect mucous membranes of the eyes, nose, and mouth during procedures and patient-care activities that are likely to generate splashes or sprays of blood, body fluids, secretions, and excretions.
- *Gown*—Wear a gown (a clean, nonsterile gown is adequate) to protect skin and to prevent soiling of clothing during procedures that are likely to generate splashes of blood, body fluids, secretions, or excretions. Select a gown that is appropriate for the activity and amount of fluid likely to be encountered (e.g., fluid-resistant in the laboratory). Remove a soiled gown before leaving the laboratory environment and sanitize hands to avoid transfer of microorganisms to other environments.
- *Respiratory hygiene and cough etiquette*—Educate health-care personnel, patients, and visitors to contain respiratory secretions to prevent droplet and fomite transmission of respiratory pathogens. Offer masks to coughing patients, distance symptomatic patients from others, and practice good hand hygiene to prevent the transmission of respiratory pathogens.
- *Needles*—Never recap used needles or otherwise manipulate them using both hands; in addition, never use any technique that involves directing the point of a needle toward any part of the body; rather, use self-sheathing needles or a mechanical device designed to conceal the needle. Do not remove unsheathed needles from disposable syringes by hand; use a mechanical device. Do not bend, break, or otherwise manipulate used needles by hand. Place used disposable syringes and needles, scalpel blades, and other sharp items in appropriate puncture-resistant containers. Place reusable syringes and needles

in a puncture-resistant container for transport to the reprocessing area. (See *Sharps Hazards* later for additional information.)

Occupational Exposure to Bloodborne Pathogens

The federal government has enacted regulations to protect health-care workers from exposure to BBPs. These regulations are monitored and enforced by OSHA. The Occupational Exposure to Bloodborne Pathogens Standard requires all employers to have a written Bloodborne Pathogen Exposure Control Plan and to provide necessary protection, free of charge, for employees. A later compliance directive called *Enforcement Procedures for the Occupational Exposure to Bloodborne Pathogens Standard* placed more emphasis on using engineering controls to prevent accidental exposure to BBPs. The components of the current Bloodborne Pathogens Exposure Control Plan that is required of all institutions are shown in the *In the Laboratory: Components of the OSHA Bloodborne Pathogen Exposure Control Plan* Box. Each health-care institution is responsible for designing and implementing its own exposure control plan.

Any accidental exposure to blood through needlestick, mucous membranes, or nonintact skin must be reported to a supervisor, and a confidential medical examination must be immediately started. Evaluation of the incident must begin right away to ensure that appropriate **postexposure prophylaxis (PEP)** is initiated within 24 hours. Needlesticks are the most frequently encountered exposure and place the laboratorian in danger of contracting HIV, hepatitis B virus (HBV), and hepatitis C virus (HCV). The CDC has recommended procedures to prevent these infections (see *In the Laboratory: Postexposure Prophylaxis* Box).

In the Laboratory

Components of the OSHA Bloodborne Pathogen Exposure Control Plan

Engineering Controls

1. Providing sharps disposal containers and needles with safety devices
2. Requiring discarding of needles with the safety device activated and the holder attached
3. Labeling all biohazardous materials and containers

Work Practice Controls

4. Requiring all employees to practice SPs
5. Prohibiting eating, drinking, smoking, and applying cosmetics in the work area
6. Establishing a daily work surface disinfection protocol

Personal Protective Equipment

7. Providing laboratory coats, gowns, face shields, and gloves to employees and laundry facilities for nondisposable protective clothing

Medical

8. Providing immunization for the hepatitis B virus free of charge
9. Providing medical follow-up to employees who have been accidentally exposed to a BBPs

Documentation

10. Documenting annual training of employees in safety standards
11. Documenting evaluations and implementation of safer needle devices
12. Involving employees in the selection and evaluation of new devices and maintaining a list of those employees and the evaluations
13. Maintaining a sharps injury log, including the type and brand of safety device, location and description of the incident, and confidential employee follow-up

From Strasinger SK, DiLorenzo MA. *The Phlebotomy Textbook.* 4th ed. Philadelphia, PA: F.A. Davis; 2018, with permission.

Biological Waste Disposal

All biological waste, except urine, must be placed in appropriate leakproof containers labeled with the **biohazard** symbol and decontaminated, usually by incineration, before disposal. This waste includes not only specimens but also the materials with which the specimens come in contact. Any supplies contaminated with blood and body fluids must also be disposed of in containers clearly marked with the biohazard symbol or with red or yellow color coding. These supplies include alcohol pads, gauze, bandages, disposable tourniquets, gloves, masks, gowns, and plastic tubes and pipettes. Urine can be discarded down the sink. The sink should be rinsed well with water and cleaned daily with a 1:10 sodium hypochlorite solution (bleach). Disposal of needles and other sharp objects is discussed in the section on sharps hazards.

Decontamination

Contaminated nondisposable equipment, blood spills, and blood and body-fluid processing areas must be disinfected regularly. Lab benches should be disinfected after every work shift and after any spill occurs. The CDC recommends the use of a 1:10 dilution of sodium hypochlorite (household bleach) prepared weekly and stored in a plastic, not glass, bottle. Other products are commercially available both in prefilled spray bottles or single-use wipes. However, one should confirm that the product is effective enough to eliminate most bacteria, including *Mycobacterium tuberculosis,* fungi, and viruses. It is also important to know the contact time needed for disinfectant chemical products to work effectively on laboratory surfaces as prescribed by the manufacturer.

When spills occur, do not mop or wipe the fluid; instead, use absorbent powder (e.g., Zorbitrol) or paper towels to remove as much fluid as possible before disinfecting. When using an absorbent powder, the liquid will solidify and can be scooped up. If paper towels are used to absorb the liquid, pour bleach over the towels. Dispose of the absorbent material and paper towels used for disinfection in the appropriate biohazard container. Disinfect the spill area with bleach or a phenol solution.

Contaminated nondisposable equipment, blood spills, and blood and body-fluid processing areas must be disinfected. The most commonly used disinfectant is a 1:10 dilution of

In the Laboratory

Postexposure Prophylaxis (PEP)

1. Draw a baseline blood specimen from the employee and test it for HBV, HCV, and HIV.
2. If possible, identify the source patient; collect a blood specimen; and test it for HBV, HCV, and HIV. Patients must usually give informed consent for these tests, and they do not become part of the patient's record. In some states, a physician's order or court order can replace patient consent because a needlestick is considered a significant exposure.
3. Testing must be completed within 24 hours for maximum benefit from PEP.

Source Patient Tests Positive for HIV

1. Employee is counseled about receiving PEP using anti-retroviral medications.
2. Medications are started within 72 hours.
3. Employee is retested at intervals of 6 weeks, 12 weeks, and 6 months.
4. Additional evaluation and counseling is needed if the source patient is unidentified or untested.

Source Patient Tests Positive for HBV

1. Unvaccinated employees can be given hepatitis B immune globulin (HBIG) and HBV vaccine.
2. Vaccinated employees are tested for immunity and receive PEP, if necessary.

Source Patient Tests Positive for HCV

1. No PEP is available.
2. Employee is monitored for early detection of HCV infection and treated appropriately.

Any exposed employee should be counseled to report any symptoms related to viral infection that occur within 12 weeks of the exposure.

From Strasinger SK, DiLorenzo MA. *The Phlebotomy Textbook*. 4th ed. Philadelphia, PA: F.A. Davis; 2018, with permission.

sodium hypochlorite (household bleach) prepared daily and stored in a plastic bottle. The bleach should be allowed to air-dry on the contaminated area before being wiped off.

Transporting Patient Specimens

If a laboratory accepts specimens from other health-care institutions, then it is important to know the regulations for packaging, transporting, and receiving these specimens. The U.S. Department of Transportation (DOT), the International Air Transport Association (IATA), and the United Nations (UN) have stringent regulations that must be followed if a laboratory is going to be involved in transporting or receiving patient specimens from another institution.

DOT and IATA Specimen Transport. Under DOT and IATA regulations, all diagnostic specimens require triple packaging **(Fig. 8–4)**. This includes the following:

- The primary container (glass, metal, or plastic) must be watertight with a positive (screw-on) cap.
- The primary container must be wrapped with enough absorbent material to be capable of absorbing all its contents. Multiple specimens must be wrapped individually before placing them in the leakproof secondary container.
- The secondary container must be placed in a sturdy outer container made of corrugated fiberboard, wood, metal, or rigid plastic. An itemized list of contents in a sealed plastic bag is also placed in the outer container. Ice packs are placed between the secondary and the outer container. Additional measures must be taken when using ice and dry ice.

Courier-Delivered Specimen Transport. Specimens transported by a hospital courier among clinics, physicians' offices, and the hospital laboratory are exempt from most DOT rules, unless they are suspected of containing an infectious substance. If specimens may contain an infectious substance, then all DOT rules apply. The transport vehicle should be used exclusively for transport of specimens and should be equipped to secure the transport containers. Minimum shipping standards for this type of transportation include:

- Leakproof, watertight specimen containers
- Tightly capped tubes placed in a rack to maintain an upright position
- Leakproof inner packaging surrounded by enough absorbent material to completely absorb all the liquid present
- A leakproof plastic or metal transport box with a secure, tight-fitting cover
- Properly labeled transport boxes accompanied by specimen data and identification forms

Specimens picked up by a courier that are to be shipped to an out-of-the-area laboratory, such as a reference laboratory, must follow DOT regulations. Many of these laboratories supply shipping containers to their clients.

Sharps Hazards

Sharp objects in the laboratory, including needles, lancets, and broken glassware, present a serious biological hazard for possible exposure to BBPs caused by accidental puncture. Although BBPs are also transmitted through contact with mucous membranes and nonintact skin, a needle or lancet used to collect blood has the capability to produce a very significant exposure to BBPs. It is essential that safety precautions be followed at all times when sharp hazards are present.

The number-one personal safety rule when handling needles is to *never* recap a needle. Many safety devices are available for needle disposal that provide a variety of safeguards. These include needle holders that become a sheath, needles that automatically resheath or become blunt, and needles with attached sheaths. All sharps must be disposed of in puncture-resistant, leakproof containers labeled with the biohazard symbol **(Fig. 8–5)**. Containers should be located in close proximity to the work area and must always be replaced when the safe capacity mark is reached. Never use any technique that involves directing the point of a needle toward any part of the body.

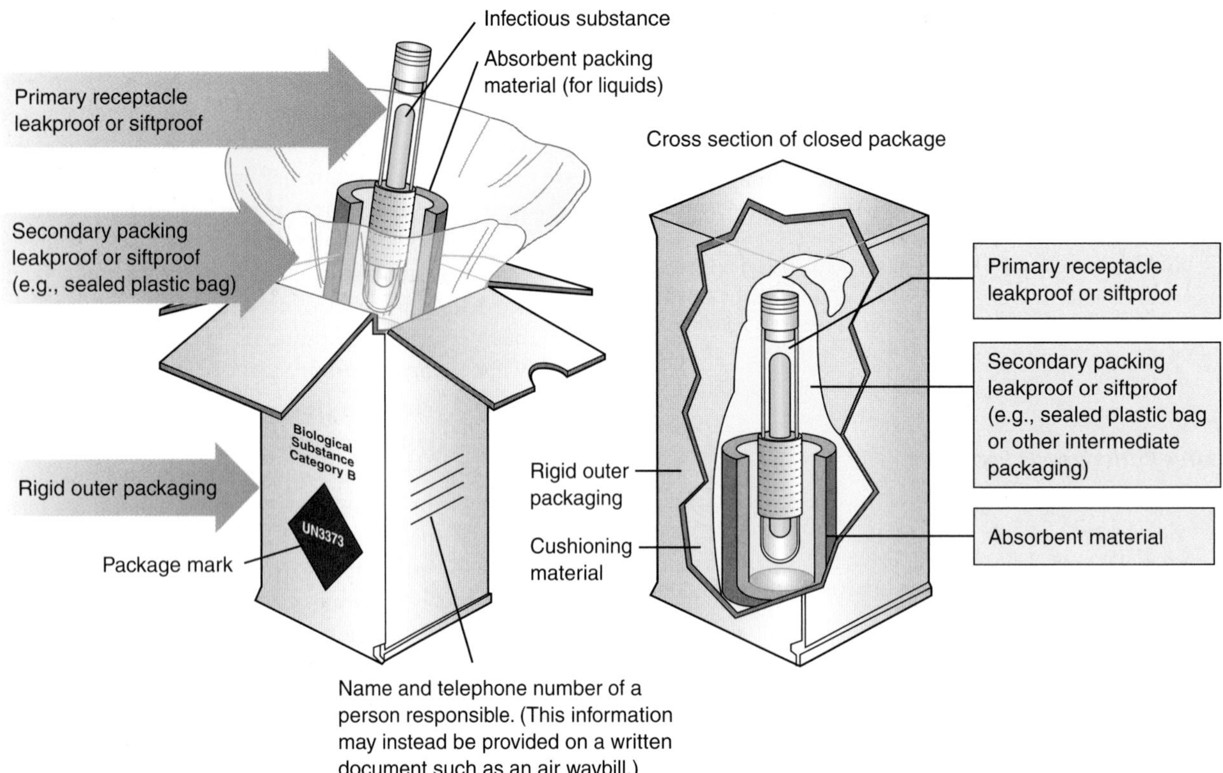

FIGURE 8–4 Packing and labeling of category B infectious substances. If multiple fragile primary receptacles are placed in a single secondary package, they must be either individually wrapped or separated to prevent contact. *(Adapted from Transporting Infectious Substances Safely, U.S. Department of Transportation. Pipeline and Hazardous Materials Safety Administration, 2006.)*

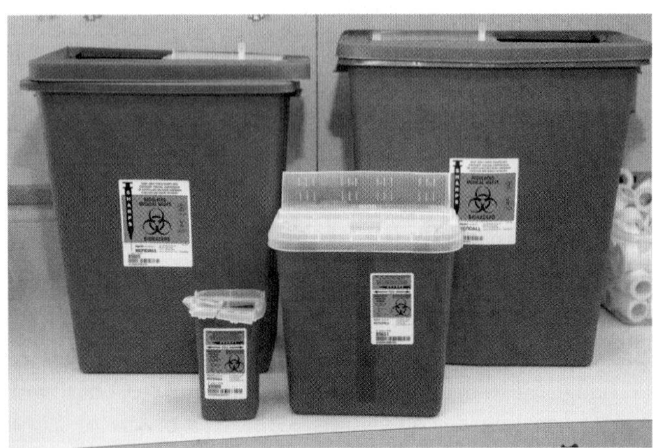

FIGURE 8–5 Examples of puncture-resistant containers. *(From Strasinger SK, DiLorenzo MS.* The Phlebotomy Textbook. *4th ed. Philadelphia, PA: F.A. Davis; 2018, with permission.)*

The Needlestick Safety and Prevention Act was signed into law in 2001. In June 2002, OSHA issued a revision to the Bloodborne Pathogens Standard compliance directive mentioned previously. In the revised directive, the agency requires that all blood holders with needles attached be immediately discarded into a sharps container after the device's safety feature is activated. The rationale for the new directive was based on the exposure of workers to the unprotected stopper-puncturing end of evacuated tube needles, the increased needle manipulation required to remove it from the holder, and the possible worker exposure from the use of contaminated holders.

Chemical Hazards

Serological testing may involve the use of chemical reagents that must be handled in a safe manner to avoid injury. The general rules for safe handling of chemicals include taking precautions to avoid getting chemicals on the body, clothes, and work area; wearing PPE such as safety goggles when pouring chemicals; observing strict labeling practices; and following instructions carefully. Preparing reagents under a fume hood is also a recommended safety precaution. Chemicals should never be mixed together unless specific instructions are followed; in addition, they must be added in the order specified. This is particularly important when combining acid and water because acid should always be added to water, rather than adding water to acid, to avoid the possibility of sudden splashing.

When skin or eye contact occurs, the best first aid is to immediately flush the area with water for at least 15 minutes and then seek medical attention. Laboratorians must know the location of the emergency shower and eyewash station in the laboratory. Do not try to neutralize chemicals spilled on the skin.

Safety Data Sheets (SDS)

All chemicals and reagents containing hazardous ingredients in a concentration greater than 1% are required by OSHA to have a **Safety Data Sheet (SDS)** on file in the work area. By law, vendors must provide these sheets to purchasers; however, it is the responsibility of the facility to obtain and keep them available to employees. An SDS contains information on physical and chemical characteristics, fire, explosion reactivity, health hazards, primary routes of entry, exposure limits and carcinogenic potential, precautions for safe handling, spill cleanup, and emergency first aid. State and federal regulations should be consulted for the disposal of chemicals. Containers of chemicals that pose a high risk must be labeled with a chemical hazard symbol representing the possible hazard, such as flammable, poison, corrosive, and so on **(Fig. 8–6).**

FIGURE 8–6 Chemical hazard symbols. *(From Strasinger SK, DiLorenzo MS.* The Phlebotomy Textbook. *4th ed. Philadelphia, PA: F.A. Davis; 2018, with permission.)*

The Globally Harmonized System (GHS) of Classification and Labeling of Chemicals

The **Globally Harmonized System (GHS)** is an international effort to standardize both the classification of hazardous chemicals and the symbols used to communicate these hazards on labels and in SDS documentation. It includes criteria for the classification of health, physical, and environmental hazards. The standard label elements include GHS pictograms, signal words, and a GHS hazard statement. The SDS under GHS provides a clear description of the data used to identify hazards and has 16 sections in a specified order **(Fig. 8–7).**

OSHA aligned its Hazard Communication Standard with the GHS and requires that all employees be trained on the new label elements and SDS format. The adoption of the GHS in the United States has increased awareness and understanding of hazards in the workplace.

Chemical Hygiene Plan

OSHA requires that all facilities that use hazardous chemicals have a written **Chemical Hygiene Plan** available to employees. The purpose of the plan is to detail the following:

- Individual chemical hygiene responsibilities
- Standard operating procedures

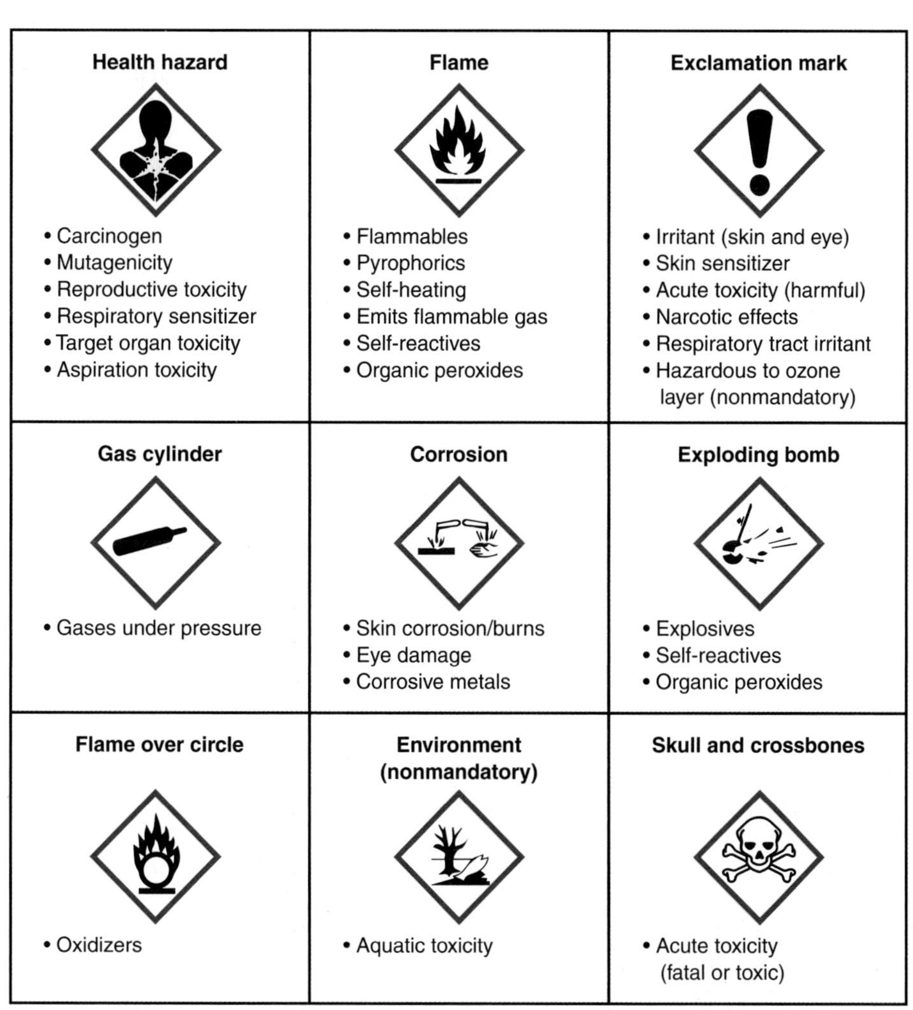

FIGURE 8–7 GHS pictograms and hazards chart. *(Courtesy of U.S. Department of Labor.)*

- PPE and apparel
- Engineering controls, such as fume hoods and safety cabinets
- Laboratory equipment
- Safety equipment
- Chemical management
- Housekeeping
- Emergency procedures for accidents and spills
- Chemical waste
- Employee training
- Safety rules and regulations
- Laboratory design and ventilation
- Exposure monitoring
- Compressed gas safety
- Medical consultation and examination

Each facility must appoint a chemical hygiene officer who is responsible for implementing and documenting compliance with the plan.

Chemical Spills

The SDS gives specific information for the appropriate action to be taken for a chemical spill. A chemical spill kit must be available in every laboratory and contains appropriate PPE (gloves and goggles), absorbent pads, disposable bags, and waste tags. Liquids are absorbed using a neutralizer, such as a sodium bicarbonate and sand mixture, or ground clay. After the liquid is absorbed, it is scooped up and placed into a waste bag and labeled appropriately for disposal. The area is then cleaned.

Chemical Waste Disposal

Any hazardous chemical waste should be disposed of per current Environmental Protection Agency (EPA) regulations. Most reagents used in the laboratory come with an SDS, mentioned previously. The SDS gives specific information for disposal of particular chemicals. All chemicals used should be disposed of by following SDS directions. Many kits used in immunologic testing often contain sodium azide as a preservative, which can be disposed of by flushing it down the drain with plenty of water. Using large amounts of water helps to avoid buildup in plumbing.

Radioactive Hazards

Laboratorians can be exposed to radioactivity when performing procedures using radioisotopes, such as radioimmunoassay. The amount of radioactivity present in most medical situations is very small and represents little danger. However, the effects of radiation are related to the length of exposure and are cumulative. Exposure to radiation is dependent on the combination of time, distance, and shielding. Persons working in a radioactive environment are required to wear measuring devices to determine the amount of radiation they are accumulating.

Laboratorians should be familiar with the radioactive symbol shown in **Figure 8–8.** This symbol must be displayed on the doors of all areas where radioactive material is present. Exposure to radiation during pregnancy presents a danger to the fetus; personnel who are or who think they may be pregnant should avoid areas with this symbol.

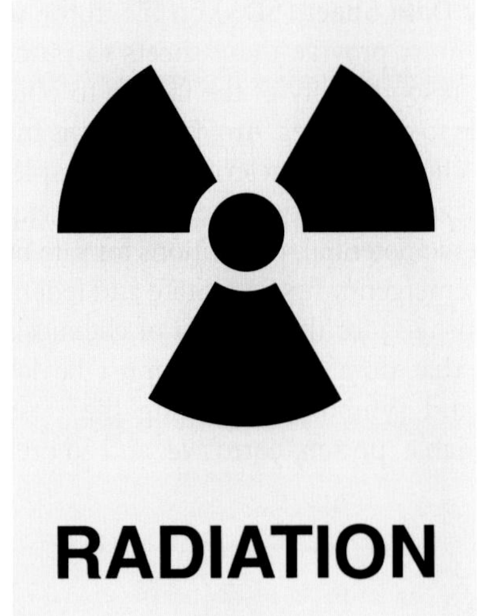

FIGURE 8–8 Radioactive symbol.

Medical Radioactive Waste Disposal

Disposal of medical radioactive waste is regulated by the Nuclear Regulatory Commission (NRC) and is also subject to local regulations. Such waste must be separated from other waste materials in the laboratory and placed in containers marked with the radioactive symbol. Disposal varies with the type of material (solid, liquid, or volatile chemical) and depends upon the amount of radioactivity present. Very few immunology laboratories use radioactivity in testing anymore, mainly because of the problem of waste disposal. If radioactivity is used, the laboratory typically contracts with a waste disposal service that picks up the radioactive waste material.

Electrical Hazards

The laboratory setting contains electrical equipment with which laboratorians have frequent contact. The same general rules of electrical safety observed outside the workplace apply in the laboratory, such as checking for frayed cords or overloaded circuits. Laboratorians also have frequent contact with water, fluids, and chemical agents; therefore, the danger of water or fluid coming in contact with equipment is greater in the laboratory setting. Equipment should not be operated with wet hands. Designated hospital personnel closely monitor electrical equipment. However, laboratory personnel should be observant for any dangerous conditions and report them to the appropriate persons.

When an accident involving electrical shock occurs, the electrical source must be removed immediately without touching the person or the equipment involved. Persons responding to the accident must avoid transferring the current to themselves by turning off the circuit breaker before unplugging the equipment or moving the equipment using a nonconductive glass or wood object. The victim should receive immediate medical assistance following discontinuation of the electricity. Cardiopulmonary resuscitation (CPR) may be necessary.

Fire and Explosive Hazards

Clinical laboratory work involves the use of potentially volatile or explosive chemicals that require special procedures for handling and storage. Flammable chemicals should be stored in safety cabinets and explosion-proof refrigerators. Cylinders of compressed gas should be located away from heat and securely fastened to a stationary device to prevent accidental tipping.

The Joint Commission (TJC), an independent body that certifies and accredits health-care organizations in the United States, requires that all health-care facilities post evacuation routes and detailed plans to follow in the event of a fire. Laboratory personnel should be familiar with these routes. When a fire is discovered, all employees are expected to take the actions described by the acronym RACE:

Rescue—rescue anyone in immediate danger.
Alarm—activate the institutional fire alarm system.
Contain—close all doors to potentially affected areas.
Extinguish or Evacuate—attempt to extinguish the fire if possible, or evacuate, closing the door.

Fire blankets should be present in the laboratory. Persons whose clothes are on fire should be wrapped in the blanket to smother the flames. The acronym PASS can be used to remember the steps in operating a fire extinguisher:

1. Pull pin.
2. Aim at the base of the fire.
3. Squeeze handles.
4. Sweep nozzle side to side.

The Standard System for the Identification of the Fire Hazard of Materials, NFPA 704, is a symbol system used to inform firefighters of the hazards they may encounter when fighting a fire in a particular area. The color-coded areas contain information relating to health hazards, flammability, reactivity, use of water, and personal protection. These symbols are placed on doors, cabinets, and reagent bottles. An example of the hazardous material symbol and information is shown in **Figure 8–9.**

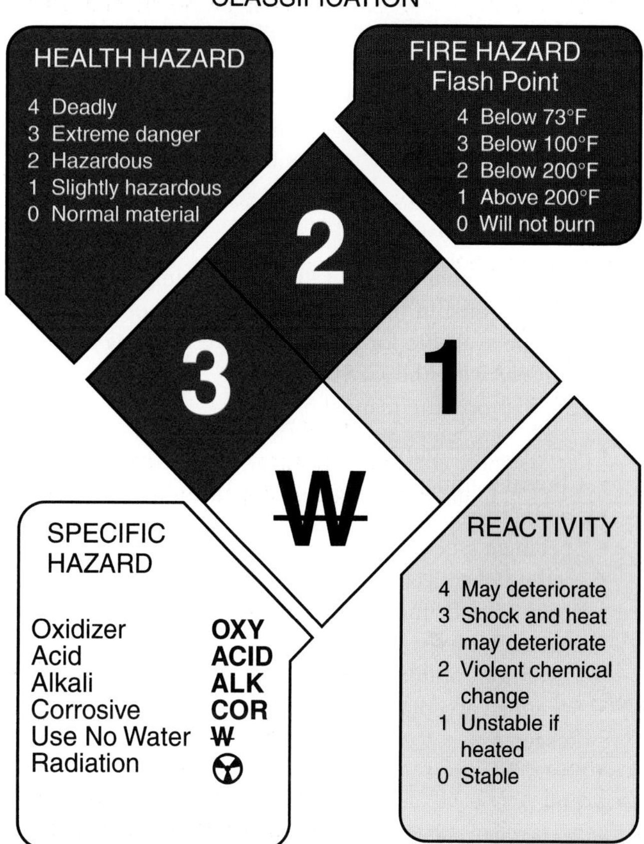

FIGURE 8–9 NFPA hazardous material symbol and classification. *(From Strasinger SK, DiLorenzo MS.* The Phlebotomy Textbook. *4th ed. Philadelphia, PA: F.A. Davis; 2018.)*

Physical Hazards

Physical hazards are not unique to the laboratory; routine precautions observed outside the workplace apply. Maintaining a clean and organized work area is essential for minimizing the hazards. General precautions to consider include not running in rooms and hallways, watching for wet floors, bending the knees when lifting heavy objects, keeping long hair pulled back, and avoiding dangling jewelry. Closed-toed shoes that provide maximum support are essential for safety and comfort.

Quality Management

The term **quality management (QM)** refers to the overall process of guaranteeing quality patient care. As it relates to the clinical laboratory, QM is the continual monitoring of the entire test process, from test ordering and specimen collection through reporting and interpreting results. Written policies and documented actions as they pertain to the patient, the laboratory, ancillary personnel, and the health-care provider are required. In addition, written remedial actions mandating the steps to take when any part of the system fails are essential to a QM program.

The **Clinical Laboratory Improvement Amendments (CLIA)** are regulations that specify required components for QM, including patient test management assessment, quality control (QC) assessment, proficiency testing assessment, comparison of test results, relationship of patient information to patient test results, patient confidentiality, specimen identification and integrity, personnel competency, personnel qualifications and evaluations, communication protocols, complaint investigations, review with staff, and maintenance of records for 2 years.

Documentation of QM procedures is required by all laboratory accreditation agencies, including TJC, the College of American Pathologists (CAP), the American Association of Blood Banks (AABB), the American Osteopathic Association (AOA), the American Society of Histocompatibility and Immunogenetics (ASHI), the American Association for Laboratory Accreditation (A2LA), and the Commission on Office Laboratory Assessment (COLA); it is also required for

Medicare and Medicaid reimbursement. Guidelines published by CAP and the **Clinical and Laboratory Standards Institute (CLSI)** provide very complete instructions for documentation and are used as a reference for the ensuing discussion of the specific areas of immunology QM. Documentation in the form of a procedure manual is required in all laboratories. This format is used as the basis for the following discussion.

Procedure Manual

A procedure manual (paper or digital) containing all the procedures performed in the immunology section of the laboratory must be available for reference in the working area and must comply with the CLSI guidelines. For each test performed, the procedure manual provides

- Principle and purpose
- Clinical significance
- Patient identification and preparation
- Specimen type
- Method of collection
- Specimen labeling
- Specimen preservation
- Conditions of transport and storage before testing
- Specimen acceptability and criteria for rejection
- Reagents
- Standards and controls acceptability and expiration policy
- Instrument calibration and maintenance protocols and schedules
- Step-by-step procedure
- Calculations
- Frequency and tolerance limits for controls and corrective actions
- Reference values and critical values
- Interpretation of results
- Common interferences
- Specific procedure notes
- Limitations of the method
- Method validation
- Confirmatory testing
- Recording of results
- References
- Effective date
- Author
- Review schedule

Current package inserts for all test kits used should be reviewed and included in the manual. The laboratory must also have a documented procedure for the correction of erroneous results.

The printed procedural manuals and electronic procedural manuals are subject to proper document control. Only authorized persons may make changes; these are dated and signed (manually or digitally). The manuals must undergo periodic review; documentation (i.e., proof) of the review is included in the manual.

Evaluating procedures and adopting new methodologies is an ongoing process in the clinical laboratory. Whenever changes are made, the written procedure in the manual should be reviewed, referenced, and signed by a person with designated authority, such as the laboratory director or section supervisor, and personnel should be notified of the changes. An annual review of all procedures by the designated authority must also be documented.

The procedure manual provides the basis for all testing in the immunology laboratory. Quality care in testing relies on strictly following procedures as written. Documentation includes every step, from specimen collection to the reporting of results. A well-documented QM program ensures quality test results and patient care.

Preexamination Variables

In a clinical laboratory, a QM program encompasses **preexamination variables** (e.g., specimen collection, handling, and storage), **examination variables** (e.g., reagent and test performance, instrument calibration and maintenance, personnel requirements, technical competence, review and interpretation), **postexamination variables** (e.g., reporting of results and specimen management), and documentation that the program is being meticulously followed.

A **variable** is defined as anything that can be changed or altered. Identification of variables throughout the testing process provides the basis for development of procedures and policies within the immunology department that are located in the procedure manual.

Preexamination variables occur before the actual testing of the specimen and include test request orders, patient preparation, time of specimen collection, specimen collection, handling and transport, and specimen storage. Health-care personnel outside the immunology department control many of these factors, such as ordering tests and collecting specimens; however, communication between departments and adequate training on the correct procedures for ordering a test, collecting a specimen, and transporting the specimen improves the **turnaround time (TAT)** of results, avoids duplication of test orders, and ensures a high-quality specimen. TAT is defined as the amount of time required between the point at which a test is ordered by the health-care provider and the results are reported to the health-care provider. The laboratory can monitor the TATs for both stat and routine tests to determine areas in the process that need improvement.

Specimen Collection and Documentation

Specific guidelines for specimen collection and handling should be stated at the beginning of each procedure listed in the manual. In addition to following the guidelines for specimen collection for each specific procedure, requisition forms and electronic entry forms should be used to document the type of specimen to be collected and the time and date of collection. The form should have space for documenting (1) the patient's first and last name, (2) the patient's identification number, (3) the patient's gender, (4) the patient's age or date of birth, (5) the name of the person requesting the test, (6) the name of the person to contact with critical results, (7) the name of the test ordered, (8) any special handling requirements, (9) the time and date of specimen collection, (10) the time the specimen was delivered to the laboratory, and (11) any additional information pertinent to laboratory interpretation. Information regarding patient preparation (e.g., fasting or elimination of interfering medications) and the type and volume of specimen required must be included in the specific procedure.

The criteria for specimen rejection for both physical characteristics and labeling errors must be present. If a specimen is rejected, the criteria for rejecting that specimen must be documented and available to the health-care provider and nursing staff. Laboratory personnel must determine the suitability of a specimen and document any problems and corrective actions taken using an internal laboratory quality improvement form (see Box: *In the Laboratory: An Example of an Internal Laboratory Quality Improvement Form*). This report enables the laboratory director to capture the information to determine the root cause of the problem and develop a preventive or corrective action plan. Laboratory information systems have the capability to electronically generate these forms for review. An acceptable specimen requires verification of the patient's identification information on the requisition form and the tube label, proper collection and processing procedures, and timely transport to the laboratory.

Examination Variables

The examination variables are the processes that directly affect the testing of specimens. They include reagents, instrumentation and equipment, testing procedure, QC, preventive maintenance (PM), access to procedure manuals, review and interpretation of results, and the competency of personnel performing the tests.

Reagents

The name and chemical formula of each reagent used, any necessary instructions for preparation or company source of prepared materials, storage requirements, and procedures for reagent QC are all found in the procedure manual. The type of water used for preparing reagents and controls must be specified. Distilled or deionized water or clinical laboratory reagent water (CLRW) must be available. A bold-type statement of any safety or health precautions associated with reagents should be present.

All reagents must be properly labeled with the date of preparation or opening, purchase and received date, expiration date, and appropriate safety information. Reagents should be checked against two levels of commercial control solutions on each shift, or at a minimum of once a day and whenever a new reagent is opened. Results of all reagent checks are properly recorded.

Instrumentation and Equipment

The procedure manual must clearly provide instructions regarding the operation, performance, frequency of calibration, and limitations of the instrumentation and equipment. The procedures to follow when limitations or linearity are exceeded, such as dilution procedures, must be included in

In the Laboratory

An Example of an Internal Laboratory Quality Improvement Form

Quality Improvement Follow-Up Report

CONFIDENTIAL

Instructions: Section I should be completed by the individual identifying the event.

Date of report: ____________ Reported by: ____________

Date of incident: ________ Date/time of discovery: ________

Patient MR#: ____________ Patient accession #: __________

Section I. Summary of Incident ____________________

Describe what happened: ______________________________

____

____

What immediate corrective action was taken? ____________

____

____

Provide the ORIGINAL to team leader or technical specialist within 24 hours of incident discovery.

Date: ____________________

To: ____________________

Forwarded for follow-up:

Date: ____________________

To: ____________________

Section II. Management Investigation: *Tracking #:* ________

Instructions: Section II should be completed by laboratory management within 72 hours.

Check the appropriate problem category.

- ☐ Unacceptable patient sample (caused by hemolysis, QNS, or contamination)
- ☐ Wrong tube type
- ☐ Equipment-related event
- ☐ Misidentified sample
- ☐ Standard operating procedure deviation
- ☐ Wrong location
- ☐ Communication problem or complaint
- ☐ Other (explain)
- ☐ Accident

Explain answers: ______________________________

____

____

Preventive or corrective action recommendations: __________

____

____

Technical specialist or team leader: ____________________
Date: ____________

Medical director review: ____________ Date: ____________

Quality assurance review: ____________ Date: ____________

FDA reportable: Yes or no ________ Date reported: ________

Adapted from Danville Regional Medical Center Laboratory, Danville, VA, with permission.

the manual, as well as instructions detailing the appropriate recording procedures.

Two levels of commercial controls must be run and recorded. Evidence of corrective action for any failed QC tests must be documented. No patient's testing may be performed until QC is acceptable. A routine PM schedule for instruments and equipment should be prepared as mandated by the TJC or CAP guidelines, and records kept of all routine and nonroutine maintenance performed.

Deionized water used for reagent preparation is quality controlled by checking its pH and purity meter resistance on a weekly basis, as well as the bacterial count on a monthly schedule. All results must be recorded on the appropriate forms.

Testing Procedures

Detailed and concise testing instructions are written in a step-by-step manner. Instructions should begin with specimen preparation, such as time and speed of centrifugation, and include types of glassware needed, time limitations and stability of specimens and reagents, calculation formulas and a sample calculation, health and safety precautions, and procedures. Additional procedure information, including reasons for special precautions, sources of error and interfering substances, helpful hints, clinical situations that influence the test, alternative procedures, and acceptable TATs for stat tests are listed under the title of Procedure Notes following the step-by-step procedure.

Reference sources should be listed. The manufacturer's package inserts may be included but cannot replace the written procedure. The laboratory director must sign and date new procedures and all modifications of procedures before they are used.

Quality Control

Quality control (QC) refers to the materials, procedures, and techniques that monitor the **accuracy, precision,** and **reliability** of a laboratory test. QC procedures are performed to ensure that acceptable standards are met during the process of patient testing. Specific QC information regarding the type of control specimen, preparation and handling, frequency of use, tolerance levels, and methods of recording should be included in the step-by-step instructions in the procedure manual for each test.

QC is performed at scheduled times, such as at the beginning of each shift or before testing patient samples, and it must always be performed if reagents are changed, an instrument malfunction has occurred, or test results are questioned by the health-care provider. Control results must be recorded in a paper or electronic log. Patient test results may not be reported until the QC is verified.

External Controls. External controls are used to verify the *accuracy* (ability to obtain the expected result) and *precision* (ability to obtain the same result on the same specimen) of a test. Reliability is the ability to maintain both precision and accuracy. The control material is tested in the same manner as the patient samples. Analysis of at least two levels of control material is required. One of these is a high-level control and the other is a low-level control. The concentrations of the controls should be at medically significant levels and should be as similar to the human specimen as possible. Documentation of QC includes dating and initialing the material when it is first opened and recording the manufacturer's lot number and the expiration date each time a control is run and a test result is obtained. U.S. Food and Drug Administration (FDA) standards require that control material test negative for HIV and HBV. External controls are tested and interpreted in the laboratory by the same person performing the patient testing.

The control data are evaluated before releasing patient results. Data obtained from repeated measurements have a Gaussian distribution or spread in the values that indicate the ability to repeat the analysis and obtain the same value. The laboratory, after repeated testing, establishes the value for each analyte and calculates the **control mean** (the average of all data points) and the **standard deviation (SD)** (a measurement statistic that describes the average distance each data point in a normal distribution is from the mean). The **coefficient of variation (CV)** is the SD expressed as a percentage of the mean. The CV indicates whether the distribution of values about the mean is in a narrow versus a broad range and should be less than 5%. *Confidence intervals* are the limits between which the specified proportion or percentage of results will lie. Control ranges are determined by setting confidence limits that are within ±2 SD or ±3 SD of the mean, which indicates that 95.5% to 99.7% of the values are expected to be within that range.

Values are plotted on Levey–Jennings control charts to visually monitor control values. Immediate decisions about patient results are based on the ability of control values to remain within a preestablished limit. Changes in the accuracy of results are indicated by either a **trend,** a gradual change in the mean in one direction that may be caused by a gradual deterioration of reagents or deterioration of instrument performance, or a **shift,** an abrupt change in the mean that may be caused by a malfunction of the instrument or a new lot number of reagents **(Fig. 8–10).** Changes in precision are shown by a large amount of scatter about the mean and an uneven distribution above and below the mean that are most often caused by errors in technique.

When control values are outside the tolerance limits, corrective action that includes the use of new reagents or controls and the verification of lot numbers and expiration dates must be taken and documented. A protocol for corrective action is shown in **Figure 8–11.** A designated supervisor reviews all the QC results.

Some laboratories may participate in a commercial QC program run by the manufacturer of the QC material. The results from the same lot of QC material are returned to the manufacturer for statistical analysis and comparison with other laboratories using the same methodology.

Internal Controls. Internal controls, also called *procedural controls*, consist of internal monitoring systems built into the test system. Internal controls monitor the sufficient addition of a patient sample or reagent, the instrument's and reagent's interaction, and for lateral flow test methods, whether the sample migrated through the test strip properly.

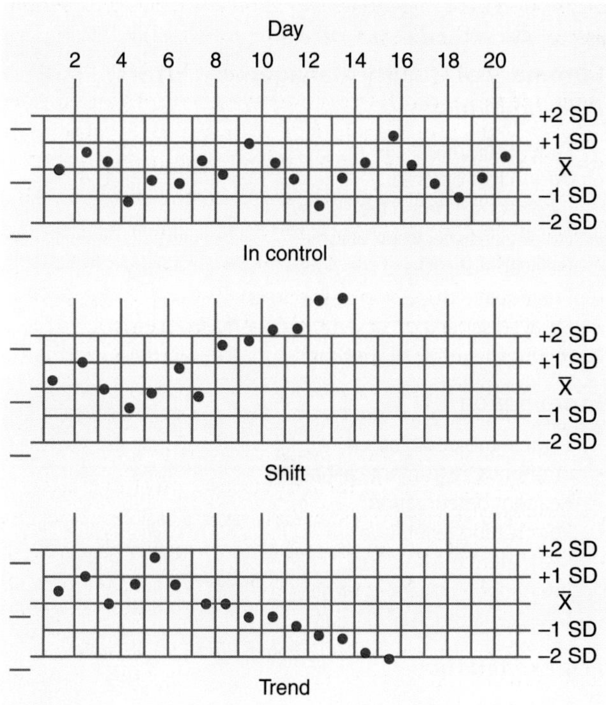

FIGURE 8–10 Levey–Jennings charts showing in–control, shift, and trend results. *(From Strasinger SK, DiLorenzo MS.* Urinalysis and Body Fluids. *6th ed. Philadelphia, PA: F.A. Davis; 2014.)*

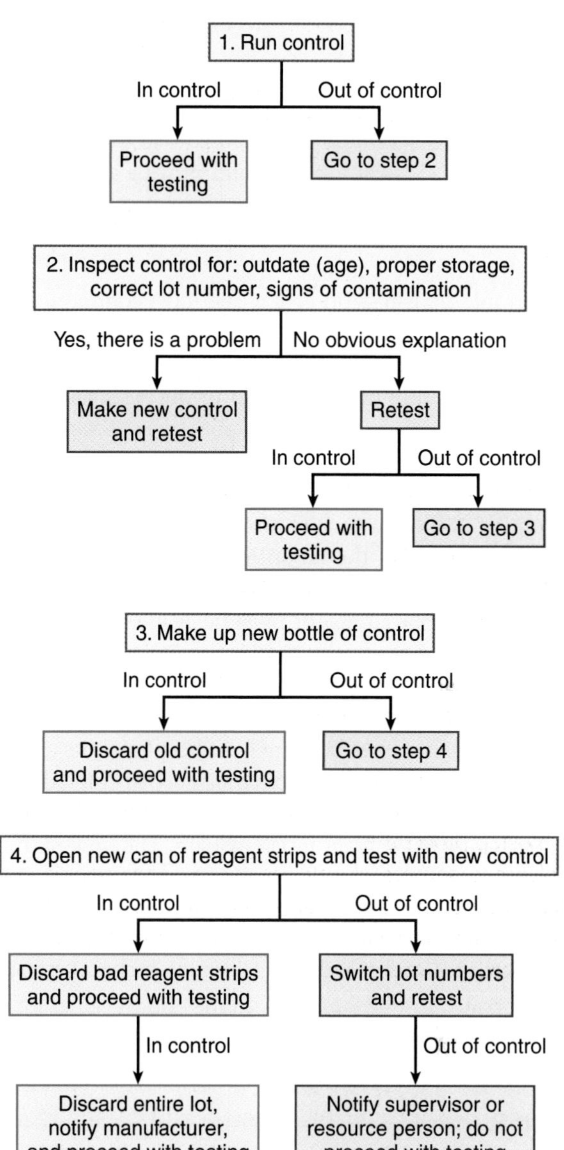

FIGURE 8–11 Procedure for "out of control" results. *(Adapted from Schweitzer SC, Schumann JL, Schumann GB. Quality assurance guidelines for the urinalysis laboratory.* J Med Technol. *1986; 3(11):567–572.*

Electronic Controls. Electronic controls use a mechanical or electrical device in place of a liquid QC specimen. This type of QC can be an internal or an external component inserted into a point-of-care (POC) instrument. Electronic controls verify the functional ability of a testing device but do not verify the integrity of the testing supplies. Many test systems use a combination of external and internal controls to verify that the entire test system is working properly.

Proficiency Testing (External Quality Assessment). Proficiency testing, or **external quality assessment (EQA),** is the testing of unknown specimens received from an outside agency. It provides unbiased validation of the accuracy, and thus quality, of patient test results. Several commercial vendors, such as the CAP, provide proficiency testing programs. Laboratories subscribing to these programs receive lyophilized or ready-to-use specimens. The results are returned to the proficiency testing vendors, where they are statistically analyzed with those from all participating laboratories. The laboratory director receives a report from the vendor, which enables the director to evaluate the laboratory's accuracy and compare it with other laboratories using the same method of analysis. The director ensures that the laboratory takes action to correct unacceptable results. The CLIA mandate comparison testing for laboratory accreditation.

Personnel and Facilities

QC is only as good as the personnel performing and monitoring it. Personnel assessment includes education and training, continuing education (CE), competency assessment, and performance appraisals. Each new employee must have documentation of training during his or her orientation to the laboratory. This documentation is a checklist of procedures and must include the date and initials of the person doing the training as well as the employee being trained. Up-to-date reference materials and atlases should be readily available, and documentation of CE must be maintained.

An adequate, uncluttered, safe working area is also essential for both quality work and personnel morale. SPs for handling body fluids must be followed at all times.

Postexamination Variables

Postexamination variables are processes that affect the reporting of results and correct interpretation of data.

Reporting Results

Standardized reporting methods minimize health-care provider confusion when reporting results. The forms for reporting results should be designed so that they present the information in a logical sequence and provide adequate space for writing. A standardized reporting format and, when applicable, reference ranges should be included with each procedure in the procedure manual.

Electronic transmission is now the most common method for reporting results. Many automated instruments have the capability for the laboratorian to electronically transmit results directly from the instrument to the designated health-care provider. It is essential that the laboratorian carefully reviews results before transmittal. Results may also be manually entered into the laboratory computer system and then transmitted to the health-care providers.

Documentation of the reporting of results is essential and required by accrediting agencies. In addition, permanent records of all reported results must be available. A method to verify the actual reporting of results also must be available and used by all employees.

The telephone is frequently used to convey results of stat tests and critical values. Personnel on hospital units and from health-care providers' offices often call requesting additional results. When telephoning results, confirm that the results are being reported to the appropriate person. The time of the call and the name of the person receiving the results must be documented according to the facility's policy. Written procedures should be available for the reporting of critical values, which are significantly abnormal results that are life-threatening. Laboratorians must be familiar with the critical values for each test and the processes for notification of attending staff in a timely manner.

Result Errors

Errors may be discovered in the laboratory through a QM procedure known as the **delta check** that compares a patient's test results with the previous results. Variation outside the established parameters alerts laboratory personnel to the possibility of an error that occurred during the testing procedure or in patient identification. Automated comparison of patient results with predetermined preapproved criteria (autoverification) is often programmed into many laboratory analyzers to expedite result delivery.

Erroneous results must be corrected in a timely manner to ensure that the patient does not receive treatment based on incorrect results. Errors can occur in patient identification, specimen labeling, or result transcription. The patient's record should be corrected as soon as the error is detected. However, the original result must not be erased in the event that the health-care provider treated the patient based on the erroneous results. Appropriate documentation of erroneous results should follow institutional protocol. The manual must contain a written procedure for reporting, reviewing, and correcting errors.

The *In the Laboratory: Summary of Quality Management Errors* Box summarizes QM errors in each phase of laboratory testing.

In the Laboratory

Summary of Quality Management Errors

Preexamination

- Patient misidentification
- Wrong test ordered
- Incorrect specimen type collected
- Insufficient specimen volume
- Delayed transport of specimen to the laboratory
- Inadequate processing of specimen
- Delayed separation of serum or plasma from cells
- Incorrect storage of specimen

Examination

- Sample misidentification
- Erroneous instrument calibration
- Reagent deterioration
- Poor testing technique
- Instrument malfunction
- Interfering substances present
- Misinterpretation of QC data

Postexamination

- Patient misidentification
- Poor handwriting
- Transcription error
- Poor quality of instrument printer
- Failure to send report
- Failure to call critical values
- Inability to identify interfering substances

Interpreting Results

The specificity and the sensitivity for each test should be included in the procedure manual for correct interpretation of results. Sensitivity and specificity vary among manufacturers. All known interfering substances should be listed for evaluation of patient test data.

Regulatory Issues

QM is regulated throughout the total testing system. The health-care regulation systems include both governmental and public agencies. All agencies have the same goal, which is to provide safe and effective health care.

Clinical Laboratory Improvement Amendments (CLIA)

The CLIA are governmental regulatory standards administered by the Centers for Medicare and Medicaid Services (CMS) and the FDA. CLIA stipulate that all laboratories that perform testing on human specimens for the purposes of diagnosis, treatment, monitoring, or screening must be licensed and obtain a certificate from the CMS. Laboratories with CLIA certification are inspected to document compliance with the regulations. The inspections may be performed by CMS personnel or an

In the Laboratory

CLIA Test Classifications

Waived Testing

- Tests considered easy to perform by following the manufacturer's instructions. These tests have little risk of error. No special training or education is required.
- Example: Whole blood infectious mononucleosis test (Monospot)

Provider-Performed Microscopy Procedures (PPMPs)

- Microscopy tests performed by a physician, midlevel practitioner, or dentist.
- Example: Microscopic urinalysis

Nonwaived Tests

- Moderate-complexity tests
  - Tests that require documentation of training in test principles, instrument calibration, periodic proficiency testing, and on-site inspections
  - Example: Automated immunoassays
- High-complexity tests
  - Tests that require sophisticated instrumentation and a high degree of interpretation
  - Proficiency testing and on-site inspections are required.
  - Example: Immunofixation electrophoresis (IFE)

accrediting agency recognized by the CMS, such as the CAP, the TJC, COLA, AABB, A2LA, ASHI, or AOA.

CLIA classifies laboratory tests into three categories: waived testing, provider-performed microscopy procedures (PPMPs), and nonwaived testing (see *In the Laboratory: CLIA Test Classifications*). Nonwaived testing is separated into the categories of moderate and high complexity with regard to requirements for personnel performing the tests. Laboratories must obtain the correct certification for the level of testing complexity performed. For each category, there is a description of the educational level necessary for personnel who may perform the test, as well as the type of quality assessment procedures that must be in place.

Clinical and Laboratory Standards Institute (CLSI)

The CLSI is a nonprofit organization that publishes recommendations by nationally recognized experts for the performance of laboratory testing. CLSI standards are considered the standard of care for laboratory procedures. The **standard of care** is the attention, caution, and prudence that a reasonable person in the same circumstances would exercise. In a legal situation, the CLSI standards would be considered the standard of care that should have been met.

The Joint Commission (TJC)

TJC is an independent, not-for-profit organization that accredits and certifies more than 21,000 health-care organizations and programs in the United States. The mission of TJC is to continuously improve the safety and quality of care provided to the public through the provision of health-care accreditation and related services that support performance improvement in health-care organizations. To maintain accreditation, organizations must pass an on-site inspection by a survey team every 3 years. Laboratories are surveyed every 2 years.

TJC has published *National Patient Safety Goals.* It is essential that health-care organizations adhere to these goals to maintain their accreditation. As of 2018, the *National Patient Safety Goals* pertaining to the laboratory are:

- *Improve the accuracy of patient identification.* Use at least two ways to identify patients who are using laboratory services. For example, use the patient's first and last name, an assigned identification number, and date of birth. The patient's room number or physical location is not used as an identifier. Label containers used for blood and other specimens in the presence of the patient.
- *Improve the effectiveness of communication among caregivers.* Get important test results to the right staff person on time. Report critical results of tests to the appropriate health-care worker on a timely basis.
- *Reduce the risk of health-care–associated infections (HAIs).* Use the current hand-hygiene guidelines from the CDC or the World Health Organization (WHO). Set goals for improving hand cleaning. Use these goals to improve hand cleaning.

College of American Pathologists (CAP)

The CAP is an organization of board-certified pathologists that advocates high-quality and cost-effective medical care. The CAP provides laboratory accreditation and proficiency testing for laboratories.

For accreditation purposes, CAP-trained pathologists and laboratory managers and technologists perform on-site laboratory inspections on a biennial basis. Inspectors examine the laboratory's records and QC of procedures for the preceding 2 years. Inspection also includes the qualifications of the laboratory staff, including CE attendance, and the laboratory's equipment, facilities, safety program, and laboratory management. CAP accreditation is accepted by both the CMS and TJC and fulfills Medicare and Medicaid requirements.

As previously described, laboratories that subscribe to this proficiency program receive periodic samples to analyze and return their results to the CAP. The laboratory receives a report on how its results compared with other laboratories performing the procedures in a similar manner. Failure to perform satisfactorily on a proficiency test can result in a laboratory losing its CLIA certificate to perform the failed test.

Quality Management Systems

A **quality management system (QMS)** incorporates many of the objectives of total QM and continuous quality improvement to ensure quality results, staff competence, and efficiency within an organization. In addition, a QMS also utilizes the concepts of the International Organization for Standardization (ISO 151189) and the Lean and Six Sigma methods. The requirements of TJC and the CAP accreditation organizations are included in a QMS.

A QMS coordinates activities to direct and control an organization with regard to quality and the reduction of medical errors. The first step in a laboratory QMS is to determine the pathway of workflow through the laboratory, as discussed previously under the preexamination, examination, and postexamination phases of testing. In each area of the pathway, all the processes and procedures that occur are determined and analyzed so that everyone knows what they are supposed to do, how they are supposed to do it, and when they are supposed to do it. Instructions must be available for each activity.

Quality System Essentials

Quality system essentials (QSEs) form the basis of a QMS. The 12 QSEs describe the management information needed for a laboratory to perform quality work **(Table 8–2).** They were developed by the former National Committee for Clinical Laboratory Standards and the current CLSI and include the methods to meet the requirements of regulatory, accreditation, and standard-setting organizations. **Quality indicators** are the measurements developed by each laboratory to determine if the QSEs are being met. They may include such items as appropriateness of the testing, correct patient identification, timely reporting of laboratory results, and correct proficiency testing results.

The Lean System

The **Lean system** originated with the automobile manufacturing industry in Japan. Its concepts have been adopted by many American industries, including the health-care industry. Lean utilizes a tool called "6S," which stands for sort, straighten, scrub, safety, standardize, and sustain. Lean focuses on the elimination of waste to allow a facility to do more with less and, at the same time, increase customer and employee satisfaction. In the health-care environment, the ability to decrease costs while providing quality health care is of primary importance. The use of the Lean tools enhances efficiency and proficiency, as described in **Table 8–3.**

Six Sigma

Six Sigma is a statistical modification of the original Plan-Do-Check-Act (PDCA) method adopted by TJC as a

Table 8–2 Description of the 12 Laboratory Quality System Essentials (QSEs)

QSE	PURPOSE	PROCESS EXAMPLES
Organization	Leadership responsibilities to meet requirements and maintain quality	• Quality planning • Management review
Customer focus	Determining customer expectations and designing processes to meet them	• Customer feedback
Facilities and safety	Physical environment, safety, and maintenance programs	• Disaster management • Health risk assessment
Personnel	Obtaining and retaining competent full staffing	• Training • Competency
Purchasing and inventory	Agreements with suppliers for products and services	• Inventory management • Supply ordering
Equipment	Selecting, installing, and maintaining equipment and instrumentation	• Preventive maintenance
Process management	Processes related to the path of workflow	• Method validation • Plan development
Documents and records	Creating, managing, and retaining documentation of policies and procedures	• Document review • Document management
Information management	Managing confidential information generated or entered into information systems	• Release of information • Downtime procedures
Nonconforming event (NCE) management	Detecting and documenting nonconformance	• Investigation of NCEs
Assessments	Verifying that processes meet requirements	• Proficiency testing • Quality indicators
Continual improvement	Identifying areas for improvement	• Lean • Root cause analysis • Six Sigma

Table 8–3 Lean 6S in the Laboratory

LEAN S	TASK	BENEFIT
Sort	Identify items in the department that can be discarded	More space and less clutter
Straighten	Identify designated areas for equipment and supplies	Less time is spent hunting for supplies
Scrub	Maintain the work area on a daily basis	Less time is spent on major cleanups
Safety	Be alert for minor areas that can be fixed before they become major	Less chance of accidents
Standardize	All work areas are stocked in the same manner	Any work area can be restocked by anyone in the department
Sustain	Everyone maintains the five other Ss on a daily basis	Less employee frustration and better outcomes

guideline for health-care organizations. It focuses on minimizing variability in process outputs that lead to wasted time and resources. Reducing variation will potentially reduce costs, improve performance, and increase profitability. The primary goal of Six Sigma is to measure, to quantify errors, and then to reduce variables and decrease errors to a level of 3.4 defects per 1 million opportunities. Attaining this goal indicates that the laboratory is addressing factors critical to customer satisfaction and quality care.

The Six Sigma methodology is represented by the acronym DMAIC:

Define goals and current processes.
Measure current processes and collect data.
Analyze the data for cause-and-effect information.
Improve the process using the data collected.
Control the correction of concerns displayed in the data.

Root Cause Analysis

Similar to Lean, **root cause analysis (RCA)** has roots in the manufacturing industry. RCA is a tool widely used in the investigation of adverse events in the health-care setting. TJC mandates the use of RCA to investigate "sentinel events," which are defined as an unexpected occurrence involving death or serious physical or psychological injury or the risk thereof. An RCA protocol begins with the investigation and reconstruction of the adverse event to determine how the event occurred. RCA focuses on the process failures, not on the individual mistakes of personnel.

By instituting quality improvement methodologies, a health-care institution can develop a structured, standardized format to systematically assess and document the quality of services to the customer.

SUMMARY

- Transmission of biological hazards that are encountered when testing patient specimens requires a chain of infection, which consists of an infectious agent, reservoir, portal of exit, mode of transmission, portal of entry, and susceptible host.
- Hand hygiene and wearing PPE are essential actions to prevent transmission of infectious organisms. Standard Precautions (SPs) should be followed at all times.
- Contaminated supplies and all specimen types except urine must be disposed of in a labeled biohazard container.
- All sharps, including needles and holders, must be disposed of in puncture-proof sharps containers. Recapping of needles is prohibited.
- The Occupational Exposure to Bloodborne Pathogens Standards are a means of providing protection from accidental exposure to BBPs through the use of engineering controls, work practice controls, and the use of PPE.
- When transporting biological specimens, the DOT and International Air Transit Association regulations must be followed. They include placing specimens in screw-cap containers; wrapping them in absorbent material; and placing them in a sturdy, leakproof container.
- Follow specific directions when mixing chemicals, and always add acid to water, rather than water to acid.
- When chemical contact with the skin or eyes occurs, immediately flush the area with water for 15 minutes.
- An SDS and a Chemical Hygiene Plan must be available to employees. Dispose of chemicals per EPA guidelines.
- The SDS contains information about the physical and chemical properties of a reagent, its flammability, explosion reactivity, health hazards, primary routes of entry, exposure limits, carcinogenic potential, precautions for safe handling, spill cleanup, and emergency first aid.
- The Globally Harmonized System (GHS) of Classification and Labelling of Chemicals is an international standardization for labeling and SDS formatting of hazards posed by chemicals.
- Dispose of radioactive material following NRC guidelines.
- Be observant for frayed cords, overloaded circuits, and improperly grounded equipment. Avoid working with electrical equipment when you are wet or the equipment is wet.
- Follow routine safety protocols and maintain a clean, organized work area to avoid physical hazards.
- The acronym RACE outlines the steps to follow when a fire is discovered: (R) rescue anyone in danger; (A) activate

the fire alarm; (C) contain the fire; (E) extinguish the fire if possible or evacuate, closing the door.

- QM is the overall process of guaranteeing quality throughout the entire testing system.
- QC involves performing individual procedures using acceptable standards and control material at various medically significant levels.
- Documentation includes a procedure manual, policies to control and monitor procedure variables, and records of competency assessment and CE.
- Preexamination variables occur before sample testing. Examination variables occur during the specimen testing. Postexamination variables occur during reporting of test results.
- Agencies and regulations regulating the laboratory include:
  - CLIA—provides requirements for persons performing waived, PPMP, moderate-complexity, and high-complexity testing.
  - TJC—provides accreditation and certification of health-care organizations.
  - CAP—provides laboratory accreditation and provision of proficiency testing.
  - CLSI—develops written standards and guidelines for specimen collection, handling and processing, and laboratory testing and reporting.
- The 12 quality essentials provide the management documentation needed to demonstrate quality work. Quality indicators are developed to monitor each phase of testing.
- The Lean system utilizes the "6S" tools (sort, straighten, scrub, safety, standardize, and sustain) to enhance efficiency and proficiency.
- The goal of the statistical Six Sigma method is to reduce variables and decrease errors to a level of 3.4 defects per 1 million opportunities.
- RCA focuses on process failures, not on the individual mistakes of personnel.

CASE STUDIES

1. Phyllis, the immunology supervisor, who has been working for the last 20 years in a small rural hospital, is training a new employee. A dilution of a patient's serum must be made to run a particular test. The supervisor is having difficulty using a serological pipette, so she removes one glove. In uncapping the serum tube, a small amount of serum splashes onto the workbench. She cleans this up with a paper towel, which she discards in the regular paper trash. She also spills a small amount onto her disposable laboratory coat. She tells the new employee that because it is such a small amount, she isn't going to worry about it and continues on to pipette the specimen. She then replaces the glove onto her ungloved hand and says that because it is almost break time, she will wait to wash her hands until then.

Questions

a. Identify all the safety violations involved.
b. What component of the chain of infection is involved?
c. How can the chain of infection be broken?

2. As the supervisor of the immunology section, you encounter the following situations. Explain whether you would accept them or take corrective action.

Situations

a. You are told that only the supervisor performs the CAP proficiency survey.
b. QC is not performed daily on the Centaur instrument.
c. The Streptozyme test reporting procedure has been recently revised.
d. Opened, unlabeled commercial QC bottles are in the refrigerator.

3. The medical laboratory scientist (MLS) working in immunology is accused of failure to report a critical result to the patient's nurse.

Questions

a. What documentation is requested from the MLS assigned to make the call?
b. What agency requires this?

REVIEW QUESTIONS

1. An MLS who observes a red rash on her hands after removing her gloves

a. should apply antimicrobial lotion to the hands.
b. may be washing the hands too frequently.
c. may have developed a latex allergy.
d. should not create friction when washing the hands.

2. In the chain of infection, a contaminated work area would serve as which of the following?

a. Reservoir
b. Means of transmission
c. Portal of entry
d. Portal of exit

3. The only biological waste that does not have to be discarded in a container with a biohazard symbol is
   a. urine.
   b. serum.
   c. feces.
   d. used serum tubes.

4. Patient specimens transported by the DOT must be labeled as a
   a. diagnostic specimen.
   b. clinical specimen.
   c. biological specimen, category b.
   d. laboratory specimen.

5. A technician places tightly capped noninfectious serum tubes in a rack and places the rack and the specimen data in a labeled, leakproof metal courier box. Is there anything wrong with this scenario?
   a. Yes, DOT requirements are not met.
   b. No, the tubes are placed in a rack.
   c. Yes, absorbent material is missing.
   d. No, the box contains the specimen data.

6. The Occupational Exposure to Bloodborne Pathogens Standard developed by OSHA requires employers to provide all of the following *except*
   a. hepatitis B immunization.
   b. safety training.
   c. hepatitis C immunization.
   d. laundry facilities for nondisposable laboratory coats.

7. An employee who receives an accidental needlestick should immediately
   a. apply sodium hypochlorite to the area.
   b. notify a supervisor.
   c. receive HIV prophylaxis.
   d. receive a hepatitis B booster shot.

8. The first thing to do when acid is spilled on the skin is to
   a. notify a supervisor.
   b. neutralize the area with a base.
   c. apply burn ointment.
   d. flush the area with water.

9. When combining acid and water,
   a. acid is added to water.
   b. water is added to acid.
   c. water is slowly added to acid.
   d. both solutions are combined simultaneously.

10. To determine the chemical characteristics of sodium azide, an employee would consult the
    a. Chemical Hygiene Plan.
    b. Merck manual.
    c. SDS.
    d. NRC guidelines.

11. The GHS requires which of the following on a chemical label?
    a. Biohazard symbol, warning sign, environmental impact
    b. Hazard pictogram, signal words, hazard statement
    c. Biological symbol, hazard pictogram, long-term effects
    d. Signal words, hazard statement, biological symbol

12. A technician who is pregnant should avoid working with
    a. organic chemicals.
    b. radioisotopes.
    c. HIV-positive serum.
    d. needles and lancets.

13. Which of the following laboratory regulatory agencies classifies laboratory tests by their complexity?
    a. OSHA
    b. CAP
    c. TJC
    d. CMS

14. Which of the following organizations publishes guidelines that are considered the standard of care for laboratory procedures?
    a. CLIA
    b. CLSI
    c. TJC
    d. CAP

15. *QM* refers to
    a. performance of two levels of testing controls.
    b. reliable control results.
    c. increased productivity.
    d. quality of specimens and patient care.

16. When external QC is run, what information must be documented?
    a. The reagent lot number
    b. Expiration date of the control
    c. Date the control was run
    d. All of the above

17. What steps are taken when the results of the QC testing are outside of the stated confidence limits?
    a. Check the expiration date of the control material.
    b. Retest the control.
    c. Open a new control bottle.
    d. All of the above

18. When a new bottle of QC material is opened, what information is placed on the label?
    a. The time the bottle was opened
    b. The supervisor's initials
    c. The lot number
    d. The date and the laboratory worker's initials

19. What is the primary goal of QMS?

a. Precise test results
b. Increased laboratory productivity
c. Improved patient outcomes and reduced medical errors
d. Reproducible test results

20. Would a control sample that has accidentally become diluted produce a trend or a shift in the Levey–Jennings chart plot?

a. Trend
b. Shift

Fill in the Blank

21. Indicate whether each of the following would be considered a (1) preexamination, (2) examination, or (3) postexamination variable by placing the appropriate number in the space.

_______ Reagent expiration date
_______ Rejection of a hemolyzed specimen
_______ Construction of a Levey–Jennings chart
_______ Telephoning a critical result to the nurse
_______ Calibrating the centrifuge
_______ Pipetting the diluent

22. A recommended way to measure and assess QSEs is to establish

a. QC.
b. quality indicators.
c. preventive maintenance.
d. quality management.

23. The basic principle of the Lean system is to increase efficiency and proficiency through

a. customized work shifts.
b. continuous quality improvement.
c. development of quality indicators.
d. elimination of waste.

24. Six Sigma is a

a. departmental evaluation of variables.
b. departmental assessment of errors and quality.
c. QC method.
d. statistical determination of variable and error reduction.

25. What is the focus of RCA?

a. Patient errors
b. Health-care provider errors
c. Process errors
d. Personnel errors

9 Principles of Serological Testing

Linda E. Miller, PhD, MB^{CM}(ASCP) SI, and Christine Dorresteyn Stevens, EdD, MT(ASCP)

LEARNING OUTCOMES

After finishing this chapter, you should be able to:

1. Describe how whole blood is processed to obtain serum for serological testing.
2. Explain the difference between a volumetric pipette and a graduated pipette.
3. Define the following: serial dilution, solute, diluent, and compound dilution.
4. Describe how accurate measurements are made using volumetric pipettes and graduated pipettes.
5. Given the volumes of diluent and solute, calculate the dilution obtained.
6. Calculate the amount of diluent or solute needed to prepare a specific dilution of a serum sample.
7. Explain how an antibody titer is determined.
8. Calculate the dilution factor required to change a given dilution to a specified new dilution.
9. Given a starting dilution and a dilution factor, determine the new dilution obtained.
10. Calculate the final dilution of a sample, given the initial dilution and all subsequent dilutions.
11. Determine how to make a specific percentage solution from a concentrate.
12. Calculate the diagnostic sensitivity and specificity of a serological test, and discuss the significance of these parameters.
13. Discuss the clinical significance of positive and negative predictive values.

CHAPTER OUTLINE

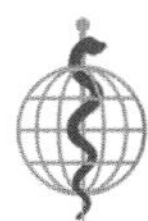

Go to FADavis.com for the laboratory exercises that accompany this text.

KEY TERMS

Blowout pipette
Diagnostic sensitivity
Diagnostic specificity
Diluent
Graduated pipettes
Micropipette
Negative predictive value
Positive predictive value
Serial dilution
Serological pipette
Serology
Serum
Solute
Titer
Volumetric pipettes

Serology is the study of the fluid components in the blood, especially antibodies. **Serum,** the liquid portion of the blood minus the coagulation factors, is the most frequently encountered specimen in immunologic testing. Knowledge of specimen collection and preparation of dilutions is essential to understanding all serological testing in the clinical laboratory.

Blood Specimen Preparation and Measuring

Blood is collected aseptically by venipuncture into a sterile tube that does not contain an anticoagulant (i.e., a red-top, gold-top, or serum separator tube). Care must be taken to avoid hemolysis, as this may produce a false-positive test. The blood specimen is allowed to clot at room temperature or at 4°C, depending upon the protocol for the specific procedure. It is then centrifuged, after which serum should be promptly separated into another tube without transferring any cellular elements **(Fig. 9–1).** Fresh serum that has not been inactivated by heating is usually recommended for testing. For some testing, however, complement must be inactivated because it interferes with test results. In this case, the serum is heated to 56°C for 30 minutes to destroy complement proteins. In either circumstance, if testing cannot be performed immediately, serum may be stored between 2°C and 8°C for up to 72 hours. If there is any additional delay in testing, the serum should be frozen at –20°C or colder.

Pipettes are commonly used to measure either serum for testing or liquid for making reagents and dilutions. The pipettes are calibrated to transfer or deliver specific volumes as marked on their surfaces. They can be categorized as either *volumetric* or *graduated.*

Volumetric pipettes are marked and calibrated to deliver only one volume of a specified liquid. These pipettes enable the user to dispense the exact measure of liquid with a small drop left behind. Pipettes are usually labeled "TD," meaning *to deliver.* The volumetric pipettes have an oval bulb in the center and a tapered dispensing end **(Fig. 9–2).** Volumetric pipettes are used with a suctioning device such as a rubber bulb. The bulb is squeezed to draw the measured amount of liquid into the pipette. Excess fluid is wiped off the outside of the pipette, and then the pipette is held vertically, with the tip against the surface of a container. The suction is released, and the liquid is allowed to flow by gravity into the container.

Graduated pipettes have markings that allow for varying amounts of liquid to be measured **(Fig. 9–3).** A graduated or measuring pipette has marks all along its length. If it is a **serological pipette,** the marks go all the way down to the

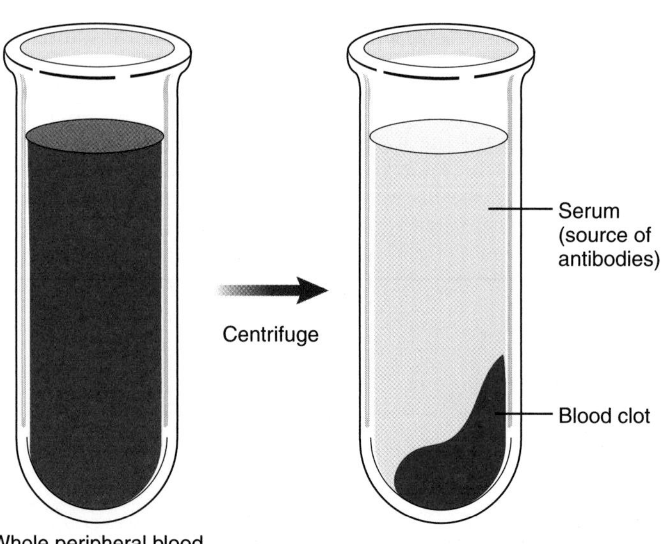

FIGURE 9–1 Serum collection.

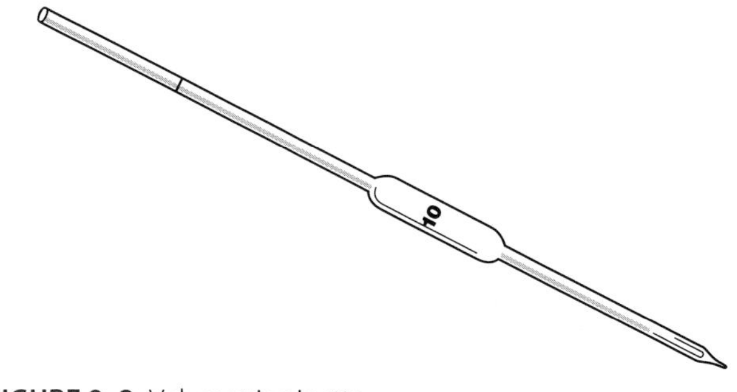

FIGURE 9–2 Volumetric pipette.

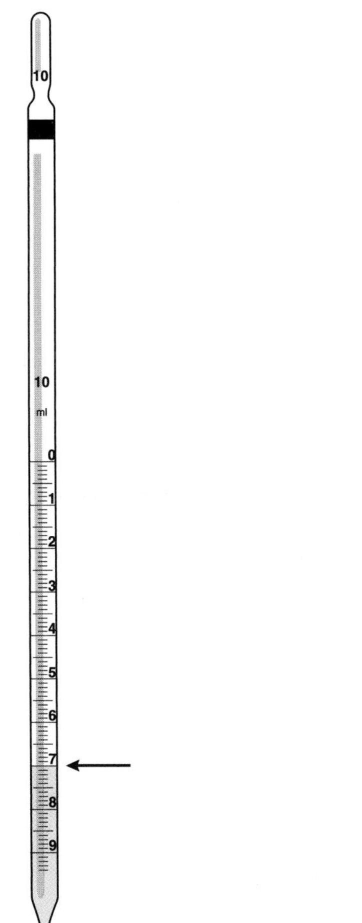

FIGURE 9–3 Graduated pipette prepared to deliver 3 mL.

tip. Some serological pipettes have a frosted band around the opening; this type is called a **blowout pipette.** These pipettes may be labeled "TC," meaning *to contain.* If they are filled to the end, the last drop of liquid must be forced out using a pipette bulb or other device to deliver an accurate volume. Alternately, a specified amount of liquid can be measured from point to point in the pipette. Keep in mind that the graduated markings may start from the top of the pipette and increase to the bottom. For example, 3 mL can be measured with a 10-mL TC pipette by filling the pipette to the 7-mL mark and dispensing down to the end rather than filling it to the 0-mL mark and allowing the liquid to flow to the 3-mL mark.

Generally, a measuring pipette is held in a vertical position when drawing up a liquid **(Fig. 9–4A).** The bottom of the meniscus should be level with the calibration line on the pipette. This is sighted at eye level (see **Fig. 9–4B**). Often, an automatic pipette filler is used with measuring pipettes to increase accuracy **(Fig. 9–5).**

In practice, volumetric and graduated pipettes are more often used to prepare reagents rather than to measure patient specimens and controls. For patient specimens, controls, and calibrators, **micropipettes** are much more accurate because they deliver volumes in the microliter (μL) range and can be used when very small volumes are needed. Micropipettes are mechanical pipettes that draw up and then release a certain volume by depressing a plunger **(Fig. 9–6).** A single-use disposable tip is used for each different specimen. Some micropipettes are adjustable and can hold a range of volumes, whereas others only hold a fixed volume.

Dilutions

In the clinical laboratory, it is often necessary to make a less concentrated solution from a reagent, such as an acid or a buffer, to be able to use the reagent in a particular procedure. In this case, either water or buffer is added to the concentrate to make the reagent the proper strength for testing. For many serology tests, it may be necessary to dilute serum with saline for a visible reaction to occur. If the relative proportions of antigen and antibody are not similar, the reaction cannot be detected (see Chapter 10).

Connections

Antigen–Antibody Equivalence

When the number of antigen molecules is in excess as compared with the number of antibody molecules, or vice versa, many of the molecules remain unbound. Therefore, only small immune complexes can form, and these may not create a visible reaction. In this case, diluting the antibody or antigen creates an equivalent number of binding sites that promotes the formation of large immune complexes. These complexes form a lattice structure that can be detected by a serological method (see Chapter 10).

When too much antibody is present, a reaction endpoint may not be reached. In this case, the serum that contains antibody must be diluted. Therefore, knowledge of dilution preparation is essential to understanding all serological testing. Accurate preparation of simple and compound dilutions and interpretation of serial dilutions are skills that are necessary for quality analysis in the serology laboratory.

Simple Dilutions

A dilution involves two entities: the **solute,** which is the substance being diluted, and the **diluent,** which is the medium making up the rest of the solution. The relationship between

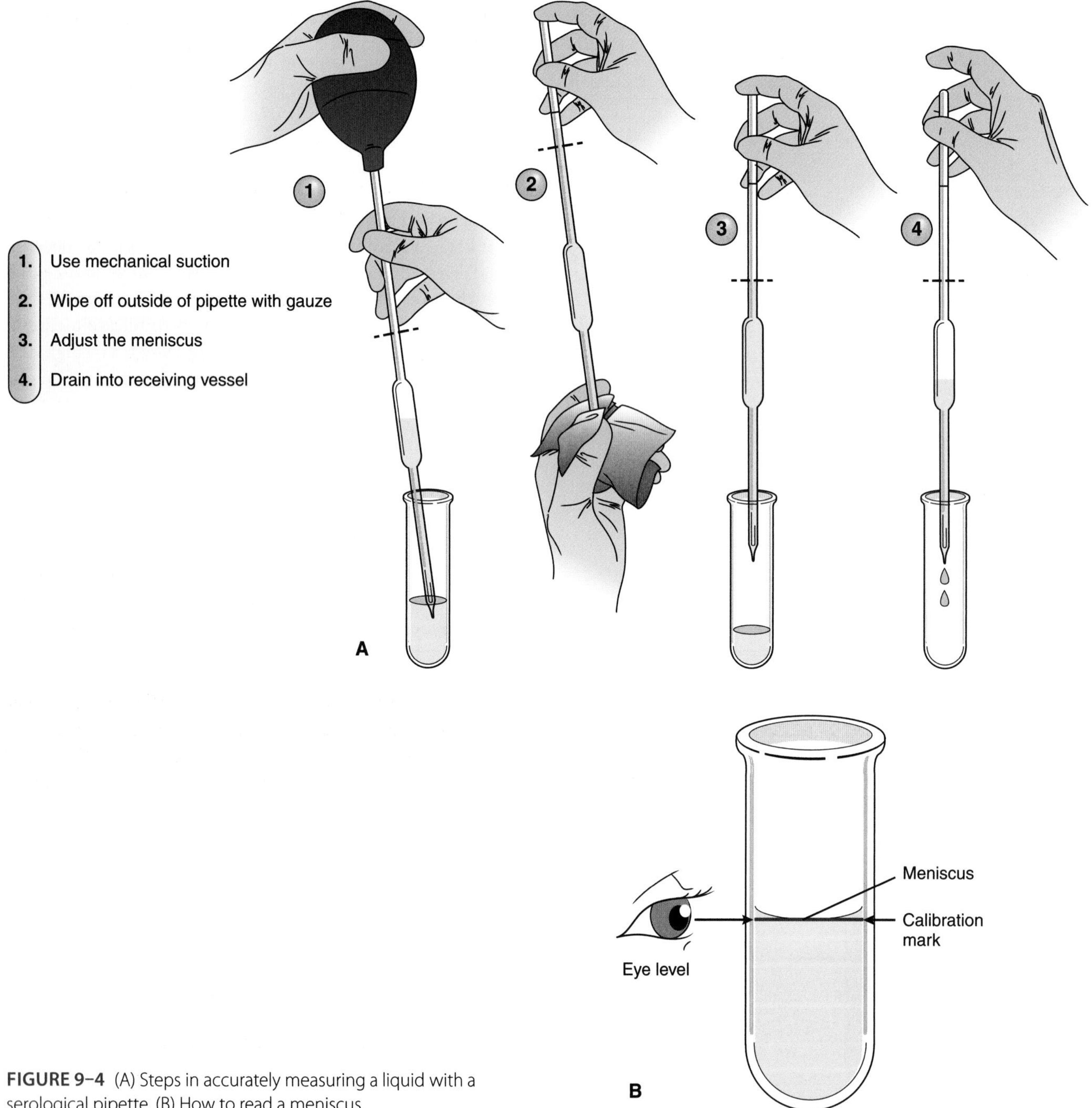
1. Use mechanical suction
2. Wipe off outside of pipette with gauze
3. Adjust the meniscus
4. Drain into receiving vessel
1
2
3
4
A
Meniscus
Calibration mark
Eye level
B

FIGURE 9–4 (A) Steps in accurately measuring a liquid with a serological pipette. (B) How to read a meniscus.

solute and diluent is a ratio that can also be expressed as a fraction. For example, a 1:20 dilution can be expressed as the fraction 1/20. This dilution implies 1 part of solute and 19 parts of diluent. The number on the bottom of the fraction is the total volume, calculated by adding the volumes of the solute and diluent together.

To create a certain volume of a specified dilution, it is necessary to know how to adjust the volumes of solute and diluent appropriately. Using the following equation, an algebraic calculation can be set up to find the total volume, the amount of solute, or the amount of diluent needed to make a dilution:

$$\frac{1}{\text{Dilution}} = \frac{\text{Amount of Solute (Often the Serum)}}{\text{Total Volume (Solute + Diluent)}}$$

Let's see how this equation can be applied by considering the following examples:

Example 1

- Suppose 2 mL of a 1:20 dilution of serum is needed to run a specific serological test. What volumes of serum and diluent are needed to make this dilution?

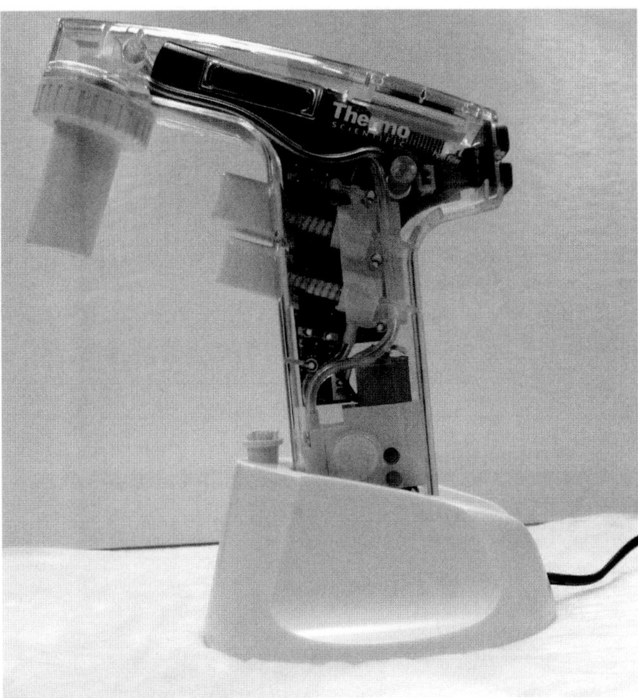

FIGURE 9–5 A pipette filler for use with serological pipettes ranging in size from 1 mL to 100 mL.

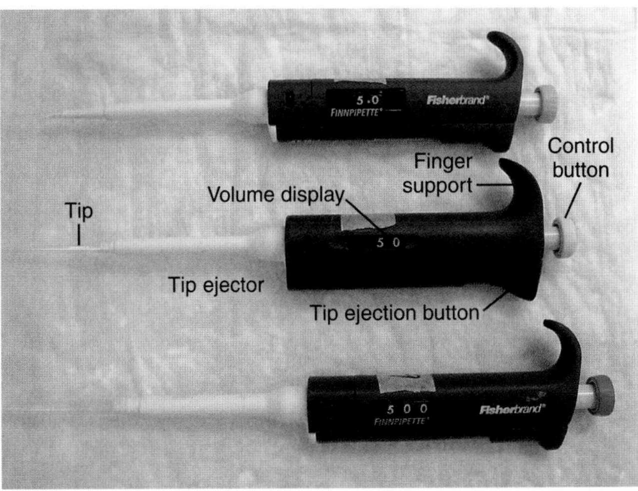

FIGURE 9–6 Micropipettes calibrated to deliver different volumes.

This problem can be solved by placing the appropriate numbers into the corresponding places in the preceding equation as follows:

$$\frac{1}{20} = \frac{x}{2\text{ mL}}$$

Note that 20 represents the total number of parts in the solution and that 2 mL is the total volume desired.

Cross-multiplying to solve this equation for x gives 0.1 mL for the amount of serum needed to make this dilution. The amount of diluent is obtained by subtracting 0.1 mL from the total volume of 2.0 mL to give 1.9 mL of diluent. To check the answer, one can set up a proportion between the amount of solute over the total volume. This should equal the dilution desired. By doing this for the preceding problem, we can see that the correct answer has been obtained:

$$\frac{0.1\text{ mL}}{(1.9\text{ mL diluent} + 0.1\text{ mL serum})} = \frac{1}{20}$$

Example 2

In this example, the amount of serum to be used is known, and the amount of diluent needed to make a specific dilution must be determined:

- Suppose a 1:5 dilution of patient serum is necessary to run a serological test. Using 0.1 mL of serum, what amount of diluent is necessary to make this dilution?

The solution to this problem can be set up in the following manner:

$$\frac{1}{5} = \frac{0.1}{(x + 0.1)}$$

Cross-multiply to get: $x + 0.1 = 0.5$

$$x = 0.4\text{ mL of diluent}$$

Note that the final volume is obtained by adding 0.1 mL of solute to 0.4 mL of diluent. Dividing the volume of the solute by the total volume of 0.5 mL yields the desired 1:5 ratio.

Example 3

- Instructions coming with a reagent bottle of concentrated buffer indicate that 1 part of buffer must be mixed with 19 parts of water for use in a serological test. What is the desired dilution, and how much water should be added to 50 mL of buffer concentrate to obtain this dilution?
- The desired dilution would be: $1/(1 + 19) = 1/20$

To determine the volume of water needed, set up the equation as follows:

$$\frac{1}{20} = \frac{50}{(50 + x)}$$

Cross-multiply to get: $50 + x = 1{,}000$

$$x = 950\text{ mL of diluent}$$

Therefore, to make the dilution, you would add 50 mL of buffer concentrate to 950 mL of water to get 1,000 mL total.

Sometimes it is necessary to dilute a concentrate to a specific percentage. A percentage is simply a different way of expressing a dilution. For instance, a 10% solution can also be expressed as 1/10. In dealing with liquids, the relationship between the solute and diluent is volume/volume. If a solid is to be dissolved in a liquid, the relationship is expressed as weight/volume. Let's look at another example to see how this type of problem would be solved:

Example 4

- Suppose you wish to dilute concentrated glacial acetic acid in water to make 500 mL of a 10% solution for a testing procedure. How much glacial acetic acid and water are needed to make the dilution?

Because the final volume and the percentage are known, we can solve for the amount of the concentrated acetic acid needed, as follows:

$$\frac{1}{10} = \frac{x}{500 \text{ mL}}$$

Cross-multiplying and solving for x gives us 50 mL of glacial acetic acid. The amount of water is determined by taking the total volume and subtracting the volume of concentrate: 500 mL − 50 mL = 450 mL of water to make up the 10% solution.

Additional problems that give more practice with dilution calculations can be found in the Review Questions section at the end of this chapter.

Compound Dilutions

The previous examples represent simple dilutions. Sometimes it is necessary to make a *compound dilution,* which involves preparation of a larger dilution from a previously prepared smaller dilution. To solve this type of problem, use the formula:

$$C1V1 = C2V2$$

In this equation, C1 is the starting concentration, C2 is the final concentration, V1 is the starting volume, and V2 is the ending volume. Let's look at an example to see how this equation would be used:

Example 1

- Suppose you wish to prepare 2.0 mL of a 1:20 dilution from an already-prepared 1:5 dilution of a solute. What volumes of the 1:5 dilution and diluent would be required?

To solve this problem, we can place the numbers into the equation, C1V1 = C2V2, to get:

$$\left(\frac{1}{5}\right)V1 = \left(\frac{1}{20}\right)2.0$$

Solving for V1, we get 0.5 mL. The volume of diluent = 2.0 − 0.5 = 1.5 mL. Thus, we have made a 1:4 dilution of the original 1:5 dilution to get a 1:20 dilution [0.5/(0.5 + 1.5)].

Occasionally, it is necessary to make a very large dilution; if so, it is more accurate and less costly to do this in several steps rather than all at once. The same approach is used as discussed in the previous example, but several dilutions are made in sequence. Consider the following example:

Example 2

Suppose a 1:500 dilution is needed. To make this dilution in a single step, one would need to mix 49.9 mL of diluent with 0.1 mL of serum. If only a small amount of solution is needed to run the test, this is wasteful. Furthermore, inaccuracy may occur if the solution is not properly mixed. Therefore, it is helpful to make several smaller dilutions.

The first step to solving a problem such as this one is to plan the number and sizes of simple dilutions necessary to reach the desired endpoint. In the preceding example, a 1:500 dilution can be made by making a 1:5 dilution of the undiluted serum, followed by a 1:10 dilution from the first dilution and a 1:10 dilution of the second dilution, as shown here:

Serum:

1:5 dilution	→	1:10 dilution	→	1:10 dilution
0.1 mL serum		0.1 mL of 1:5 dilution		0.1 mL of 1:10 dilution
0.4 mL diluent		0.9 mL diluent		0.9 mL diluent

Multiplying 5 × 10 × 10 equals 500, or the total dilution. Each of the simple dilutions is calculated individually by doing mental arithmetic or by using the formula given for simple dilutions. In this example, the 1:500 dilution was made using very little diluent in a series of test tubes, rather than having to use a larger volume in a flask. The volumes were kept small enough so that mixing could take place easily. The final volume of 1.0 mL is all that is necessary to perform the test.

Serial Dilutions

If the dilution factor is exactly the same in each step of the dilution, this is known as a **serial dilution.** To prepare a serial dilution, a series of test tubes is set up with exactly the same amount of diluent in each **(Fig. 9–7).** Each tube in the series contains 1/*n* the concentration of the preceding sample. The series of tubes illustrated in Figure 9–7 is an example of a two-fold serial dilution system, in which each tube is one-half as concentrated as the tube before it. The series, 1:5, 1:25, 1:125, 1:625, 1:3125, is an example of a five-fold serial dilution system, in which each tube is diluted five times as much as the preceding tube. Serial dilutions are often used to obtain an antibody **titer,** which is an indicator of the amount of antibody present in the original serum sample. Once the serum has been serially diluted, a constant amount of the corresponding antigen is added to each tube, and the tubes are observed for an antigen–antibody reaction. The antibody titer

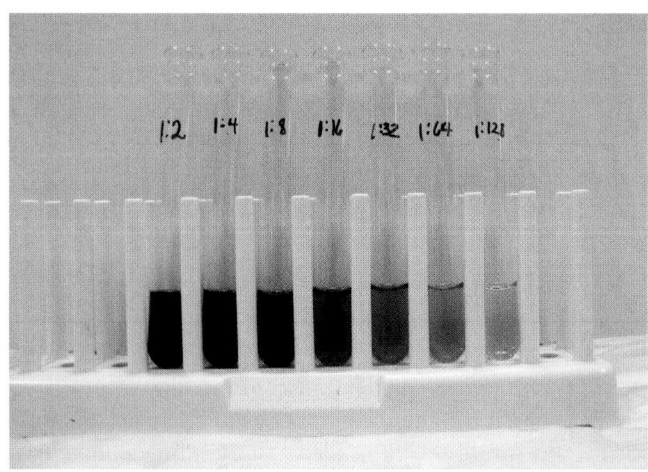

FIGURE 9–7 Serial dilution. Each tube contains the same amount of diluent and a blue dye. Each time a dilution is made, the amount of dye is cut in half in each successive tube. The final volume of each tube should be exactly the same. The color becomes visibly lighter with each dilution.

Connections

Agglutination

A common type of reaction used in a serial dilution system is agglutination. In agglutination, antibodies combine with particulate antigens, such as red blood cells, to form large lattice structures that become visible as aggregates. In direct and passive agglutination tests (see Chapter 10), the reciprocal of the last dilution at which agglutination can be observed is reported as the antibody titer.

is the reciprocal of the last dilution in the series that demonstrates the desired reaction. For example, if the last tube to show a visible reaction contained a 1:125 dilution, the titer would be stated as 125.

The antibody dilutions in each tube of a serial dilution system can be calculated by using a series of four steps. It is also helpful to visualize the problem by making a drawing of the setup before performing the calculations. Let's proceed to solve the following example by using this process.

Example: Serial Dilution

Suppose you set up a series of 10 tubes. You pipet 0.8 mL of saline into tube 1 and 0.4 mL of saline into tubes 2 to 10. Next, 0.2 mL of a serum sample is added to tube 1. The tube is mixed, and 0.4 mL is serially transferred through tube 10. Finally, 0.1 mL of antigen is added to all the tubes. What is the final titer of tube 4?

A drawing illustrating the set-up for this problem is shown in **Figure 9-8**.

Step 1

The first step to solving such a problem is to determine the dilution of serum in tube 1. This is equal to

$$\frac{0.2}{(0.2+0.8)}=\frac{1}{5}$$

Step 2

The second step in such a problem is to determine the dilution fold, which can be calculated using the following formula:

$$\frac{1}{\text{Dilution Fold (df)}}=\frac{\text{Volume Transferred}}{\text{Total Volume}}$$

The total volume is equal to the volume transferred from one tube to the next in the series plus the volume of diluent in the tube. To determine the dilution fold, it is best to use the volumes in any tube except tube 1, which may sometimes have a different volume of diluent than the other tubes.

In this example, the 1/df is equal to

$$\frac{0.4}{(0.4+0.4)}=\frac{1}{2}$$

Step 3

Once the dilution of tube 1 and the dilution fold are determined, these numbers can be used to calculate the dilutions in the remaining tubes before the addition of antigen. The dilution of each tube can be determined using the following formula:

$$\text{Dilution of Tube } n = \text{Dilution of Tube 1} \times \left(\frac{1}{\text{Dilution Fold}}\right)^{(n-1)}$$

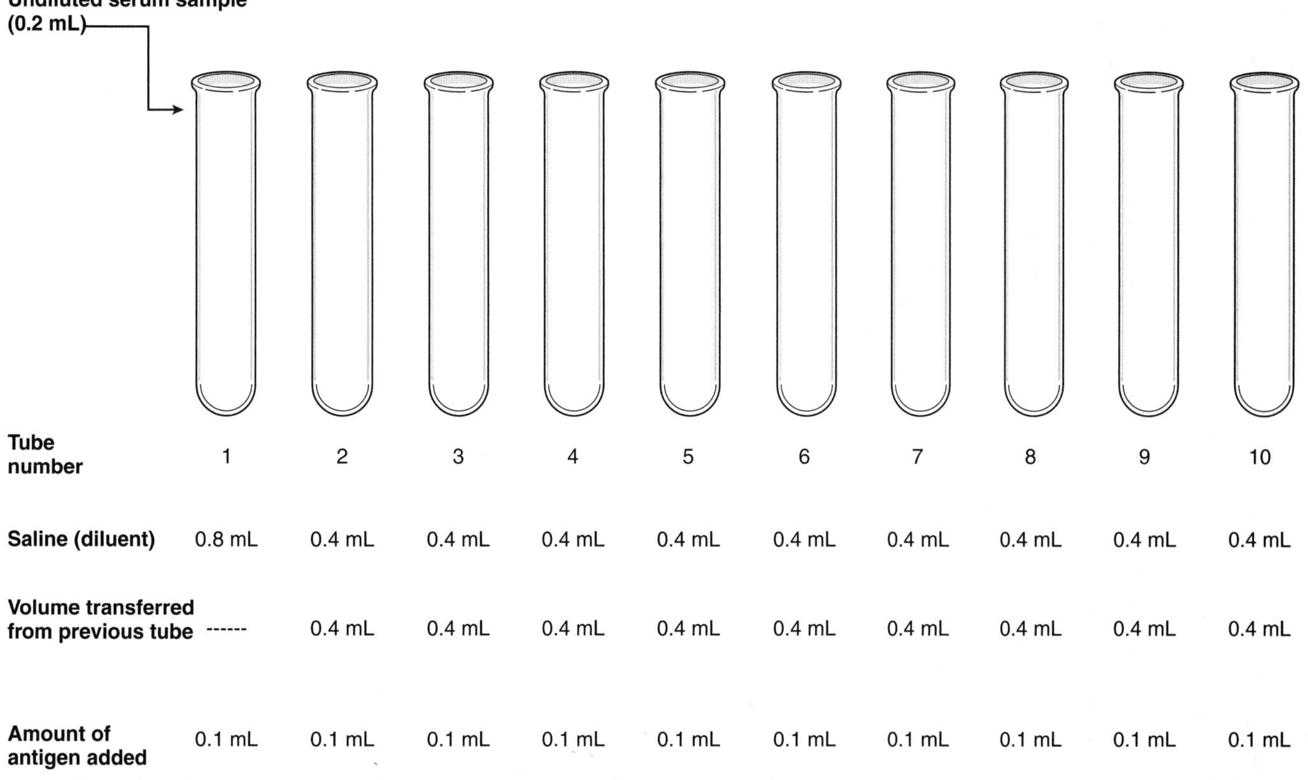

FIGURE 9–8 Sample serial dilution problem.

By placing the numbers in this example into this formula, the dilution of tube 4 would be calculated as follows: $1/5 \times [1/2]^{(4-1)} = 1/5 \times ½ \times ½ \times ½ = 1/40$

Step 4

The final titer is then calculated by incorporating the amount of antigen added to the tube, using the equation C1V1 = C2V2, where C1 and V1 refer to the tube before the addition of antigen, and C2 and V2 refer to the tube after to the addition of antigen. V1 is the volume in the tube after the serial dilution has been performed (i.e., volume of diluent plus volume transferred from the previous tube, minus volume transferred to the next tube). In this example, C1 = 1/40, V1 = 0.4 mL, and V2 = 0.5 mL. The final dilution of tube 4 (C2) can be calculated as follows:

$$1/40 \times 0.4 = C2 \times 0.5$$

$$C2 = 1/40 \times 0.4/0.5 = 1/50$$

The antibody titer in tube 4 is the reciprocal of this number, or 50. This titer would be reported by the laboratory if tube 4 was the last tube demonstrating a visible antigen–antibody reaction.

Test Parameters

A question sometimes arises as to whether or not a patient actually has the condition or disease being tested for when the results are obtained from a laboratory test. To make such a judgment, it is important to know the diagnostic sensitivity and specificity of a particular test. **Diagnostic sensitivity** can be defined as the proportion of people who have a specific disease or condition and who have a positive test result. Diagnostic sensitivity is a measure of the true-positive results and can be calculated using the following formula:

$$\text{Sensitivity (\%)} = \frac{\text{True Positives}}{\text{True Positives + False Negatives}} \times 100$$

The *diagnostic sensitivity* refers to the ability of a laboratory test to identify individuals with a given disease or condition. This is not to be confused with the *analytic sensitivity,* which refers to the lower limit of detection for the analyte measured by a laboratory test (see Chapter 11).

Diagnostic specificity refers to the proportion of people who do not have a disease or condition and who have a negative test. Diagnostic specificity is a measure of the true-negative results and can be calculated using the following formula:

$$\text{Specificity (\%)} = \frac{\text{True Negatives}}{\text{True Negatives + False Positives}} \times 100$$

The *diagnostic specificity* refers to the ability of a laboratory test to correctly identify individuals in whom a particular disease or condition is absent. This is not to be confused with the *analytic specificity,* which refers to the ability of a laboratory method to only detect the analyte it is designed to measure, without detecting other related (i.e., cross-reacting) substances.

Let's look at an example of test results to see how the diagnostic sensitivity and specificity are calculated.

Example

Suppose a new laboratory test was used with a particular population. The following results were obtained after 200 patients were tested: For the patients with the disease, 160 gave a positive test result (true positives), and 1 gave a negative result (false negative); for the patients without the disease, 14 gave a positive test result (false positives), and 25 gave a negative result (true negatives). Calculate the diagnostic sensitivity and specificity of the test.

Solution

To help clarify the problem, a table containing the given results can be constructed:

	NUMBER OF PATIENTS WITH DISEASE	NUMBER OF PATIENTS WITHOUT DISEASE
Positive test result	160 (true positives)	14 (false positives)
Negative test result	1 (false negative)	25 (true negatives)

The diagnostic sensitivity and specificity can then be calculated by placing these numbers into the formulas previously discussed:

$$\text{Sensitivity (\%)} = [160 \div (160 + 1)] \times 100 = 99.4\%$$

$$\text{Specificity (\%)} = [25 \div (25 + 14)] \times 100 = 64.1\%$$

This particular test is highly sensitive, detecting 99.4% of people who have the disease being tested for. However, the test is not very specific because it gives true-negative results in only 64.1% of people without the disease, and the remaining 35.9% without the disease have false-positive results.

Sensitivity and specificity are characteristics of the test itself. However, to determine the probability that a person with a particular test result actually has the disease or not, it is important to consider how often the disease occurs in the population being tested. The parameters used to make this determination are called *predictive values.* The **positive predictive value** is the probability that a person with a positive test actually has the disease being tested for. The positive predictive value is determined by dividing the true-positive results by the true-positive and the false-positive results added together:

$$\text{Positive Predictive Value (\%)} = \frac{\text{True Positives}}{\text{True Positives + False Positives}} \times 100$$

In the example given earlier, out of 200 patients, 160 were truly positive and 14 were falsely positive. Using these values in the equation gives us:

$$\text{Positive Predictive Value (\%)} = [160 \div (160 + 14)] \times 100 = 91.95\%$$

Thus, in this case, if an individual tests positive for a certain disease, there is approximately a 92% probability that the individual has that disease.

Likewise, the **negative predictive value** is the probability that a person with a negative screening test does not have the disease. It can be determined using the following formula:

$$\text{Negative Predictive Value (\%)} = \frac{\text{True Negatives}}{\text{True Negatives} + \text{False Negatives}} \times 100$$

Now let's use this formula to calculate the negative predictive value for the test results discussed in the previous example:

$$\text{Negative Predictive Value (\%)} = [25 \div (25 + 1)] \times 100 = 96.2\%$$

In this case, there is a 96.2% probability that a person with a negative test result does not have the disease in question. These values can help clinicians make a decision about an individual patient based on his or her test results and the prevalence of the disease in that particular population.

SUMMARY

- Serum for serological testing is obtained by allowing a sterile tube of blood to clot at either room temperature or 4°C and then carefully removing the serum from the clot after centrifugation has taken place.
- Volumetric pipettes hold a specified amount of liquid and are calibrated to deliver (TD) that exact amount.
- Serological pipettes are calibrated all the way to the bottom of the pipette. The liquid remaining in such a pipette must be blown out to deliver the exact amount of liquid required. These pipettes are labeled "TC" (to contain).
- A dilution is prepared by adding a liquid (called the *diluent*) to either a reagent or a sample of patient serum (the solute) to make a weaker solution. It is often necessary to make a dilution for a visible endpoint to occur in antigen–antibody reactions.
- In serological testing, an antibody in a sample of patient serum can be made less concentrated by adding diluent. The resulting dilution can be expressed as a ratio (e.g., 1:20) or as a fraction—for example, 1/20.
- When a series of dilutions is made using a constant dilution factor, this is called a *serial dilution*.
- Serial dilutions are used to determine the titer, or strength, of an antibody. The last tube in which a visible reaction is seen is considered the endpoint.
- *Diagnostic sensitivity* is defined as the proportion of people who have a specific disease or condition and have a positive test result for that disease or condition.
- *Diagnostic specificity* refers to the proportion of people who do not have the disease or condition and who have a negative test result for that disease or condition.
- If a test is highly sensitive and highly specific, it is a good indicator that a patient has the disease or condition if positive results are obtained.
- The positive predictive value is the likelihood that a person with a positive screening test actually has the disease.
- The negative predictive value is the probability that a person with a negative screening test does not have the disease.
- Positive and negative predictive values help clinicians determine whether a positive or a negative test is likely to be a true result based on a specific test population.

CASE STUDY

1. A serology supervisor who has worked for the last 20 years in a small rural hospital is training a new employee. A dilution of a patient's serum must be made to run a particular test. The supervisor is showing the new employee how to pipette the serum specimen. The amount needed is 0.1 mL. Using a serological pipette, she draws up the patient specimen to the 0.9-mL mark. She then lets it drain out. There is a tiny drop left in the pipette, but she explains to the new person that this is close enough. She then adds 1.9 mL of diluent to the tube with the serum. She needs a 1:40 dilution of the serum to run the test.

Questions

a. Explain any mistakes the supervisor may have made during her demonstration.
b. Was the dilution prepared correctly? If not, indicate how the dilution should be prepared, showing your calculations.

REVIEW QUESTIONS

1. If serum is not tested immediately, how should it be treated?
   a. It can be left at room temperature for 24 hours.
   b. It can be stored in the refrigerator for up to 72 hours.
   c. It can be stored in the refrigerator for up to 48 hours.
   d. It needs to be frozen immediately.

2. A 1:750 dilution of serum is needed to perform a serological test. Which of the following series of dilutions would be correct to use in this situation?
   a. 1:5, 1:15, 1:10
   b. 1:5, 1:10, 1:5
   c. 1:15, 1:10, 1:3
   d. 1:15, 1:3, 1:5

3. How much diluent needs to be added to 0.2 mL of serum to make a 1:20 dilution?
   a. 19.8 mL
   b. 4.0 mL
   c. 3.8 mL
   d. 10.0 mL

4. If glacial acetic acid needs to be diluted with water to make a 10% solution, what does the glacial acetic acid represent?
   a. Solute
   b. Diluent
   c. Titer
   d. Serial dilution

5. A pipette that has markings all the way down to its tip is called a
   a. volumetric pipette.
   b. serial pipette.
   c. graduated pipette.
   d. micropipette.

6. A serological test requires 5 mL of a 1:50 dilution. How much serum is required to make this dilution?
   a. 0.5 mL
   b. 0.01 mL
   c. 1.0 mL
   d. 0.1 mL

7. If 0.02 mL of serum is diluted with 0.08 mL of diluent, what dilution of serum does this represent?
   a. 1:4
   b. 1:5
   c. 1:10
   d. 1:20

8. A tube containing a 1:40 dilution is accidentally dropped. A 1:2 dilution of the specimen is still available. A volume of 4 mL is needed to run the test. How much of the 1:2 dilution is needed to remake 4 mL of a 1:40 dilution?
   a. 0.2 mL
   b. 0.4 mL
   c. 0.5 mL
   d. 1.0 mL

9. If 0.4 mL of serum is mixed with 15.6 mL of diluent, what dilution of serum does this represent?
   a. 1:4
   b. 1:40
   c. 2:70
   d. 1:80

10. How much diluent needs to be added to 0.1 mL of serum to make a 1:15 dilution?
    a. 1.4 mL
    b. 1.5 mL
    c. 5.0 mL
    d. 15 mL

11. Which of the following choices would be considered a serial dilution?
    a. 1:5, 1:15, 1:20
    b. 1:2, 1:10, 1:25
    c. 1:15, 1:30, 1:40
    d. 1:5, 1:15, 1:45

12. The following dilutions were set up to titer an antibody. The following results were obtained: 1:4 +, 1:8 +, 1:16 +, 1:32 +, 1:64 –. How should the titer be reported out?
    a. 4
    b. 16
    c. 32
    d. 64

13. If a serological test is positive for an individual who does not have a particular disease, the result was caused by a problem with
    a. sensitivity.
    b. specificity.
    c. accuracy.
    d. poor pipetting.

14. Which of the following would be the correct way to make a 5% solution of hydrochloric acid from concentrated hydrochloric acid?
    a. 0.5 mL of acid and 9.5 mL of water
    b. 0.5 mL of acid and 95 mL of water
    c. 0.1 mL of acid and 9.9 mL of water
    d. 0.1 mL of acid and 4.9 mL of water

15. What is the final dilution of serum obtained from the following serial dilutions: 1:4, 1:4, 1:4, 1:4, 1:4, 1:4?
    a. 1:24
    b. 1:256
    c. 1:1,024
    d. 1:4,096

16. Suppose you set up a row of 10 tubes. You pipet 0.4 mL of saline into tube 1 and 0.6 mL of saline into tubes 2 to 10. Next, you add 0.4 mL of patient serum to tube 1. Then, you serially transfer 0.2 mL from one tube to the next, discarding 0.2 mL from tube 10. What is the dilution of tube 4?
    a. 1:16
    b. 1:54
    c. 1:128
    d. 1:256

17. Suppose you set up a row of 10 tubes. You pipet 0.8 mL of saline in tube 1 and 0.9 mL of saline in tubes 2 to 10. You add 0.2 mL of patient serum to tube 1, and serially transfer 0.1 mL through tube 10. Finally, you add 0.9 mL of antigen to each tube. What is the final titer of tube 3?
    a. 1:500
    b. 1:1,000
    c. 1:5,000
    d. 1:10,000

18. A new laboratory assay gave the following results: number of patients tested = 100; number of true positives = 54, number of true negatives = 42; number of false positives = 2; number of false negatives = 2. What is the specificity of this assay in whole numbers?
    a. 75%
    b. 85%
    c. 95%
    d. 98%

19. What is the sensitivity of the assay in Question 18?
    a. 84%
    b. 90%
    c. 92%
    d. 96%

20. A screening test gave the following results: number of patients tested = 150; number of true positives = 50; number of true negatives = 85; number of false positives = 5; number of false negatives = 10. What is the positive predictive value rounded off to a whole number for a patient whose test is positive?
    a. 91%
    b. 83%
    c. 89%
    d. 56%

10 Precipitation and Agglutination Reactions

Christine Dorresteyn Stevens, EdD, MT(ASCP), and Linda E. Miller, PhD, MB^{CM}(ASCP)SI

LEARNING OUTCOMES

After finishing this chapter, you should be able to:

1. Discuss affinity and avidity and their influence on antigen–antibody reactions.
2. Describe how the law of mass action relates to antigen–antibody binding.
3. Define precipitation and agglutination and differentiate between the two types of reactions.
4. Describe the relative concentrations of antigen and antibody in the three zones of the precipitin curve and discuss why optimal precipitation occurs in the zone of equivalence.
5. Differentiate between immunoturbidimetry and nephelometry and discuss the role of each in the measurement of precipitation reactions.
6. Compare single diffusion to double diffusion.
7. Summarize the principle of the endpoint method of radial immunodiffusion (RID).
8. Determine the relationship between two antigens by looking at the pattern of precipitation resulting from Ouchterlony immunodiffusion.
9. Describe the principle of immunofixation electrophoresis (IFE).
10. Recognize how immunoglobulin M (IgM) and immunoglobulin G (IgG) differ in their ability to participate in agglutination reactions.
11. Describe physiological conditions that can be altered to enhance agglutination.
12. Define and give an example of each of the following: (a) direct agglutination, (b) passive agglutination, (c) reverse passive agglutination, (d) agglutination inhibition, and (e) hemagglutination inhibition.
13. Describe the principle of measurement used in particle-enhanced turbidimetric inhibition immunoassay (PETINIA).
14. Identify conditions that must be met for optimal results in agglutination testing.

CHAPTER OUTLINE

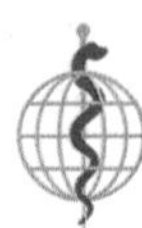

Go to FADavis.com for the laboratory exercises that accompany this text.

KEY TERMS

Affinity
Agglutination
Agglutination inhibition
Agglutinins
Avidity
Coombs reagent
Cross-reactivity
Direct agglutination
Electrophoresis
Endpoint method
Hemagglutination
Hemagglutination inhibition
Immunofixation electrophoresis (IFE)
Immunoturbidimetry
Lattice
Law of mass action
Nephelometry
Ouchterlony double diffusion
Passive agglutination
Passive immunodiffusion
Postzone
Precipitation
Prozone
Radial immunodiffusion (RID)
Rate nephelometry
Reverse passive agglutination
Sensitization
Zone of equivalence

The combination of an antigen with a specific antibody plays an important role in the laboratory in diagnosing many different diseases. Immunoassays have been developed to detect either antigen or antibody and vary from easily performed manual tests to highly complex automated assays. The first such assays were based on the principles of precipitation or agglutination. **Precipitation** involves combining soluble antigen with soluble antibody to produce insoluble complexes that are visible. **Agglutination** is the process by which particulate antigens, such as cells, aggregate to form larger complexes when a specific antibody is present. Precipitation and agglutination are considered unlabeled assays because a marker label is not needed to detect the reaction. Labeled assays, which were developed much later, will be considered in Chapter 11.

Precipitation was first noted in 1897 by Kraus, who found that culture filtrates of enteric bacteria would precipitate when they were mixed with specific antibodies. For such reactions to occur, both the antigen and antibody must have multiple binding sites for one another, and the relative concentration of each must be equal. Binding characteristics of antibodies, called *affinity* and *avidity*, also play a major role in generating a precipitation reaction.

> **Connections**
>
> **Epitope**
>
> Recall from Chapter 3 that an epitope (also known as an *antigenic determinant*) is the part of an antigen that binds to the antigen-binding site of an antibody.

Antigen–Antibody Binding

The primary union of binding sites on an antibody with specific epitopes on an antigen depends on two characteristics of antibody known as *affinity* and *avidity*. These characteristics are important because they relate to the sensitivity and specificity of testing in the clinical laboratory.

Affinity

Affinity is the initial force of attraction that exists between a single Fab site on an antibody molecule and a single epitope or determinant site on the corresponding antigen. As the epitope and binding site come into close proximity to each other, they are held together by weak bonds occurring over a short distance of approximately 1×10^{-7} mm.

The strength of attraction depends on the specificity of antibody for a particular antigen. One antibody molecule may initially attract numerous different antigens, but it is the epitope's shape and the way it fits together with the binding sites on an antibody molecule that determine whether the bonding will be stable. Antibodies are also capable of reacting with antigens resembling the original antigen that induced antibody production, a phenomenon known as **cross-reactivity.** The more the cross-reacting antigen resembles the original antigen, the stronger the bond will be between the antigen and the binding site. However, if the epitope and the binding site have a perfect lock-and-key fit, as is the case with the original antigen, the affinity will be maximal **(Fig. 10–1).** When the affinity is higher, the assay reaction is more sensitive because more antigen–antibody complexes will be formed and visualized more easily.

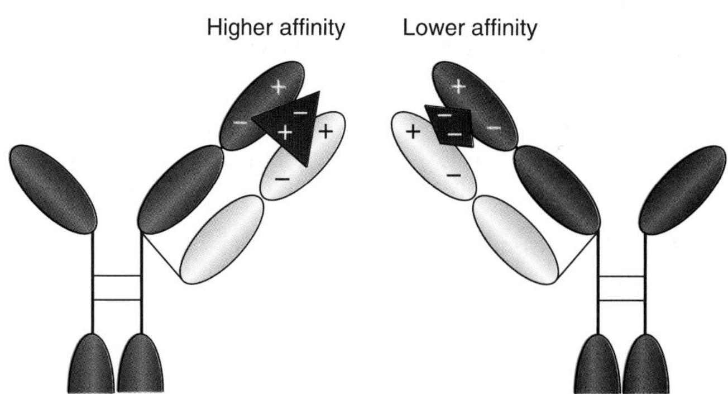

FIGURE 10–1 Affinity is determined by the three-dimensional fit and molecular attractions between one antigenic determinant and one antibody-binding site. The antigenic determinant on the left has a better fit and charge distribution than the epitope on the right and hence will have a higher affinity for the antibody.

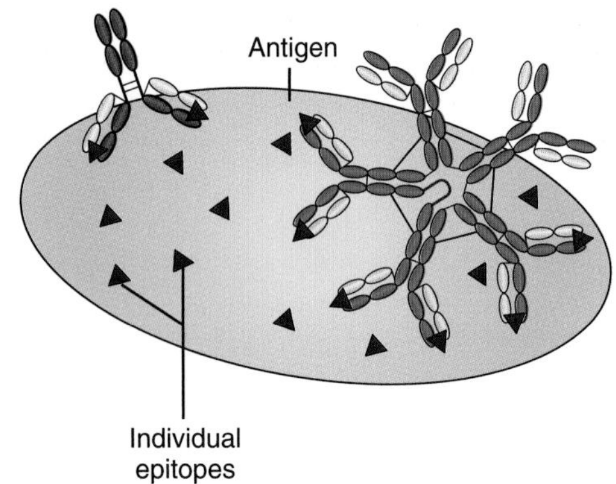

FIGURE 10–2 Avidity is the sum of the forces binding multivalent antigens to multivalent antibodies. In a comparison between immunoglobulin G (IgG) and IgM, IgM has the most potential binding sites for antigen and thus a higher avidity. Note that the monomer subunits in IgM can swing up or down in order to bind antigen more effectively.

Avidity

Avidity represents the overall strength of antigen–antibody binding and is the sum of the affinities of all the individual antibody–antigen combining sites. *Avidity* refers to the strength with which a multivalent antibody binds a multivalent antigen and is a measure of the overall stability of an antigen–antibody complex. In other words, avidity is the force that keeps the molecules together after binding has occurred. A high avidity can actually compensate for a low affinity. Different classes of antibodies differ in their avidities. The more bonds that form between antigen and antibody, the higher the avidity is. Immunoglobulin M (IgM), for instance, has a higher avidity than IgG because IgM has the potential to bind 10 different antigens **(Fig. 10–2).** Both affinity and avidity contribute to the stability of the antigen–antibody complexes, which is essential to detecting the presence of an unknown, whether it is antigen or antibody.

Law of Mass Action

All antigen–antibody binding is reversible and is governed by the **law of mass action.** This law states that free reactants are in equilibrium with bound reactants. The equilibrium constant K represents the difference in the rates of the forward and reverse reactions according to the following equation:

$$K = [AgAb]/[Ab][Ag]$$

where [AgAb] = concentration of the antigen–antibody complex (mol/L), [Ab] = concentration of free antibody (mol/L), and [Ag] = concentration of free antigen (mol/L).

The value of K depends on the strength of binding between antibody and antigen. As the strength of binding, or avidity, increases, the tendency of the antigen–antibody complexes to dissociate decreases, thus increasing the value of K. When the value of K is higher, the amount of antigen–antibody complex is larger, and the assay reaction is more visible or easily detectable. The ideal conditions in the clinical laboratory would be to have an antibody with a high affinity, or initial force of attraction, and a high avidity, or strength of binding. The higher the values are for both affinity and avidity, the more antigen–antibody complexes that are formed, and the more sensitive the test.

Precipitation Curve

In addition to the affinity and avidity of the antibody involved, precipitation depends on the relative proportions of antigen and antibody present. Optimal precipitation occurs when the relative amounts of antigen- and antibody-binding sites are equivalent, and neither is in excess as compared with the other. This relationship was discovered in 1932 by Heidelberger and Kendall, who set up a series of tubes containing a constant amount of antibody and increasing amounts of the corresponding antigen. As you can see in **Figure 10–3,** when the concentration of antigen is plotted on the *x*-axis of a graph and the number of antigen–antibody complexes is plotted on the *y*-axis, a bell-shaped curve results. The curve can be divided into three zones: the zone of antibody excess, the zone of antigen excess, and the zone of equivalence.

Three Zones of the Precipitation Reaction

In the *zone of antibody excess,* the concentration of antibody molecules is greater than the concentration of antigen

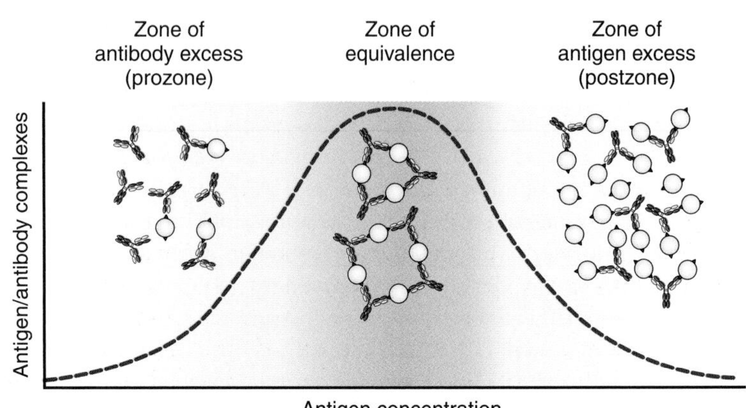

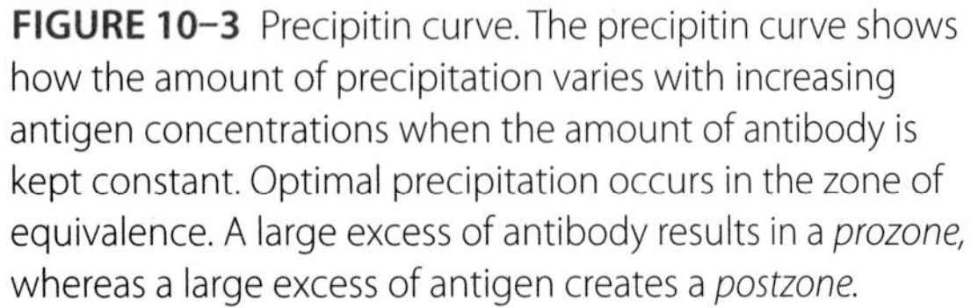
FIGURE 10–3 Precipitin curve. The precipitin curve shows how the amount of precipitation varies with increasing antigen concentrations when the amount of antibody is kept constant. Optimal precipitation occurs in the zone of equivalence. A large excess of antibody results in a *prozone,* whereas a large excess of antigen creates a *postzone.*

molecules. This results in the formation of small immune complexes, with little or no precipitation. Likewise, in the *zone of antigen excess,* the concentration of antigen molecules is greater than the concentration of antibody molecules. Again, little or no precipitation results, and the reaction is less than optimal.

In the **zone of equivalence** seen in the middle of the curve, the number of multivalent sites of antigen and antibody are approximately equal. In this zone, precipitation is the result of random, reversible reactions whereby each antibody binds to more than one antigen, and vice versa, forming a stable network or **lattice.** The concept of lattice formation, as formulated by Dr. Philippa Marrack, is based on the assumptions that each antibody molecule must have at least two binding sites and the antigen must be multivalent. As antigen and antibody combine, a multimolecular lattice forms that increases in size until it precipitates out of solution.

As illustrated in Figure 10–3, when the same amount of soluble antigen is added to increasing dilutions of antibody, the amount of precipitation increases until the zone of equivalence is reached. When the amount of antigen becomes greater than the number of antibody-binding sites present, precipitation begins to decline because fewer lattice networks are formed. Thus, optimal precipitation occurs in the zone of equivalence. It is important to note that the relationship between the amounts of antigen and antibody and the formation of immune complexes also applies to immunologic reactions other than precipitation and is the basis for all serological testing.

Prozone and Postzone

As seen in the precipitin curve, precipitation declines on either side of the equivalence zone because of an excess of either antigen or antibody. When antibody excess is large, a **prozone** occurs, in which antigen combines with only one or two antibody molecules, and no cross-linkages are formed. In the prozone, usually only one site on an antibody molecule is used, many free antibody molecules remain in solution, and precipitation is undetectable.

At the other side of the curve, where there is a large antigen excess, a **postzone** occurs in which small aggregates are surrounded by excess antigen. In this case, every available antibody site is bound to a single antigen, and no cross-links are formed. Again, no lattice network is formed, and precipitation does not occur (see Fig. 10–3).

The prozone and postzone phenomena must be considered in the clinical laboratory because negative reactions occur in both. A false-negative reaction may take place in the prozone because of a high antibody concentration in the unknown sample, such as patient serum. If it is suspected that the reaction is a false negative, diluting out the antibody until equivalence is reached and performing the test again can produce a positive result. In the postzone, excess antigen may obscure the presence of a small amount of antibody. If the antigen to be detected is in the patient sample, the sample can be diluted to reach equivalence with the antibody reagent. If the antigen is the reagent in the test, the test may be repeated with another sample from the patient collected about a week later. The extra time would allow for the further production of antibody by the patient. If the repeated test is negative, it is unlikely that the patient has that particular antibody.

Immunoturbidimetry and Nephelometry

Precipitation is one of the simplest methods of detecting antigen–antibody reactions because most antigens are multivalent and therefore capable of forming aggregates in the presence of the corresponding antibody. When antigen and antibody solutions are mixed, the antigen cross-links with numerous antibody molecules, and the lattice networks become so large that they precipitate out of solution. Although the oldest methods to measure precipitation were manual, in today's clinical laboratory, precipitation reactions are most commonly measured by automated methods based on immunoturbidimetry or nephelometry.

Immunoturbidimetry involves measurement of the *turbidity* or cloudiness of a solution. A detection device is placed 180 degrees from an incident light, collecting the light after it has passed through the solution **(Fig. 10–4).** This device measures the reduction in light intensity caused by reflection, absorption, or scatter of light as immune complexes are formed. The result is recorded in absorbance units, a measure of the ratio of incident light to that of transmitted light. The measurements are made using a spectrophotometer or an automated clinical chemistry analyzer.

Nephelometry measures the light that is scattered at a particular angle from the incident beam as it passes through a suspension (see Fig. 10–4). Scattering occurs when a beam of light passes through a solution, encounters molecules in its

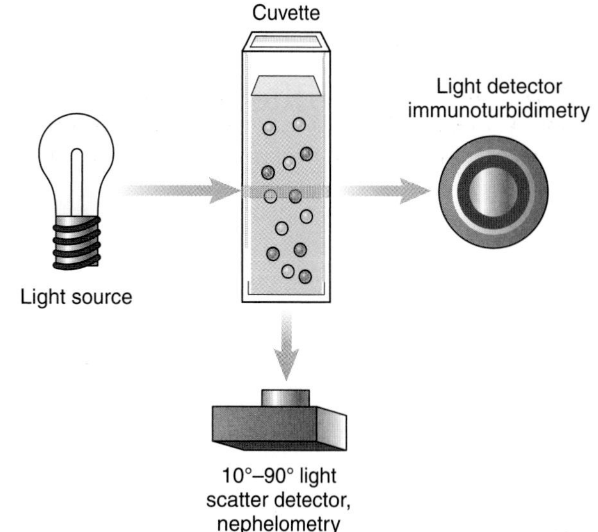

FIGURE 10-4 Principles of nephelometry and immunoturbidimetry. In nephelometry, the light-detection device is at an angle to the incident light, in contrast to immunoturbidimetry, which measures light rays passing directly through the solution.

path, and bounces off the molecules. The light travels in all directions and is measured by an instrument called a *nephelometer,* which contains a photodetector located between 30 and 90 degrees from the light source. The amount of light scatter is proportional to the size, shape, and concentration of molecules in solution, in this case, free antigen, free antibody, and antigen–antibody complexes. Thus, light scatter increases as the number of immune complexes increases and is an index of the concentration of antigen or antibody in solution.

Clinical instruments use a technique called **rate nephelometry** for the measurement of serum proteins. In this instance, patient serum contains the antigen, and a reagent containing the corresponding antibody is added to the reaction cuvette. For example, to measure C-reactive protein (CRP) in patient serum, an anti-CRP reagent is added. The rate of light scatter increase is measured immediately after adding the reagent antibody; thus, several samples can be assayed in just a few minutes. The concentration of antibody is kept constant, and the rate of light scatter increase is directly related to the antigen concentration in the patient serum. Light scatter is extrapolated by a computer to give the concentration of antigen in the patient sample in milligrams per deciliter (mg/dL) or international units per milliliter (IU/mL), based on established values of standards.

Rate nephelometry and immunoturbidimetry are commonly used to quantify the immunoglobulins IgG, immunoglobulin A (IgA), IgM, and immunoglobulin E (IgE), as well as kappa and lambda light chains. Other serum proteins measured by these methods include complement components such as C3 and C4, CRP, haptoglobin, and ceruloplasmin. Nephelometry and immunoturbidimetry provide accurate and precise quantitation of serum proteins, and because of automation, the cost per test is typically lower than manual methods. Additionally, very small sample volumes can be analyzed. In general, nephelometry is more sensitive than immunoturbidimetry, with a lower limit of detection of 1 to 10 mg/L, although the sensitivity of immunoturbidimetry methods has increased.

Passive Immunodiffusion Techniques

The precipitation of antigen–antibody complexes can also be detected by manual methods that use a support medium, such as a gel. Agarose, a purified high-molecular-weight complex polysaccharide derived from seaweed, is used for this purpose. When antigen and antibody diffuse toward one another in a gel matrix, visible lines of precipitation will form. Agarose helps stabilize the diffusion process and allow visualization of the precipitin bands.

Antigen and antibody are added to wells cut into the gel, diffuse through the gel medium, and combine with each other. This process is known as **passive immunodiffusion** when no electrical current is used to speed up the migration of the reactants. The rate of diffusion is affected by several factors, including the size of the particles (larger particles migrate slower than smaller ones), the temperature (warmer temperatures speed up the reaction), and the gel viscosity (molecules travel slower when the gel is more viscous and less hydrated). Immunodiffusion reactions can be classified according to the number of reactants diffusing in the gel and the direction of diffusion.

Radial Immunodiffusion

Radial immunodiffusion (RID) is a single-diffusion technique involving migration of antigen only. In this method, reagent antibody is uniformly mixed into the support gel, and antigen contained in commercial standards or the patient sample is applied to wells cut into the gel. During incubation, the antigen diffuses out from each well and combines with specific antibody in the agarose to form rings of precipitation around the wells. The rings expand in size until the zone of equivalence is reached and a stable lattice network is formed. The area of the ring obtained is a measure of the antigen concentration in a particular well. The antigen concentration within a patient sample can be derived from a standard curve obtained by using antigens of known concentrations. **Figure 10–5** depicts typical RID results.

One technique for the measurement of RID was developed by Mancini and is known as the **endpoint method.** In this technique, antigen is allowed to diffuse to completion; when equivalence is reached, there is no further change in the ring diameter. Equivalence occurs between 24 and 72 hours. The square of the ring diameter is directly proportional to the concentration of the antigen. When concentrations of antigen standards are plotted on the *x*-axis and the ring diameter is squared on the *y*-axis, a linear graph connecting the points

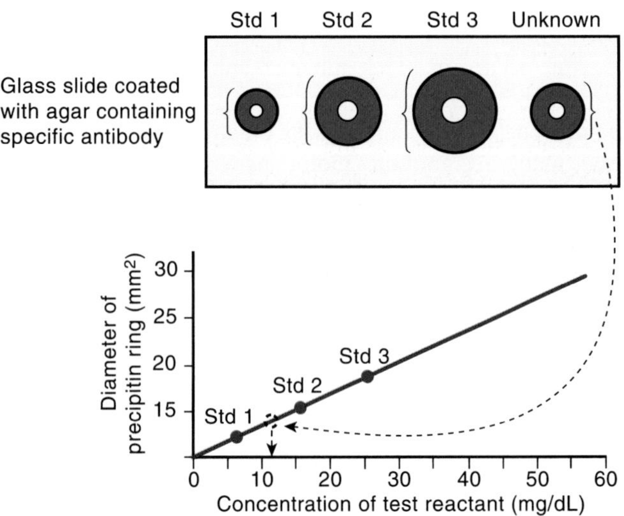

FIGURE 10–5 Radial immunodiffusion. The amount of precipitate formed is in proportion to the antigen present in the sample. In the Mancini endpoint method, antigen concentration is in proportion to the diameter squared. The concentration of the test reactant in the unknown sample can be determined from a standard curve generated from standards with known concentrations of the reactant.

is created. The major drawback to this method is the time it takes to obtain results. Another method, the kinetic or Fahey method, uses ring-diameter readings taken at about 19 hours before equivalence is reached. In this case, the ring diameter is proportional to the log of the antigen concentration, and a graph is plotted using semi-log paper. The diameter is plotted on the *x*-axis and the antigen concentration is on the *y*-axis, automatically giving a log value. Commercial kits may also contain a chart provided by the manufacturer that indicates concentration relative to the ring diameter.

The precision of the assay is directly related to accurate measurement of samples and standards. Sources of error include overfilling or underfilling the wells with sample, nicking the side of the wells when filling, spilling sample outside the wells, improper incubation time and temperature, and incorrect measurement of ring diameters. Similar to nephelometry and immunoturbidimetry, RID has been used to measure immunoglobulin classes and subclasses as well as complement components and other serum proteins. Immunodiffusion is simple to perform and requires no instrumentation but requires expensive reagents, has a long turnaround time to results, and is subject to technical artifacts. For these reasons, it has been largely replaced by automated techniques in the clinical laboratory.

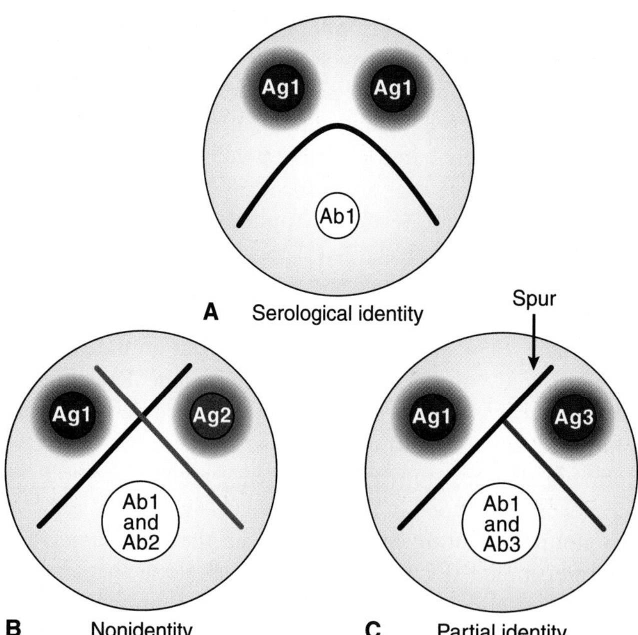

FIGURE 10–6 The three Ouchterlony diffusion patterns. An antibody mixture is placed in the central well. Unknown antigens are placed in the outside wells. The antibodies (Ab) and antigens (Ag) diffuse radially out of the wells. (A) Serological identity. If the antigens are identical, they will react with the same antibody, and the precipitate line forms a continuous arc. (B) Nonidentity. If the antigens share no identical determinants, they will react with different antibodies, and two crossed lines are formed. (C) Partial identity. Antibodies react with two similar antigens, forming two lines and a spur that points to the simpler antigen (the antigen that reacts least with the antibody). For example, suppose antigen 3 has an epitope in common with antigen 1, and there are two antibodies in the center well (anti-1 and anti-3). One of the antibodies reacts with the epitope common to both antigens. The other antibody reacts with a different epitope on antigen 1 (that is absent on antigen 3). Two precipitin lines form, with a spur pointing toward antigen 3.

Ouchterlony Double Diffusion

One of the older, classic immunochemical techniques is **Ouchterlony double diffusion.** In this technique, both antigen and antibody diffuse independently through a semisolid medium in two dimensions, horizontally and vertically. Wells are cut into a gel, and reactants are added to the wells. Most Ouchterlony plates are set up with a central well surrounded by four to six equidistant outer wells. Antibodies are placed in the central well, and different antigens are placed in the surrounding wells to determine if the antigens share identical epitopes. Diffusion takes place radially from the wells. After an incubation period of between 12 and 48 hours in a moist chamber, precipitin lines form where the moving front of antigen meets that of antibody and the point of equivalence is reached. The density of the lines reflects the amount of immune complex formed.

The position of the precipitin bands between wells allows for the antigens to be compared with one another. Three patterns of precipitation are possible (see **Fig. 10–6**):

1. *Identity*—fusion of the lines at their junction to form an arc represents serological identity or the presence of a common epitope.
2. *Non-identity*—a pattern of crossed lines demonstrates two separate reactions and indicates that the compared antigens share no common epitopes.
3. *Partial identity*—indicated by fusion of two lines with a spur. In the case of partial identity, the two antigens share a common epitope, but some antibody molecules are not captured by the simpler antigen and travel through the initial precipitin line to combine with additional epitopes found in the more complex antigen. Therefore, the spur always points to the simpler antigen.

Although of more limited use because it is labor intensive and requires experience to read, Ouchterlony double diffusion is still used to identify antibodies to some fungal organisms, such as *Aspergillus, Blastomyces, Coccidioides,* and *Candida.*

Electrophoretic Techniques

Diffusion can be combined with electrophoresis to speed up or sharpen the results. **Electrophoresis** separates molecules according to differences in their electric charge when they are placed in an electric field. A direct current is forced through the gel, causing antigen, antibody, or both to migrate. As diffusion takes place, distinct precipitin bands are formed. Through the years, several precipitation techniques have been combined with electrophoresis, including immunoelectrophoresis, counter immunoelectrophoresis, rocket immunoelectrophoresis, and immunofixation electrophoresis. Currently, immunofixation electrophoresis is routinely used in the clinical laboratory.

Immunofixation electrophoresis (IFE), as first described by Alper and Johnson, involves an initial electrophoresis step to separate proteins in patient serum on an agarose or cellulose acetate gel. Because diffusion occurs across a thin gel (approximately 1 mm), separation takes place in less than 1 hour.

Typically, patient serum is applied to six lanes of the gel. After electrophoresis, five lanes are overlaid with one of each of the following reagent antibodies: antibody to gamma, alpha, or mu heavy chains and to kappa or lambda light chains. The sixth lane is overlaid with antibody to all serum proteins and serves as the reference lane. Reactions in each of the five lanes are compared with the reference lane. Immunoprecipitates form only where a specific antigen–antibody combination has taken place and the complexes have become trapped in the gel. The gel is washed to remove any nonprecipitating proteins and can then be stained for easier visibility. IFE is a qualitative technique that can be used to visualize increases or decreases in immunoglobulin production and to differentiate monoclonal from polyclonal immunoglobulins. Hypogammaglobulinemias, which are characterized by low antibody production, exhibit faintly staining bands, whereas polyclonal hypergammaglobulinemias (overproduction of antibody) show darkly staining bands in the gamma region. The presence of monoclonal antibody, such as those found in certain malignancies of the immune system, results in dark, narrow bands in specific lanes **(Fig. 10–7)**.

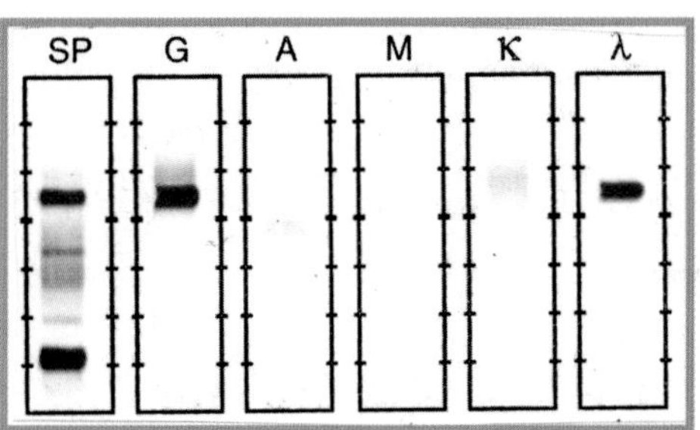

FIGURE 10–7 Immunofixation electrophoresis. A complex antigen mixture such as serum proteins is separated by electrophoresis. An antiserum template is aligned over the gel. Then protein fixative and monospecific antisera, IgG, IgA, IgM, **κ**, and **λ** are applied to the gel. After incubating for 30 minutes, the gel is stained and examined for the presence of abnormal immunoglobulins. Precipitates form where specific antigen–antibody combination has taken place. In this case, the patient has an IgG monoclonal antibody with **λ** chains. *(Courtesy of Helena Laboratories, Beaumont, TX.)*

Comparison of Precipitation Techniques

Each type of precipitation technique has distinct advantages and disadvantages. Some techniques are technically more demanding, whereas others are more automated. Each type of precipitation testing has particular applications for which it is best suited. **Table 10–1** presents a comparison of the precipitation techniques discussed in this chapter.

Clinical Correlations

Immunoproliferative Diseases

Normally, the immune system produces polyclonal immunoglobulins, generated by many clones of B cells as they respond to different antigens in our environment. Patients with cancers involving B cells or plasma cells produce high levels of a monoclonal antibody that originate from the single malignant clone. These conditions are referred to as *immunoproliferative diseases* and include multiple myeloma, which is most commonly characterized by the production of monoclonal IgG, IgA, or free light chains, and Waldenström macroglobulinemia, in which patients produce monoclonal IgM. See Chapter 18 for details.

Table 10–1 Comparison of Precipitation Techniques

TECHNIQUE	APPLICATIONS	SENSITIVITY (μg Ab/mL)	PRINCIPLE
Nephelometry	Immunoglobulins, complement, CRP, other serum proteins	1–10	Light that is scattered at an angle is measured, indicating the amount of antigen or antibody present.
Radial immunodiffusion (RID)	Immunoglobulins, complement	10–50	Antigen diffuses out into a gel that is infused with antibody. Measurement of the precipitin ring diameter indicates the concentration of the antigen.
Ouchterlony double diffusion	Antibodies to complex antigens, such as fungal antigens	20–200	Both antigen and antibody diffuse out from wells in a gel. The patterns of precipitate lines formed indicate the relationship of the antibodies.
Immunofixation electrophoresis (IFE)	Over- or underproduction of antibody; presence of monoclonal antibody	Variable	Electrophoresis of serum followed by direct application of reagent antisera to the gel.

Principles of Agglutination Reactions

Whereas precipitation reactions involve soluble antigens, agglutination is the visible aggregation of particles caused by combination with specific antibody. Antibodies that produce such reactions are often called **agglutinins.** Because this reaction takes place on the surface of the particle, antigen must be exposed and be able to bind with antibody. Types of particles participating in such reactions include erythrocytes, bacterial cells, and inert carriers such as latex particles. Each particle must have multiple antigenic determinant sites, which are cross-linked to sites on other particles through the formation of antibody bridges.

In 1896, Gruber and Durham published the first report about the ability of antibody to clump cells, based on observations of agglutination of bacteria by serum. This finding gave rise to the use of serology as a tool in the diagnosis of disease and also led to the discovery of the ABO blood groups. Widal and Sicard developed one of the earliest diagnostic tests in 1896 for the detection of antibodies occurring in typhoid fever, brucellosis, and tularemia. Agglutination reactions have had a wide variety of applications in the detection of both antigens and antibodies over the years. Such testing is simple to perform, and the endpoints can easily be read visually.

Agglutination, similar to precipitation, is a two-step process that results in the formation of a stable lattice network. The first step, called **sensitization**, involves antigen–antibody combination through single antigenic determinants on the particle. Sensitization is rapid and reversible. The second step, *lattice formation,* involves the development of cross-links that form visible aggregates. Lattice formation represents the stabilization of antigen–antibody complexes with the binding together of multiple antigenic determinants **(Fig. 10–8).**

Sensitization is affected by the nature of the antigens on the agglutinating particles. If epitopes are sparse or obscured by other surface molecules, they are less likely to interact with antibody. Additionally, red blood cells (RBCs) and bacterial cells have a slightly negative surface charge; because like charges tend to repel one another, it is sometimes difficult to bring such cells together into a lattice formation.

The class of immunoglobulin is also important; because IgM has a potential valence of 10, it is more than 700 times more efficient in agglutination than is IgG, which has a valence of 2. (See Fig. 10–2 for a comparison of IgG versus IgM.) Antibodies of the IgG class often cannot bridge the distance between particles because their small size and restricted flexibility at the hinge region may prohibit multivalent binding. IgM antibodies, on the other hand, are strong agglutinins because of their larger size.

Achieving visible reactions with IgG often requires the use of enhancement techniques that vary physicochemical conditions, such as the ionic strength of the solution, the pH, and the temperature. Antibodies belonging to the IgG class agglutinate best at 30°C to 37°C and are referred to as *warm-reacting antibodies*, whereas IgM antibodies are cold-reacting, working best at temperatures between 4°C and 27°C. Because naturally occurring antibodies against the ABO blood groups belong to the IgM class, these reactions are best run at room temperature. Antibodies to other human blood groups usually belong to the IgG class; reactions involving these must be run at 37°C. These latter reactions are the most important to consider in selecting compatible blood for a transfusion because these are the ones that will actually occur in the body.

In addition to temperature considerations, detection of IgG antibodies often requires the use of a second antibody, anti-human immunoglobulin, to visualize a reaction. Anti-human immunoglobulin is also known as **Coombs reagent** and is used frequently in blood bank testing. Coombs reagent attaches to the Fc portion of IgG and helps to bridge the gap between RBCs so that a visible agglutination reaction can occur. **Figure 10–9** demonstrates how Coombs reagent works.

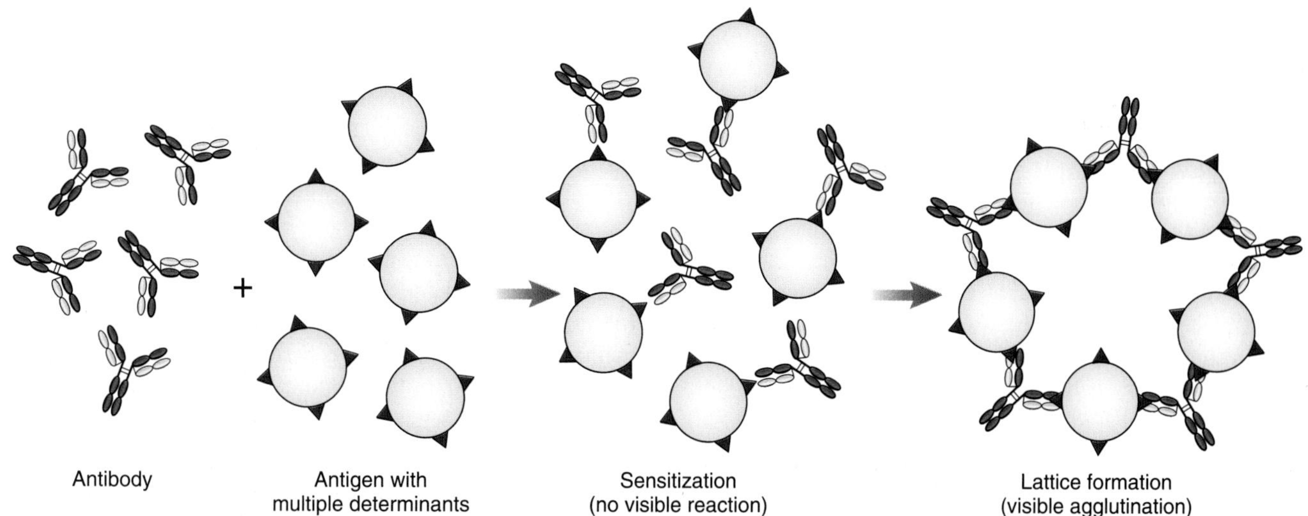

FIGURE 10–8 Phases of agglutination. Sensitization: Single epitopes on the antigen bind to antibody. Lattice formation: Multiple antigen and antibody molecules bind together to form a stable lattice.

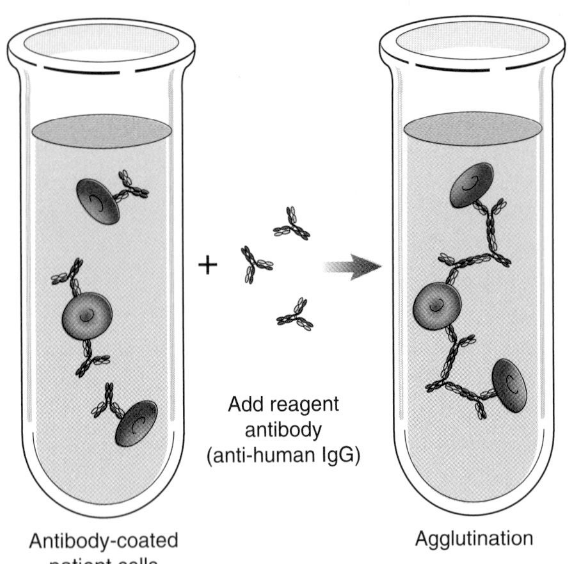

FIGURE 10–9 Coombs reagent. Coombs reagent is anti-human immunoglobulin used to enhance agglutination reactions by attaching to the Fc portion of IgG found on antibody-coated RBCs. Coombs reagent helps to bridge the gap between RBCs so that a visible agglutination reaction will occur.

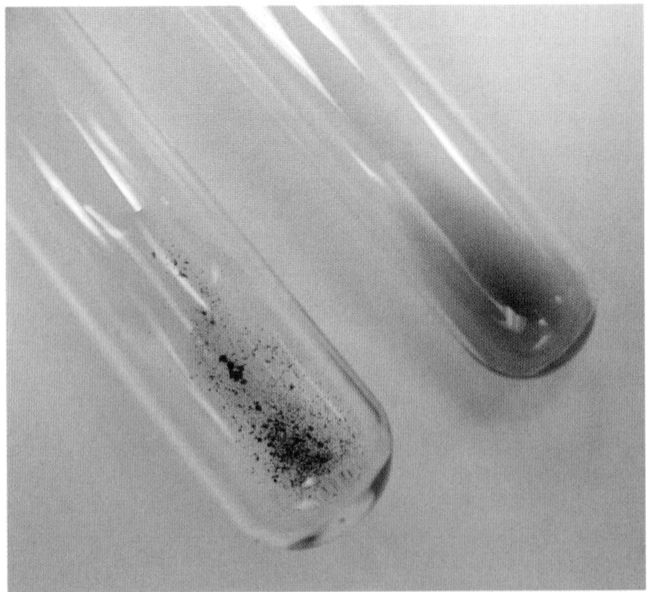

FIGURE 10–10 RBC agglutination. The tube on the left is a positive test for RBC agglutination, whereas the tube on the right is a negative test showing that the RBCs have remained in a smooth suspension. *(Courtesy Linda Miller.)*

Types of Agglutination Reactions

Agglutination tests are easy to carry out, require no complicated equipment, and can be performed as needed in the laboratory without having to batch specimens. Many kits are available for standard testing, so reagent preparation is minimal. Agglutination reactions can be used to identify either antigen or antibody. Typically, most agglutination tests are qualitative, simply indicating the absence or presence of antigen or antibody, but dilutions can be made to obtain semiquantitative results. Many variations exist that can be categorized according to the type of particle used in the reaction and whether antigen or antibody is attached to it.

Direct Agglutination

Direct agglutination occurs when antigens are found naturally on a particle. One of the earliest types of direct agglutination testing developed involves the use of known bacterial antigens to test for the presence of bacterial antibodies in a patient. Typically, patient serum is diluted into a series of tubes or wells on a slide and reacted with bacterial antigens specific for the suspected disease. Detection of antibodies is primarily used in the diagnosis of diseases for which the bacterial agents are extremely difficult to culture. One such example is the Widal test, a rapid screening test for antibodies to *Salmonella typhi* antigens, which has been used to help detect typhoid fever. A significant finding is a fourfold increase in antibody titer through time when paired dilutions of serum samples are tested with any of these antigens. Although more specific tests are now available, the Widal test is still considered useful in diagnosing typhoid fever in developing countries and remains in use in many areas throughout the world.

If an agglutination reaction involves RBCs, then it is called **hemagglutination.** The best example of this occurs in ABO blood group typing of human RBCs, one of the world's most frequently used immunoassays. Patient RBCs mixed with antisera of the IgM type can be used to determine the presence or absence of the A and B antigens; this reaction is usually performed at room temperature, without the need for any enhancement techniques. Group A RBCs will agglutinate with anti-A antibody, and Group B RBCs will agglutinate with anti-B antibody. This type of agglutination reaction is simple to perform, relatively sensitive, and easy to read **(Fig. 10–10).**

Other examples of direct hemagglutination tests are some versions of the Monospot test and cold agglutinins testing. The Monospot test is used to detect the heterophile antibody characteristic of infectious mononucleosis by its ability to agglutinate horse or bovine RBCs. Cold agglutinins, produced by patients with certain autoimmune disorders, malignancies, or infections, are antibodies that agglutinate human type O RBCs when incubated at cold temperatures. See Chapters 14 and 23 for details.

A titer that yields semiquantitative results can be performed in test tubes or microtiter plates by making serial dilutions of the antibody. The reciprocal of the last dilution still exhibiting a visible reaction is the titer, indicating the antibody's strength. Interpretation of the test is done on the basis of the cell sedimentation pattern. If the test is performed in a microtiter plate, a dark red, smooth button at the bottom of the microtiter well indicates that the result is negative. A positive result will have cells that are spread across the well's bottom because of formation of an antigen–antibody lattice, which may be smooth or have a jagged pattern with an irregular edge. Test tubes also can be centrifuged and then shaken to see if the cell button can be evenly resuspended. If it is resuspended with no visible

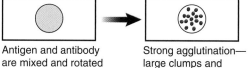

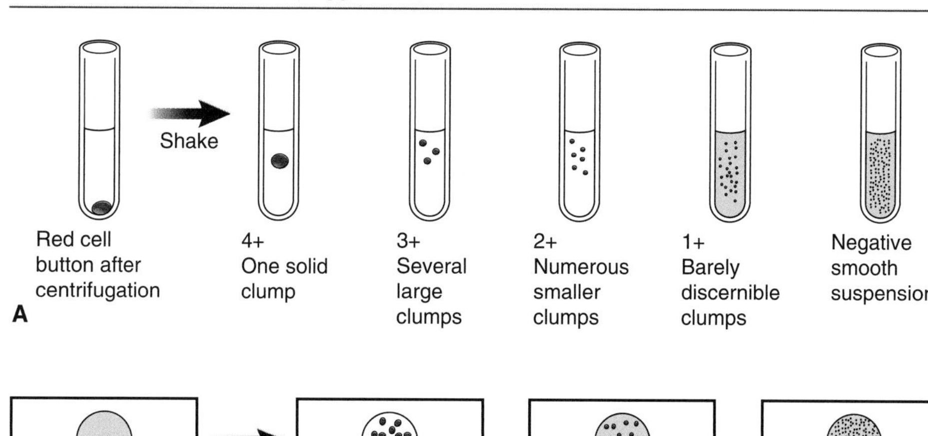

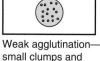

FIGURE 10–11 Grading of agglutination reactions: (A) Tube method. If tubes are centrifuged and shaken to resuspend the button, reactions can be graded from negative to 4+, depending on the size of the clumps observed. (B) Rapid slide method.

clumping, then the result is negative. Positive reactions can be graded to indicate the strength of the reaction **(Fig. 10–11).**

Passive Agglutination

Passive, or indirect, **agglutination** employs particles that are coated with antigens not normally found on their surfaces. A variety of particles, including erythrocytes, latex, and gelatin, are used for passive agglutination. The use of synthetic beads or particles provides the advantages of consistency and uniformity. Reactions are easy to read visually and give rapid results. Many antigens, especially polysaccharides, adsorb to RBCs spontaneously, so they are also relatively easy to manipulate. Particle sizes vary from 7 mm for RBCs down to 0.8 mm for fine latex particles.

In 1955, Singer and Plotz found by happenstance that IgG was naturally adsorbed to the surface of polystyrene latex particles. Latex particles are inexpensive, relatively stable, and not subject to cross-reactivity with other antibodies. A large number of antibody molecules can be bound to the surface of latex particles, so the number of antigen-binding sites is large. Additionally, the large particle size facilitates reading of the test. Passive latex agglutination tests have been used to detect many antibodies, including rheumatoid factor (an anti-IgG found in some autoimmune disorders), antibodies to Group A *Streptococcus* antigens, and antibodies to viruses such as cytomegalovirus and rubella.

Because many of these kits are designed to detect IgM antibody, there is a risk of nonspecific agglutination caused by the presence of other IgM antibodies, and reactions must be carefully controlled and interpreted. Commercial tests are usually performed on disposable plastic slide cards or glass slides. Kits contain positive and negative controls; if the controls do not give the expected results, the test is not valid. Such tests are typically used as screening tools, which are followed by more extensive testing if the results are positive.

> **Clinical Correlations**
>
> **Passive Agglutination Tests for Syphilis**
>
> A hemagglutination test called the *microhemagglutination assay for* Treponema pallidum *antibodies* (MHA-TP) was developed to detect antibodies to *T. pallidum,* the cause of syphilis, but has been replaced by a more sensitive gel particle agglutination method, the TP-PA. In this test, patient serum is incubated with gel particles coated with *T. pallidum* antigen in microtiter plate wells. A positive test is indicated by a smooth mat of particles (lattice) covering the well and is seen in patients who currently have syphilis or had syphilis in the past. See Chapter 21 for details.

Reverse Passive Agglutination

In **reverse passive agglutination,** antibody rather than antigen is attached to a carrier particle. The antibody must still be reactive and is joined in such a manner that the active sites are facing outward. Adsorption may be spontaneous, or it may require some of the same manipulation as is used for antigen attachment. This type of testing is often used to detect microbial antigens. **Figure 10–12** shows the differences between passive and reverse passive agglutination.

Numerous kits are available for the rapid identification of antigens from such infectious agents as Group A *Streptococcus,* Group B *Streptococcus, Staphylococcus aureus,* rotavirus, and *Cryptococcus neoformans.* Rapid agglutination tests have found the widest application in detecting soluble antigens in urine, spinal fluid, and serum. The principle is the same for all these tests: Latex particles coated with antibody are reacted with a patient sample containing the suspected antigen. In some cases, an extraction step is necessary to isolate antigen before the reagent latex particles are added. Organisms can be identified in a few minutes with fairly high sensitivity

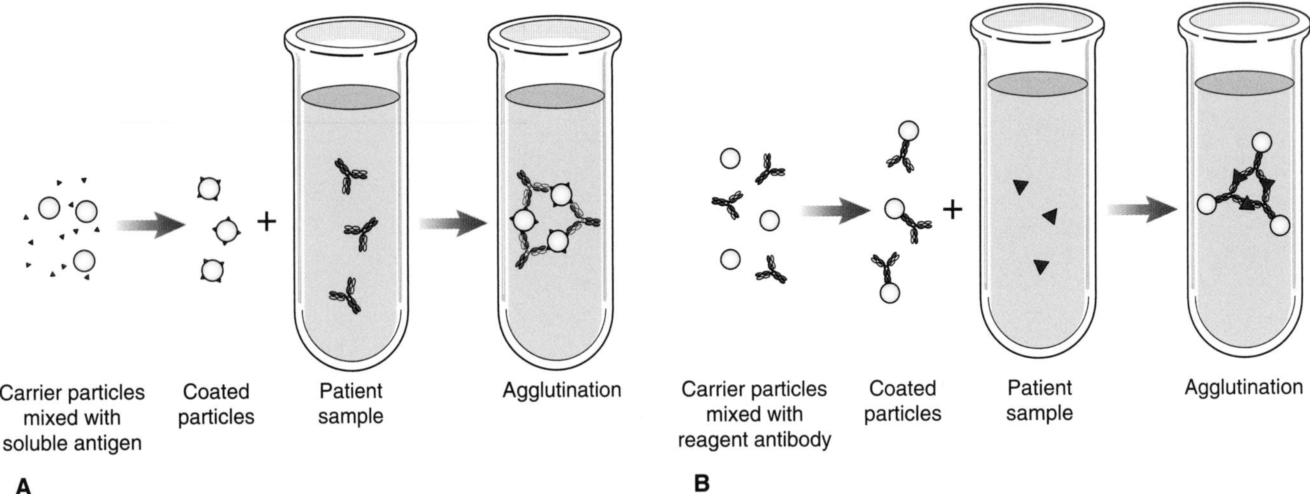

FIGURE 10–12 Passive and reverse passive agglutination. (A) Passive agglutination. Antigen is attached to the carrier particle; agglutination occurs if patient antibody is present. (B) Reverse passive agglutination. Antibody is attached to the carrier particle; agglutination occurs if patient antigen is present.

and specificity, although this varies for different organisms. The use of monoclonal antibodies has greatly reduced cross-reactivity, but there is still the possibility of interference or nonspecific agglutination.

Such tests are most often used to detect infections with organisms that are difficult to grow in the laboratory or for instances when rapid identification will allow treatment to be initiated more promptly. Reverse passive agglutination testing has also been used to measure levels of certain therapeutic drugs, hormones, and plasma proteins such as haptoglobin and CRP.

Agglutination Inhibition

Agglutination inhibition reactions are based on competition between particulate and soluble antigens for limited antibody-combining sites. Typically, this type of reaction involves haptens that are complexed to proteins; the hapten–protein conjugate is then attached to a carrier particle. The patient sample is first reacted with a limited amount of reagent antibody that is specific for the hapten being tested. Indicator particles that contain the same hapten one wishes to measure in the sample are then added. If the patient sample has no free hapten, the reagent antibody is able to combine with the carrier particles and produce a visible agglutination. Agglutination is a negative reaction, indicating that the patient did not have sufficient hapten to inhibit the secondary reaction **(Fig. 10–13).** In contrast, if the patient sample contains a significant concentration of hapten, it will bind to the reagent antibody and inhibit agglutination; thus, a lack of agglutination indicates a positive reaction.

Either antigen or antibody can be attached to the particles. The sensitivity of the reaction is governed by the avidity of the antibody itself. It can be a sensitive assay capable of detecting small quantities of antigen. Tests used to detect illicit drugs such as cocaine or heroin are examples of agglutination inhibition tests.

Hemagglutination inhibition reactions use the same principle, except RBCs are the indicator particles. This type of testing has been used to detect antibodies to certain viruses, such as rubella, influenza, and respiratory syncytial virus (RSV). RBCs have naturally occurring receptors for these viruses. When virus is present, spontaneous agglutination occurs because the virus particles link the RBCs together. Presence of patient antibody inhibits the agglutination reaction **(Fig. 10–14).**

To perform a hemagglutination inhibition test, dilutions of patient serum are incubated with a viral preparation. Then RBCs that the virus is known to agglutinate are added to the mixture. If antibody is present, it will attach to the viral particles and prevent agglutination, so a lack of or reduction in agglutination indicates the presence of patient antibody. Controls are necessary because there may be a factor in the serum that causes agglutination, or the virus may have lost its ability to agglutinate RBCs.

Instrumentation

Although agglutination reactions require no complicated instrumentation to read, several chemistry analyzers have been developed using automation to increase sensitivity. Nephelometry and immunoturbidimetry have been applied to the reading of agglutination reactions, and the term *particle-enhanced immunoassay* is used to describe such reactions. When particles are used, the sensitivity can be increased to nanograms/mL. For this type of reaction, small latex particles with a diameter smaller than 1 mm are used. Latex particles are coated with antigen, whole antibody molecules, or with $F(ab')_2$ fragments. Use of the latter reduces interference and nonspecific agglutination.

An example of an assay that involves automated measurement of agglutinated particles is a homogeneous competitive immunoassay called "PETINIA" (particle-enhanced

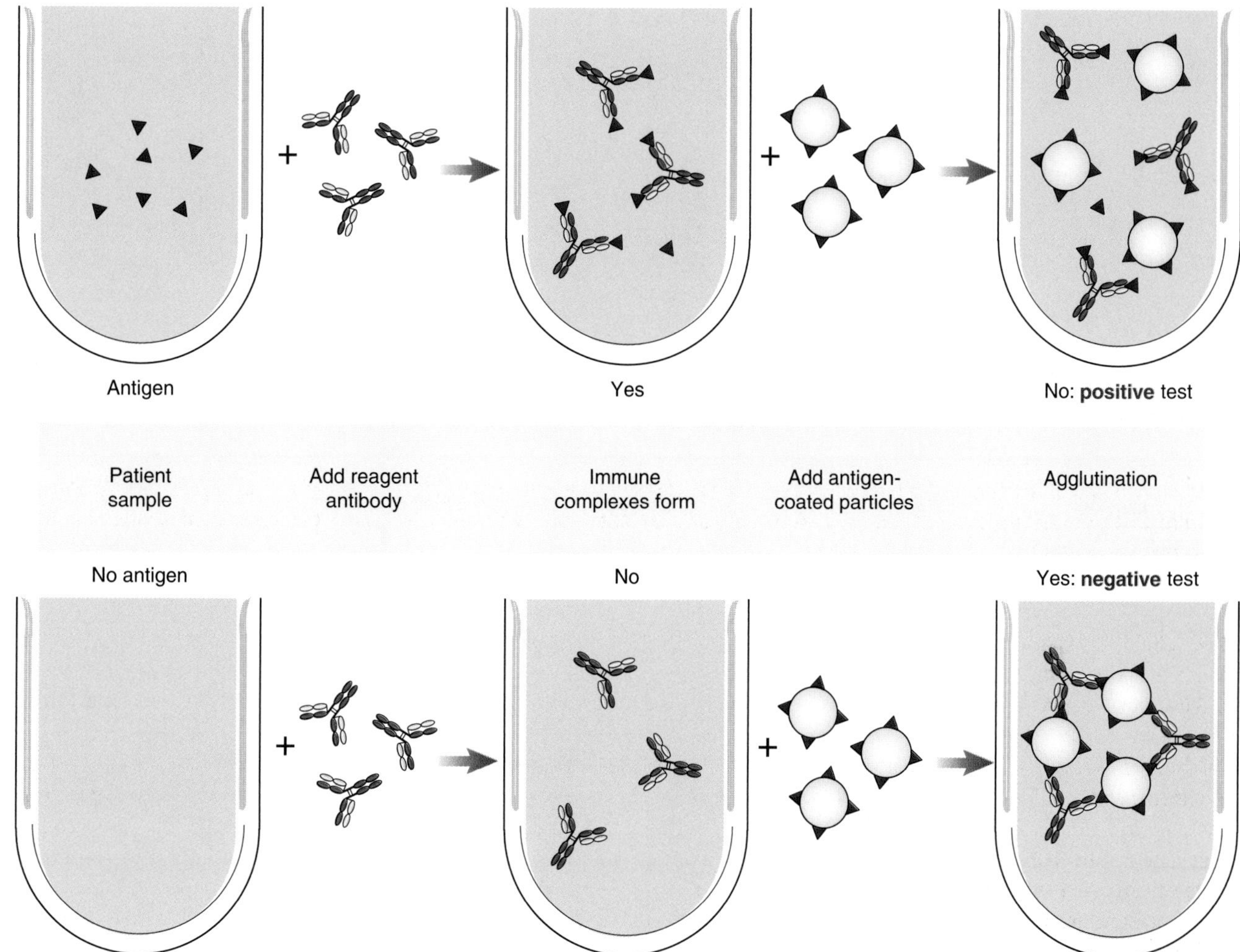

FIGURE 10–13 Agglutination inhibition. Reagent antibody is added to the patient sample. If patient antigen is present, antigen–antibody combination results. When antigen-coated particles are added, no agglutination occurs, which is a positive test. If no patient antigen is present, the reagent antibody combines with the particles, and agglutination results, which is a negative test.

Clinical Correlations

Anti-Streptolysin O (ASO) Detection by Nephelometry

ASO is an antibody that is measured in the laboratory to detect acute rheumatic fever or post-streptococcal glomerulonephritis, sequelae of Group A *Streptococcal* infections (see Chapter 20). ASO is routinely measured by a nephelometric method in which patient serum is mixed with Streptolysin O antigen that has been attached to particles made from a synthetic polymer. The rate of light scatter increases with the formation of immune complexes formed during the antigen–antibody reaction and is an indication of the concentration of ASO in the patient sample.

turbidimetric inhibition immunoassay). In this method, the specimen is incubated with latex beads coated with the analyte of interest and a reagent antibody to the analyte. If a low amount of analyte is present in the sample, the reagent antibody will bind to the latex beads, resulting in aggregate formation and a high level of turbidity. In contrast, when the concentration of the analyte in the patient sample is high, the analyte will bind to the reagent antibody and prevent it from binding to the latex beads, resulting in less turbidity. This method is commonly used to measure small analytes, such as therapeutic drugs (e.g., digoxin), in a sample. The amount of turbidity is inversely proportional to the concentration of the drug analyte in the sample.

Quality Control and Result Interpretation

Although agglutination reactions are simple to perform, interpretation must be carefully done. Techniques must be standardized regarding the concentration of antigen, incubation time, temperature, diluent, and the method of reading. The possibility of cross-reactivity and interfering antibody should always be considered. Cross-reactivity is caused by the presence of antigenic determinants that resemble one another so

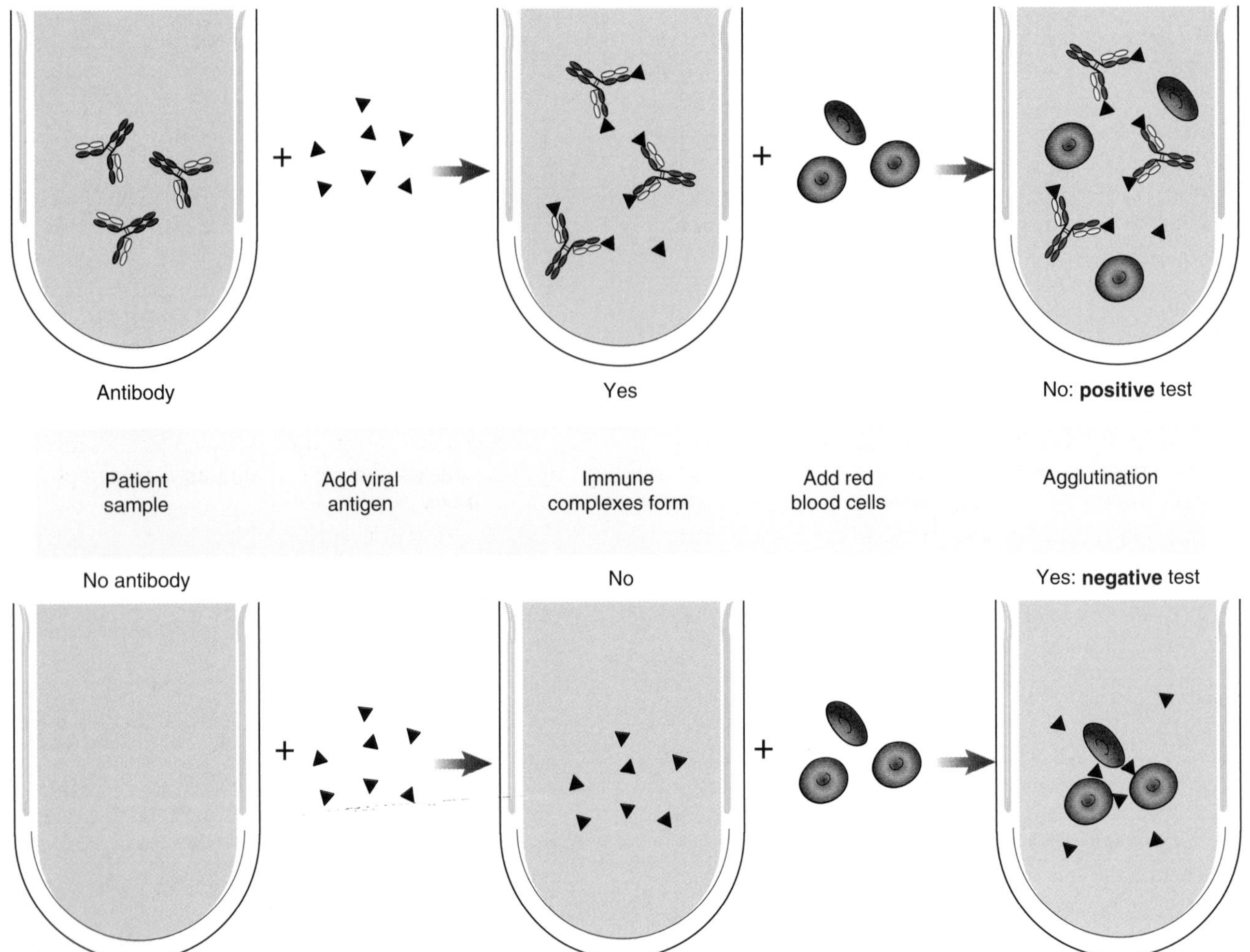

FIGURE 10–14 Hemagglutination inhibition. In the presence of certain viruses, RBCs spontaneously agglutinate. However, if patient antibody is present, then agglutination is inhibited. Thus, a lack of agglutination indicates the presence of antibody.

closely that antibody formed against one will react with the other. Most cross-reactivity can be avoided through the use of monoclonal antibody directed against an antigenic determinant that is unique to a particular antigen.

Other considerations include proper storage of reagents and close attention to expiration dates. Reagents should never be used beyond the expiration date. Each new lot should be evaluated before use, and the manufacturer's instructions for each kit should always be followed. The sensitivity and specificity of different kits may vary and thus must be taken into account.

Advantages of agglutination reactions include rapidity; relative sensitivity; and the fact that if the sample contains a microorganism, the organism does not need to be viable. In addition, most tests are simple to perform and require no expensive equipment. Tests are conducted on cards, tubes, and microtiter plates, all of which are extremely portable. A wide variety of antigens and antibodies can be tested for in this manner. It must be kept in mind, however, that a negative result does not rule out the presence of the disease or the antigen. The quantity of antigen or antibody may be below the sensitivity of the test system. Although the number of agglutination tests has decreased in recent years, they continue to play an important role in the identification of rare pathogens such as *Francisella* and *Brucella* and more common organisms such as rotavirus and *Cryptococcus*, for which other testing is complex or unavailable.

SUMMARY

- Precipitation involves the combination of soluble antigen with soluble antibody to produce insoluble complexes that are visible.
- Union of antigen and antibody depends on *affinity*, or the force of attraction that exists between one antibody-binding site and a single epitope on an antigen.
- *Avidity* is the sum of all attractive forces occurring between multiple binding sites on antigen and antibody.
- Maximum binding of antigen and antibody occurs when the aggregate number of multivalent sites of antigen and antibody are approximately equal.

- The concentrations of antigen and antibody that yield maximum binding represent the zone of equivalence. In this zone, the multivalent sites of antigen and antibody are approximately equal.
- In the prozone, when antibody is being tested for against a standard concentration of antigen, antibody is in excess as compared with antigen, and precipitation or agglutination cannot be detected.
- In the postzone, antigen is in excess compared with the concentration of antibody, so manifestations of antigen–antibody combination, such as precipitation and agglutination, are undetectable.
- Immunoturbidimetry is an automated method that measures the reduction in light intensity because of the formation of immune complexes.
- Nephelometry is an automated technique that measures the amount of light scattered at a particular angle from an incident beam from free antigen or antibody molecules and from antigen–antibody complexes in solution.
- RID is a single-diffusion technique in which antibody is incorporated into a gel. Antigen is placed in wells in the gel and diffuses out and reacts with the antibody, forming rings of precipitation around the wells. The diameter of each precipitate ring is directly related to the amount of antigen in the well.
- In Ouchterlony double diffusion, both antigen and antibody diffuse from wells and travel toward each other. Precipitin lines may indicate identity, nonidentity, or partial identity, depending on the pattern formed between a known antigen or antibody and an unknown antigen or antibody.
- In IFE, antibody is applied directly to a gel after electrophoresis of antigens has taken place. IFE is commonly used to detect monoclonal immunoglobulins produced by patients with immunoproliferative diseases such as multiple myeloma.
- Agglutination is the process by which particulate antigens, such as latex beads, RBCs, or gel particles, react with specific antibody to form large aggregates or clumps.
- The process of agglutination can be divided into two steps: (1) *sensitization,* or initial binding of antigen and antibody, which depends on the nature of the antibody and the antigen-bearing surface, and (2) *lattice formation,* which is governed by such factors as pH, ionic strength, and temperature.
- Because of its larger size, IgM is usually able to mediate lattice formation with antigen without additional enhancement. In contrast, agglutination reactions involving IgG require enhancement techniques that vary physicochemical conditions and the addition of an anti-human immunoglobulin (Coombs reagent) in order to see a visible reaction.
- In direct agglutination tests, patient serum is incubated with antigens that are found naturally on the indicator particles.
- In passive agglutination tests, patient serum is reacted with antigens that are artificially attached to such particles.
- Reverse passive agglutination is so called because antibody, rather than antigen, is attached to the indicator particles.
- Agglutination inhibition is based on competition between antigen-coated particles and soluble patient antigen for a limited number of antibody sites. It is the only instance in which agglutination represents a negative test.
- Agglutination reactions are typically used as rapid screening tests. They are sensitive and can yield valuable information when interpreted correctly.

Study Guide: Comparison of Agglutination Reactions

TYPE OF REACTION	PRINCIPLE	RESULTS
Direct agglutination	Patient serum is reacted with antigen that is naturally found on a particle.	Agglutination indicates the presence of patient antibody to a natural antigen.
Indirect (passive) agglutination	Patient sample is reacted with particles coated with antigens not normally found on their surfaces.	Agglutination indicates the presence of patient antibody to an artificially attached antigen.
Reverse passive	Patient sample is reacted with particles that are coated with reagent antibody.	Agglutination indicates the presence of specific antigen in the patient sample.
Agglutination inhibition	Haptens are attached to carrier particles. Particles compete with patient antigens for a limited number of antibody sites.	Lack of agglutination is a positive test, indicating the presence of antigen in the patient sample.
Hemagglutination inhibition	RBCs spontaneously agglutinate if viral particles are present.	Lack of agglutination is a positive test, indicating the presence of patient antibody.

CASE STUDIES

1. A 4-year-old female was hospitalized for pneumonia. She had a history of upper respiratory tract infections and several bouts of diarrhea since infancy. Because of her recurring infections, the physician decided to measure her immunoglobulin levels. The following results were obtained by nephelometry:

Immunoglobulin	Normal Level (3–5 Yrs) (mg/dL)	Patient Level (mg/dL)
IgG	550–1,700	800
IgA	50–280	20
IgM	25–120	75

Questions

a. What do these results indicate?
b. How do they explain the patient's symptoms? (You may want to refer back to Chapter 5 for a discussion of the function of different classes of antibody.)
c. How do nephelometry measurements compare with the use of RID?

2. A 30-year-old man visits his physician because of a generalized skin rash, malaise, and fatigue. His doctor notes that the patient had an active sexual history. Among other tests, the doctor orders a *T. pallidum* particle agglutination assay (TP-PA) test to check for syphilis. The test result showed the presence of a smooth mat of particles covering the well of the microtiter plate when a 1:80 dilution of patient serum was used.

Questions

a. Does the smooth mat of particles indicate a positive or negative result? Explain your answer.
b. Suppose a 1:40 dilution of patient serum was used, and the result was negative. How can the discrepancy between the 1:40 and 1:80 results be explained?
c. Does the test result mean that the patient has an active case of syphilis?

REVIEW QUESTIONS

1. In a precipitation reaction, how can the ideal antibody be characterized?
   a. Low affinity and low avidity
   b. High affinity and low avidity
   c. High affinity and high avidity
   d. Low affinity and high avidity

2. Precipitation differs from agglutination in which way?
   a. Precipitation can only be measured by an automated instrument.
   b. Precipitation occurs with univalent antigen, whereas agglutination requires multivalent antigen.
   c. Precipitation does not readily occur because few antibodies can form aggregates with antigen.
   d. Precipitation involves a soluble antigen, whereas agglutination involves a particulate antigen.

3. When soluble antigens diffuse in a gel that contains antibody, in which zone does optimal precipitation occur?
   a. Prozone
   b. Zone of equivalence
   c. Postzone
   d. Prezone

4. Which of the following statements applies to rate nephelometry?
   a. Readings are taken before equivalence is reached.
   b. It is more sensitive than immunoturbidimetry.
   c. Measurements are time dependent.
   d. All of the above apply.

5. Which of the following is characteristic of the endpoint method of RID?
   a. Readings are taken before equivalence.
   b. The antigen concentration is directly in proportion to the square of the ring diameter.
   c. The ring diameter is plotted against the log of the concentration.
   d. It is primarily a qualitative rather than a quantitative method.

6. In which zone might an antibody-screening test be false negative?
   a. Prozone
   b. Zone of equivalence
   c. Postzone
   d. None of the above

7. How does immunoturbidimetry differ from nephelometry?
   a. Immunoturbidimetry measures the increase in light after it passes through a solution.
   b. Nephelometry measures light that is scattered at an angle.
   c. Immunoturbidimetry deals with univalent antigens only.
   d. Nephelometry is not affected by large particles falling out of solution.

8. Which of the following refers to the force of attraction between an antibody and a single antigenic determinant?
   a. Affinity
   b. Avidity
   c. Van der Waals attraction
   d. Covalence

9. If crossed lines result in an Ouchterlony immunodiffusion reaction with antigens 1 and 2, what does this indicate?
   a. Antigens 1 and 2 are identical.
   b. Antigen 2 is simpler than antigen 1.
   c. Antigen 2 is more complex than antigen 1.
   d. The two antigens are unrelated.

10. Which technique represents a single-diffusion reaction?
    a. Radial immunodiffusion
    b. Ouchterlony diffusion
    c. Counter immunoelectrophoresis
    d. Immunofixation electrophoresis

11. Which best describes the law of mass action?
    a. Once antigen–antibody binding takes place, it is irreversible.
    b. The equilibrium constant depends only on the forward reaction.
    c. The equilibrium constant is related to the strength of antigen–antibody binding.
    d. If an antibody has a high avidity, it will dissociate from antigen easily.

12. Agglutination of dyed bacterial cells represents which type of reaction?
    a. Direct agglutination
    b. Passive agglutination
    c. Reverse passive agglutination
    d. Agglutination inhibition

13. If a single IgM molecule can bind many more antigens than a molecule of IgG, which of the following is higher?
    a. Affinity
    b. Initial force of attraction
    c. Avidity
    d. Initial sensitization

14. Agglutination inhibition could best be used for which of the following types of antigens?
    a. Large cellular antigens, such as erythrocytes
    b. Soluble haptens
    c. Bacterial cells
    d. Coated latex particles

15. Which of the following correctly describes reverse passive agglutination?
    a. It is a negative test.
    b. It can be used to detect autoantibodies.
    c. It is used for identification of antigens.
    d. It is used to detect sensitization of RBCs.

16. Reactions involving IgG may need to be enhanced for which reason?
    a. IgG is only active at 25°C.
    b. IgG may be too small to produce lattice formation.
    c. IgG has only one antigen-binding site.
    d. IgG is only able to produce visible precipitation reactions.

17. For which of the following tests is a lack of agglutination a positive reaction?
    a. Hemagglutination
    b. Passive agglutination
    c. Reverse passive agglutination
    d. Agglutination inhibition

18. Typing of RBCs with reagent antiserum represents which type of reaction?
    a. Direct hemagglutination
    b. Passive hemagglutination
    c. Hemagglutination inhibition
    d. Reverse passive hemagglutination

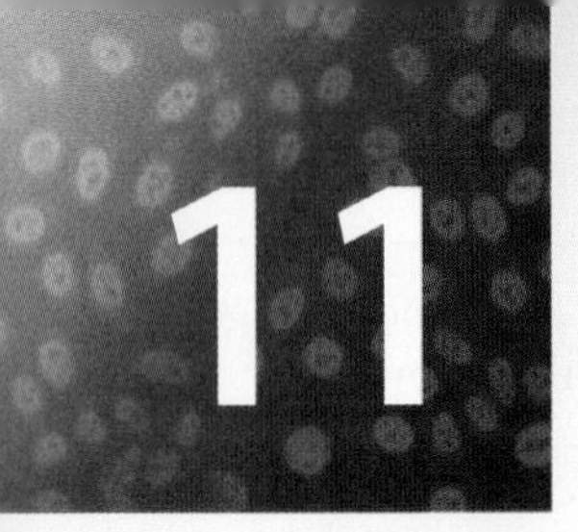

11 Labeled Immunoassays

Paul R. Johnson, PhD, MBA, MT(ASCP), DABCC

LEARNING OUTCOMES

After finishing this chapter, you should be able to:

1. Describe the difference between competitive and noncompetitive immunoassays.
2. Distinguish between heterogeneous and homogeneous immunoassays.
3. Describe major characteristics of colorimetric, chemiluminescent, radioactive, and fluorescent labels.
4. Explain the principle of competitive binding in immunoassay design.
5. Recognize common enzymes used in enzyme immunoassays (EIAs).
6. Explain the principle of biotin-streptavidin labeling and its applications in immunoassays.
7. Outline the steps of a noncompetitive indirect enzyme-linked immunosorbent assay (ELISA) to detect an antibody in a patient sample.
8. Outline the steps of a sandwich, capture, or immunometric assay to detect an antigen in a patient sample.
9. Discuss clinical applications for homogeneous EIAs.
10. Describe basic principles and clinical uses for rapid immunoassays.
11. Compare and contrast the analytical sensitivity of immunoassays using different labels.
12. Describe the difference between direct and indirect immunofluorescence techniques.
13. State the principles of the enzyme-multiplied immunoassay technique (EMIT), cloned enzyme donor immunoassay (CEDIA), multiplex immunoassay (MIA), and fluorescence polarization immunoassay (FPIA).
14. Review advantages and disadvantages of immunoassays, based on each method design.
15. Choose an appropriate immunoassay for a particular analyte.
16. Discuss interfering factors and other technical concerns that may contribute to false-positive or false-negative immunoassay results.

CHAPTER OUTLINE

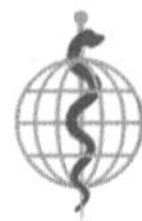

Go to FADavis.com for the laboratory exercises that accompany this text.

KEY TERMS

Analyte
Analytical sensitivity
Analytical specificity
Biotin
Capture immunoassay
Chemiluminescence
Chemiluminescent immunoassay
Chemiluminescent microparticle immunoassay (CMIA)
Cloned-enzyme donor immunoassay (CEDIA)
Competitive immunoassay
Direct immunofluorescence assay
Electrochemiluminescence immunoassay (ECLIA)
Enzyme
Enzyme immunoassay (EIA)
Enzyme-linked immunosorbent assay (ELISA)
Enzyme-multiplied immunoassay technique (EMIT)
Flow cytometry
Fluorescence polarization immunoassay (FPIA)
Fluorochrome
Fluorophores
Heterogeneous immunoassay
Heterophile antibodies
High-dose hook effect
Homogeneous immunoassay
Immunochromatography
Immunofluorescence assay (IFA)
Immunometric assay
Indirect ELISA
Indirect immunofluorescence (IIF) assay
Multiplex immunoassay (MIA)
Noncompetitive immunoassay
Radioimmunoassay (RIA)
Rapid immunoassays
Sandwich immunoassay
Single-step, competitive, immunochromatographic method
Streptavidin (SAv)

Unlabeled immunoassays, such as the precipitation and agglutination reactions that were discussed in Chapter 10, are fairly simple techniques that are often performed without the need for sophisticated equipment. However, one limitation of these techniques is they have a relatively poor analytical sensitivity because visualizing a macroscopic reaction requires sufficiently high sample concentration of the biomarker analyte. In contrast, labeled immunoassays are designed to improve analytical sensitivity, which allows for detecting substances at much lower concentrations using instrumentation equipped with sensitive detectors. Labeled immunoassay techniques are commonly used in the clinical laboratory to measure a wide variety of substances found in blood, urine, and tissues. The substance measured is often called the **analyte** (or biomarker). Analytes discussed in this chapter broadly include antigens and antibodies. Biological analytes measured by immunoassay techniques include proteins, peptides, hormones, tumor markers, immunoglobulins, and microbial antigens. Small-molecule antigens, or haptens, can also be measured with immunoassays; examples include steroid hormones or drugs. In certain clinical situations, it may be of interest to detect and quantify antibody levels rather than antigen levels to support a clinical diagnosis. The methods by which antigens or antibodies are measured varies extensively, depending on individual immunoassay techniques developed across different *in vitro* diagnostic (IVD) test manufacturers.

In general, the analyte of interest is a protein substance. The analyte can be either antigen or antibody, depending on clinical need. Anti-human immunoglobulin is designed to react specifically with the analyte if the protein being detected is an antibody from patient serum. The anti-human immunoglobulin used in such a test system is derived from another species (mouse, rabbit, or goat). One reactant, either antigen or antibody, will contain a label as a detection marker so that the amount of binding can be monitored. Affinity and avidity of the antigen–antibody pair is important to achieve optimal reaction conditions, and this largely influences the specificity of the reaction. High **analytical specificity** implies that only the analyte of interest is detected and measured. On the other hand, **analytical sensitivity** defines the lowest measurable concentration of analyte, usually described as the lower limit of detection (LoD). The detection limits of immunoassays are determined by several variables, including the label used as well as the antigen–antibody affinity and avidity. As a general rule, analytical sensitivity is optimal when using a chemiluminescent substrate, followed by a fluorophore. A colorimetric product is the least sensitive. Radioisotopes generally have sensitivity close to that achieved by fluorescent labels. In principle, each label may be coupled to any assay design.

Connections

Affinity and Avidity

Recall from Chapter 10 that *affinity* refers to the initial force of attraction between a single antigen-binding site on an antibody molecule and a single epitope of the corresponding antigen. *Avidity* describes the overall strength of antigen–antibody binding produced by the sum of the binding affinities between sites on a multivalent antibody and a multivalent antigen.

The development of rapid, specific, and sensitive immunoassays to determine the presence of important biological molecules has ushered in a new era of testing in the clinical laboratory. The ability to detect very small quantities of antigen or antibody has revolutionized the diagnosis and monitoring of numerous diseases, leading to more prompt treatment for many such conditions.

Immunoassay Labels

Labeled immunoassays differ from unlabeled techniques by including a detection molecule (label) in the test system. Most current techniques utilize non-isotopic labels to generate a light signal. Depending on manufacturer design, labels may include a colorimetric substrate, fluorescent compound (fluorophore), or luminescent molecule. Earlier generation immunoassays used radioactive isotope elements as the label, but these techniques are less commonly used in clinical laboratories today. Generation of the detection signal also varies across manufacturers. Labels are sometimes referred to as "tracer" molecules because they allow for tracing of the detection signal. One technique common to many labeled immunoassay methods is enzyme-mediated catalysis of a reagent substrate to generate a light signal.

A wide variety of test designs have been developed by different manufacturers, and the selection of the label is aimed at the testing needs for measuring the analyte of interest. Each of these labels will be described in detail within the discussion of each immunoassay format.

General Immunoassay Formats

Heterogeneous Versus Homogeneous Immunoassays

There are two major formats for all labeled immunoassays, *heterogeneous* and *homogeneous*. Separation of bound and free tracer label before signal measurement is a requirement in all immunoassay designs. The approaches to achieve this can be broadly categorized as heterogeneous or homogeneous. In **heterogeneous immunoassays,** physical separation of bound and free components is required. Separation of components is achieved by a variety of methods, including centrifugation, binding to solid-phase material, or magnetic separation. Solid-phase materials are the most common and include polystyrene reaction wells, microparticle beads, latex beads, and plastic tubes.

Immunoassay methods that do not require a physical separation step are termed **homogeneous immunoassays.** Although homogeneous immunoassay designs have this property in common, the methods by which they measure the detection signal and patient analyte concentration can vary extensively across manufacturers.

Additional subclassifications are made to describe whether immunoassay method designs are *competitive* or *noncompetitive,* based on the principle of the test reaction. The immunoassays discussed in this chapter, along with their classification, are listed in **Table 11–1**.

Competitive Versus Noncompetitive Immunoassays

Competitive Immunoassays

In **competitive immunoassays,** the test system reagents consist of limited antibody (Ab), tracer or labeled antigen (Ag*), and reagent substrate. The only variable in the reaction is the concentration of patient antigen (Ag), which is the analyte of interest. All the reactants are mixed together simultaneously; labeled tracer antigen (Ag*) competes with unlabeled patient antigen (Ag) for a limited number of binding sites for antibody (Ab). The concentration of the labeled analyte (Ag*) is in excess to ensure all binding sites on the antibody will be occupied whether or not sample antigen is present. After washing to remove unbound label, the amount of antibody-bound label (Ag*Ab) is measured and used to determine the amount of patient antigen present. If patient antigen is present, some binding sites will be occupied with unlabeled analyte, thus decreasing the amount of bound label detected **(Fig. 11–1).** Therefore, the amount of bound label is inversely proportional to the concentration of the labeled antigen, which means that the more labeled antigen detected, the less antigen is present in the patient sample.

Table 11–1 Homogeneous and Heterogeneous Immunoassay Formats

HOMOGENEOUS	HETEROGENEOUS	OTHER (TISSUE/CELL BASED)
Enzyme-multiplied immunoassay technique (EMIT)	Enzyme immunoassay (EIA)	Direct immunofluorescence assay
Cloned-enzyme donor immunoassay (CEDIA)	Enzyme-linked immunosorbent assay (ELISA)	Indirect immunofluorescence assay
Fluorescence polarization immunoassay (FPIA)	Chemiluminescent microparticle immunoassay (CMIA)	Multiplex immunoassay (MIA)
	Electrochemiluminescence immunoassay (ECLIA)	
	Radioimmunoassay (RIA)	
	Fluorescence immunoassay (FIA)	
	Rapid immunoassays (immunochromatography)	

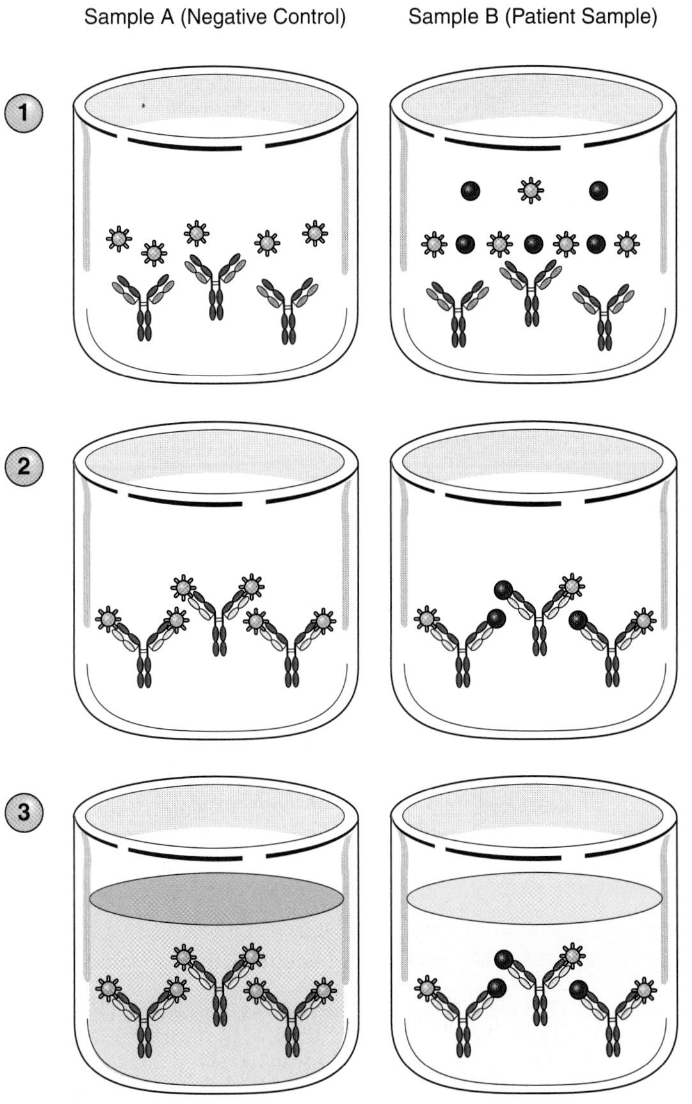

1. Unknown concentration of analyte in patient sample (red dots) competes with labeled analyte (yellow stars) for binding sites on immobilized antibody.
2. Wash to remove unbound materials.
3. After substrate is added, a colored product (signal) is generated with an intensity proportional to the amount of enzyme-labeled analyte bound to the antibody.

The signal strength is usually **inversely** related to the analyte concentration.

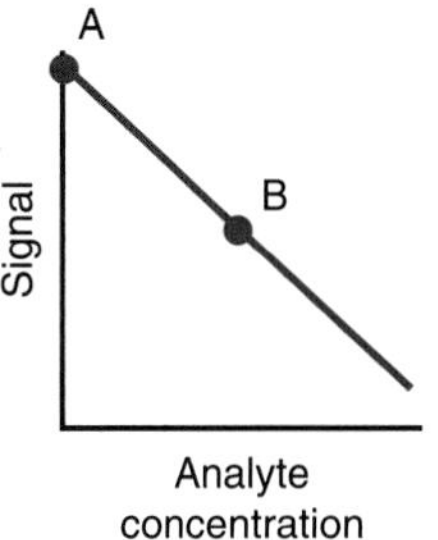

FIGURE 11–1 Principle of a competitive immunoassay.

This relationship can be illustrated by considering the ratio of tracer-bound antigen to sample antigen (analyte) in the example that follows.

Suppose labeled antigen (Ag*) and unlabeled antigen (Ag) occur in three different ratios: 2:1, 1:1, and 1:2. Binding to a limited number of antibody sites will take place in the same ratios. The reaction between the antigens and their corresponding antibody can be depicted in an equation where the reactants are listed on the left side of the arrow and the products on the right. Labeled antigen (Ag*) and reagent antibody (Ab) are held constant, at 100 units and 50 units, respectively. By altering the patient antigen (Ag) concentration, the amount of labeled antigen bound to antibody will change according to the patient antigen concentration. Thus, on the right side of the equation, one-third (33%) of binding sites are occupied by labeled antigen (Ag*Ab) at a 2:1 Ag*:Ag ratio, 25% of binding sites are occupied at a 1:1 ratio, and 17% at a 1:2 ratio. Additional ratio values of labeled antigen (Ag*) to patient antigen (Ag) help to further illustrate this relationship, as depicted in **Figure 11–2**. It can be observed that the detection signal is inversely proportional to the patient antigen concentration on a nonlinear scale. The relationship can be mathematically linearized to generate a standard curve, using calibrators with known amounts of antigen, in order to extrapolate the signal to the concentration of antigen in the patient sample.

Noncompetitive Immunoassays

In a standard **noncompetitive immunoassay,** reagent antibody (often called *capture antibody*) is first passively absorbed onto a solid-phase material, such as microtiter plates, nitrocellulose membranes, or plastic beads. Excess capture antibody is present to ensure that any patient antigen present will be bound. Unknown patient antigen reacts with (i.e., is captured by) the solid-phase antibody. After washing to physically remove unbound antigen, a labeled antibody, directed

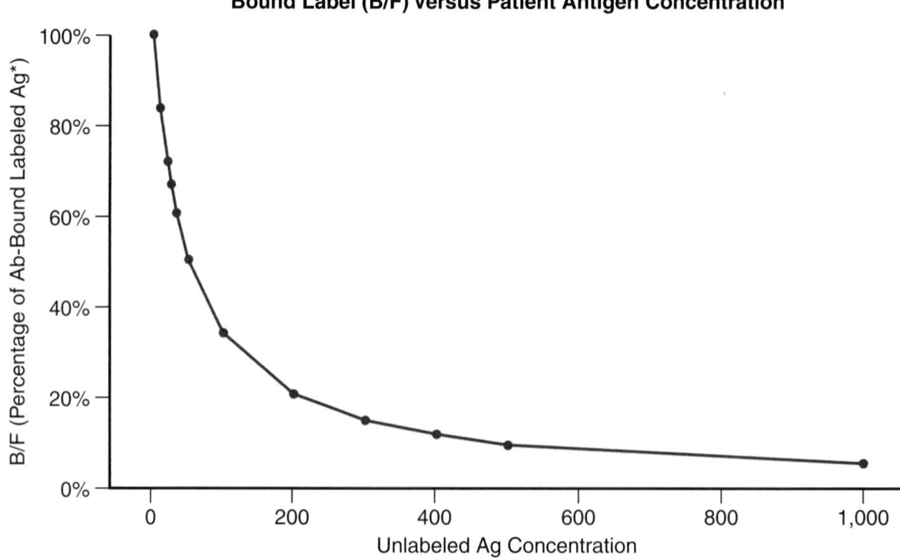

C1	C2	C3	C4	C5	C6	C7	C8	C9
Ratio of Labeled Ag*/Patient Ag	Patient Ag Concentration	Labeled Ag* Concentration	Ab	AgAb	Ag*Ab	% Bound (C6/C3)	Free Ag* (C3–C6)	B/F C6/C8
2:1	50	100	50	17	33	33%	67	49%
1:1	100	100	50	25	25	25%	75	33%
1:2	200	100	50	33	17	17%	83	20%

FIGURE 11–2 Example of the effect of the ratio of labeled antigen to unlabeled antigen on the percentage of labeled antigen bound to antibody in a competitive immunoassay. *(Figure courtesy of Dr. Paul Johnson.)*

against a different epitope of the antigen, is added to the reaction **(Fig. 11–3)**. The amount of label measured is directly proportional to the amount of patient antigen present and is represented by a mathematical linear relationship.

Radioimmunoassay (RIA)

The original immunoassay developed was based on a competitive principle, using a radioisotope label. This technique, called **radioimmunoassay (RIA)**, was pioneered by Yalow and Berson in the late 1950s, who developed the immunoassay to measure insulin hormone levels in humans. Yalow was honored with the 1977 Nobel Prize in Physiology or Medicine for her groundbreaking work. The success of this original immunoassay design ultimately led researchers to develop additional RIA methods to measure other clinical analytes, including several hormones (e.g., aldosterone, cortisol), serum proteins, drugs, viral antigens, and immunoglobulins.

Radioactive elements have nuclei that decay spontaneously into other elements and, in the process, release energy, which is measured by detectors such as a gamma counter. Depending on the immunoassay design, radiolabeled antigens can be tagged with various radioactive elements, including tritium (^{3}H), carbon (^{14}C), or iodine (^{125}I or ^{131}I). Detectors are able to measure very low quantities of radioactivity, which gives these immunoassays extremely high analytical sensitivity.

However, the chief disadvantages of RIA methods include health hazards involved in working with radioactive substances, radioactive waste disposal problems, and the limited shelf life of some elements (for example, ^{125}I has a half-life of about 60 days). For these reasons, RIA testing in clinical laboratories has become limited.

Enzyme Immunoassays (EIAs)

Enzyme immunoassays (EIAs), using enzymes as labels, were developed as alternatives to RIA. **Enzymes** are naturally occurring molecules that catalyze biochemical reactions. When used in a test system, they convert reagent substrates to produce chemically modified products that can be detected. Substances produced and detected in this method include colored or visible light, ultraviolet (UV) light, fluorescent light, and luminescence. These methods have sufficient analytical sensitivity for many clinical tests and eliminate the concerns of disposal problems or health hazards associated with radioactive isotopes. Because one molecule of enzyme can generate many molecules of product, the addition of an enzyme label further improves analytical sensitivity.

Enzymes used as labels for immunoassays are chosen according to their physical properties, including the number of substrate molecules converted per molecule of enzyme, ease and speed of detection, and stability. The availability and

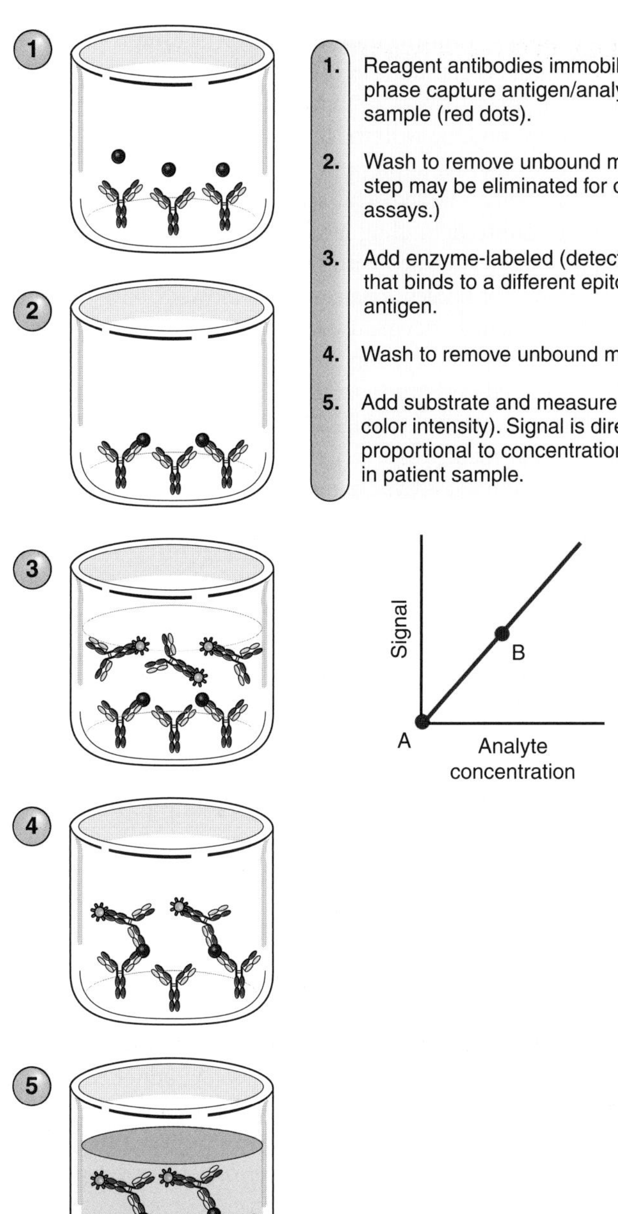

1
2
3
4
5
1. Reagent antibodies immobilized on solid phase capture antigen/analyte in patient sample (red dots).
2. Wash to remove unbound materials. (This step may be eliminated for one-step assays.)
3. Add enzyme-labeled (detection) antibody that binds to a different epitope on the antigen.
4. Wash to remove unbound materials.
5. Add substrate and measure signal (e.g., color intensity). Signal is directly proportional to concentration of antigen in patient sample.
Signal
B
A
Analyte concentration

FIGURE 11–3 Capture, sandwich, or immunometric assay.

cost of the enzyme and substrate may factor into the design of a particular enzyme reagent. Common enzymes used as labels in EIA include horseradish peroxidase (HRP), alkaline phosphatase (ALP), β-D-galactosidase, and glucose-6-phosphate dehydrogenase (G6PDH). EIAs can be further classified as either heterogeneous or homogeneous on the basis of whether a separation step is necessary, as previously mentioned.

Heterogeneous Enzyme Immunoassays

Competitive Enzyme Immunoassays

The first EIAs, developed by Eva Engvall and Peter Perlmann in 1971, were based on the competitive principles of RIA. Capture antibodies were adsorbed onto plastic tubes, which led these investigators to name this new method **enzyme-linked immunosorbent assay (ELISA).** Alkaline phosphatase (enzyme) was conjugated to the antigen of interest. In competitive ELISAs, sample antigen competes with enzyme-conjugated antigen for a limited number of binding sites on antibody molecules attached to a solid phase, such as plastic tubes or microtiter plate wells. After careful washing to remove unbound antigen, enzyme activity present in the final reaction catalyzes the conversion of the substrate to a detectable product. The product signal is inversely proportional to the concentration of the test substance. In the original ELISA method, sample antigen was accurately detected at a concentration as low as 1 ng/mL, achieving comparable analytical sensitivity to RIA. Since the time that ELISA methods were introduced, they have dramatically increased in popularity and have become a mainstay of testing in research and clinical laboratories. In practice, an ELISA is an EIA, so these terms may be used interchangeably.

Noncompetitive Enzyme Immunoassays

Alternately, ELISA/EIA methodology may be based on a noncompetitive design. Noncompetitive immunoassay formats can be used to detect the presence of either an antigen or an antibody in the test sample. Immunoassays that detect antibody are most commonly **indirect ELISAs**, whereas those that detect antigen are termed "capture immunoassays." ELISA test kit procedures often use 96-well microtiter plates as the solid phase. In addition to microtiter plates, a variety of solid-phase supports have been developed, including plastic reaction well tubes, plastic beads, magnetic particles, and latex particles. Most automated immunoassays in the laboratory today are designed on similar noncompetitive principles. This type of immunoassay is one of the most frequently used immunoassays in the clinical laboratory because of its sensitivity, specificity, and simplicity of use.

Indirect ELISAs

Indirect ELISAs are most commonly used to detect a patient antibody of interest. They are termed "indirect" because the enzyme-labeled reagent does not participate in the initial antigen–antibody reaction. In these immunoassays, the associated antigen is bound to the solid phase, and patient serum with an unknown antibody concentration is added. Incubation time allows for specific interaction between solid-phase antigen and patient antibody. After a wash step, an enzyme-labeled anti-globulin, or secondary antibody, is added. This second antibody reacts with any patient antibody that is bound to the solid phase. If no patient antibody is bound to the solid phase, the second labeled antibody will not be bound and will be removed during a second wash step. This is followed by incubation with the enzyme substrate, and finally, a stop solution to cease enzyme activity after a specified period of time. The amount of color, fluorescence, or luminescence generated by action of the enzyme label on the substrate is measured using a detection device and is compared with known amounts of antigen according to a standard curve. In the noncompetitive format, signal detection is directly proportional to the amount of antibody in the specimen **(Figs. 11–4 and 11–5).** Clinical applications include measurement of antibody production to infectious agents that are difficult to isolate in the laboratory; for example, this technique is useful as a screening tool for detecting patient antibodies to viruses such as HIV, hepatitis B, and hepatitis C. Another clinical application is detection of autoantibody production as the cause of a disease; for example, detection of autoantibodies to insulin and glutamate decarboxylase helps to support a diagnosis of type 1 diabetes mellitus.

Capture (Sandwich) Immunoassays

When antigen is the analyte of interest, antibody is bound to the solid phase. These immunoassays are also termed **sandwich immunoassays, capture immunoassays,** or **immunometric assays.** Antigens captured in these immunoassays must have multiple epitopes. Excess antibody attached to the solid phase is allowed to combine with the test sample to capture any antigen present. After an appropriate incubation period, enzyme-labeled antibody is added. This secondary antibody recognizes a different epitope or binding site than the solid-phase antibody. The final complex formed with sample antigen in between the two reagent antibodies creates the "sandwich." Depending upon the particular enzyme used, either a colored, fluorescent, or chemiluminescent reaction product is detected. Product formation is directly proportional to the amount of antigen present in the test sample (see Fig. 11–3). The use of monoclonal antibodies has made this a very sensitive test system.

Capture immunoassays are best suited to antigens that have multiple determinants, such as cytokines, proteins, tumor markers, and microorganism antigens. When used to detect microorganisms, the epitope must be unique to the organism being tested and ideally, must be present in all strains of that organism. Another use of capture immunoassays is in the measurement of immunoglobulins, especially those of certain classes. For instance, the presence of immunoglobulin M (IgM) can help indicate an acute infection. When capture immunoassays are used to measure immunoglobulins, the specific immunoglobulin class being detected is technically acting as the antigen, and the reagent antibody is anti-human immunoglobulin.

Biotin-Avidin Labeling

One way to achieve increased analytical sensitivity of labeled immunoassays is by complexing biotin to the capture antibody and streptavidin to the solid-phase material. **Biotin,** also known as vitamin B_7 or vitamin H, is a vitamin of the B-complex family, whereas avidin is a protein enriched in egg yolks. The discovery of this interaction led researchers to isolate a bacterial version of avidin, called **streptavidin (SAv),** which was demonstrated to have stronger binding affinity for biotin. The formation of biotin-SAv complexes is the rationale for using these molecules in immunoassay design, especially as each molecule of SAv has multiple high-affinity binding sites for biotin. The end result is signal amplification with enhanced detection when coupled to one of the previously discussed non-isotopic labels. Biotin-SAv labeling can be used in both indirect ELISAs and capture immunoassays. When a biotin-SAv design is used in a capture immunoassay, it is sometimes referred to as a *delayed capture immunoassay* because the final incubation step includes binding of the sandwich complex to SAv on the solid phase.

Although all these immunoassay formats are useful in measuring antigen or antibody levels in patients, there are certain limitations for which the clinical laboratorian must be aware. Commonly encountered immunoassay test interferences are described in detail in the subsequent section.

Interferences in Immunoassays

False-positive or false-negative results in immunoassays may occur for a variety of reasons. They can be produced simply

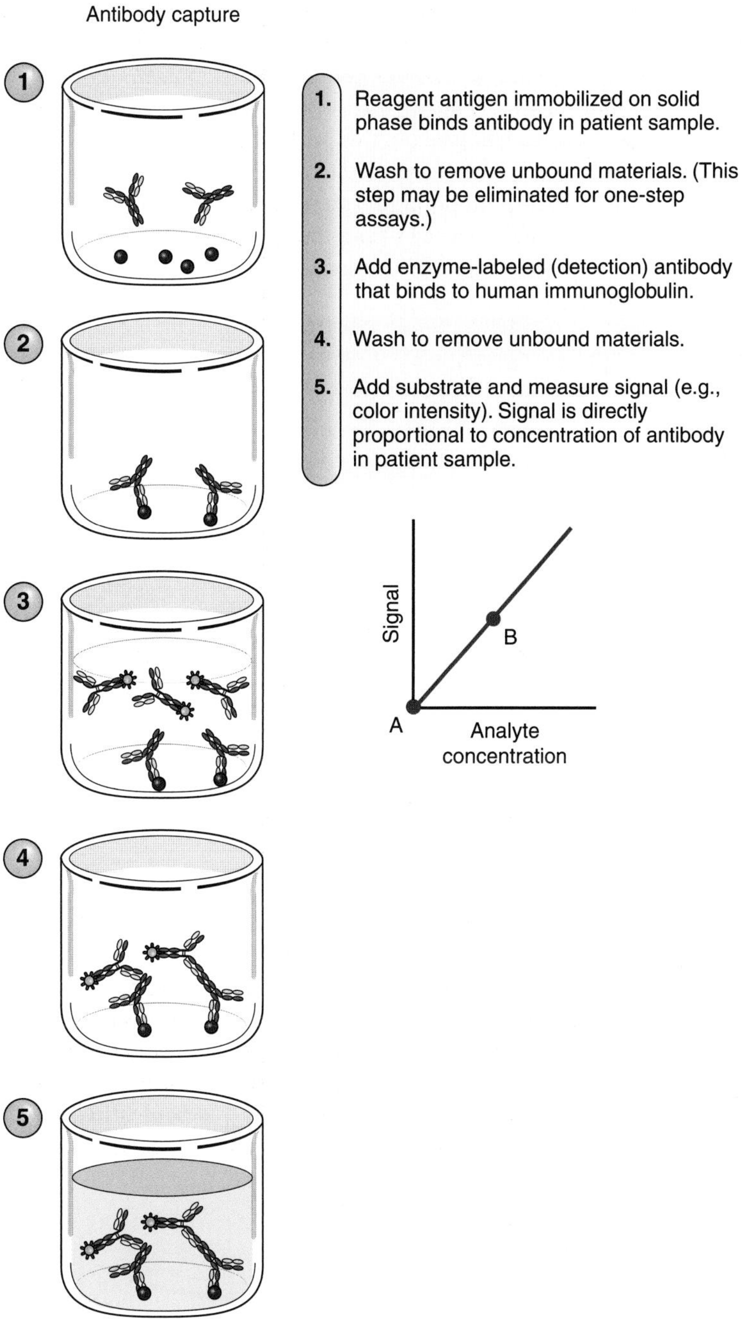

Antibody capture

1. Reagent antigen immobilized on solid phase binds antibody in patient sample.
2. Wash to remove unbound materials. (This step may be eliminated for one-step assays.)
3. Add enzyme-labeled (detection) antibody that binds to human immunoglobulin.
4. Wash to remove unbound materials.
5. Add substrate and measure signal (e.g., color intensity). Signal is directly proportional to concentration of antibody in patient sample.

Signal
B
A
Analyte concentration

FIGURE 11–4 Noncompetitive, indirect immunoassay.

because of certain physical properties of the specimen itself, as some biological materials such as urine or plasma may cause quenching of light emission or exhibit background fluorescence. However, additional test interferences may occur for several different reasons related to immunoassay design. Most of the interferences described are predominantly observed when heterogeneous methods are used to measure the test analyte, rather than homogeneous methods.

Antigen Interference

The improved turnaround time, speed, and sensitivity of capture immunoassays have made them excellent tools for measuring several biological substances. However, they are subject to certain limitations. The most commonly observed of these is the **high-dose hook effect,** or *postzone* effect, where excess patient antigen causes falsely decreased detection, leading to an analyte concentration that appears to be low or normal. This effect is illustrated in **Figure 11–6.** Note that the curve that depicts the relationship between the analyte and the intensity of the reaction signal takes on the shape of a "hook." The high-dose hook effect occurs predominantly when there are not enough capture antibody sites for antigen binding because the majority of binding sites are filled, so the remainder of patient antigen has no place to bind and gets removed during the wash step. When a hook effect is suspected, the technologist should dilute the sample to the point where the

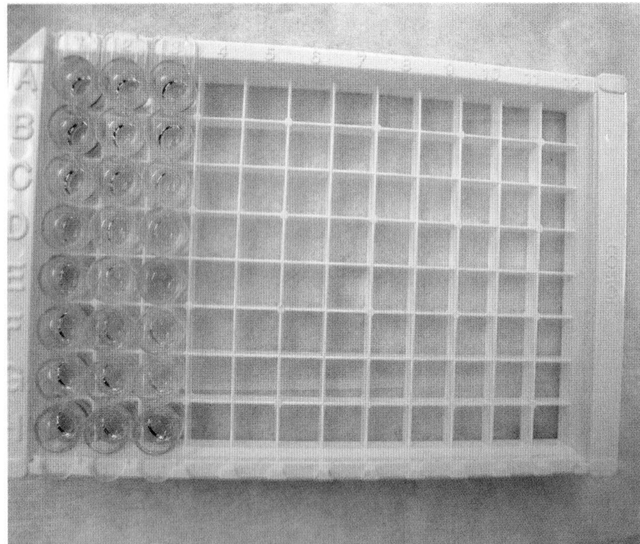

FIGURE 11–5 Sample wells from indirect ELISA to detect patient antibody (in this example, antibody to the rubella virus). Well A1 is the reagent blank; well B1 is the positive control; well C1 is the negative control; and wells D1, E1, and F1 are calibrators run in triplicate. The remaining wells are individual patient samples. Note that the negative wells remain colorless, whereas wells containing samples that are positive for the antibody produce a yellow color following addition of the stop solution. Actual absorbance values are read on a spectrophotometer. *(Figure courtesy of Dr. Linda Miller.)*

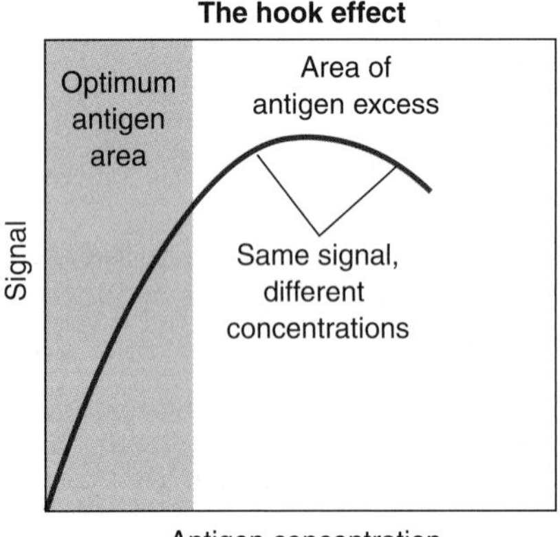

FIGURE 11–6 The high-dose hook effect. Antigen excess can saturate antibodies, and the intended "sandwich" configurations cannot form, leading to a false decrease in signal.

concentration is within the analytical measuring range (calibration range). Increased antigen concentration after dilution provides evidence that a hook effect was present in the original undiluted sample.

Antibody Interference

Autoantibodies

Antibodies produced in vivo may interfere with immunoassays whenever the antibody produced is similar to that of the test kit reagent. Production of autoantibodies (antibodies directed against self-antigens) by individuals with an autoimmune disease is one possible source of interference. A clinical example is in patients with rheumatoid arthritis who test positive for rheumatoid factor (RF). If present, RF can cause false-positive results in clinical tests that use immunoglobulin G (IgG) antibodies. If this is suspected, serum can be pretreated with a blocking reagent to avoid this problem. As an example, animal IgG antibodies may be added to the patient sample to bind RF before testing. Importantly, these "blocking antibodies" must be of a different species than the capture and detection antibodies used in the immunoassay test.

Clinical Correlations

Rheumatoid Factor (RF)

RF is an antibody directed against the Fc portion of IgG molecules. It is produced by a significant number of patients with systemic autoimmune diseases that affect the joints, although it can be found in individuals who do not have these conditions (see Chapter 15). Most commonly, the RF is an IgM antibody. The IgM anti-IgG can bind to IgG molecules in immunoassays and produce false-positive results.

Heterophile Antibodies

Similar interference mechanisms may occur in individuals who have **heterophile antibodies** that react with animal proteins because the detection antibodies used in test reagents are generated in nonhuman species (mouse, rabbit, goat). Heterophile antibodies may be produced by patients with certain infections, patients who have received therapeutic animal globulins, or patients who have frequent contact with animals.

Heterophile interference occurs when the individual produces antibodies similar to those used in the test reagent kit, such as anti-mouse, -rabbit, or -goat antibodies. Heterophile antibodies will often cross-link reagent capture and detection antibodies in the absence of antigen (test analyte) to produce a falsely increased test signal **(Fig. 11–7).** In rarer

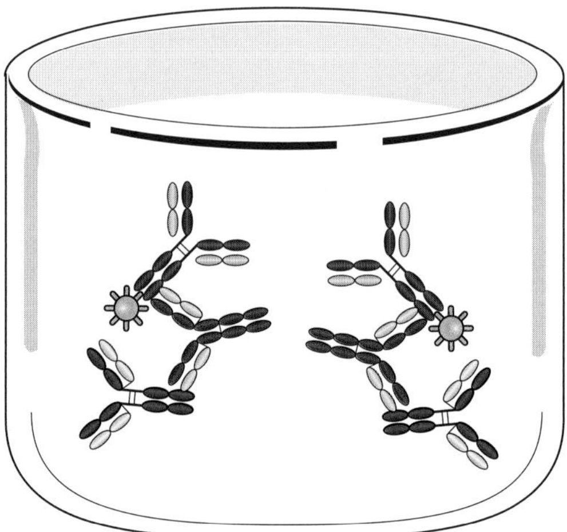

FIGURE 11–7 Interference by heterophile or anti-animal antibodies. Heterophile or anti-animal antibodies (red) can cause both false decreases and false increases, depending on their reactivity against the antibody species used in an immunoassay. However, false increases caused by linking the capture antibodies (blue) and the detection antibodies (black) together are most likely, as shown.

Clinical Correlations

Human Anti-Mouse Antibodies (HAMAs)

Human anti-mouse antibodies (HAMAs) are a type of heterophile antibody that commonly causes interference in immunoassays. These antibodies are often produced by patients who receive mouse monoclonal antibodies as therapeutic agents for diseases such as cancer and autoimmune disorders (see Chapter 25).

cases, heterophile antibodies can cause a falsely decreased test result by binding to the antigen of interest or by binding to the labeled detector antibody, preventing the formation of an immune complex.

Biotin Interference

When test reagent kits also use a biotin-SAv complex, even more unpredictable interferences can occur. The most pressing concern facing clinical laboratorians using this immunoassay format is when the individual being tested has recently taken high-dose biotin as a nutritional supplement or medication (usually at a dose equal to or greater than 1 milligram/1,000 micrograms). The ingested biotin causes interference in the immunoassay, and depending on the immunoassay design, test results may be falsely increased (competitive design) or decreased (noncompetitive immunoassay). Such interference is usually discovered when reported test results are found to be inconsistent with the clinical picture. For example, a markedly abnormal thyroid-stimulating hormone (TSH) test result may be observed in a person with no other evidence of pituitary or thyroid disease. Fortunately, the solution to correct or prevent this problem is often quite simple, by having the patient refrain from taking biotin for at least 8 to 48 hours before blood sample collection. Alternatively, measuring the same analyte on a different platform that does not use the biotin-SAv reaction could be performed on the sample to obtain reliable results. Biotin interference in the original test result would be suspected if the result on the re-tested sample normalizes when the alternative method is used.

Other Technical Concerns

Cross-reactivity describes detection of a substance other than the analyte of interest. This often occurs because of similar structure to the analyte(s) used to calibrate the test method immunoassay. When cross-reactivity occurs, it is typically observed as a false-positive result. Multiple case reports of cross-reactivity in drug immunoassays have been reported in the literature. One case example was a false-positive opiate immunoassay screen result in which naloxone (an opiate antagonist) was detected as an opiate by a homogeneous EIA method (CEDIA, described in a later section). In such instances, an alternative method must be used to confirm the initial result obtained by the immunoassay.

Finally, the clinical laboratorian must be cautious whenever interpreting immunoassay test results across different manufacturers, as direct comparisons may not be possible. Because test manufacturers often develop capture and detection antibodies to slightly different epitopes, the reference interval (normal range) established for an immunoassay can vary widely across manufacturers, even for the same clinical test. This is especially critical when serial measurements of tumor marker proteins are being performed to monitor medical treatment of cancer patients.

Homogeneous Enzyme Immunoassays

The chief use of homogeneous immunoassays has been in the determination of low-molecular-weight analytes (haptens), such as hormones, therapeutic drugs, and drugs of abuse, in both serum and urine. Homogeneous immunoassays **(Fig. 11–8)** may provide quicker test results because wash steps are not required, and as mentioned, these immunoassays

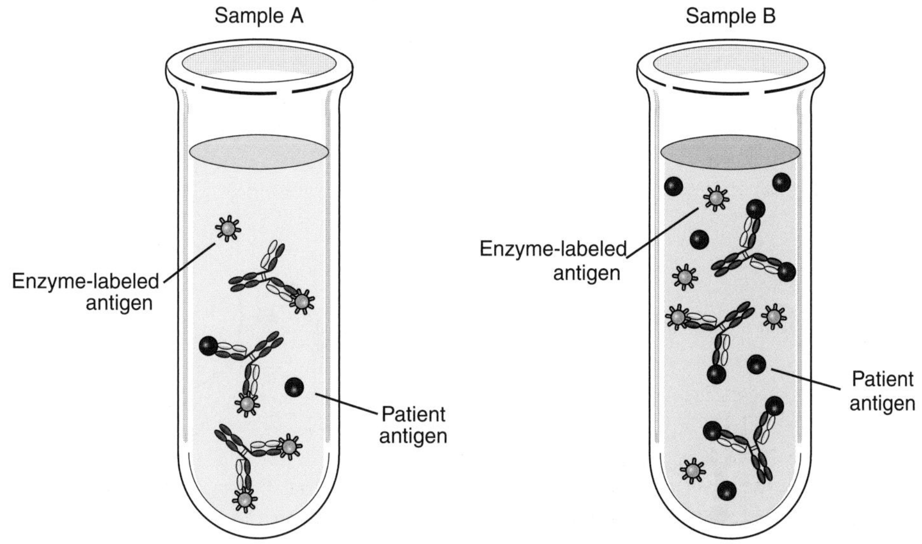

FIGURE 11–8 Homogeneous immunoassay. Reagent antibody is in solution. Patient antigen and enzyme-labeled antigen are added to the test tube. Patient antigen and enzyme-labeled antigen compete for a limited number of binding sites on the antibodies. When patient antigen is present, the enzyme label on the reagent antigen is not blocked, so color development is observed. Sample A has a low concentration of patient antigen, whereas Sample B contains more patient antigen and has stronger color development.

Connections

Haptens

Recall from Chapter 3 that haptens are small molecules that are unable to elicit an immune response on their own but will induce a response if complexed to a large carrier molecule, such as a protein.

tend to be less prone to analytical interferences. Despite the advantages of homogeneous immunoassays, their analytical sensitivity is not as robust as heterogeneous immunoassays.

The original homogeneous immunoassay design, which is still in use today on multiple platforms, is the **enzyme-multiplied immunoassay technique (EMIT)** first developed by the Syva Corporation (now part of Siemens). The EMIT immunoassay is based on the principle of change in enzyme activity as specific antigen–antibody interaction occurs in solution. Reagent antigen is bound to an enzyme tag, commonly glucose-6-phosphate dehydrogenase (G6PDH). When reagent antibody binds to specific determinant sites on the enzyme–antigen pair, the active site on the enzyme is blocked, resulting in a measurable loss of activity. Free analyte (antigen in the patient sample) competes with enzyme-labeled analyte for a limited number of antibody-binding sites. G6PDH catalyzes the reduction of NAD+ to NADH, leading to increased absorbance in the UV-wavelength region (340 nm). The resulting enzyme activity and signal generated are directly proportional to the concentration of patient antigen or hapten present in the test solution **(Fig. 11–9).**

The **cloned-enzyme donor immunoassay (CEDIA)** is another example of a homogeneous immunoassay. CEDIA was developed using genetic engineering techniques to produce the β-galactosidase enzyme in two parts: acceptor and donor. When separated, the enzyme is not fully formed, and there is no enzymatic activity; when the acceptor–donor pair combine, enzymatic activity is restored, and reagent substrate is catalyzed to generate a product signal that is measured by photometry. To achieve this reaction, the hapten antigen (Ag) is attached to the enzyme donor piece. The enzyme-donor Ag competes with patient Ag (analyte) for limited antibody-binding spots. As patient Ag binds to reagent Ab, it leaves the enzyme donor free to bind with the enzyme-acceptor molecule. Therefore, enzymatic activity and signal are directly proportional to patient Ag concentration. This reaction occurs in solution without need of a solid-phase material, which makes it a homogeneous immunoassay. Its most common clinical use is to detect or quantitate drug levels (both therapeutic and abused).

Chemiluminescent Immunoassays

The majority of immunometric assays on the market today are based on chemiluminescent label detection. These are collectively referred to as **chemiluminescent immunoassays. Chemiluminescence** is the emission of light caused by a chemical reaction, typically an oxidation reaction, producing an excited molecule that releases light during return to its original ground state. Large numbers of molecules are capable of chemiluminescence, and some of the most common substances used in test systems are luminol, acridinium esters, ruthenium derivatives, and nitrophenyl oxalates. When these substances are oxidized, intermediates are produced that are of a higher energy state. These intermediates spontaneously return to their original ground state, emitting photon energy (light) in the process. Light emissions range from a rapid flash of light to a more continuous glow that can last for hours. For example, when acridinium esters are oxidized by hydrogen peroxide under alkaline conditions, they emit a quick flash of light. When luminol is used in the reaction, the light signal remains for a longer time period.

Chemiluminescent technology is the basis for several types of automated immunoassays, which are used to detect a wide variety of clinical analytes, including antigens and antibodies. The design can be applied to heterogeneous or homogeneous immunoassay formats. Haptens such as therapeutic drugs and

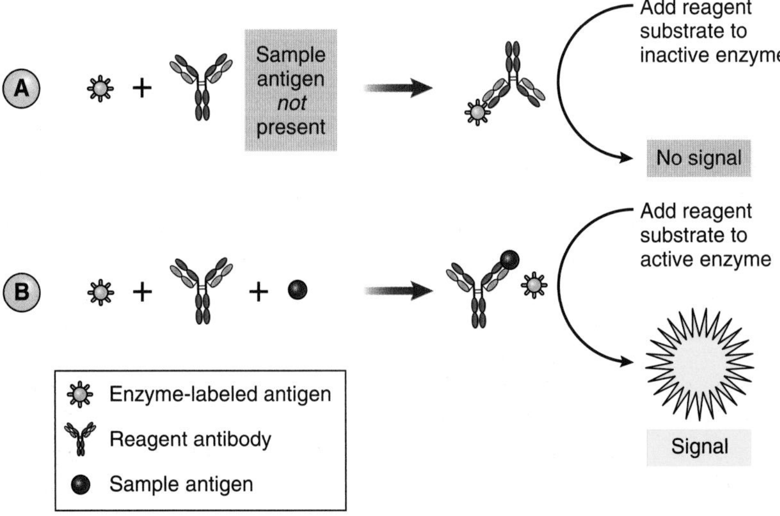

FIGURE 11–9 EMIT immunoassay design. *(Figure courtesy of Dr. Paul Johnson.)*

steroid hormones are measured using competitive immunoassays, whereas the sandwich or capture format is used for larger analytes such as protein hormones. These immunoassays also demonstrate excellent analytical properties for measurement of serum antibodies produced in several types of infectious diseases and autoimmune disorders.

Chemiluminescent immunoassays have superior analytical sensitivity and a wide dynamic range, the latter implying that the immunoassay performs well at both very low and very high analyte concentrations. This provides excellent sensitivity to detect very low levels while also reducing the need for sample dilution because extremely elevated results can be accurately measured. Detecting high antigen concentration without need for sample dilution can be especially useful when measuring tumor markers or autoantibodies in diseased patients, where concentration levels can be 10-fold or greater than the upper limit of the normal cutoff value.

Chemiluminescent Microparticle Immunoassay

In the **chemiluminescent microparticle immunoassay (CMIA)** design, antibody-coated microparticles are used in the reagent. In this method, patient antigen competes with a hapten (Ag) labeled with an acridinium ester. Magnets are used to attract the microparticles for physical separation and allow for unbound substances to be washed off. As such, CMIA is a heterogeneous immunoassay because the particles are physically separated by magnets. As antigen concentration increases in the patient sample, it prevents labeled Ag molecules from binding to the Ab-coated microparticles. Conversely, low patient antigen causes more labeled Ag to bind to the microparticles. A final test signal is generated by adding hydrogen peroxide to the alkaline solution, which destabilizes the acridinium ester, resulting in a flash of light (chemiluminescence). The resulting signal is indirectly proportional to the antigen concentration in the patient sample. CMIA technology has been largely applied for use in drug measurements, for example, phenytoin, a common anti-epileptic drug measured in therapeutic drug monitoring (TDM), to ensure the patient's drug levels are within the effective dose range, and are not at toxic or subtherapeutic levels.

Electrochemiluminescence Immunoassay

A newer modification of the traditional chemiluminescent immunoassay is the **electrochemiluminescence immunoassay (ECLIA).** Ruthenium, a chemical substance used as an indicator, can be conjugated to antibody used in capture immunoassays. It undergoes an electrochemiluminescent reaction with another chemical substance, tripropylamine (TPA), at the surface of an electrode. When the ruthenium is oxidized and then returned to its reduced state through interaction with TPA, it gives off light that can be measured by a photomultiplier tube. Magnetic beads or microparticles are often used as the solid phase to capture the labeled antibody.

Fluorescent Immunoassays

In 1941, Albert Coons demonstrated that antibodies could be labeled with molecules that fluoresce. These fluorescent compounds, called **fluorophores** or **fluorochromes,** can absorb energy from an incident light source and convert that energy into light of a longer wavelength and lower energy as the excited electrons return to the ground state. Fluorophores are typically organic molecules with a ring structure; each has a characteristic optimal absorption range. The time interval between absorption of energy and emission of fluorescence is very short and can be measured in nanoseconds.

Ideally, a fluorescent probe should exhibit high intensity, remain stable in solution, and be distinguished from background sample fluorescence. The two compounds most often used are fluorescein and rhodamine, usually in the form of isothiocyanates, because these can be readily coupled to antigen or antibody. Fluorescein absorbs maximally at 490 to 495 nm and emits a green color at 520 nm. It has high intensity, good photostability, and a high quantum yield. Tetramethylrhodamine absorbs at 550 nm and emits red light at 585 nm. Because their absorbance and emission patterns differ, fluorescein and rhodamine can be used together.

Fluorescent-labeled antibodies or antigens have been used in a variety of immunoassays, including direct and indirect immunofluorescence assays, multiplex immunoassays (MIAs), and fluorescence polarization immunoassays (FPIAs). In contrast to the "reagent-based" systems discussed in preceding sections, some fluorescent immunoassays take place on a microscope slide or on the surface of live cells. These techniques are called **immunofluorescence assays (IFAs).** The principles of laboratory methods that use fluorescent labels and examples of their clinical applications are presented in the text that follows.

Direct Immunofluorescence Assays

Fluorescent staining methods can be categorized as either direct or indirect, depending on whether the antibody specific for the antigen has a fluorescent tag attached to it. **Figure 11–10** depicts the difference between the two techniques.

Direct immunofluorescence assays may be used to detect antigens on tissue sections fixed onto a microscopic slide or in live cell suspensions. In a direct IFA performed on a microscope slide, antibody that is conjugated with a fluorescent tag is added directly to sample antigen fixed onto the slide. After incubation and a wash step to remove unbound antibody, the slide is read using a fluorescence microscope. The bound fluorescent probe is detected under UV light (see **Fig. 11–10A**). In this manner, multiple antigens can be detected with a high degree of sensitivity and specificity. Antigens are typically visualized as bright-apple-green or orange-yellow objects against a dark background. Examples of antigens detected by direct IFA methods include bacterial pathogens such as *Legionella pneumophila* and *Chlamydia trachomatis.*

Cell-based IFA methods combine the principles of hematology cell counters with fluorescent-labeled antibodies to better classify cells. An important application of direct IFA is to

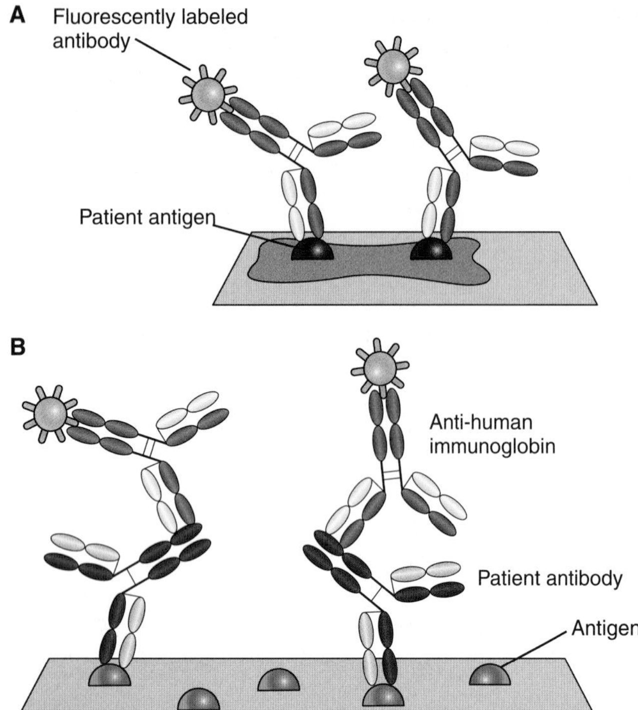

FIGURE 11–10 Direct versus indirect immunofluorescent assays. (A) In a direct fluorescent immunoassay, the patient antigen is fixed to a microscope slide and incubated directly with a fluorescent-labeled antibody. The slide is washed to remove unbound antibody. If specific antigen is present in the patient sample, fluorescence will be observed. (B) In indirect immunofluorescence, well-characterized tissues or cells are fixed to slides. Specific antibody in patient serum (red) binds to the antigens on the slides. A wash step is performed, and a labeled anti-human immunoglobulin is added. After a second wash step to remove any uncombined anti-immunoglobulin, the fluorescence of the sample is determined. The amount of fluorescence is directly in proportion to the amount of patient antibody present.

differentiate cell populations of the immune system, such as T and B lymphocytes, based on their cluster of differentiation (CD) antigens by incubation of the cells with fluorescent-labeled antibodies specific for those markers. For example, this assay is very useful in the detection and quantitation of abnormal cell populations observed in leukemias. The results are analyzed by automated **flow cytometry** (see Chapter 13 for a complete discussion of the principles of flow cytometry).

Alternatively, more recent advances in flow cytometry include *mass cytometry* profiling of cells based on CD marker identification. In this method, fluorescent labels are replaced with metal isotope labels for detection. Metal isotopes provide for simultaneous detection of a greater number of cellular markers as compared with traditional fluorescent labels.

Indirect Immunofluorescence Assays

In general, a direct immunofluorescence assay is only used for antigen detection in cells or tissues, whereas **indirect immunofluorescence (IIF) assays** can be used for either antigen or antibody identification, depending on the intended clinical application. IIF assays involve two steps, in a manner similar to reagent-based capture immunoassays. In the first step of IIF assays used to detect antibody, patient serum is incubated on a microscope slide to which a known antigen has been attached. Tissue antigen is usually affixed to the slide; for example, human epithelial cells are used for anti-nuclear antibody (ANA) testing. The slide is then washed, and an anti-human immunoglobulin containing a fluorescent tag is added. This labeled immunoglobulin combines with the first antibody to form a sandwich, which localizes the fluorescence (see **Fig. 11–10B**). In this manner, one antibody conjugate can be used for many different types of reactions, eliminating the need for numerous purified, labeled reagent antibodies.

IIF assays generate increased staining because multiple molecules can bind to each primary molecule, making this a more sensitive technique. Such immunoassays are especially useful in antibody identification and have been used in syphilis testing to detect treponemal antibodies, viral antibodies, and autoantibodies such as ANAs and anti-neutrophil cytoplasmic antibodies (ANCAs). Reading immunofluorescent slides is partly a subjective interpretation because the technologist reports results based on the visual presence or absence of signal as well as signal intensity in positive samples. Technical experience is essential for accurate and reliable reporting of slide test results. For example, there are several nuclear patterns observed in ANA testing that the technologist must be able to distinguish when interpreting slide results (see Chapter 15).

Multiplex Immunoassay (MIA)

A more recently developed platform, based on fluorescent labeling and detection, is the **multiplex immunoassay (MIA).** This high-throughput, automated method has improved ease of clinical testing, especially in testing for autoimmune diseases. Polystyrene beads are used as the solid phase. When the technique is used to detect antibodies in patient serum, beads conjugated to different antigens are used. These beads can be distinguished by their unique shade of red, created by a specific combination of infrared and fluorescent dyes. Patient sample is added to the bead mixture, and antibodies in the sample are detected with a fluorescent-tagged anti-human immunoglobulin. The beads containing the immune complexes are identified by flow cytometry (see Chapter 13). A benefit of MIA technology is that it allows for multiple antibodies to be detected simultaneously. Clinical applications of MIA include ANA testing (see Chapter 15) and detection of antibodies in transplant patients to donor antigens (see Chapter 16 and Fig. 16–7). MIA can also be used to simultaneously detect multiple antigens in a test sample when the polystyrene beads are coated with the corresponding antibodies. One application is the detection of cytokines produced by cells cultured under different conditions.

Fluorescence Polarization Immunoassays

Application of fluorescent labels for homogeneous immunoassay designs led to the development of the **fluorescence polarization immunoassay (FPIA).** This technique is of more historical interest today because in 2008 the manufacturer (Abbott) announced it was discontinuing its FPIA-based instruments. The company has since changed many of its previous platforms to chemiluminescent technology (discussed in an earlier section). Students should remain aware of FPIA technology; however, owing to reduced availability and manufacturer support for FPIA methods, their use has rapidly declined.

The FPIA method was based on the change in polarization of fluorescent light emitted from a labeled molecule when it is bound to antibody. Incident light directed at the specimen is polarized with a lens or prism so that the waves are aligned in one plane. If a molecule is small, it will rotate quickly, causing the emitted light to become unpolarized. If, however, the labeled molecule is bound to antibody, the molecule is unable to tumble rapidly, and light will remain polarized. Thus, the degree of polarized light detected corresponds to the amount of antibody-labeled antigen complex formed in solution. As the method is based on a competitive design, where labeled antigen competes with patient sample antigen for a limited number of antibody-binding sites, the fluorescence polarization detected is inversely proportional to the sample analyte concentration.

Rapid Immunoassays

Rapid immunoassays are membrane-based tests that are easy to perform and give reproducible results. Although designed primarily for point-of-care testing, many of these have found use within clinical laboratories because of their faster turnaround time of results, ease of use, and little space needed for setup. These tests are used on urine or serum samples and are designed as single-use, disposable immunoassays in a plastic cartridge.

The original rapid immunoassays are based on a flow-through design. The membrane and its large surface area enhance immunofiltration of the sample to provide speed and a high level of sensitivity. This method is a two-step immunoassay in which antigen or antibody in the patient sample is first absorbed onto the membrane containing the corresponding antibody or antigen. Following a wash step, a detection reagent is added. The reaction is then read by looking for the presence of a colored reaction product.

Newer **immunochromatography** methods combine all the previously mentioned steps into one step. The analyte is applied at one end of the strip and migrates toward the distal end, where there is an absorbent pad to maintain a constant capillary flow rate. The labeling and detection zones are set between the two ends. Sample is added to an application point; the application point also contains a labeled antigen or antibody conjugated to colored latex or colloidal gold particles. The sample reconstitutes the conjugate, where the two form a complex that migrates across the membrane. An antigen or antibody immobilized in the detection zone captures the immune complex and forms a colored line for a positive test when the immunoassay is of a noncompetitive format **(Fig. 11–11)**. This type of test device has been used to detect

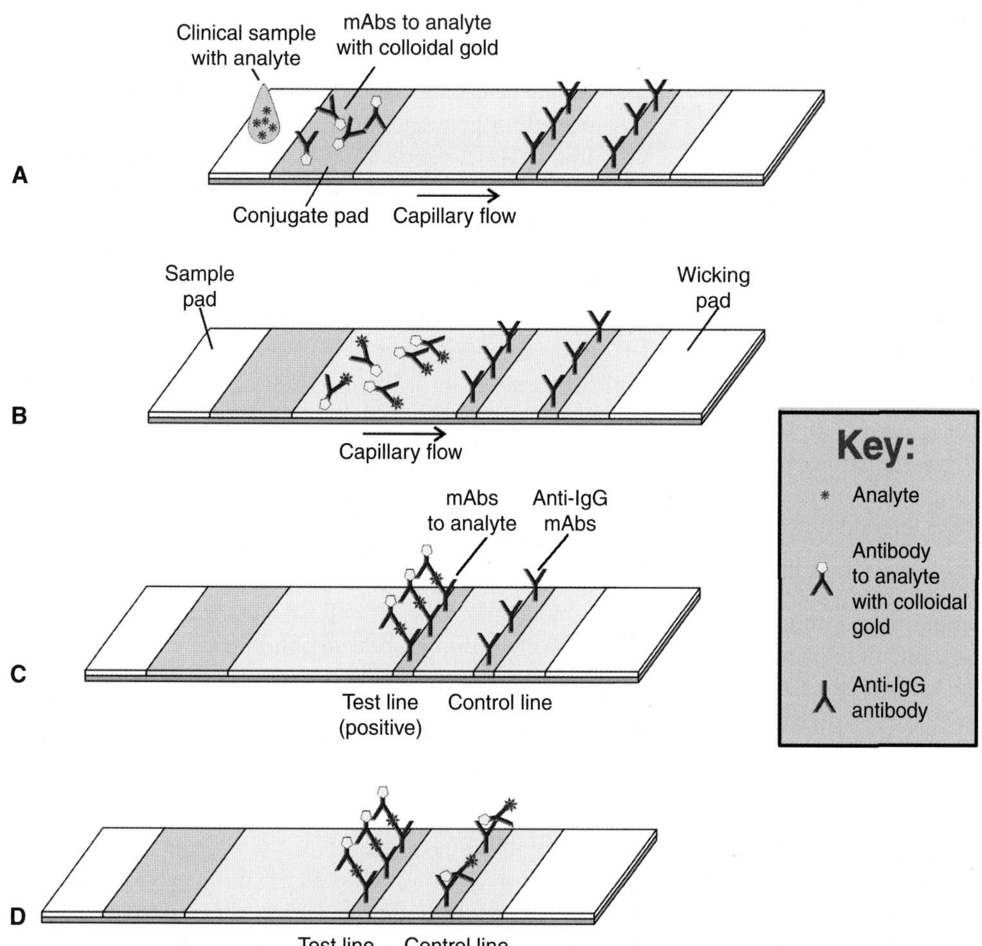

FIGURE 11–11 Immunochromatographic assay (noncompetitive). (A) Patient sample is added to a cassette containing antibody labeled with colloidal gold. (B) Sample combines with antibody and is moved along by capillary flow. (C) Monoclonal antibody to the analyte captures the patient antigen attached to gold-labeled antibody. (D) Control line has antibody that captures the colloidal gold-labeled antibody. *(Courtesy of University of Nevada School of Medicine.)*

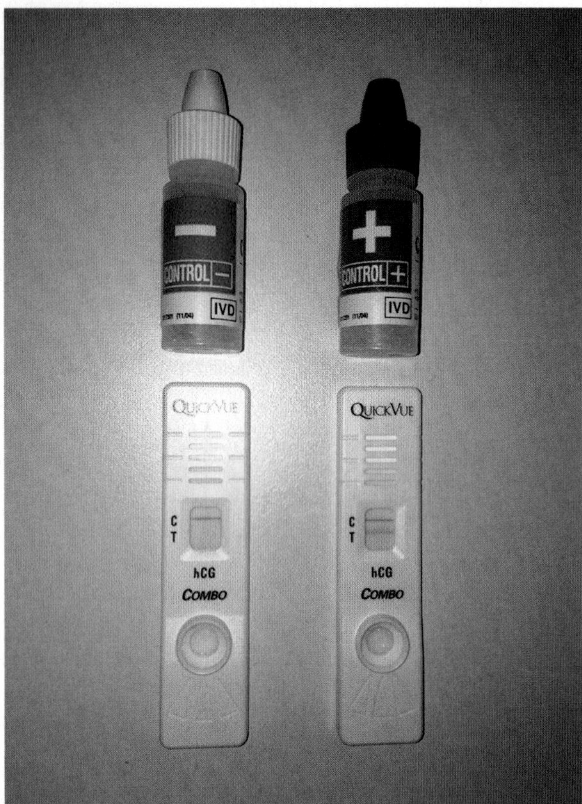

FIGURE 11–12 Rapid immunoassay for human chorionic gonadotropin (hCG). The negative control (left) has a line in the control region only. The positive control (right) has lines in both the control (C) region and the test (T) region. The control line must be present for the results to be valid, regardless of the test result. *(Photo courtesy of Dr. Paul Johnson.)*

diverse analytes of interest. Prototypical examples of rapid immunoassay uses include detection of the human chorionic gonadotropin (hCG) hormone as an indicator of pregnancy **(Fig. 11–12)**; identification of microorganisms such as *Streptococcus pyogenes,* the cause of streptococcal pharyngitis (see Fig. 20–13); and cardiac troponin to diagnose a heart attack.

The immunochromatographic design illustrated in Figure 11–11 is based on a capture or noncompetitive design. Some newer test systems, which still use similar materials, are based on a competitive format. These results must be carefully interpreted because the observed line indicates a negative result, and absence of the line is a positive result. Rapid screening tests to detect drugs of abuse provide one example of this format. A **single-step, competitive, immunochromatographic method** contains detection antibody adsorbed onto colloidal gold particles, which is then dried onto the entire membrane surface. Drug conjugates (drug bound to bovine serum albumin) are made for each drug of detection, all of which are immobilized to a unique test-line position on the membrane. When the sample (urine) is added, it wicks along the entire surface of the white membrane. As it passes along each test lane, drug-free urine sample dissolves the antibody–gold particle complex at each lane, resulting in observation of purple-red colored lines. Any drug present in the sample will inhibit that reaction, such that no line will be observed on the white membrane background. As this method is based on a competitive design, it may lead to initial confusion when interpreting test results. This is because the color line indicator is observed only when there is no antigen or drug present in the sample (negative result), while the absence of the line indicator is a positive result. The test system may also include use of a strip-reading device, which aids the laboratorian in interpreting the final results. In addition, all single-use test kit immunoassays include a control line to ensure the test kit cartridge is functioning properly before reporting out results (see Fig. 11–12).

SUMMARY

- Labeled immunoassays were developed to measure antigens and antibodies that may be small in size or present in very low concentrations.
- The substance that is being measured is called the *analyte*.
- Labeling techniques include the use of radioactivity, enzymes, fluorescence, chemiluminescence, and chromatography.
- The two major formats of immunoassays are heterogeneous and homogeneous. In heterogeneous immunoassays, physical separation of bound and free components is required. Homogeneous immunoassays do not require a physical separation step.
- Additional subclassifications describe whether immunoassay method designs are competitive or noncompetitive. In competitive immunoassays, all the reactants are added at the same time, and labeled antigen competes with patient antigen for a limited number of antibody-binding sites.
- In competitive immunoassays, the amount of bound label is inversely proportional to the concentration of the labeled antigen. In other words, the greater the amount of labeled antigen detected, the less antigen is present in the patient sample.
- In noncompetitive immunoassays, reagent antibody is passively absorbed onto a solid-phase material. Excess capture antibody is present to ensure that any patient antigen will be bound. A labeled antibody, directed against a different epitope of the antigen, is added.
- In noncompetitive immunoassays, the amount of the label detected is directly proportional to the amount of patient antigen present.

- Antibodies used in immunoassays must be very specific and have a high affinity for the antigen in question. Specificity helps to reduce cross-reactivity, and the affinity determines how stable the binding is between antigen and antibody. These two factors help to determine the sensitivity of such immunoassays.
- Radioimmunoassays (RIAs) are based on a competitive principle, using a radioisotope label. These assays have extremely high analytical sensitivity but come with the disadvantages inherent in using radioactive substances.
- Enzyme immunoassays (EIAs) use enzymes that catalyze biochemical reactions. They convert reagent substrates to produce chemically modified products that can be detected.
- In competitive enzyme-linked immunosorbent assays (ELISAs), antigen in the sample competes with enzyme-conjugated antigen for a limited number of binding sites on antibody molecules attached to a solid phase. Enzyme activity present in the final reaction catalyzes the conversion of the substrate to a detectable product.
- Indirect ELISAs are a type of noncompetitive immunoassay. These immunoassays are termed *indirect* because the enzyme-labeled reagent does not participate in the initial antigen–antibody reaction. The associated antigen is bound to the solid phase. Patient serum with an unknown antibody concentration is added. A second antibody reacts with any patient antibody that is bound to the solid phase.
- Immunoassays that detect antigen are termed *capture immunoassays*. In capture or sandwich immunoassays, the antibody is bound to a solid phase, and any patient antigen is allowed to bind or be captured. A second enzyme-labeled antibody is added. The final complex formed with sample antigen in between the two reagent antibodies creates the "sandwich."
- Homogeneous enzyme immunoassays require no separation step. They are based on the principle that enzyme activity changes as specific antigen–antibody binding occurs. When antibody binds to enzyme-labeled antigen, steric hindrance results in a loss of enzyme activity.
- Increased analytical sensitivity of labeled immunoassays can be achieved by complexing biotin to the capture antibody and streptavidin to the solid-phase material. Biotin-SAv labeling can be used in both indirect ELISAs and capture immunoassays.
- The most commonly observed limitation of capture immunoassays is the high-dose hook effect, or *postzone* effect. Excess patient antigen causes falsely decreased detection, leading to an analyte concentration that appears to be low or normal.
- Antibodies produced in vivo may interfere with immunoassays whenever the antibody produced is similar to that of a test reagent. Heterophile interference occurs when the individual produces antibodies similar to those used in the test reagent kit, such as anti-mouse, -rabbit, or -goat antibodies. Test kits using a biotin-SAv complex can cause unpredictable interferences.
- *Cross-reactivity* describes detection of a substance other than the analyte of interest. It is typically observed as a false-positive result.
- Homogeneous immunoassays are used for the detection of low-molecular-weight analytes, such as hormones, therapeutic drugs, and drugs of abuse. The cloned-enzyme donor immunoassay (CEDIA) is an example of a homogeneous immunoassay.
- One-step, easy-to-interpret formats have been developed for heterogeneous enzyme immunoassays. Rapid immunochromatographic test devices are able to capture antigen or antibody in a specific location on a membrane.
- The majority of immunometric assays are based on chemiluminescent label detection. Chemiluminescence is produced by certain compounds when oxidized. Substances that do this can be used as markers in reactions that are similar to RIA and EIAs.
- Fluorochromes are fluorescent compounds that absorb energy from an incident light source and convert that energy to light of a longer wavelength.
- Direct immunofluorescence assays involve antigen detection through a specific antibody that is labeled with a fluorescent tag. The presence of fluorescence is detected with a fluorescent microscope that utilizes UV light.
- In indirect immunofluorescent assays, the original antibody is unlabeled. Incubation with antigen is followed by addition of a second fluorescent-labeled anti-immunoglobulin that detects antigen–antibody complexes.
- Multiplex immunoassay (MIA) involves using polystyrene beads as the solid phase. To detect antibodies in patient serum, beads conjugated to different antigens are used. MIA technology allows for multiple antibodies or antigens to be detected simultaneously.
- Fluorescence polarization immunoassay (FPIA) was a type of homogeneous fluorescent immunoassay. It was based on the principle that when an antigen is bound to antibody, polarization of light increases.
- Newer, single use disposable immunoassays are rapid tests based on immunochromatography that are designed to detect analytes such as hCG and drugs in urine.

Study Guide: Labeled Immunoassays

TYPE OF IMMUNOASSAY	PRINCIPLE	RESULTS
Homogeneous EIA	No physical separation step of bound and labeled antigens required. Patient antigen and labeled antigen react with reagent antibody in solution. Enzyme label is inactivated when reagent antigen binds to antibody.	Patient antigen concentration is directly proportional to the signal.
Heterogeneous	Requires solid-phase material to allow for antigen or antibody binding. Includes both competitive and noncompetitive immunoassay designs.	In a noncompetitive immunoassay, the concentration of patient antigen is directly proportional to the signal. In a competitive immunoassay, patient antigen concentration is indirectly proportional to the signal.
Competitive	Patient antigen (Ag) competes with labeled antigen (Ag*) for limited antibody-binding (Ab) sites. Final detected signal is Ag*Ab (labeled antigen bound to antibody), as shown in the reaction: $Ag, Ag^*, Ab \rightarrow Ag^*Ab + AgAb$	Inverse ratio: The more patient antigen is present, the less label is detected.
Noncompetitive, indirect ELISA for antibody detection	Excess solid-phase antigen binds patient antibody, and a second labeled antibody (anti-human immunoglobulin) is added.	All patient antibody is allowed to bind. Amount of label is directly proportional to the amount of patient antibody present.
Capture or sandwich	Excess solid-phase antibody binds patient antigen, and a second labeled antibody (to the antigen) is added after a wash step.	All patient antigen is allowed to bind. Amount of label is directly proportional to the amount of patient antigen present.
Enzyme-multiplied immunoassay technique (EMIT)	Reagent antigen is bound to an enzyme tag. Change in enzyme activity is observed as specific antigen–antibody interaction occurs in solution. If reagent antibody binds to the enzyme–antigen pair, enzyme activity is blocked. Otherwise, enzyme is active. Active enzyme (commonly glucose-6-phosphate dehydrogenase) catalyzes the reduction of NAD+ to NADH, leading to increased absorbance in the UV-wavelength region.	All patient antigen is allowed to bind. Amount of signal generated is directly proportional to the amount of patient antigen present.
Direct immunofluorescence	Patient sample (e.g., tissue) is attached to a slide. Specific fluorescent-labeled antibody is added. In cell-based immunoassays, patient cells are incubated with fluorescent-labeled antibody to a cell surface antigen.	If fluorescence is detected, patient sample is positive for the antigen. Fluorescence on cell surface indicates that the cell is positive for the antigen.
Indirect immunofluorescence	To detect patient antibody, reagent antigen is attached to a slide and incubated with the patient sample. A second fluorescent-labeled antibody (anti-human immunoglobulin) is added. To detect antigen, patient sample is fixed to a slide and incubated with antibody to the antigen (primary antibody), followed by labeled secondary antibody, directed against the primary antibody.	If fluorescence is detected, antibody or antigen is present in the sample, and the test is positive.
Fluorescence polarization	Fluorescent-labeled antigen competes with patient antigen for a limited number of soluble antibody-binding sites.	When patient antigen binds to antibody, less reagent-labeled antigen binds, and less polarized light will be detected. Inverse ratio between patient antigen and amount of polarization.
Rapid Immunochromatographic	Patient sample is added to a test strip and migrates through the strip. Patient antigen complexes to antibody-labeled particles or competes with antigen-labeled particles across individual test lanes at unique detection zones.	Presence of test line may indicate either positive or negative result, depending on manufacturer design.

CASE STUDY

1. A 60-year-old male presented to his primary care physician with fatigue, loss of appetite, weight loss, and abdominal pain. His urine was dark in color. The physician suspected the patient may have pancreatic cancer based on family history of the disease. Ultrasonography of the abdominal region identified a large mass, which appeared localized to the pancreas. A computed tomography (CT) scan was ordered to confirm and identify the large mass. The CT scan results supported the presence of a pancreatic tumor, and a diagnosis of pancreatic cancer was made. Before initiating chemotherapy and radiation therapy treatments, his physician ordered a serum CA 19-9 tumor marker immunoassay to establish a baseline value, then reordered the test at the patient's follow-up visit 3 months later. The baseline sample was sent to a hospital laboratory that uses Instrument Manufacturer "A." The test result at the patient's 3-month office visit was sent to the regional testing laboratory, which uses Instrument Manufacturer "B."

Test results are included in the table that follows:

CA 19-9 TEST RESULT	TESTING NOTES	REFERENCE INTERVAL CUT-OFF	DATE OF RESULT	INSTRUMENT USED
1,250 U/mL	Final result reported after sample dilution	< 38 U/mL	Just before initiation of treatment regimen	"A"
110 U/mL	Undiluted sample result	< 55 U/mL	3 months after treatment was initiated	"B"
950 U/mL	Instrument result of 95 U/mL after 1:10 dilution of sample	< 55 U/mL	3 months after treatment was initiated	"B"

Questions

a. Based on the patient's baseline test value, what technical concern should the technologist have upon seeing the most recent test result (at 3 months post-treatment)?
b. What procedure could the technologist perform to verify that the test result is correct?
c. What is the disadvantage of monitoring a patient's tumor marker immunoassay test result when immunoassays developed by different manufacturers are used?
d. If the need to send the patient's blood sample to another clinical laboratory using a different immunoassay instrument could not be avoided, what is the best course of action to interpret the test result?

REVIEW QUESTIONS

1. Which of the following statements accurately describes heterogeneous competitive binding immunoassays?
   a. Excess binding sites for the analyte are provided.
   b. Test signal is generated in solution without the need of a solid-phase support material.
   c. The concentration of patient analyte is inversely proportional to bound label.
   d. All the patient analyte is bound in the reaction.

2. How do heterogeneous immunoassays differ from homogeneous immunoassays?
   a. Heterogeneous immunoassays require a separation step.
   b. Heterogeneous immunoassays require less technical skill to perform than homogeneous immunoassays.
   c. For noncompetitive immunoassays, the concentration of patient analyte is indirectly proportional to bound label in heterogeneous immunoassays.
   d. Homogeneous immunoassays have better analytical sensitivity compared with heterogeneous immunoassays.

3. Which of the following responses characterizes a capture or sandwich enzyme immunoassay?
   a. Less analytically sensitive than competitive enzyme immunoassays
   b. Labeled antigen attached to a solid phase
   c. Best for small antigens with a single epitope determinant
   d. Excess number of antibody sites on solid-phase material

4. Which of the following is an advantage of enzyme immunoassay over radioimmunoassay?
   a. Decrease in hazardous waste
   b. Shorter shelf life of kit reagents
   c. No interference by biological inhibitors
   d. Must be read manually

5. Which of the following is characteristic of direct fluorescence immunoassays?
   a. The anti-immunoglobulin has the fluorescent tag.
   b. Antibody is attached to a solid phase.
   c. This method can be used for rapid identification of microbial antigens.
   d. The amount of color is inversely proportional to the amount of antigen present.

6. Which of the following is true of the enzyme-multiplied immunoassay technique (EMIT)?
   a. It is classified as a heterogeneous method.
   b. Nicotinamide adenine dinucleotide (NAD+) is a substrate used in the test reaction.
   c. When the patient sample antigen concentration is high, the final test signal will be low.
   d. Patient sample antigen blocks the enzyme active site in the test reaction.

7. A fluorescent substance is best described as one in which
   a. light energy is absorbed and converted to a longer wavelength.
   b. the emitted wavelength can be seen under normal white light.
   c. there is a long time between the absorption and emission of light.
   d. it spontaneously decays and emits light.

8. In a noncompetitive ELISA, if a negative control shows the presence of signal, which of the following might be a possible explanation?
   a. No reagent was added.
   b. Washing steps were incomplete.
   c. The enzyme was inactivated.
   d. No substrate was present.

9. Which of the following best characterizes chemiluminescent immunoassays?
   a. Only the antigen can be labeled.
   b. Tests can be read manually.
   c. These are only homogeneous immunoassays.
   d. A chemical is oxidized to produce light.

10. Immunofluorescence assays may be difficult to interpret for which reason?
    a. Autofluorescence of substances in serum
    b. Nonspecific binding to serum proteins
    c. Subjectivity in reading results
    d. Any of the above

11. Which statement best describes rapid immunochromatographic assays?
    a. Test results are always reported as quantitative values.
    b. They are designed primarily for point-of-care testing.
    c. Urine is the only acceptable sample type.
    d. Formation of a colored line always indicates a positive result.

12. Which of the following is characteristic of an indirect enzyme immunoassay?
    a. The first antibody has the enzyme label.
    b. Only one antibody is required.
    c. Color is directly proportional to the amount of patient antibody present.
    d. Enzyme specificity is not essential.

13. In an indirect ELISA, what would be the outcome of an improper wash after the antibody–enzyme conjugate is added?
    a. Results will be falsely decreased.
    b. Results will be falsely increased.
    c. Results will be unaffected.
    d. No wash step is required in the ELISA procedure.

14. In a heterogeneous enzyme immunoassay, if the patient sample produces more signal than the highest positive control, what action should be taken?
    a. Report the results out as determined.
    b. Dilute the patient sample.
    c. Repeat the immunoassay using one-half the volume of the patient sample.
    d. Report the results as falsely positive.

15. Which of the following can uniquely cause interferences in immunoassays designed with streptavidin bound to the solid-phase surface?
    a. Elevated concentration of biotin in the patient test sample can cause falsely increased results.
    b. Heterophile antibodies present in the patient sample cause falsely decreased results.
    c. Antibody excess in the patient sample leads to a hook effect.
    d. Solid-phase particles will dissolve easily if the reaction temperature is increased.

12 Molecular Diagnostic Techniques

Lela Buckingham, PhD, MB(ASCP), DLM(ASCP)

LEARNING OUTCOMES

After finishing this chapter, you should be able to:

1. Describe the structure of DNA and RNA.
2. Deduce complementary nucleic acid sequences.
3. Define *hybridization*.
4. Interpret results from gel or capillary electrophoresis.
5. Describe how restriction enzymes work.
6. Explain the basic steps of the polymerase chain reaction (PCR).
7. Discuss the principles of modified PCR methods, including quantitative PCR (qPCR), reverse transcriptase PCR (RT-PCR), sequence-specific primer PCR (SSP-PCR), and digital droplet PCR.
8. Assess template quantity by qPCR.
9. Discuss isothermal DNA and RNA amplification methods.
10. Explain the basis of DNA chain termination (Sanger) sequencing and pyrosequencing.
11. Describe two next-generation sequencing (NGS) technologies.
12. Differentiate between targeted sequencing, whole exome sequencing, and whole genome sequencing.
13. Discuss the applications of basic bioinformatics to the assessment of DNA sequence variants.

CHAPTER OUTLINE

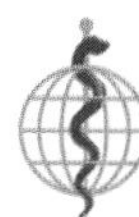

Go to FADavis.com for the laboratory exercises that accompany this text.

KEY TERMS

Amplification
Bioinformatics
Branched DNA (bDNA)
Cell cycle
Chain termination sequencing
Chromosome
Digital droplet PCR
DNA
Electrophoresis
Epigenetics
Fluorescence in situ hybridization (FISH)
Genes
Genome
Genomics
Hybridization
Immunohistochemistry
In situ hybridization (ISH)
Microarray
Mutation
Next-generation sequencing (NGS)
Nucleic acid
Nucleotide
Polymerase chain reaction (PCR)
Polymorphism
Primers
Probe
Pyrosequencing
Quantitative PCR (qPCR)
Restriction endonuclease
Restriction fragment length polymorphisms (RFLPs)
Reverse transcriptase
RNA
Single-nucleotide polymorphisms (SNPs)
Transcription
Translation
Variant
Western blot

Nucleic acids carry genetic information that codes for protein structure. Primary characteristics of nucleic acids, such as nucleic acid complementarity and melting temperature, form the basis of specificity for almost all nucleic acid–based tests. Methods of analysis are under continual development, with gel and capillary electrophoresis, nucleic acid amplification techniques, spectrophotometry, and fluorescent labeling in common use and DNA sequencing increasingly implemented in laboratories. Such techniques are especially advantageous in infectious disease testing because nucleic acids can be detected earlier than antibodies during the course of an illness. Today, molecular diagnostics make important contributions to therapeutic decisions, transplant selection, drug efficacy, forensics, diagnosis of infections, and disease prognosis. We begin this chapter with an overview of nucleic acid structure and proceed to discuss the molecular techniques by which changes in DNA sequence can be detected and applied to the diagnosis of disease.

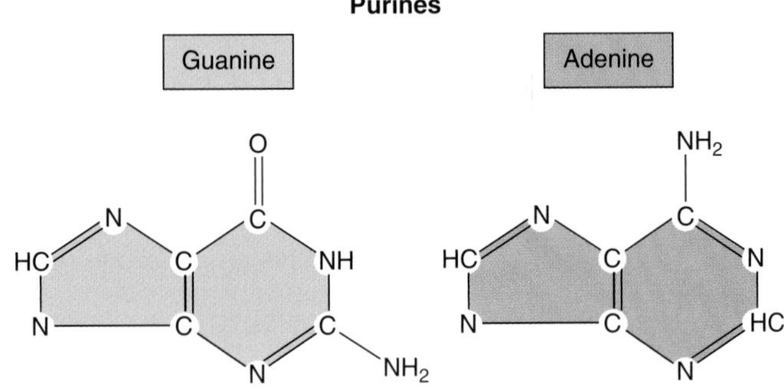

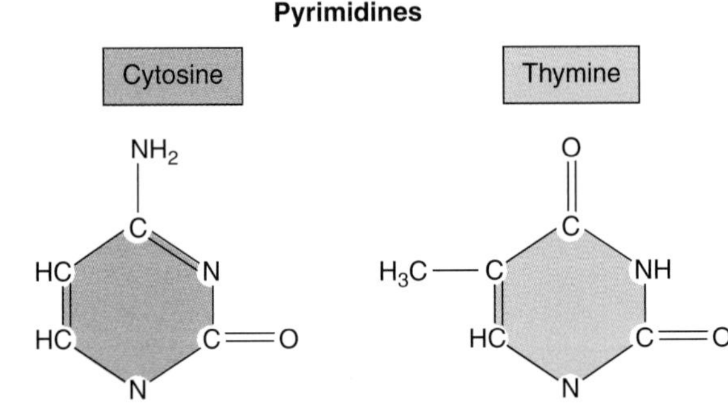

FIGURE 12–1 DNA is composed of polymers of four nucleotides: deoxyguanosine triphosphate (dGTP), deoxyadenosine triphosphate (dATP), deoxythymidine triphosphate, and deoxycytidine triphosphate (dCTP). A nucleoside is an unphosphorylated (deoxy) ribose sugar carrying a nitrogen base. *(Adapted from Buckingham L. Molecular Diagnostics. 2nd ed. Philadelphia, PA: F.A. Davis; 2011, with permission.)*

DNA and RNA

The two main kinds of nucleic acids are **DNA** and **RNA.** DNA carries the primary genetic information within chromosomes found in each cell. There are different types of RNA, including messenger RNA (mRNA), transfer RNA (tRNA), ribosomal RNA (rRNA), and noncoding RNA. The functions of these different RNA molecules in translating the genetic code of DNA into proteins and in regulating the expression of the genetic code will be discussed in sections that follow. DNA and RNA are macromolecules of nucleotides. A **nucleotide** is composed of a phosphorylated deoxyribose or ribose sugar and a nitrogen base. There are five nitrogen bases that make up the majority of nucleic acids found in nature: adenine (A), cytosine (C), guanine (G), thymine (T, found in DNA), and uracil (U; found only in RNA **[Fig. 12–1]**).

Positions in the deoxyribose and nitrogen base rings are numbered as shown in **Figure 12–2.** The nitrogen base of a nucleotide, either guanine, adenine, cytosine, or thymine, is attached to the 1′ carbon of the deoxyribose sugar. The

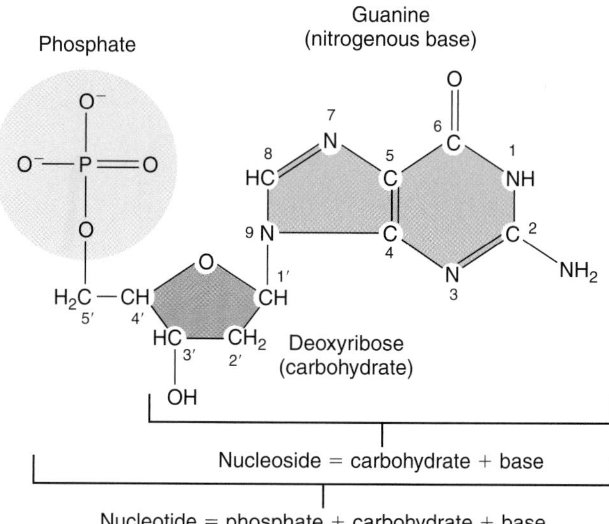

FIGURE 12–2 Nucleotide structure. Nitrogen base ring positions are numbered ordinally, and the ribose ring positions are numbered with prime numbers. *(Adapted from Buckingham L.* Molecular Diagnostics. *2nd ed. Philadelphia, PA: F.A. Davis; 2011, with permission.)*

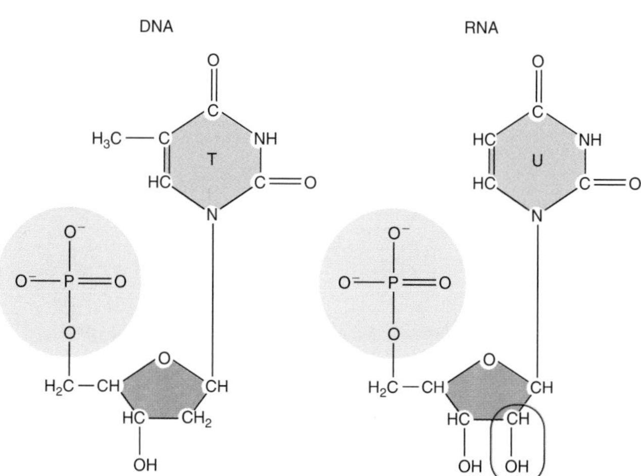

FIGURE 12–3 The ribose sugar in RNA is hydroxylated on the 2′ and 3′ carbons (right), whereas in DNA, it's only hydroxylated at the 3′ carbon (left). The nitrogen base uracil, found in RNA (right), is analogous to thymine found in DNA (left). *(Adapted from Buckingham L.* Molecular Diagnostics. *2nd ed. Philadelphia, PA: F.A. Davis; 2011, with permission.)*

deoxyribose 5′ carbon may be bound to one, two, or three phosphate groups. The deoxyribose 3′ carbon carries a hydroxyl group (OH).

In contrast to the deoxyribose sugar in DNA, nitrogen bases are attached to a ribose sugar in RNA. RNA contains adenine, cytosine, and guanine but has uracil nucleotides in place of the thymines found in DNA. Unlike deoxyribonucleotides, which are hydroxylated on the 3′ carbon, the phosphorylated ribose sugar in RNA carries hydroxyl groups on both the 2′ and 3′ carbons **(Fig. 12–3)**.

Substituted Nucleotides

Natural modifications of the nucleotide structure include methylation, deamination, additions, substitutions, and other chemical modifications. These modifications may be enzymatically catalyzed in the cell or spontaneous reactions.

Nucleotide modifications can also result in nucleotides with new properties. Addition and removal of methyl groups (–CH3) to DNA affect gene function. Nucleotide base modifications are also caused by environmental insults such as chemicals or radiation. These changes can lead to undesirable effects such as dysregulated cell proliferation as seen in cancer.

Gram-negative bacteria use modified nucleotides in a type of immune system, the restriction modification (rm) system. The bacterium adds methyl groups to its own DNA to distinguish it from that of invaders, such as bacterial viruses. Recognizing its own DNA in this way, the bacterium can target the invader's DNA for enzymatic degradation. Bacteria can also copy invading nucleic acid sequences for degradation by the Cas9 enzyme in another type of defense called *clustered regularly interspaced short palindromic repeats* or CRISPR-Cas9, which will be discussed in a later section.

> **Clinical Correlations**
>
> **Modified Nucleotides**
>
> Modified nucleotides are used in the clinic as well as in the laboratory. Azidothymidine (Zidovudine, Retrovir) and acyclovir (Zovirax) are modified nucleotides that are potent antiviral agents used against HIV and herpes viruses. Another modified nucleotide, 5-fluorouracil, is an anticancer drug. Dideoxynucleotides, which lack the second hydroxyl group on the ribose sugar, are used in chain termination sequencing (see later section).

The Nucleic Acid Polymer

Nucleotides are polymerized into nucleic acids by attachment of the 3′ hydroxyl groups on the deoxyribose or ribose sugar to the 5′ phosphate group of the adjacent nucleotide, forming a phosphodiester bond. A chain of nucleotides makes up one strand of DNA or RNA. Although most (but not all) RNA exists as a single-stranded molecule without a partner strand, DNA is mostly double-stranded, arranged in a double helix **(Fig. 12–4)**. The double helix is formed by two single DNA chains wrapped around each other. There is a complementary relationship between the two linear polymers (strands) of the double helix. All C's are across from G's in the partner strand, and all A's are across from T's.

The hydroxyl group on the 3′ carbon and the phosphate group on the 5′ carbon that participate in the formation of the DNA polymer through phosphodiester bonds give the DNA strands polarity, that is, a 5′ phosphate end and a 3′ hydroxyl end. Sequences are by convention ordered in the 5′ to 3′ direction. In the double helix, complementary strands hydrogen-bond together in an antiparallel arrangement, with the 5′ phosphates of the two strands at opposite ends of the helix **(Fig. 12–5)**.

The two chains (strands) of the DNA double helix are held together by hydrogen bonds between their nucleotide bases. Guanine (G) and cytosine (C) are complementary; that is,

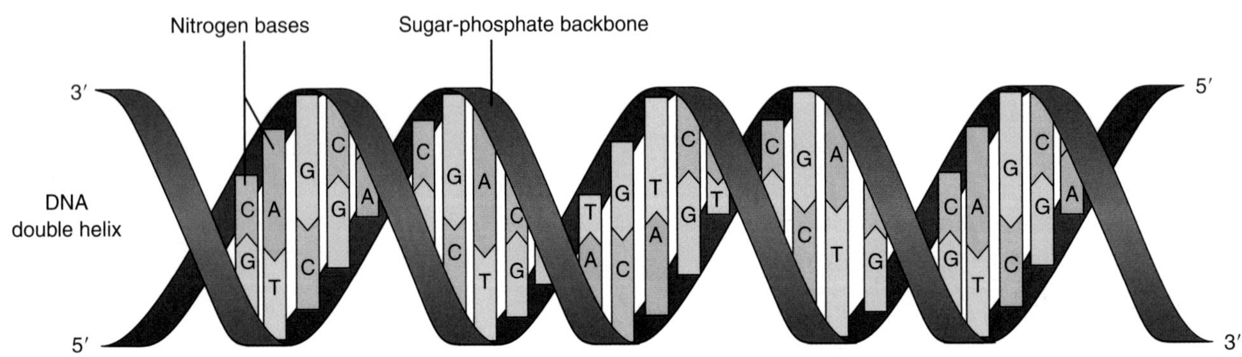

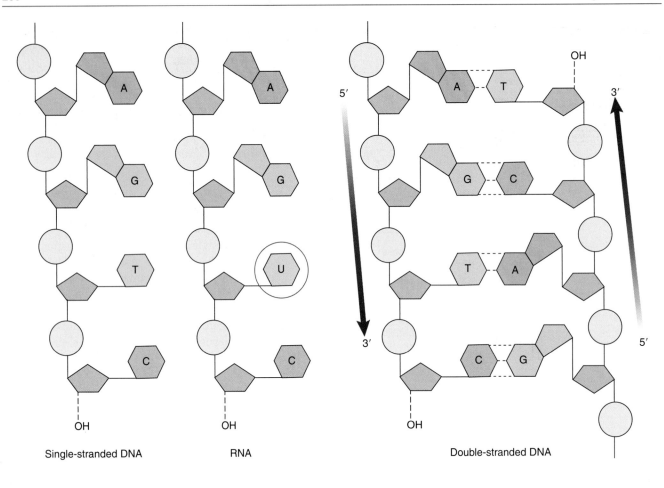

FIGURE 12–4 Nucleic acids are composed of a sequence of covalently attached nucleotides. The sugar-phosphate groups of adjacent nucleotides form the backbone of the molecule. RNA is single stranded and has uracil nucleotides rather than thymines. DNA forms a double-stranded helix with the base pairs in the center of the two complementary strands. *(Adapted from Buckingham L.* Molecular Diagnostics. *2nd ed. Philadelphia, PA: F.A. Davis; 2011, with permission.)*

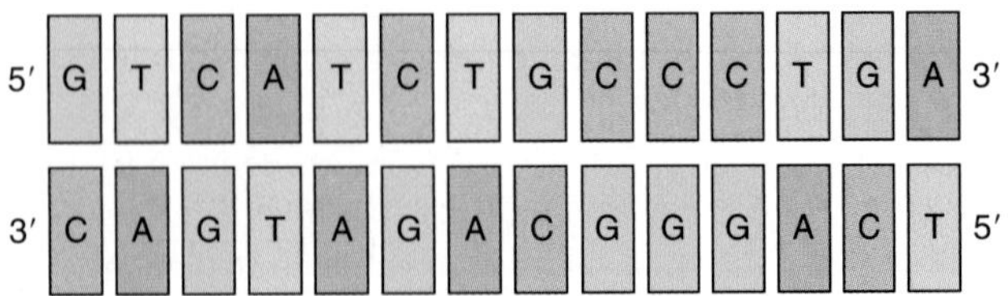

FIGURE 12–5 Complementary sequences are not identical. In each nucleotide chain, G nucleotides always hydrogen-bond to C nucleotides, and A nucleotides bond with T nucleotides in the complementary chain. Complementary sequences hybridize in an antiparallel arrangement.

they will only hydrogen-bond with each other. Adenine (A) and thymine (T) are complementary to each other as well. G pairs with C by three hydrogen bonds, and A pairs with T by two hydrogen bonds. Two bases joined together in this way are called a *base pair* (bp). The length of a double-stranded DNA macromolecule is measured in bp. The length of a single strand of RNA (or DNA) is measured in bases (b). Metric prefixes are used to describe long strands of DNA or RNA, for example, 1,000 bp or b comprise a kilobase pair (kbp) or kilobase (kb), respectively. One million bp or b comprise a megabase pair (Mbp) or megabase (Mb), respectively.

Most microorganisms contain one double helix, usually in circular form and a few Mbp in size. Viruses may carry a double- or single-stranded DNA or RNA molecule. In plants and animals, DNA is separated into multiple chromosomes per cell. Each **chromosome** is a double helix of DNA. In humans, there are 46 chromosomes contained in the cell nucleus, two copies of each of the 22 autosomes or non-sex chromosomes (1–22) and two copies of the X chromosome in females (designated 46,XX) or one copy each of the X and Y chromosome in males (designated 46,XY). The autosomes are numbered according to size from the largest, chromosome 1 (246 Mbp), to the smallest, chromosome 22 (47 Mbp). The X chromosome, 154 Mbp, is much larger than the Y chromosome (57 Mbp). **Genes** are sequences of nucleotides in chromosomes that carry information for either a protein or a non-coding RNA molecule. There are more than 21,000 protein-coding genes carried on the 23 chromosomes, with two copies of each gene making up the diploid genome (two copies of each of the 23 chromosomes per cell or 46 chromosomes). Bacterial and animal cells may also carry extra-chromosomal DNA in the form of small, usually circular plasmids, which are several thousands of bp in size. Human cells also carry mitochondrial DNA outside of the nucleus.

With the development of array and sequencing technology, it is possible to investigate the entirety of DNA in the cell **(genome)** or a population of microorganisms in a host (microbiome). In contrast to tests for a single gene at a time, these -omic studies are designed to analyze whole microbial populations, multiple genes, gene regions, or all the genes to assess the status of an organism or population of organisms.

DNA Replication

Chromosomes in bacteria carry a defined sequence of nucleotides called the *origin of replication* for DNA replication to begin. Replication proceeds through the chromosome, followed by binary fission of the bacterial cell. Some bacteria, such as *Escherichia coli* and *Bacillus subtilis,* have replication at two, four, or eight origins, depending on the growth rate, which allows for shorter cell doubling times in rich growth environments. The timing of replication ensures that initiation occurs simultaneously at all origins once per generation.

Eukaryotic cells have multiple chromosomes, and their replication must be coordinated. As these cells divide, they undergo a series of events in which they increase in size and duplicate their DNA. This process, called the **cell cycle,** consists of four stages: G1, S, G2, and M **(Fig. 12–6).** DNA replication takes place during the S phase of the cell cycle. At the end of the S phase, the DNA complement of the cell is doubled. This is the G2 phase. One complement of chromosomes is divided into each of two daughter cells during the M phase. Each daughter cell will then be in the G1 phase. Movement of the cell cycle from G1 to S is strictly regulated, as is movement from G2 to M. Loss of control at these "checkpoints" occurs in cancer.

Replication of DNA is semiconservative; that is, the two strands of the DNA duplex are separated, and each single strand serves as a template for a newly synthesized complementary strand. DNA replication proceeds with the formation of phosphodiester bonds between the 5′ phosphate of an incoming nucleotide and the 3′ hydroxyl group of the previously added nucleotide **(Fig. 12–7).** This reaction is catalyzed by a DNA polymerase enzyme. The parental template strand is read from the 3′ to 5′ direction, whereas synthesis proceeds from 5′ to 3′, making the completely replicated strands antiparallel.

DNA synthesis cannot begin without a preexisting 3′ hydroxyl group. To begin synthesis *in vivo*, a **primer** of RNA is synthesized by an RNA polymerase (primase) enzyme. This aspect of DNA synthesis is useful in the laboratory for directing

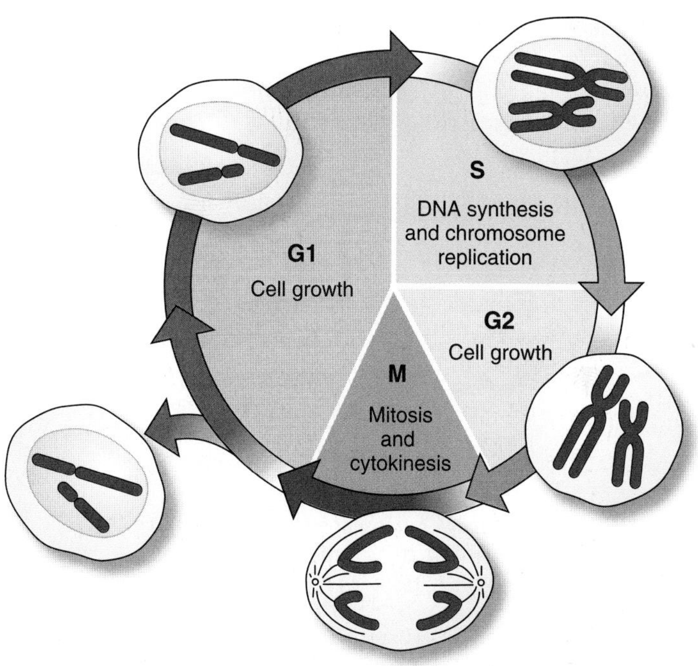

FIGURE 12-6 The cell cycle consists of four phases: G1, S, G2, and M. G1 and G2 are stages that prepare the cell to divide. DNA replication takes place during the S phase of the cell cycle in diploid organisms. In mitosis (M), the cell divides, and one chromosome set moves to each daughter cell. Mitosis has four main stages: prophase, metaphase, anaphase, and telophase. Before and after mitosis, cells are said to be in interphase. *(Adapted from Buckingham L.* Molecular Diagnostics. *3rd ed. Philadelphia, PA: F.A. Davis; 2019, with permission.)*

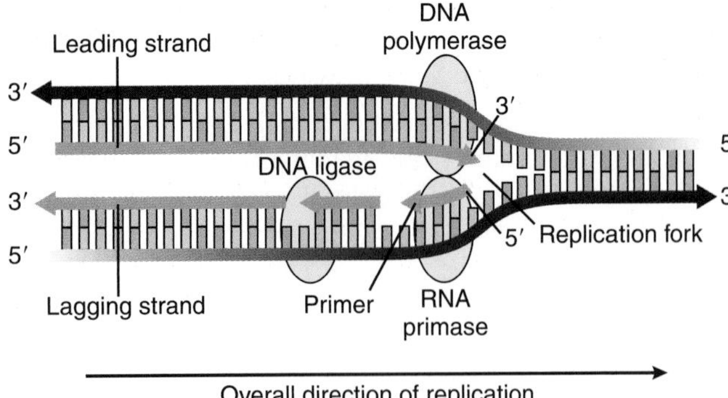

FIGURE 12–7 DNA is replicated in a semiconservative manner where each parent strand of the double helix serves as a template or guide for addition of new nucleotides to the newly synthesized strand. DNA polymerase forms a phosphodiester bond between the 3′ hydroxyl group of the previously added nucleotide to one phosphate of the incoming nucleotide, releasing the remaining two phosphates (pyrophosphate).

synthesis to a specific place in DNA. Synthetic single-stranded DNA primers are used routinely to direct copying of specific regions of DNA by the **polymerase chain reaction (PCR)** and other nucleic acid–amplification methods.

The double helix is copied in a single pass such that DNA undergoing replication can be observed by electron microscopy as a replication fork. The requirement for DNA synthesis to read the template strand in a 3′ to 5′ direction is not consistent with copying of both strands simultaneously in the same direction. To accommodate this arrangement, one strand, termed the *lagging strand*, is copied discontinuously toward the replication fork, whereas the other strand, called the *leading strand*, is copied continuously in the direction of replication; see Figure 12–7.

RNA Synthesis

RNA synthesis proceeds in a manner that is chemically similar to that of DNA synthesis, with some exceptions. RNA synthesis is catalyzed by RNA polymerase, which begins polymerization of RNA by binding to its recognition start site in DNA (promoter). Unlike DNA synthesis, RNA synthesis can start *de novo* without a primer. RNA synthesis is catalyzed by RNA polymerase, a more error-prone, slower polymerase (50–100 bases/second) than DNA polymerase (1,000 bases/second). There are more start sites for RNA polymerization than for DNA synthesis in the cell. The bulk of DNA synthesis takes place in the S phase of the cell cycle, whereas RNA synthesis occurs throughout the cell cycle and varies, depending on the cellular requirements.

RNA is copied from almost all the genome; however, only about 2% of the RNA-coding regions are translated into protein. Some genes code for transfer RNA and ribosomal RNA, which are required for translation of protein-coding messenger RNA into protein (see section that follows). Large portions of the genome are occupied by retrotransposons, DNA elements that can move from one location to another through an RNA intermediate. The remaining noncoding RNA, initially thought to be spontaneous and randomly initiated RNA synthesis, is now known to be composed of regulatory RNA molecules that affect both transcription and translation of the protein-coding genes. These RNAs include microRNA and long noncoding RNA.

Noncoding RNA, along with methylated nucleotides and modified histone proteins associated with DNA, are considered epigenetic mechanisms. In contrast to genetics, which is based on the order or sequence of nucleotides, **epigenetics** involves chemical changes in histone proteins, modification of DNA such as base methylation, and noncoding RNA activities that can influence the expression of genes independent of the nucleotide sequence.

Protein Synthesis

The central dogma of genetics states that genetic information flows from DNA to mRNA, the process of **transcription,** and from mRNA to protein, the process called **translation (Fig. 12–8).** Proteins are directly responsible for the *phenotype,* or observable properties, of an organism, such as eye color, height, and enzyme activity.

After DNA is transcribed by RNA polymerase into mRNA, the mRNA transcripts of protein-coding genes are translated

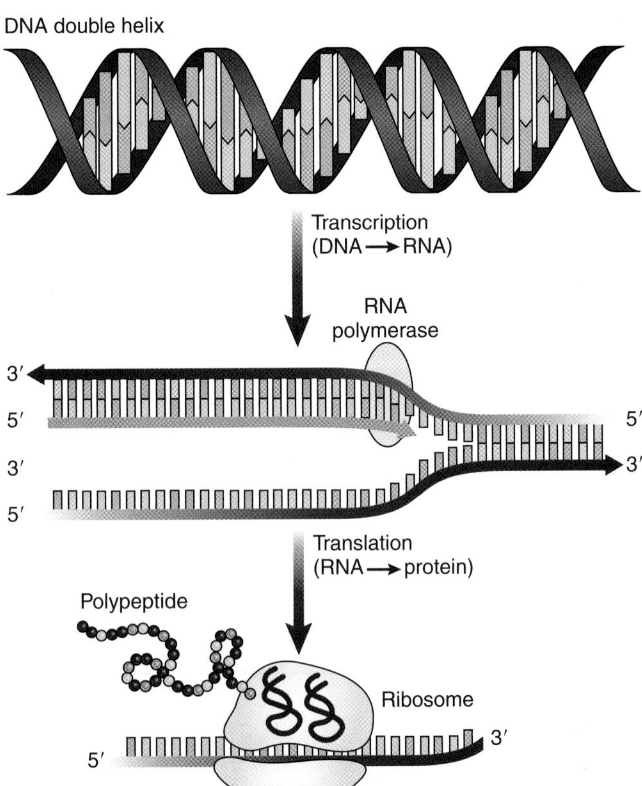

FIGURE 12–8 mRNA is transcribed from DNA using RNA polymerase. The mRNA delivers the information to ribosomes, where protein synthesis takes place. As each amino acid is added, the peptide chain continues to grow. This process, known as *translation*, is accomplished with the help of *tRNA*, which brings in individual amino acids.

into protein. Each mRNA is marked by a guanidine nucleotide covalently attached to its 5′ end in an unusual 5′–5′ bond (cap) and 2 to 20 adenines at the 3′ end (polyadenylation). These structures maintain the stability of the mRNA and allow its recognition by the ribosomes. Ribosomes are organelles that are composed of ribosomal proteins and ribosomal RNA (rRNA). Ribosomes assemble on the mRNA for protein synthesis.

Translation means converting information from one language to another. The language held in the order or sequence of the four nucleotides in the DNA chains must be translated into the order or sequence of the 20 amino acids making up a protein chain. The nucleotide sequence of mRNA contains a 3-base recognition sequence called a *codon* for each of the 20 amino acids, that is, the genetic code **(Table 12–1).** The codons are carried from the nucleus to the cytoplasm in mRNA to be translated into protein. Molecules of tRNA serve as adaptors between the nucleotide sequence in the RNA and the amino acid sequence in proteins. There are distinct tRNAs for each of the 20 amino acids. Each tRNA, folded into an inverted "L"-like structure, carries an amino acid at the 3′ end and a 3-base complementary sequence (anti-codon) to the codon of that amino acid. The 5′ ends of the tRNAs are covalently attached to their corresponding amino acids (charged) by aminoacyl-tRNA synthetase enzymes.

The charged tRNAs assemble with the ribosome and mRNA to initiate protein synthesis. Within the ribosome, the anti-codon hydrogen-bonds to the codon on the mRNA, holding the amino acid in place to be covalently attached to the growing peptide by peptidyl transferase activity. Synthesis proceeds as the ribosome moves in three base steps along the mRNA as each charged tRNA binds. Synthesis terminates when the ribosome encounters a stop codon in the mRNA. Multiple initiation, elongation, and termination factors participate in this process. Newly synthesized proteins are directed through the endoplasmic reticulum of the cell to their final destination.

DNA Sequence Changes

A change in the nucleotide sequence in DNA is called a **mutation** or **variant.** Depending on its frequency of occurrence, a nucleotide sequence change may also be referred to as a *polymorphism*. The term *variant* is recommended for nucleotide

Table 12–1 The Genetic Code Connects the 4-Base Nucleotide Sequence to the 20 Amino Acids

AMINO ACID	ABBREVIATION	SINGLE LETTER CODE	CODONS*
Alanine	Ala	A	GCU, GCG, GCC, GCA
Arginine	Arg	R	AGA, AGG, CGU, CGC, CGA, CGG
Asparagine	Asn	N	AAC, AAU
Aspartic acid	Asp	D	GAU, GAC
Cysteine	Cys	C	UGU, UGC
Glutamine	Gln	Q	CAA, CAG
Glutamic acid	Glu	E	GAA, GAG
Glycine	Gly	G	GGU, GGA, GGC, GGG
Histidine	His	H	CAU, CAC
Isoleucine	Ile	I	AUU, AUC, AUA
Leucine	Leu	L	UUA, UUG, CUA, CUC, CUG, CUU
Lysine	Lys	K	AAA, AAG
Methionine	Met	M	AUG
Phenylalanine	Phe	F	UUU, UUC
Proline	Pro	P	CCU, CCA, CCC, CCG
Serine	Ser	S	AGU, AGC, UCU, UCC, UCA, UCG
Threonine	Thr	T	ACU, ACA, ACG, ACC
Tryptophan	Trp	W	UGG
Tyrosine	Tyr	Y	UAU, UAC
Valine	Val	V	GUU, GUA, GUC, GUG
(Stop codons)†		X	UAA, UAG, UGA

**Each amino acid has at least one associated 3-base sequence (codon) carried in mRNA.*

†Stop codons direct mRNA synthesis to stop.

Table 12–2 DNA Changes Affect Amino Acid Sequences

MUTATION TYPE	DESCRIPTION	EXAMPLE: CODON (mRNA) CHANGE	EXAMPLE: AMINO ACID CHANGE
Conservative substitution	Nucleotide base substitution that results in an amino acid with similar properties as compared with the original	AUC → CUC	Isoleucine → Leucine
Nonconservative substitution	Nucleotide base substitution that results in an amino acid with dissimilar properties as compared with the original	CAU → CCU	Histidine → Proline
Silent	Nucleotide base substitution that results in the same amino acid	UAU → UAC	Tyrosine → Tyrosine
Nonsense	Nucleotide base substitution that results in creation of a stop codon	CAA → UAA	Glutamine → Stop
Frameshift	Insertion or deletion of a nucleotide base that causes a shift in the codon reading frame	UGU AAC CAG → UGU AAA CCA G . . .	Cys Asn Gln → Cys Lys Pro . . .

sequence changes that are inherited (germline), whereas *mutation* is a more general term for spontaneous changes in DNA (somatic). These alterations may range in size from a single base pair to millions of base pairs that result in chromosomal structural abnormalities. Point mutations involve one or a few base pairs and are classified by their effect on the amino acid sequence **(Table 12–2).** Conservative and silent mutations do not affect phenotype, whereas nonconservative, nonsense, and frameshift mutations will likely affect protein structure or function, depending on their location in the protein sequence. Mutations early in the gene sequence will likely have a greater effect on protein function than mutations that occur toward the end of the protein.

There is a recommended nomenclature for naming nucleotide changes in clinical reports. Mutations are indicated by the location of the change in the nucleotide sequence, followed by the original nucleotide, an arrow, and finally, the replacement nucleotide. For example, a mutation that replaces a guanidine with an adenosine nucleotide at position 2175 would be expressed as: 2175G→A. The term may be preceded by further notations (g., c., r.) to indicate whether the mutation is in genomic DNA, complementary DNA from the mRNA sequence, or RNA, respectively. For example, in large databases, the mutation just described might be denoted as: c.G2175A.

Changes in the amino acid sequence are indicated by the original amino acid and the location in the protein, followed by the substituted amino acid. For example, a replacement of a glycine with a valine at the 339th amino acid in a protein would be expressed as G339V or p.G339V, using the single letter code for the amino acids (see Table 12–1). These expressions are designed to avoid confusion when referring to amino acid or nucleotide changes because the letters A, C, G, and T are also used in the single-letter amino acid codes.

Polymorphisms

Structurally, mutations, variants, and polymorphisms are the same thing—changes in the reference amino acid or nucleotide sequence. Alterations in DNA or protein sequences shared by at least 2% of a natural population are considered **polymorphisms.** The different versions of the affected sequences are referred to as *alleles*. Polymorphisms can involve a single base pair **(single-nucleotide polymorphisms or SNPs)** or millions of base pairs. Polymorphic changes may or may not have phenotypic effects. Deleterious phenotypic changes are usually limited so that they do not reach the required frequency in a population; however, some polymorphisms are maintained because they are also associated with a beneficial phenotypic effect. A well-known example of this is the A to T base substitution in the beta-globin gene on chromosome 11 that causes sickle cell anemia. This DNA substitution results in the replacement of glutamic acid (E) with valine (V) at position 6 in the protein sequence (E6V). The mutation results in abnormal red blood cells that do not circulate efficiently. The deleterious effect has likely been maintained in the population because it is balanced by a beneficial phenotype of resistance to *Plasmodium* species, which cause malaria.

A highly polymorphic region in the human genome is the major histocompatibility (MHC) locus on chromosome 6. The different nucleotide sequences result in multiple versions or alleles of the human leukocyte antigen (HLA) genes in the human population. These alleles differ by nucleotide sequence at the DNA level (polymorphisms) and by amino acid sequence. Each person will have a particular group of HLA alleles, which are inherited from his or her parents. The HLA proteins coded for by these alleles play important roles in the immune response and allow the immune system to differentiate "self" from "non-self" (see Chapter 3). The recommended nomenclature for HLA alleles is discussed in Chapter 16.

Other highly polymorphic areas of the genome include the genes coding for the antibody proteins and antigen receptor proteins in B cells and T cells, respectively. Polymorphisms are introduced in each cell through cell-specific genetic events (gene rearrangements), followed by enzymatically catalyzed sequence changes (somatic hypermutation). These sequences differ from cell to cell, allowing for the generation of a large repertoire of antibodies and antigen receptors to better match any foreign antigen (see Chapters 4 and 5).

Polymorphisms are found all over the human genome. Although there are millions of SNPs, larger polymorphic differences occur less frequently. Polymorphisms that create, destroy, or otherwise affect sequences in DNA that are recognized by nuclease enzymes (restriction enzymes isolated from bacteria) are detected as **restriction fragment length variations** or **polymorphisms (RFLPs)** that differ among individuals. Repeat-sequence polymorphisms, such as short tandem repeats (STRs) and variable-number tandem repeats (VNTRs), are head-to-tail repeats of a single base pair to more than 100 bp repeat units. STRs and VNTRs can be detected as RFLPs or by using amplification procedures. STR testing has replaced RFLP testing for human identification (DNA fingerprinting in forensics) and HLA typing for parentage testing. STRs and VNTRs are the markers commonly used to follow engraftment of donor cells into recipient blood and bone marrow after allogeneic bone marrow transplantation.

In addition to the nuclear genome, mitochondria, located in the cytoplasm of eukaryotic cells, carry their own genome. The mitochondrial genome is circular, containing about 16,500 bp. Polymorphisms are also found in two regions of mitochondrial DNA sequences (hypervariable regions). These polymorphisms are not transcribed into RNA and do not affect protein structures. They are used for maternal lineage testing, because all maternal relatives share the same mitochondria and so have the same mitochondrial polymorphisms.

Electrophoresis

Analysis of DNA for mutations and polymorphisms is performed in a variety of ways. Many of these laboratory procedures use electrophoresis to observe the sizes or amounts of nucleic acid. **Electrophoresis** is the movement of particles under the force of an electric current. Particles can move through gas, liquid, or even solid phases.

Gel Electrophoresis

For nucleic acids, a semisolid matrix or gel is used to sieve the nucleic acid polymers. There are two types of gels used for nucleic acid analysis: agarose and polyacrylamide. Agarose gels are natural polymers of agarobiose, a disaccharide found in plants. Polyacrylamide gels are synthetic polymers of acrylamide and bis-acrylamide. These synthetic polymers are more precisely designed for high-resolution separation, that is, distinguishing differences in nucleic acids as small as one nucleotide. Polyacrylamide gels are also used for protein resolution by size or charge. In contrast, agarose gels do not have such high resolution but are less expensive and less toxic to use than acrylamide. Agarose gels are useful for standard laboratory separations of nucleic acids of 50 bp or more. Agarose in low concentrations is used to separate very large nucleic acids of tens of thousands of base pairs.

Under the force of an electric current, nucleic acids, which are negatively charged, will move from the negative pole (cathode) to the positive pole (anode). Smaller (shorter) nucleic acid chains will move faster through the gel matrix than larger ones. The shorter chains will appear below longer ones when the nucleic acid samples are visualized in the gel by staining. A standard molecular weight marker of nucleic acid chains of known sizes run with the test samples can be used to estimate the size in bases or base pairs of the test nucleic acids.

The proper type and concentration of gel are determined based on the expected sizes of the nucleic acids to be separated. Agarose gels are frequently prepared from powdered agarose dissolved and melted in a buffer solution that will carry the electric current (running buffer). There are a variety of buffer solutions used for different types of nucleic acids and different gel types. The agarose suspension is heated to a clear liquid, poured into a mold, and allowed to cool and polymerize. Because powdered acrylamide is toxic, most laboratories purchase predissolved acrylamide solutions or polymerized gels. Liquid acrylamide solutions require the addition of a nucleating agent and catalyst in order to solidify. For both agarose and polyacrylamide gels, a comb is placed in the liquid gel to form wells at one end of the gel for loading of the samples.

After solidifying, the gels are placed in a bath of running buffer. To detect the nucleic acid, a fluorescent stain (ethidium bromide, SYBR green, or others) can be mixed with the gel solution, placed in the gel bath, or used to soak the gel after the electrophoresis is complete. The nucleic acid sample to be separated is mixed with a loading solution that contains a density agent (glycerol or Ficoll) and a visual dye, such as bromophenol blue. The density agent allows loading of the sample into the wells of the gel submerged in the running buffer. The visual dye aids in seeing the sample while loading into the well and during electrophoresis. The gel bath is connected to a power supply that will establish a current between platinum wires at the top and bottom of the gel, the two poles of the gel bath. The nucleic acids will move under the force of the current, working their way through the gel matrix at a speed that depends on their size.

After electrophoresis, the nucleic acids can be visualized through the fluorescent dye excited by ultraviolet light. Nucleic acid chains will appear as lines or bands on the gel **(Fig. 12–9A).** The distance from the loading well to the band will be inversely proportional to the size of the nucleic acid.

Capillary Electrophoresis

Capillary electrophoresis is a more sensitive, semiautomated type of electrophoresis, separating particles in a gas, liquid, or gel. Because nucleic acids do not resolve in solution, a gel or polymer is inserted into the capillary to sieve the nucleic acids (capillary gel electrophoresis). Capillary gel electrophoresis instruments range from a single capillary to 96 capillaries. Multiple samples can run through each capillary, as the instruments are capable of detecting fluorescent signals at more than one wavelength.

For detection, DNA chains must carry a fluorescent label (a covalently attached molecule that emits fluorescence). A laser

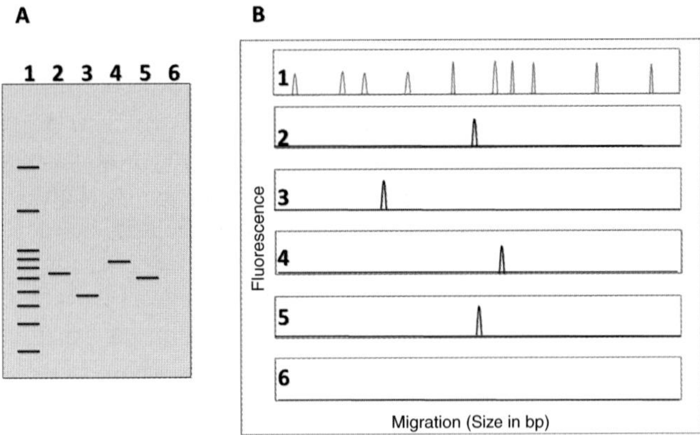

FIGURE 12–9 After gel electrophoresis (A), nucleic acids are visualized by detection of a nucleic acid–specific fluorescent dye, such as ethidium bromide or SYBR green. The agarose gel shown has six lanes, where samples were loaded. The first lane (1) shows the molecular weight standard. Lanes 2 to 5 show sample DNA. The size of the DNA fragments can be estimated by comparing how far they migrated in the gel compared with the molecular weight standard. A negative (blank) control is in lane 6. In capillary electrophoresis (B), the gel is replaced by an electropherogram. Instead of bands, peaks appear, representing the nucleic acid fragments (top four rows). The last row on the electropherogram shown is the negative control. Peaks of a molecular weight standard are shown at the top. From it, the instrument computes and displays the lengths of the nucleic acid fragments in base pairs (boxes beneath each peak). All the fragments shown and the molecular weight marker were run simultaneously through a single capillary.

inside of the capillary instrument excites the fluorescent labels as they move through the capillary. The dyes emit fluorescence that is detected and transferred to a computer as an electrical signal. The signals are displayed as peaks of fluorescence **(Fig. 12–9B).**

The preparation of capillary gel electrophoresis involves loading premixed polymer solution and buffers into the electrophoresis instrument along with the capillary (or array of capillaries for multicapillary systems). The polymer is automatically injected into the capillary by the instrument. Nucleic acid samples are diluted in formamide to denature the DNA into single strands, and the molecular weight standard is added directly to the sample. The samples are placed into the instrument either in separate tubes or in a plate format. Molecular weight standards are mixed with each sample. The samples enter the capillary by an electrokinetic process that attracts the negatively charged DNA to the end of the capillary submerged into the tube or plate well containing the sample. During electrophoresis, the nucleic acids sieve through the capillary as they would in a gel. The shorter fragments move faster than the longer ones. As each labeled nucleic acid chain passes by the detector, a peak is generated by the computer. The molecular weight markers move through the same capillary with the sample, enabling the instrument to automatically assess the size of the fragments in base pairs.

Molecular Analysis

Nucleic acid tests are designed to detect changes in the DNA sequence (mutations and polymorphisms) or to measure differences in amounts of RNA synthesized. There are four main approaches to nucleic acid analysis: strand cleavage methods, hybridization methods, amplification methods, and sequencing.

Strand Cleavage Methods

Specific Procedures

Restriction Enzymes

One of the first methods for analysis of DNA was restriction enzyme mapping. Restriction enzymes are endonucleases that will separate the phosphodiester bonds between nucleotides in DNA. These endonucleases recognize and bind to specific nucleotide sequences in the DNA so that they will only separate the DNA at those locations.

Restriction enzymes used in clinical laboratory methods recognize palindromic sites, that is, nucleotide sequences that read the same 5′ to 3′ on both strands of the DNA, for example:

5′GAATTC3′
3′CTTAAG5′

which is the recognition site for the restriction enzyme EcoR1.

Restriction enzymes are isolated from bacteria, where they serve as part of a primitive immune system that allows the bacteria to recognize their own DNA and degrade any incoming foreign DNA. Restriction enzymes are named for the organisms from which they are isolated. EcoR1 was the first enzyme isolated from *E. coli*, strain R. HindIII is the third enzyme isolated from *Haemophilus influenzae*, strain d.

There are hundreds of restriction enzymes with unique binding and cleavage sites. DNA is characterized based on the pattern of fragments produced after incubation with restriction enzymes and electrophoresis. DNA with a different sequence will yield different-sized fragments characteristic of that DNA **(Fig. 12–10).** Early work in recombinant DNA technology relied on these types of studies. Today, RFLP analysis is applied to epidemiological studies of microorganisms

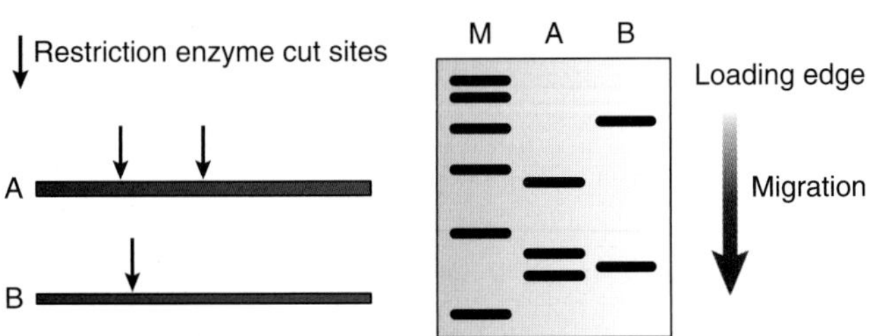

FIGURE 12–10 Restriction enzyme mapping characterizes DNA by the pattern of fragments generated when the DNA is cut with restriction enzymes. DNA sample A has two restriction sites (arrows), whereas the DNA sample B has only one. When these two DNAs are digested with the restriction enzyme, DNA A will yield three fragments, and DNA B will yield two. These band patterns are a characteristic of the two DNAs. (M = molecular weight standard, used for sizing the DNA fragments)

and identification of resistance factors carried on extrachromosomal DNA (plasmids) in the cell.

CRISPR-Cas9

DNA analysis using restriction enzymes is limited to sequences recognized by these enzymes. Another type of restriction system found in archaea, gram-negative, and gram-positive bacteria uses a common enzyme guided by RNA to specific sites. Clustered regularly interspaced short palindromic repeats (CRISPRs) are classes of repeated DNA sequences found in microbial DNA. The repeated sequences are interrupted by spacer sequences matching regions extracted from invading plasmids or viruses. These spacer sequences serve as adaptive immunity with memory of the invading DNA. The locus also encodes the CRISPR-associated protein (Cas) enzyme. To fend off an invader, short RNA sequences transcribed from the CRISPR spacer regions guide the Cas enzyme to the matching invading DNA.

CRISPR/Cas9 has been used in the laboratory to alter DNA at user-defined locations by substituting synthetic RNA of a desired sequence to guide the Cas enzyme. The synthetic RNA leads the Cas9 endonuclease to the site of choice, providing the specificity of restriction enzymes with the versatility of guiding cuts to any sequence site. CRISPR RNA can also lead transcription activators, repressors, gene promoters, or reporter molecules to target sequences. CRISPR has been utilized for DNA analysis, gene therapy, and genome editing. Clinical applications of this system are under development.

Other types of cleaving enzymes, such as those that only digest single-stranded nucleic acids or those that recognize folded nucleic acids, are also used to screen for mutations and polymorphisms.

Hybridization Methods

Specific Procedures

Restriction enzyme cleavage methods are highly informative for investigating small genomes, such as those of microorganisms or plasmids. For complex genomes, such as human DNA, such analyses are not practical, as the DNA is too large and complex to generate readable fragment patterns. How does one analyze specific DNA regions in a complex genome by RFLP without first cloning the region of interest? This question was addressed by Edwin Southern in the mid-1970s. The significance of his invention, the Southern blot, was that informative studies could be performed directly on large and complex genomes by cleaving the DNA into smaller fragments with restriction enzymes, separating the fragments by gel electrophoresis, and identifying the region of interest through hybridization with labeled **probes** (short nucleic acids that bind to complementary sequences). **Hybridization** involves the binding of two complementary strands of nucleic acids, in this case, the template strand and a probe. A variation of the Southern blot, called the *northern blot*, was subsequently developed to analyze RNA structure and expression. Northern blots were mostly research tools and not used routinely for diagnostic purposes.

Clinical Correlations

Western Blot

The western blot was used for many years as a confirmatory test for the presence of antibodies to HIV, the cause of AIDS, and to *Borrelia burgdorferi*, the cause of Lyme disease. Although the western blot has been replaced by less labor-intensive methods in the clinical laboratory, this highly specific method is still widely used in research laboratories for protein analysis (see Chapters 21 and 24).

Detection of proteins and protein modifications can be done by a method known as the **western blot.** In the western blot procedure, serum, cell lysate, or extracted proteins are separated by gel electrophoresis and blotted to a membrane. The probes for western blot are polyclonal or monoclonal antibodies specific for the proteins of interest. Western blots may also be probed with biological fluids such as serum to detect the presence of antibodies produced in response to infection. Detection is performed with secondary antibody–enzyme conjugates and color- or light-producing substrates.

Array Methods

Southern blotting and its variations allowed assessment of one or a few molecular targets on as many samples as the gel system would allow. As knowledge of genetic networks and pathways grew, it became apparent that informative studies should include simultaneous analysis of many genes or proteins to assess the true biological state of a cell or an organism. Thus began the study of genomics. **Genomics** refers to the analysis of hundreds to thousands of targets or whole genomes, rather than single genes.

The first methodology to perform these studies involved reverse-dot-blot hybridization, that is, hybridization of a labeled sample to unlabeled immobilized probes spotted or arrayed on a solid support. Modern arrays can carry up to hundreds of thousands of probes. There are three basic types of arrays: comparative genomic arrays, RNA expression arrays, and high-density oligonucleotide or SNP arrays. Comparative genomic hybridization arrays are used to detect amplifications or deletions in DNA **(Fig. 12–11).** Gene expression (mRNA synthesis) is measured using expression arrays, where mRNA from the test material is converted into labeled cDNA, which is hybridized to the probes. SNP arrays have single-nucleotide resolution and can even be used to determine DNA nucleotide sequence. Generally, thousands of targets with probes bound to a very small area, such as a microscope slide, is referred to as a **microarray.**

Microarrays use highly specific unlabeled probes attached directly to a solid support. The support can be glass slides or beads (bead arrays). The test sample (nucleic acids or proteins isolated from cultures, cells, or body fluids) is labeled and hybridized to the many immobilized probes. Microarrays are used for a variety of applications, including detection of chromosome microdeletions by virtual karyotyping and gene-expression profiling. In the former method, genomic DNA is

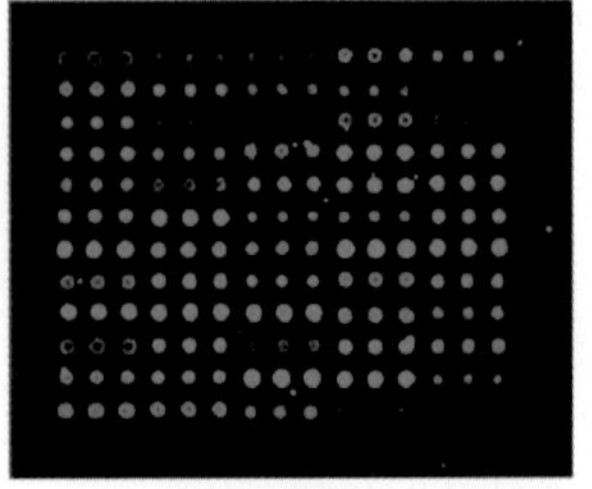
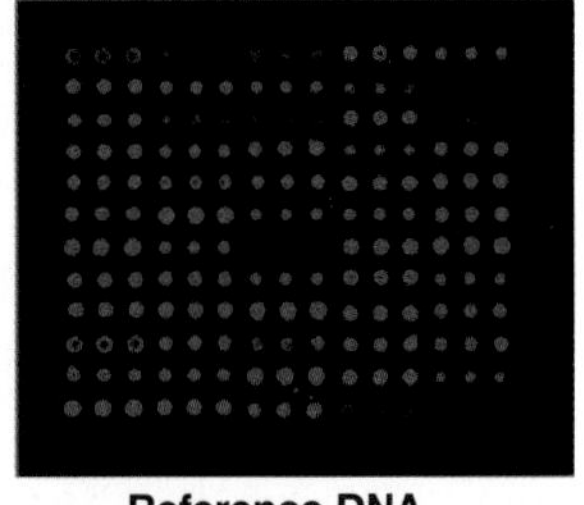

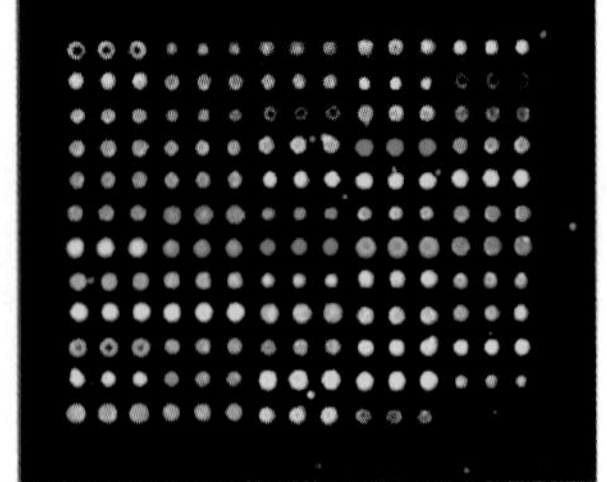

FIGURE 12–11 For array analysis, unlabeled probes are immobilized and hybridized to labeled sample material (green). A reference material (red) is hybridized to the same array. The results of the array are relative test:reference colors. In this example, a green color indicates amplified gene regions, and the neutral yellow colors indicate no amplification or deletion of those regions. A lack of red color, which would indicate deletion of a gene region, is seen.

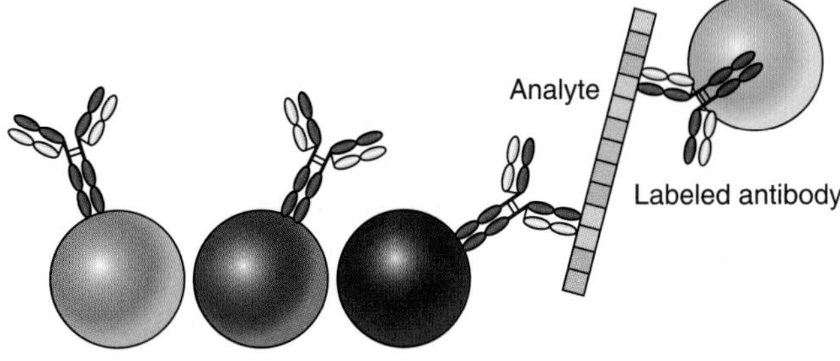

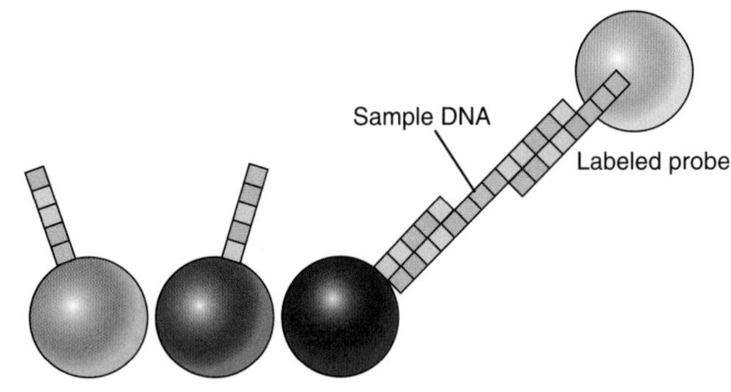

FIGURE 12–12 (A) Three of 100 to 400 bead colors, each with antibody to a different analyte. The presence of multiple targets can be detected by the unique colors of the beads that have associated fluorescence from the secondary antibody. Flow cytometry is used to assay each bead separately for bound fluorescence. (B) For nucleic acid analysis, bead array antibodies are replaced with single-stranded oligonucleotides complementary to the test nucleic acid. If present, biotinylated sample DNA will hybridize to the sequences, and the biotin-specific conjugate will generate a signal.

assessed for loss or gain of genetic material at specific chromosomal locations compared with a normal reference sample. In the latter method, the levels of mRNA transcribed from thousands of genes are compared with normal reference samples to look for up- or down-regulation of gene transcription.

For array analysis, sample labeling is fluorescent, allowing dual detection of the test sample and a reference sample that is hybridized to the array along with it (see Fig. 12–11). This results in measurement of increased or decreased amounts of test material relative to the normal reference. In bead array systems, beads carry fluorescent labels specific to the probe they carry so that bound sample, if present, can be detected in a flow cytometric method.

Bead array assays are based on preparations of fluorescent beads of 100 to 400 different fluorescent "colors." Each color bead is attached to an antibody or a nucleic acid probe that will bind specifically to the target protein or nucleic acid sequences. The target nucleic acid molecules may be directly labeled, or for protein targets, a secondary antibody conjugated to a fluorescent signal may be used to detect the presence of the target **(Fig. 12–12)**. Because many beads are used, each bound to a different antibody or probe, multiple targets can simultaneously be detected in a single assay run; in other words, a multiplex assay is performed. Clinical applications include HLA typing (see Chapter 16) and respiratory virus panels.

In Situ Hybridization

In situ hybridization (ISH) refers to detection of targets in place as they appear in tissues, cells, and subcellular structures. Labeled probes are used to bind or hybridize to the targets. ISH is frequently used in pathology studies of tissue and cell suspensions. **Immunohistochemistry** is a type of ISH using labeled antibodies to detect the presence of clinically significant protein targets, such as those expressed by tumor cells. Probes for these tests are monoclonal antibodies linked to enzymes, such as horseradish peroxidase, that produce visible signals from chromogenic substrates. Alternatively, enzyme-linked secondary antibodies recognizing the primary antibody isotype may be used.

Positive and negative controls must be included in ISH testing to ensure accuracy of the results. Normal tissue that expresses the protein target should serve as the positive control, whereas an adjacent section cut from the test tissue without the addition of the primary antibody and tumor tissues that do not express the antigen should serve as negative controls. Ideally, the control tissues are processed with the test

Clinical Correlations

Programmed Cell Death Ligand (PD-L1)

The programmed cell death ligand (PD-L1) is a transmembrane protein that suppresses the adaptive immune response when it is bound to a receptor on activated lymphocytes and dendritic cells called *programmed cell death protein 1* (PD-1). PD-L1 is found on some tumor cells and is thought to block recognition of the abnormal cells by lymphocytes that express PD-1. Detection of PD-L1 by immunohistochemistry guides the use of immunotherapy for those tumors that express the ligand.

tissue. Control tissues processed differently from the test tissue validate reagent performance but do not verify the tissue preparation. If staining of positive control tissue is not satisfactory, or if unwanted staining occurs in negative controls, all results with the patient specimen should be considered invalid.

Fluorescence in situ hybridization (FISH) methods use fluorescently labeled probes and require specialized microscopes equipped to detect the emitted fluorescent signals. FISH is commonly performed to detect specific chromosome abnormalities, such as microdeletions or gene amplifications. In these methods, probes ranging in size from a few thousand to hundreds of thousands of bases long are covalently attached to the fluorescent dye. FISH can be performed on nondividing (or interphase) cells or directly on metaphase chromosomes from dividing cells. The DNA from the sample is denatured into single strands. The probes are applied to prepared slides of the cells or chromosomes, where they hybridize to their complementary sequences. The resulting signals indicate if the targeted gene or region is abnormal. In addition to the test probes, reference probes that target the centromeres of selected chromosomes are used to identify the chromosomes of interest while assessing deletion or amplification (**Fig. 12–13**).

ISH methods are sensitive to the buffer and temperature conditions of hybridization, a concept referred to as *stringency*. Protocols must be strictly followed to avoid false-positive results caused by nonspecific binding of probes or false negatives caused by failure of the probe to bind. Array methods (comparative genome hybridization) complement FISH testing in cases of multiple or complex genetic abnormalities as well as deletions and amplification of genes.

Amplification Methods

Specific Procedures

The most frequently used methods in molecular diagnostics involve some aspect of **amplification,** that is, copying of nucleic acids. Previously performed *in vivo* using replication of plasmids carrying cloned fragments in bacteria, the development of the *in vitro* PCR by Kerry Mullis greatly facilitated and broadened the potential applications of gene amplification. PCR was quickly followed by other target-amplification methods, such as **reverse transcriptase** PCR (RT-PCR), transcription-mediated amplification (TMA), and strand displacement amplification (SDA). PCR has also facilitated the development of DNA sequencing assays.

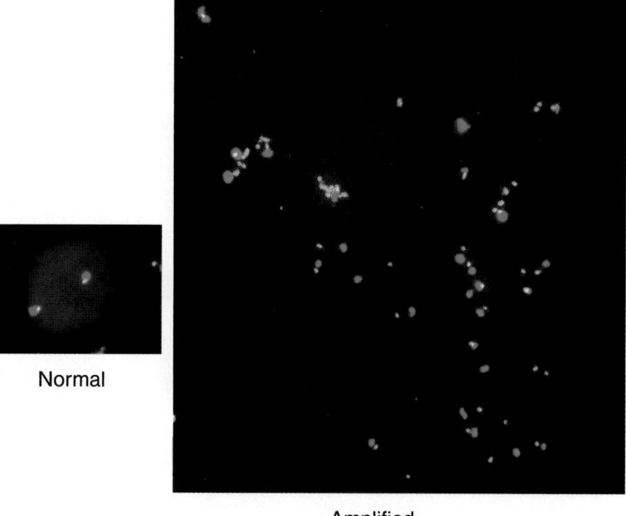

FIGURE 12–13 FISH analysis of the epidermal growth factor receptor gene. The gene probe is labeled orange, whereas a probe complementary to the centromere of chromosome 7 is labeled green. Normally, there are two chromosomes, each carrying one gene in each nucleus (left). The image on the right shows gene amplification with multiple orange signals associated with single green signals.

Polymerase Chain Reaction (PCR)

PCR is an *in vitro* DNA replication procedure. A PCR reaction includes all the necessary components required for DNA replication: the sample containing the DNA template to be copied, oligonucleotide primers to prime the synthesis of the copies, the four deoxyribonucleotides (dNTPs), DNA polymerase to covalently join the dNTPs, and buffer containing mono- and divalent cations with a pH optimal for the polymerase activity. The oligonucleotide primers are key components to the specificity of the PCR reaction. Primers are synthetic single-stranded nucleic acids, usually 18 to 30 b in length. They are complementary to sequences flanking the region of the template DNA to be copied **(Fig. 12–14).**

For many procedures, premixed PCR reagents (deoxyribonucleotides, primers, and buffer) are supplied from manufacturers to which only the template DNA and, in some cases, enzyme are added. The PCR reaction mix is subjected to an amplification program consisting of a designated number of cycles. A cycle is comprised of temperature changes. A standard three-step PCR cycle includes (1) a denaturation step to separate the double-stranded DNA into single strands (94°C–96°C), (2) an annealing step to allow binding of the primers (50°C–70°C), and (3) an extension step in which complementary nucleotides are added to the 3′ end of the primers to complete DNA synthesis (68°C–72°C). In a standard cycle, each of these temperatures will be held for 30 to 60 seconds. PCR cycles vary, depending on the target DNA and the protocol. The cycle is repeated 20 to 50 times

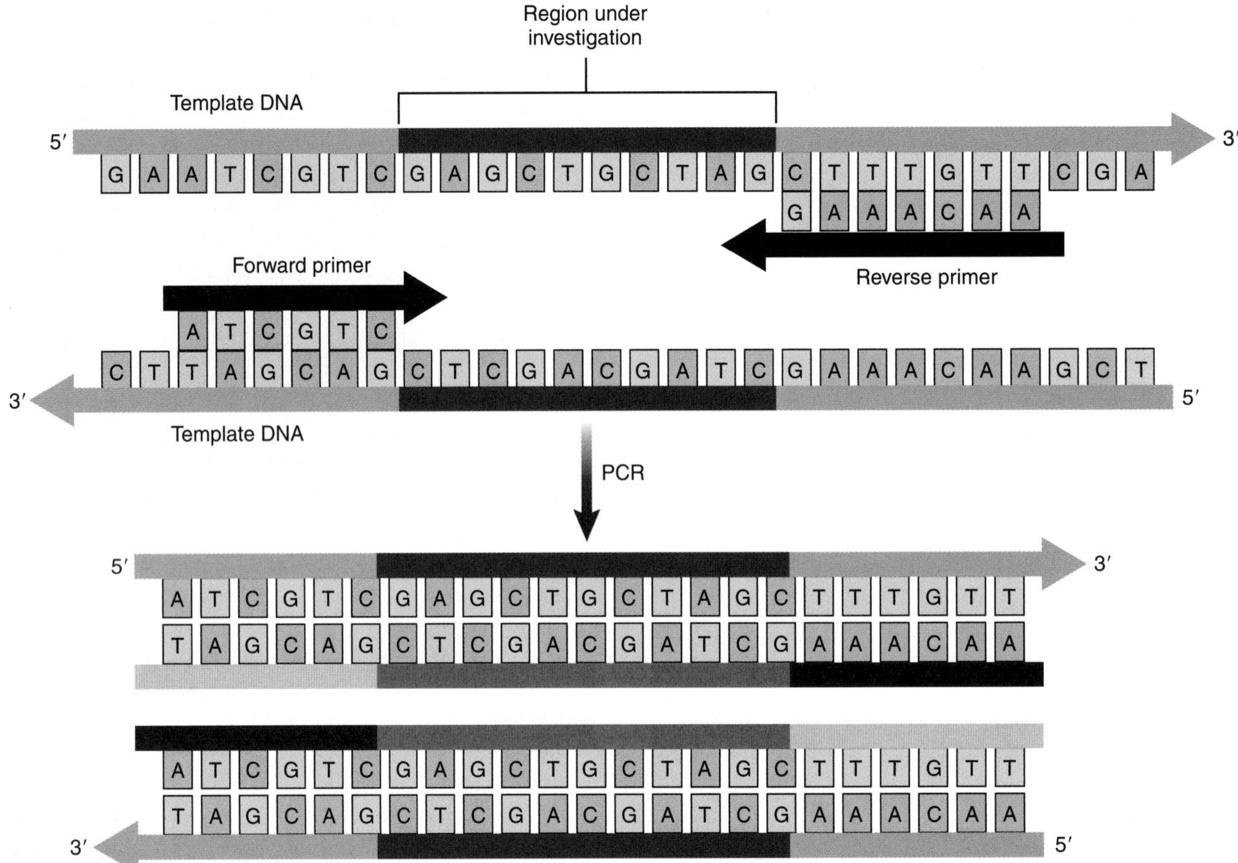

FIGURE 12–14 In the PCR reaction, short, single-stranded primers hydrogen-bond to complementary sequences flanking the region of interest. The PCR reaction will produce millions of copies of the desired sequences. Note: The image is shortened. Primers are usually 18 to 30 b long, and the PCR products range from 50 to more than 1,000 bp.

depending on the assay. The set of repeated cycles makes up the PCR program. The program may also include an initial 5- to 15-minute incubation at the denaturation temperature to activate specialized DNA polymerases, which are designed to remain inactive at room temperature. A final 7- to 10-minute step at the extension temperature may also be included after the last cycle to allow complete copying of the products. For convenience, a hold at 4°C is usually added to the end of the amplification program.

The instrument used to carry out the amplification program is called a *thermal cycler*. There are a variety of thermal cyclers configured for different applications. In general, thermal cyclers are either chamber-based or block-based. In chamber-based cyclers, the sample tubes are subjected to the amplification program temperatures through the surrounding air in the chamber. In block cyclers, sample tubes are placed in a metal block that is heated and cooled according to the amplification program. Amplification programs may include the time it takes to achieve the different temperatures (ramp speed). Ramp speed will affect the efficiency of the amplification as well as the time required to complete the program.

PCR amplification produces millions of copies or amplicons of the DNA region of interest. At 100% PCR efficiency, the number of copies will be 2^n, where n is the number of cycles (20–50) in the amplification program. The products of the PCR reaction are visualized by gel or capillary gel electrophoresis, as the last part of a PCR procedure **(Fig. 12–15).** For many tests, the presence, absence, or size of a PCR product is the test result. For other applications, PCR products are directly placed into subsequent reactions, such as restriction enzyme analysis or sequencing.

A variety of modifications have been made to the PCR reaction. RT-PCR starts with an RNA template. Complementary or copy DNA (cDNA) is synthesized from the RNA in a separate step using reverse transcriptase, an RNA-dependent DNA polymerase. The cDNA serves as the template for the PCR reaction. Alternatively, enzymes that copy both RNA and DNA are used in simultaneous RT and PCR reactions that do not require a separate RT step. RT-PCR is a method of analysis for cellular RNA or qualitative detection of RNA viruses, such as HIV and hepatitis C virus (HCV).

PCR primer design introduces additional flexibility into the PCR reaction. In sequence-specific primer PCR (SSP-PCR, also called *amplification refractory mutation system PCR,* or ARMS-PCR), primers are designed so that they will end on a potentially mutated or polymorphic base pair. Annealing of the last base at the 3′ end of the primer is critical for polymerase activity. If the last base of the primer is not complementary to the template, the DNA polymerase will not recognize the primer as a substrate for extension, and no PCR product will

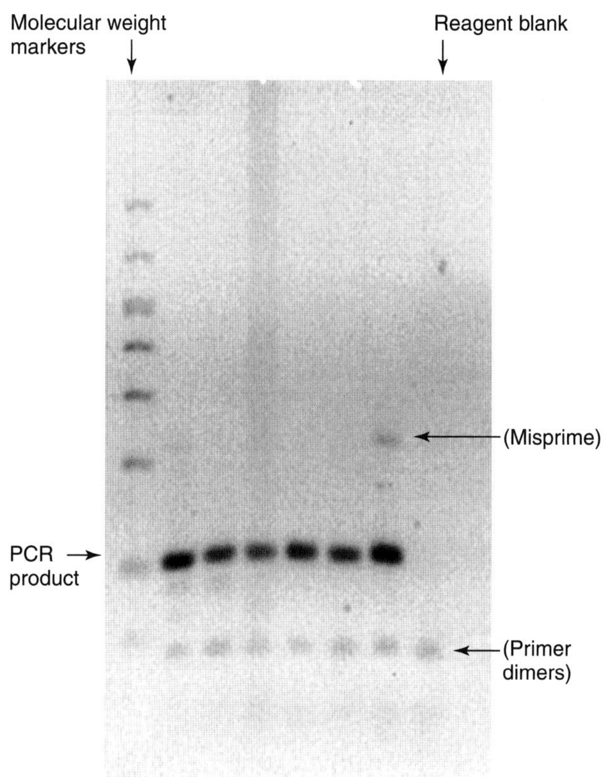

FIGURE 12–15 Detection of PCR products by gel electrophoresis. The first lane (left) contains molecular weight markers (fragments of known size). The next six lanes are PCR products, followed by a reagent blank control for contamination (lane 8). *(From Buckingham L. Molecular Diagnostics. 2nd ed. Philadelphia, PA: F.A. Davis; 2011, with permission.)*

be produced. SSP-PCR is a common approach used to detect mutations and polymorphisms, such as in HLA typing (see Chapter 16).

Unlike the 3′ end of primers, the 5′ end does not have to be complementary to the template. This allows attachment of noncomplementary sequences containing restriction enzyme recognition sites or RNA polymerase-binding sites to PCR products. The amplicons can then be conveniently inserted into plasmids for biological analyses or transcribed into RNA and translated into in vitro transcription or translation systems. Labels in the form of fluorescent molecules, biotin, or other molecules may also be covalently attached to the 5′ end of primers. This allows capture immobilization of the PCR products or detection in capillary electrophoresis systems **(Fig. 12–16).**

Quantitative PCR (qPCR). Standard PCR results are interpreted as the presence, absence, or size of the PCR product, but quantification of starting material is not easily measured. In 1993, Higuchi et al. demonstrated that target quantification could be achieved by observing the accumulation of PCR product in real time during amplification. Both DNA and RNA targets can be measured by qPCR. For RNA, complementary DNA made from the RNA using reverse transcriptase as the input material. Although originally termed "real-time PCR" or "RT-PCR," the preferred term is now **quantitative PCR** or **qPCR** to avoid confusion with reverse transcriptase PCR (also RT-PCR).

To be detected in real time, the qPCR product was followed initially by photography and then by using a fluorescent dye specific for double-stranded DNA (ethidium bromide) at intervals during the amplification program. A less toxic DNA-specific dye, SYBR green, is now used for this purpose. While primers determine the intended target, more specific detection of a product is achieved with probes rather than DNA binding dyes.

There are four types of probes in general use: fluorescence resonance energy transfer (FRET), TaqMan, molecular beacon, and scorpion probes **(Fig. 12–17).** These probes hybridize by sequence complementarity in order to generate fluorescent signals from the accumulating PCR products. SYBR green is not specific to the sequence, so artifacts of the PCR reaction (misprimes and primer dimers from primer self-amplification) will also produce a signal. Because the probes are sequence-specific, they provide higher specificity for the intended product than SYBR green.

Accumulation of PCR product detected by TaqMan probes through 50 PCR cycles is shown in **Figure 12–18.** The fluorescence depicted on the *y*-axis is the fluorescence signal from the dye or probe. The fluorescence plotted versus cycle number generates a curve similar to a bacterial growth curve, with a lag phase, a log phase, a linear phase, and a stationary phase. The length of the lag phase is assessed by counting the number of PCR cycles required to reach a threshold level of fluorescence. The cycle at which the sample fluorescence reaches this value is called the *threshold cycle* or *Ct*.

As seen in a standard curve of dilutions of known target nucleic acid shown in **Figure 12–19,** there is an inverse relationship between the amount of target and the Ct value. For test samples, target is quantified by converting its Ct to the number of DNA copies in the starting sample using the standard curve.

An internal amplification control is included in each reaction. This control is a gene target that is always present at a constant level. For qPCR and RT-qPCR, internal controls confirm that negative results are true negatives and are not because of amplification failure during the PCR. In RT-qPCR, the level of target quantified in this way is expressed relative to an internal amplification control.

Just as PCR stimulated a wide variety of test methods and applications, qPCR has also been modified to address a variety of clinical questions. Widely used applications of qPCR and RT-qPCR include detection of microorganisms, especially viruses and other pathogens that are difficult or dangerous to culture in the laboratory; tumor-associated gene expression; and tissue typing.

Multiplex qPCR methods are performed to assess multiple targets simultaneously, such as in the analysis of expression of multiple genes. qPCR testing can also be applied to the measurement of donor bone marrow in the recipient after a bone marrow transplant.

Digital Droplet PCR. Another approach to qPCR is **digital droplet PCR**. Unlike the relative quantification of qPCR,

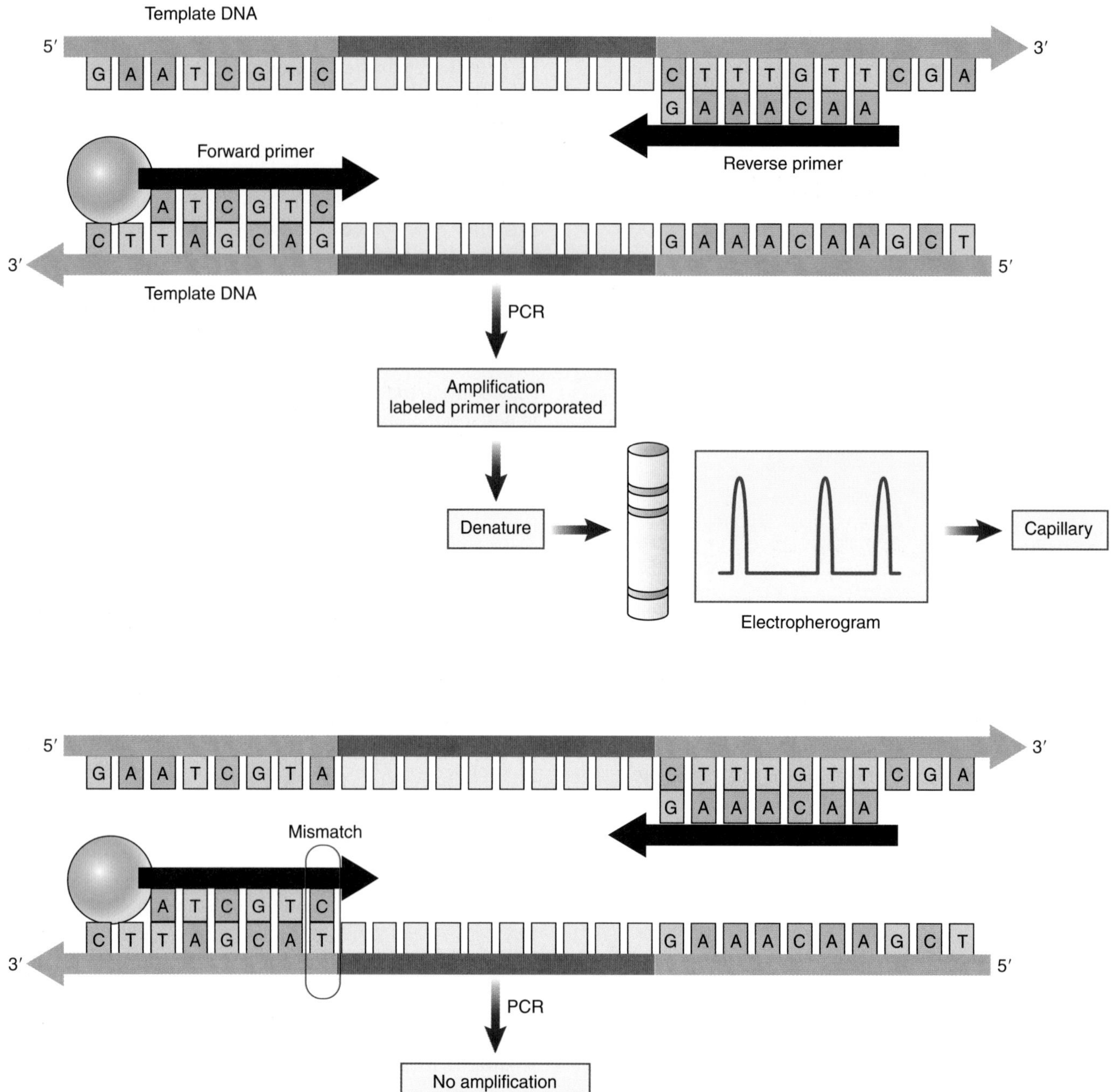

FIGURE 12–16 Detection of PCR products by capillary gel electrophoresis. One PCR primer (forward or reverse) is covalently attached to a fluorescent dye, such as fluorescein. The double-stranded products are denatured and diluted (left). Only the single strand of the PCR product with labeled primer will be detected (center). The output from the capillary instrument is an electropherogram (right) showing peaks of fluorescence that are analogous to band patterns on gel electrophoresis.

digital droplet PCR provides absolute quantification; that is, there is a numerical expression of the number of molecules in the sample (in contrast to the number of molecules relative to a control). Furthermore, digital droplet PCR measurements are made after the amplification program has finished (endpoint), and therefore, they are not affected by variations in PCR efficiencies that may be encountered with different primers and targets.

Digital droplet PCR is based on preparing a limiting dilution of sample template molecules into individual droplets of reaction buffer in oil, followed by separate amplification of each molecule **(Fig. 12–20)**. When sample template DNA in an aqueous reaction mix is added to inert oil, an emulsion forms. The droplets in oil act as individual reaction chambers. The emulsion is then subjected to a PCR amplification program. After amplification, droplets that received a template molecule will contain product, and droplets without template will not. The droplets in the oil emulsion are counted by microfluidics to determine how many of the droplets contained template and how many did not. Instrument software

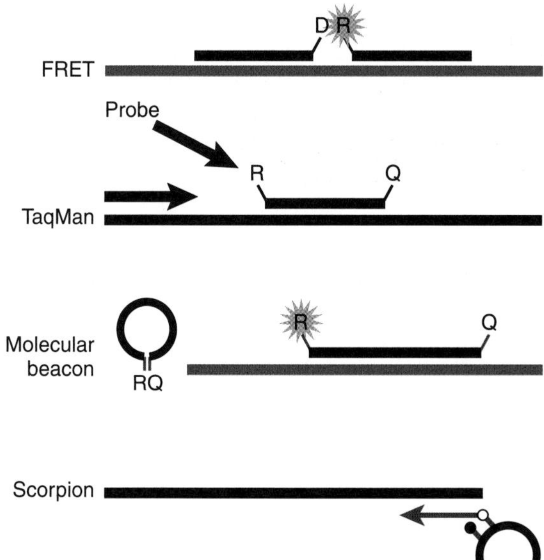

FIGURE 12–17 Probe systems for real-time quantitative PCR (qPCR). FRET probes generate a signal when target (or copies of target) sequences are present. When the donor (D) and reporter (R) probes bind, energy provided to the reporter dye by the donor dye generates a fluorescent signal. TaqMan probes generate a signal as the target DNA is copied. This results in the degradation of the probe, releasing the reporter dye (R) from the quencher (Q), allowing the reporter dye to fluoresce. Molecular beacons also contain a reporter (R) and quencher (Q), which are separated in the presence of target sequences; these hybridize to the probe and separate the reporter and quencher. The bottom part of the figure shows a scorpion probe covalently attached to a primer. With each replication of target, the scorpion probe is opened, releasing a reporter from a quencher dye and generating a signal. Unlike the other probes, the scorpion signal is covalently attached to the product.

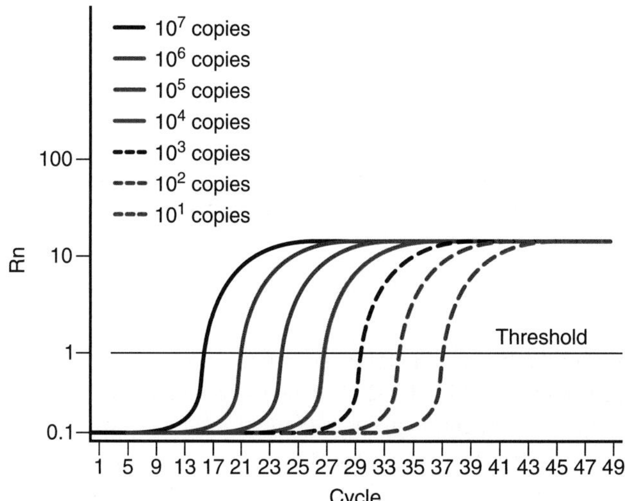

FIGURE 12–18 Real-time quantitative PCR signal generated from a TaqMan probe. The normalized fluorescence (ΔRn) is plotted against PCR cycles 1 to 50. The threshold cycle is indicated by the green line. The length of the lag phase is inversely correlated with the amount of starting material.

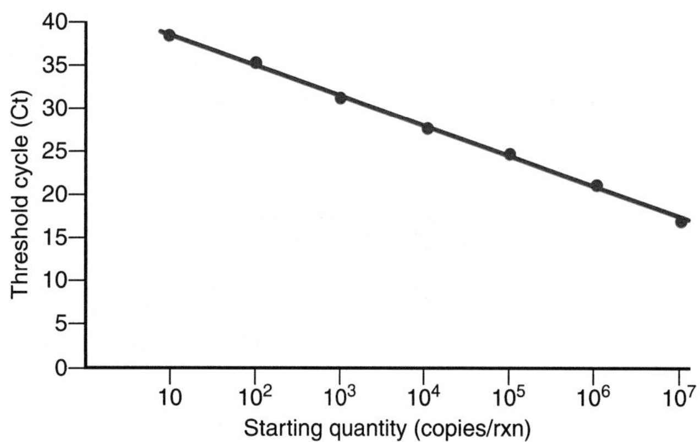

FIGURE 12–19 Ct values (*y*-axis) were determined for serial 10-fold dilutions of a synthetic target of known concentration (*x*-axis). The resulting standard curve is used to convert Ct values of test samples to concentration.

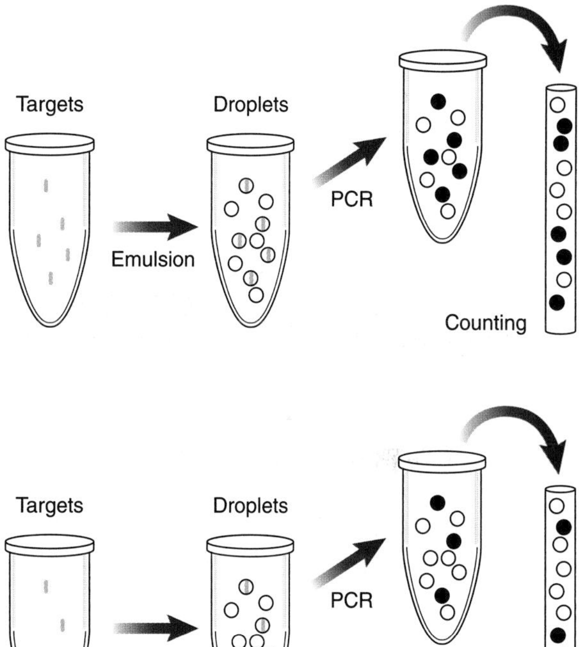

FIGURE 12–20 Digital droplet PCR quantifies the absolute number of target molecules (left) by limiting dilution into an emulsion of individual aqueous droplets, each containing one or no template molecules. After the PCR, droplets with product are counted, and the ratio of empty droplets to product-containing droplets is calculated to determine the absolute number of molecules in the specimen. Top: high concentration of template; bottom: low concentration of template.

translates the positive and negative droplet ratio to the absolute number of target molecules.

The linear response of the digital PCR quantification allows the detection of small changes in target number that is not possible by qPCR. Digital PCR has been applied to analysis of gene copy number variation, detection of rare mutations, and infectious disease.

Transcription-Based Amplification

A variety of amplification methods have been developed since the introduction of PCR. An advantage of several of these methods is that temperature cycling is not required. Kwoh and colleagues developed a transcription-based amplification system in 1989. Commercial variations of this process include transcription-mediated amplification (TMA), nucleic acid sequence–based amplification (NASBA), and self-sustaining sequence replication (3SR). The methods are similar, with variations in enzyme systems.

For transcription-based amplification systems, RNA is the target as well as the primary product. A complementary DNA copy (cDNA) is synthesized from the target RNA, and then transcription of the cDNA produces millions of copies of RNA products. The RNA products transcribed from the cDNA can also serve as target RNA for synthesis of more cDNA **(Fig. 12–21)**. The RNA products are detected by chemiluminescence with acridinium ester or, in the case of NASBA, molecular beacon probes.

In contrast to PCR, TMA is an isothermal process, which does not involve the repeated heating and cooling required for PCR. Targeting RNA allows for the direct detection of RNA viruses, such as HCV and HIV. Targeting the RNA of organisms with DNA genomes, such as *Mycobacterium tuberculosis*, is more sensitive than targeting the DNA because each microorganism makes multiple copies of RNA, whereas it has only one copy of DNA per cell. Detection of *Chlamydia trachomatis* in genital specimens and cytomegalovirus (CMV) quantification in blood are additional applications for TMA. The high sensitivity of TMA also makes it suitable for screening for viral infections in donor blood.

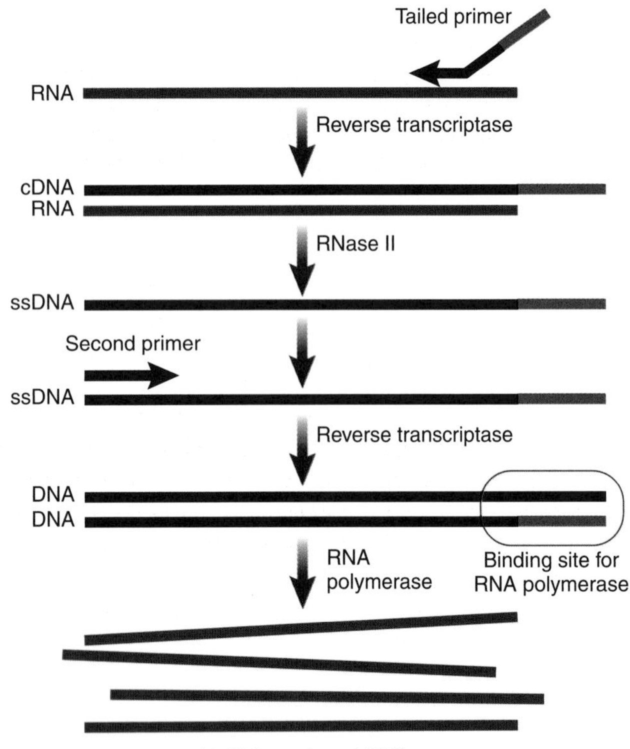

FIGURE 12–21 Transcription-mediated amplification (TMA) targets RNA. In the first step, a cDNA:RNA hybrid is synthesized by reverse transcriptase using a primer with a tail (that will ultimately form the binding site for a later enzyme). Hybridized (but not single-stranded) RNA is degraded by RNase II, leaving single-stranded DNA. This ssDNA serves as a template for reverse transcriptase to synthesize a complementary strand of DNA, including the primer tail, to complete the binding site for RNA polymerase. The RNA polymerase uses dsDNA as a template to synthesize many copies of RNA. This new RNA can cycle back to step one and repeat the process, resulting in a large amplification of product.

Probe Amplification

In probe amplification, the number of target nucleic acid sequences in a sample is not changed. Rather, primers are extended or ligated into many copies of detectable probes. Examples of probe amplification are strand displacement amplification (SDA), loop-mediated isothermal amplification (LAMP), and molecular inversion probe amplification (MIP).

Strand Displacement Amplification (SDA). SDA is an isothermal amplification process. After an initial denaturation step, the reaction proceeds at one temperature. In SDA, the amplification products are the probes rather than the target DNA. After the target DNA is denatured by heating to 95°C, two primers—an outer and an inner primer—bind close to each other **(Fig. 12–22)**. As the outer primer is extended by DNA polymerase, it displaces the product formed by the simultaneous extension of the inner primer (probe). The probe becomes the target DNA for the next stage of the process. The second stage of the reaction is the exponential probe amplification phase, which involves extension from a nick formed in the strand by a **restriction endonuclease** enzyme.

Loop-Mediated Isothermal Amplification (LAMP). The LAMP system has high specificity and sensitivity for target DNA. In this process, PCR primers carry sequences at the 5′ end that will self-hybridize, forming loops that self-prime in a cyclic manner. An advantage of this process is the shortened run time (fewer than 30 minutes). LAMP methods are used to detect HIV, cytomegalovirus, *Staphylococcus aureus*, and *E. coli*.

Molecular Inversion Probe (MIP). MIP (also called *padlock probe*) is another isothermal, highly sensitive detection system. In this method, the ends of the probes bind to target sequences so that, in the presence of target, the probe ends are brought together and ligated to form circles. Circularized probes accumulate based on the amount of target present and are detected by gel electrophoresis. These probes can be further PCR-amplified to increase sensitivity. MIP methods have been applied to detection of *S. aureus*, *Streptococcus mutans*, influenza virus, and to RNA typing.

Signal Amplification

In signal amplification, large amounts of signal are bound to the target sequences that are present in the sample. Branched DNA is an example of a commercially available signal amplification method.

Branched DNA. In **branched DNA (bDNA)** amplification, a series of short, single-stranded DNA probes are used to capture the target nucleic acid and to bind to multiple reporter molecules, loading the target nucleic acid with signal **(Fig. 12–23)**.

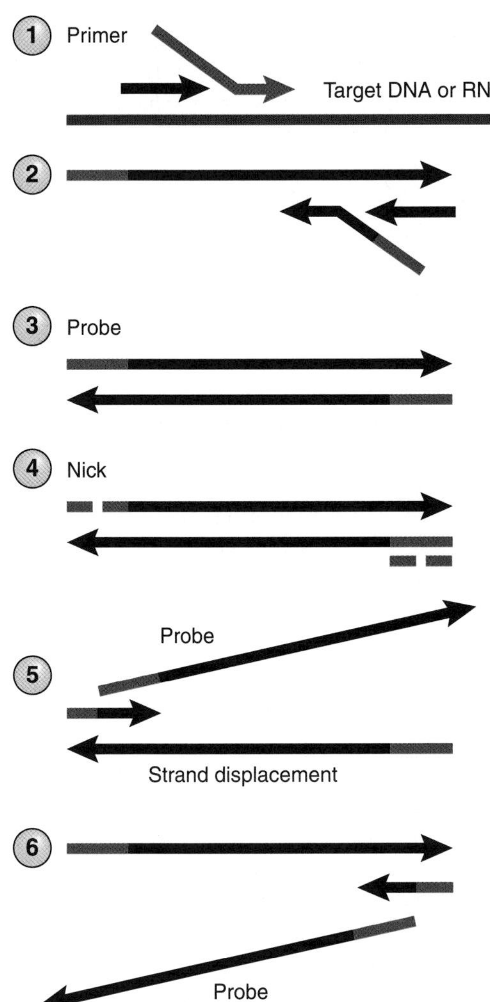

FIGURE 12–22 SDA showing one target strand. (1) Primers bind to single-stranded DNA at a complementary sequence. (2) A polymerase extends the primer from the 3′ end. (3) The extended primer forms a double-stranded DNA segment containing a site for a restriction enzyme at each end. (4) The enzyme binds double-stranded DNA at the restriction site and forms a nick (cutting only one strand of the double helix). (5) The DNA polymerase recognizes the nick and extends the strand from that site, displacing the previously created strand. (6) Each strand can then anneal and continue the process.

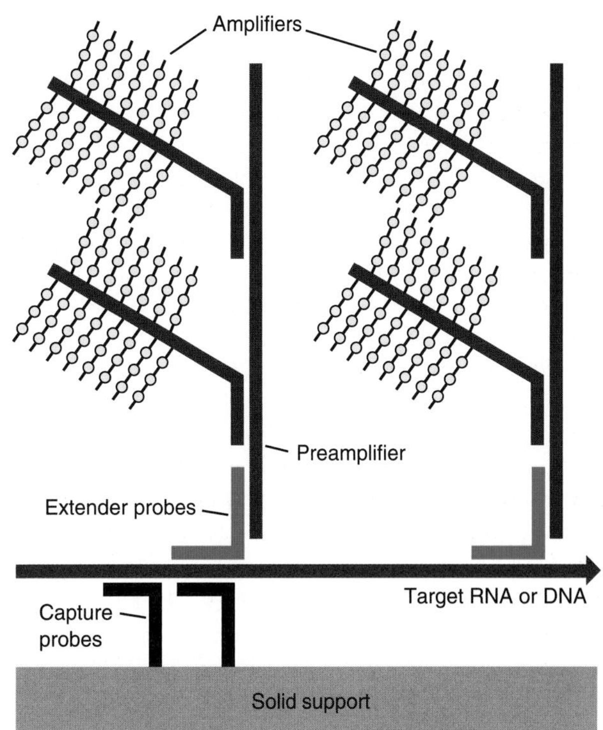

FIGURE 12–23 In branched DNA, signal is amplified through hybridization of complementary probes to the target DNA or RNA. Branched DNA molecules carry multiple signals for each target molecule. A second generation of the method has increased sensitivity because of the binding of additional signals. *(Adapted from Buckingham L.* Molecular Diagnostics. *2nd ed. Philadelphia, PA: F.A. Davis; 2011, with permission.)*

Because multiple probes hybridize to the target sequences in bDNA, its specificity is enhanced over methods using a single probe or primer to bind to the target. This allows for multiple genotypes of the same virus to be detected by incorporating different probes that recognize slightly different sequences. The bDNA signal amplification assay has been applied to the qualitative and quantitative detection of hepatitis B virus (HBV), HCV, and HIV-1.

DNA Sequencing

Specific Procedures

The function of DNA is to store genetic information. That information is stored in the form of the order or sequence of the four nucleotide bases in the DNA chain. Early in the history of recombinant DNA technology, the idea of sequencing or detecting the nucleotide order of the nucleic acids was actively pursued. Two sequencing methods emerged in the mid-1970s: the Maxam–Gilbert chain breakage method and the chain termination sequencing method developed by Dr. Fred Sanger and colleagues. Sanger or chain termination sequencing quickly gained popularity, as it was not subject to the toxic chemicals and complex interpretation required by the Maxam–Gilbert method. Alternative sequencing methods have since been developed, including pyrosequencing and next-generation sequencing.

Chain Termination (Sanger) Sequencing

Direct determination of the order, or sequence, of nucleotides in a DNA chain is the most explicit method for identifying genetic mutations or polymorphisms, especially when looking for changes affecting only one or two nucleotides. **Chain termination sequencing** is a modification of the DNA replication process. It uses modified nucleotide bases called *dideoxynucleotide triphosphates* (ddNTPs), which differ from dNTPs in that they do not have an OH group at the 3′ carbon of the deoxyribose sugar **(Fig. 12–24).**

In a standard Sanger sequencing reaction, the DNA template to be copied is denatured into single strands, and similar

Nitrogen base Nitrogen base

dNTP ddNTP

FIGURE 12–24 Dideoxyribonucleotides lack the 3′ hydroxyl group necessary for formation of the phosphodiester bond during DNA replication. *(Adapted from Buckingham L.* Molecular Diagnostics. *2nd ed. Philadelphia, PA: F.A. Davis; 2011, with permission.)*

to PCR, all components required for DNA synthesis are added: a primer pair to outline the target DNA, DNA polymerase enzyme, and the four dNTPs. In addition, the four ddNTPs (ddATP, ddTTP, ddCTP, and ddGTP) are added to the mixture. Each ddNTP is labeled with a different fluorescent dye (ddATP green, ddCTP blue, ddGTP black, ddTTP red) so that the products of the sequencing reaction can be distinguished by color. Synthesis will stop if a ddNTP is incorporated into the growing DNA chain (chain termination) because without the hydroxyl group at the 3′ sugar carbon, the 5′-3′ phosphodiester bond cannot be made. Each newly synthesized chain will terminate, therefore, with a ddNTP **(Fig. 12–25).** The result of the sequencing reaction is a collection of fragments of various sizes, or DNA ladder.

The fluorescently labeled DNA ladder is resolved by gel or capillary gel electrophoresis. Gel-based resolution will result in a series of bands of different sizes. The DNA sequence is read from the bottom to the top of the gel by which ddNTP terminated each fragment. Sequencing results from capillary gel electrophoresis are a series of fluorescent peaks, termed an *electropherogram* **(Fig. 12–26).**

Accuracy of interpretation of sequencing data from a dye terminator reaction depends on the quality of the template (free of residual PCR components), the efficiency of the sequencing reaction, and the purity of the sequencing ladder. Clear, clean sequencing ladders are read accurately by sequencing software, and a text sequence is generated. Software programs

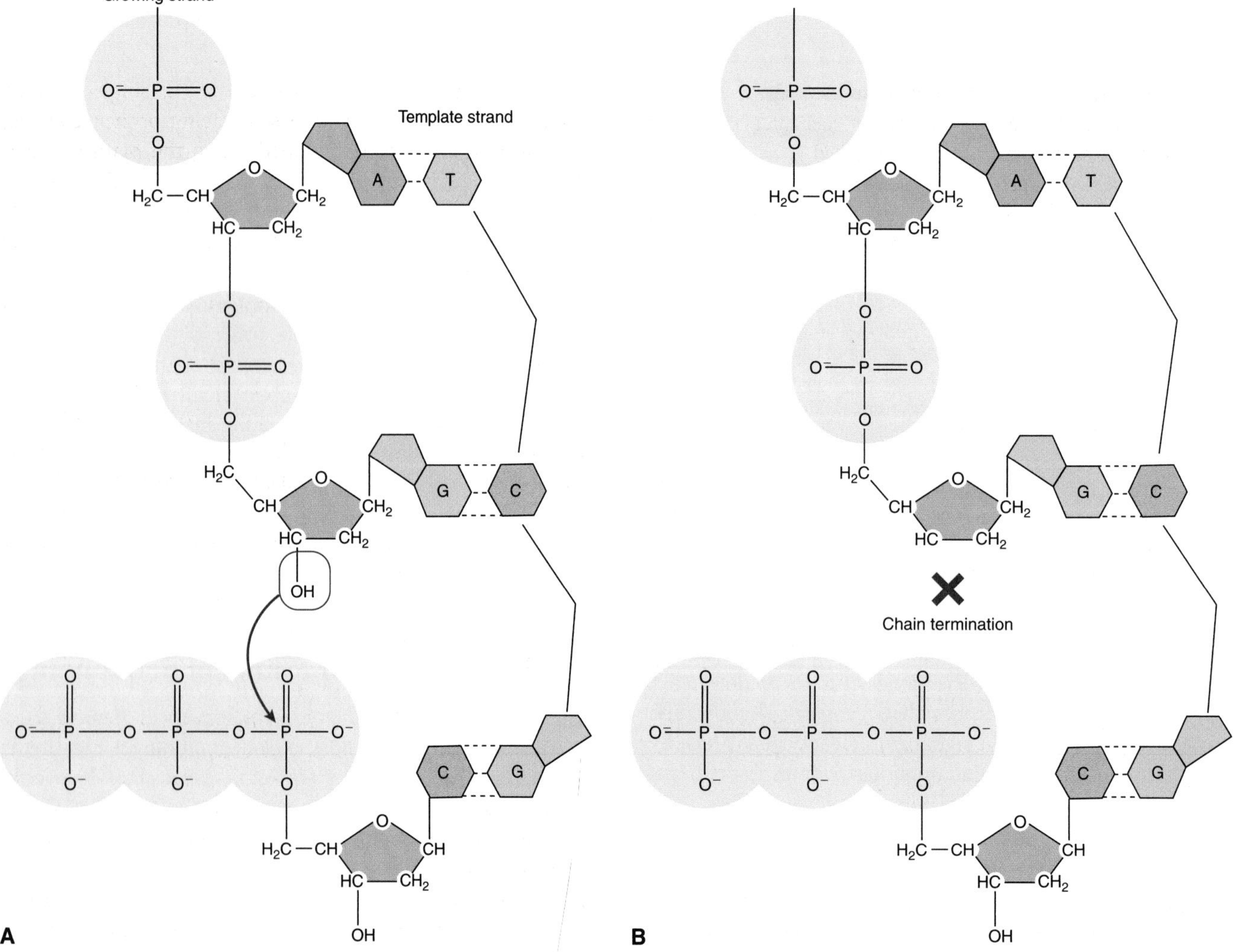

FIGURE 12–25 (A) DNA synthesis proceeds by formation of a phosphodiester bond between the ribose 3′OH of a previous nucleotide and the ribose 5′ phosphate group of the incoming nucleotide. (B) If the 3′OH is missing, as in ddNTP, synthesis terminates (right). *(Adapted from Buckingham L.* Molecular Diagnostics. *2nd ed. Philadelphia, PA: F.A. Davis; 2011, with permission.)*

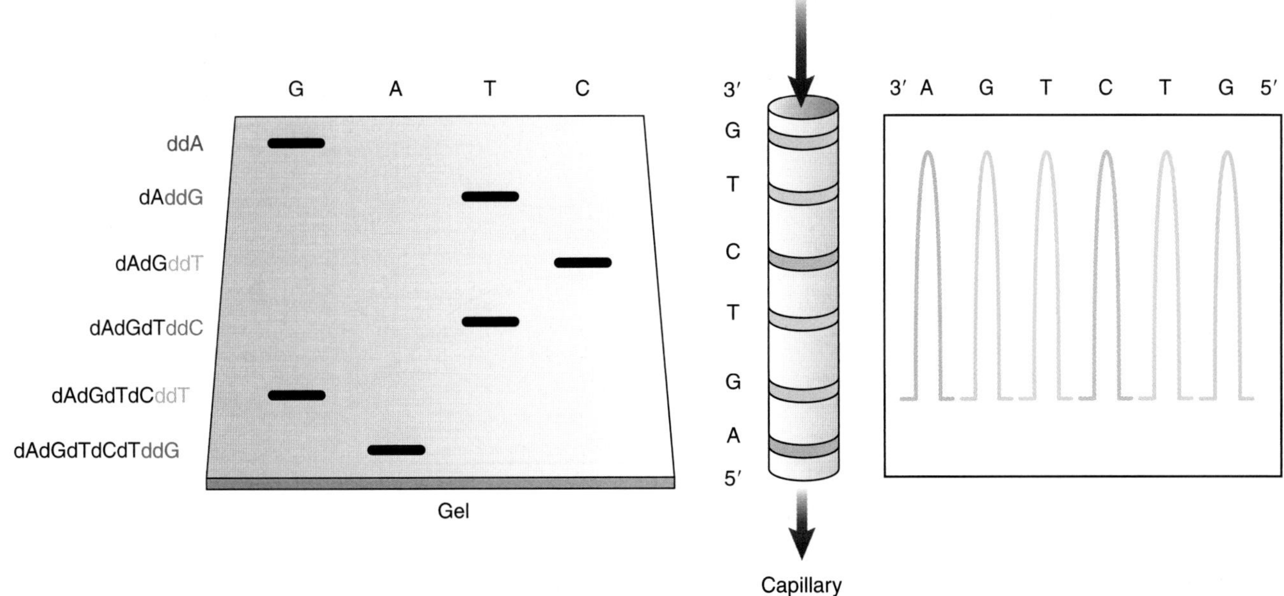

FIGURE 12–26 A DNA ladder (left) resolved by gel electrophoresis is read from the bottom of the gel to the top of the gel (shortest fragment to the longest). The terminating base is determined by its tube (gel lane). In dye terminator sequencing, the sequence is read automatically as fluorescently labeled fragments migrate through the gel or capillary. Each fragment passes a detector that will generate an electropherogram of fluorescent peaks (right). Sequencing software will produce a text report of the DNA sequence.

report the certainty of each nucleotide base in the sequence and compare test sequences with reference sequences to identify mutations or polymorphisms in the DNA.

Sequencing and re-sequencing of known DNA regions are routine laboratory methods where mutations are not always in predicted locations in genes, requiring a survey of most or all of the gene sequences. Sequencing is used extensively in genetics and oncology for definitive identification of gene abnormalities. It is also used for sequence-based tissue typing.

Germline or inherited variations in the DNA sequence are readily detected, usually from blood specimens. Somatic (non-inherited) mutations in clinical specimens, such as cancerous tumors, are sometimes difficult to detect, as they may be diluted by normal sequences that mask the somatic change.

A Sanger sequencing reaction is performed on a single DNA strand. When a sequence change is detected, the alteration is confirmed by sequencing the complementary strand of the DNA by priming the synthesis reaction on the strand opposite the strand that was sequenced. Alterations affecting a single base pair may be subtle on an electropherogram, especially if the alteration is in the heterozygous form or mixed with a normal reference sequence. For this reason, standard Sanger sequencing is less sensitive for the detection of DNA sequence changes than other methods.

Pyrosequencing

Pyrosequencing is a sequencing method first developed in the 1980s. The procedure relies on the generation of light (luminescence) when nucleotides are added to a growing strand of DNA. With this system, there are no gels, fluorescent dyes, or ddNTPs.

In the pyrosequencing reaction mix, a single-stranded DNA template is mixed with a sequencing primer, enzyme, and substrate. In a predetermined order, the pyrosequencer introduces dNTPs sequentially to the reaction. If the introduced nucleotide is complementary to the base in the template strand next to the 3′ end of the primer, DNA polymerase forms a phosphodiester bond between the primer and the nucleotide, releasing pyrophosphate (PPi) **(Fig. 12–27).** The released PPi is converted to ATP in the presence of adenosine 5′ phosphosulfate (APS) to energize generation of a luminescent signal. This signal indicates that the introduced nucleotide is the correct base in the sequence. If the dNTP is not complementary to the template, no phosphodiester bond is formed, and no signal is produced. Unincorporated dNTPs are enzymatically removed before the introduction of the next dNTP. The pyrosequencing reaction generates a pyrogram of luminescent peaks associated with the addition of the complementary nucleotides (see Fig. 12–27, bottom panel).

Because pyrosequencing produces short- to moderate-length sequence information (up to 100 bases), it is not as versatile as Sanger sequencing, which can produce reads longer than 1,000 bases, especially for sequencing long unknown regions of DNA. Two factors have kept pyrosequencing in use. With increasing identification of clinically important, frequently recurring variants in known gene locations ("hot spots"), it became necessary only to sequence targeted areas, the immediate regions around the nucleotide base change. Because pyrosequencing is less labor intensive than Sanger sequencing, it is more convenient for these types of short sequence analyses. Second, some instruments developed for genomic or **next-generation sequencing (NGS)** utilize the pyrosequencing chemistry.

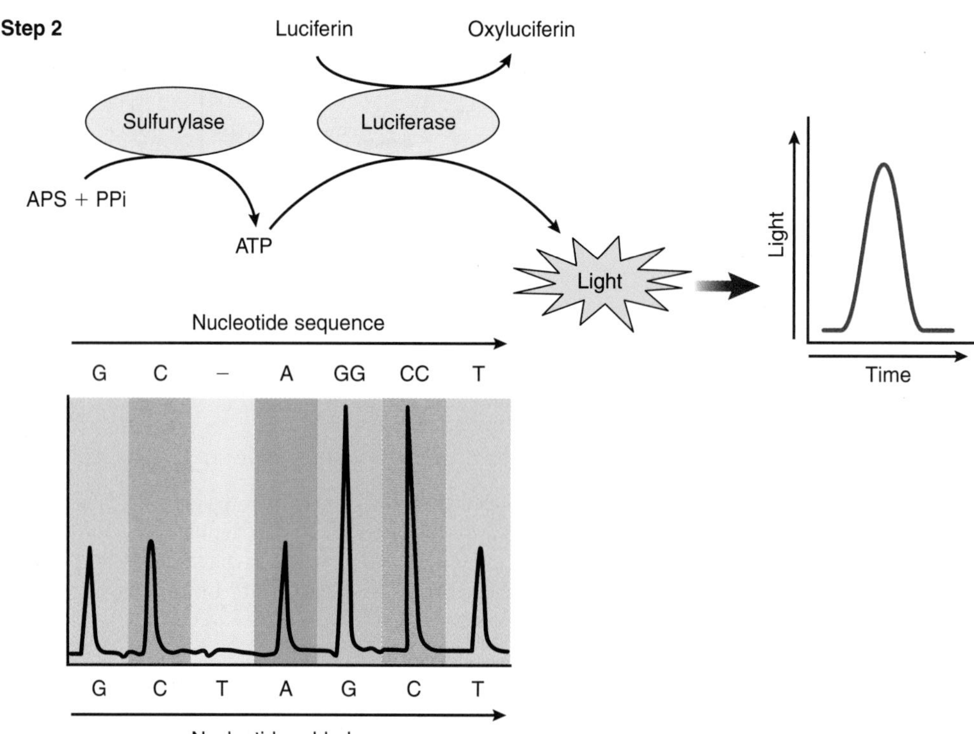

FIGURE 12–27 Pyrosequencing detects nucleotide sequence by introducing dNTPs in a predetermined order to the sequencing reaction. If the nucleotide is not complementary to the template sequence, no reaction occurs, and the nucleotide is then degraded. If the nucleotide is complementary to the sequence, polymerase forms a phosphodiester bond extending the primer and releasing pyrophosphate (PPi, Step 1). The pyrophosphate then goes through a series of reactions to ultimately produce a chemiluminescent signal (Step 2). The pyrosequencing output is a pyrogram, as shown on bottom. *(Adapted from Buckingham L.* Molecular Diagnostics. *2nd ed. Philadelphia, PA: F.A. Davis; 2011, with permission.)*

Next-Generation Sequencing

The first human genome was sequenced by chain termination (Sanger) sequencing. The 7-year project involved hundreds of capillary electrophoresis instruments and bioinformatics experts and cost billions of dollars. With NGS technologies, a human genome can now be sequenced by a single sequencer in a few hours. NGS is designed to sequence large numbers of templates simultaneously (massively parallel sequencing), yielding hundreds of thousands of sequences in a single run. These short sequences are then assembled into a complete sequence. NGS is also a metagenomic technology, involving simultaneous sequencing of multiple small genomes, such as mixed populations of microorganisms in the environment or in body fluids.

A goal that stimulated the development of NGS technologies was to sequence the human genome for a minimal cost (less than $1,000), bringing the expense of genomic studies into the realm of clinical analysis. Production of the "$1,000 genome" has been achieved, and thousands of genomes have been sequenced as part of the 1,000 Genome Project. Not initially included in the sequencing cost were challenges of interpretation, reporting, and data storage. These issues are now included for implementation of NGS in clinical analysis.

The first mass-marketed technologies of NGS included pyrosequencing, sequencing by synthesis with reversible dyes, ion conductance, and sequencing by ligation. Pyrosequencing, reversible dye sequencing, and ion conductance sequencing have most frequently been applied to clinical applications.

In contrast to chain termination sequencing of PCR products or long templates in large plasmids, NGS procedures begin with short DNA templates, less than 1 kb, usually less than 500 bp. Methods of template preparation include amplification with multiple primer pairs to select regions of interest in multiplex PCR reactions or using emulsion PCR. Alternatively, a set of short fragments can be prepared from enzymatically digested or sonicated genomic DNA. Fragments generated by these methods comprise a library. A library can include selected genes or gene regions (known as *targeted libraries* or *gene panels*), only coding DNA or exons (whole exome sequencing), or whole genomes (whole genome sequencing).

PCR primers or probes are used to select targeted libraries and exomes. For example, analysis of the MHC locus by NGS begins with PCR selection and amplification of Class I and Class II genes. The PCR products are templates for sequencing. Probes are used similar to primers to select and copy targeted regions for sequencing **(Fig. 12–28).**

Fragmented DNA is prepared from whole genomes or from larger (>1,000 bp) PCR-selected gene regions. The ends of the DNA fragments are ligated to adapters, that is, short synthetic double-stranded DNA sequences carrying PCR primer-binding sites. The primer-binding sites allow unbiased

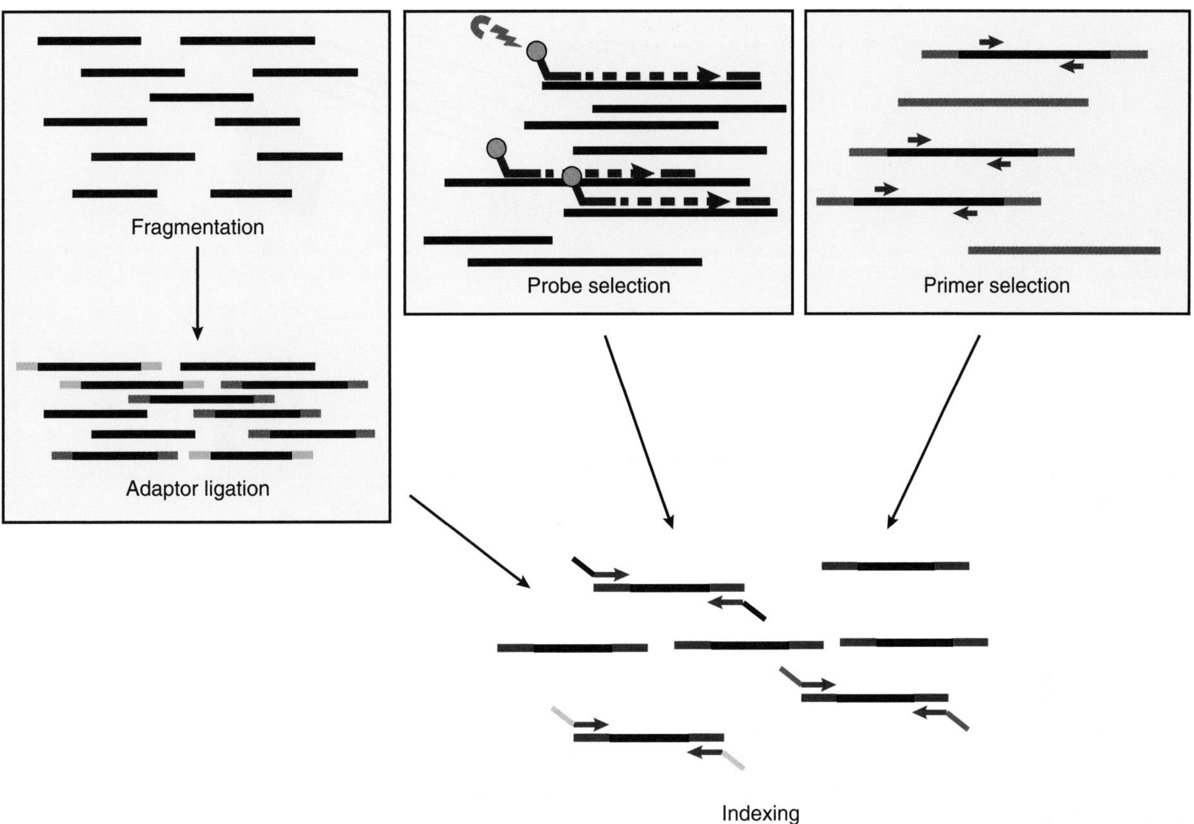

FIGURE 12–28 DNA libraries are prepared using fragmentation, probe, or primer selection of specific genes or gene regions. Adaptors carrying primer-binding sites are added to the ends of fragmented DNA. In a second PCR reaction, primers carry short index DNA sequences to identify each sample, as all samples in a run are pooled and sequenced simultaneously.

amplification to occur for all the genomic fragments using a single primer pair.

Amplification of the adapter-ligated library is performed with indexing primers. On the 5′ end of indexing primers are short sequences or "bar codes" to assist in organization of the sequence data. A bar code or index is a 6- to 10-b sequence assigned to each sample and gene region in the library. With multiple samples sequenced together in a run, bar codes are used in post-run analysis to associate samples and gene regions with their sequences.

After library amplification and indexing, the PCR products are cleaned of residual reaction products, pooled, and introduced to the sequencer. Depending on the sequencing technology, the sequencing may be in solution or immobilized on a solid support.

For NGS by pyrosequencing, libraries are generated by emulsion PCR. One primer in each PCR reaction is bound to a solid support (bead). After the PCR reaction, the products are denatured, and the beads carry one strand of the PCR product as sequencing templates into hundreds of thousands of wells of a picoplate. Reagents and nucleotides are introduced into the plate, and independent sequencing reactions result in the release of PPi, which simultaneously generates light signals, as previously described.

In ion conductance sequencing, nucleotide order is determined through release of hydrogen ions (analogous to release of PPi in pyrosequencing) by DNA synthesis. Bead-attached library templates prepared as previously described are loaded with sequencing reagents onto a semiconductor or ion chip. When a nucleotide complementary to a template is introduced and incorporated, the release of the hydrogen ion is detected by a pH change in the reaction **(Fig. 12–29).** The ion chip contains sensors for more than one million wells, which allow parallel, simultaneous detection of hundreds of thousands of independent sequencing reactions. Ion conductance sequencing is faster than other methods that require optical sensing (images).

In the reversible dye terminator technology, libraries carry sequences complementary to immobilized primers on a solid support (flow cell). After introduction of the sample to the flow cell, the libraries are amplified by bridge PCR, forming clusters of templates across the flow cell. Sequencing occurs at hundreds of thousands of cluster locations by addition, detection, and removal of each of the four nucleotide labels **(Fig. 12–30).**

For all NGS variations, sequence data in the form of processed images or electrical pulses are collected by instrument software. The sequence quality is assessed and then the sequence is determined. Variants, polymorphisms, or the sequence itself are identified by comparison with stored reference sequences. After a successful NGS run, areas of interest will have been sequenced from a few to thousands of times.

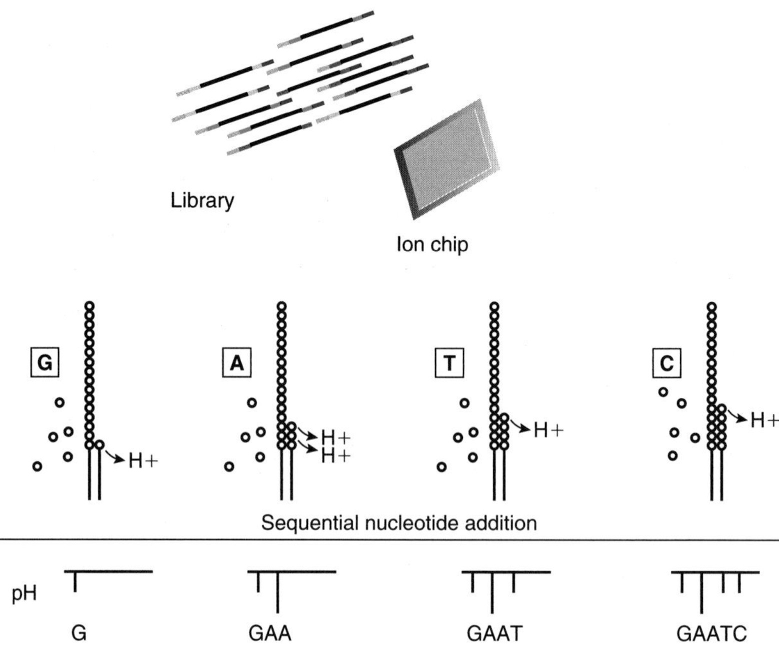

FIGURE 12–29 In ion chip sequencing, the pooled, indexed DNA libraries and sequencing primers are applied to an ion chip in individual micro-DNA synthesis reactions. Nucleotides are introduced sequentially to the chip, and if the introduced nucleotide is complementary to the template sequence, a phosphodiester bond is formed, releasing a hydrogen ion. A sensor detects the resulting pH change correlated with addition of each nucleotide base.

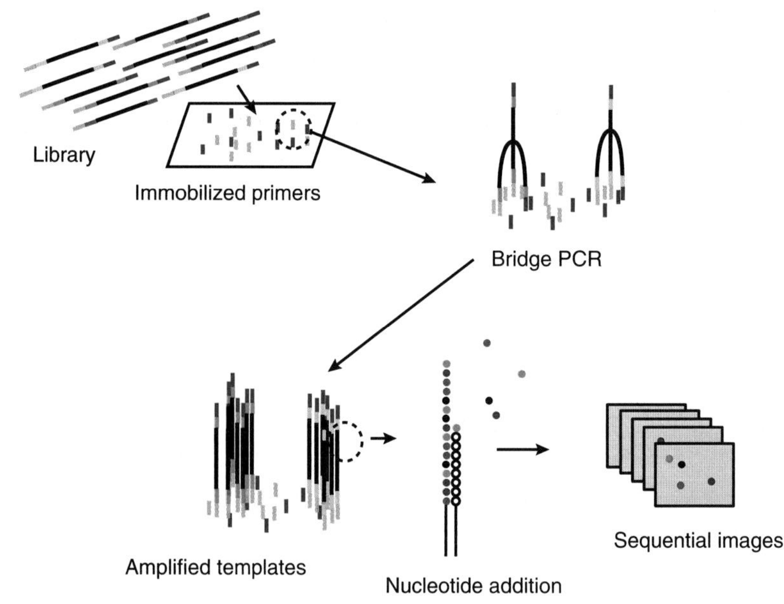

FIGURE 12–30 For reversible dye terminator sequencing, the pooled, indexed libraries are hybridized to immobilized primers at millions of positions on a solid support (flow cell). Each molecule of DNA is then amplified in place by bridge PCR. The amplified templates are sequenced by synthesis with simultaneous addition of the four fluorescently labeled nucleotides. Nucleotides complementary to each amplified template are added to the end of the growing chain, and an image is made of the flow cell. The fluorescent signals from the nucleotides are removed, followed by addition of the next round of nucleotides. The sequential images are converted to sequence information for each template.

The number of times a region is sequenced is called the *coverage*. Whole human genomes will have lower coverage (30X to 40X, 3 billion bp sequenced) than whole exome sequencing (sequencing of only protein-coding regions; 50X to 100X, 30 to 50 million bp sequenced). Gene panels of a few hundred targeted genes are sequenced with higher coverage than genomes or exomes, depending on the number of genes included in the panel. At least 500X coverage is required to call rare variants, such as those in mixed tissue samples (tumor DNA containing lymphocytes or other normal tissue). Cost is the limiting factor for the degree of coverage used.

A sequence variant (difference from the reference sequence) may be present in some or all of the copies of the sequence covered. The percentage of sequences carrying the variant is the allele frequency in the sample. Somatic variants tend to have low allele frequencies, whereas germline (inherited) sequence changes will comprise 50% or 100% of the covered sequences.

In the clinical laboratory, targeted NGS has been most commonly applied to genetics (including pharmacogenomics), oncology, and HLA typing. NGS has advanced the accuracy and extent of HLA typing. NGS is used for typing of the HLA Class I HLA-A, -B, and -C and Class II HLA-DRB1/3/4/5, HLA-DQA1, HLA-DQB1, HLA-DPA1, and HLA-DPB1 genes. The increased amount of information and throughput of NGS allows resolution of ambiguities that were not possible with previous molecular methods, including Sanger sequencing.

Clinical Correlations

The Cancer Genome Atlas (TCGA)

The Cancer Genome Atlas (TCGA) is a national program in which NGS has been used to sequence the nucleic acid isolated from tumors of thousands of patients. The large amount of data has been catalogued and analyzed by bioinformatics to identify common themes among cancer types. The information obtained continues to increase our understanding of cancer and has had a large clinical impact by improving the ways in which cancer is being diagnosed and treated (see Chapter 17).

Ambiguities in HLA typing arise from polymorphisms outside of sequenced areas and from closely spaced polymorphisms that may be on one or separate chromosomes.

Whole exome sequencing has been used to identify variants responsible for inherited disease conditions. Whole genome sequencing is primarily a research tool. Unlike other methods, massive parallel sequencing has the capacity to investigate all known genetic loci for clinically significant alterations. Tumor mutational burden (number of mutations/Mb of sequenced DNA) has been identified as a biomarker for some types of cancer. DNA alterations increase the antigenicity of the tumor, which can affect treatment strategy decisions and disease prognosis.

Genetic data have been amassed in large databases, facilitating future sequence analysis. There are also growing databases of somatic variant data used in diagnosis and treatment strategies for cancer and other diseases.

Bioinformatics

Information technology has had to accommodate the vast amount of data arising from molecular analyses such as high-throughput sequencing and arrays. **Bioinformatics** merges this biological data with information technology. The interpretation of data such as that generated by NGS requires massive storage space and contributes to continual renewal of previously stored data in organized databases. This database information can then be used to refine interpretation of newly collected data.

In NGS, powerful computer data assembly systems are required to organize the short sequence information generated from sequence libraries and identify variants. Several factors affect the identification of sequences and sequence variants. Adequate sample DNA is required to provide the required coverage of regions of interest. The quality of the sequence must be sufficient for confidence in identifying each base at each position of the sequence. For clinical sequencing, a 1/1,000 probability of error is recommended.

For targeted gene panels, manufacturers have developed programs to produce a finished report with variants identified automatically directly from the sequencer. Software programs independent of the sequencer have been designed to generate spreadsheet files that allow the user to apply quality, variant type, allele frequency (what percentage of the coverage contains the variant), and other parameters in a process called *filtering*. Nucleotide or protein sequence data at this stage may be stored as text files in the FASTA or FASTQ format (named after a DNA and protein sequence alignment software package first described in 1985). FASTA files are the text of nucleotide sequences only. FASTQ files include a quality symbol for each base.

NGS tends to be more error-prone than Sanger sequencing, mostly because of the library preparation. Errors must be distinguished from true sequence variants in a sample. Variants occurring with a frequency of less than 2% are suggested to be indicators of sequence error. Errors are detected and minimized with adequate coverage, database information, and software design.

Once variants are identified, further assessment is required to find their biological significance. Intronic or silent exonic mutations that do not affect protein sequence or conservative changes that do not affect protein structure are not biologically significant. Variants that change protein structure or affect protein epitopes may be, but are not always, significant.

For clinical applications, the medical significance of variants and the genes in which they are found must be determined. Variants are classified based on historical sequence database information. Large databases of previously observed variants and phenotypic associations are used for annotating the variants and identifying those that are significant and reportable. In some cases, such as germline genetic disease associations, standard chain termination sequencing is recommended for confirmation of critical variants. A standard nomenclature system developed by the International Union of Pure and Applied Chemistry and the International Union of Biochemistry and Molecular Biology is used to express sequence information so that clear communication and organized storage of sequence data are possible.

SUMMARY

- The two main types of nucleic acids are DNA and RNA. They are polymers made up of chains of nucleotides.
- Nucleotides of DNA contain a deoxyribose sugar with one of the following bases: adenine, guanine, thymine, or cytosine.
- RNA is made up of nucleotides containing a ribose sugar bonded to one of four nitrogen bases: adenine, guanine, cytosine, or uracil (instead of thymine).
- DNA is double stranded and arranged in a double helix, whereas RNA is typically single stranded.
- In a DNA molecule, specific base pairing occurs: adenine pairs with thymine, and guanine pairs with cytosine.
- When a DNA molecule replicates, the two daughter strands separate; each is a template for a newly synthesized complementary strand.
- The high specificity of detection of nucleic acid sequences through complementary base pairing is the basis of all molecular diagnostic testing.

- The central dogma of molecular biology refers to the fact that DNA serves as the template for messenger RNA, which in turn codes for proteins.
- Mutations and polymorphisms are changes in nucleotide sequences that may affect specific protein structure and function.
- Gel and capillary electrophoresis are used in many molecular methods. In these techniques, the negatively charged DNA fragments are separated by size under the force of an electric current in a semisolid gel or polymer solution.
- Restriction fragment length polymorphisms (RFLPs) are changes in DNA that result in different size pieces when cleaved by restriction enzymes.
- CRISPR-Cas9 is a gene-editing system that can be used to alter DNA at specific locations.
- Hybridization is the very specific binding of two complementary DNA strands or a DNA strand and an RNA strand. Often a probe, which has a short known nucleic acid sequence, is used to detect an unknown nucleic acid sequence in a sample.
- Hybridization techniques include Southern blot analysis, microarray technology for simultaneous assessment of multiple genes, and fluorescent in situ hybridization of specific genetic regions.
- Amplification involves making many copies of a specific nucleic acid sequence to obtain enough material for laboratory identification.
- Amplification methods include polymerase chain reaction (PCR), reverse transcriptase PCR (RT-PCR), quantitative PCR (qPCR), and digital PCR. All these methods amplify the target DNA.
- In transcription-mediated amplification (TMA), the target is RNA instead of DNA. A cDNA copy is made of the original RNA and used to produce millions of RNA copies.
- Strand displacement amplification (SDA) involves amplification of a probe rather than the original target DNA. Other probe amplification methods are loop-mediated amplification (LAMP) and the molecular inversion probe (MIP) method.
- Branched DNA represents a signal amplification method in which multiple probes attach to the original target sequence DNA.
- DNA sequencing involves determining the order of nucleotides in a DNA chain and is the most specific way of detecting polymorphisms and mutations.
- The Sanger chain termination sequencing method involves replicating a single DNA strand in the presence of fluorescent-labeled modified nucleotide bases called *dideoxy nucleotide triphosphates*. DNA fragments of various sizes are generated from the original template, and the sequence is determined by detecting the fluorescent labels.
- Pyrosequencing is an alternate sequencing method that relies on the generation of light when nucleotides are added to a growing DNA chain.
- Next-generation sequencing (NGS) methods allow for rapid sequencing of a large number of small DNA templates at one time. The short sequences are then assembled into a complete sequence. NGS can be used to determine the sequence of specific genes using targeted gene panels, the sequence of only the coding regions within DNA (whole exome sequencing), or the sequence of an entire genome (whole genome sequencing) to identify mutations associated with a variety of diseases.
- Bioinformatics uses information technology to analyze the vast amount of data generated by NGS testing and interprets the data for clinical relevance by comparison with known databases.

CASE STUDIES

1. A patient with a diagnosis of stage III lung cancer underwent surgery, and the tumor tissue was submitted for PD-L1 testing by immunohistochemistry (IHC). A section of tumor was placed in 10% buffered formalin for 24 hours, embedded in paraffin, and thin (4 micron) sections were cut from the fixed tissue in the paraffin block. The tissue sections were tested by IHC in an automated immunostainer using rabbit IgG anti-human PD-L1 primary antibody. Bound primary antibody was detected with an anti-rabbit isotype secondary antibody conjugated to an enzyme-labeled polymer to generate a color stain. Upon pathology review of the stained sections, it was determined that 60% of the tumor cells expressed PD-L1.

Questions

a. Describe positive and negative controls that would be used for the detection of PD-L1.
b. What is the immunologic role of PD-L1?
c. What is the clinical significance of the test results, and should the patient in this case receive immunotherapy?

2. A blood sample from a patient under treatment for HIV infection was submitted for testing. A laboratory test for the presence of HIV by qPCR was performed. The test can detect 50 to 1,000,000 viral copies per mL of plasma. Previous results had shown the presence of the virus at levels of 1,500, 600, 500, 220, and

100 copies per mL during the course of treatment. The results of the qPCR test for the current specimen were negative; however, the internal amplification control for the qPCR test was also negative.

Questions

a. How would you interpret these results?
   1. The results are negative, consistent with the patient history.
   2. The results are not interpretable because the amplification control is negative.
   3. The amplification control confirms that there is no contamination.
   4. The results are not correct, based on the previous positive results.

b. The test was repeated, and this time the target (HIV) amplification was negative, whereas the amplification control was positive. How would you interpret these results?
   1. The results show a true negative.
   2. The results are not interpretable because of contamination.
   3. The results are not correct, based on the previous positive results.
   4. The amplification control confirms the presence of HIV.

c. To prepare the test report, the results are entered along with the sensitivity of the test (50 copies/mL). Should these results be reported as 0 copies/mL because nothing was detected by this qPCR test?

REVIEW QUESTIONS

1. Which is associated only with RNA synthesis?
   a. Promoter
   b. Cytosine
   c. S phase
   d. Primer
2. The speed at which nucleic acids migrate in gel electrophoresis is determined by which property?
   a. Charge
   b. Fluorescence
   c. Absorption
   d. Size
3. What is the function of restriction endonucleases?
   a. They splice short DNA pieces together.
   b. They cleave DNA at specific sites.
   c. They make RNA copies of DNA.
   d. They make DNA copies from RNA.
4. Which of the following techniques uses RNA-guided enzymes?
   a. Microarray
   b. CRISPR
   c. Immunohistochemistry
   d. Restriction fragment mapping
5. To what does *in situ hybridization* refer?
   a. Probes react with intact cells within tissues.
   b. Probes are protected from degradation if hybridized.
   c. RNA polymerase copies messenger RNA.
   d. Hybridization takes place in solution.
6. Which probe sequence will hybridize to 5′AGTCGATCGATGC3′?
   a. 5′TCAGCTAGCTACG3′
   b. 5′GCATCGATCGACT3′
   c. 5′AGTCGATCGATGC3′
   d. 5′CGTAGCTAGCTGA3′
7. Which best describes the principle of microarrays?
   a. Arrays contain multiple unlabeled probes on a solid support.
   b. Arrays contain multiple copies of one unique probe.
   c. The sample is labeled with a fluorescent tag.
   d. Hybridization is detected by the presence of radioactivity.
8. Which best describes PCR?
   a. Probes are joined by a ligating enzyme.
   b. RNA copies of the original DNA are made.
   c. Extender probes are used to detect a positive reaction.
   d. Primers are used to make multiple DNA copies.
9. During PCR, what happens in the annealing step?
   a. The primers bind to the target DNA.
   b. Strands are separated by heating.
   c. An RNA copy is made.
   d. Protein is made from the DNA strands.

10. What is the purpose of an amplification control in qPCR?
    a. To avoid false positives
    b. To ensure accuracy of target detection
    c. To avoid contamination
    d. To avoid false negatives

11. Which technique is based on RNA amplification?
    a. PCR
    b. TMA
    c. dPCR
    d. SDA

12. Which is used in Sanger sequencing?
    a. UNG
    b. ddNTP
    c. ePCR
    d. FRET

13. What type of signal is generated in pyrosequencing?
    a. Light
    b. Fluorescence
    c. Ionic conductance
    d. Color

14. What is an NGS sequencing library?
    a. A database of clinically significant sequences
    b. A collection of software programs used for sequence analysis
    c. A collection of short templates to be sequenced simultaneously
    d. A list of all variants found in a sequencing run

15. In NGS, what is coverage?
    a. The percentage of sequences carrying a variant
    b. The number of genes sequenced
    c. The number of times a region is sequenced
    d. The percentage of the genome represented

13 Flow Cytometry and Laboratory Automation

Jeannie Guglielmo, MS, MAT, MLS [CM](ASCP), and Songkai Hu, MA, MLS [CM](ASCP)

LEARNING OUTCOMES

After finishing this chapter, you should be able to:

1. List and describe the function of each of the major components of a flow cytometer.
2. Compare intrinsic and extrinsic parameters in flow cytometry.
3. Discuss the advantages and disadvantages of automated testing in a clinical immunology laboratory.
4. Summarize the principle of hydrodynamic focusing within the flow cytometer.
5. Define the concept of fluorescence in flow cytometry.
6. Explain the difference between forward light scatter (FSC) and side scatter (SSC) and the cellular properties they identify.
7. Describe the difference between analyzing flow cytometry data using single-parameter histograms and dual-parameter dot plots.
8. Discuss clinical applications of flow cytometry.
9. Apply knowledge of T- and B-cell surface antigens to identify various cell populations.
10. Compare the advantages and disadvantages of automated immunoassay analyzers.
11. Explain the difference between a random-access analyzer and a batch analyzer.
12. Define accuracy, precision, reportable range, analytic sensitivity, analytic specificity, and reference interval.

CHAPTER OUTLINE

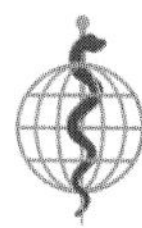

Go to FADavis.com for the laboratory exercises that accompany this text.

KEY TERMS

Accuracy
Analytic sensitivity
Analytic specificity
Automatic sampling
Batch analyzers
Dual-parameter dot plot
Extrinsic parameters
Flow cytometry
Fluorochrome
Forward scatter (FSC)
Gate
Immunophenotyping
Intrinsic parameters
Precision
Random-access analyzers
Reference interval
Reportable range
Side scatter (SSC)
Single-parameter histogram

Flow Cytometry

Flow cytometry is a system in which single cells (or beads) in a fluid suspension are analyzed in terms of their intrinsic light-scattering characteristics. The cells are simultaneously evaluated for their extrinsic properties (i.e., the presence of specific surface or cytoplasmic proteins) using fluorescent-labeled antibodies or probes. Flow cytometers, originally developed in the 1960s, did not make their way into the clinical laboratory until the early 1980s. At that point, physicians started seeing patients with a new mysterious disease characterized by a decrease in circulating T helper (Th) cells. Since that time, flow cytometry has been routinely used for monitoring HIV infection status, as well as **immunophenotyping** cells, or identifying their surface and cytoplasmic antigen expression.

Flow cytometers can simultaneously measure multiple cellular or bead properties by using several different fluorochromes. A **fluorochrome,** or fluorescent molecule, is one that absorbs light across a spectrum of wavelengths and emits light of lower energy across a spectrum of longer wavelengths. Each fluorochrome has a distinctive spectral pattern of absorption (excitation) and emission. By using laser light, different populations of cells or particles can be analyzed and identified on the basis of their size, shape, and antigenic properties.

Flow cytometry is frequently used in leukemia and lymphoma characterizations as well as in the identification of immunodeficiency diseases such as AIDS (see Chapters 18, 19, and 24). Flow cytometry is also used to enumerate hematopoietic stem cells, detect human leukocyte antigen (HLA) antibodies in transplantation, and identify cells undergoing apoptosis. In addition, flow cytometry has been applied in functional assays for chronic granulomatous disease (CGD) and leukocyte adhesion deficiency, fetal red blood cell (RBC) and F-cell identification in maternal blood, and identification of paroxysmal nocturnal hemoglobinuria (PNH), to give just a few examples. A significant advantage of flow cytometry is that because the flow rate of cells within the cytometer is so rapid, thousands of events can be analyzed in seconds, allowing for the accurate detection of cells that are present in very small numbers.

Instrumentation

The major components of a flow cytometer include the fluidics, the laser light source, and the optics and photodetectors. Data analysis and management are performed by computers.

Fluidics

For cellular parameters to be accurately measured in the flow cytometer, it is crucial that cells pass through the laser light one cell at a time. Cells are processed into a suspension; the cytometer draws up the cell suspension and injects the sample inside a carrier stream of isotonic saline (sheath fluid) to form a laminar flow. The sample stream is constrained by the carrier stream and is thus hydrodynamically focused so that the cells pass single file through the intersection of the laser light source **(Fig. 13–1).** Each time a cell passes in front of a laser beam, light is scattered, and the interruption of the laser signal is recorded.

Laser Light Source

Solid-state diode lasers are typically used as light sources. The wavelength of monochromatic light emitted by a laser in turn dictates which fluorochromes can be used in an assay. Not all fluorochromes can be used with all lasers because each fluorochrome has distinct spectral characteristics. Newer instruments have up to five lasers—red, blue, violet, ultraviolet (UV), and yellow-green—each of which produces different colors when exciting a particular fluorochrome. This allows for as many as 20 fluorochromes, or colors, to be analyzed in a single tube at one time.

Because of a cell passing through the laser, light is scattered in many directions. The amount and type of light scatter (LS) can provide valuable information about a cell's physical properties. Light at two specific angles is measured by the flow cytometer: (1) **forward scatter (FSC)** and (2) **side scatter (SSC),** also called *right-angle* LS. FSC is considered an indicator of size, whereas the SSC signal is indicative of granularity or the intracellular complexity of the cell. Thus, these two values can be used to characterize different cell types based on their inherent properties and are considered **intrinsic parameters.** If one looks at a sample of whole blood on a flow cytometer where all the RBCs have been lysed, the three major populations of white blood cells (WBCs)—lymphocytes, monocytes, and neutrophils—can be roughly differentiated from each other based solely on their intrinsic parameters (FSC and SSC) **(Fig. 13–2).**

Unlike FSC and SSC, which represent light-scattering properties that are intrinsic to the cell, **extrinsic parameters** require the addition of a fluorescent probe for their detection. Fluorescent-labeled antibodies bound to the cell can be detected with the laser. By using fluorescent molecules

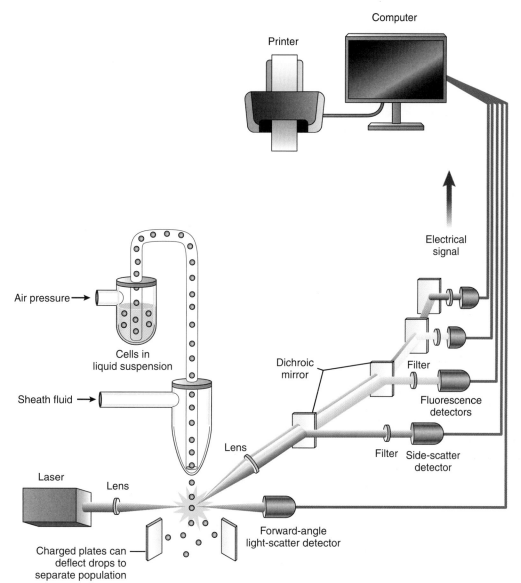

FIGURE 13–1 Flow cytometry. Components of a laser-based flow cytometer include the fluidics system for cell transportation, a laser for cell illumination, photodetectors for signal detection, and a computer-based data management system. Both forward and 90-degree LS are measured, indicating cell size and type.

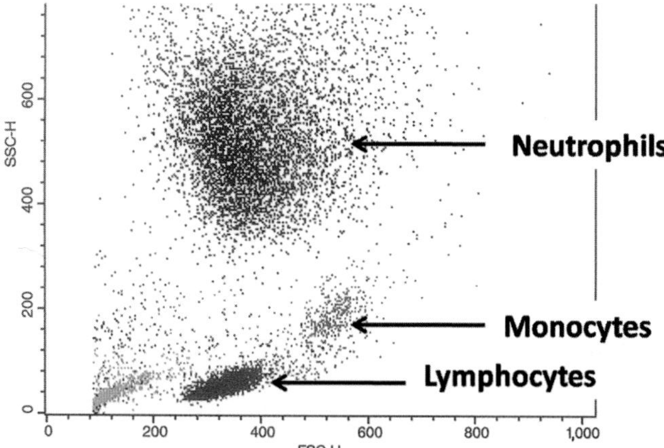

FIGURE 13–2 Peripheral blood leukocyte analysis by simultaneous evaluation of forward light scatter (FSC) and 90-degree LS (SSC). Based on the intrinsic characteristics of size (FSC) and complexity/granularity (SSC), the three main populations of WBCs (lymphocytes, monocytes, and neutrophils) can be discriminated into individual populations.

with various emission wavelengths, laboratory scientists can simultaneously evaluate an individual cell for several extrinsic properties. The clinical utility of such multicolor analysis is enhanced when the fluorescent data are analyzed in conjunction with FSC and SSC to enable more accurate subtyping. The combination of data allows for characterization of cells according to size, granularity, DNA and RNA content, antigens, total protein, and cell surface receptors.

Optics and Photodetectors

The various signals (light scatter and fluorescence) generated by the cells' interaction with the laser are detected by photodiodes for FSC and by photomultiplier tubes for fluorescence. The number of fluorochromes capable of being measured simultaneously depends upon the number of photomultiplier tubes in the flow cytometer. The specificity of each photomultiplier tube for a given band length of wavelengths is achieved through the arrangement of a series of optical filters that are designed to maximize collection of light derived from a specific fluorochrome while minimizing interference of light from other fluorochromes. The newer flow cytometers use fiber-optic cables to direct light to the detectors.

When fluorescence from labeled antibodies bound to cell surfaces reaches the photomultiplier tubes, it creates an electrical current that is converted into a voltage pulse. The voltage pulse is then converted into a digital signal using various methods, depending on the manufacturer. The digital signals are proportional to the intensity of light detected. The intensity of these converted signals is measured on a relative scale that is generally set into 1 to 256 channels, from the lowest energy level or pulse to the highest level.

Sample Preparation

Samples commonly used for analysis include whole blood, bone marrow, and fluid aspirates. Whole blood should be collected into ethylenediaminetetraacetic acid (EDTA), the anticoagulant of choice for samples processed within 30 hours of collection. Heparin can also be used for whole blood and bone marrow and can provide improved stability in samples for up to 48 hours. Blood should be stored at room temperature (20°C to 25°C) before processing and should be well mixed before being pipetted into staining tubes. Hemolyzed or clotted specimens should be rejected.

Peripheral blood, bone marrow, and other samples with large numbers of RBCs require erythrocyte removal to allow for efficient analysis of WBCs. Historically, density gradient centrifugation with Ficoll-Hypaque (Sigma, St. Louis, MO) was used to generate a cell suspension enriched for lymphocytes or lymphoblasts. However, this method results in selective loss of some cell populations and is time-consuming. Density-gradient centrifugation has mainly been replaced by erythrocyte lysis techniques, both commercial and non-commercial. Samples are treated with lysing buffers to destroy the erythrocytes while leaving the WBCs intact.

Tissue specimens such as lymph nodes should be collected and transported in tissue culture medium (RPMI 1640) at either room temperature (if analysis is imminent) or 4°C (if analysis will be delayed). The specimen is then disaggregated to form a single cell suspension, either by mechanical dissociation or enzymatic digestion. Mechanical disaggregation, or "teasing," is preferred and is accomplished by the use of a scalpel and forceps, a needle and syringe, or a wire mesh screen. Antibodies are then added to the resulting cellular preparation and the samples are processed for analysis. The antibodies used are typically monoclonal, each labeled with a different fluorescent tag.

Data Acquisition and Analysis

Once the intrinsic and extrinsic properties of the cells have been collected, the data are digitized and ready for analysis. Typically 10,000 to 20,000 "events" are collected for each sample. Each parameter can be analyzed independently or in any combination. Graphics of the data can be represented in multiple ways. The first level of representation is the **single-parameter histogram,** which plots a chosen parameter (generally fluorescence) on the *x*-axis versus the number of events on the *y*-axis; thus, only a single parameter is analyzed using this type of graph **(Fig. 13–3).** The operator can then set a marker to differentiate cells that have low levels of fluorescence (negative) from cells that have high levels of fluorescence (positive) for a particular fluorochrome-labeled antibody. The computer will then calculate the percentage of "negative" and "positive" events from the total number of events collected.

The next level of representation is the bivariate histogram, or **dual-parameter dot plot,** where each dot represents an individual cell or event. Two parameters, one on each axis, are plotted against each other. Each parameter to be analyzed is determined by the operator. Using dual-parameter dot plots, the operator can draw a "**gate**" around a population of interest and analyze various extrinsic and intrinsic parameters of the cells contained within the gated region **(Fig. 13–4).** The gate allows the operator to screen out debris and isolate subpopulations of cells of interest. Gates can be thought of as a set of filtering rules for analyzing a very large database. The operator

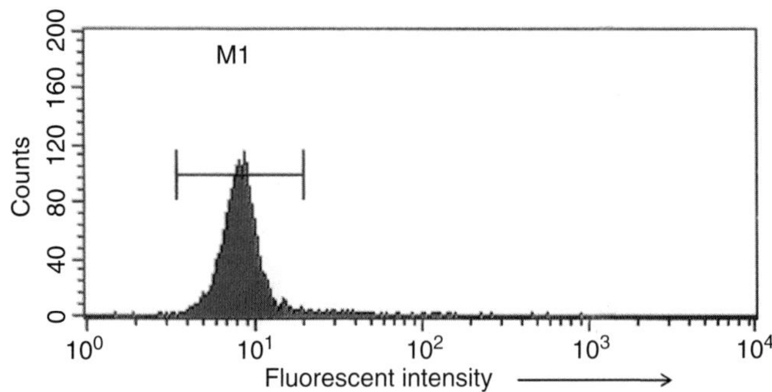

FIGURE 13–3 Example of a single-parameter flow histogram. The *y*-axis consists of the number of events. The *x*-axis is the parameter to be analyzed, which is chosen by the operator; it is usually an extrinsic parameter, such as a fluorescence. The operator can then set a marker to isolate the positive events. The computer will then calculate the percentage of positive events within the designated markers.

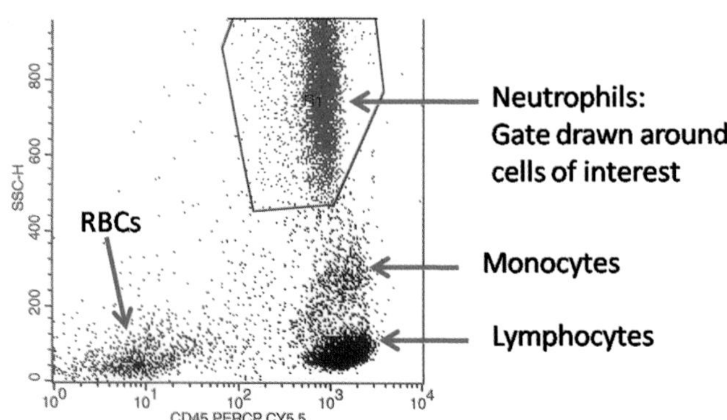

FIGURE 13–4 A dual-parameter dot plot. Both parameters on the *x*- and *y*-axes are chosen by the operator. In this case, lysed whole blood is analyzed for CD45 (*x*-axis) and SSC (*y*-axis). The operator then draws a "gate" to isolate the population of interest (e.g., granulocytes) for further analysis.

can filter the data in any way and set multiple or sequential filters (or gates).

When analyzing a population of cells using a dual-parameter dot plot, the operator chooses which parameters to analyze on both the *x*- and *y*-axes, divides the dot plot into four quadrants, and separates the positive events from the negative events in each axis **(Fig. 13–5)**. Quadrant 1 consists of cells that are positive for fluorescence on the *y*-axis and negative for fluorescence on the *x*-axis. Quadrant 2 consists of cells that are positive for fluorescence on both the *x*- and *y*-axes. Quadrant 3 consists of cells that are negative for fluorescence on both the *x*- and *y*-axes. Quadrant 4 consists of cells that are positive for fluorescence on the *x*-axis and negative for fluorescence on the *y*-axis. The computer and specialized software will calculate the percentage of cells in each quadrant based on the total number of events counted.

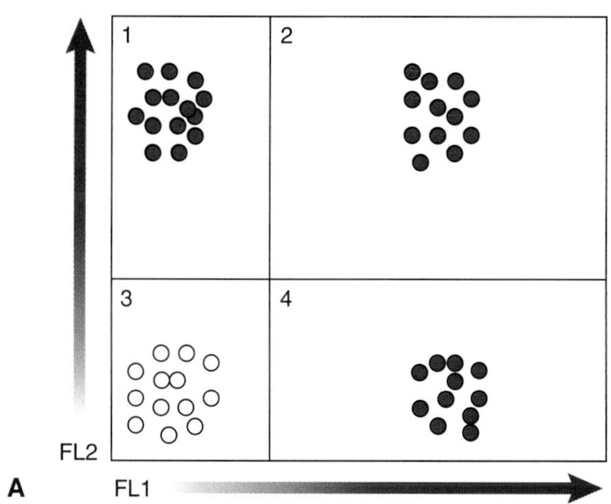

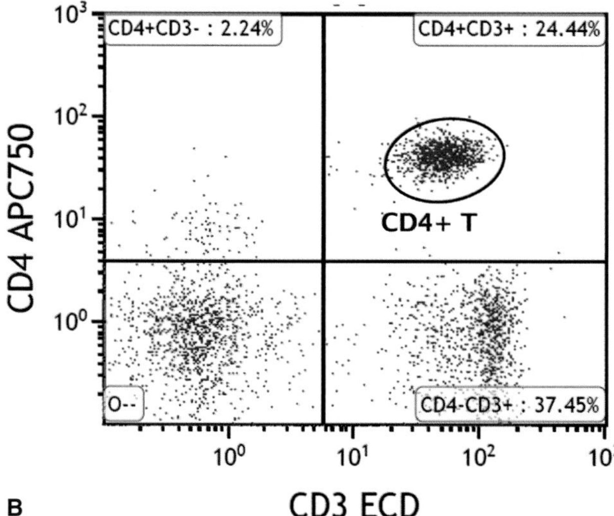

FIGURE 13–5 Quadrant analysis of a dual-parameter dot plot. The operator chooses which parameters to analyze on each axis. (A) On each axis, there are fluorescence positive and fluorescence negative cells. (B) Example of a dual-parameter dot plot to identify CD4+ T cells: CD3 on the *x*-axis and CD4 on the *y*-axis. The cells in quadrant 2 that are positive for both CD3 and CD4 are true CD4+ T cells.

A gate can be drawn around a population of cells based on their FSC versus SSC characteristics, and the extrinsic characteristics of the gated population can then be analyzed. For example, lymphocytes can be gated, after which the T-cell subpopulations (CD3+, CD4+ or CD3+, CD8+) and B cells (CD38+, CD3–) can be analyzed **(Fig. 13–6)**. The absolute count of a particular cell type—for instance, CD4+ T lymphocytes—can be obtained by multiplying the absolute cell count of the population of interest (e.g., lymphocytes) derived by a hematology analyzer by the percentage of the fluorescent-positive cells in the sample CD3+, CD4+ lymphocytes. This method is considered a dual-platform analysis. The disadvantage to this type of analysis is that it has a greater potential for added error associated with the use of two distinct methods to derive the absolute count. The single platform is now the method of choice to eliminate this type of error. Single platforms can be achieved by two types of methods: bead-based or volumetric. In the bead-based method, a known quantity of fluorescent beads is added to the flow cytometry tubes, and a simple mathematic calculation allows the absolute WBC numbers to be directly determined from the individual flow cytometry tubes. In the volumetric method, the precise volume of the sample can be used to calculate the absolute number of events.

Detailed phenotypic analysis can determine the lineage and clonality, as well as the degree of differentiation and activation, of a specific cell population. This information is useful for differential diagnosis or clarification of closely related lymphoproliferative disorders (see Chapter 18). Immunophenotyping requires careful selection of combinations of individual markers based on a given cell lineage and maturation stage. Attempts to standardize individual marker panels, especially by European laboratory groups, are ongoing; however, the markers selected for inclusion in testing panels vary from institution to institution.

Clinical Applications

Routine applications of flow cytometry in the clinical laboratory can be divided into two categories: nonmalignant immunophenotyping and malignant immunophenotyping. Nonmalignant immunophenotyping includes the characterization and enumeration of normal lymphocytes, such as CD4+ T cells and CD34+ stem cells. *Malignant immunophenotyping* refers to immunophenotypic characterization of leukemias, lymphomas, and other hematopoietic disorders.

Immunophenotyping by flow cytometry has become an important component of initial evaluation and subsequent post-therapeutic monitoring in leukemia and lymphoma management. Flow cytometric findings have been incorporated into current leukemia and lymphoma classifications, beginning with the Revised European-American Lymphoma (REAL) classification in 1994 and, more recently, in the World Health Organization (WHO) classifications. One of the most important components of flow cytometric analysis is the stratification of hematopoietic malignancies by their lineage (i.e., B cell, T cell, or myeloid) and degree of differentiation.

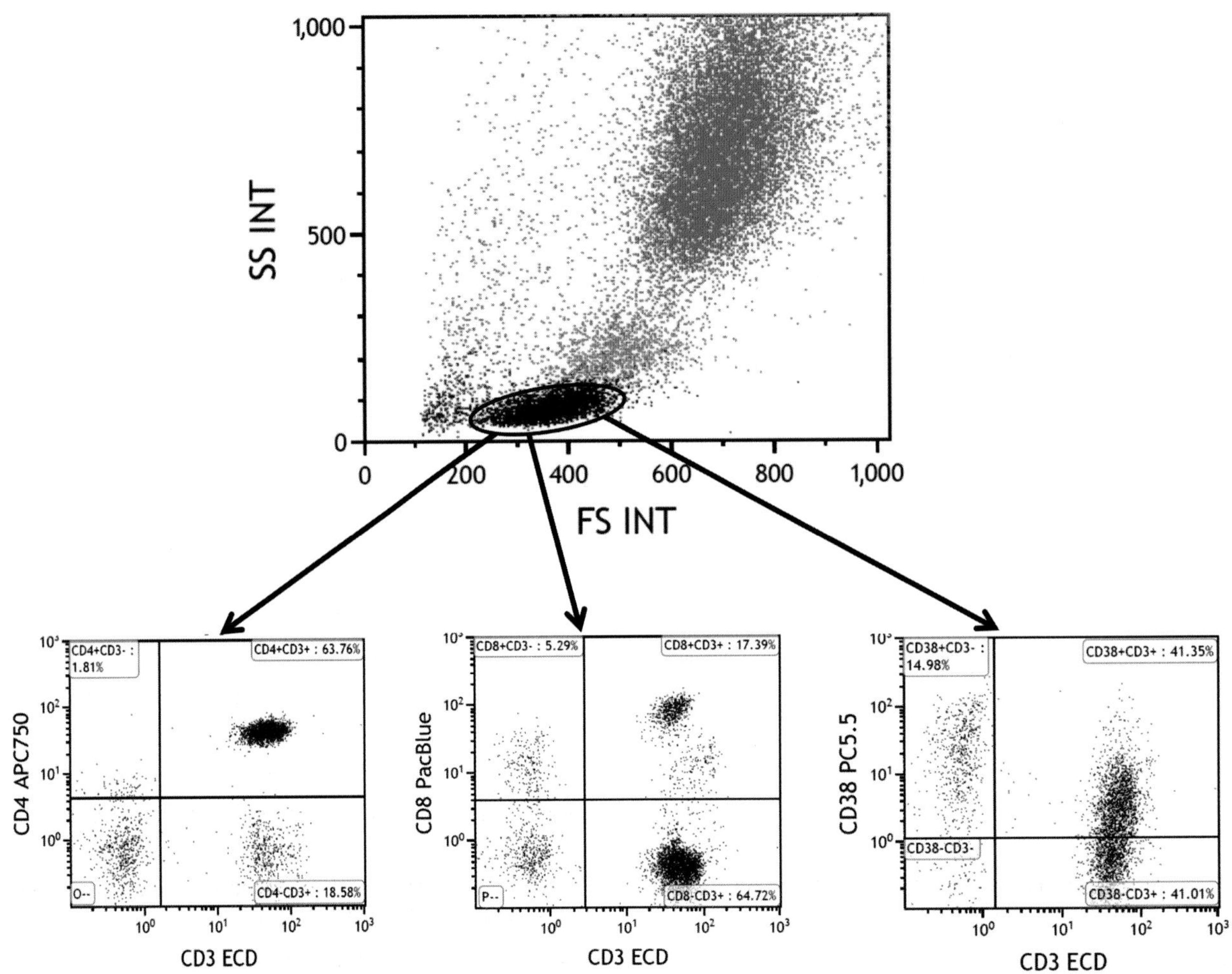

FIGURE 13–6 Gating strategy to analyze lymphocyte subsets in a sample of whole blood. Whole blood is incubated with fluorescent-labeled antibodies specific for CD3, CD4, CD8, and HLA-DR. The sample is washed, RBCs are lysed, and the sample is analyzed on the flow cytometer. To analyze using gating strategies, the sample is first plotted using FSC versus SSC. (A) A gate, or region, is drawn around the lymphocyte population. (B) On the subsequent plots of fluorescent markers, only the lymphocyte population is analyzed. The dot plot is divided into four quadrants to isolate positive from negative populations. The computer calculates the percentage of positive cells in each quadrant. The three flow contour plots are analyzing two different cell surface markers. In the first dot plot, quadrant 2 (upper right) identifies CD4+ CD3+ T-helper-cell lymphocytes. Quadrant 3 (lower left) includes B lymphocytes and natural killer (NK) cells. Quadrant 4 (lower right) identifies CD3+ CD4– T-cell lymphocytes. In the second dot plot, quadrant 1 (upper left) identifies low-intensity CD8+ CD3– NK cells. Quadrant 2 identifies CD3+ CD8+ T-cytotoxic lymphocytes. Quadrant 3 contains any lymphocyte that is not CD8+, CD3+ (B-cell lymphocytes). Quadrant 4 contains CD3+ CD8– T helper cell lymphocytes. In the third contour plot, quadrant 1 identifies CD38+ CD3– B cells, quadrant 2 identifies CD38+ CD3+ activated T cells, quadrant 3 contains CD38– CD3– cells, and quadrant 4 identifies CD3+ CD38– T cells, not activated.

Some of the more common cell-differentiation antigens are listed in **Table 13–1.**

Knowing the unique characteristics of leukemias and lymphomas and pairing the specific markers that identify these characteristics can be useful in making a more reliable diagnosis. For example, in chronic lymphocytic leukemia (CLL), typically CD5 (a T-cell lymphocyte marker) is paired with CD20 (a B-cell lymphocyte marker) for analysis. The presence of a significant number of cells that are both CD5+ and CD20+ is an indication of CLL or mantle cell lymphoma. Common marker combinations are shown in **Table 13–2.**

CD45 is a pan-leukocyte marker present on all WBCs but with varying levels of expression based on the cell's maturity as well as lineage. This variance in expression results in different levels of fluorescence. Blasts express lower levels of CD45 (low fluorescence) but show an increase of CD45 expression as the cell matures; therefore, mature WBCs have much brighter CD45 fluorescence compared with their earlier progenitor stages. The analysis of CD45 expression levels is useful in differentiating various populations of WBCs and, in combination with SSC, has replaced gating by FSC and SSC in many laboratories. However, it is always a good idea to examine the FSC and SSC plot to be sure a population is not being missed.

Immunophenotyping of WBC populations is also essential when an immunodeficiency is suspected. Patient values are compared with reference ranges established by the clinical laboratory performing the testing. Typical ranges for B cells, T-cell subsets, and natural killer (NK) cells are listed in **Table 13–3.**

Table 13–1 Surface Markers on Leukocytes

ANTIGEN	CELL TYPE	FUNCTION
CD2	Thymocytes, T cells, NK cells	Involved in T-cell activation
CD3	Thymocytes, T cells	Associated with T-cell antigen receptor; role in TCR signal transduction
CD4	T helper cells, monocytes, macrophages	Co-receptor for class II MHC; receptor for HIV
CD5	Mature T cells, thymocytes, subset of B cells (B1 cells)	Positive or negative modulation of T- and B-cell receptor signaling
CD7	T cells, thymocytes, NK cells, pre-B cells	Regulates peripheral T-cell and NK cell cytokine production
CD8	Thymocyte subsets, cytotoxic T cells	Co-receptor for class I MHC
CD10	Bone marrow stromal cells	Protease; marker for pre-B cells; CALLA
CD11b	Myeloid and NK cells	αM subunit of integrin CR3, binds complement component iC3b, myeloid cell adhesion
CD13	Myelomonocytic cells	Zinc metalloproteinase
CD14	Monocytic cells	Lipopolysaccharide receptor
CD15	Neutrophils, eosinophils, monocytes	Terminal trisaccharide expressed on glycolipids
CD16	Macrophages, NK cells, neutrophils	Low-affinity Fc receptor, mediates phagocytosis and ADCC
CD19	B cells, follicular dendritic cells	Part of B-cell co-receptor, signal transduction molecule that regulates B-cell development and activation
CD20	B cells, T-cell subsets	Binding activates signaling pathways, regulates B-cell activation
CD21	B cells, follicular dendritic cells, subset of immature thymocytes	Receptor for complement component C3d; part of B-cell co-receptor with CD19
CD22	B cells, B-ALL (surface and cytoplasmic), B-CLL, HCL, PLL	Involved in B-cell adhesion and B-cell signaling
CD23	B cells, monocytes, follicular dendritic cells	Regulation of IgE synthesis; triggers release of IL-1, IL-6, and GM-CSF from monocytes
CD25	Activated T cells, B cells, monocytes	Receptor for IL-2
CD33	Myeloid cell, monocytes, macrophages, granulocytes (weak), myeloid-Pro, myeloid leukemia, AML	Cell adhesion and signaling; receptor that inhibits proliferation of myeloid cells
CD34	Hematopoietic progenitor cells, endothelial cells, immature leukemias	Cell adhesion, hematopoiesis
CD38	Plasma cells, thymocytes, NK cells, early B lymphocytes, monocytes, multiple myeloma, ALL, acute myeloblastic leukemia	Regulates cell adhesion, activation, and proliferation
CD44	Most leukocytes	Adhesion molecule mediating homing to peripheral lymphoid organs
CD45	All hematopoietic cells	Tyrosine phosphatase, augments signaling
CD56	NK cells, subsets of T cells, neural tissue	Cell adhesion
CD57	NK cells, subsets of T cells	NK cell subsets, T-cell subsets, small cell lung carcinoma
CD94	NK cells, subsets of T cells	Subunit of NKG2-A complex involved in inhibition of NK cell cytotoxicity
CD103	Intraepithelial lymphocytes, HCL, adult T-cell leukemia	Ligand for E-cadherin, an adhesion molecule on epithelial cells
CD138	Plasma cells, pre-B cells, epithelial cells, neural cells, breast cancer cells	Transmembrane proteoglycans that play a role in cell adhesion, migration, and proliferation

(continued)

Table 13–1 Surface Markers on Leukocytes—cont'd

ANTIGEN	CELL TYPE	FUNCTION
HLA-DR	B lymphocytes, activated T lymphocytes, monocytes; lack of expression is diagnostic of M3 myeloid leukemia	T-cell activation
FCM7	B-cell subset, mantle lymphoma	In vitro response to antigens or mitogens
Kappa chains	B cells	Light-chain part of antibody molecule on B cells
Lambda chains	B cells	Light-chain part of antibody molecule on B cells

ADCC = antibody-dependent cellular cytotoxicity; ALL= acute lymphocytic leukemia; AML= acute myeloid leukemia; CALLA = common acute lymphoblastic leukemia antigen; CLL= chronic lymphocytic leukemia; Fc = fragment crystallizable; GM-CSF = granulocyte-macrophage colony-stimulating factor; HCL = hairy cell leukemia; IgE = immunoglobulin E; IL = interleukin; MHC = major histocompatibility class; NK = natural killer; PLL= prolymphocytic leukemia; TCR = CD3-αβ receptor complex.

Table 13–2 Common Markers Used for Lymphoproliferative and Myeloproliferative Studies in Clinical Flow Cytometry

DISEASE	ANTIBODIES PAIRED	INTERPRETATION
Chronic lymphocytic leukemia (CLL) and prolymphocytic leukemia	FMC7 with CD23	FMC7 negative and CD23 positive in CLL, CD23 negative and FMC7 positive in mantle cell lymphoma
	CD5 with CD20	When a cell is both CD5 positive and CD20 positive: characteristic of CLL and well-differentiated lymphocytic lymphoma (WDLL), as well as mantle cell lymphoma
	CD19 with kappa CD19 with lambda	CD19 positive with only one light chain (kappa or lambda) is expressed in low intensity; occasionally light chains are not detected
	CD45 with CD14	CD45 fluorescence is brightly expressed and CD14 negative
	(anti-glycophorin added to bone marrows)	Used to determine erythroid component of the specimen
Hairy cell leukemia (HCL)	CD3 with CD23	CD3 negative and CD23 negative
	CD11c with CD22	Brightly expressed CD11c and CD22, unlike CLL
	CD20 with CD5	CD20 positive and CD5 negative (occasionally weak expression of CD5)
	CD19 with kappa	CD19 positive with one monoclonal light chain expressed
	CD103 with CD25	CD103 is highly specific for HCL, and CD25 is usually expressed; hairy cell variants may be negative for these two markers
	CD21 with HLA-DR	CD21 negative and DR positive
	CD45 with CD14	CD45 is brightly expressed and CD14 negative
	(anti-glycophorin added to bone marrows)	To determine erythroid component of the specimen, CD10 (CALLA) is weakly expressed in 26% of cases
B-cell acute lymphocytic leukemia (ALL)	CD3 with HLA-DR	CD3 (T-cell receptor) negative and HLA-DR positive
	CD5 with CD20	CD5 negative and CD20 variably positive (low intensity or negative on precursor B-cell ALL, positive on more mature B-cell ALL)
	CD19 with kappa CD19 with lambda	CD19 positive (stem cell is negative) and surface Ig negative (a mature B-cell ALL may have surface immunoglobulin)
	CD34 with CD38	CD34 positive ALL correlates with good prognosis in pediatric patients and poor prognosis in adults; CD38 is positive from stem cell to pre-B ALL
	TdT with CD10	TdT and CD10 (CALLA) positive in common ALL and pre-B ALL; CD10 positivity is associated with favorable complete treatment response and disease-free survival; CD10 is usually high intensity
	TdT with CD33	CD33 negative; however, very early B-ALL may be positive
	CD45 with CD14	CD45 dimly expressed and CD14 negative
	(anti-glycophorin added to bone marrows)	Used to determine erythroid component of the specimen

(continued)

Table 13–2 Common Markers Used for Lymphoproliferative and Myeloproliferative Studies in Clinical Flow Cytometry—cont'd

DISEASE	ANTIBODIES PAIRED	INTERPRETATION
Myeloma plasmacytoid leukemia or lymphoma	CD3 with HLA-DR	CD3 negative; most are HLA-DR negative, although some early plasmacytoid cells may be DR positive
	CD5 with CD20	CD5 and CD20 negative
	CD19 with kappa CD19 with lambda	CD19 and surface Ig negative; occasionally surface Ig is positive; cytoplasmic Ig positive
	CD45 with CD38	CD45 negative or low intensity; CD38 is high-intensity positive
	CD40 with CD56	Usually CD40 positive; CD56 has been reported to be positive on myeloma cells but negative on normal plasma cells
	CD10	CD10 positivity indicates poor prognosis
	CD138	Syndecan-1 positive in mature plasma cells
	CD45 with CD14	CD14 negative
T-cell acute lymphoblastic leukemia (ALL)	CD1a with CD3	CD1a positivity associated with longer disease-free survival in adult T-cell ALL; CD3 is negative in 99% of cases (exception is mature medullary thymocyte T-cell ALL)
	CD2 with CD25	CD2 variably expressed and CD25 negative
	CD38 with CD7	CD38 and CD7 are positive
	CD4 with CD8	CD4 and CD8 variably expressed depending on maturity; dual expression is common
	CD5 with CD20	CD5 positive except for prothymocyte stage T-cell ALL, CD20 negative
	CD45 with CD14	CD45 positive and CD14 negative
	HLA-DR with CD34	DR positive T-cell ALL associated with a worse prognosis; CD34 in pediatric patients associated with CNS involvement and poor prognosis and predicts myeloid expression
	TdT with CD10	TdT is positive; CD10 positive T-cell ALL associated with prolonged disease-free survival
	CD19 and kappa	Negative
	CD19 with lambda	Negative
	(anti-glycophorin added to bone marrows)	To determine erythroid component to the specimen
Post-thymic T-cell leukemia or lymphoma	CD1a with CD3	CD1a negative, CD3 positive; note: peripheral T-cell lymphomas lack 1 or more pan–T-cell antigens (CD3, CD2, CD5, or CD7) 75% of the time
Peripheral T-cell leukemia	CD2 with CD25	CD2 positive; CD25 positive in adult T-cell leukemias and some peripheral T-cell lymphomas
Adult T-cell leukemia	CD5 with CD7	CD5 positive; CD7 positive except in adult T-cell leukemia
	CD4 with CD8	Variable expression
	CD19 with kappa	Negative
	CD19 with lambda	Negative
	CD45 with CD14	CD45 positive and CD14 negative
	TdT with CD10	Negative
	(anti-glycophorin added to bone marrows)	To determine erythroid component of the specimen
Tγ proliferative disease (NK-like T-cell leukemia) NK-like T-cell lymphoma	CD2 with CD57	NK-like T-cell lymphoma tends to be CD56 positive, CD57 negative and is usually clinically aggressive; NK cell leukemias tend to be CD56 or CD16 positive, CD57 negative and are usually clinically aggressive; Tγ proliferative disease is CD56 negative, CD57 positive and exhibits a chronic indolent course; CD2 is usually positive for all, but there are variants
NK cell leukemia	CD3 with CD56, CD16	Surface CD3 is positive in Tγ proliferative disease and NK-like T-cell lymphoma; CD3 is negative in NK cell leukemia; for CD56 and CD57, see above
	CD11c with CD11b	Usually positive
	CD4 with CD8	Usually CD8 positive, CD4 negative; however, dual staining and CD4 positivity have been reported
	CD19	Negative
	CD45 with CD14	CD45 positive and CD14 negative

(continued)

Table 13–2 Common Markers Used for Lymphoproliferative and Myeloproliferative Studies in Clinical Flow Cytometry—cont'd

DISEASE	ANTIBODIES PAIRED	INTERPRETATION
Acute myelogenous leukemia (AML)	CD11c with CD11b	CD11c positive on mature myeloid cells; CD11b positive on myelomonocytic cells, eosinophilic myelocytes, eosinophils, and neutrophils; differentiated AML usually expresses mature markers
	CD13 with CD15	Poorly differentiated AML usually lacks CD15, CD11c, CD11b, but positive for CD13
	CD33 with TdT	CD33 in the absence of CD34, HLA-DR, or CD13 suggests immature acute basophilic or mast cell leukemia; TdT is often expressed in low intensity in poorly differentiated AML
	CD14 with CD64	CD14 on early promonocytes to mature monocytes; high expression of CD14 and CD11b predicts poor outcome; CD64 on immature and mature monocytes
	CD3 with CD7	CD3 negative; some immature AML expresses CD7
	CD19 with kappa	CD19 occasionally expressed on some primitive AML
	CD19 with lambda	Surface Ig negative
	CD34 with HLA-DR	Poorly differentiated AML often expresses CD34; high-intensity CD34 has worse prognosis; CD34 coexpressed with HLA-DR has worse prognosis; lack of HLA-DR indicates either APL or very immature AML
	CD10 with TdT	CD10 is present on neutrophils
	(anti-glycophorin added to bone marrows)	To determine erythroid component present in the specimen
	MPO with CD117	Myeloperoxidase (MPO) is found on fairly mature AMLs, whereas CD117 is a myeloid blast marker

ADCC = antibody-dependent cell cytotoxicity; CALLA = common acute lymphoblastic leukemia antigen; Fc = fragment crystallizable; GM-CSF = granulocyte-macrophage colony-stimulating factor; IgE = immunoglobulin E; MHC = major histocompatibility class; NK = natural killer; TCR = CD3-αβ receptor complex; TdT = terminal deoxynucleotidyl transferase.

Table 13–3 Reference Ranges for Lymphocyte Populations in Peripheral Blood*

MARKER	CELL POPULATION	% OF TOTAL LYMPHOCYTES	ABSOLUTE NUMBER OF LYMPHOCYTES (CELLS/≮L)
CD19	B lymphocytes	6–23	91–610
CD3	Total T lymphocytes	62–87	570–2,400
CD4	Helper T cells**	32–64	430–1,800
CD8	Cytotoxic T cells**	15–46	210–1,200
CD16/CD56	NK cells	4–26	78–470

**Reference values vary by age and testing laboratory. Values in table were obtained from ARUP Laboratories for individuals aged 16 to 64 years (http://ltd.aruplab.com/Tests/Pub/0095892).*

***The ARUP reference range for the ratio of helper T to cytotoxic T cells (CD4:CD8) for persons 16 to 64 years is 0.80 to 3.90.*

Flow cytometry is essential to the evaluation of immunodeficiency resulting from infection with HIV, which can lead to AIDS. Enumeration of peripheral blood CD4+ T cells in HIV-infected patients by the flow cytometry laboratory is used to classify stages of HIV disease and determine treatment options (see Chapter 24). HIV type 1 (HIV-1) infections cause a rapid, profound decrease in CD4+ T-cell numbers and an expansion of CD8+ T-cell levels during the early course of the illness (12 to 18 months). Some individuals continue to rapidly lose CD4+ T cells and progress to AIDS, whereas others maintain relatively stable CD4+ T-cell counts and remain AIDS-free for years. During the chronic phase of HIV-1 disease, there can be a slow decline in CD4+ T cells throughout many years because of available therapies and maintenance of homeostatic mechanisms in the patient. If these mechanisms fail, further declines in CD4+ T and CD8+ T cells occur, leading to the development of AIDS.

Connections

CD4 T- Cell Counts and Staging of HIV Infection

CD4+ T-cell numbers are used to stage HIV disease progression and are prognostic for the development of AIDS. CD4 T-cell counts are also used to monitor patient response to antiretroviral therapy; numbers of CD4 T cells will increase if therapy is successful. Table 24–2 (Chapter 24) shows the incorporation of CD4 values in defining stages of HIV infection, per the Centers for Disease Control and Prevention (CDC) guidelines.

Flow cytometry is also the method of choice for the diagnosis of several inherited immunodeficiency diseases such as Bruton's tyrosine kinase deficiency, which is characterized by a lack of circulating mature B cells (CD19+). Another example is chronic granulomatous disease, an X-linked or autosomal recessive disease in which neutrophils are defective in their oxidative burst. In this case, neutrophils are exposed to the dye dihydrorhodamine 123, which is not fluorescent until oxidized. When normal neutrophils are stimulated in vitro, the dye is oxidized and becomes intensely fluorescent. Neutrophils from patients with CGD are unable to oxidize the dye and do not become fluorescent after stimulation.

Another example is paroxysmal nocturnal hemoglobinuria (PNH), an inherited disease characterized by hemolytic anemia. The RBCs, neutrophils, monocytes, and other cells of patients with PNH lack the glycosylphosphatidylinositol (GPI) anchors by which many surface proteins are attached to the cell membrane. Therefore, the RBCs are fragile. Hemolysis occurs during pH changes in the blood, typically at night. Several flow cytometry tests are available to detect this defect. One test looks for the antigens that use the GPI anchor because these antigens will be missing or reduced in patients with PNH. Another test detects the GPI anchor itself by its ability to bind to fluorescent aerolysin (FLAER). Normal granulocytes and monocytes will be fluorescent because they possess the anchor, whereas the fluorescence in PNH cells missing the anchor will be reduced or absent.

Immunophenotyping has also become an essential test in the diagnosis and monitoring of patients with leukemias and lymphomas (see Chapter 18). Finding a small number of abnormal cells in a particular cell population can be easily accomplished by flow cytometry. Patients who have been treated for leukemia or lymphoma can be monitored for "minimal residual disease" (MRD) because statistically significant rare cell events can be easily detected. Likewise, in the case of a fetal-maternal hemorrhage, using flow cytometry to detect hemoglobin F-positive cells is much more sensitive than the traditional Kleihauer–Betke method.

Additional examples of flow cytometry use include the determination of DNA content or ploidy status of tumor cells. This analysis can provide physicians with important prognostic information. Ploidy analysis is also useful in examining products of conception for molar pregnancies.

Flow cytometry also has applications in transplant immunology. HLA typing and cross-matching for solid-organ transplantation can be performed by flow cytometry much faster and more accurately than other serological methods (see Chapter 16).

Finally, other important uses for flow technology in clinical diagnosis involve cytometric bead arrays. In this technology, beads of various sizes and different fluorescent levels are used to identify multiple analytes at the same time. Theoretically, this technology has the potential to detect 100 analytes from a single blood sample.

For example, in testing for anti-nuclear antibodies, different colored beads can be coated with different nuclear antigens. Patient serum is then added, followed by fluorescent anti-IgG. If the patient has a particular anti-nuclear antibody, the respective bead will fluoresce and can be identified and quantitated (see Chapter 15). Similarly, molecular techniques such as polymerase chain reaction (PCR) and hybridization can be performed on cytometric beads to detect viral nucleic acids and various genetic mutations (see Chapter 12 for a discussion of molecular methods).

Flow cytometry relies on the use of fluorescent-labeled monoclonal and polyclonal antibodies. Monoclonal antibodies are preferable to polyclonal antibodies for immunophenotyping. The commercial availability of monoclonal antibody reagents has contributed greatly to the accuracy of flow cytometry and has widened its use.

Connections

Monoclonal Antibodies

Recall from Chapter 5 that monoclonal antibodies are produced through hybridoma and recombinant DNA techniques. Because these antibodies are directed against a single epitope on an antigen, they are highly specific. Monoclonal antibodies against the CD antigens are commercially available and are used routinely in immunophenotyping to identify various leukocyte populations.

Immunoassay Automation

In addition to flow cytometry, the use of automated technology has become more prevalent in clinical immunology laboratories with the advent of immunoassay analyzers. Reliable immunoassay instrumentation, excluding radioimmunoassay, was first available in the early 1990s. Using a solid support for separating free and bound analytes, these instruments have made it possible to automate heterogeneous immunoassays even for low-level peptides such as peptide hormones. Currently, there are more than 60 different automated immunoassay analyzers that are capable of performing almost all common diagnostic immunoassays; they have largely replaced manual testing, especially in larger laboratories.

The driving motivation for the development of immunoassay analyzers has been the need to create an automated system capable of reducing or eliminating the many manual tasks required to perform analytical procedures and the demand to handle large volumes of samples. Eliminating manual steps decreases the likelihood of error by reducing the potential error caused by fatigue or erroneous sampling. Laboratory professionals are also trying to streamline test performance to reduce turnaround time and cost per test. Automation, in some cases, is much more accurate and precise compared with manual methods; depending on the assay platform, it may be more sensitive as well. Other potential benefits of immunoassay automation include the ability to provide more services with less staff, saving on controls, avoiding duplicate and repeat testing, longer shelf life of reagents and less disposal because of outdating, and sample delivery with bar codes for better sample identification.

Because of the wide variety of automated immunoassay analyzers available, it can be difficult to determine the best instrument for any given laboratory. **Table 13–4** offers a partial list of the many factors to consider in determining what type of analyzer will fulfill a laboratory's needs. It is important for all those involved in the instrument's selection to prioritize the properties of any analyzer to meet the demands of the laboratory.

There are currently two main types of immunoassay analyzers on the market: batch analyzers and random-access analyzers **(Table 13–5)**. **Batch analyzers** can examine multiple samples and provide access to the test samples for the formation of subsequent reaction mixtures. However, such batch analyzers permit only one type of analysis at a time. In some cases, this may be considered a drawback; stat samples cannot be loaded randomly, and there cannot be multiple analyses on any one sample. Partially for those reasons, the next generation of analyzers was designed in a modular system that could be configured to measure numerous analytes from multiple samples. These types of analyzers are called **random-access analyzers;** in these analyzers, many test samples can be analyzed, and several different tests can be performed on any one sample.

Automation can and does occur in all three stages of laboratory testing: the preanalytical, analytical, and post-analytical stages. For the purposes of this section, discussion is limited to automation within the analytical stage of testing.

The tasks of the analytical stage include introducing a sample, adding reagent, mixing the reagent and sample, incubating, detecting, calculating, and reporting the readout or results. All or some of these tasks may be automated on various immunoassay analyzers. **Automatic sampling** can be accomplished by several different methods; peristaltic pumps (older technology) and positive-liquid displacement pipettes (newer technology) are two examples. In most systems, samples are pipetted using thin, stainless-steel probes. Such probes have clot detectors that will automatically reject a sample if a clot is detected. They also have a liquid-level sensor that can detect the lack of sample in a tube, usually because of a short draw. Samples without the proper amount of liquid in them are also rejected. An issue associated with reusable pipette probes is carryover or contamination of one

Table 13–4 Factors for Consideration in Selecting an Automated Immunoassay Instrument

CATEGORY	FACTOR
Analytical	Sensitivity Precision Accuracy and test standardization Linearity Interferences Carryover effects
Economic	Purchase cost Lease options Shipping and installation fees Maintenance costs Reagent costs Operator time and costs Disposable costs Training for personnel Warranty
Instrument	Maintenance requirements Automation compatibility/LIMS compatibility Space requirements Utility requirements (electrical and HVAC) Reliability Clot error detection Hardware costs Nonwarranty service
Manufacturer	Future product plans Speed of service response Reputation Technical support Menu expansion plans Purchase of a warranty/service contract
Operational	Test menu Throughput Reagent capacity Reagent stability Stat capability Reflex testing ability Reagent kit size/availability Training requirements Operating complexity Waste requirements Reagent storage requirements Reagent performance Downtime plans

HVAC = heating, ventilation, and air conditioning; LIMS = laboratory information management systems; STAT = From the Latin word statum, meaning 'immediately; in other words, testing should be done immediately- this is a common abbreviation.

Adapted from Remaley AT, Hortin GL. Protein analysis for diagnostic applications. In: Detrick B, Hamilton RG, Folds JD, et al., eds. Manual of Molecular and Clinical Laboratory Immunology. *7th ed. Washington, DC: American Society for Microbiology; 2006:15; and Appold K. Checklist for buying a chemistry analyzer. Clin Lab Products. Nov. 2013:12–15.*

Table 13-5 Automated Immunoassay Analyzers

MANUFACTURER	INSTRUMENT	OPERATIONAL TYPE	ASSAY PRINCIPLE
Abbott Diagnostics	AxSYM	Continuous random-access stat processing	FPIA, MEIA
Abbott Diagnostics	Architect Series: Ci4100, Ci8200, Ci6200, i1000SR, i2000SR, i4000SR	Batch, random access, continuous random access	Enhanced chemiluminescence
DYNEX Technologies	Agility DS2 DSX	Batch	EIA
Awareness Technology	ChemWell	Batch, random access	EIA
Beckman Coulter	Access UniCel DXI 800 Access UniCel DXI 600 Access	Continuous random access, stat capability (up to 400 tests/hr) (up to 200 tests/hr)	Chemiluminescence, EIA
BioMérieux	VIDAS miniVIDAS (multiparametric IA)	Batch, random-access stat capability	FEIA-coated SPR Solid-phase receptacle SPR pipetting device
Bio-Rad Laboratories, Clinical Diagnosis Group	BioPlex 2200 Multiplex Testing PhD System	Continuous random access Batch	Bead flow cytometric (multiplex) EIA
Diamedix Corporation	Mago 4S Automated Immunoassay System Mago Plus Automated EIA Processor	Batch, random access	EIA ELISA and IFA
DiaSorin, Inc.	ETI-MAX (Germany/Italy)	Batch, random access	EIA
Dynex	DS2	Batch	EIA
Hycor Biomedical, Inc.	HYTEC 288 Plus	Random batches	EIA
Inova	BIO-FLASH Ds2	Batch, continued random access	Chemiluminescence
Inverness Medical Professional Diagnostics	AIMS (Automated IA Multiplexing System)	Batch	EIA, multiplexing or bead diagnostics
Ortho Clinical Diagnostics, a J&J Co.	VITROS 3600	Continuous random access	Chemiluminescence (enhanced)
Phadia Thermo Fisher Scientific-Phadia	ImmunoCAP Phadia Laboratory System	Continuous random access	FEIA
Siemens Medical Solutions Diagnostics	ADVIA Centaur Dimension EXL Dimension Vista 1500 IMMULITE	Continuous random access Batch, random access, continuous random access Continuous random access	Chemiluminescence Chemiluminescence, EIA Chemiluminescence
TOSOH Bioscience, Inc.	AIA	Continuous random access	Fluorescence, EIA

EIA = enzyme immunoassay; ELISA = enzyme-linked immunosorbent assay; FEIA = fluoroenzyme immunoassay; FPIA = fluorescent polarization immunoassay; IFA = indirect fluorescent antibody; MEIA = microparticle enzyme immunoassay; SPR = solid-phase receptacle.

sample with material from the previous samples. Various methods have been developed to reduce carryover, including the use of disposable pipette tips to initially transfer samples and flushing the internal and external surfaces of sample probes with diluent.

Reagent usage in automated immunoassay analyzers requires consideration of the following factors: handling, preparing and storing, and dispensing. Some reagents come ready for use; if they do not, the analyzer must be able to properly dilute reagents before they can be used. Most reagents come with bar codes that are read by the analyzer to reduce operator error; if the wrong reagent is loaded into the analyzer by mistake, the analyzer will detect the error and generate an error message. For many analyzers, reagents must be stored in laboratory refrigerators; however, in larger systems, there is a reagent storage compartment within the analyzer itself.

Table 13–6 CLIA-Related Websites

AGENCY	WEBSITE
Centers for Disease Control and Prevention	http://www.cdc.gov
Centers for Medicare and Medicaid Services	https://www.cms.gov/Center/Provider-Type/Clinical-Labs-Center.html
U.S. Food and Drug Administration	http://www.fda.gov
The College of American Pathologists Laboratory Accreditation Program Inspection Checklist for Chemistry	https://www.cap.org/laboratory-improvement/accreditation/laboratory-accreditation-program
Clinical Laboratory Standards Institute Evaluation Standards	http://clsi.org

After reagents have been added to the samples, the next concern is proper mixing to obtain reliable results. Analyzers use different methods for mixing, including magnetic stirring, rotation paddles, forceful dispensing, and vigorous lateral shaking. Whichever method is used, it is imperative that no splashing between sample wells occurs to prevent erroneous results.

Timed incubation is then carried out at ambient temperatures. Some analyzers have built-in incubators for temperature-controlled incubation. Heated metal blocks are widely used to incubate reagent wells or cuvettes.

Detection of the final analyte depends upon the chemistry involved in the immunoassay. In the past, colorimetric absorption spectroscopy has been the principal means of measurement because of its ability to measure a wide variety of compounds. Other methods of detection include fluorescence and chemiluminescence, both of which require fluorescence detectors. With the growing trend to offer flexibility in an automated analyzer, several companies have developed analyzers that have the ability to combine chemistry and immunoassay testing on a single platform. Two examples are Beckman Coulter's UniCel DXC chemistry systems and Roche Diagnostics' COBAS analyzer series.

Instrumentation can reduce turnaround time for testing, remove the possibility of manual errors, and allow for greater sensitivity in determining the presence of low-level analytes. Batch analyzers may work best if only one type of testing is performed on a large scale. Random-access analyzers allow for more flexibility and include rapid processing of stat samples. In either case, any new instrument requires extensive validation before patient results can be reported with confidence.

Validation

Regardless of the instrumentation considered, proper validation of new instrumentation or methodology must always be performed. The laboratory needs to determine how it will meet the Clinical Laboratory Improvement Amendments (CLIA) regulations for verifying the manufacturer's performance specifications. The regulations apply to each nonwaived test or test system brought into the laboratory for the first time. Validation of the new instrument or method must be completed before patient results can be reported. There are multiple resources available on the topic of method validation. The Centers for Medicare and Medicaid Services has an overview of the CLIA (available at https://www.cms.gov/CLIA). The specific requirements for method validation for nonwaived and modified tests can be found at https://www.cms.gov/Regulations-and-Guidance/Legislation/CLIA/Categorization_of_Tests.html. **Table 13–6** lists other websites with information regarding method and instrument validation. In addition, it is imperative that laboratories must comply with their individual state's regulatory agency standards.

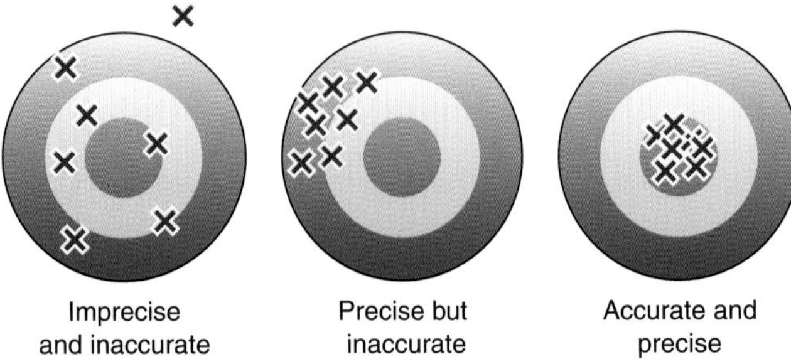

FIGURE 13–7 Pictorial representation of the difference between accuracy and precision.

As designated by CLIA, the required verifications to be determined for a new method are accuracy, precision, analytic sensitivity, and analytic specificity, including interfering substances, reportable range, and reference intervals. **Accuracy** refers to the test's ability to actually measure what it claims to measure. For example, the assay may be tested using previously known positives or negatives as provided by proficiency testing or interlaboratory exchange. Also, parallel testing with an alternative method or technology is a form of accuracy testing. **Precision** refers to the ability to consistently reproduce the same result on repeated testing of the same sample. See **Figure 13–7** for a pictorial representation of the difference between accuracy and precision. CLIA '88 specifies that the standard deviation and coefficient of variation should be calculated from 10 to 20 day-to-day quality control results. At least one normal and one abnormal control should be included in the analysis. **Analytic sensitivity** is defined as the lowest measurable amount of an analyte, whereas **analytic specificity** is the assay's ability to generate a negative result when the analyte is not present. The **reportable range** is defined as the range of values that will generate a positive result for the specimens assayed by the test procedure. Note that this may not include the entire dynamic range of the analytic instrument used to produce the result. Finally, the **reference interval** is the range of values found in healthy individuals, which is used as a guideline for clinical interpretation.

SUMMARY

- Flow cytometry, a powerful tool to identify and enumerate various cell populations, was first used in clinical laboratories to perform CD4+ T-cell counts in HIV-infected individuals.
- A flow cytometer measures multiple properties of cells suspended in a moving fluid medium.
- As each cell or particle passes single file through a laser light source, it produces a characteristic light pattern that is measured by multiple detectors for scattered light (forward and 90 degrees) and fluorescent emissions if the cell is stained with a fluorochrome.
- Scattered light in a forward direction is a measure of cell size, whereas the side scatter determines a cell's internal complexity or granularity.
- A single-parameter histogram shows a chosen parameter (on the *x*-axis) versus the number of events (on the *y*-axis).
- A dual-parameter dot plot displays two parameters against each other.
- A gate isolates a particular region of cells for further analysis.
- Immunophenotyping is a laboratory technique that uses antibodies to identify cells by their characteristic antigen expression.
- Quantification of an individual's lymphocyte populations is essential in diagnosing such conditions as lymphomas, immunodeficiency diseases, unexplained infections, or acquired immune diseases such as AIDS.
- Lymphoid and myeloid cells are identified using monoclonal antibodies directed against specific surface antigens. Flow cytometry is the most commonly used method for immunophenotyping of lymphoid and myeloid populations.
- Clinical immunology laboratories have replaced many manual immunoassay procedures with a variety of automated immunoassay analyzers to allow for more accurate, precise, and sensitive testing of many analytes.
- There are many factors to consider in determining which analyzer will fill the needs of a particular laboratory, including deciding whether a batch analyzer or a random-access analyzer can best serve testing needs.
- Automation is incorporated in all stages of laboratory testing: preanalytical, analytical, and post-analytical.
- Once an analyzer has been purchased, a thorough validation of all assays to be performed must be done to ensure quality. Validation should include a determination of accuracy, precision, reportable range, reference range, analytic sensitivity, and analytic specificity.
- *Accuracy* refers to a test's ability to measure what it actually claims to measure.
- Precision is the ability to consistently reproduce the same result on a particular sample.
- Automated analyzers are costly; however, they can reduce turnaround time and errors in the testing process.

CASE STUDIES

1. A laboratory has just purchased a new immunoassay analyzer, and validation is being done before patient results can be reported out. Twenty random patient samples are run by both the old and new methodology. According to the newer instrumentation, three samples that were negative by the old method are positive by the new instrument.

Questions

a. What sort of possible error—that is, sensitivity, specificity, accuracy, or precision—does this represent?
b. What steps should be taken to resolve this discrepancy?

2. A 3-year-old female is sent for immunologic testing because of recurring respiratory infections, including several bouts of pneumonia. The results show decreased immunoglobulin levels, especially of immunoglobulin G (IgG). Although her WBC count was within the normal range, her lymphocyte count was low. Flow cytometry was performed to determine if a particular subset of lymphocytes was low or missing. **Figure 13–8** shows the flow cytometry results obtained.

Questions

a. What do the flow cytometry patterns indicate about the population of lymphocytes affected?
b. How can this account for the child's recurring infections?
c. What further type of testing might be indicated?

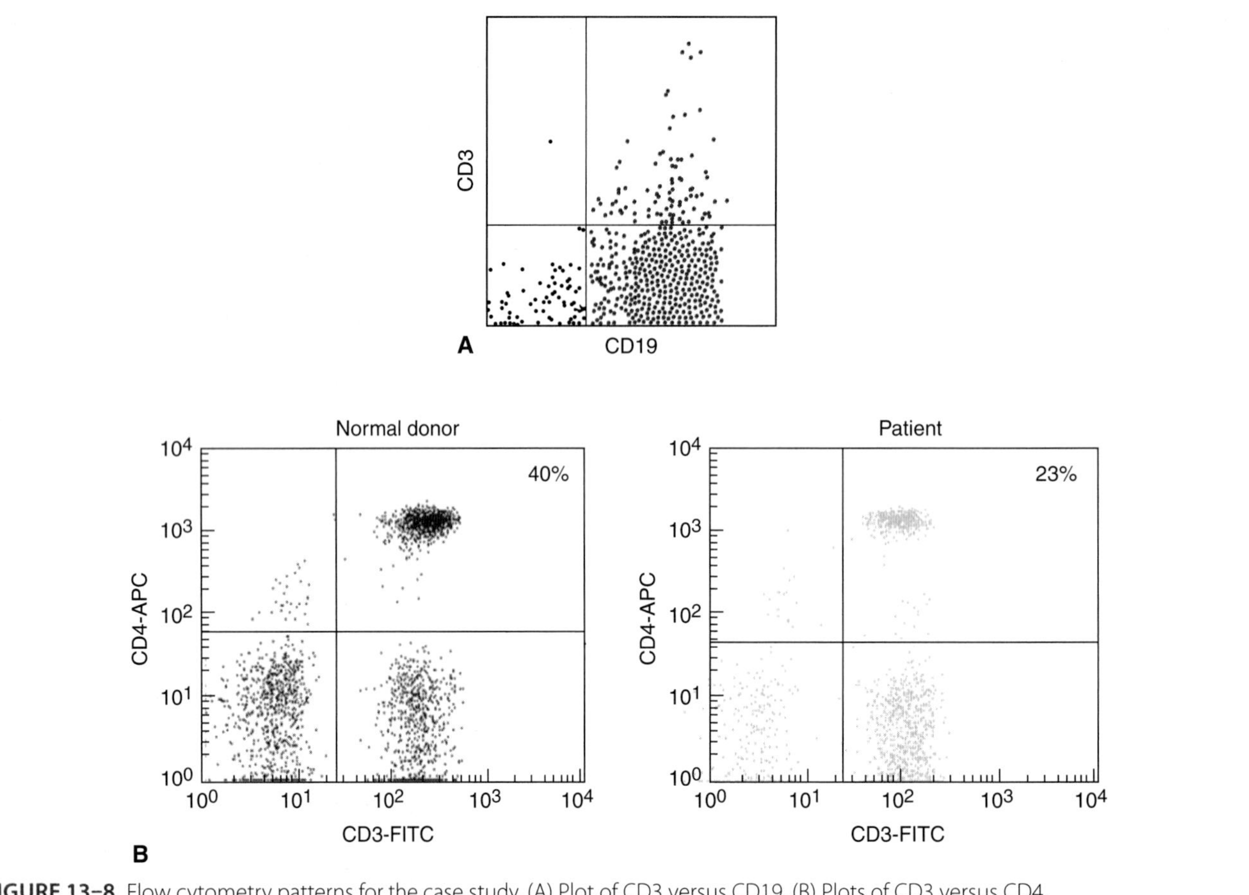

FIGURE 13–8 Flow cytometry patterns for the case study. (A) Plot of CD3 versus CD19. (B) Plots of CD3 versus CD4.

REVIEW QUESTIONS

1. Flow cytometry characterizes cells based on all of the following *except*
   a. forward scatter of an interrupted beam of light.
   b. side scatter of the interrupted beam of light.
   c. fluorescence emitted from the cells.
   d. the transmittance of light by cells in solution.

2. Forward light scatter is an indicator of a cell's
   a. granularity.
   b. density.
   c. size.
   d. number.

3. What is the single most important requirement for samples to be analyzed on a flow cytometer?
   a. Whole blood is collected into a serum separator tube.
   b. Cells must be in a single-cell suspension.
   c. Samples must be fixed in formaldehyde before processing.
   d. Blood must be kept refrigerated while processing.

4. Which statement represents the best explanation for a flow cytometer's ability to detect several cell surface markers at the same time?
   a. The forward scatter can separate out cells on the basis of complexity.
   b. One detector can be used to detect many different wavelengths.
   c. For each marker, a specific fluorochrome–antibody combination is used.
   d. Intrinsic parameters are separated out on the basis of the amount of side scatter.

5. Which of the following cell surface markers would be present on a population of T helper (Th) cells?
   a. CD3 and CD4
   b. CD3 and CD8
   c. CD3 only
   d. CD4 only

6. If an analyzer consistently indicates a positive test when the analyte in question is not present, this represents a problem with
   a. sensitivity.
   b. specificity.
   c. reportable range.
   d. precision.

7. All of the following are clinical applications for flow cytometry *except*
   a. fetal hemoglobin.
   b. immunophenotyping of lymphocyte subpopulations.
   c. HIV viral load analysis.
   d. enumeration of stem cells in a peripheral blood mononuclear cell product.

8. The various signals generated by cells intersecting with a flow cytometry laser are captured by
   a. bandwidth waves.
   b. wave channels.
   c. photomultiplier tubes.
   d. flow cells.

9. Analysis of flow cytometer data of cells can be filtered in many ways by using a method of
   a. "gating" in a dot plot.
   b. banding of a histogram.
   c. single-parameter histogram monitoring.
   d. automatic sampling.

10. A newer flow cytometry technology that has the potential to detect 100 analytes from one sample of blood is called a/an
    a. RBC fragmentation assay.
    b. Dihydrorhodamine 123.
    c. sucrose test.
    d. cytometric bead array.

11. Many flow cytometry laboratories now use the CD45 marker in combination with SSC in differentiating various populations of WBCs to replace which of the following combinations?
    a. CD4 + SSC
    b. CD4 + FSC
    c. FSC + SSC
    d. FSC + CD45

12. Which cell surface marker is present on cells seen in hairy cell leukemia?
    a. CD138
    b. CD33
    c. CD103
    d. CD34

13. CD45 is a pan-leukocyte marker expressed on WBCs in varying levels or amounts of expression, based on the
    a. size of a cell.
    b. granularity of a cell.
    c. maturity and lineage of a cell.
    d. malignancy of a cell.

14. Which of the following statements best describes a single-parameter histogram?
    a. Each event is represented by a dot.
    b. Data are distributed in four quadrants.
    c. Positive and negative events are plotted on the *x*- and *y*-axes.
    d. A chosen parameter is plotted versus the number of events.

15. Which of the following statements regarding PNH is NOT correct?
    a. PNH could affect RBC and WBC counts.
    b. Patients with PNH usually present with symptoms such as hemolytic anemia.
    c. Flow cytometry can diagnose PNH by detecting missing anchor proteins.
    d. PNH is an immunodeficiency disease that is caused by environmental factors.

16. Which type of analyzer allows one to measure multiple analytes from numerous samples, loaded at any time?
    a. Batch analyzer
    b. Random-access analyzer
    c. Front-end-loaded analyzer
    d. Sequential access analyzer

17. Operational considerations when selecting automated analyzers for a laboratory include which of the following?
    a. Reagent stability
    b. Test menu
    c. Stat capability
    d. All of the above

18. Analyzers use different methods for mixing, including magnetic stirring, rotation paddles, and forceful dispensing. Whichever method is used, it is imperative that
    a. reagents should always be kept refrigerated.
    b. there is no splashing or carryover between samples.
    c. samples are kept at room temperature.
    d. multiple methods are not used simultaneously.

19. All of the following are benefits of automation *except*
    a. greater accuracy.
    b. reduced turnaround time.
    c. savings on reagents.
    d. controls are no longer needed.

20. If an analyzer gets different results each time the same sample is tested, what type of problem does this represent?
    a. Sensitivity
    b. Specificity
    c. Accuracy
    d. Precision

Immune Disorders

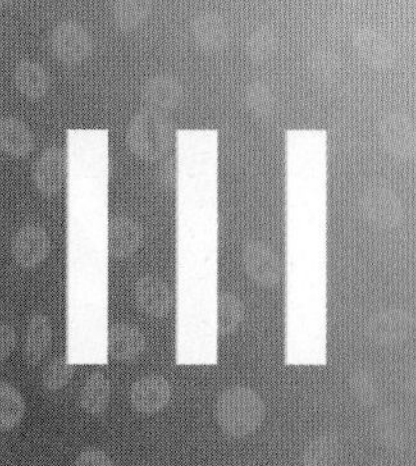

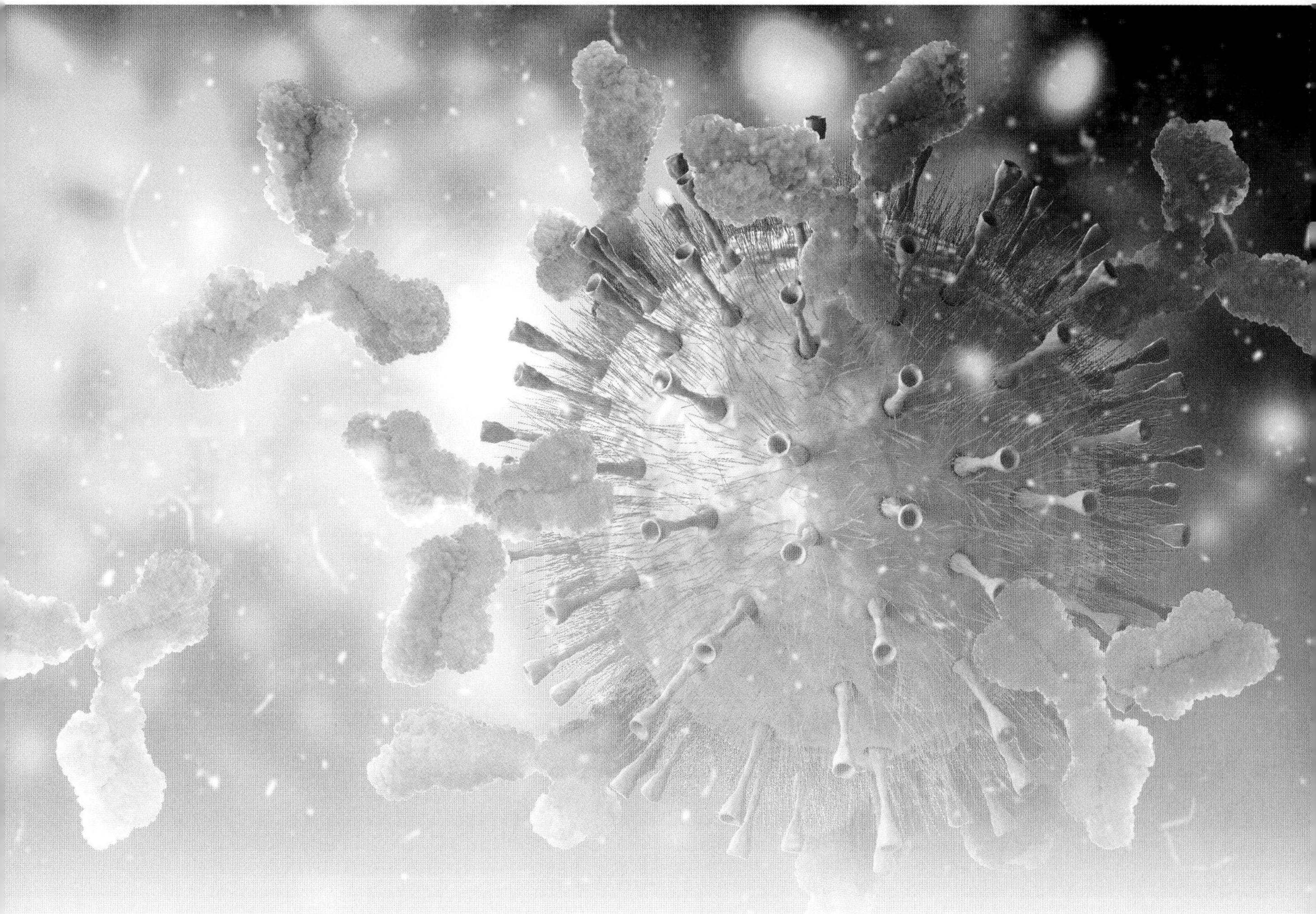

14 Hypersensitivity

Linda E. Miller, PhD, MB^CM(ASCP)SI

LEARNING OUTCOMES

After finishing this chapter, you should be able to:

1. Explain the concept of hypersensitivity.
2. Differentiate between the four types of hypersensitivity reactions in terms of antibody involvement, complement involvement, antigen triggers, and timing of the response.
3. Associate specific examples of clinical manifestations with each type of hypersensitivity.
4. Discuss the immunologic mechanisms involved in each of the four types of hypersensitivity reactions.
5. Provide examples of preformed and newly synthesized mediators released from immunoglobulin E (IgE)-sensitized mast cells and basophils and discuss their effects.
6. Discuss the influence of genetic and environmental factors on susceptibility to type I hypersensitivity responses.
7. Discuss the types of reactions that can result from latex sensitivity and their clinical manifestations.
8. Explain the underlying mechanisms of pharmacological therapy, monoclonal anti-IgE therapy, and allergy immunotherapy (AIT) in the treatment of allergies.
9. Discuss the procedure, clinical applications, advantages, and limitations of skin testing for type I hypersensitivity.
10. Discuss the principles and clinical applications of allergen-specific and total-IgE testing.
11. Explain how hemolytic disease of the fetus and newborn (HDFN) arises.
12. Explain the principles and clinical uses of the direct antiglobulin test (DAT) and the indirect antiglobulin test (IAT).
13. Discuss the principle of cold agglutinins testing and associate the presence of a positive result with specific disorders.
14. Discuss how skin testing for delayed hypersensitivity is performed, its clinical applications, and how to interpret the results.
15. Explain the principle of interferon gamma release assays (IGRA) and as well as their clinical utility, advantages, and limitations.

CHAPTER OUTLINE

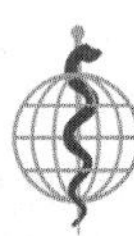

Go to FADavis.com for the laboratory exercises that accompany this text.

KEY TERMS

Allergen
Allergy immunotherapy (AIT)
Anaphylaxis
Anergy
Arthus reaction
Atopy
Autoimmune hemolytic anemia
Cold agglutinins
Contact dermatitis
Delayed hypersensitivity
Direct antiglobulin test (DAT)
Granulomas
Hemolytic disease of the fetus and newborn (HDFN)
Histamine
Hypersensitivity
Immediate hypersensitivity
Indirect antiglobulin test (IAT)
Isohemagglutinins
Leukotrienes (LT)
Paroxysmal cold hemoglobinuria
Serum sickness
Type I hypersensitivity
Type II hypersensitivity
Type III hypersensitivity
Type IV hypersensitivity

In previous chapters, immune responses have been described as defense mechanisms by which the body rids itself of potentially harmful antigens. However, in some cases, the antigen can persist, and the immune response can cause damage to the host. This type of reaction is termed **hypersensitivity,** which is defined as an exaggerated response to a typically harmless antigen that results in tissue injury, disease, or even death.

In the 1960s, British immunologists Philip Gell and Robin Coombs devised a classification system for these reactions based on their immunologic mechanisms. In this widely used system, hypersensitivity reactions are classified into four categories:

- **Type I hypersensitivity**—also known as *anaphylactic* hypersensitivity
- **Type II hypersensitivity**—also known as *antibody-mediated cytotoxic* hypersensitivity
- **Type III hypersensitivity**—also known as *complex-mediated* hypersensitivity
- **Type IV hypersensitivity**—also known as *cell-mediated* hypersensitivity

Hypersensitivity types I, II, and III are mediated by antibodies. Because symptoms of these types develop within a few minutes to a few hours after exposure to the inducing antigen, they are also known as **immediate hypersensitivity** reactions. In contrast, sensitized T cells, rather than antibodies, are responsible for type IV hypersensitivity. Clinical manifestations of type IV hypersensitivity do not appear until 24 to 48 hours after contact with antigen; therefore, this type is sometimes referred to as **delayed hypersensitivity.**

The four main types of hypersensitivity are discussed in more detail in the sections that follow. Although some disease manifestations may overlap among these types, knowledge of the general characteristics of each type will help you understand the immune processes that trigger tissue damage. In this chapter, we will review the nature of the immune reactants, clinical examples, and relevant testing for each of the four types of hypersensitivity.

Type I Hypersensitivity

Type I hypersensitivity reactions are commonly thought of as *allergies*. Some examples of these reactions are hay fever, allergic asthma, hives, and systemic anaphylaxis. The antigens that trigger type I hypersensitivity are called **allergens.** Examples of common allergens include peanuts, eggs, and pollen. A distinguishing feature of type I hypersensitivity is the short time span, usually minutes, between exposure to allergen and the onset of clinical symptoms.

The first clue about the cause of type I hypersensitivity was provided by Carl Wilhelm Prausnitz and Heinz Küstner, who showed that a serum factor was responsible. In their historic experiment, serum from Küstner, who was allergic to fish, was injected into Prausnitz. A later exposure to fish antigen at the same site resulted in redness and swelling. This type of reaction is known as *passive cutaneous anaphylaxis*. It occurs when serum is transferred from an allergic individual to a non-allergic individual, and the second individual is challenged at a later time with the specific allergen. Although this experiment was conducted in 1921, it was not until 1967 that the serum factor responsible for this reaction was identified as immunoglobulin E (IgE).

Connections

Immunoglobulin E

Recall from Chapter 5 that IgE is the least abundant antibody class in the serum, normally accounting for less than 1% of all the immunoglobulins. This is likely because IgE is not involved in typical immune responses such as complement fixation and opsonization. IgE is unique in its ability to bind to specific receptors on mast cells and basophils. This property enables IgE to play a major role in type I hypersensitivity allergic reactions and in defense against parasites (see Chapter 22). Patients with these conditions typically have increased concentrations of IgE in the bloodstream.

Typically, patients who exhibit allergic hypersensitivity reactions produce a large amount of IgE antibody in response to a small concentration of allergen. IgE levels appear to depend on the interaction of both genetic and environmental factors. **Atopy,** a term derived from the Greek word *atopos* (meaning "out of place"), refers to an inherited tendency to develop classic allergic responses to naturally occurring inhaled or ingested allergens. The section that follows will provide details about the immunologic mechanism that occurs in susceptible individuals to produce the symptoms of type I hypersensitivity reactions.

Immunologic Mechanism

Type I hypersensitivity is also known as *anaphylactic hypersensitivity,* based on its immunologic mechanism. The key immunologic components involved in this hypersensitivity type are IgE antibody, mast cells, basophils, and eosinophils. These components act together to produce an immediate type of reaction, which typically occurs within 30 to 60 minutes after antigen exposure. Type I hypersensitivity has two major phases: sensitization and activation **(Fig. 14–1)**. A late-phase reaction may also occur in some individuals.

Sensitization Phase

The response begins when a susceptible individual is exposed to an allergen and produces specific IgE antibody. IgE is primarily synthesized by B cells and plasma cells in the lymphoid tissue of the respiratory and gastrointestinal tracts, as well as the lymph nodes. Langerhans and dendritic cells internalize and process allergens from the environment and transport the allergen-major histocompatibility complex (MHC) class II complex to T helper cells in the local lymphoid tissue.

The regulation of IgE production appears to be a function of the type 2 helper T cells (Th2; see Chapter 4). In a normal immune response to microorganisms and other antigens, there is an appropriate balance between the activity of the Th2 cells and the type 1 helper T cells (Th1), which results in protective immunity that does not harm the host. However, in people with allergies, the immune response is shifted so that Th2 cells predominate. This Th2 type of response results in the production of several cytokines, including interleukin 4 (IL-4) and interleukin (IL-13). These cytokines are responsible for the final differentiation that occurs in B cells, initiating the transcription of the gene that codes for the epsilon heavy chain of immunoglobulin molecules belonging to the IgE class.

In the sensitization phase, the IgE antibody produced attaches to high-affinity receptors called *FcεRI*, which bind the fragment crystallizable (Fc) region of the epsilon heavy chain. Large numbers of these receptors are found on mast cells and basophils, with a single cell having as many as 200,000 such receptors. Binding of IgE to cell membranes increases the half-life of the antibody from 2 or 3 days to at least 10 days. Once bound, IgE functions as an antigen receptor on mast cells and basophils.

Mast cells are the principal effector cells of immediate hypersensitivity. These cells are found throughout the body, and in most organs, tend to be concentrated around the small blood vessels, the lymphatics, the nerves, and the glandular tissue. Mast cells have abundant cytoplasmic granules that store numerous preformed inflammatory mediators. They are long-lived, residing for months in the tissues (see Chapter 1). Basophils are similar to, but distinct from mast cells in terms of their appearance and function. They are present in the peripheral blood, where they represent less than 1% of the total white blood cells (WBCs). They have fewer, but larger granules than mast cells, and the concentrations of inflammatory substances in the basophil granules differ from those of the mast cell. Basophils respond to chemotactic stimuli during inflammation and accumulate in the tissues, where they can persist for a few days.

Activation Phase

Upon repeated exposure to the allergen, the sensitized mast cells and basophils become activated and release chemicals that induce the symptoms of allergy. In the activation phase of the response, adjacent cell-bound IgE molecules are cross-linked by a bivalent or multivalent antigen, causing aggregation of the surface FcεRI receptors. This action, in turn, initiates complex intracellular signaling events involving multiple phosphorylation reactions, an influx of calcium, and the secretion of cytokines. The increase in intracellular calcium triggers rapid degranulation of the mast cells and basophils, which release chemical mediators that have been previously made and stored in the granules (Fig. 14-1B).

The most abundant preformed mediator is **histamine,** which comprises approximately 10% of the total weight of the granules in mast cells. These preformed substances are referred to as *primary* mediators. Other primary mediators include heparin, eosinophil chemotactic factor of anaphylaxis (ECF-A), neutrophil chemotactic factor, and proteases. The effects of these mediators are summarized in **Table 14–1.** Release of these substances is responsible for the early-phase symptoms seen in allergic reactions, which occur within 30 to 60 minutes after exposure to the allergen. The chemical mediators bind to receptors on target organs, most notably the skin, respiratory tract, and gastrointestinal tract, producing symptoms characteristic of an allergic response. The clinical manifestations depend on the target tissue and type of receptors activated. For example, in the skin, local swelling and redness, sometimes referred to as a *wheal-and-flare* reaction, can develop. Contraction of the smooth muscle in the

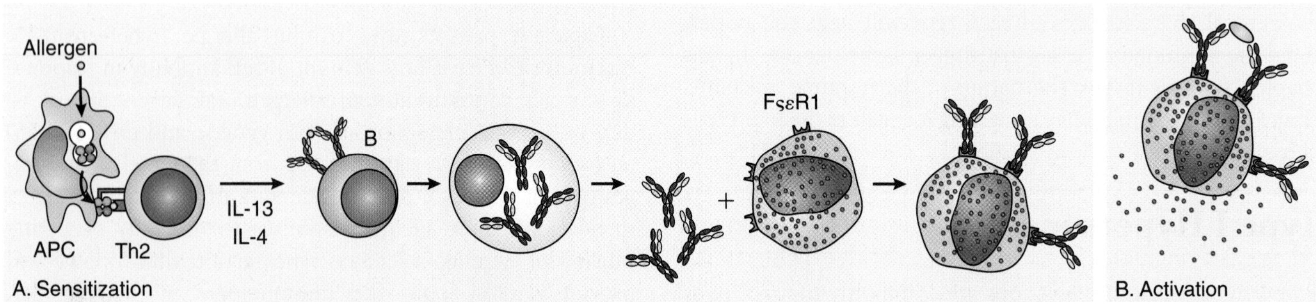

FIGURE 14–1 Type I hypersensitivity. (A) Sensitization: Formation of antigen-specific IgE that attaches to mast cells and basophils. (B) Activation: Reexposure to the same antigen, causing degranulation of mast cells and basophils and release of mediators.

Table 14–1 Mediators of Type I Hypersensitivity

	MEDIATOR	ACTIONS
Primary (Preformed)	Histamine	Smooth muscle contraction, vasodilation, increased vascular permeability
	Heparin	Smooth muscle contraction, vasodilation, increased vascular permeability
	Eosinophil chemotactic factor of anaphylaxis (ECF-A)	Chemotactic for eosinophils
	Neutrophil chemotactic factor of anaphylaxis (NCF-A)	Chemotactic for neutrophils
	Proteases (e.g., tryptase, chymase)	Convert C3 to C3b, stimulate mucus production, activate cytokines
Secondary (Newly Synthesized)	Prostaglandin PGD_2	Vasodilation, increased vascular permeability
	Leukotriene LTB_4	Chemotactic for neutrophils, eosinophils
	Leukotrienes LTC_4, LTD_4, LTE_4	Increased vascular permeability, bronchoconstriction, mucus secretion
	Platelet-activating factor (PAF)	Platelet aggregation
	Cytokines IL-1, IL-3, IL-4, IL-5, IL-6, IL-9, IL-13, IL-14, IL-16, tumor necrosis factor-α (TNF- α), granulocyte-macrophage colony-stimulating factor (GM-CSF)	Increase inflammatory cells in area, and increase IgE production

bronchioles may result in airflow obstruction. Increased vascular permeability can cause hypotension or shock. Depending on the route by which an individual is exposed to the triggering allergen, one or more of these effects may be seen.

Late Phase

In addition to immediate release of preformed mediators, mast cells and basophils are triggered to synthesize other reactants from the breakdown of phospholipids in the cell membrane. These newly formed, or *secondary,* mediators include platelet-activating factor (PAF); prostaglandin (PG) D_2; **leukotrienes (LT)** B_4, C_4, D_4, and E_4; and cytokines (see Table 14–1). These products are more potent than the primary mediators and are responsible for a late-phase allergic reaction that can be seen in some individuals 6 to 8 hours after exposure to the antigen. In this phase of the reaction, numerous cells, including eosinophils, neutrophils, Th2 cells, mast cells, basophils, and macrophages, exit the circulation and infiltrate the allergen-filled tissue. They release additional mediators that prolong hyperactivity and cause further tissue damage.

Eosinophils play an important role in the late-phase reaction. These cells normally comprise 1% to 3% of the circulating WBCs. During allergic reactions, interleukin-5 (IL-5) and other cytokines released from the Th2 cells stimulate the bone marrow to increase production of eosinophils, and the number in the peripheral blood increases, producing eosinophilia. The number of FcεRI receptors on eosinophils increases during the allergic response, and the eosinophils are stimulated to release a variety of toxic molecules and inflammatory mediators from their granules. These mediators are believed to contribute to the ongoing damage that occurs during chronic allergic conditions.

In individuals with persistent inflammation resulting from the late-phase reaction, such as those with chronic asthma, tissue remodeling can result. This involves structural changes, such as thickening of smooth muscle, as well as changes in connective tissue, blood and lymphatic vessels, mucus glands, and nerves.

Genetic and Environmental Influences on Type I Hypersensitivity

The development of IgE responses and allergy appears to depend on complex interactions between genetic factors and environmental triggers. Several hundred genes associated with susceptibility to developing allergies have been identified. These genes affect different aspects of the immune response that contribute to the pathogenesis of the type I hypersensitivity response. Some of these genes affect the structure of the epithelium lining in places where allergens can enter the body, such as the skin, gastrointestinal tract, and respiratory tract. Certain polymorphisms in these genes can result in altered ability of the body's protective barriers to prevent penetration of microbes and potential allergens. Another group of genes plays a role in recognition of the antigen by the innate immune system once it has entered through the epithelial barriers. Defects in these genes, which code for pattern recognition receptors such as CD14 and the Toll-like receptors (TLRs), can affect cell interactions with antigens in the initial phases of immune defense. A third group of genes can influence susceptibility to allergic disorders by affecting aspects of the adaptive immune response, such as cytokine production and the ability of T cells to differentiate into Th1 cells,

Th2 cells, and T regulatory cells. Aberrations in these genes can result in dysregulation of the immune response, inducing production of cytokines that promote IgE synthesis, such as IL-4 and IL-13. In addition, allergy and asthma appear to be associated with certain human leukocyte antigen (HLA) class II genes. The HLA-D molecules coded for by these histocompatibility genes are known to play a role in antigen presentation and may influence the tendency to respond to specific allergens (see Chapter 3). Finally, genes that play a role in modulating the inflammatory response can influence the long-term consequences of allergies by affecting the process of tissue remodeling and repair.

Many environmental influences on the allergic response have also been identified. Exposure to infectious organisms appears to play a key role in the development of allergic disease. The increased prevalence of allergy in industrialized regions may be due, in part, to increased hygiene practices and use of antibiotics, with a consequent decrease in exposure to microbes. This, in turn, could have significant effects on the immune system by altering the microbial constituent of the gut and decreasing microbial diversity in the body. Multiple studies indicate that in utero or early life exposure to the diverse microbial populations in a farming environment provides protection against allergies by inducing the development of regulatory T cells and by directing the immune system toward beneficial Th1 responses and away from Th2 atopic reactions. In addition, exposure to stress, variations in physical factors such as temperature, and contact with environmental pollutants such as cigarette smoke and diesel exhaust fumes can intensify clinical manifestations of allergy in susceptible individuals.

Clinical Manifestations of Type I Hypersensitivity

Clinical manifestations of type I hypersensitivity are common. The prevalence of allergic diseases has been increasing in developed countries for more than 50 years, and it is estimated that up to 40% of the world's population has allergic sensitization to common environmental antigens such as pollen or peanuts. More than 50 million people are affected in the United States alone, where allergies are the sixth-leading cause of chronic illness.

The clinical manifestations caused by the release of inflammatory mediators from mast cells and basophils vary from a localized skin reaction to a severe systemic response known as **anaphylaxis.** Symptoms depend on such variables as route of antigen exposure, dose of allergen, and frequency of exposure. If an allergen is inhaled, it is most likely to cause respiratory symptoms such as asthma or rhinitis. Ingestion of an allergen may result in gastrointestinal symptoms, whereas injection into the bloodstream can trigger a systemic response.

Allergic Rhinitis

Rhinitis is the most common form of atopy, or allergy, affecting between 10% and 30% of populations worldwide. Symptoms include paroxysmal sneezing; rhinorrhea, or runny nose; nasal congestion; and itching of the nose and eyes. Although the condition itself is merely annoying, complications such as sinusitis, otitis media (ear infection), eustachian tube dysfunction, and sleep disturbances may result. Pollen, mold spores, animal dander, and particulate matter from house dust mites are examples of airborne foreign particles that act directly on the mast cells in the conjunctiva and respiratory mucous membranes to trigger rhinitis. Seasonal allergic rhinitis, triggered by tree and grass pollens in the air during the spring in temperate climates, is called "hay fever."

Allergic Asthma

Asthma, derived from the Greek word for "panting" or "breathlessness," is caused by inhalation of small particles such as pollen, dust, or fumes that reach the lower respiratory tract. It can be defined clinically as recurrent airflow obstruction that leads to intermittent sneezing, breathlessness, and occasionally, a cough with sputum production. The airflow obstruction is caused by bronchial smooth muscle contraction, mucosal edema, and heavy mucus secretion. All these changes lead to an increase in airway resistance, making it difficult for inspired air to leave the lungs. This trapped air creates the sense of breathlessness.

Food Allergies

Food allergies are another example of type I immediate hypersensitivity reactions. Some of the most common food allergies are caused by cow's milk, eggs, nuts, soy, wheat, fish, and shellfish. Symptoms limited to the gastrointestinal tract include cramping, vomiting, and diarrhea, whereas spread of antigen through the bloodstream may cause hives and angioedema on the skin, asthma, rhinitis, or anaphylaxis (see the text that follows).

Skin Reactions

Local inflammation of the skin, or *dermatitis,* can also be caused by type I immediate hypersensitivity reactions. These reactions manifest as either acute urticaria or eczema. *Urticaria,* or hives, appear within minutes after exposure to the allergen and are characterized by severe itching, erythema (redness) caused by local vasodilation, leakage of fluid into the surrounding area, and a spreading area of redness around the center of the lesion **(Fig. 14–2).** Commonly called a *wheal-and-flare reaction,* this reaction is caused by the release of vasoactive mediators from mast cells in the skin following contact with allergens such as pet dander or insect venom.

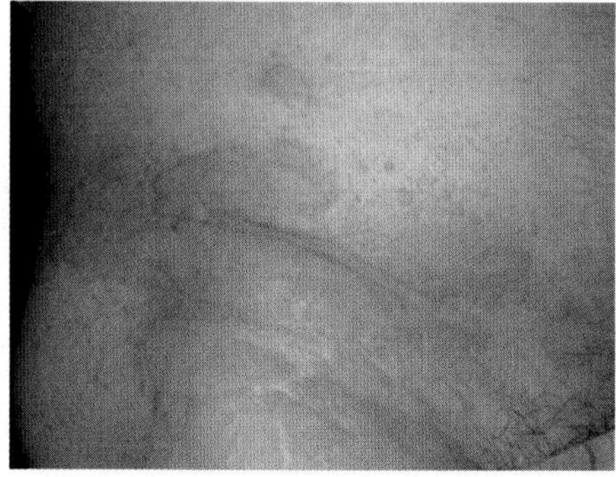

FIGURE 14–2 Urticaria (hives) caused by an immediate hypersensitivity reaction to a medication. *(From Barankin B, Freiman A.* Derm Notes. *Philadelphia, PA: F.A. Davis; 2006, with permission.)*

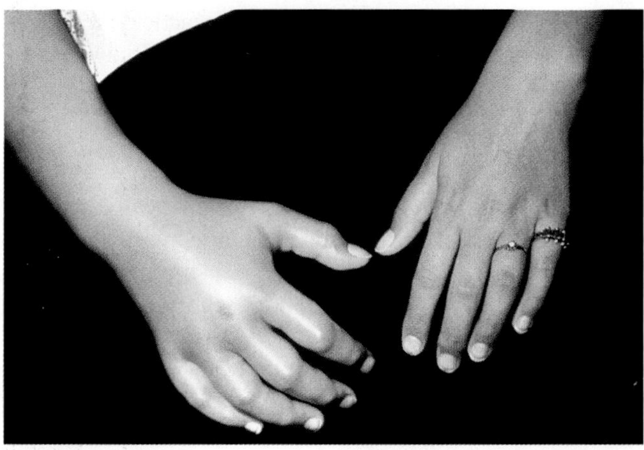

FIGURE 14–3 Angioedema caused by a yellow jacket sting on the right hand just above the middle finger. *(Courtesy of CDC/Margaret A. Parsons, Public Health Image Library.)*

When these reactions occur deeper in the dermal tissues, they are known as *angioedema* **(Fig. 14–3)**. Urticaria can also appear because of other clinical manifestations, such as anaphylaxis and food allergies. Atopic eczema can take on a variety of forms, from erythematous, oozing vesicles to thickened, scaly skin, depending on the stage of activity and age of the individual. It is a chronic, itchy skin rash that usually develops during infancy, persists during childhood, and is strongly associated with allergic rhinitis and asthma.

Anaphylaxis

Anaphylaxis is the most severe type of allergic response because it is an acute reaction that simultaneously involves multiple organs. It may be fatal if not treated promptly. Coined by biologists Paul Portier and Charles Richet in 1902, the term literally means "without protection." Anaphylactic reactions are typically triggered by glycoproteins or large polypeptides. Smaller molecules, such as penicillin, can trigger anaphylaxis by acting as haptens that may become immunogenic by combining with host cells or proteins. Typical agents that induce anaphylaxis include venom from bees, wasps, and hornets; drugs such as penicillin; and foods such as shellfish, peanuts, and dairy products.

Clinical signs of anaphylaxis begin within minutes after antigenic challenge and may include bronchospasm and laryngeal edema, vascular congestion, skin manifestations such as urticaria (hives) and angioedema, diarrhea or vomiting, and intractable shock because of the effect on blood vessels and smooth muscle of the circulatory system. The severity of the reaction depends on the number of previous exposures to the antigen. This is because multiple exposures result in additional accumulation of IgE on the surface of the mast cells and basophils. Massive release of reactants, especially histamine, from the granules is responsible for the ensuing symptoms. Death may result from asphyxiation because of upper-airway edema and congestion, irreversible shock, or a combination of these symptoms.

Latex Sensitivity

Latex sensitivity became a significant problem in the late 1980s after the implementation of Universal Precautions by the Centers for Disease Control and Prevention (CDC) and regulations by the Occupational Safety and Health Administration (OSHA) that required health-care workers to wear gloves when performing laboratory procedures and working with patients. Reactions to antigens in natural rubber latex include type I hypersensitivity and contact dermatitis caused by skin irritation or type IV hypersensitivity. Type I hypersensitivity reactions can manifest as urticaria, rhinoconjunctivitis, asthma, angioedema, or anaphylaxis. Sensitization to latex can occur because of direct skin contact or inhalation of airborne latex particles released when gloves are donned and removed. The risk of the latter occurring is increased when cornstarch powder is used in gloves because residual latex proteins can bind to the powder particles.

Groups at particular risk for latex allergy include health-care workers, rubber industry workers, patients who have had multiple surgeries, and individuals who are allergic to certain foods that cross-react with latex allergens. The prevalence of latex sensitivity in the general population is estimated to be 1% to 6%, whereas it is thought to range from 8% to 12% in health-care workers and more than 60% in patients who have undergone multiple surgeries early in life. The incidence of latex sensitization has decreased in recent years in countries where policies to avoid contact with latex have been implemented. These policies may include the use of low-protein, powder-free gloves or gloves made from non-latex materials, such as nitrile, neoprene, vinyl, or synthetic polyisoprene rubber.

Treatment of Type I Hypersensitivity

Avoidance of known allergens is the first line of defense. Individuals can employ environmental interventions such as encasing mattresses and pillows in allergen-proof covers and removing a harmful food from the diet. However, it is not always possible to completely eliminate contact with allergens. In these cases, pharmacological therapy is necessary to relieve acute symptoms, control chronic allergy manifestations, and in some cases, modulate the immune response to the allergen.

Drugs used to treat immediate hypersensitivity vary with the severity of the reaction. Localized allergic reactions, such as hay fever, hives, or rhinitis, can be treated with antihistamines and decongestants. Asthma is often treated with a combination of therapeutic reagents, including antihistamines and bronchodilators. In cases of persistent asthma, LT receptor antagonists and mast cell stabilizers are also used; in severe cases, corticosteroids can be added to block recruitment of inflammatory cells and their ability to cause tissue damage. Systemic anaphylaxis is a medical emergency that requires timely injection of epinephrine, a powerful vasoconstrictor, to quickly reverse symptoms that could potentially be fatal.

Another treatment approach is aimed at modulating the type I hypersensitivity response through the use of monoclonal antibodies. Omalizumab, the first anti-IgE monoclonal antibody to be approved for clinical use, is a recombinant humanized antibody composed of human immunoglobulin G (IgG) framework genes recombined with complementarity-determining region genes from mouse anti-human IgE. This antibody binds to the Cε3 domain of human IgE, which is the site that IgE normally uses to bind to FcεRI receptors. Blocking this site prevents circulating IgE from binding to mast cells and basophils and sensitizing them. In addition, treatment with omalizumab has been shown to downregulate cellular expression of FcεRI receptors. Anti-IgE monoclonal antibodies have been used successfully to treat patients with moderate to severe asthma when added to conventional drug therapy. Another monoclonal antibody, mepolizumab, has been approved for the treatment of severe asthma. This humanized antibody is directed against IL-5, a cytokine that plays a major role in the development and activation of eosinophils; thus, treatment results in reduced eosinophil number and activity. A third example of a monoclonal antibody therapy for type I hypersensitivity is dupilumab, which is used to treat patients with moderate-to-severe atopic dermatitis. This antibody targets a subunit of the IL-4 receptor and blocks intracellular signaling by IL-4 and IL-13.

If environmental control and drug therapy are not successful in managing the symptoms in an individual with allergies, **allergy immunotherapy (AIT)** may be considered. The goal of AIT is to induce immune tolerance to a specific allergen by administering gradually increasing doses of the allergen over time. This therapy is believed to shift the patient's immune response to the allergen to a Th1-type response and to induce the development of allergen-specific T regulatory cells (Tregs) that release interleukin-10 (IL-10) and other immunosuppressive cytokines. These cytokines regulate T- and B-cell responses to the allergen and redirect the immune system to produce allergen-specific IgG4 "blocking" antibodies that combine with the antigen before it can attach to IgE-coated cells. Therefore, decreased activation of mast cells and basophils occurs, along with inhibition of eosinophil responses.

Connections

Immune Tolerance

As we will discuss in Chapter 15, *immune tolerance* is defined as a state of immune unresponsiveness directed against a specific antigen. The development of immune tolerance to an allergen means that the type I hypersensitivity response to the allergen is inhibited. This is achieved by AIT.

The standard practice for AIT has been to administer allergens subcutaneously (i.e., under the skin) through a period of 3 to 5 years. This practice has been shown to significantly reduce symptoms in patients with allergic rhinitis or asthma; however, it has the potential to induce anaphylaxis and must be administered in a physician's office. More recently, other routes of administration that pose a decreased risk of severe adverse reactions have been used, namely, oral and sublingual (placement of allergen extract under the tongue). These methods of delivery have been shown to reduce symptoms associated with allergic asthma and rhinitis and to significantly decrease or eliminate allergic reactions to certain food allergens, such as peanuts. Researchers also are investigating the use of purified, recombinant allergens and allergoids, which have been chemically altered to reduce reactivity with IgE. These approaches may further increase the effectiveness of AIT while decreasing the associated risk of severe reactions.

Testing for Type I Hypersensitivity

Evaluation of patients with an allergy begins with a medical history and physical examination to assess clinical symptoms. These assessments are followed by specific *in vivo* skin tests and *in vitro* tests for IgE antibodies to confirm the presence of an allergy and to determine the allergens to which a patient is sensitized. There are several types of *in vitro* IgE tests: allergen-specific IgE, allergen component IgE (also known as *molecular-based allergy diagnostics*), point-of-care rapid tests, and total IgE.

In Vivo Skin Tests

Testing for allergies typically begins with direct skin testing because this procedure is less expensive than serological testing and provides immediate results. Two types of skin tests are used in clinical practice: percutaneous tests (also known as *prick* or *puncture tests*) and intradermal tests. Percutaneous tests can detect hypersensitivity to a wide variety of inhaled or food allergens. In these tests, the clinician uses a needle or pricking device to introduce a small drop of allergen extract into the upper layers of the individual's skin in the inner forearm or the back. A panel of allergens is routinely used, with each applied to separate sites 2 to 2.5 cm apart. A negative control, consisting of the diluent used for the allergy extract, and a positive control of histamine are also included. After 15 to 20 minutes, the clinician examines the testing spots and records the reaction. In a positive test, a wheal-and-flare reaction will appear at the site where the allergen was applied **(Fig. 14–4)**. Scoring of the reaction is based on the presence or absence of erythema and the diameter of the wheal, with a diameter larger than 3 to 4 mm correlating best with the presence of allergy.

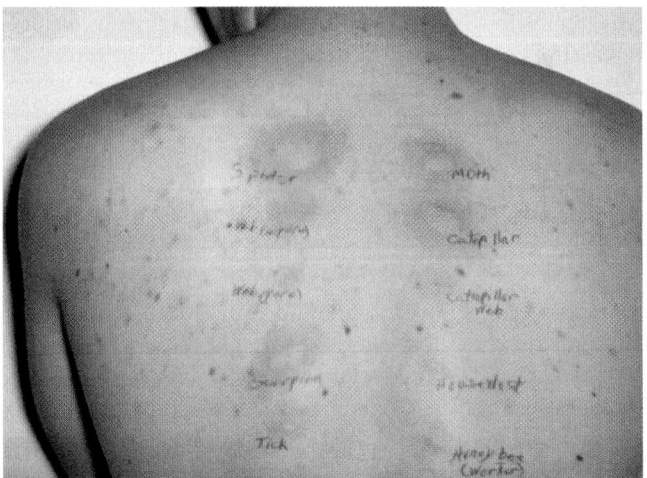

FIGURE 14–4 This individual is undergoing an allergen sensitivity test. The strongest positive reactions are to spider, moth, scorpion, caterpillar, and tick allergens, as indicated by the wheal-and-flare reactions at the sites of injection. *(Courtesy of the CDC/Dr. Frank Perlman and M.A. Parsons. Public Health Image Library.)*

Intradermal tests use a greater amount of antigen and are more sensitive than cutaneous tests. However, they are usually performed only if prick tests are negative and allergy is still suspected because they carry a larger risk (0.05%) for anaphylactic reaction than prick tests (0.03%). In intradermal testing, a 1-mL tuberculin syringe is used to administer 0.01 to 0.05 mL of test solution between layers of the skin. The test allergen is diluted 100 to 1,000 times more than the solution used for cutaneous testing. This test is performed on the inner forearm or upper arm so that if a systemic reaction occurs, a tourniquet can be applied to the arm to help stop the reaction. After 15 to 20 minutes, the site is inspected for erythema and wheal formation, and the wheal diameter is measured to determine a score.

Although skin testing is sensitive as well as relatively simple and inexpensive to perform, it has some important limitations. Antihistamines and certain other medications must be discontinued a few days before testing because they can decrease or inhibit the skin reaction. Improper technique or use of an inappropriate dilution or improperly stored allergen extract can also lead to false-negative results. False-positive results can also occur; these may be caused by the patient's reaction to the diluent, preservative, or contaminants in the allergen extract or to physical trauma to the skin in patients with severe skin dermatographism or eczema. In addition, there is the danger that a systemic reaction can be triggered. In cases where the risk of a harmful reaction is too large, skin disorders are present, or patients cannot discontinue medications before testing, serological testing for allergen-specific IgE antibodies is indicated.

Allergen-Specific IgE Testing

Allergen-specific IgE tests are safer to perform than skin testing. They are easier on some patients, especially children or apprehensive adults, and have excellent analytical sensitivity. These tests are useful in detecting allergies to several common triggers, including ragweed, trees, grasses, molds, animal dander, foods, and insect venom.

The original commercial testing method for determining specific IgE, the *radioallergosorbent test (RAST),* was introduced in 1972. In this radioimmunoassay, patient serum was incubated with a paper disk to which various allergens were covalently linked. Following a washing step to remove unbound antibody, bound IgE was detected by adding a radiolabeled anti-IgE. After a second wash step, the amount of radioactivity detected was measured by a gamma counter and was proportional to the amount of allergen-specific IgE in the patient's sample.

The principles of current immunoassays for serum IgE remain the same, but the newer, automated methods use enzyme labels that react with substrates to produce fluorescence, chemiluminescence, or colorimetric reactions rather than radioactive labels. **Figure 14–5** illustrates the principle of these tests. The tests can be run with a single allergen or as a multiallergen screen using a panel of allergens in a single run. A commercial noncompetitive fluoroimmunoassay is considered by most allergy specialists to be the method of choice. In this assay, patient serum is incubated with an allergen-coated cellulose sponge that has a high binding capacity for IgE antibody. After a wash step, an enzyme-labeled anti-IgE reagent is added; following incubation, another washing step is performed to remove unbound materials. The corresponding

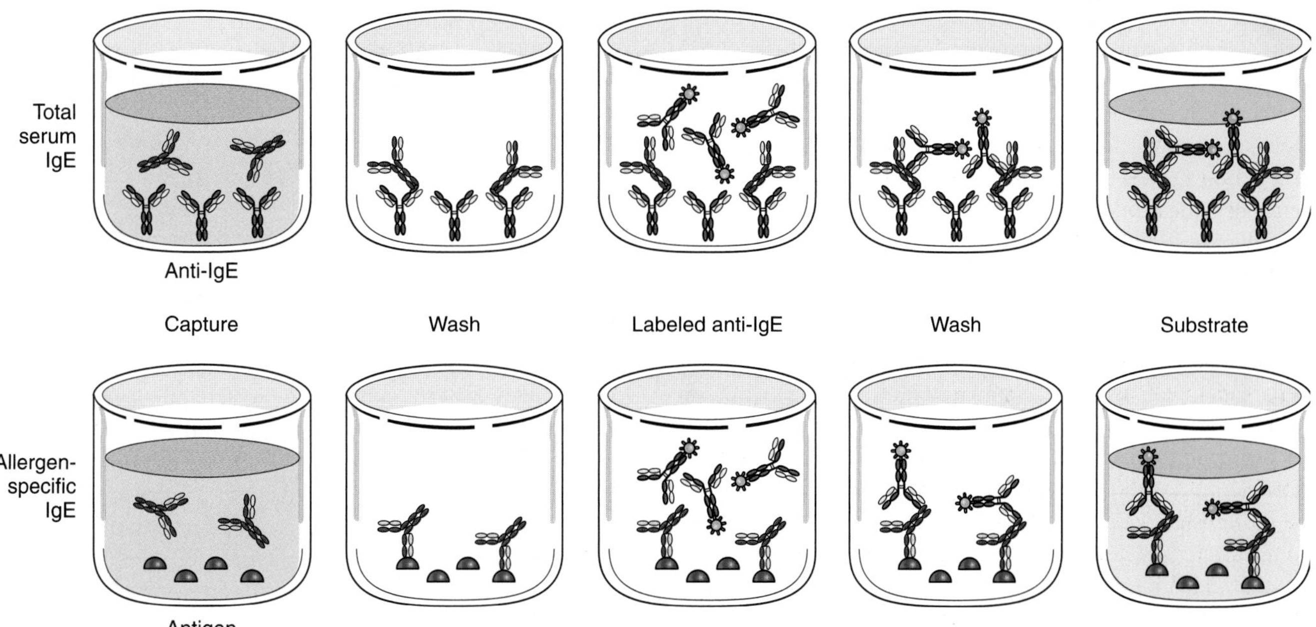

FIGURE 14–5 Comparison of noncompetitive immunoassays for total serum IgE (formerly known as *RIST*) and allergen-specific IgE (formerly known as *RAST*). IgE in the patient serum is shown in red for both tests. Total IgE is measured by capturing the antibody with an anti-IgE bound to a solid phase. A second anti-IgE immunoglobulin with an enzyme label is used to produce a visible reaction. Antigen-specific IgE is measured by using solid-phase antigen to capture patient antibody. Then a second antibody, enzyme-labeled anti-IgE immunoglobulin, is added. This combines with any bound IgE to produce a visible reaction in the presence of substrate.

substrate is added, and fluorescence is produced in proportion to the amount of allergen-specific IgE in the sample. Patient results are derived from a standard calibration curve that is linked to the World Health Organization (WHO) IgE standard. Allergen-specific IgE values are reported in kilo international units (IU) of allergen-specific antibody per liter (kUa/L), where 1 unit is equal to 2.42 ng/mL of IgE. The method can detect IgE antibodies in the range of 0 to 100 kU/L, and 0.35 kU/L is commonly used as the cutoff for a positive test.

The results obtained by different immunoassays are not interchangeable because of differences in the composition of the allergen reagents. Some assays use extracts of whole, natural allergens that contain both allergenic and non-allergenic proteins. Although these tests are highly sensitive, reactivity to clinically insignificant antigens may be detected. This limitation has stimulated the development of recombinant allergen components produced by cloning the genes coding for these proteins and purifying the allergenic substances produced by the genetically modified cells. Recombinant allergens are being incorporated into existing assay formats and increase the diagnostic specificity of allergy testing.

Using advanced biochemical and molecular techniques, scientists have been able to characterize more than 900 allergens. This knowledge has led to the development of molecular-based allergy diagnostics that allow for parallel detection of IgE antibodies to numerous allergens using microarray or macroarray formats. In these systems, patient serum is incubated with a biochip or nitrocellulose membrane containing miniature spots to which either allergen extracts or purified allergenic components have been applied. The spots contain a wide variety of antigens, from foods to pollens, molds, fungi, latex, and insect venom. If allergen-specific IgE is present, it will bind to the appropriate spots. After washing, a fluorescent- or enzyme-labeled anti-IgE is added. After another wash step and addition of substrate, the intensity of the reaction is recorded for each spot. Molecular-based allergy diagnostics, also known as *component IgE testing*, is highly specific but very costly and may detect sensitization that is not clinically significant. For these reasons, the WHO recommends reserving the use of component IgE testing for special situations, when there is a need to distinguish between responses to true allergens and cross-reactivity, predict the severity of clinical allergic responses, or select patients for specific allergen immunotherapy. The use of these tests has been especially helpful in the evaluation of peanut allergies.

Another development in IgE testing is a point-of-care lateral flow assay that can be used by primary care physicians to screen for reactivity to a few common allergens. In this assay, the allergen extracts are coated onto nitrocellulose strips encased in a cassette. A drop of blood from a finger prick is added to one well in the cassette, and a color-developing solution is added to a second well, driving the blood toward the antigen zone. In this semiquantitative test, the presence of allergen-specific IgE is indicated by a colored line in the corresponding allergen position. Patients with positive results can be referred to an allergist for further evaluation.

Regardless of the format of the specific IgE test used, the results should always be interpreted in light of the patient's medical history and clinical symptoms. This is because the presence of allergen-specific IgE antibody indicates sensitization to the allergen but not necessarily the presence of a clinical allergy.

In Vitro Tests: Total IgE

The first test for the measurement of total serum IgE was the competitive *radioimmunosorbent test (RIST)*. The RIST used radiolabeled IgE to compete with patient IgE for binding sites on a solid phase coated with anti-IgE. Because of the expense and difficulty of working with radioactivity, RIST has largely been replaced by noncompetitive solid-phase immunoassays or nephelometry assays with enhanced sensitivity.

In the noncompetitive solid-phase immunoassays, anti-human IgE is bound to a solid phase, such as cellulose, a paper disk, or a microtiter well. Patient serum is added and allowed to react, and then an enzyme-labeled anti-IgE is added to detect the bound patient IgE. The second anti-IgE antibody recognizes a different epitope than that recognized by the first antibody. The resulting "sandwich" of solid-phase anti-IgE, serum IgE, and labeled anti-IgE is washed; a colorimetric, fluorometric, or chemiluminescent substrate is then added. The amount of reactivity detected is directly proportional to the IgE content of the serum (see Fig. 14–5).

Total IgE values are reported in kilo international units (IU) per liter. One IU is equal to a concentration of 2.4 ng of protein per milliliter. IgE concentration varies with the individual's age and exposure to allergens. The total IgE concentration is typically lower than 1 kU/L in cord blood, and serum IgE usually reaches adult levels at about 10 years of age. In adults, a cutoff value of 100 kU/L is considered the upper limit of normal. Levels above 100 kU/L are common in individuals with allergies. However, measurement of total serum IgE is not recommended for the routine clinical evaluation of patients with suspected allergies because values vary widely among patients and do not necessarily correlate with the presence of allergy. Patients with slightly elevated IgE levels may not have an allergy, and many patients with allergies have a total serum IgE concentration that falls within the reference range. Thus, allergen-specific IgE tests are considered to have more value in the diagnosis of allergies.

Total serum IgE testing is more beneficial in evaluating patients with other conditions in which IgE levels may be elevated, such as helminth infections, and certain immunodeficiencies, such as Wiskott–Aldrich syndrome, DiGeorge syndrome, and hyper-IgE syndrome. Children living in areas where parasitic infections are endemic typically have serum IgE concentrations greater than 1,000 kU/L, whereas patients with hyper-IgE syndrome have extremely high IgE levels (2,000 to 50,000 kU/L). Measurement of total serum IgE is also helpful in monitoring patients undergoing allergen immunotherapy or treatment with monoclonal anti-IgE antibody. Successful treatment results in significant reductions in total serum IgE levels and in the ratio of allergen-specific IgE to total IgE.

Type II Hypersensitivity

Type II hypersensitivity is also known as *antibody-mediated cytotoxic* hypersensitivity. It is an immediate form of hypersensitivity that typically occurs a few hours after exposure to antigen. The key components involved in these reactions are IgG and IgM antibodies, as well as complement.

Immunologic Mechanism

In type II hypersensitivity, IgG and IgM antibodies are produced against antigens found on cell surfaces. These antigens may be self-antigens, as in the case of autoimmune hemolytic anemia, or heteroantigens, such as red blood cell antigens that stimulate transfusion reactions. Binding of the antibody to a cell can have one of three major effects, depending on the situation **(Fig. 14–6)**:

1. The cell can be destroyed.
2. The function of the cell can be inhibited.
3. The function of the cell can be increased above normal.

Cell damage can occur by several different mechanisms, some of which involve complement as well as antibodies: (1) Activation of the classical pathway of complement can lead to the formation of the membrane attack complex and cell lysis. (2) Coating of the cell surface by antibodies can promote opsonization and subsequent phagocytosis of the cells. Opsonization can occur either through binding of IgG antibody to Fc receptors on macrophages and neutrophils or binding of cell surface C3b to complement receptors on

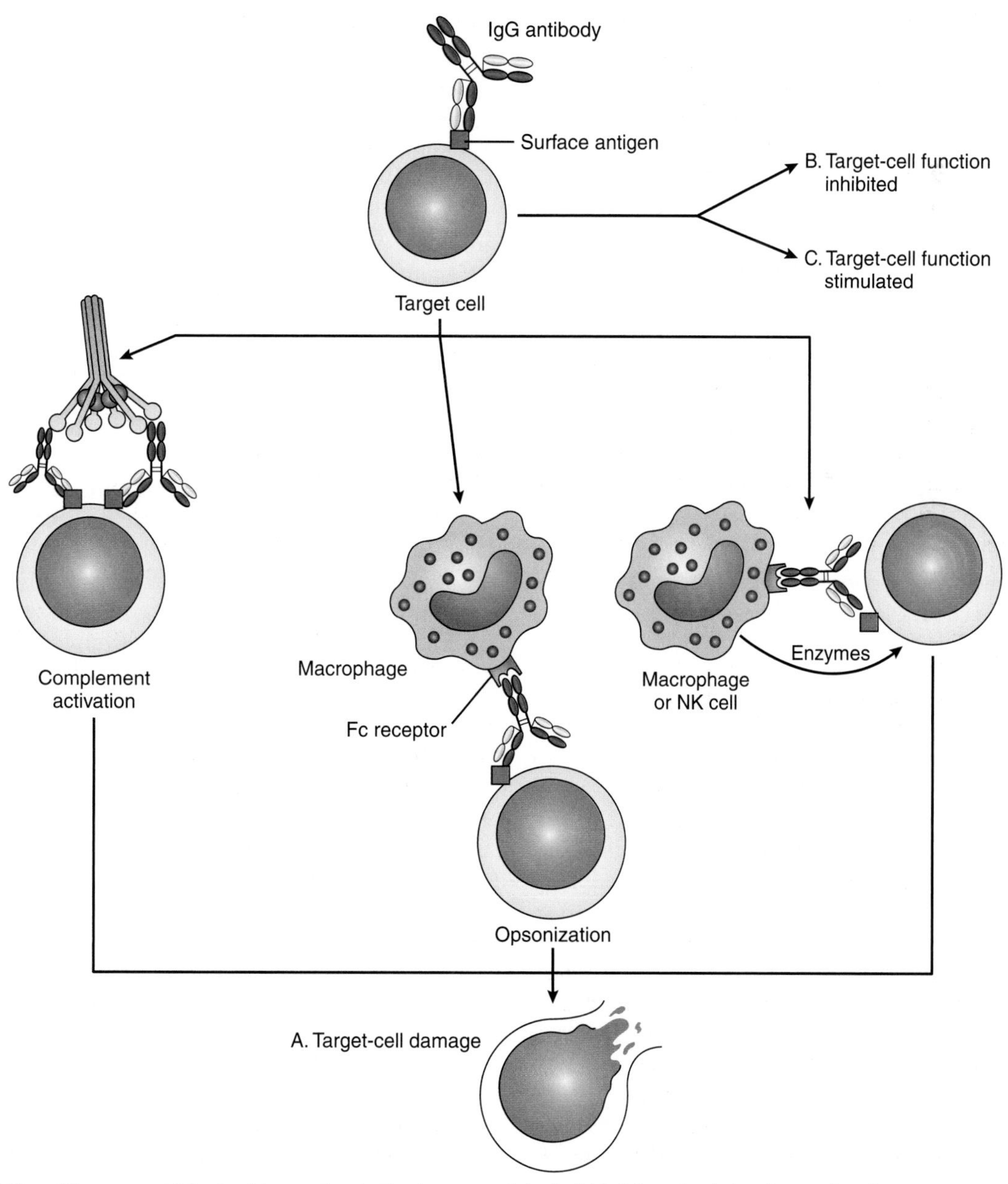

FIGURE 14–6 Type II hypersensitivity. In this reaction, IgG or immunoglobulin M (IgM) antibody binds to cell surface receptors, resulting in (A) cell damage through complement activation, opsonization, or antibody-dependent cellular cytotoxicity (ADCC); (B) inhibition of cell function; or (C) stimulation of cell function.

phagocytic cells. (3) Cell damage can result from the mechanism of antibody-dependent cellular cytotoxicity (ADCC). ADCC is mediated through binding of IgG antibody to its corresponding antigen on the target cell and to Fc receptors on macrophages or natural killer (NK) cells. This binding stimulates the release of cytotoxic enzymes that destroy the cell. Clinical examples that involve destruction of cells by type II hypersensitivity include blood transfusion reactions, hemolytic disease of the newborn, and autoimmune hemolytic anemia. These conditions are discussed in the sections that follow.

A second possible effect of type II hypersensitivity is that the cell surface antibody can inhibit the function of a cell. This can occur when antibody blocks the binding of a physiological ligand to its receptor, resulting in dysfunction of the cell. An example of this effect occurs in the autoimmune disease myasthenia gravis, which affects the neuromuscular junctions. Patients with this disease produce autoantibodies to receptors on muscle cells for the neurotransmitter acetylcholine (ACH). Normally, ACH is released from the nerve endings and binds to its corresponding receptors on muscle cells, stimulating contraction in the muscle fibers and muscle movement. However, in myasthenia gravis, attachment of the autoantibody to the ACH receptor blocks the binding of ACH, leading to muscle weakness (see Chapter 15).

Sometimes, binding of an antibody to a self-antigen can have the opposite effect, stimulating the cell instead of inhibiting its function. This results in overproduction of the cell's product, such as a hormone. The classic example of this effect is an autoimmune disorder of the thyroid gland called Graves' disease. Patients with Graves' disease produce antibodies against the receptor for the thyroid-stimulating hormone (TSH) on thyroid cells. TSH, a hormone produced by the pituitary gland in the brain, binds to the TSH receptors and stimulates the thyroid cells to produce hormones that increase metabolism. Normally, this process is carefully regulated by a feedback loop that signals the pituitary gland to make less TSH in the presence of high levels of thyroid hormones. However, in Graves' disease, the autoantibody binds to the TSH receptor, resulting in unregulated production of thyroid hormones. This leads to symptoms associated with increased metabolism, known as *hyperthyroidism* (see Chapter 15).

Clinical Examples of Type II Hypersensitivity

Transfusion Reactions

Transfusion reactions are examples of cell destruction that results from antibodies combining with heteroantigens. There are 36 different blood group systems with more than 380 different red blood cell (RBC) antigens. Some antigens are stronger than others and are more likely to stimulate antibody production. Major groups involved in transfusion reactions include the ABO, Rh, Kell, Duffy, Kidd, MNS, and Diego blood group systems. Antibodies to some of these antigens are produced naturally with no prior exposure to RBCs, whereas other antibodies are produced only after contact with cells carrying that antigen.

The ABO blood group is of primary importance in considering transfusions. Anti-A and anti-B antibodies are naturally occurring antibodies, or **isohemagglutinins,** which are probably triggered by contact with similar antigenic determinants on microorganisms or environmental agents such as pollen. Individuals do not make these antibodies to their own RBCs. Thus, a person who has type A blood has anti-B in the serum and a person with type B blood has anti-A antibodies. An individual with type O blood has both anti-A and anti-B in the serum because O cells have neither of these two antigens. The antibody formed typically belongs to the IgM class, but IgG may also be made.

If a patient is given blood for which antibodies are already present, a transfusion reaction occurs. This reaction can range from acute massive intravascular hemolysis to an undetected decrease in RBC survival. The extent of the reaction depends on several factors, including the temperature at which the antibody is most active, the plasma concentration of the antibody, the immunoglobulin class involved, the extent of complement activation, the density of the antigen on the RBC, and the number of RBCs transfused. It is most important to detect antibodies that react at 37°C. If a reaction occurs only below 30°C, it is not clinically significant because antigen–antibody complexes formed at colder temperatures tend to dissociate at 37°C.

Acute hemolytic transfusion reactions may occur within minutes or hours after receipt of incompatible blood. In this case, the individual has been exposed to the antigen before the transfusion (e.g., through previous transfusion or pregnancy) and has preformed antibodies to it. Reactions that begin immediately are most often associated with ABO blood group incompatibilities, and the antibodies are of the IgM class. As soon as cells bearing the antigen are introduced into the patient, intravascular hemolysis occurs because of complement activation, resulting in the release of hemoglobin and vasoactive and procoagulant substances into the plasma. This may induce disseminated intravascular coagulation (DIC), vascular collapse, and renal failure. Symptoms in the patient may include fever, chills, nausea, lower back pain, tachycardia, shock, and hemoglobin in the urine.

Delayed hemolytic reactions occur days to weeks following a transfusion and are caused by an anamnestic response to the antigen to which the patient has previously been exposed. The type of antibody responsible is IgG, which was initially present in such low titer that it was not detectable with an antibody screen. Antigens most involved in delayed reactions include those in the Rh, Kell, Duffy, and Kidd blood groups. The Rh, Kell, and Duffy antigens may also be involved in immediate transfusion reactions. In a delayed reaction, antibody-coated RBCs are removed extravascularly in the spleen or in the liver. The patient may experience a mild fever, low hemoglobin, mild jaundice, and anemia. Intravascular hemolysis does not take place to any great extent because IgG is not as efficient as IgM in activating complement. (See Chapter 5 for further details.)

Hemolytic Disease of the Fetus and Newborn

Hemolytic disease of the fetus and newborn (HDFN) appears in infants whose mothers have been exposed to blood-group antigens on the baby's cells that differ from their own. The mother makes IgG antibodies in response to these antigens; these antibodies cross the placenta and destroy the fetal RBCs. When anemia becomes severe, erythropoiesis increases and immature red blood cells are released from the bone marrow into the fetal circulation; thus, severe HDFN may be called *erythroblastosis fetalis*. A major cause of severe reactions is the D antigen, a member of the Rh blood group. HDFN caused by ABO incompatibility is actually more common; however, the disease is milder, probably because the A and B antigens on the fetus's RBCs are more poorly developed or reduced in number. Antibodies to more than 50 non-ABO blood group antigens have been associated with HDFN, including anti-c, anti-C, anti-E, and anti-e and antibodies to the Kell, Duffy, MNS, and Kidd blood groups.

Sensitization of the mother to paternal blood group antigens may occur during pregnancy but to a larger extent during the birth process, when fetal cells leak into the mother's circulation. Typically, the first child is unaffected; however, the second and later children have an increased risk of the disease because of an anamnestic response. The extent of the first fetal–maternal bleed influences whether antibodies will be produced. If enough of the baby's RBCs enter the mother's circulation, memory B cells develop. These cells become activated upon reexposure to the same RBC antigen, resulting in the production of IgG. This antibody crosses the placenta and attaches to the fetal RBCs in a subsequent pregnancy.

Depending on the degree of antibody production in the mother, the fetus may be aborted, stillborn, or born with evidence of hemolytic disease, as indicated by jaundice. As RBCs are lysed and free hemoglobin released, this is converted to bilirubin, which builds up in the plasma. There is too much of it to be conjugated in the liver, so it accumulates in the tissues. Excessive bilirubin may deposit in the brain and result in a severe neurological condition known as *kernicterus*. Treatment for severe HDN involves an exchange transfusion to replace antibody-coated RBCs. If serum antibody titrations during the pregnancy indicate a high level of circulating antibody, intrauterine transfusions can be performed.

To prevent the consequences of HDFN, all women should be screened at the onset of pregnancy. If they are Rh-negative, they should be tested for the presence of anti-D antibodies on a monthly basis. In current practice, a commercially prepared product consisting of purified anti-D, called *Rh-immune globulin* or *RhIg*, is administered prophylactically at 28 weeks of gestation and within 72 hours following delivery. The mechanism by which RhIg works is not completely known, but it is thought to facilitate clearance of the fetal RBCs through opsonization and therefore suppress the production of maternal antibody **(Fig. 14–7)**. This practice has dramatically reduced the incidence of HDFN cases caused by anti-D antibodies to less than 0.1% in countries where RhIg is routinely used. In these countries, antibodies to the Kell antigens are emerging as a leading cause of HDFN.

Autoimmune Hemolytic Anemia

Autoimmune hemolytic anemia is an example of a type II hypersensitivity reaction directed against self-antigens

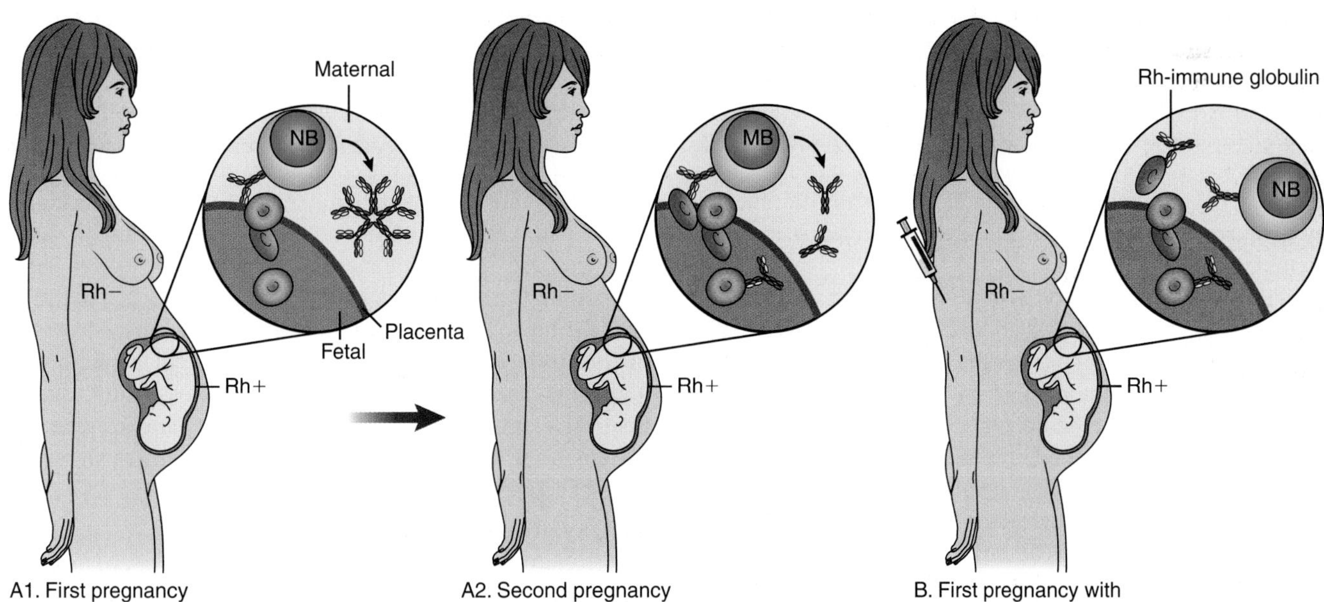

FIGURE 14–7 HDFN can develop in Rh-positive babies who are born to Rh-negative mothers if no treatment is administered. (A1) An Rh-negative mother may produce anti-Rh antibodies if an Rh-positive baby's RBCs enter her circulation late in gestation or during the birth process. In this primary immune response, naïve B cells (NB) differentiate, into plasma cells that secrete mainly anti-Rh IgM, which does not cross the placenta; therefore, a healthy baby is delivered. However, memory B cells (MB) are also produced, and (A2) if the mother becomes pregnant with another Rh-positive baby, these memory cells produce a stronger secondary immune response and secrete mainly anti-Rh IgG, which crosses the placenta and destroys the baby's RBCs, resulting in HDFN. (B) Alternatively, passive vaccination of the mother with an anti-Rh IgG during pregnancy and upon delivery prevents the mother from mounting an active immune response, allowing her future Rh-positive children to be born normally.

because individuals with this disease form antibodies to their own RBCs. Symptoms include malaise, lightheadedness, weakness, unexplained fever, pallor, and possibly mild jaundice. Such antibodies can be categorized into two groups: warm reactive antibodies, which react at 37°C, and cold reactive antibodies, which only react below 30°C. Autoimmune hemolytic anemia has been estimated to occur in 1 in 50,000 to 80,000 individuals.

Warm autoimmune hemolytic anemia accounts for more than 70% of autoimmune anemias and is characterized by the formation of IgG antibody, which reacts most strongly at 37°C. Some of these antibodies may be primary with no other disease association; others may be secondary to another disease process. Associated diseases may include viral or respiratory infections—such as infectious mononucleosis, cytomegalovirus, or chronic active hepatitis—or immunoproliferative diseases, such as chronic lymphocytic leukemia (CLL) and lymphomas. Often, the underlying cause of antibody production is unknown; this is referred to as *idiopathic autoimmune hemolytic anemia.*

In addition, certain drugs can induce the production of antibodies that can cause hemolytic anemia. These drugs are capable of attaching to the RBCs directly or of forming immune complexes that attach to the RBCs. Damage to the RBCs is believed to occur through several mechanisms. Some drugs, such as the penicillins and cephalosporins, can act as haptens after binding to proteins on the RBC membrane. These drugs stimulate the production of anti-drug antibodies that destroy the RBCs, primarily through extravascular hemolysis. The cephalosporins are also thought to modify the RBC membrane by facilitating binding of immunoglobulins and complement. Other drugs, such as quinidine and phenacetin, can stimulate the production of anti-drug antibodies that bind to the drug to form soluble immune complexes. The complexes attach loosely to the surface of the RBCs, which are cleared by intravascular hemolysis after binding of complement. Other drugs, such as methyldopa, can induce hemolytic anemia by stimulating production of autoantibodies against the RBC membrane.

Typically, patients exhibit symptoms of anemia because of the clearance of antibody-coated RBCs by macrophages in the liver and spleen. Hemolysis is primarily extravascular because IgG is not as efficient as IgM in activating complement; however, intravascular hemolysis can also occur if complement does become activated. The severity of the hemolysis is affected by the subclass of IgG involved, with IgG3 and IgG1 being most destructive to the RBCs because they are efficient at binding complement. Patients with warm autoimmune hemolytic anemia are usually treated with corticosteroids to reduce antibody synthesis or, in more serious cases, with a splenectomy to decrease RBC clearance. Treatment with monoclonal anti-CD 20 (rituximab) can be used for cases that are refractory to corticosteroids. This antibody attaches to B cells and causes a decrease in antibody production.

Cold Agglutinin Antibodies

Cold agglutinins are a less frequent cause of immune hemolytic anemias. By definition, cold agglutinins are autoantibodies that react with antigens on the RBC membrane at cold temperatures. The reaction is reversible upon exposure to a warm temperature. These cold-reacting antibodies belong to the IgM class, and most are specific for the Ii blood groups on RBCs. Cold agglutinins may be transient or chronic, depending on the cause. Polyclonal cold agglutinins can be produced secondary to certain infections, most notably *Mycoplasma* pneumonia and infectious mononucleosis but also respiratory viruses and HIV. In most cases, cold agglutinin production is transient and resolves in 2 to 3 weeks. Persistent, high-titer, monoclonal cold agglutinins have been associated with B-cell or plasma cell lymphoproliferative disorders, including B-cell CLL, B-cell lymphomas, Hodgkin disease, and Waldenström macroglobulinemia, as well as autoimmune diseases such as systemic lupus erythematosus (SLE). Chronic cold agglutinins can also be produced as a primary characteristic of a disease entity of unknown origin, which is known as *chronic cold agglutinin disease* (CCAD) or *chronic hemagglutinin disease* (CHD). CHD typically occurs in persons older than the age of 50 and is responsible for about 20% of autoimmune hemolytic anemia cases.

Cold agglutinins do not cause clinical symptoms unless the individual is exposed to the cold and usually have their maximal effect when the temperature in the peripheral circulation falls below 30°C. Under these conditions, the antibodies can bind to the RBCs to form lattices, which can obstruct the small capillaries in the skin. The areas of the body most affected are those having the greatest exposure to the cold, most notably the fingers, toes, earlobes, and nose. These areas develop a blue coloration known as *acrocyanosis* and become numb, stiff, and slightly painful. The symptoms are quickly reversible when the patient returns to warm surroundings; however, in severe cases, peripheral necrosis may result.

Another consequence of cold agglutinins results from the fixation of complement. Although complement activation cannot be completed in the cold, it can proceed once the cells recirculate and reach body temperature. If the RBCs become coated with C3b, opsonization can facilitate binding to macrophages and rapid clearance of the cells by the liver. Less commonly, the entire classical pathway is activated, and intravascular hemolysis occurs. Both processes lead to destruction of the RBCs and corresponding symptoms of autoimmune hemolytic anemia. Patients with this disease are usually treated by simply avoiding cold temperatures and keeping the extremities warm; drug therapy is only used if these measures are ineffective.

Paroxysmal Cold Hemoglobinuria

A rare condition known as **paroxysmal cold hemoglobinuria** can also cause autoimmune hemolytic anemia. This condition occurs most often after infection with certain viral illnesses, including measles, mumps, chickenpox, and infectious mononucleosis. Patients produce a biphasic autoantibody that binds to the RBCs at cold temperatures and activates complement at 37°C to produce an intermittent hemolysis. Consequently, an acute, rapidly progressing anemia with hemoglobin in the urine is seen. The condition occurs most often as a transient disorder in children and young adults.

Type II Reactions Involving Tissue Antigens

All the reactions that have been discussed so far deal with individual cells that are destroyed when a specific antigen–antibody combination takes place. Some type II reactions involve destruction of tissues because of their combination with antibody. Organ-specific autoimmune diseases in which antibody is directed against a particular tissue are in this category. Anti-glomerular basement membrane (anti-GBM) disease, formerly known as *Goodpasture's syndrome*, is an example of such a disease (see Chapter 15 for details). The antibody produced during the course of this disease reacts with basement membrane protein. Usually the glomeruli in the renal and pulmonary alveolar membranes are affected. Antibody binds to glomerular and alveolar capillaries; this triggers the complement cascade, which provokes inflammation. An evenly bound linear deposition of IgG in the glomerular basement membrane, which can be detected with fluorescent-labeled anti-IgG, is indicative of anti-GBM disease. Treatment usually involves the use of corticosteroids or other drugs to suppress the immune response.

Other examples of type II hypersensitivity reactions to tissue antigens include the organ-specific autoimmune disorders, Hashimoto's disease, myasthenia gravis, and insulin-dependent diabetes mellitus. Immunologic manifestations and detection of these diseases are presented in Chapter 15.

Testing for Type II Hypersensitivity

In 1945, Coombs, Mourant, and Race developed antiglobulin testing, which detects binding between RBC antigens and their corresponding antibodies by producing agglutination. The **direct antiglobulin test (DAT)** detects RBCs that have been sensitized with antibody or complement in vivo. The DAT is performed to detect transfusion reactions, HDFN, autoimmune hemolytic anemia, and drug-induced hemolytic anemia. In this technique, patient RBCs are initially incubated with polyspecific anti-human globulin, which is a mixture of antibodies to IgG and complement components such as C3b and C3d. If the test is positive for RBC agglutination, it is repeated using monospecific anti-IgG, anti-C3b, and anti-C3d to determine which of these is present. If the antibody attached to the RBCs is IgM, only the tests for complement components would be positive. (Refer to the exercise by going to FADavis.com for the laboratory exercises that accompany this text for more detail.)

The **indirect antiglobulin test (IAT)** is used in the cross-matching of blood to prevent a transfusion reaction. It is also used to determine the presence of a particular antibody in patient plasma or to type patient RBCs for specific blood group antigens. The method detects in vitro binding of antibody to RBCs rather than in vivo binding. This method is a two-step process in which RBCs and antibody are allowed to combine at 37°C and then the cells are carefully washed to remove any unbound antibody. Anti-human globulin is added, and a visible agglutination reaction occurs if antibody has been specifically bound. Any negative tests are confirmed by quality-control cells that are coated with antibody.

To determine the titer of a cold agglutinin antibody, the patient serum can be serially diluted and incubated overnight at 4°C with a dilute suspension of washed human type O RBCs. The tubes are then gently shaken and observed for agglutination. The last tube with agglutination represents the titer. Titers of 64 or higher are considered to be clinically significant. The agglutination should disappear after warming the tubes briefly in a 37°C water bath. Before testing, it is important to use prewarmed blood to separate the serum or plasma from the patient's RBCs. Failure to do so can result in binding of the cold agglutinins to the patient's own RBCs, producing false-negative results when the patient's serum is assayed for cold agglutinin reactivity against the reagent type O cells.

Type III Hypersensitivity

Type III hypersensitivity is also known as *complex-mediated* hypersensitivity. It is an immediate form of hypersensitivity that typically occurs a few hours after exposure to antigen. Type III hypersensitivity reactions are similar to type II reactions in that IgG or IgM is involved and destruction is complement-mediated. However, in the case of type III–associated diseases, the antigen is soluble.

Immunologic Mechanism

When soluble antigen combines with antibody, complexes are formed that precipitate out of the blood. Normally, such complexes are cleared by phagocytic cells; however, if the immune system is overwhelmed, these complexes deposit in the tissues. There, they bind complement, causing damage to the involved tissue. Deposition of antigen–antibody complexes is influenced by the relative concentration of both components. If a large excess of antigen is present, sites on antibody molecules become filled before cross-links can be formed. In antibody excess, a lattice cannot be formed because of the relative scarcity of antigenic determinant sites (see Fig. 10–3). The small complexes that are produced in either of the preceding cases remain suspended in the blood or may pass directly into the urine. Precipitating complexes, on the other hand, occur in mild antigen excess and are the ones most likely to deposit in the tissues. Sites in which this typically occurs include the glomerular basement membrane, vascular endothelium, joint linings, and pulmonary alveolar membranes.

Complement binds to the complexes in the tissues, causing the release of mediators that increase vasodilation and vasopermeability, attract macrophages and neutrophils, and enhance binding of phagocytic cells by C3b-mediated opsonization. If the target cells are large and cannot be engulfed for phagocytosis to take place, granule and lysosome contents are released by a process known as *exocytosis*. This process results in the damage to host tissue that is typified by type III reactions. Long-term changes include loss of tissue elements that cannot regenerate and accumulation of scar tissue. The mechanism of type III hypersensitivity is illustrated in **Figure 14–8.** Type III hypersensitivity reactions can be local or systemic, depending on where the immune complexes deposit in the body.

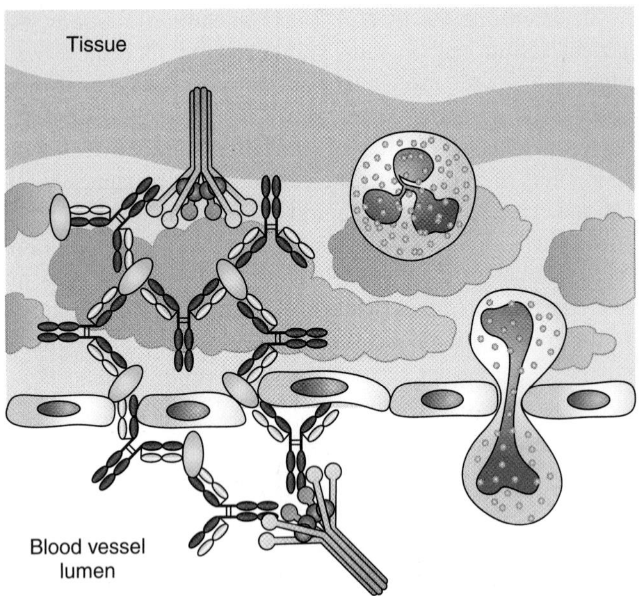

FIGURE 14–8 Type III hypersensitivity. Antigen and antibody combine to form immune complexes that deposit on the walls of blood vessels and tissues and activate complement. Complement-generated anaphylatoxins cause vasodilation, increased vascular permeability, edema, and accumulation of neutrophils.

Clinical Examples of Type III Hypersensitivity

Arthus Reaction

The classic example of a localized type III reaction is the **Arthus reaction,** demonstrated by Maurice Arthus in 1903. Using rabbits that had been immunized to produce an abundance of circulating antibodies, Arthus showed that when these rabbits were challenged with an intradermal injection of the antigen, a localized inflammatory reaction resulted. The reaction, which is characterized by erythema and edema, peaks within 3 to 8 hours and is followed by a hemorrhagic necrotic lesion that may ulcerate. The inflammatory response is caused by a combination of antigen and antibody to form immune complexes that deposit in small dermal blood vessels. Complement is fixed, attracting neutrophils and causing aggregation of platelets. Neutrophils release toxic products, such as oxygen-containing free radicals and proteolytic enzymes. Activation of complement is essential for the Arthus reaction because the C3a and C5a that are generated activate mast cells to release permeability factors; consequently, immune complexes localize along the endothelial cell basement membrane. The Arthus reaction can sometimes be seen in humans following booster injections with tetanus, diphtheria, or measles vaccines.

Serum Sickness

Serum sickness is a generalized type III hypersensitivity reaction that results from passive immunization of humans with animal serum. Before the advent of antibiotics and vaccines, serum sickness was observed more often because horse antiserums were used to treat infections such as diphtheria, tetanus, and pneumonia. These anti-sera were produced by immunizing horses with the corresponding antigen and provided immediate immunity to the individuals receiving them. Today, horse anti-venoms are still used to treat people who have been bitten by poisonous snakes. Serum sickness can also occur after treatment of patients with mouse monoclonal antibodies for diseases such as cancer or autoimmune disorders. Patients exposed to such animal sera can produce antibodies against the foreign animal proteins. These can combine with their corresponding antigen to form immune complexes that can deposit in the tissues and trigger the type III hypersensitivity response.

Generalized symptoms of serum sickness appear 7 to 21 days after injection of the animal serum and include headache, fever, nausea, vomiting, joint pain, rashes, and lymphadenopathy. Usually this is a self-limiting disease, and recovery takes a few weeks after the offending antigen is eliminated. However, previous exposure to animal serum can result in a more rapid reaction with increased severity.

Autoimmune Diseases and Other Causes of Type III Hypersensitivity

Type III hypersensitivity reactions can also be triggered by autologous antigens, as seen in several of the autoimmune diseases. SLE and rheumatoid arthritis (RA) are two such examples. Patients with these diseases commonly produce antibodies against nuclear constituents such as DNA and histones. They may also produce an antibody against IgG called *rheumatoid factor.* The autoantibodies combine with their corresponding antigen to produce immune complexes that trigger the type III hypersensitivity response. In SLE, immune complex deposition involves multiple organs; however, the main damage occurs to the joints, skin, and kidneys. In rheumatoid arthritis, immune complexes primarily cause damage to the joints. Complement enhances tissue destruction in both diseases. See Chapter 15 for a more detailed discussion of these two conditions.

Type III hypersensitivity can also be caused by several other factors. These include components of vaccines, bee stings, treatment with certain drugs (e.g., penicillin and sulfonamides), and infections such as viral hepatitis and Group A *Streptococcus*.

Testing for Type III Hypersensitivity

The laboratory methods associated with type III hypersensitivity are varied and depend on the condition being detected. In autoimmune diseases such as SLE and RA, the presence of antinuclear antibodies can be detected by a variety of methods, including indirect immunofluorescence, enzyme-linked immunosorbent assay (ELISA), and fluorescent microsphere multiplex immunoassays (see Chapter 15 for details). Fluorescent staining of tissue sections has also been used to determine deposition of immune complexes in the tissues. The staining pattern seen and the particular tissue affected help to identify the disease and determine its severity. Rheumatoid factor can be detected by latex agglutination, nephelometry, or other immunoassays (see Chapter 15).

A more general method of evaluating immune complex diseases is by measuring complement levels. During periods of high disease activity, complement levels in the serum may be decreased because of binding of some of the complement to the antigen–antibody complexes. The results should be interpreted in conjunction with other clinical findings. Refer to Chapter 7 for a discussion of complement testing.

Type IV Hypersensitivity

Type IV hypersensitivity was first described in 1890 by Robert Koch. He observed that individuals infected with *Mycobacterium tuberculosis* developed a localized inflammatory response after receiving intradermal injections of a filtrate from the organism. Type IV hypersensitivity differs from the other three types of hypersensitivity in that sensitized T cells, rather than antibodies, play the major role in its manifestations. It is therefore known as *cell-mediated* hypersensitivity. Because symptoms peak between 48 and 72 hours after exposure to antigen, this reaction is also referred to as *delayed hypersensitivity.*

Immunologic Mechanism

Although there are different mechanisms involved in type IV hypersensitivity, the classic type IV response involves the Th1 subclass of T helper (Th) cells. There is an initial sensitization phase of 1 to 2 weeks that takes place after the first contact with antigen. During this phase, Langerhans cells in the skin and macrophages in the tissues capture antigen and migrate to nearby lymph nodes, where they present the antigen to naïve Th cells. The antigen-presenting cells (APCs) also release cytokines that promote differentiation of the naïve T cells into Th1 cells and other T-cell subsets and induce their proliferation. The expanded Th1 cells then migrate to the site where the antigen is located, and the effector phase of the response begins. At the site, the activated Th1 cells release cytokines. Interleukin 3 (IL-3) and granulocyte-macrophage colony-stimulating factor (GM-CSF) induce hematopoiesis of cells of the granulocyte-macrophage lineage, and chemokines such as monocyte chemotactic protein (MCP-1/CCL2) recruit macrophages to the site. In the tissues, the monocytes differentiate into macrophages and are activated by interferon gamma (IFN-γ) and tumor necrosis factor-β (TNF-β). These activated macrophages release reactive oxygen species, nitric oxide, and proinflammatory mediators that recruit more macrophages to the site and stimulate them to become effective APCs, thus perpetuating the response. The immunologic mechanism of type IV hypersensitivity is illustrated in **Figure 14–9.**

Chronic persistence of antigen leads to the development of organized clusters of cells called **granulomas,** which consist of epithelioid-shaped and multinucleated fused macrophages with an infiltrate of lymphocytes or other WBCs. Many of these macrophages contain engulfed antigens, such as intracellular bacteria. Thus, the granuloma can function to wall off the organism in a contained area, preventing its spread to other parts of the body. However, cells in the granuloma can release large amounts of lytic enzymes that can destroy surrounding tissue and promote fibrin deposition. Cytotoxic T cells are also recruited, and they bind with antigen-coated target cells to cause further tissue destruction.

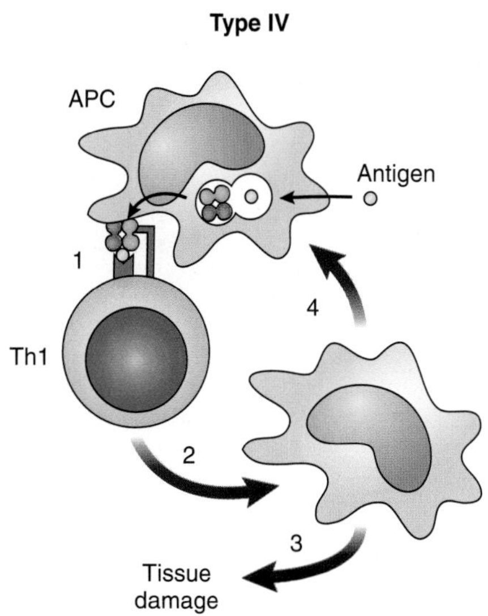

FIGURE 14–9 Type IV hypersensitivity. APCs take up antigen and activate Th1 T helper cells. The Th1 cells produce cytokines that stimulate macrophages to elicit an inflammatory response and, in some cases, activate cytotoxic T cells to cause tissue damage (latter not shown).

The antigens that can trigger type IV hypersensitivity are generally one of two types: intracellular pathogens or contact antigens. The intracellular pathogens can be bacteria, fungi, parasites, or viruses. Pathogens that commonly induce delayed hypersensitivity include *M. tuberculosis, Mycobacterium leprae, Pneumocystis carinii, Leishmania* species, and herpes simplex virus. Contact antigens are those that come into direct contact with the skin. They include plants such as poison ivy and poison oak, metals such as nickel salts, and components of hair dyes and cosmetics. Clinical manifestations of type IV hypersensitivity induced by these antigens are discussed in the sections that follow.

Clinical Manifestations of Type IV Hypersensitivity

Contact Dermatitis

Contact dermatitis is among the most prevalent skin disorders, affecting an estimated 15% to 20% of the general population. Reactions are usually caused by low-molecular-weight compounds that touch the skin. The most common causes include poison ivy, poison oak, and poison sumac, all of which release the chemical urushiol in the plant sap and on the leaves. Allergic dermatitis caused by contact with these plants affects millions of Americans every year. Other common compounds that produce allergic skin manifestations include nickel; rubber; formaldehyde; hair dyes and fabric finishes; cosmetics; and medications applied to the skin, such as topical anesthetics, antiseptics, and antibiotics. In addition, latex sensitization has been reported as a cause of contact dermatitis in a significant number of health-care workers (see the previous text).

Most of these substances probably function as haptens that bind to glycoproteins on skin cells. Langerhans cells in the

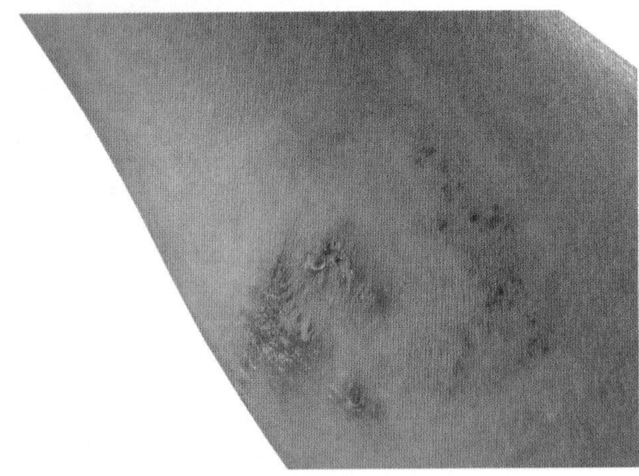

FIGURE 14–10 Contact hypersensitivity. Formation of papules occurs after exposure to poison ivy. *(Courtesy of Yong Choi/ Thinkstock.)*

skin are thought to process the hapten–protein complexes and migrate to the regional lymph nodes, where they present the antigen to Th1 cells. Sensitization of the Th cells takes several days; however, once it occurs, its effects can last for years because of immunologic memory. Cytokine production by the Th1 cells causes macrophages to accumulate and release cytokines and other substances that produce a local inflammatory response.

Contact dermatitis produces a skin eruption characterized by erythema, swelling, and the formation of papules that appears from 6 hours to several days after the exposure **(Fig. 14–10)**. The papules may become vesicular, with blistering, peeling, and weeping. The site usually itches. The dermatitis is first limited to skin sites exposed to the antigen, but then it spreads to adjoining areas. The duration of the reaction depends upon the degree of sensitization and the concentration of antigen absorbed. Dermatitis can last for 3 to 4 weeks after the antigen has been removed. Simple redness may fade of its own accord within several days. If the area is small and localized, a topical steroid may be used for treatment. Otherwise, systemic corticosteroids may be administered. Patients also need to avoid contact with the offending allergen.

Hypersensitivity Pneumonitis

Hypersensitivity pneumonitis is mediated predominantly by sensitized T lymphocytes that respond to inhaled allergens. IgG and IgM antibodies are formed, but these are thought to play only a minor role in the pathogenesis of this disorder. Hypersensitivity pneumonitis is an allergic disease of the lung parenchyma characterized by inflammation of the alveoli and interstitial spaces. It is caused by chronic inhalation of a wide variety of antigens and is most often seen in individuals who are engaged in work or hobbies involving exposure to the implicated antigen.

Depending on the occupation and the particular antigen, the disease goes by several names: *farmer's lung, bird breeder's lung disease,* and *humidifier* or *air-conditioner lung disease.* The reaction is most likely caused by microorganisms, especially bacterial and fungal spores, to which individuals are exposed when working with moldy hay, pigeon droppings, compost, moldy tobacco, infested flour, and moldy cheese, to name just a few examples. Symptoms include a dry cough, shortness of breath, fever, chills, weight loss, and general malaise, which may begin 6 to 8 hours after exposure to a high dose of the offending antigen. Alveolar macrophages and lymphocytes trigger a chronic condition characterized by interstitial fibrosis with alveolar inflammation. Systemic corticosteroid therapy is used for treatment.

Skin Testing for Delayed Hypersensitivity

Skin testing is used clinically to detect delayed hypersensitivity responses to a variety of antigens. The tests are based on a T-cell–mediated memory response. When antigen is injected intradermally or applied to the surface of the skin, previously sensitized individuals develop a reaction at the application site. This reaction results from infiltration of T lymphocytes and macrophages into the area. Blood vessels in the vicinity become lined with mononuclear cells, and the reaction reaches a peak by 72 hours after exposure. Skin testing has been used to determine allergen sensitivity in contact dermatitis, assess exposure to *M. tuberculosis,* and evaluate the competency of cell-mediated immune responses in patients with immune deficiency diseases. Each of these applications is discussed in the text that follows.

The patch test is considered the gold standard in testing for contact dermatitis. This test must be done when the patient is free of symptoms or at least has a clear test site. A nonabsorbent adhesive patch containing the suspected contact allergen is applied on the patient's back, and the skin is checked for a reaction during the next 48 hours. Redness with papules or tiny blisters is considered a positive test. Final evaluation is conducted at 96 to 120 hours. All readings should be done by a skilled evaluator. False negatives can result from inadequate contact with the skin.

Skin testing for exposure to tuberculosis (TB) is a classic example of a delayed hypersensitivity reaction. The test is based on the principle that soluble antigens from *M. tuberculosis* induce a reaction in people who currently have TB or have been exposed to *M. tuberculosis* in the past. The tuberculin skin test uses an *M. tuberculosis* antigen extract prepared from a purified filtrate of the organism's cell wall, called a *purified protein derivative* (PPD). The test is routinely performed by the Mantoux method, in which 0.1 mL of 5 tuberculin units (TU) of PPD is injected intradermally into the inner surface of the forearm using a fine needle and syringe **(Fig. 14–11)**. The test site is examined between 48 and 72 hours for the presence of a hardened, raised area called *induration.* Interpretation of the reaction depends on the particular group in which the individual is categorized. An induration reaction of 15 mm or more is considered a positive test in individuals with no risk factors, whereas a reaction of 10 mm or greater is considered positive in recent immigrants from high-prevalence countries, intravenous drug users, employees of health-care and other high-risk facilities, persons with certain clinical conditions, and children younger than 5 years of age. An induration reaction of 5 mm or more is considered positive in persons who

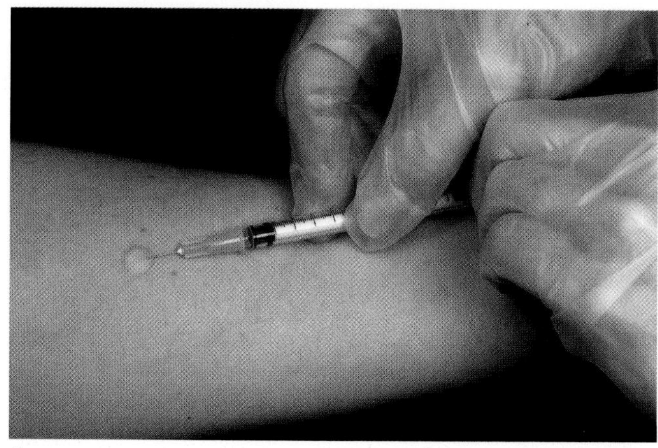

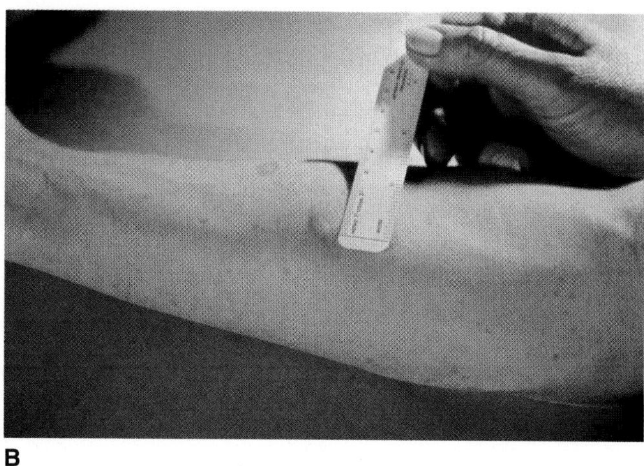

A B

FIGURE 14–11 The Mantoux test. (A) PPD is injected into an individual's forearm, which causes a wheal (i.e., a raised area of the skin surface) to form at the injection site. (B) After 48 hours, the individual presented with an induration (hardened, raised area), indicating a positive reaction. *(A. Courtesy of the CDC/Gabrielle Benenson and Greg Knobloch, Public Health Image Library. B. Courtesy of the CDC/Donald Kopanoff, Public Health Image Library.)*

have HIV infection or other forms of immunosuppression, features on a chest x-ray consistent with TB, or recent contact with TB patients. A positive tuberculin skin test indicates that the individual has previously been exposed to *M. tuberculosis* or a related organism, but it does not necessarily mean that he or she has an active TB infection. Positive test results also occur in persons who have previously received the Bacillus Calmette-Guerin (BCG) vaccine for TB. The test has been an important screening tool to detect exposure in health-care workers and other individuals at risk for the infection.

Skin testing can also be used to determine whether the cell-mediated arm of the immune system is functioning properly in individuals suspected of having immunodeficiency disorders. Antigens typically used for testing are from sources to which individuals have been commonly exposed, such as *Candida albicans,* tetanus toxoid, *Streptococcus* bacteria, and fungal antigens such as trichophyton and histoplasmin. The antigens are injected intradermally by the Mantoux method; the injection sites are then examined at 48 hours for redness and induration. Normal individuals should mount a memory response and develop a positive skin reaction to at least one of the antigens tested. Those with deficient cell-mediated immunity will display **anergy,** or the absence of positive reactions for all the common antigens used in the skin test.

Interferon Gamma Release Assays (IGRAs)

Most people exposed to *M. tuberculosis* and related bacteria develop a latent infection that is asymptomatic; however, they have an increased risk (5% to 10%) of developing active TB disease with serious respiratory and other symptoms throughout the course of their lives. The tuberculin skin test has been used for more than 100 years to identify individuals infected with bacteria of the *M. tuberculosis* complex. However, this test has important limitations, as discussed in the previous section. False-positive results can occur in people who have received the BCG vaccine or who have been infected with nontuberculous mycobacteria. In addition, the test requires a second visit from the patient to read the skin reaction that develops as a memory response 48 to 72 hours after the PPD injection.

Interferon gamma release assays (IGRA) have been developed as an alternative to tuberculin skin testing to detect latent TB infection. These tests are based on detecting a cell-mediated immune response by measuring the production of IFN-γ by patient T cells that have been stimulated with *M. tuberculosis*–specific antigens. Currently, there are two commercially available IGRAs that have been approved by the U.S. Food and Drug Administration (FDA): the Quantiferon TB Gold Plus assay and the T-SPOT.TB test.

In the Quantiferon TB Gold Plus assay, patient blood is drawn into specialized collection tubes containing peptides that are highly specific for *M. tuberculosis* (ESAT-6 and CFP-10). These antigens are not found in most strains of nontuberculous mycobacteria or in the bacteria used to make the BCG vaccine. A negative control tube that does not contain the TB antigens and a positive control tube containing the T-cell mitogen, phytohemagglutinin (PHA), are also set up. Patient blood is incubated in the tubes at 37°C for 16 to 24 hours. During the incubation, T cells from patients who have been infected with *M. tuberculosis* will respond to the TB antigens by producing the cytokine, IFN-γ. The tubes are then centrifuged to collect patient plasma, and the amount of IFN-γ in the plasma is measured by an ELISA.

The T-SPOT.TB test is based on the enzyme-linked immunospot (Elispot) technique. In this test, mononuclear cells are isolated from patient peripheral blood and placed into wells of a microtiter plate that have been precoated with antibody to IFN-γ. *M. tuberculosis*–specific antigens (ESAT-6 and CFP-10) are added to the wells, and the contents are incubated at 37°C for 16 to 20 hours in the presence of 5% CO_2. Positive and negative control wells are also included in the assay. During the incubation, T cells from patients exposed to *M. tuberculosis* release IFN-γ in their vicinity. After a wash step, an enzyme-labeled antibody to IFN-γ is added, and after another incubation and wash, substrate is added to the wells. Dark blue spots are produced where the IFN-γ–secreting cells were located in the wells, and the number of spots is counted under a magnifying glass or stereomicroscope (see Fig. 6-7).

The CDC recommends using either IGRA method to detect latent TB in people who are at high risk of developing active disease, including those who were recently infected, those with HIV infection or certain medical conditions, those receiving immunosuppressive drugs, and infants and children younger than 5 years of age. Both IGRA methods are more sensitive and specific than the tuberculin skin test and provide more objective results that are easier to interpret and available sooner. In addition, IGRAs can be used in people who have received the BCG vaccine and require only a single patient visit to the clinic. However, none of the methods can differentiate between latent and active TB or predict which patients with latent infection will progress to develop active TB disease.

SUMMARY

- Hypersensitivity is an exaggerated immune response to antigens that are usually not harmful. It results in cell destruction and tissue injury.
- Gell and Coombs devised a system for classifying hypersensitivity reactions into four types based on the immunologic mechanism involved and the nature of the triggering antigen.
- Hypersensitivity types I, II, and III are antibody-mediated. Because they occur within minutes to hours after exposure to antigen, they are referred to as *immediate reactions*.
- Type IV hypersensitivity is a cell-mediated response involving T lymphocytes. Because the clinical manifestations do not appear until 24 to 72 hours after contact with the antigen, the type IV response is also referred to as *delayed hypersensitivity*.
- Type I hypersensitivity involves the production of IgE antibody to an allergen. In the sensitization phase of this response, the IgE binds to high-affinity FcεRI receptors on mast cells and basophils. In the activation phase, the receptors become cross-linked when the allergen binds to adjacent IgE molecules. Degranulation of the mast cells and basophils occurs, with the release of preformed and newly synthesized chemical mediators that cause an inflammatory response. Cytokines produced during the response can cause a late-phase response of prolonged inflammation.
- Preformed mediators that are released from mast cells and basophils include histamine, eosinophil chemotactic factor of anaphylaxis, neutrophil chemotactic factor, and proteolytic enzymes such as tryptase. These factors cause contraction of smooth muscle in the bronchioles, blood vessels, and intestines; increased capillary permeability; chemotaxis of eosinophils and neutrophils; and decreased blood coagulability. Newly synthesized mediators such as prostaglandins, leukotrienes, and PAF potentiate the effects of histamine and other preformed mediators.
- Clinical manifestations of type I hypersensitivity include localized wheal-and-flare skin reactions (i.e., urticaria or hives), rhinitis, allergic asthma, and a life-threatening condition called *systemic anaphylaxis*.
- Susceptibility to allergies is based on a combination of genetic factors that affect the immune response and environmental influences, such as exposure to infectious organisms.
- Allergies can be treated with drugs such as antihistamines, decongestants, and corticosteroids. Monoclonal anti-IgE antibodies such as omalizumab have been used to block the binding of IgE to mast cells and basophils in patients with moderate to severe asthma.
- Allergen immunotherapy (AIT) can be administered to patients for whom drug therapy and environmental control measures are not successful. The goal of AIT is to induce immune tolerance by administering gradually increasing doses of the allergen through time.
- The preferred method of screening for allergies is an in vivo skin prick test, in which very small amounts of potential allergens are injected under the skin. A positive test produces a wheal-and-flare reaction within 20 minutes.
- In patients unable to tolerate skin testing, in vitro testing by noncompetitive solid-phase immunoassays for allergen-specific IgE can be performed. In these assays, patient serum is incubated with a solid phase to which a specific allergen has been attached. Binding is detected with an enzyme-labeled anti-human IgE antibody and a colorimetric, fluorescent, or chemiluminescent substrate.
- Solid-phase immunoassays for total serum IgE can be used to monitor patients undergoing treatment with AIT or monoclonal anti-IgE or to detect patients with certain diseases characterized by elevated IgE levels. The principle of these tests is the same as that for allergen-specific IgE tests except that anti-IgE, rather than allergen, is attached to the solid phase.
- Type II hypersensitivity involves the production of IgG or IgM antibodies to antigens on the surface of host cells. These antibodies can destroy the cells through complement-mediated cytolysis, opsonization and phagocytosis, or antibody-dependent cellular cytotoxicity (ADCC). In other cases, binding of the antibody to the cell surface antigen can result in dysfunction or overstimulation of the cell.
- Examples of type II reactions that involve cell damage include autoimmune hemolytic anemia, transfusion reactions, and hemolytic disease of the fetus and newborn (HDFN). Myasthenia gravis is an example of a type II disorder in which the antibody blocks binding of a ligand to cell receptors, causing dysfunction of the cells. In contrast, antibodies in Graves' disease stimulate cells after binding to their receptors.
- The direct antiglobulin test (DAT) is used to screen for transfusion reactions, autoimmune hemolytic anemia, and HDFN. In this test, washed patient RBCs are combined with anti-human globulin and observed for agglutination, indicating the presence of IgG or complement components on the cells.
- The indirect antiglobulin test (IAT) is used in antibody screening and identification and in crossmatching of blood to prevent transfusion reactions. It is also used to type patient RBCs for specific blood group antigens. The

method detects in vitro binding of antibody to RBCs after addition of anti-human globulin to cause a visible agglutination reaction.

- Cold agglutinin antibodies bind to RBCs at temperatures below 30°C and cause microocclusions of small blood vessels or destruction of the RBCs, mainly through opsonization and extravascular clearance by macrophages in the liver. Production of cold agglutinins may be from unknown causes or may be associated with certain infections or B cell/plasma cell lymphoproliferative disorders. Cold agglutinin titers can be determined by incubating patient serum with a dilute suspension of human type O RBCs overnight at 4°C and observing for agglutination.
- Type III hypersensitivity involves the formation of IgG or IgM antibody that reacts with soluble antigen under conditions of slight antigen excess to form small complexes that precipitate in the tissues. These complexes activate complement, resulting in the migration of neutrophils to the site, with subsequent release of lysosomal enzymes that produce damage to the surrounding tissues.
- The Arthus reaction, characterized by deposition of antigen–antibody complexes in the blood vessels of the skin, is a classic example of a type III reaction. Other examples include serum sickness and autoimmune diseases such as SLE and RA.
- Type IV hypersensitivity is a cell-mediated mechanism that involves the activation of Th1 cells to release cytokines. Therefore, macrophages and other immune cells are recruited to the area, where they induce an inflammatory reaction. Cytotoxic T cells may also cause damage to the target cells involved.
- Contact dermatitis is an example of a type IV hypersensitivity reaction. It results from exposure to chemicals released by plants such as poison ivy and poison oak, metals such as nickel, or components of hair dyes and cosmetics that act as haptens when bound to self-proteins. Hypersensitivity pneumonitis is a type IV hypersensitivity response that results mainly from occupational exposure to inhaled antigens.
- Skin testing is used to detect the type IV hypersensitivity responses in contact dermatitis and tuberculin (PPD) testing. It is also used to test for functional cell-mediated immunity to common antigens in patients suspected of having immunodeficiency diseases. Positive test results appear in 48 to 72 hours and indicate sensitization to the antigen(s) used in the test.
- Interferon gamma release assays (IGRAs) provide an alternative to tuberculin skin testing to detect latent *M. tuberculosis* infection. The IGRAs have several advantages compared with skin testing, including increased specificity, clearer result interpretation, and faster turnaround time to results.
- All four types of hypersensitivity represent defense mechanisms that stimulate an inflammatory response to cope with and react to an antigen that is seen as foreign. In many cases, the antigen is not harmful, but the response to it results in tissue damage.

Study Guide: Comparison of Hypersensitivity Reactions

	TYPE I	TYPE II	TYPE III	TYPE IV
Immune Mediators	IgE	IgG or IgM	IgG or IgM	T cells
Synonym	Anaphylactic	Antibody-mediated cytotoxic	Complex-mediated	Cell-mediated or delayed type
Timing	Immediate	Immediate	Immediate	Delayed
Antigen	Heterologous	Cell surface: autologous or heterologous	Soluble: autologous or heterologous	Autologous or heterologous
Complement Involvement	No	Yes	Yes	No
Immune Mechanism	Release of mediators from IgE-sensitized mast cells and basophils	Cell destruction caused by antibody and complement, opsonization, or ADCC Cell function inhibited by antibody binding Cell function stimulated by antibody binding	Antigen–antibody complexes activate complement proteins. Neutrophils are recruited and release lysosomal enzymes that cause tissue damage.	Antigen-sensitized Th1 cells release cytokines that recruit macrophages and induce inflammation or activate cytotoxic T cells to cause direct cell damage.
Clinical Examples	Anaphylaxis, allergic rhinitis, allergic asthma, food allergies, urticaria	Transfusion reactions, autoimmune hemolytic anemia, hemolytic disease of the fetus and newborn, drug reactions, myasthenia gravis, Anti-GBM disease, Graves' disease	Serum sickness, Arthus reaction, lupus erythematosus, rheumatoid arthritis, drug reactions	Contact dermatitis, tuberculin and anergy skin tests, hypersensitivity pneumonitis

CASE STUDIES

1. A 13-year-old male had numerous absences from school in the spring because of cold symptoms that included head congestion and cough. He had received antibiotic treatment twice, but he seemed to get one cold after another. A complete blood count (CBC) showed no overall increase in WBCs, but a mild eosinophilia was present. Because he had no fever or other signs of infection, his physician suggested that allergy testing be run.

Questions

a. What would account for the eosinophilia noted?
b. What tests should be run for this patient?
c. If the patient was treated with allergy immunotherapy, what test could be used to monitor his response through time?

2. A 55-year-old male went to his physician complaining of feeling tired and run down. Two months previously, he had pneumonia and was concerned that he might not have completely recovered. He indicated that his symptoms only become noticeable if he goes out in the cold. A CBC count was performed, showing that his WBC count was within normal limits; however, his RBC count was just below normal. A DAT performed on his RBCs was weakly positive after incubating at room temperature for 5 minutes. When the DAT was repeated with monospecific reagents, the tube with anti-C3d was the only one that was positive.

Questions

a. What does a positive DAT indicate?
b. What is the most likely class of the antibody causing the reaction?
c. Why was the DAT positive only with anti-C3d when monospecific reagents were used?

REVIEW QUESTIONS

1. Which of the following is a general characteristic of hypersensitivity reactions?
   a. The immune responsiveness is depressed.
   b. Antibodies are involved in all reactions.
   c. An exaggerated immune response to an antigen occurs.
   d. The antigen triggering the reaction is a harmful one.

2. Which of the following is associated with an increase in IgE production?
   a. Transfusion reaction
   b. Activation of Th2 cells
   c. Reaction to poison ivy
   d. Hemolytic disease of the fetus and newborn

3. Which of the following would cause a positive DAT test?
   a. Presence of IgG on RBCs
   b. Presence of C3b or C3d on RBCs
   c. A transfusion reaction caused by preformed antibody
   d. Any of the above

4. All of the following are associated with type I hypersensitivity *except*
   a. release of preformed mediators from mast cells.
   b. activation of complement.
   c. cell-bound antibody bridged by antigen.
   d. an inherited tendency to respond to allergens.

5. Which of the following is associated with anaphylaxis?
   a. Buildup of IgE on mast cells
   b. Activation of complement
   c. Increase in cytotoxic T cells
   d. Large amount of circulating IgG

6. To determine if a patient is allergic to ryegrass, the best test to perform is the
   a. total IgE test.
   b. skin prick test.
   c. DAT.
   d. complement fixation.

7. Which condition would result in hemolytic disease of the fetus and newborn?
   a. Buildup of IgE on mother's cells
   b. Sensitization of cytotoxic T cells
   c. Exposure to antigen found on both mother and baby RBCs
   d. Prior exposure to foreign RBC antigen

8. What is the immune mechanism involved in type III hypersensitivity reactions?
   a. Cellular antigens are involved.
   b. Deposition of immune complexes occurs in antibody excess.
   c. Only heterologous antigens are involved.
   d. Tissue damage results from complement-mediated lysis.

9. What is the immune phenomenon associated with the Arthus reaction?
   a. Tissue destruction by cytotoxic T cells
   b. Removal of antibody-coated RBCs
   c. Deposition of immune complexes in blood vessels
   d. Release of histamine from mast cells

10. Which of the following conclusions can be drawn about a patient whose total IgE level was determined to be 150 IU/mL?
    a. The patient definitely has allergic tendencies.
    b. The patient may be subject to anaphylactic shock.
    c. Antigen-specific testing should be done.
    d. The patient will never have an allergic reaction.

11. Which of the following explains the difference between type II and type III hypersensitivity reactions?
    a. Type II involves cellular antigens.
    b. Type III involves IgE.
    c. IgG is involved only in type III reactions.
    d. Type II reactions involve no antibody.

12. Two days after administration of the tuberculin skin test, a female health-care worker developed an area of redness and induration 12 mm in size at the injection site. This result means that she has
    a. an active case of TB.
    b. been exposed to *M. tuberculosis*.
    c. developed protective immunity against TB.
    d. a result in the normal range for her risk group.

13. A young woman developed red, itchy papules on her wrist 2 days after wearing a new bracelet. This reaction was caused by
    a. IgE-sensitized mast cells in the skin.
    b. antigen–antibody complexes in the skin.
    c. damage to the skin cells by antibodies and complement.
    d. an inflammatory response induced by cytokines released from Th1 cells.

14. Reactions to latex are caused by
    a. type I hypersensitivity.
    b. type IV hypersensitivity.
    c. skin irritation.
    d. all of the above.

15. To determine a cold agglutinin titer,
    a. patient serum should be separated from whole blood at 4°C and tested at 4°C.
    b. patient serum should be separated from whole blood at 4°C and tested at 37°C.
    c. patient serum should be separated from whole blood at 37°C and tested at 4°C.
    d. patient serum should be separated from whole blood at 37°C and tested at 37°C.

16. In vitro methods to detect a cell-mediated response to *M. tuberculosis* measure production of which of the following immunologic components?
    a. IgE antibody
    b. Interleukin-1
    c. Interleukin-2
    d. Interferon gamma

15 Autoimmunity

Linda E. Miller, PhD, MB^{CM}(ASCP)SI

LEARNING OUTCOMES

After finishing this chapter, you should be able to:

1. Explain the mechanisms of central and peripheral tolerance that are essential in preventing the development of autoimmunity.
2. Discuss genetic and environmental factors that are thought to contribute to the development of autoimmunity.
3. Explain the relationship between microbial infections and the development of autoimmune disease.
4. Distinguish between organ-specific and systemic autoimmune diseases, providing examples of each and their associated target tissues.
5. Discuss the immunopathology and clinical manifestations of each of the following diseases: systemic lupus erythematosus (SLE), rheumatoid arthritis (RA), granulomatosis with polyangiitis (Wegener's granulomatosis), Graves' disease, Hashimoto's thyroiditis, type 1 diabetes mellitus, celiac disease, autoimmune hepatitis (AIH), primary biliary cirrhosis, multiple sclerosis (MS), myasthenia gravis (MG), and anti-glomerular basement membrane disease.
6. Associate each of the diseases listed in Learning Outcome 5 with its corresponding autoantibodies and laboratory findings.
7. Identify autoantibodies associated with Sjögren's syndrome, systemic sclerosis (SSc), mixed connective tissue disease (MCTD), and the inflammatory myopathies.
8. Explain the principles of laboratory methods used to screen for and confirm the presence of anti-nuclear antibodies (ANAs).
9. Describe common immunofluorescence patterns seen in the indirect immunofluorescence (IIF) test for ANAs and their clinical significance.
10. Describe the c-ANCA and p-ANCA patterns seen in the IIF test for ANCAs and their clinical significance.
11. Discuss the composition and clinical significance of rheumatoid factor (RF) and anti-cyclic citrullinated peptide (anti-CCP).

CHAPTER OUTLINE

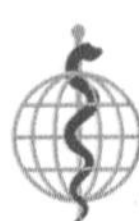

Go to FADavis.com for the laboratory exercises that accompany this text.

KEY TERMS

Anergy
Anti-centromere antibodies
Anti-cyclic citrullinated peptide (anti-CCP or ACPA)
Anti-glomerular basement membrane (anti-GBM) disease
Anti-histone antibodies
Anti-neutrophil cytoplasmic antibody (ANCA)
Anti-nuclear antibodies (ANAs)
Anti-phospholipid antibodies
Anti-RNP antibody
Autoantibodies
Autoimmune diseases
Autoimmune hepatitis (AIH)
Autoimmune liver disease
Autoimmune thyroid diseases (AITDs)
Celiac disease
Central tolerance
CREST syndrome
Dermatomyositis (DM)
Double-stranded DNA (dsDNA) antibodies
Epigenetics
Epitope spreading
Extractable nuclear antigens (ENAs)
Fluorescent anti-nuclear antibody (FANA) testing
Goodpasture's syndrome
Granulomatosis with polyangiitis (PGA)
Graves' disease
Hashimoto's thyroiditis
Immunologic tolerance
Inflammatory myopathies (IMs)
Mixed connective tissue disease (MCTD)
Molecular mimicry
Multiple sclerosis (MS)
Myasthenia gravis (MG)
Nucleolus
Nucleosome antibodies
Peripheral tolerance
Polymyositis (PM)
Primary biliary cholangitis (PBC; primary biliary cirrhosis)
Rheumatoid arthritis (RA)
Rheumatoid factor (RF)
Self-tolerance
Sjögren's syndrome
Sm antigen
SS-A/Ro
SS-B/La
Superantigens
Systemic lupus erythematosus (SLE)
Systemic sclerosis (SSc)
Thyroglobulin (Tg)
Thyroid peroxidase (TPO)
Thyroid-stimulating hormone (TSH)
Thyroid-stimulating hormone receptor antibodies (TRAbs)
Thyroid-stimulating immunoglobulins (TSIs)
Thyrotoxicosis
Thyrotropin-releasing hormone (TRH)
Tissue transglutaminase (tTG)
Type 1 diabetes mellitus (T1D)
Wegener's granulomatosis (WG)

In the early 1900s, Paul Ehrlich noted that the immune system could attack the very host it was intended to protect, a phenomenon he referred to as "horror autotoxicus," or "fear of self-poisoning." Conditions in which this phenomenon occurred later became known as *autoimmune diseases*. **Autoimmune diseases** are disorders in which immune responses are targeted toward self-antigens and result in damage to organs and tissues in the body. These harmful effects can be caused by T-cell–mediated immune responses or **autoantibodies** that are directed against host antigens. More than 100 autoimmune diseases have been discovered, and these can involve various organ systems. Autoimmune diseases are a leading cause of chronic illness and death, affecting about 5% of the world's population, including more than 20 million people in the United States alone. This chapter will begin by discussing the factors that are thought to contribute to the development of autoimmunity so that the student can gain a better understanding of the underlying pathology of autoimmune disease. The discussion will then proceed to the clinical manifestations and immunopathology of specific autoimmune diseases, as well as the laboratory tests that are used in their diagnosis.

Etiology of Autoimmune Disease

Self-Tolerance

Under normal circumstances, the immune system is able to differentiate between "self" and "nonself" or "foreign" so that self-antigens are not destroyed. This fundamental concept was introduced in Chapter 3. Central to this phenomenon is **self-tolerance,** or the ability of the immune system to accept self-antigens and not initiate a response against them. Autoimmune disease is thought to result from a loss of self-tolerance.

Self-tolerance is a type of **immunologic tolerance,** or a state of immune unresponsiveness that is directed against a specific antigen, in this case, a self-antigen. In order for self-tolerance to develop, lymphocytes must be "educated" so that they can distinguish between self-antigens and foreign antigens. This education takes place at two levels: central and peripheral.

Central tolerance occurs in the central or primary lymphoid organs, the thymus and the bone marrow. As T cells mature in the thymus, they encounter self-antigens that are normally present on the surface of the thymic epithelial cells. In a process called *negative selection*, T cells that express T-cell receptors (TCRs) with a strong affinity for these self-antigens are deleted by apoptosis, a physiological form of cell death (see Chapter 4 and **Fig. 15–1**). Negative selection occurs with both the immature, double-positive CD4+/CD8+ cells in the cortex and with the more mature, single-positive CD4+ or CD8+ cells in the medulla. During this process, some of the self-reactive CD4+ T cells are not deleted but instead differentiate into T regulatory (Treg) cells that can specifically inhibit immune responses to self-antigens. Similarly, as B cells mature in the bone marrow, those with receptors having a strong affinity for self-antigens are eliminated by apoptosis. Some self-reactive B cells are not deleted; rather, they are stimulated to rearrange their immunoglobulin genes so that their B-cell receptors are no longer antigen specific. This process is known as *receptor editing*. B cells

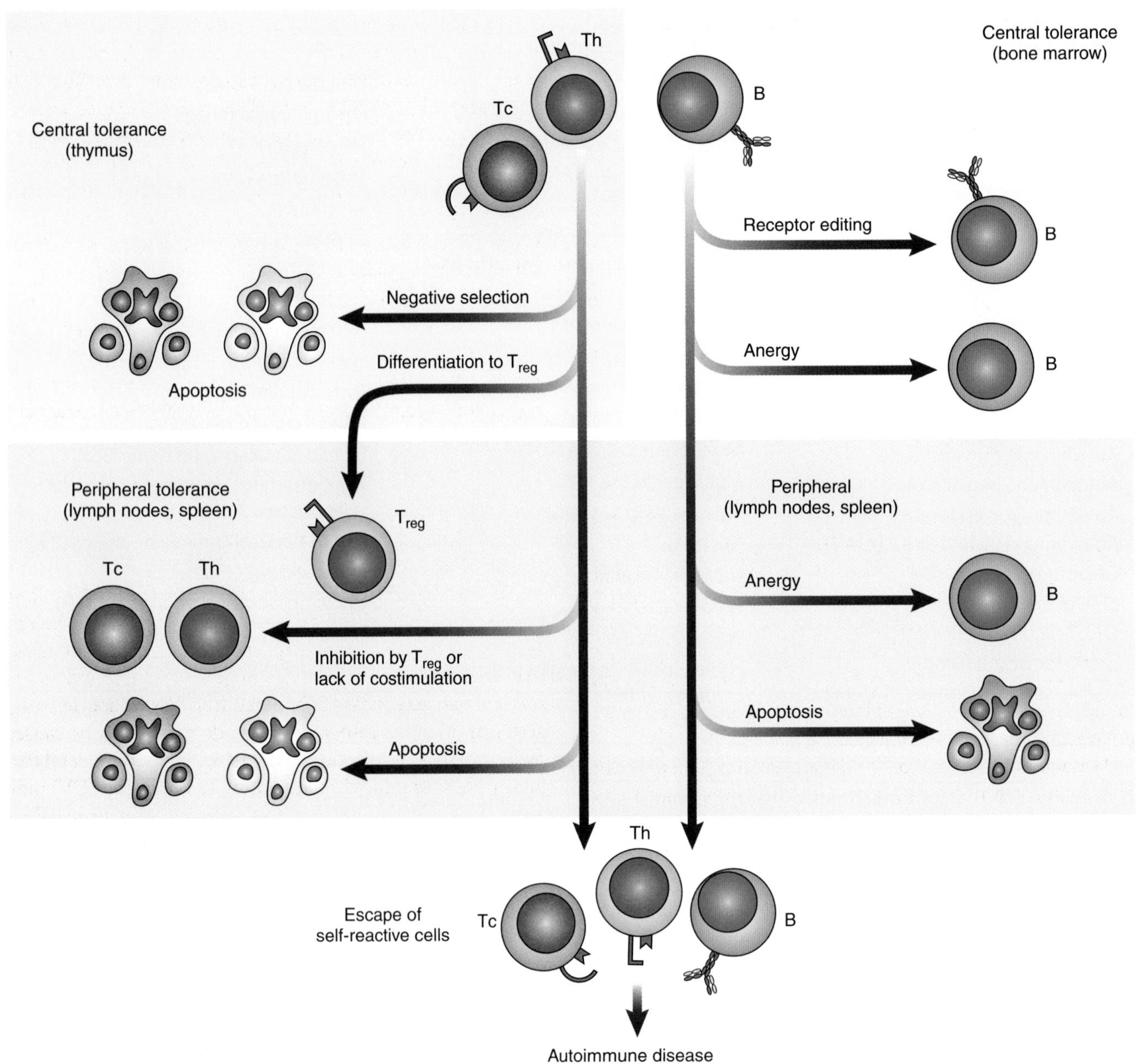

FIGURE 15–1 Mechanisms of central and peripheral tolerance.

that possess receptors that only weakly recognize self-antigens are induced to downregulate the expression of their receptors and develop a specific state of unresponsiveness to the antigens known as **anergy.**

Thus, there are several ways in which the central tolerance of T and B cells can be achieved. This process is not totally effective, however, and some self-reactive lymphocytes manage to escape to the secondary lymphoid organs, such as the lymph nodes and spleen. Therefore, a second level of protection is needed. In **peripheral tolerance,** lymphocytes that recognize self-antigens in the secondary lymphoid organs are rendered incapable of reacting with those antigens. Peripheral tolerance of T cells can result from anergy caused by the absence of a costimulatory signal from an antigen-presenting cell (APC) or binding of inhibitory receptors such as CTLA-4 (a molecule that prevents T-cell activation). Peripheral T-cell tolerance can also result from inhibition by Tregs or death by apoptosis. Self-reactive B cells in the periphery can be deleted by apoptosis, be rendered anergic after repeated stimulation with self-antigens, or receive inhibitory signals through receptors such as CD22.

In some individuals, self-tolerance can fail even after this second layer of protection; if this happens, autoimmunity can arise. The development of autoimmune disease is thought to be caused by complex interactions between genetics, exposure to environmental factors, and defects in immune regulation. Some of the major factors that are believed to contribute to autoimmunity will be discussed in the text that follows.

Genetics

There is much evidence supporting a genetic basis for autoimmune disease. Autoimmune diseases are often more prevalent among family members than among unrelated individuals and are more prevalent among monozygotic (genetically identical) twins than dizygotic (non-identical) twins or siblings. Researchers conducting molecular studies continue to identify specific genetic polymorphisms or mutations that are associated with autoimmune diseases.

Most of the research concerning humans has focused on genes in the major histocompatibility complex (MHC) (see Chapter 3). Investigators have found that there is an association between the presence of certain human leukocyte antigen (HLA) types and the risk of developing a particular autoimmune disorder. The strongest link found is between the HLA-B27 allele and the development of ankylosing spondylitis, an autoinflammatory disease that affects the spine. Individuals who possess HLA-B27 have about a 100 times greater chance of developing the disease than individuals who do not have that allele. Other associations with specific MHC genes are discussed in the sections on particular autoimmune diseases in this chapter. Differences in MHC genes are thought to influence the development of autoimmune disease because the specific structure of the MHC molecule can determine whether or not a self-antigen can attach to the peptide-binding cleft of the molecule and subsequently be processed and presented to T cells. In addition, class II MHC molecules can sometimes be abnormally expressed on cells where they are not typically found, resulting in the presentation of self-antigens for which no tolerance has been established.

Genome-wide association studies are revealing that polymorphisms in some non-MHC genes can also be associated with the development of autoimmune disease. Many of these genes influence the development and regulation of immune responses. Examples include the *PTPN22* gene, which has a role in T- and B-cell receptor signaling; the *IL2RA* gene, which is involved in T-cell activation and maintenance of Tregs; the *CTLA4* gene, which has an inhibitory effect on T-cell activation; the *BLK* gene, which is involved in B-cell activation and development; and the *AIRE* (autoimmune regulator) gene, which promotes the development of T-cell tolerance in the thymus. Although most autoimmune diseases involve multiple genes (~20 to 30), single-gene mutations that can be inherited in a Mendelian fashion have been associated with rare autoimmune disorders.

Inheritance of specific genes may make an individual more susceptible to a particular autoimmune disease, but genetic makeup is not totally responsible because the majority of people with a particular gene will not develop autoimmunity. Environmental and other factors are also thought to play a role in the development of autoimmune disease. A discussion of some of the major factors that are believed to trigger autoimmune responses follows.

Other Endogenous and Environmental Factors

Hormonal Influence

Women are 2.7 times more likely to acquire an autoimmune disease than men; in fact, about 78% of patients with autoimmune diseases are of female gender. Women also tend to develop autoimmunity at an earlier age and have a higher risk for acquiring more than one autoimmune disease as compared with men. Furthermore, females have been found to have higher absolute CD4+ T-cell counts and higher levels of circulating antibodies than men. These observations suggest that there is a hormonal influence on the development of autoimmunity. Studies on the effects of hormones have shown that estrogens tend to direct the immune system in favor of a type 2 helper cell (Th2) response, resulting in more B-cell activation and antibody production, whereas androgens favor a type 1 helper cell (Th1) response with activation of CD8+ T cells. Prolactin, a hormone that stimulates the production of breast milk in pregnant and nursing women, can stimulate both humoral and cell-mediated immune responses. The stimulatory effects of female hormones may place women at a greater risk for developing autoimmune disease.

Tissue Trauma and Release of Cryptic Antigens

When immunologic tolerance to self-antigens occurs during the early development of lymphocytes in the thymus and bone marrow, some self-antigens may be *cryptic,* or hidden within the tissues of the host. T and B lymphocytes are shielded from these sequestered antigens and are not educated to become tolerant to them. At a later time in life, inflammation or tissue trauma could cause the cryptic antigens to be released and to suddenly be accessible to the uneducated lymphocytes, triggering an immune response. Tissue damage could be caused by factors such as infections, contact with environmental toxins, or physical injury from exposure to ultraviolet (UV) radiation. This concept has also been referred to as *immunologic ignorance* and may be responsible for the production of autoantibodies to the lens of the eye following an ocular injury, autoantibodies to sperm after a vasectomy, and autoantibodies to DNA following damage to skin cells by overexposure to UV rays from the sun.

Microbial Infections

Scientists have been very interested in the association of microbial infections with the development of autoimmune disease. Bacteria, viruses, and other infectious pathogens may be able to trigger autoimmune responses in a variety of ways. A principal means by which microbes are thought to accomplish this is through molecular mimicry. **Molecular mimicry** refers to the fact that many bacterial or viral agents contain antigens that closely resemble the structure or amino acid sequence of self-antigens. Exposure to such foreign antigens may trigger immune responses that cross-react with similar self-antigens. Molecular mimicry has been postulated as a mechanism for several human autoimmune diseases. The best-known example involves the association between the gram-positive bacterium *Streptococcus pyogenes* and rheumatic fever, an autoimmune disorder that primarily affects the joints and the heart. Some patients who have acquired scarlet fever or pharyngitis because of infection with *S. pyogenes* will proceed to develop rheumatic fever if they are not treated adequately with antibiotics (see Chapter 20). Symptoms develop 2 to 4 weeks after the infection and are thought to be caused by the production of antibodies to the M protein and N-acetyl glucosamine components of the bacteria, which cross-react with cardiac myosin, causing damage to the heart.

A second way that microbes might trigger autoimmunity is through a *bystander effect*. In this mechanism, the microbial organism does not have to share structurally similar antigens with the host. Instead, the microorganism can induce a local inflammatory response that recruits leukocytes and stimulates APCs to release cytokines that nonspecifically activate T cells. Some of the T cells that are activated may have specificity for self-antigens. This expansion of the immune response to unrelated antigens has also been termed "**epitope spreading.**"

A third way that microorganisms might induce autoimmunity is through superantigens. **Superantigens** are proteins that are produced by various microbes that have the ability to bind to both class II MHC molecules and TCRs, regardless of their antigen specificity. Examples are the staphylococcal enterotoxins that cause food poisoning and toxic shock syndrome. These superantigens can act as potent T-cell mitogens by activating a large number of T cells with different antigen specificities. If some of these T cells possess specificity for a self-antigen, autoimmune responses might result. Likewise, some viruses, including the Epstein-Barr virus (EBV) and cytomegalovirus (CMV), can cause polyclonal activation of B cells.

Scientists have also been very interested in the complex relationship between microbiota, or normal flora, and the immune system. Research has shown that the presence of certain strains of endogenous bacteria may be associated with a greater risk for autoimmune disease. These strains, as well as pathogenic microorganisms, may stimulate innate immune responses through interaction with pattern recognition receptors, such as the Toll-like receptors (TLRs). This interaction triggers cell-signaling pathways that result in the production of cytokines such as interferon alpha (IFN-α), which can stimulate cells of the adaptive immune system, some of which are directed toward self-antigens. A decrease in the number and function of Tregs can perpetuate the activity of autoreactive cytotoxic T cells and hyperactive B cells that produce autoantibodies. The activated lymphocytes, in turn, produce proinflammatory cytokines that provide signals to stimulate cells of the innate system, thus producing a vicious cycle that amplifies the immune response and sustains autoimmunity.

Epigenetics and Modification of Self-Antigens

Investigators have done much research in the area of epigenetics and how it may relate to the development of autoimmunity. **Epigenetics** refers to modifications in gene expression that are *not* caused by changes in the original DNA sequence. These alterations are stable and can be inherited. They are thought to be triggered by exposure to environmental toxins, ingestion of harmful foods or drugs, or the aging process. These factors can induce epigenetic changes by increasing or decreasing methylation of cytosine bases, modifying histones, and causing abnormal regulation by microRNAs. These modifications can result in changes in the level at which genes are expressed by affecting their ability to be transcribed into mRNA, which is subsequently translated into proteins that will influence the phenotype of an individual. Over- or underexpression of certain genes in the immune system may result in homeostatic imbalances and a breakdown of self-tolerance, leading to autoimmunity.

Sometimes, exposure to environmental factors can lead to changes at the protein level. These changes, known as *post-translational modifications,* may involve biochemical processes such as acetylation, lipidation, citrullination, and glycosylation. These modifications can alter the immunogenicity of an antigen, affecting its ability to be processed by APCs and presented to T cells. Such alterations of self-antigens can make them more immunogenic, leading to autoimmune responses. For example, citrullination of collagen might play a role in the pathogenesis of **rheumatoid arthritis (RA)**, and glycosylation of myelin may be involved in the pathology of multiple sclerosis (MS; see the *Rheumatoid Arthritis* and *Multiple Sclerosis* sections in the text that follows).

Interactions Between Factors

Although the precise etiology of autoimmunity is unknown, there is much evidence that suggests that this heterogeneous disease entity is caused by complex interactions between genetic and environmental factors **(Fig. 15–2).** Certain genes are thought to make individuals more susceptible to immune responses against self-antigens but are not sufficient by themselves

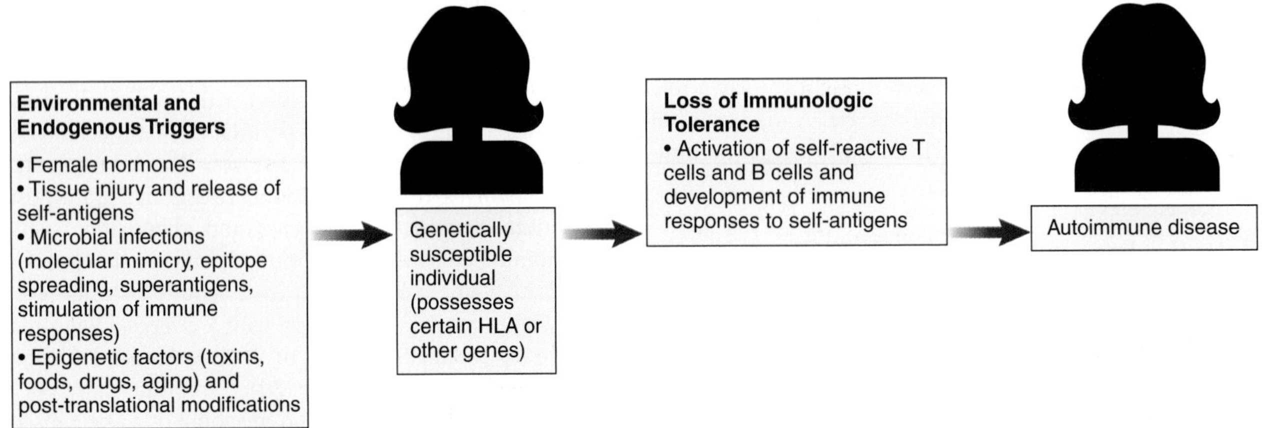
Environmental and Endogenous Triggers
• Female hormones
• Tissue injury and release of self-antigens
• Microbial infections (molecular mimicry, epitope spreading, superantigens, stimulation of immune responses)
• Epigenetic factors (toxins, foods, drugs, aging) and post-translational modifications
Genetically susceptible individual (possesses certain HLA or other genes)
Loss of Immunologic Tolerance
• Activation of self-reactive T cells and B cells and development of immune responses to self-antigens
Autoimmune disease

FIGURE 15–2 Interactions between genetic and environmental factors in the development of autoimmunity.

to cause autoimmune disease. The gender of the individual, tissue injury, and exposure to infectious microorganisms or other environmental agents are all believed to have significant effects on the immune system that can trigger autoimmune responses in susceptible individuals. Because of this break in immunologic tolerance, autoreactive T cells recognize and proliferate in response to self-antigens, and B cells develop into plasma cells that secrete autoantibodies. This can result in the release of proinflammatory cytokines, which, together with dysfunctions in immune-regulatory cells, perpetuates the autoimmune responses. If these responses are not held in check, they can culminate in autoimmune disease. Tissue injury in these disorders results from hypersensitivity reactions that involve autoantibodies to cell surface receptors, deposition of immune complexes that contain self-antigens, and cell-mediated cytotoxicity. The immunopathological mechanisms vary with specific autoimmune diseases and will be discussed in the text that follows.

Systemic Autoimmune Diseases

Autoimmune diseases can be classified as systemic or organ-specific, depending on the extent of pathology in the body. The systemic diseases affect multiple organs and tissues, whereas the organ-specific diseases mainly involve a single organ or gland. Two important groups of systemic diseases are the systemic autoimmune rheumatic diseases (SARDs), which involve inflammation of the joints and their associated structures, and the anti-neutrophil cytoplasmic antibodies (ANCA)-associated vasculitides, which are characterized by inflammation of the blood vessels. **Table 15–1** lists examples of systemic autoimmune diseases, along with their corresponding target tissues and associated autoantibodies. The sections that follow discuss selected systemic autoimmune diseases and the laboratory tests that are essential to their diagnosis.

Systemic Lupus Erythematosus (SLE)

Systemic lupus erythematosus (SLE) is a chronic systemic inflammatory disease that affects between 40 and more than 200 persons per 100,000, depending on the population. The peak age of onset is usually between 20 and 40 years. Women are much more likely to be affected than men, by a ratio of about 9 to 1. SLE is also more common in African Americans and Hispanics than in Caucasians. With earlier diagnosis and improved treatments, the 5-year survival rate has increased from 50% in the 1950s to 95% today.

Etiology

SLE appears to originate from complex interactions between environmental factors, genetic susceptibility, and abnormalities within the immune system. Environmental factors thought to play a role in SLE include UV light, certain medications, and possibly infectious agents. Exposure to sunlight is a well-known trigger of the photosensitive skin rashes seen in many lupus patients. Certain drugs, such as procainamide (used to treat abnormal heart rhythms), hydralazine (used for high blood pressure), and the tuberculosis drug isoniazid, can induce a transient lupus-like syndrome that resolves once the drug is stopped. Hormones are also important, as indicated by the significantly higher incidence of lupus in females and an increased risk of developing lupus in women who have used estrogen-containing contraceptives or hormone replacement therapy. Hormones may be important because they may help

Table 15–1 Systemic Autoimmune Diseases

DISEASE	TARGET CELLS AND TISSUES	ASSOCIATED AUTOANTIBODIES
Systemic lupus erythematosus (SLE)	Multiple cells and organs throughout the body, including the skin, joints, kidneys, brain, heart, lungs	Anti-nuclear antibodies (ANAs) (e.g., anti-dsDNA, anti-Sm) Phospholipid antibodies Antibody to RBCs Antibody to platelets Antibody to lymphocytes Antibody to ribosomal components Antibody to endothelium Rheumatoid factor
Rheumatoid arthritis (RA)	Joints, bone; other tissues in some cases	Anti-CCP (cyclic citrullinated protein) Rheumatoid factor ANAs
Sjögren's syndrome	Eyes, mouth	ANAs, rheumatoid factor, anti-salivary duct antibodies, anti-lacrimal gland antibodies
Systemic sclerosis	Connective tissue	ANAs: anti-Scl-70, anti-centromere antibody
Polymyositis/ Dermatomyositis	Muscles, skin	ANAs (e.g., anti-Jo-1)
Granulomatosis with polyangiitis (Wegener's granulomatosis)	Upper respiratory system, lungs, blood vessels	Anti-neutrophil cytoplasmic antibodies (ANCA); c-ANCA pattern Rheumatoid factor ANAs

regulate the transcription of genes that are central to the expression of SLE.

The majority of individuals exposed to the environmental factors mentioned previously do not develop lupus, and genetic makeup is believed to play an important role in susceptibility to SLE, which is thought to be caused by interactions between multiple genes. More than 60 genetic loci associated with lupus in humans have been discovered. People with certain HLA types, especially HLA-A1, B8, and DR3, have an increased chance of developing lupus. Another group of genes that has been associated with increased susceptibility to SLE plays a role in the clearance of immune complexes (see the text that follows). Other lupus-associated genes include polymorphisms in genes associated with immune function, genes coding for various cytokines, and genes involved in signaling of innate immune responses. These defects are thought to result in uncontrolled autoreactivity of T and B cells, which leads to the production of numerous autoantibodies.

Immunopathology

Over 100 autoantibodies associated with SLE have been discovered. These include antibodies to double-stranded DNA (dsDNA), histones, and other nuclear components, as well as autoantibodies to lymphocytes, erythrocytes, platelets, phospholipids, ribosomal components, and endothelium. The typical patient has several circulating autoantibodies.

B cells and the autoantibodies they produce are believed to play a central role in the pathogenic mechanisms that are responsible for this complex disease. In fact, the presence of autoantibodies can precede the onset of disease by several years. Abnormal apoptosis of certain types of cells may occur, releasing excess amounts of cellular constituents such as DNA and ribonucleic acid (RNA). Dysfunctional removal of cellular debris by phagocytes may allow these cellular components to persist, increasing the chances for autoantibody production.

Antibodies to dsDNA are present in 70% of patients with lupus and are highly specific for the disease. Anti-dsDNA and complement proteins have been found in immune complexes that are deposited in organs such as the kidneys and skin and are thought to play a major role in the pathogenesis of SLE. Accumulation of IgG to dsDNA seems to be the most pathogenic because it forms complexes of an intermediate size that become deposited in the glomerular basement membrane (GBM).

Once immune complexes are formed, they cannot be cleared efficiently because of other possible deficiencies in lupus patients. These include defects in complement receptors on phagocytic cells; defects in receptors for the Fc portion of immunoglobulins; or rarely, deficiencies of early complement components such as C1q, C2, or C4 (see Chapter 7). The immune complexes activate complement and initiate an inflammatory response. Leukocytes are attracted to the sites of inflammation and release cytokines that perpetuate the response, resulting in tissue damage by a type III hypersensitivity mechanism (see Chapter 14).

Autoantibodies to nuclear and nonnuclear antigens can also cause cellular destruction by other mechanisms. For example, antibodies to red blood cells (RBCs) can cause hemolytic anemia, and antibodies to platelets can cause thrombocytopenia by antibody-dependent cellular cytotoxicity (type II hypersensitivity). Antibodies to endothelial cells can cause inflammation of the blood vessels and vascular damage in lupus, which may be responsible for the vasculitis and neuropsychiatric symptoms seen in some SLE patients. Phospholipid antibodies are associated with increased miscarriage, stillbirth, and preterm delivery in pregnant women with lupus. Neonatal lupus, which occurs in up to 8% of babies born to pregnant women with SLE, is associated with antibodies to the nuclear antigens, **SS-A/Ro** and **SS-B/La.** Symptoms are transient and resolve at 6 to 8 months of age when the maternal antibodies have cleared from the infant's circulation. In utero heart block is a serious complication that occurs in 2% of fetuses whose mothers have anti–SS-A antibodies.

Connections

Type III Hypersensitivity

The immune complexes generated in SLE activate complement, inducing the generation of chemotaxins such as C5a. The activation of complement results in the recruitment of neutrophils, which release lysosomal enzymes that cause injury to the surrounding tissues. This is an example of a type III hypersensitivity response, which was discussed in Chapter 14.

Clinical Signs and Symptoms

The clinical symptoms of SLE are extremely diverse, varying in terms of severity and the areas of the body that are affected. Nonspecific symptoms such as fatigue, weight loss, malaise, fever, and anorexia are often the first to appear. The disease is marked by alternating relapses or flares and periods of remission. Joint involvement seems to be the most frequently reported manifestation because over 90% of patients with SLE have polyarthralgias or arthritis. Typically, the arthritis is symmetric and involves the small joints of the hands, wrists, and knees.

After joint involvement, the next most common signs are skin manifestations. These can present in various forms and are experienced by about 80% of patients with lupus. An erythematous rash may appear on any area of the body exposed to UV light. Less common but perhaps more dramatic is the classic butterfly rash across the nose and cheeks that appears in some SLE patients **(Fig. 15–3).** This rash is responsible for the name *lupus,* derived from the Latin term meaning "wolf-like." In discoid lupus, skin lesions have central atrophy and scarring.

Evidence of renal involvement is present in about half of all patients with lupus; nephritis is a major cause of illness and death. There are several types of lesions, but the most dangerous is diffuse proliferative glomerulonephritis, characterized by cell proliferation in the glomeruli that can lead to end-stage renal disease. Other conditions involving the kidneys may include deposition of immune complexes in the subendothelial tissue and thickening of the basement membrane, all of which can lead to renal failure.

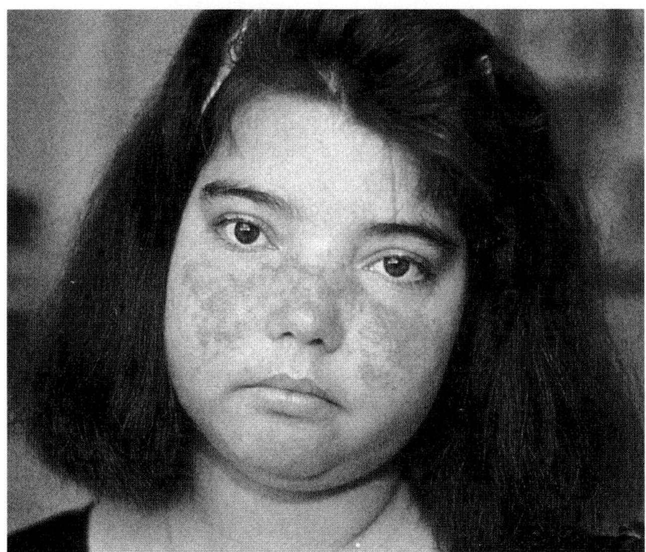

FIGURE 15–3 Butterfly rash in SLE. Characteristic rash over the cheekbones and forehead is diagnostic of SLE. The disease often begins in young adulthood and may eventually involve many organ systems. *(From Steinman L. Autoimmune disease.* Sci Am. *1993;269:107, with permission.)*

Other systemic effects may include cardiac involvement with pericarditis, tachycardia, or ventricular enlargement; pleuritis with chest pain; and neuropsychiatric manifestations such as seizures, mild cognitive dysfunction, psychoses, or depression. Hematologic abnormalities such as anemia, leukopenia, thrombocytopenia, or lymphopenia can also be present.

Drug-induced lupus differs from the more chronic form of the disease, in that symptoms usually disappear once the drug is discontinued. The most common drugs implicated are procainamide, hydralazine, chlorpromazine, isoniazid, quinidine, anticonvulsants such as methyldopa, and possibly oral contraceptives. Typically, this is a milder form of the disease and is usually manifested as fever, arthritis, or rashes; rarely are the kidneys involved.

In 1982, the American College of Rheumatology (ACR) established a set of clinical and immunologic criteria that could be used to define SLE for the purposes of research and surveillance. Revisions in the criteria were published in 1997, 2012, and 2019. The 2019 criteria, developed through collaboration of the ACR and the European League Against Rheumatism (EULAR), have a high level of sensitivity and specificity for the disease. These criteria begin with an absolute requirement that the patient has a current or previously positive ANA with a titer of at least 1:80 by indirect immunofluorescence (IIF) on HEp-2 cells (see discussion on *Anti-Nuclear Antibodies* that follows). If the patient meets this initial criterion, he or she is further evaluated in seven clinical domains (constitutional, hematologic, neuropsychiatric, mucocutaneous, serosal, musculoskeletal, and renal) and three immunologic domains (anti-phospholipid antibodies, C3 and C4 complement protein levels, and SLE-specific antibodies—anti-dsDNA and anti-Sm). The domains are weighted, and the patient is classified as having SLE if he or she meets at least one of the clinical criteria and has a total score of 10 or higher. It is likely that the criteria will continue to evolve as molecular studies identify new biomarkers that are associated with SLE.

Although these criteria are not meant to be used for diagnosis, they reflect the major clinical and laboratory features that are associated with SLE and are useful in identifying patients who qualify for research studies and clinical trials. Some of the main laboratory tests that are helpful in diagnosis are discussed in the *Laboratory Diagnosis of Systemic Lupus Erythematosus* section later in this chapter.

Treatment

The anti-malarial drug hydroxychloroquine is recommended for all SLE patients because it has immunomodulatory and anti-thrombotic effects. Systemic glucocorticoid and other immunosuppressive drugs are used to treat serious complications, such as acute fulminant (severe and sudden) lupus, lupus nephritis, or central nervous system (CNS) manifestations, because they suppress the immune response and lower antibody titers. Patients must be monitored closely for side effects and drug doses tapered as clinical symptoms subside. The monoclonal antibodies, belimumab (directed against soluble B lymphocyte stimulator [BlyS]) or rituximab (anti-CD20), which affect B-cell activity, may be used for patients who have not responded adequately to the previous treatments. New biological drugs continue to be evaluated for the treatment of SLE.

The most common causes of death in lupus patients are renal failure and infection, followed by heart disease. The key to successful treatment is to prevent organ damage and achieve remission. Overall, the treatments of today have come a long way in achieving this goal, as the 5-year survival rate has increased to about 95%, and 20-year survival to nearly 80%.

Laboratory Diagnosis of Systemic Lupus Erythematosus

General laboratory tests that can be used in the initial evaluation of patients include a complete blood count (CBC), a platelet count, creatinine levels, and urinalysis to assess renal function. Some of the first laboratory findings in lupus patients are leukopenia and possible anemia and thrombocytopenia. In addition, the erythrocyte sedimentation rate (ESR) may be elevated even though the C-reactive protein (CRP) level tends to be low or normal.

When SLE is suspected, the first test typically done is a screening test for **anti-nuclear antibodies (ANAs)** because these are present in the majority of patients with the disease. When the screen is positive, further tests are done to differentiate the type of ANA. Antibodies to dsDNA and antibodies to the Sm nuclear antigen are highly specific for SLE. ANAs and the methods used to detect them are discussed in more detail in the section that follows. Phospholipid antibodies are present in some patients with lupus and are discussed in a later section.

Once the diagnosis has been made, further tests are performed to monitor disease activity. Antibody to dsDNA can be measured in those patients who are positive for this antibody, as titers often increase before a disease flare. Quantification of complement proteins such as C3 and C4 is also helpful for disease monitoring because serum complement levels decrease during disease flares because of complement consumption by immune complexes. Additional laboratory tests are ordered based on the patient's clinical symptoms.

Anti-Nuclear Antibodies (ANAs)

Types of Anti-Nuclear Antibodies

ANAs are autoantibodies that are directed against antigens in the nuclei of mammalian cells. ANAs are present in over 95% of patients with active lupus and are used as a major marker for the disease. However, ANAs are not specific for SLE because they can also be detected in a significant percentage of patients with other SARDs, including RA, mixed connective tissue disease (MCTD), Sjögren's syndrome, scleroderma, and polymyositis-dermatomyositis. They can also be found in some individuals with other conditions, including chronic infections, cancer, and pregnancy. Furthermore, up to 5% of healthy persons and up to 30% of elderly individuals are ANA-positive.

ANAs are a heterogeneous group of antibodies that have different antigen specificities. The nuclear antigens they are directed against include dsDNA and single-stranded DNA (ssDNA), histones, nucleosomes (DNA–histone complexes), centromere proteins, and extractable nuclear antigens (ENAs). Some of the more common ANAs and their associated features are discussed in the text that follows and listed in **Table 15–2.**

Double-stranded DNA (dsDNA) antibodies are the most specific for SLE because they are mainly seen in patients with lupus, and their levels correlate with disease activity. Although they are found in only 40% to 70% of patients, the presence of these antibodies is considered diagnostic for SLE, especially when they are found in combination with low levels of the complement component C3. Antibodies to dsDNA typically produce a homogeneous staining pattern on IIF. See the *Indirect Immunofluorescence (IIF)* section for further explanation.

Anti-histone antibodies can also be found in lupus patients. Histones are nucleoproteins that are essential components of chromatin. There are five major classes of histones: H1, H2A,

Table 15–2 Common Anti-Nuclear Antibodies

AUTOANTIBODY	ANTIGEN (S)	IMMUNOFLUORESCENT PATTERN	DISEASE ASSOCIATION
Anti-dsDNA	dsDNA	Homogeneous	SLE
Anti-ssDNA	Related to purines and pyrimidines	Not detected on routine screen	SLE, many other diseases
Anti-histone	Different classes of histones	Homogeneous	Drug-induced SLE, other diseases
Anti-DNP	DNA–histone complex (nucleosomes)	Homogeneous	SLE, drug-induced SLE
Anti-Sm	Extractable nuclear antigen (uridine-rich RNA component)	Coarse speckled	Diagnostic for SLE
Anti-RNP	Proteins complexed with small nuclear RNA	Coarse speckled	SLE, mixed connective tissue diseases
Anti–SS-A/Ro	Proteins complexed to RNA	Finely speckled	SLE, Sjögren's syndrome, others
Anti–SS-B/La	Phosphoprotein complexed to RNA polymerase	Finely speckled	SLE, Sjögren's syndrome, others
Anti-nucleolar	RNA polymerase, fibrillarin, PM-1	Prominent staining of nucleoli (can be smooth, clumpy, or speckled)	SLE, systemic sclerosis
Anti–Scl-70	DNA topoisomerase I	Compound pattern with speckling	Systemic sclerosis, scleroderma
Anti–Jo-1	Histidyl-tRNA synthetase	Fine cytoplasmic speckling	Polymyositis
Anti-centromere	CENP-A/B/C in the chromosome centromeres	Discrete speckled	CREST syndrome (limited cutaneous systemic sclerosis)
DSF70/LEDGF	Lens epithelium-derived growth factor/transcription co-activator p75	Dense fine speckled	Usually indicates absence of SARDs

Adapted from Dellavance A, de Melo Cruvinel W, Francescantonio PLC, Andrade LEC. Antinuclear antibody tests. In: Detrick B, Hamilton RG, Folds, JD, eds. Manual of Molecular and Clinical Laboratory Immunology. *8th ed. Washington, DC: ASM Press; 2016:843–858.*

CREST = calcinosis cutis, Raynaud's phenomenon, esophageal dysmotility, sclerodactyly, and telangiectasia; DNP = deoxyribonucleoprotein; dsDNA = double-stranded DNA; RNA = ribonucleic acid; RNP = ribonucleoprotein; SARDs = systemic autoimmune rheumatic diseases; SLE = systemic lupus erythematosus; ssDNA = single-stranded DNA.

H2B, H3, and H4. Antibodies to H2A and H2B can be detected in almost all patients with drug-induced lupus. The presence of anti-histone antibody alone or combined with antibody to ssDNA supports the diagnosis of drug-induced lupus. Although other patients with SLE have elevated levels of anti-histone antibodies, the titers are usually fairly low. High levels of anti-histone antibodies tend to be associated with more active and severe SLE. Anti-histone antibodies are also found in other SARDs, but the levels are usually lower. Anti-histone antibodies typically produce a homogeneous pattern in the IIF assay.

Nucleosome antibodies are stimulated by DNA–histone complexes, known as *nucleosomes*, or deoxyribonucleoprotein (DNP). These antibodies are directed only against the complexes and not against DNA or the individual histones. Nucleosome antibodies are found in about 85% of patients with SLE, and their levels correlate with disease severity. They typically produce a homogeneous pattern in the IIF assay.

Extractable nuclear antigens (ENAs) are a group of nuclear antigens that were so named because they were isolated in saline extracts of mammalian tissues. These antigens represent a family of small nuclear proteins associated with uridine-rich RNA. The ENAs include ribonucleoproteins (RNPs), the Sm antigen, the SS-A/Ro and SS-B/La antigens, Scl-70, Jo-1, and PM-1.

Antibody to the **Sm antigen** is specific for lupus because it is not found in other autoimmune diseases. However, it is found in only 20% to 40% of patients with SLE, depending on the race of the population. Antibody to a preparation of this ENA was first described in a patient named Smith, hence the name *anti-Sm antibody*. The anti-Sm antibody produces a coarse speckled pattern of nuclear fluorescence on IIF.

Anti-RNP antibody is directed against RNP, which consists of several nonhistone proteins complexed to a small nuclear RNA called *U1-snRNP* (*U* for "uridine-rich"). RNP forms complexes with the Sm antigen in the nucleus, and antisera to these antigens produce a pattern of partial identity when they are reacted in the Ouchterlony double-immunodiffusion test (see discussion and Fig. 15–7 in the text that follows). In the IIF assay, anti-nRNP produces a coarse speckled pattern. Antibodies to RNP are detected in about one-fourth of patients with SLE but are also found at a high titer in individuals with MCTD and in lower levels in patients with other SARDs such as systemic sclerosis (SSc), Sjögren's syndrome, and RA.

Lupus patients can also produce antibodies to another family of ENAs called SS-A/Ro and SS-B/La. These antigens consist of small, uridine-rich RNAs complexed to cellular proteins and were given the prefix of SS- because a large percentage of patients with Sjögren's syndrome possess antibodies to the antigens. Anti–SS-A/Ro also appears in some patients with SLE and has been closely associated with the presence of nephritis, vasculitis, lymphadenopathy, photosensitivity, and hematologic manifestations such as leukopenia. Antibodies to SS-B/La are found in a small percentage of patients with SLE, and all of these have anti–SS-A/Ro. The SS-B/La antibody is most often found in patients who have cutaneous manifestations of SLE, especially photosensitivity dermatitis. Antibodies to both SS-A/Ro and SS-B/La can cross the placenta and have been associated with neonatal lupus. Newborns who have anti–SS-A/Ro are more likely to develop cardiac manifestations, whereas those who have anti–SS-B/La are more likely to have other symptoms, such as skin lesions. To detect the presence of these antibodies on IIF, human tissue culture cells such as HEp-2 (human epithelial) must be used because SS-A/Ro and SS-B/La antigens are not found in mouse or rat liver and kidneys. A finely speckled pattern is evident. Antibodies to the SS-A/Ro antigen are best detected on IIF using a special cell line, HEp-2000, which has been genetically transfected so that the cells hyperexpress the antigen.

The **nucleolus** is a prominent structure within the nucleus where transcription and processing of ribosomal RNA and assembly of the ribosomes takes place. Staining of the nucleolus in IIF is mainly caused by antibodies to one of three nucleolar components: fibrillarin, RNA polymerase I, and PM-1. Antibody to fibrillarin is common in **systemic sclerosis** (**SSc**; also known as *scleroderma*) and is indicated by clumpy nucleolar fluorescence in the IIF assay. SSc is an autoimmune disease that primarily involves the skin and the blood vessels. Antibodies to RNA polymerase are also associated with SSc but produce a speckled nucleolar pattern in IIF. Homogeneous staining of the nucleolus is associated with antibodies to the PM-1 antigen (also known as *PM/Scl*) and is found in polymyositis and SSc.

Anti-centromere antibodies bind to proteins in the middle region of a chromosome where the sister chromatids are joined. These antibodies are directed against three centromere proteins called *CENP-A*, *CENP-B*, and *CENP-C*. They are found in over half of patients with the **CREST syndrome,** a subset of scleroderma named after its five major features: calcinosis, Raynaud's phenomenon, esophageal dysmotility, sclerodactyly, and telangiectasia. In the IIF assay, centromere antibodies produce discrete speckled staining in the nuclei of the cells.

Methods of ANA Detection

A variety of methods have been developed to detect ANAs in patient serum, including IIF, enzyme-linked immunosorbent assay (ELISA), microsphere multiplex immunoassays (MIA), and immunodiffusion. These assays are discussed in the text that follows.

Indirect Immunofluorescence (IIF)

Fluorescent anti-nuclear antibody (FANA) testing has been the most widely used and accepted test because it is highly sensitive, detects a wide range of antibodies, and is inexpensive and easy to perform. In addition, the antigens are in their original form and location within the cells used in the test. This test has three main applications: It has been used (1) as an initial test to determine the presence or absence of ANAs in patients who have symptoms of SARDs, aiding in their diagnosis; (2) to provide guidance in the selection of follow-up tests based on the immunofluorescence patterns obtained; and (3) to determine ANA titer because moderate to high titers have been better correlated with disease, whereas low titers are seen more often in the general population.

The IIF test uses a commercially prepared microscope slide onto which nucleated cells have been fixed. The human epithelial cell line, HEp-2, is the standard substrate for clinical laboratories worldwide. HEp-2 cells are used because they

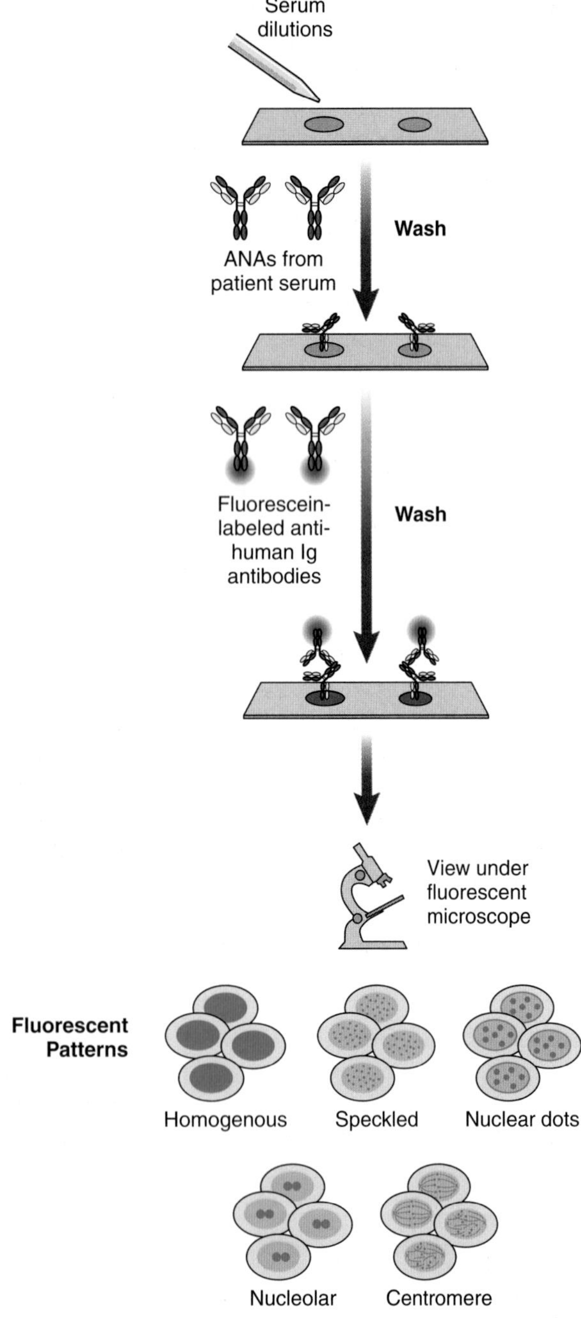

FIGURE 15–4 Fluorescent ANA test principle. Patient serum (containing anti-nuclear antibodies) is diluted and incubated on a microscope slide coated with HEp-2 cells. After washing, fluorescein-labeled anti-human Ig is added to detect bound autoantibodies. After a final wash, the slide is read under a fluorescent microscope. Five typical patterns in nondividing cells are shown.

have large nuclei with high antigen expression, allowing for high sensitivity and facilitating visualization of results. Patient serum is incubated with the HEp-2 cell-coated slide, washed to remove unbound antibodies, and then allowed to react with an anti-human immunoglobulin (Ig) labeled with a fluorescent tag to detect bound immunoglobulin G (IgG) or total immunoglobulins. Following a second incubation and wash, the slide is mounted and viewed under a fluorescent microscope using 400× magnification (40× objective and 10× eyepiece). The principle of this assay is shown in **Figure 15–4.**

The screening test is commonly performed with a 1:80 or 1:160 dilution of patient serum in order to avoid detecting low positive titers that may be seen in healthy persons, although the exact dilution used for screening may vary with the laboratory and population being tested. A titer of 160 or more is generally considered to be clinically significant. Patient samples that are positive on the ANA screen are serially diluted and tested to determine the antibody titer, specified as the highest dilution to show nuclear fluorescence. Inclusion of a 1+ endpoint control serum can help to standardize the readings by setting the minimum level of fluorescence that is considered positive.

In addition to the antibody titer, the pattern of fluorescence is also reported because it can provide clues about the autoantibody present and associated diseases. In 2015, an International Consensus on ANA Patterns (ICAP) was established by a committee of the International Union of Immunological Societies (IUIS) in conjunction with the Centers for Disease Control and Prevention (CDC). The ICAP classification is available on the website https://www.anapatterns.org/index.php and is periodically updated. The committee recognized that fluorescence may be detected not only within the nucleus but also in the cytoplasm or mitotic structures of the cell. Currently, 15 nuclear patterns, 9 cytoplasmic patterns, and 5 mitotic patterns have been identified and agreed upon. The nuclear patterns have been classified into seven major groups and are further categorized into subgroups. The five most common nuclear groups are described in the bulleted list that follows and are depicted in **Figure 15–5.**

- **Homogeneous**—This pattern is characterized by uniform staining of the entire nucleus in interphase (nondividing) cells and of the condensed chromosomal region in metaphase cells. It is associated with antibodies to dsDNA, histones, and nucleosomes. The homogeneous pattern is found in patients with SLE, drug-induced lupus, chronic **autoimmune hepatitis (AIH),** and juvenile idiopathic arthritis.
- **Speckled**—These patterns are characterized by discrete, fluorescent specks throughout the nuclei of interphase cells. The speckled group is divided into three subgroups depending on whether the specks are dense fine, tiny/fine, or large/coarse. In the fine and coarse subgroups, staining is variable in the nucleolus and absent in the chromatin region of dividing cells. The fine and coarse speckled patterns are associated with antibodies to ENAs and can be found in patients with SLE, Sjögren's syndrome, SSc, and other SARDs. The dense fine speckled pattern is associated with antibodies to the DFS70/LEDGF (lens epidermal-derived growth factor) antigen and is correlated with absence of a SARD upon confirmatory testing.
- **Centromere**—Numerous discrete speckles are seen in the nuclei of interphase cells and the chromatin of dividing cells. Most cells have 46 speckles, representing the number of chromosomes. This pattern is caused by antibodies to proteins in the centromeres of the chromosomes and is found mainly in patients with the CREST syndrome (also known as *limited cutaneous SSc*).
- **Nucleolar**—Prominent staining of the nucleoli within the nuclei of interphase cells is seen in this pattern. The

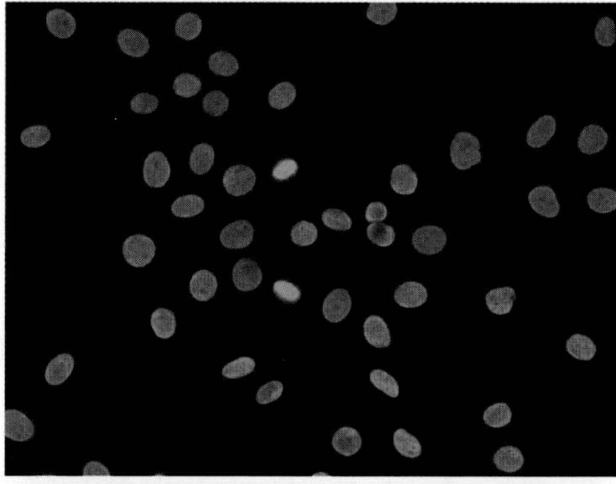
Homogeneous pattern

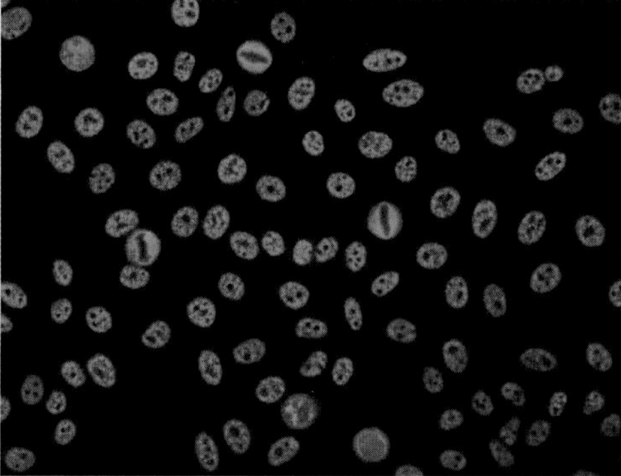
Speckled pattern

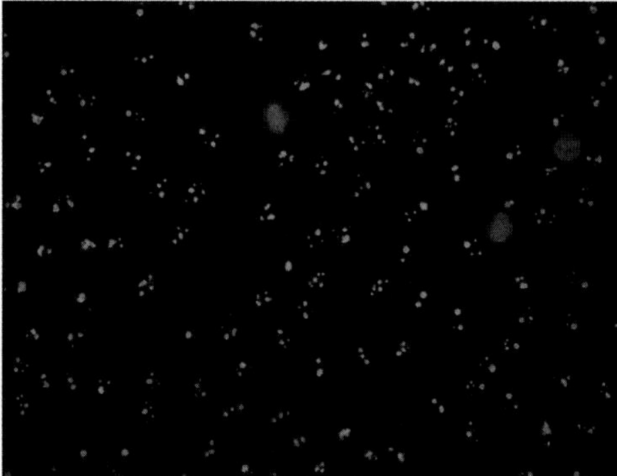
Nucleolar pattern

FIGURE 15–5 Photomicrographs showing three patterns of immunofluorescent staining for anti-nuclear antibodies. Examples of common staining patterns obtained are homogeneous—staining of the entire nucleus; speckled pattern—staining throughout the nucleus; and nucleolar pattern—staining of the nucleolus. *(Courtesy of DiaSorin, Inc., with permission.)*

size, shape, and number of the nucleoli per cell are variable, and staining can be smooth, clumpy, or speckled, depending on the type of antibody present. Staining may or may not be present in the dividing cells. The nucleolar patterns are primarily caused by antibodies to RNA and RNP and are seen mainly in patients with SSc but can also be present in patients with other SARDs.

- **Discrete Nuclear Dots**—This group is characterized by the presence of 1 to 6 or 6 to 20 discrete nuclear dots per cell, depending on the subgroup. The multiple nuclear dot subgroup can be attributed to presence of antibodies to the Sp-100, PML (promyelocytic leukemia) proteins, and MJ/NXP-2 antigens. This pattern has been associated with a broad spectrum of autoimmune diseases, including primary biliary cholangitis and dermatomyositis. The few nuclear dot subgroup pattern has not been strongly associated with any disease.

Mixed patterns can also be observed; in some cases, one pattern may totally or partially obscure another (for example, a homogeneous pattern might mask a speckled pattern). In these cases, titration of the patient serum can help to distinguish between the separate patterns, and an antibody titer would be reported for each one. If the FANA test is negative, no clearly discernable fluorescent pattern is observed in the nuclei of the cells. Up to 5% of SLE patients test negative, so this test cannot be used to absolutely rule out SLE.

Although FANA is the method of choice for ANA screening by many laboratories, it has some important limitations. The test is time-consuming and requires a significant amount of technical expertise to correctly identify the fluorescent patterns. Discrepancy in results can be caused by variations in the buffers, conjugate, and mounting medium supplied by different manufacturers of IIF assays and the use of different fluorescent microscopes. The use of a microscope with an LED light source can help to enhance the images. Automated IIF ANA assays have been developed that may help to reduce subjectivity in result interpretation and also allow for storage and retrieval of the fluorescent images. Although automated IFA systems are being used increasingly by clinical laboratories, interpretation of the results may vary between different instruments, and further standardization is needed. In addition, the autoantibodies present cannot be precisely identified on the basis of the fluorescent patterns alone, and supplemental tests are needed. Some of the tests commonly used to further characterize ANAs are described in the section that follows.

Other Assays for ANA

Solid Phase Immunoassays. Several solid-phase methods have been developed for the detection of ANAs, in the format of ELISA, chemiluminescence immunoassay (CLIA), and (microsphere multiplex immunoassay [MIA]) (see Chapter 11 for details). These assays use polystyrene microtiter plates, nitrocellulose strips, or synthetic beads as the solid phase to which the potential autoantigens are attached. The antigens used in commercial kits are derived from tissue extracts, or are produced by recombinant technology. Patient serum is incubated with the solid phase; then, following a wash step, bound autoantibodies are detected with anti-human immunoglobulin reagents to which an enzyme, fluorochrome, or chemiluminescent dye has been attached. They can be designed to test for a broad range of antibodies if multiple antigens are coated onto the solid phase, or for specific ANAs if each microtiter well or bead is coated with a single antigen. For the latter application, arrays of the following antigens are often used: dsDNA, Sm, U1-RNP, SS-A/Ro, SS-B/La, Jo-1, Scl-70, PM/Scl, Mi-2, CENP-B, and histones.

Solid-phase assays have the advantages of automation, ease of performance, and yielding objective results. Because of these advantages, these assays have been especially suited for high-volume testing laboratories. However, because of the antigen preparation used, the sensitivity of solid-phase assays is generally less than the IIF, and false-negative results may occur

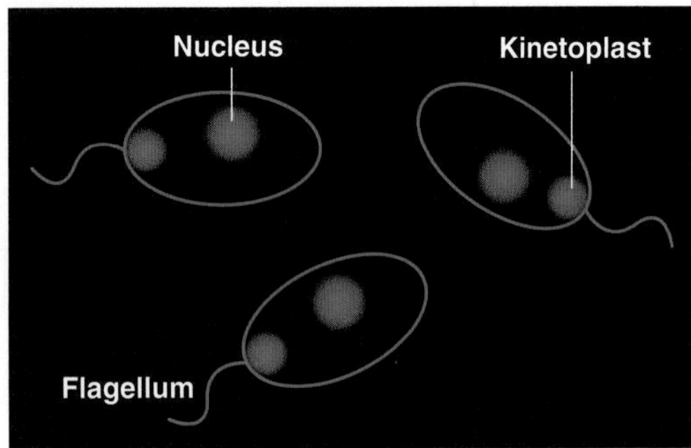

FIGURE 15–6 An illustration of *Crithidia luciliae* fixed to a microscope slide. A positive test for dsDNA will show green fluorescence in the nucleus and kinetoplast.

when they are used to screen patients for ANAs. Therefore, the ACR has recommended that the IIF test remain the gold standard for ANA testing (although this may change in the future as solid-phase designs continue to improve) and that clinical laboratories should specify the method they used when they are reporting results. When solid-phase assays are used in conjunction with IIF, they can confirm the presence of ANAs and identify individual ANAs, thus increasing specificity of the results and enhancing the probability of their clinical relevance.

Immunofluorescence Using *Crithidia luciliae*. This IIF assay is used to detect antibodies to dsDNA. In testing for these antibodies, a purified antigen preparation that is free from ssDNA must be used because antibodies to ssDNA occur in many individuals with other autoimmune or inflammatory diseases. One particularly sensitive assay for dsDNA is an IIF test using a hemoflagellate organism called *Crithidia luciliae* as the substrate. This trypanosome has a circular organelle called a *kinetoplast* that is composed mainly of dsDNA **(Fig. 15–6)**. In this test, patient serum is incubated on a microscope slide coated with *C. luciliae* organisms, and binding is detected with a fluorescent-labeled anti-Ig conjugate. Washing of the slide is performed after each step to remove unbound antibody. A positive test is indicated by a brightly stained kinetoplast.

Ouchterlony Test. ANAs can also be detected by immunodiffusion. This method can be used to determine the immunologic specificity of a positive FANA test, particularly when a speckled pattern is observed. Ouchterlony double diffusion detects antibody to several of the small nuclear proteins, or ENAs. These include antibodies to Sm, RNP, SS-A/Ro, SS-B/La, Scl-70 (DNA topoisomerase I), and Jo-1 (see the previous descriptions and Table 15–2). A solution containing ENA antigens is placed in a central well of an agarose plate, and patient samples and controls are placed in the surrounding wells, as indicated in **Figure 15–7**. A visible precipitate is formed between the ENA well and each surrounding well that contains antibodies to any of the ENAs present (e.g., anti-Sm, anti-RNP, or antibodies to other ENAs). If an outer well does not contain antibodies to any of the ENAs, no precipitate is formed between that well and the center well. Samples in the outer wells are identified as containing antibody to a particular ENA by comparing their reactivity patterns of identity, nonidentity, or partial identity to control sera containing specific ENA antibodies. A positive reaction is indicated by immunoprecipitation lines of serological identity. (Refer to Chapter 10 for a discussion of Ouchterlony test principles.) Although this type of testing is highly specific, it is not as sensitive and has a longer turnaround time to results as compared with the other techniques described.

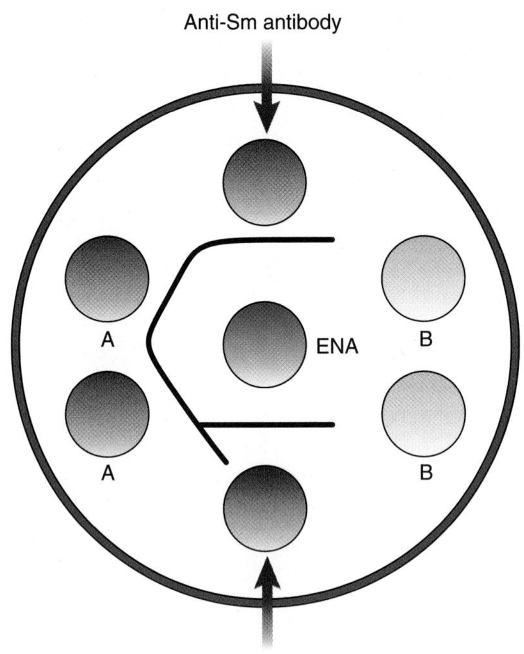

FIGURE 15–7 Extractable nuclear antibody immunodiffusion pattern. A mixture of ENAs, including RNP, Sm, and other soluble nuclear antigens, is placed in a central well in an agarose gel. Sm antibody and RNP antibody are run as positive controls and patient samples A and B are placed between the controls. The pattern of precipitin lines formed indicates the antibodies present in patient serum. The arc of serological identity formed between Sm and serum from patient A indicates that serum A contains anti-Sm antibodies. The arc of partial identity formed between serum A and RNP occurs because RNP is always found complexed to Sm antigen. RNP antibodies are not present. Serum B contains neither Sm nor RNP antibody.

Anti-Phospholipid Antibodies

Anti-phospholipid antibodies are a heterogeneous group of antibodies that bind to phospholipids alone or phospholipids complexed with protein. They can affect every organ in the body, but they are especially associated with deep-vein and arterial thrombosis and with recurrent pregnancy loss. Anti-phospholipid antibodies have been found in up to 60% of patients with lupus, but they are also associated with several other disease states. They can be identified by their ability to cause false-positive results in nontreponemal tests for syphilis, the lupus anticoagulant assay, and immunoassays for antibodies to cardiolipin or other phospholipids.

The lupus anticoagulant, one of several types of anti-phospholipid antibodies, was so named because it produces a prolonged activated partial thromboplastin time (APTT) and prothrombin time (PT). In patients with anti-phospholipid antibodies, the APTT may be prolonged, but it is not corrected by mixing with normal plasma. Ironically, patients with this antibody have an increased risk of clotting and spontaneous abortion. Platelet function may also be affected, and thrombocytopenia may be present. In addition to determining the APTT and PT, a noncompetitive ELISA can be used to detect anti-phospholipid antibodies. If these antibodies are suspected, factor assays may also need to be performed to rule out any factor deficiencies or factor-specific inhibitors.

Rheumatoid Arthritis (RA)

RA is another example of a systemic autoimmune disorder. It affects about 0.5% to 1.0% of the adult population, but prevalence varies with ethnicity and geographic location. Typically, it strikes individuals between the ages of 25 and 55. Women are three times as likely to be affected as men; in addition, the prevalence of the disease is highest in women who are more than 65 years of age. RA can be characterized as a chronic, symmetric, and erosive arthritis of the peripheral joints that can also affect multiple organs such as the heart and the lungs. Progress of the disease varies because there may be spontaneous remissions, or an increasingly active disease in some individuals that rapidly progresses to joint deformity and disability. In recent years, RA patients have experienced less disability and a better quality of life because of advances in therapy and earlier treatment (see the *Treatment* section in the text that follows).

Etiology

Associations of RA with more than 100 genetic regions have been discovered. The strongest associations have been between a subset of patients with RA and specific HLA-DRB1 alleles or *PTPN22* gene polymorphisms. These patients are positive for **rheumatoid factor (RF)** or antibodies to CCP (see the section on *Laboratory Diagnosis*). Epigenetic factors, such as altered DNA methylation affecting the transcription of critical genes, are also believed to play a role in the pathogenesis of RA. The strongest environmental risk factor for RA is believed to be cigarette smoking, which doubles the risk of developing the disease. Other factors have also been implicated, but their associations are weaker. Numerous infectious agents have been proposed as possible triggering antigens for RA, but a cause–effect relationship has not been proven.

Immunopathology

The pathology of RA is caused by an inflammatory process that results in the destruction of bone and cartilage. The lesions in rheumatoid joints show an increase in cells lining the synovial membrane and formation of a *pannus,* a sheet of inflammatory granulation tissue that grows into the joint space and invades the cartilage. Infiltration of the inflamed synovium with T and B lymphocytes, plasma cells, dendritic cells, mast cells, and granulocytes is evidence of immunologic activity within the joint.

The balance between proinflammatory and anti-inflammatory cytokines in RA appears to be tipped toward continual inflammation. Proinflammatory cytokines found in synovial fluid that contribute to inflammation include interleukin (IL)-1, IL-6, IL-17, and tumor necrosis factor alpha (TNF-α) (see Chapter 6). TNF-α plays a key role in the inflammatory process by stimulating the production of other cytokines and facilitating the transport of white blood cells (WBCs) to the affected areas. The proinflammatory cytokines trigger the release of matrix metalloproteinases from fibroblasts and macrophages; these enzymes degrade important structural proteins in the cartilage.

Local bone erosion is another feature that is characteristic of the pathology in RA. Multinucleated giant cells called osteoclasts are central to the structural damage that is seen in the bones. Osteoclasts absorb bone as part of the normal bone-remodeling process that occurs in the body in response to growth and repair of damaged bone. Normally, there is a good balance between bone production and destruction. However, in RA, the osteoclasts become overly activated in the inflammatory environment of the joints. TNF-α, in conjunction with other cytokines and a molecule called *RANKL* (receptor activator of nuclear factor kappa-B ligand), induces the differentiation of osteoclasts and inhibits bone formation. Significant local bone destruction occurs and there is also generalized osteoporosis throughout the body.

The production of autoantibodies is thought to be induced by the overproduction of cytokines. Two key antibodies found in the disease are RF and anti-CCP. RF is an antibody that is most often of the immunoglobulin m (IgM) class and is directed against the Fc portion of IgG. It has been postulated that RFs may play a role in the pathogenesis of RA by increasing macrophage activity and enhancing antigen presentation to T cells by APCs.

Antibodies to cyclic citrullinated proteins **(anti-cyclic citrullinated peptide antibody [anti-CCP or ACPA])** are a second major type of antibody associated with RA. Citrullinated proteins contain an atypical amino acid called *citrulline,* which is generated when the enzyme peptidyl arginine deiminase (PAD) modifies the amino acid arginine by replacing an NH_2 group with a neutral oxygen. This enzyme is associated with granulocytes, monocytes, and macrophages, as well as other types of cells. Death of granulocytes and macrophages triggers production of citrullinated proteins; overexpression of these antigens may provoke an immune response in individuals with certain HLA-DRB1 alleles. These antibodies can react with citrulline-containing components of the matrix, including filaggrin, keratin, fibrinogen, and vimentin, and are thought to correlate with the pathogenesis of RA. ANAs are also present in some RA patients (see the previous *Anti-Nuclear Antibodies* section).

In RA, autoantibodies such as RF and anti-CCP are thought to combine with their specified antigen, and the resulting immune complexes become deposited in the joints, resulting in a type III (or immune complex) hypersensitivity reaction. The complement protein C1 binds to the immune complexes, activating the classical complement cascade. During this process, C3a and C5a are generated, which act as chemotactic factors for neutrophils and macrophages. The continual presence of these cells and their associated cytokines leads to chronic inflammation, which damages the synovium itself.

Clinical Signs and Symptoms

The initial symptoms of RA involve the joints, tendons, and bursae. The RA patient commonly experiences nonspecific symptoms such as malaise, fatigue, fever, weight loss, and transient joint pain that begin in the small joints of the hands and feet. The joints are typically affected in a symmetric fashion. Joint stiffness and pain are usually present in the morning and improve during the day. The disease can progress to the larger joints, often affecting the knees, hips, elbows, shoulders, and cervical spine. Joint pain can lead to muscle spasms and limitation of motion. The ongoing inflammation, if left untreated, results in permanent joint dysfunction and deformity. Osteoporosis (bone erosion) occurs in about 20% to 30% of RA patients because of the inflammatory environment of the joints and activation of osteoclasts.

A significant number of patients with RA develop extra-articular manifestations, which occur outside of the joints. These patients are most likely to have had a history of smoking, have early disease onset, and test positive for anti-CCP or RF. Extra-articular manifestations include the formation of subcutaneous nodules, pericarditis, lymphadenopathy, splenomegaly, interstitial lung disease, or vasculitis. Some patients have small masses of tissue called *nodules* over the bones. Nodules can also be found in the myocardium, pericardium, heart valves, pleura, lungs, spleen, and larynx. About 10% of patients with RA develop secondary Sjögren's syndrome, an autoimmune disorder characterized by the presence of dry eyes and dry mouth in addition to connective tissue disease. A small percentage will develop Felty's syndrome, a combination of chronic, nodular RA coupled with neutropenia and splenomegaly. The most common cause of death in RA is cardiovascular disease, presumably because of the acceleration of arteriosclerosis by proinflammatory cytokines released during the disease process.

Diagnostic classification criteria for RA were established by the ACR in 1987 to standardize identification of RA patients for clinical trials. These criteria were revised in 2010 in collaboration with the EULAR in order to improve the identification of patients in the early stages of disease who could benefit from new treatments. The criteria are based on the number and types of joints involved, duration of symptoms, serology results for RF and anti-CCP, serum level of the acute-phase reactant, CRP, and the ESR. These important laboratory tests will be discussed in more detail.

Treatment

In the past, therapy for RA was primarily based on NSAIDs such as salicylates (aspirin) and ibuprofen. Although these agents can be used to reduce local swelling and pain, they are no longer the dominant treatment for RA. The discovery that joint destruction occurs early in the disease has prompted more aggressive treatment and the development of new drugs to prevent disease progression. Disease-modifying anti-rheumatic drugs (DMARDs), most notably methotrexate, are now prescribed at the time of diagnosis. Methotrexate is thought to act by inhibiting adenosine metabolism and T-cell activation. If methotrexate alone does not work, it can be combined with other conventional DMARDs or with biological DMARDs. Short-term therapy with glucocorticoids such as prednisone can also be used in initial treatment or during acute disease flares.

Biological DMARDs have revolutionized the way that RA is treated because they target components of the immune system that are central to the pathogenesis of the disease. Several key therapies for RA block the activity of the cytokine TNF-α. Agents that act against TNF-α are classified into two categories: (1) monoclonal antibodies to TNF-α (e.g., infliximab, adalimumab, certolizumab, golimumab) and (2) TNF-α receptors fused to an IgG molecule (etanercept). All of these agents specifically target and neutralize TNF-α and have demonstrated effectiveness in halting joint damage. Additional biological therapies that target other immunologic components involved in RA pathogenesis may also be used.

DMARDs have become the mainstay of RA treatment because they act on specific components of the inflammatory response and are effective in slowing the progression of joint erosion. The use of these treatments has resulted in higher rates of disease-free periods (remission) and has dramatically improved the quality of life and prognosis of RA patients. Although these agents are effective in treating RA, patients must be monitored closely because they are at greater risk for infection.

Laboratory Diagnosis of Rheumatoid Arthritis

Diagnosis of RA is based on a combination of clinical manifestations, radiographic findings, and laboratory testing. RF is the antibody that is most often tested for when making the initial diagnosis. The importance of testing for the presence of RF is also reflected in the fact that it is one of the classification criteria for RA. Recall that RF is an autoantibody, usually of the IgM class, that reacts with the Fc portion of IgG. Approximately 70% to 90% of patients with RA test positive for RF. Thus, a negative result does not rule out the presence of RA. Conversely, a positive test result is not specific for RA because RF is also present in about 5% of healthy individuals and in 10% to 25% of those over the age of 65. In addition, RF can be found in patients with other SARDs, such as SLE, Sjögren's syndrome, scleroderma, and MCTD, as well as in people with some chronic infections.

Manual agglutination tests using charcoal or latex particles coated with IgG have been used for many years to detect RF. These tests, however, only detect the IgM isotype, found in about 75% of patients, and have been largely replaced by ELISA, CLIA, and nephelometric methods, which are automated, have greater precision and sensitivity, and can also detect other RF isotypes. Testing for IgG and immunoglobulin A (IgA) RFs increases test specificity. The presence of both IgM and IgA, or of all three isotypes, rarely occurs in other disease states, which may help in making a differential diagnosis. In addition, testing for specific RF isotypes may have some prognostic value.

Laboratory testing for antibody to cyclic citrullinated peptides (anti-CCP) has been added to the classification criteria to increase the specificity for RA and is widely available. These assays are performed mainly by ELISA and use a circular synthetic form of citrullinated peptides to increase test sensitivity. A significant number of RF-negative patients are positive for anti-CCP, and the presence of anti-CCP precedes the onset of RA by several years, making it a better marker for early disease. The presence of anti-CCP is also associated with an increased likelihood of developing clinically significant disease activity with a worse prognosis. Importantly, specificity of anti-CCP for RA is higher than RF, about 95%. Furthermore, the combination of anti-CCP and RF testing has a specificity of 98% to 100%, providing for a more accurate diagnosis of RA by allowing for better differentiation from other forms of arthritis.

Low titers of ANAs are present in about 40% of patients. The pattern most frequently identified is the speckled pattern directed against RNP. The significance of this group of autoantibodies remains unclear because they do not appear to be directly related to pathogenesis.

Once a diagnosis of RA is made, the most helpful tests for following the progress of the disease are general indicators of inflammation, such as measurement of ESR, CRP, and complement components. Typically, CRP and ESR are elevated and the levels of serum complement components are normal or increased because of increased acute-phase reactivity. CRP levels correlate well with disease activity because levels reflect the intensity of the inflammatory response.

Other Systemic Autoimmune Rheumatic Diseases (SARDs)

Other SARDs include Sjögren's syndrome, SSc, MCTD, and the inflammatory myopathies. **Sjögren's syndrome** is characterized by chronic inflammation of the exocrine glands, most notably the ocular and salivary glands. This produces symptoms of dry eyes and a dry mouth, also known as "sicca syndrome." The syndrome can be broadly classified into two groups, primary Sjögren's syndrome, which occurs in the absence of other diseases, and secondary Sjögren's syndrome, which occurs in patients who also have other diseases, most commonly SLE or rheumatoid arthritis. The majority of patients with the primary form of the disease test positive for RF and ANAs, exhibiting a fine speckled pattern of fluorescence that is indicative of anti–SS-A/Ro and/or anti–SS-B/La. The presence of antibodies to SS-A/Ro is one component of the 2016 criteria established by the ACR and EULAR for the classification of primary Sjögren's syndrome.

SSc, also known as *scleroderma,* is a rare SARD that is characterized by excessive fibrosis and vascular abnormalities that affect the skin and joints and progress over time to involve internal organs, most commonly the esophagus, lower gastrointestinal tract, lungs, heart, and kidneys. Symptoms include tightening and hardening of the skin, musculoskeletal pain, Raynaud's phenomenon, and heartburn. The combination of calcinosis cutis, Raynaud's phenomenon, esophageal dysmotility, sclerodactyly, and telangiectasia has been referred to as the *CREST syndrome.* Complications involving the internal organs often result in functional impairment, leading to death. Cases can be classified into one of two major groups, depending on the extent of skin involvement. The first group, *diffuse cutaneous systemic sclerosis,* involves the skin, extending from the fingers to the trunk of the body; patients with this form are at risk of more rapid involvement of the internal organs. In the second group, *limited cutaneous systemic sclerosis,* skin involvement is restricted to the fingers, distal parts of the arms and legs, and face and does not affect the trunk of the body; progression to the internal organs is typically slower.

At least 10 different types of ANAs have been identified in patients with SSc. Three of these are useful to determine the diagnosis, subgrouping, and prognosis of patients with the disease and are included in the ACR/EULAR classification criteria for SSc. Anti-centromere antibodies are found only in patients with limited cutaneous SSc and correlate with a better survival rate, antibodies to topoisomerase I (also known as Scl-70) are associated with diffuse cutaneous SSc and a poor prognosis, and antibodies to RNA polymerase III are associated with the diffuse form of the disease and rapid thickening of the skin but have a better prognosis than those with anti–Scl-70. Thus, these three ANAs are important biomarkers for SSc.

Mixed connective tissue disease (MCTD) is an overlap syndrome of limited cutaneous SSc combined with clinical features of SLE, polymyositis, and RA. MCTD is typically associated with high titers of autoantibodies to U1-RNP but the absence of anti-centromere antibodies and generally has a better prognosis than limited cutaneous SSc.

The **inflammatory myopathies (IMs)** are a group of diseases characterized by chronic inflammation of the skeletal muscles ("myositis") and progressive muscle weakness. The muscles closest to the trunk of the body are generally affected first. Other organs, such as the skin, heart, lungs, gastrointestinal tract, and joints, are also frequently involved, and patients have an increased risk of malignancy. Two examples of IM are **polymyositis (PM)** and **dermatomyositis (DM).** DM differs from PM in that DM can present in children as well as adults and is characterized by the presence of a skin rash in addition to muscle involvement. Patients with DM and PM and other IMs can produce antibodies to a variety of cellular antigens, some of which are myositis-associated and found in other SARDs (e.g., SS-A/Ro, SS-B/La, PM-Scl, snRNPs) and others that are myositis-specific, including antibodies to tRNA anti-synthetases, the most common being anti–Jo-1, which produces a fine speckled pattern in the cytoplasm of HEp-2 cells in the FANA test.

Granulomatosis With Polyangiitis (Wegener's Granulomatosis)

Granulomatosis with polyangiitis (GPA), formerly known as **Wegener's granulomatosis** or **WG,** is a rare autoimmune disease involving inflammation of the small- to medium-sized blood vessels, or *vasculitis.* The disease usually begins with a localized inflammation of the upper and lower respiratory tract. General symptoms include fever, malaise, arthralgias, anorexia, and weight loss. The majority of patients progress to develop a more systemic form of the disease that can affect any organ system.

Virtually all patients have symptoms that affect the upper respiratory system and lungs. Symptoms of the upper airway include severe or persistent rhinorrhea ("runny nose"), rhinitis, sinusitis, oral or nasal ulcers, and gingivitis. Damage to the nasal mucosa leads to drying of the nasal membranes, which become susceptible to infection and frequent bleeding. Chronic otitis media can cause perforation and scarring of the eardrums, leading to hearing loss. Tissue damage can lead to perforation of the nasal septum or collapse of the bridge of the nose. Pulmonary infiltrates are commonly observed upon x-ray of the lungs. Although patients can experience coughing, shortness of breath, chest pain, or hemoptysis (coughing up blood), they may be asymptomatic.

As the disease progresses, other organ systems become involved. The majority of patients have renal involvement, which can range from mild glomerulonephritis with little functional impairment to severe glomerulonephritis that can rapidly lead to kidney failure. Most patients experience pain and arthritis of the large joints, which is usually symmetric but not deforming. Skin lesions may occur in patients with GPA. Many patients have ocular manifestations that can potentially lead to vision loss. Other areas of the body that can be affected include the nervous system, heart, and thyroid gland. Without treatment, the majority of patients will die within 2 years of diagnosis.

The etiology of GPA is unknown, but multiple genes are thought to be involved. The HLA-DPB1*0401 allele has been found to have a strong association with GPA in Caucasian patients, whereas the HLA-DRB1*0901 and HLA-DRB* 1501 alleles are associated with increased risk in Asian and African American populations, respectively. Although environmental factors have not been definitively identified, chronic nasal infection with *Staphylococcus aureus* bacteria has been associated with a greater rate of relapse in patients with WG. *S. aureus* may induce molecular mimicry because it contains peptides that bear similarity to the proteinase 3 (PR3) autoantigen. Exposure to silica or to certain drugs, such as hydralazine and penicillamine, may also be risk factors.

Most patients with GPA have antibodies to neutrophil cytoplasmic antigens; in 80% of these, the antibody is directed against an enzyme found in the azurophilic granules of neutrophils called *PR3*. Antibody to the PR3 antigen is thought to play a role in the pathophysiology of the systemic vasculitis seen in GPA. Events such as chronic infections can result in the release of the proinflammatory cytokine TNF-α, which stimulates neutrophils and results in migration of the PR3 antigen from the granules to the neutrophil membrane. Binding of PR3 antibodies to the PR3 antigen and Fcγ-receptors on the cell surface result in activation of the neutrophils, which adhere to the endothelial cells lining the blood vessels. There, they release reactive oxygen species and proteolytic enzymes that damage the vascular endothelium. A Th1 response follows, with release of cytokines that induce macrophage maturation and the formation of granulomatous lesions. Chronic activation of T cells within these lesions is thought to induce differentiation of autoreactive B cells into plasma cells that produce antibodies to PR3, thus perpetuating the response.

Therapy for GPA is directed toward suppression of this inflammatory response. Patients with severe forms of GPA are treated initially with a combination of glucocorticoid drugs and cyclophosphamide, which produces remission with resolution of the inflammatory lesions in most patients. Biological agents, especially the anti-CD20 monoclonal antibody rituximab, may also be used. Patients must then be maintained on a less potent immunosuppressive drug regimen. Immunosuppressive therapy has greatly improved patient outcomes and survival.

Laboratory Diagnosis

General laboratory findings include a normochromic, normocytic anemia; leukocytosis; eosinophilia; and an elevated ESR. In addition, there may be a decreased concentration of albumin in the blood and mild to severe renal insufficiency. Urinalysis typically shows microhematuria, proteinuria, and cellular casts.

A key diagnostic aid is the presence of a positive anti-neutrophil cytoplasmic antibody (ANCA) test result, specifically antibody to proteinase 3 (see the following section). Other serological findings include an elevated CRP; elevated immunoglobulin levels; and possibly other autoantibodies, such as RF and ANAs.

Anti-Neutrophil Cytoplasmic Antibodies (ANCAs)

Anti-neutrophil cytoplasmic antibodies (ANCAs) are autoantibodies that are produced against proteins that are present in the neutrophil granules. These antibodies are strongly associated with three syndromes involving vascular inflammation: GPA (WG), microscopic polyangiitis (MPA), and eosinophilic granulomatosis with polyangiitis (EGPA; formerly known as *Churg-Strauss syndrome*); these syndromes are collectively known as *ANCA-associated vasculitides (AAVs)*. In patients with GPA, ANCAs are mainly directed against the PR3 antigen, whereas in MPA and EGPA, they are usually specific for myeloperoxidase (MPO).

International consensus guidelines for ANCA testing published in 1999 recommended that patient sera be screened for ANCAs by IIF using ethanol-fixed leukocytes as the cellular substrate. Ethanol treatment permeabilizes the granule membranes, allowing for migration of the contents. In this method, patient serum is incubated with a microscope slide containing ethanol-fixed leukocytes. Following incubation, the slide is washed to remove unbound serum, and an anti-human IgG, fluorescein isothiocyanate (FITC)-labeled conjugate, is added. Following a second incubation and wash step, the slide is viewed under a fluorescent microscope for staining of the neutrophils. Lymphocyte staining should not be present; if it is, it should be minimal.

Two patterns of fluorescence can be observed: *cytoplasmic,* also known as *c-ANCA,* and *perinuclear,* or *p-ANCA*. The c-ANCA pattern is primarily caused by PR3-ANCA and appears as a diffuse, granular staining in the cytoplasm of the neutrophils **(Fig. 15–8A).** Staining is most intense in the center of the cell between the nuclear lobes and gradually fades at the outer edges of the cytoplasm. In the p-ANCA pattern, fluorescence surrounds the lobes of the nucleus, blending them together so that individual lobes cannot be distinguished (**Fig. 15–8B**). This is because the p-ANCA pattern is caused by antibodies against positively charged antigens such as MPO that migrate out of the granules after ethanol fixation and are attracted toward the negatively charged nucleus. **Table 15–3** summarizes the main features of ANCAs.

It is important to distinguish the p-ANCA pattern from ANAs, which can also stain the nuclei of the neutrophils. With ANAs, the nuclear lobes may be more clearly separated, speckled staining may be present, and the nuclei of the lymphocytes will also be stained. In addition, if a true p-ANCA pattern is present, ANA testing using HEp-2 cells as the substrate in IIF should be negative. For more definitive differentiation, the test can be repeated using microscope slides with formalin-fixed

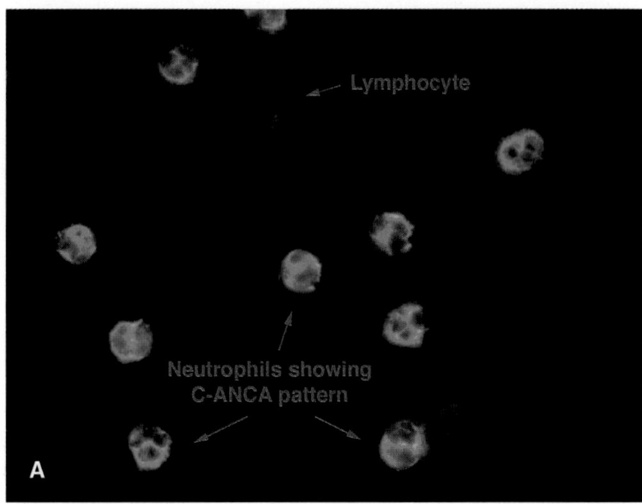

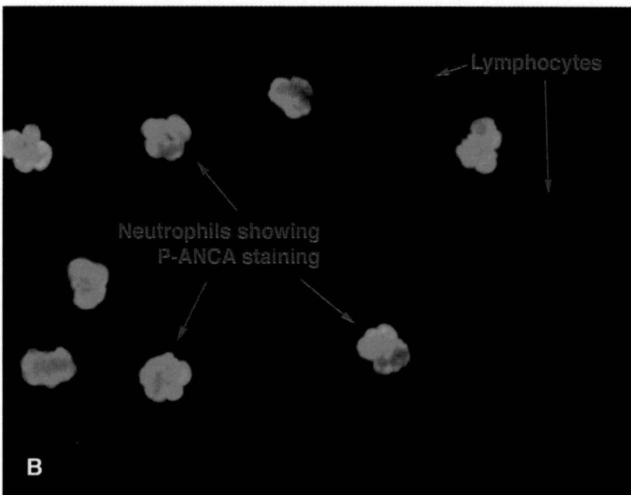

FIGURE 15–8 c-ANCA and p-ANCA fluorescent patterns. (A) c-ANCA (cytoplasmic pattern). Note the granular staining of the primary granules in the cytoplasm of the neutrophils and the more intense fluorescence between the lobes of each nucleus. The lymphocytes have negative staining. This pattern can be seen with either ethanol-fixed or formalin-fixed neutrophils. (B) p-ANCA (fluorescent pattern). This pattern is characterized by smooth or homogeneous staining of the multilobed nuclei in ethanol-fixed neutrophils as shown. (On formalin-fixed neutrophils, these antibodies would produce a granular cytoplasmic staining.) The lymphocytes are not stained. (Reprinted with permission from Immuno Concepts.)

Table 15–3 Anti-Neutrophil Cytoplasmic Antibodies (ANCAs)

PATTERN ON INDIRECT IMMUNOFLUORESCENCE WITH ETHANOL-FIXED LEUKOCYTES	APPEARANCE	AUTOANTIGENS	ASSOCIATED DISEASES
c-ANCA	Diffuse, granular staining in the cytoplasm of the neutrophils, fading toward the outer edges of the cells	PR3 antigen	Granulomatosis with polyangiitis (GPA; Wegener's granulomatosis)
p-ANCA	Fluorescence surrounding the lobes of the neutrophil nuclei, blending them together	Positively charged antigens, including myeloperoxidase (MPO)	Microscopic polyangiitis (MPA) Eosinophilic granulomatosis with polyangiitis (EGPA; Churg-Strauss syndrome)

c-ANCA = cytoplasmic anti-neutrophil cytoplasmic antibody; p-ANCA = perinuclear anti-neutrophil cytoplasmic antibody.

leukocytes. Formalin is a cross-linking fixative that prevents the migration of antigens out of the granules. Therefore, in the presence of antibodies to MPO or other positively charged proteins, perinuclear staining will be prevented, and intense, granular staining of the cytoplasm will be seen that resembles c-ANCA.

ANCA detection by IIF has a sensitivity of more than 90% for the AAVs but has a lower specificity (80% or less) because ANCAs, especially those producing the p-ANCA pattern, can be found in other conditions. Therefore, experts recommend that samples that are positive through initial testing with IIF should be confirmed by PR3- and MPO-specific immunoassays whenever possible to increase clinical significance of the results.

Although IIF has been widely used by clinical laboratories to test for ANCA, automated immunoassays have been developed in a variety of formats, including ELISA, CLIA, and fluorescent microbead immunoassays; and have improved in quality over the years. This development prompted experts to propose a revised International Consensus on ANCA testing in 2017. The revised consensus guidelines recommend screening for ANCA with an automated immunoassay for antibodies to PR3 and MPO instead of an IIF. If the test result is negative but small-vessel vasculitis is still suspected, a second immunoassay or an IIF can be performed. It is important to note that failure to detect ANCAs does not completely rule out the presence of AAV, and experts recommend that biopsies of affected organs be performed in ANCA-negative patients who are suspected of having an AAV.

It is also important to understand that ANCAs are not diagnostic for AAV and can be found in a variety of other disorders, including other types of vasculitis; SARDs such as SLE and RA; autoimmune gastrointestinal and liver diseases, certain infections, including HIV and hepatitis C; malignancy; and other diseases. Patients with these conditions often have ANCAs directed toward neutrophil antigens other than PR3 or MPO, which can also be detected by IIF. High ANCA titers correlate better with presence of disease and are useful in monitoring disease activity. Thus, a positive ANCA test must be combined with clinical manifestations and histological findings of biopsy tissue to make an accurate diagnosis. The clinical value of an ANCA test result is increased when the test is only performed on patients with specific clinical indications of AAV to reduce the probability of false-positive results.

Organ-Specific Autoimmune Diseases

This chapter will refer to organ-specific autoimmune diseases as those diseases in which the immune response is directed against self-antigens that are mainly found in a single organ or gland. Although the clinical manifestations are largely related to the target area, systemic effects may sometimes also occur. Examples of organ-specific autoimmune diseases are listed in **Table 15–4**; several of these will be discussed in more detail here.

Autoimmune Thyroid Diseases (AITDs)

Autoimmune thyroid diseases (AITDs) encompass several different clinical conditions, the most notable of which are Hashimoto's thyroiditis and Graves' disease. Although these conditions have distinctly different symptoms, both interfere with thyroid function, and they share some of the same antibodies. The thyroid gland is a bilobed, butterfly-shaped organ located in the anterior region of the neck and is normally between 12 and 20 grams in size. It is essential in regulating the body's metabolism, thus controlling heart, muscle, and

Table 15–4 Organ-Specific Autoimmune Diseases

DISEASE	TARGET CELLS OR TISSUES	ASSOCIATED AUTOANTIBODIES
Addison's disease	Adrenal glands	Antibody to adrenal cells
Autoimmune hemolytic anemia	Red blood cells (RBCs)	Antibody to RBCs
Autoimmune hepatitis (AIH)	Liver	AIH-1—smooth muscle antibodies; anti-nuclear antibodies (ANAs) AIH-2—anti-liver kidney microsomal antibody (anti-LKM-1); anti-liver cytosol type 1 antibody (anti-LC-1)
Autoimmune thrombocytopenic purpura	Platelets	Anti-platelet antibody
Celiac disease	Small intestine and other organs	Anti-transglutaminase (tTG) Antibodies to deamidated gliadin peptides (DGPs) Endomysial antibodies
Anti-glomerular basement membrane disease (Goodpasture's syndrome)	Kidneys, lungs	Antibody to an antigen in the renal and pulmonary basement membranes
Graves' disease	Thyroid gland	Thyroid-stimulating hormone receptor antibodies (TRAbs) Anti-thyroglobulin Anti-thyroid peroxidase (TPO)
Hashimoto's thyroiditis	Thyroid gland	Anti-thyroglobulin Anti-thyroid peroxidase (TPO)
Multiple sclerosis	Myelin sheath of nerves	Antibodies to myelin basic protein
Myasthenia gravis	Nerve-muscle synapses	Antibodies to acetylcholine receptors (AChR) Anti–muscle-specific kinase (MuSK) Antibody to the lipoprotein LRP4
Pernicious anemia	Stomach	Parietal cell antibody, intrinsic factor antibody
Poststreptococcal glomerulonephritis	Kidneys	Streptococcal antibodies that cross-react with kidney tissue
Primary biliary cholangitis	Intrahepatic bile ducts	Anti-mitochondrial antibodies (AMA)
Rheumatic fever	Heart	Streptococcal antibodies that cross-react with cardiac tissue
Type 1 diabetes mellitus	Pancreas	Anti-insulin Islet cell antibodies Anti–IA-2 and anti–IA-2βA Antibody to glutamic acid phosphatase (GAD)

digestive functions; it also controls neurological development and maintenance of bone structure.

The thyroid gland consists of units called *follicles* that are spherical in shape and lined with cuboidal epithelial cells. Follicles are filled with material called *colloid*. The primary constituent of colloid is **thyroglobulin (Tg)**, a large iodinated glycoprotein from which the active thyroid hormone triiodothyronine (T3) and its precursor, thyroxine (T4), are synthesized. The enzyme **thyroid peroxidase (TPO)** plays an important role in the synthesis of these hormones by oxidizing iodine ions, allowing for their incorporation into the tyrosine residues of thyroglobulin to produce the building blocks for the hormones.

Under normal conditions, the synthesis of T3 and T4 is tightly regulated by an endocrine feedback loop called the *hypothalamic–pituitary–thyroid axis* **(Fig. 15–9)**. **Thyrotropin-releasing hormone (TRH)** is secreted by the hypothalamus to initiate the process that eventually causes release of hormones from the thyroid. TRH acts on the pituitary gland to induce release of **thyroid-stimulating hormone** (**TSH**), which is also known as *thyrotropin*. TSH, in turn, binds to receptors on the cells of the thyroid gland, causing thyroglobulin to be broken down into secretabal T3 and T4. If the concentrations of T3 and T4 in the blood are too low, TRH and TSH secretion increases in order to stimulate hormone production by the thyroid gland. In contrast, if the levels of T3 and T4 become too high, they feed back to the hypothalamus and pituitary to inhibit release of TRH and TSH, resulting in decreased production of the thyroid hormones. The presence of autoantibodies to components of the thyroid gland interferes with this process and causes under- or overactivity of the gland.

Etiology

The genes thought to be associated with a predisposition to thyroid autoimmunity are related to immune function or are thyroid specific. A strong association between HLA-DR3 and Graves' disease has been observed. The association of Hashimoto's thyroiditis with the inheritance of HLA antigens DR3, DR4, DR5, and DQ7 has been reported in Caucasians, but this is not consistent among different ethnic populations. A unique feature of both Graves' and Hashimoto's diseases is that HLA-DR antigens are expressed on the surface of thyroid epithelial cells, perhaps increasing the autoimmune response. Mutations in the thyroglobulin gene may allow for interaction of the protein with HLA-DR antigens, resulting in anti-thyroglobulin antibodies. These can be found in both Graves' and Hashimoto's disease. Additionally, in Graves' disease, modifications in the TSH receptor gene may allow the immune system to recognize the receptor and produce antibodies against it.

Possible environmental triggers of AITDs include infections, certain medications, smoking, psychological stress, and pregnancy, but the strongest link is thought to be between high iodine intake and development of Hashimoto's disease. Highly iodinated thyroglobulin is thought to be more immunogenic, possibly creating or exposing more epitopes and facilitating the antigen uptake and processing step of the adaptive immune response (see Chapter 4).

Clinical Signs and Immunopathology of Hashimoto's Thyroiditis

Hashimoto's thyroiditis, also known as *chronic lymphocytic thyroiditis*, was discovered in Japan in 1912 by Dr. Hakaru Hashimoto. It is a common autoimmune disease, affecting about 8 out of every 1,000 individuals. The disease is most often seen in middle-aged women; in addition, women are 5 to 10 times more likely to develop the disease than men. Patients develop an enlarged thyroid called a *goiter*, which is irregular and rubbery. Patients also produce thyroid-specific autoantibodies and cytotoxic T cells. Immune destruction of

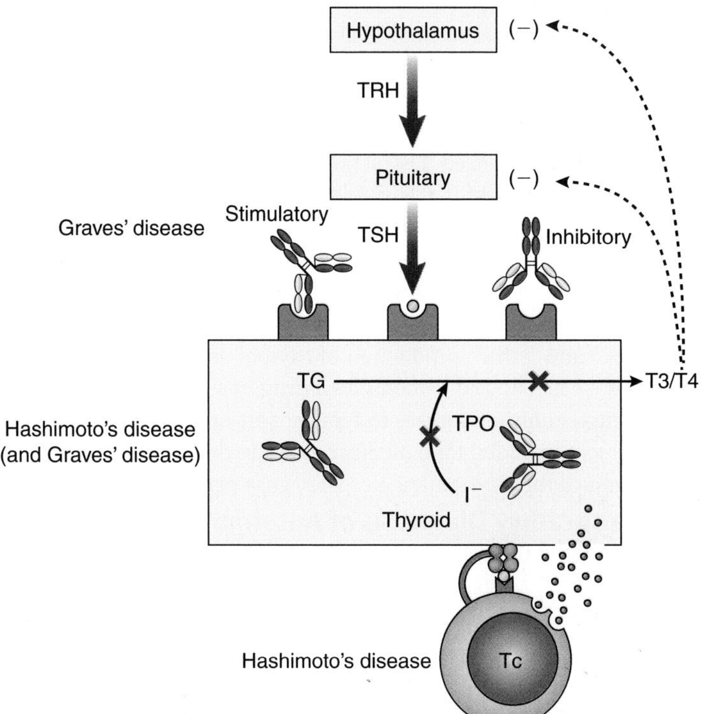

FIGURE 15–9 Autoimmune disorders in thyroid hormone synthesis and regulation. The actions of autoantibodies and cytotoxic T cells in the pathogenesis of Graves' disease and Hashimoto's disease is shown. Solid arrows = stimulation; dotted arrows = feedback inhibition.

the thyroid gland occurs, which results in a state of decreased thyroid function called *hypothyroidism*. Symptoms of hypothyroidism include dry skin, decreased sweating, puffy face with edematous eyelids, pallor with a yellow tinge, weight gain, fatigue, and dry and brittle hair.

Several forms of Hashimoto's disease have been described, each with distinct pathological features. In the classic form of the disease, the thyroid shows hyperplasia with an increased number of lymphocytes. Cellular types present include activated T and B cells (with T cells predominating), macrophages, and plasma cells. Pathology to the thyroid gland is mediated primarily by CD8+ cytotoxic T cells, which bind to the thyroid cells and destroy them by releasing enzymes that cause apoptosis or necrosis. Production of the cytokines TNF-α, IL-1, and interferon gamma (IFN-γ) is thought to promote inflammation and contribute to destruction of the thyroid cells. The immune response also results in the development of germinal centers that almost completely replace the normal glandular architecture of the thyroid and progressively destroy the thyroid gland. Many patients produce antibodies to Tg and TPO; these antibodies have the ability to fix complement, and this may result in an inflammatory response that perpetuates the tissue damage. A smaller percentage of patients produce antibodies against the TSH receptor that prevent binding of TSH. Injury to the thyroid gland and inhibition of its function result in the symptoms associated with hypothyroidism.

Clinical Signs and Immunopathology of Graves' Disease

Graves' disease, in contrast to Hashimoto's thyroiditis, is characterized by *hyperthyroidism,* a state of excessive thyroid function. Graves' disease is, in fact, one of the most frequently occurring autoimmune diseases and the most common cause of hyperthyroidism. Women exhibit greater susceptibility to Graves' disease, by a margin of about 5 to 1, and most often present with the disease in the fifth and sixth decades of life.

The disease is manifested as **thyrotoxicosis,** or an excess of thyroid hormones, with a diffusely enlarged goiter that is firm instead of rubbery. Clinical symptoms include nervousness, insomnia, depression, weight loss, heat intolerance, sweating, rapid heartbeat, palpitations, breathlessness, fatigue, cardiac dysrhythmias, and restlessness. Another sign, present in approximately one-third of patients, is exophthalmos, in which hypertrophy of the eye muscles and increased connective tissue in the orbit cause the eyeball to bulge out so that the patient has a large-eyed, staring expression **(Fig. 15–10).** There is evidence that orbital fibroblasts express TSH receptor-like proteins that are affected by thyroid-stimulating immunoglobulin just as the thyroid is (see discussion that follows). Localized edema in the lower legs can also occur.

The thyroid shows uniform hyperplasia with a patchy lymphocytic infiltration. The follicles have little colloid but are filled with hyperplastic epithelium. A large number of these cells express HLA-DR antigens on their surface in response to IFN-γ produced by infiltrating T cells. This allows presentation of self-antigens, such as the thyrotropin receptor, to activated T cells. B cells, in turn, are stimulated to produce antibody.

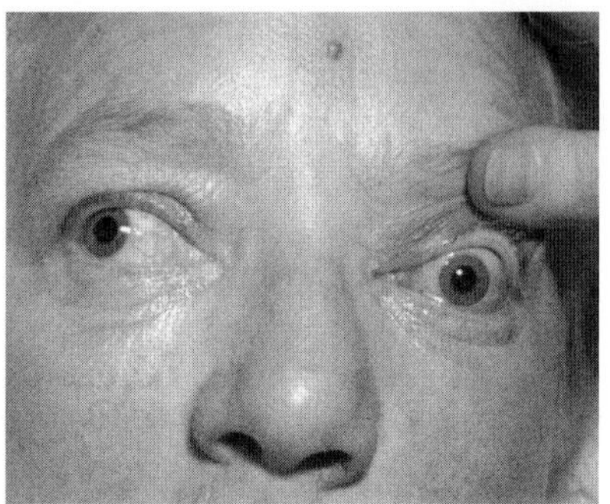

FIGURE 15–10 Exophthalmos indicative of Graves' disease. *(Courtesy of CDC/Dr. Sellers/Emory University.)*

The main antibodies involved in the pathogenesis of Graves' disease are the **thyroid-stimulating hormone receptor antibodies (TRAbs)**. There are two main types of TRAbs. The type responsible for the hyperthyroidism seen in Graves' disease are called **thyroid-stimulating immunoglobulins (TSIs)**. When TSIs bind to the TSH receptor, they mimic the action of TSH, resulting in uncontrolled receptor stimulation with excessive release of thyroid hormones (see Fig. 15–9). Another type of TRAb, the thyroid-blocking antibodies (TBAbs), prevent TSH from binding to its receptor and cause decreased thyroid function. Other antibodies present include anti-Tg and anti-TPO. Depending on the relative activity of stimulating and blocking autoantibodies, patient symptoms may vary from hyperthyroidism to euthyroidism (the state of normal thyroid function) to hypothyroidism, which may confound the patient's diagnosis.

Treatment of Autoimmune Thyroid Diseases

Treatment for Hashimoto's disease consists of daily oral thyroid hormone replacement therapy, with levothyroxine (T4) being the preferred drug. TSH levels should be monitored throughout treatment and are used in adjusting the dose of the drug so that normal TSH levels are maintained.

Several different protocols are used in the treatment of Graves' disease. In the United States, the first line of treatment usually involves radioactive iodine, which emits beta particles that cause localized destruction of the thyroid cells. The iodine is administered for 1 to 2 years and results in a long-term remission in many individuals. Some patients, however, develop hypothyroidism within 5 years; therefore, continued monitoring is essential. In Europe and Japan, patients are typically first placed on anti-thyroid medications that inhibit the function of TPO and reduce production of thyroid antibodies. This initial course is followed by continued drug treatment, radioactive iodine therapy, or surgery to remove part of the thyroid. Surgery is recommended for patients resistant to drug treatment but can damage the laryngeal nerves and cause permanent hoarseness.

Laboratory Diagnosis of Autoimmune Thyroid Diseases

Initial screening for AITDs involves measurement of circulating TSH levels. Recall that because of the hypothalamic–pituitary–thyroid axis, the TSH level is inversely related to the levels of T3 and T4. TSH is routinely measured with highly sensitive chemiluminescent immunoassays that can detect

Table 15–5 Typical Laboratory Findings in Autoimmune Thyroid Diseases

DISEASE	TSH LEVEL	FREE T4 (FT4) LEVEL	AUTOANTIBODIES
Hashimoto's thyroiditis	Normal or elevated	Decreased	Anti-thyroglobulin Anti-thyroid peroxidase (TPO)
Graves' disease	Decreased or undetectable	Elevated	Thyroid-stimulating hormone receptor antibodies (TRAbs)* Anti-thyroglobulin Anti-thyroid peroxidase (TPO)

*Diagnostic.

down to 0.01 mU/L. A normal TSH level indicates normal thyroid function, with rare exceptions. If the TSH level is abnormally high or low, laboratory tests for circulating thyroid hormone levels must be performed. Although immunoassays for total serum T3 and T4 are available, the majority of these hormones are protein-bound, and alterations in these hormone-binding proteins can affect test results. Therefore, it is more useful to measure unbound thyroid hormone, usually free T4 (FT4). **Table 15–5** summarizes some of the main laboratory findings in Hashimoto's disease and Graves' disease.

Patients with Hashimoto's thyroiditis will have normal or high TSH levels and low FT4 levels. To establish an autoimmune etiology for the hypothyroidism, it is necessary to follow these findings by testing for thyroid antibodies. These antibodies are most commonly detected by sensitive ELISA and chemiluminescent immunoassays. Antibodies to TPO are the best indicator of the disease because they are found in up to 95% of patients with Hashimoto's disease but in only 10% to 15% of the general population. Antibodies to Tg are less sensitive and specific because they are detected in only 60% to 80% of patients with the disease and are found more frequently than TPO antibodies in healthy persons. Because anti-Tg antibodies are not found in all patients, a negative test result does not necessarily rule out Hashimoto's disease.

In contrast, patients with Graves' disease characteristically have low or undetectable levels of TSH and increased levels of FT4. Increased uptake of radioactive iodine also helps to confirm the diagnosis. Although antibodies to TPO and Tg are found in the majority of patients, they are generally not useful in making the diagnosis. TRAbs, on the other hand, are highly indicative of Graves' disease because they are present in 98% to 100% of patients; TRAbs are therefore included as one component of the diagnostic criteria for Graves' disease.

There are two types of tests for TRAbs: binding assays and bioassays. In binding assays, such as automated solid-phase ELISA or chemiluminescent immunoassays, a labeled TRAb reagent competes with the patient antibody for TSH receptor bound to a solid phase. These assays can be performed by routine clinical laboratories but are unable to distinguish between TSI and TBAb. Bioassays require tissue culture and are difficult to perform. However, these assays specifically measure the function of TSI. Current bioassays detect the ability of TSI to bind to TSH receptors on live cells and trigger cyclic adenosine monophosphate (cAMP)-dependent luciferase activity. These assays may be performed by reference laboratories to evaluate patient response to therapy by monitoring TSI titers, clarify cases that are difficult to diagnose, and predict the risk of thyroid dysfunction in newborns born to mothers with Graves' disease.

Type 1 Diabetes Mellitus (T1D)

Diabetes mellitus is a group of common endocrine disorders that are characterized by *hyperglycemia* (a high level of glucose in the blood). The American Diabetes Association (ADA) has classified diabetes into four main categories based on the etiology of the disease: type 1 diabetes, type 2 diabetes, gestational diabetes, and diabetes because of other causes (e.g., neonatal diabetes, pancreatitis). The majority of patients have type 2 diabetes, which is characterized by insulin resistance and occurs most commonly in obese individuals over the age of 40. About 5% to 10% of patients with diabetes mellitus are classified as having **type 1 diabetes mellitus (T1D)**, which is characterized by a complete or nearly complete deficiency in insulin. Of these patients, 90% have an immune-mediated form of the disease known as *type 1A diabetes*, whereas the remaining 10% are idiopathic cases with no identifiable cause (type 1B diabetes). Gestational diabetes develops in some women during pregnancy. This section will focus on type 1A diabetes, which will be referred to as *T1D*. T1D was previously known as *insulin-dependent diabetes* or *juvenile-onset diabetes* because it requires treatment with insulin and usually develops in children or in young adults before the age of 30.

T1D is a chronic autoimmune disease that involves selective destruction of the beta cells of the pancreas. These cells are located in clusters called the *islets of Langerhans* and are responsible for the production and secretion of the hormone insulin. Insulin plays a vital role in regulating the amount of glucose in the circulation by promoting its absorption by skeletal muscles and fat tissue so that it can be converted into energy needed by our cells. The autoimmune destruction of beta cells in T1D results in insufficient insulin production, hyperglycemia, and toxic effects on the body. Long-term effects include cardiovascular complications, renal disease, nerve damage, blindness, and infections of the lower extremities, which can lead to amputation. Patients require lifelong insulin injections to control glucose levels and lower the risk of these complications.

Family studies indicate that there is an inherited genetic susceptibility to the disease, probably attributable to multiple genes. Most people with T1D carry the *HLA-DR3* or *DR4* gene, and there is an increased risk when both of these genes are present. There is also a strong correlation between certain HLA-DQ haplotypes and T1D. Environmental factors have not been clearly defined, but possible influences include certain viral infections, proteins in cow's milk, and obesity.

Immunopathology

Progressive inflammation of the islets of Langerhans in the pancreas leads to fibrosis and destruction of most beta cells. The subclinical period may last for years. Hyperglycemia does not become evident until 80% or more of the beta cells are destroyed. Immunohistochemical staining of inflamed islets shows a preponderance of CD8+ lymphocytes, along with plasma cells and macrophages. B cells themselves may act as APCs, stimulating activation of CD4+ lymphocytes. A shift to a Th1 response causes production of certain cytokines, including TNF-α, IFN-γ, and IL-1. The generalized inflammation that results is responsible for the destruction of the beta cells. Cell death is likely caused by nitric acid metabolites, attack by cytotoxic lymphocytes, and apoptosis.

Autoantibody production has been found to precede the development of clinically evident T1D by several years. Autoantibodies are produced against various components of the pancreatic islet cells and are present in newly diagnosed patients and in prediabetic individuals who are being monitored because they have a high risk of developing diabetes. Antibody production diminishes with time, however. Among the antibodies found are antibodies to two tyrosine phosphatase–like transmembrane proteins called *insulinoma antigen 2 (IA-2,* also known as *ICA-512)* and *IA-2βA (phogrin); anti-insulin and anti-proinsulin antibodies;* antibodies to the enzyme *glutamic acid decarboxylase (GAD-65);* antibodies to *zinc transporter 8 (ZnT8);* and antibodies to various other islet cell proteins, called *islet cell antibodies (ICAs).* Many of these antigens are components of the regulated pathway that is essential for the secretion of insulin.

Treatment

The primary therapy for T1D involves multiple daily injections of insulin, with the goal of achieving normal levels of glucose in the blood as much as possible. The insulin is prepared by recombinant DNA technology and consists of the amino acid sequence of human insulin or variations that have been genetically modified to improve absorption and function. Clinical trials are investigating the use of immunosuppressive drugs and biological agents to inhibit the autoimmune responses that lead to beta cell destruction and prevent disease progression in T1D patients. Transplantation of the whole pancreas or pancreatic beta islet cells has been used for T1D patients who have poor glucose control, but this treatment requires continual immunosuppressive therapy to prevent rejection, and the number of suitable donors is limited. New technologies, such as the use of stem cells to produce islet cells in vitro and methods to induce immunologic tolerance in recipients, offer hope that islet cell transplantation may encounter fewer obstacles in the future.

Laboratory Diagnosis of Type 1 Diabetes Mellitus

According to the ADA, a person is considered to have diabetes if he or she meets one of four criteria: (1) a fasting glucose greater than 126 mg/dL on more than one occasion (normal value is lower than 100 mg/dL); (2) a random plasma glucose level of 200 mg/dL or more with classic symptoms of diabetes; (3) an oral glucose tolerance test of 200 mg/dL or more in a 2-hour sample with a 75 g glucose load; or (4) a hemoglobin A1c value (HbA1c) greater than 6.5%. HbA1c is a glycated form of hemoglobin that is made when the RBC protein combines with glucose in the blood. The HbA1c plasma level is proportional to the life span of the circulating RBCs (up to 120 days) and reflects the average plasma glucose concentration over the previous 2 to 3 months.

Although T1D is usually diagnosed by demonstrating its prime characteristic of hyperglycemia, it may be useful to perform serological tests to distinguish T1D from type 2 diabetes, as ICAs have been found in the sera of the majority of patients who have been newly diagnosed with T1D. When T1D is suspected, tests for antibodies to glutamic acid decarboxylase (GAD) and IA-2A can be done to confirm the diagnosis. If these results are negative, they can be followed by testing for ICA in children and for insulin antibodies in adults. Another use of serological testing is to predict the risk of developing T1D in children who possess genetic factors that predispose them to the disease. Studies have shown that the presence of two or more pertinent autoantibodies is associated with a high risk of developing T1D in these children.

Antibodies to islet cells have traditionally been detected by IIF using frozen sections of human pancreas. However, such assays are rather cumbersome to perform, and other methods are available, including ELISA, radioimmunoassay, radio-immunoprecipitation assays, Western blotting, and mass spectrometry. These methods can also be used to detect antibodies to other pancreatic antigens, such as insulin, GAD, and IA-2. Combined screening for IA-2A, ICA, and GAD antibodies appears to have the most sensitivity and best positive predictive value for T1D in high-risk populations.

Celiac Disease

Celiac disease is an autoimmune disease affecting the small intestine and other organs. It affects 1% to 1.5% of the world's population, but this number is thought to be an underestimate because many cases go undiagnosed. Celiac disease is unique in that it is associated with a known environmental trigger—dietary gluten. Gluten is a protein complex found in wheat, barley, and rye that is poorly digested by the upper gastrointestinal system. It contains an alcohol-soluble component called *gliadin* that is rich in the amino acids glutamine and proline. Gliadin is resistant to digestive enzymes in the stomach, pancreas, and small intestine and therefore remains intact in the lumen, or space within the intestines, after ingestion. If there is an increase in the permeability of the intestinal walls, possibly because of an infection, undigested gliadin is able to pass through the epithelial barrier of the intestine and triggers an inappropriate immune response. The immunogenicity of gliadin is enhanced when it is acted on by **tissue transglutaminase (tTG),** an intestinal enzyme that converts the glutamine residues in gliadin to glutamic acid.

Immunogenic peptides are generated that specifically react with HLA-DQ2 or HLA-DQ8 molecules on APCs. In fact, the vast majority of patients with celiac disease possess one of these two HLA haplotypes. Most patients have an HLA-DQ2 allele, whereas almost all of the remaining patients are positive for HLA-DQ8. The gliadin peptides that are picked up by the APC are presented to antigen-specific CD4+ T cells, which produce cytokines that activate CD8+ T cells and trigger an inflammatory response that damages the architecture of the intestinal mucosa and causes injury to the villi. In addition, B cells are stimulated to produce antibodies to the deamidated gliadin peptides (DGPs), tTG, and endomysium (a layer of connective tissue surrounding the intestinal muscles).

Environmental factors believed to play a role in the development of celiac disease include administration of gluten in the diet of an infant younger than 4 months in the absence of breastfeeding, rotavirus infection, and overgrowth of pathogenic bacteria in the gut. In addition, the disease is found more often in women than in men (ratio, 2:1 to 3:1) and among those who have selective IgA deficiency, Down syndrome, Turner syndrome, or certain autoimmune diseases. Several non-HLA genes involved in immune function are also thought to contribute to this autoimmune response.

Clinical Symptoms and Treatment

The clinical symptoms of celiac disease vary with age. Infants typically present with diarrhea, abdominal distention, and failure to thrive but may also experience vomiting, irritability, anorexia, and constipation. Older children, teenagers, and adults may have the classic symptoms of diarrhea and abdominal pain or discomfort but often have extraintestinal manifestations that make the condition difficult to diagnose. These include short stature, arthritis or arthralgia, osteoporosis, neurological symptoms, iron-deficiency anemia, and dermatitis herpetiformis (a skin disorder with itchy blistering).

Treatment of celiac disease involves placing patients on a gluten-free diet. Elimination of gluten from the diet usually results in improvement of clinical symptoms within days or weeks and healing of intestinal damage in 6 months to 2 years. However, a significant number of patients do not adhere to a gluten-free diet because of expense, inconvenience, or social stigma; in addition, some patients have persistent symptoms despite adherence to the diet. Alternative treatments, such as the use of recombinant enzymes to digest the toxic gliadin, are being investigated.

Laboratory Diagnosis of Celiac Disease

Diagnosis of celiac disease is based on clinical symptoms, serological findings, duodenal biopsy, and the presence of the HLA-DQ2 or HLA-DQ8 haplotype. Serological testing is the initial approach taken to evaluate patients suspected of having celiac disease and helps to differentiate these patients from those having conditions with similar symptoms, such as gluten sensitivity or wheat allergy. It is recommended that patients follow a regular diet before serological testing because false-negative antibody results can occur in individuals on a gluten-free diet.

The first serological test for celiac disease was produced in the 1980s and measured antibodies to gliadin. However, this test was associated with a significant number of false-positive results and has been replaced with testing for anti-DGP (see discussion that follows).

Currently, detection of IgA antibodies to tTG is the serological method of choice for initial testing. This is because highly sensitive, automated, ELISA-based assays using purified human or recombinant tTG antigen have been developed. Rapid point-of-care enzyme immunoassay (EIA) tests are also available for the detection of antibodies to tTG but may not perform as well as the ELISA tests. Serum IgA levels should be concurrently measured in individuals suspected of having celiac disease because a significant number of patients also have selective IgA deficiency and will therefore test negative in IgA-based assays. In patients who are IgA deficient, testing for IgG anti-tTG or for IgG antibodies to DGPs can be performed. Automated ELISA tests for anti-DGPs show an especially high sensitivity in children under the age of 2 to 3 years, who may test negative for other antibodies.

Despite their high specificity, false-positive results for anti-tTG can occur in patients with other autoimmune diseases and a variety of other conditions. Therefore, positive anti-tTG results should be confirmed by repeat testing or by another method. Detection of endomysial antibodies (EMAs), which are directed against the tissue that surrounds smooth muscle fibers, can be used for confirmation. EMA tests are highly specific for celiac disease but are costly and labor-intensive because they are based on IIF assays using monkey esophagus or human umbilical cord tissue as the substrate; therefore, they are not performed as commonly as anti-tTG. Newer markers, such as antibodies to epitopes exposed on tTG-modified gliadin, are also being studied for their clinical utility.

Because serology testing has limitations, biopsy of the small intestine should be performed to confirm the diagnosis in adults. Initial biopsy results can also provide a baseline for comparing future samples for intestinal injury. Histological examination of biopsy tissue characteristically shows an increase in the number of intraepithelial lymphocytes, elongation of the intestinal crypts, and partial to total atrophy of the villi (**Fig. 15–11**). Determination of the T lymphocyte count by CD3 staining as well as observation of IgA transglutaminase antibody deposits in the tissue can provide additional information to support the diagnosis. In order to minimize the occurrence of false-negative results, multiple biopsies should be obtained from different parts of the duodenum because mucosal injury may be patchy.

HLA typing is also useful in differentiating celiac disease from other conditions, especially when serological tests and biopsy results are borderline. The absence of HLA-DQ2 or HLA-DQ8 virtually excludes a diagnosis of celiac disease because individuals who are negative for these haplotypes are highly unlikely to have the disease.

Following proper diagnosis and maintenance of patients with celiac disease on a gluten-free diet, clinical symptoms usually improve, antibody titers revert to negative, and histology

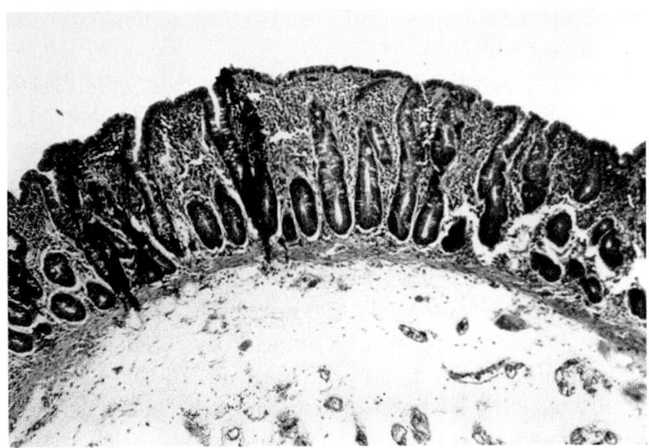

FIGURE 15–11 This photomicrograph depicts the cyto-architecture exhibited by a section of intestinal epithelial mucosa that had been excised from an individual with gluten-induced enteropathy. Note the thickened, fused, and blunted morphology of the intestinal villi. *(Courtesy of CDC Public Health Image Library.)*

can return to normal. However, about 5% of patients fail to improve, usually because of nonadherence to the diet (which can sometimes be unintentional) but sometimes caused by refractory disease, incorrect diagnosis, complications of celiac disease, or simultaneous gastrointestinal disorders.

Autoimmune Liver Diseases

There are three major forms of **autoimmune liver disease:** autoimmune hepatitis (AIH), **primary biliary cholangitis (PBC**; formerly known as *primary biliary cirrhosis*), and primary sclerosing cholangitis (PSC). In AIH, the autoimmune process targets the hepatocytes; in PBC, it affects the small interlobular bile ducts; and in PSC, it affects the medium-sized intra- and extrahepatic bile ducts. There can also be overlap syndromes that combine features of these diseases. Many patients also have other autoimmune disorders, such as autoimmune thyroiditis or ulcerative colitis. This section will discuss two of these diseases, AIH and PBC, and the serological tests that are used in their diagnosis in more detail.

Connections

Hepatitis

It is important to differentiate autoimmune liver diseases from infectious hepatitis, which presents with similar symptoms and elevated liver enzymes. The three most common hepatitis viruses are hepatitis A, which is transmitted by the fecal-oral route; hepatitis B; and hepatitis C, the latter two being bloodborne pathogens (see Chapter 23).

Autoimmune Hepatitis (AIH)

AIH, formerly known as *chronic active hepatitis,* is an immune-mediated liver disease that can lead to end-stage liver failure if left untreated. It can affect children and adults of all ages and is more common in females than in males. The clinical features of AIH can be quite variable. About 25% of individuals are asymptomatic and are diagnosed only after abnormal liver function tests are found coincidentally when blood work is performed. Adults usually present with an unexpected onset of vague symptoms, including fatigue, nausea, weight loss, abdominal pain, itching, and maculopapular rashes. Less often, patients have symptoms of portal hypertension, such as gastrointestinal bleeding or hypersplenism. Jaundice may also be present. Rarely, the initial presentation is fulminant liver failure requiring liver transplantation.

Two types of AIH can be differentiated on the basis of its autoantibody specificity (see the text that follows); these are referred to as *AIH-1* and *AIH-2*. AIH-1 accounts for two-thirds of all AIH cases and has a female:male ratio of 4:1. AIH-2 has a female:male ratio of 10:1 and is seen mostly in children.

A higher risk of developing type I AIH has been associated with presence of HLA-DR-3 and HLA-DR4 in Caucasians, whereas certain HLA-DRB1 and HLA-DQB1 alleles are associated with type II AIH. The frequency of these alleles varies in different ethnic populations. Exposure to certain drugs or viruses, the most notable being hepatitis C, has been suggested to play a role in triggering AIH, possibly through molecular mimicry and cross-reactivity between their epitopes and liver antigens.

Common laboratory findings include elevated levels of the liver enzymes aspartate aminotransferase (AST) and alanine aminotransferase (ALT), with less prominent increases in serum bilirubin and alkaline phosphatase. Serum immunoglobulin levels, particularly IgG, are high; in adults, various autoantibodies are present, including RF, ANAs, ANCAs, smooth muscle antibodies (SMAs), anti-liver kidney microsomal antibody (anti-LKM-1), anti-liver cytosol type 1 antibody (anti-LC-1), and anti-mitochondrial antibodies (AMAs).

Autoantibody profiles can distinguish between AIH-1 and AIH-2. AIH-1 patients are characteristically positive for SMA or ANA. Patients may also exhibit an atypical p-ANCA. ANAs most commonly produce a homogeneous pattern on IIF but can sometimes produce a speckled pattern. The SMAs are directed against actin and other components of the cytoskeleton. They can be detected by IIF on rodent kidney, stomach, or liver sections, where they produce fluorescent staining of the smooth muscle in the artery walls and other components, such as the glomeruli and tubules of the kidneys. Antibody titers are usually 1:80 or higher in adults but can be as low as 1:20 in children.

In contrast, patients with AIH-2 characteristically produce antibodies against LKM-1, which are directed against cytochrome P450 2D6, or against LC-1. LKM antibodies can be detected by IIF, competitive ELISA, or immunoblotting methods. On IIF using rodent tissue substrates, anti-LKM-1 stains the cytoplasm of the hepatocytes and the P3 portion of the kidney tubules. The resulting immunofluorescent pattern appears similar to that produced by mitochondrial antibodies but can be distinguished by experts when testing is performed on multiple tissue substrates and the intensity of fluorescent staining of different components of the substrates is carefully examined. Clinically significant titers are considered to be 1:40 in adults and 1:10 in children; antibody titers correlate with disease activity. Antibodies to LC-1 are directed against a folate-metabolizing enzyme in the liver and stain the cytoplasm of liver cells in IIF. These antibodies can be masked by anti-LKM-1 if they are also present, and other methods, such as immunodiffusion, may be required to detect them.

Liver biopsy is necessary to confirm the diagnosis of AIH and to assess the extent of liver damage. Inflammation at the portal–parenchymal boundary, known as *interface hepatitis*, is typical of AIH and is characterized by an infiltrate of lymphocytes, plasma cells, and histiocytes surrounding dying hepatocytes. Histological findings, along with detection of pertinent autoantibodies, elevated IgG, and exclusion of viral hepatitis, comprise a widely used simplified set of criteria recommended by the International Autoimmune Hepatitis Group for the diagnosis of AIH.

Laboratory findings are essential for early diagnosis, and treatment should be started promptly once the diagnosis is made. Most patients respond to the standard immunosuppressive treatment of prednisolone (+/– azathioprine) to induce remission, followed by azathioprine alone to maintain remission. However, patients must be monitored carefully because they are at increased risk of developing cirrhosis and possibly hepatocellular carcinoma. If untreated, AIH usually progresses to liver failure, at which point liver transplantation is required.

Primary Biliary Cholangitis (PBC)

PBC, formerly known as *primary biliary cirrhosis*, is the most common autoimmune liver disease, occurring about 10 times as often in females as in males. There is a genetic link with certain HLA-DRB1, HLA-DQA1, HLA-DPB1, and HLA-DQB1 haplotypes. PBC is an autoimmune disease that involves progressive destruction of the intrahepatic bile ducts. The destruction leads to chronic *cholestasis* (a condition in which the flow of bile is slowed or blocked), inflammation of the portal vein in the liver, and accumulation of scar tissue that can ultimately lead to cirrhosis and liver failure. Individual patients can be asymptomatic or have slowly or rapidly progressing disease. Symptoms include fatigue, pruritis (itchy skin), abdominal pain, and dry eyes and mouth; in the later stages, patients experience jaundice, ascites, and greasy stools. The standard initial therapy for PBC is ursodeoxycholic acid (UDCA), a bile acid that helps move bile through the liver. The use of UDCA has helped to slow down disease progression and increase patient survival; other drugs may be used for patients who do not respond to UDCA. Liver transplantation is the only effective treatment for patients who have reached end-stage liver disease.

AMAs are found in the majority of patients with PBC, and their presence is one of three diagnostic criteria for the disease. The other two criteria are a serum alkaline phosphatase level elevated at least 1.5 times the upper limit of normal for 6 months or more and liver biopsy showing nonsuppurative destructive cholangitis (inflammation of the bile duct system) and interlobular bile duct injury. A diagnosis of PBC can be made if at least two out of three of these criteria are met. In addition, patients commonly have elevated levels of aminotransferases and serum immunoglobulins, especially IgM, because of polyclonal activation of B cells. ANAs may also be positive and, depending on the antibodies present, can produce various patterns on FANA, including multiple nuclear dots (because of anti-Sp100), smooth nuclear envelope, or centromere.

Different methods have been developed to detect AMAs, including IIF, immunoblotting with mitochondrial preparations from mammalian tissue, ELISA, and fluorescent microbead immunoassay. Traditionally, AMAs have been detected by IIF with mitochondria-rich tissue substrates such as rodent liver, kidney, or stomach sections. These antibodies produce a bright, uniform granular cytoplasmic fluorescence in the distal renal tubules, gastric parietal cells, thyroid epithelial cells, and cardiac muscle. IIF uses antigens in their natural configuration and has fairly high levels of sensitivity and specificity; however, the method is manual, is time-consuming, and requires a high level of expertise to correctly interpret the pattern. In addition, a small percentage of PBC patients test negative for AMAs on IIF or may give atypical staining patterns that are difficult to interpret. ELISA testing for antibodies to the nuclear antigens GP210 or SP100 may be beneficial to the diagnosis of PBC in AMA-negative patients.

Since the development of IIF, the target antigens of AMAs have been identified as components of the 2-oxo-acid dehydrogenase complexes that are involved in mitochondrial energy-producing pathways. Identification of these antigens allowed for the development of solid-phase ELISA and fluorescence microbead immunoassays. The mitochondrial antigens employed in these solid-phase assays consist of preparations of porcine or bovine heart, mixtures of recombinant subunits of pertinent antigens, designer antigens composed of particular subunits, or mixtures of native and designer antigens, depending on the commercial manufacturer. they have the advantages of automation and provision of objective results, but their performance can vary because they generally do not include the full spectrum of antigenic epitopes available by IIF.

A cost-effective approach to testing may be to screen samples for AMAs and other autoantibodies by IIF, then follow-up with an AMA ELISA assay for confirmation. This approach would also be helpful in identifying AMAs in those patients who test negative through IIF. This testing strategy would facilitate an earlier diagnosis for PBC patients, allowing the initiation of treatment that could slow down disease progression and improve patient survival. It is important to note that a diagnosis of PBC cannot be based on the presence of AMAs alone because these antibodies have also been observed in patients with other conditions, such as SLE, RA, and graft-versus-host disease, as well as a small percentage of healthy persons.

Multiple Sclerosis (MS)

Multiple sclerosis (MS) is an autoimmune disorder involving inflammation and destruction of the CNS. It affects more than 900,000 Americans and millions of individuals worldwide. The disease most often begins in young and middle-aged adults between the ages of 20 and 50 and is twice as common in women as in men. Multiple genes are thought to contribute to the development of MS, but the disease is most closely associated with inheritance of the HLA allele, DRB1*1501. Environmental factors that have been associated with MS include reduced exposure to sunlight, vitamin D deficiency, cigarette smoking, and infection with EBV after early childhood.

MS is characterized by the formation of lesions called *plaques* in the white matter of the brain and spinal cord, resulting in the progressive destruction of the myelin sheath of axons. Within the plaques, T cells and macrophages predominate; these are believed to orchestrate demyelination. Antibody binds to the myelin membrane and may initiate the immune response, stimulating macrophages and specialized phagocytes called *microglial cells.* The cascade of immunologic events results in acute inflammation, injury to axons and glia, structural repair with recovery of some function, and then postinflammatory neurodegeneration. The Th1 cytokines IL-1, TNF-α, and IFN-γ are believed to be central to the pathogenesis of the disease, promoting changes in the endothelial cells that facilitate adherence of activated T cells and their migration across the blood–brain barrier. Th17 cells are also thought to play an important role in the inflammatory response of the CNS. A Th2 response, characterized by production of IL-4, IL-5, and IL-10, may also contribute to pathogenesis.

Clinical Symptoms and Treatment

Damage to the tissue of the CNS can cause visual disturbances, weakness or diminished dexterity in one or more limbs, locomotor incoordination, dizziness, facial palsy, and numerous sensory abnormalities, such as tingling or "pins and needles" that run down the spine or extremities, as well as flashes of light seen on eye movement. MS can be classified into four major subtypes based on the clinical course of the disease. More than 80% of patients fall into the first subtype, relapsing-remitting MS, which is characterized by clearly defined episodes of neurological attacks with periods of full or partial recovery in between. Most patients with MS eventually develop progressive deterioration of the CNS and functional disability.

Treatment for MS is aimed at easing recovery from acute attacks and reducing the risk of future relapses. Acute exacerbations can be treated with glucocorticoids to reduce inflammation. Numerous disease-modifying therapies that affect various functions of the immune system have been approved to treat MS for the long term. These agents have had a large impact on reducing the severity of MS symptoms and improving the long-term prognosis of MS. Two examples of such therapies are the humanized monoclonal antibodies, ocrelizumab, which binds to CD20 and depletes mature B cells from the blood, and natalizumab, which is directed against an adhesion molecule of lymphocytes, preventing them from binding to endothelial cells and crossing the blood–brain barrier. Experimental therapies such as high-dose biotin to improve disability, agents to promote remyelination, and stem cell transplantation hold promise for the future.

Laboratory Diagnosis of Multiple Sclerosis

The diagnosis of MS is based primarily on clinical symptoms, demonstration of disseminated lesions in the white matter of the brain and spinal cord by magnetic resonance imaging (MRI), and exclusion of other possible causes. Several laboratory tests can be used in combination to support the diagnosis, especially in cases in which the patient's symptoms or MRI findings do not meet the diagnostic criteria for MS. Immunoglobulins are increased in the spinal fluid in the majority of patients with MS, producing two or more distinct bands on protein electrophoresis that are not seen in the serum. These bands are referred to as *oligoclonal* and can be identified by isoelectric focusing with immunoblotting, a more sensitive technique than protein electrophoresis. The IgG index, a calculated ratio of cerebral spinal fluid (CSF) IgG/albumin ÷ serum IgG/albumin, is typically elevated and may also be used in making a diagnosis, even though it is not specific for MS. Although there is not one specific antibody that is diagnostic for MS, a large percentage of patients produce antibody directed against a myelin basic protein peptide. Other antibodies are directed against components of oligodendrocytes and against myelin membranes.

Myasthenia Gravis (MG)

Myasthenia gravis (MG) is an autoimmune disease that affects the neuromuscular junction. It is characterized by weakness and fatigability of skeletal muscles. It has a prevalence of 150 to 200 people per 1,000,000, depending on the population. The disease is heterogeneous in terms of its age of onset and gender involvement. Early-onset MG (EOMG) occurs before the age of 50 and affects predominantly females, whereas the late-onset form of the disease (LOMG) occurs after the age of 50 and is seen more often in males.

In MG, antibody-mediated damage to the acetylcholine receptors in skeletal muscle or to other proteins in the neuromuscular junction leads to progressive muscle weakness. Early signs are *ptosis* (drooping of the eyelids), *diplopia* (double vision), and the inability to retract the corners of the mouth, often resulting in a snarling appearance. In the majority of patients, the disease progresses to a generalized form that involves more muscle groups. In patients with generalized MG, muscle weakness is most noticeable in the upper limbs. These patients can also experience difficulty in speaking, chewing, and swallowing and may be unable to maintain support of the trunk, neck, or head. If respiratory muscle weakness occurs, it can be life threatening. Onset of symptoms can be acute or they may develop and worsen over time.

Immunopathogenesis

Approximately 85% of patients have antibodies to acetylcholine (ACh) receptors (AChRs), which appear to contribute to the pathogenesis of the disease by three mechanisms (referred to as *blocking*, *binding*, and *modulating*). Normally, ACH is released from nerve endings to generate an action potential that causes the muscle fiber to contract. When blocking antibodies combine with the receptor site, binding of ACh is thought to be prevented **(Fig. 15–12)**. Binding antibodies can

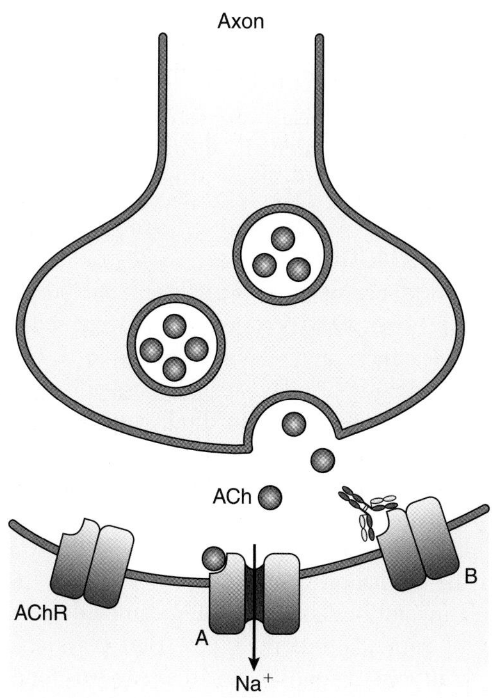

FIGURE 15–12 Mechanism of immunologic injury in MG. (A) Normal nerve impulse transmission: Ach is released from axon vesicles and binds to AchRs on the postsynaptic membrane, opening channels and allowing sodium ions to enter. (B) In MG, antibodies to the AChRs are formed, blocking transmission of nerve impulses.

interact with complement to damage the postsynaptic muscle membrane, whereas modulating antibodies promote rapid endocytosis of the AChRs, resulting in reduced numbers on the muscle cell membranes.

Patients lacking anti-AChR may produce antibodies to other proteins involved in the neuromuscular junction. About 6% of patients, mostly young females, have antibodies against muscle-specific kinase (MuSK), an enzyme that plays an important role in the development of the neuromuscular junction and in the clustering of AChRs on the muscle cell membrane, which enhances the transmission of the signals from the nerve cells. Consequently, there is fragmentation of the postsynaptic AChR clusters, resulting in muscle weakness and atrophy. Symptoms are usually severe, involving the facial, bulbar, and respiratory muscles. About 2% of patients with generalized MG have antibodies against LRP4, a lipoprotein involved in the activation of MuSK. These patients are typically young females who have a mild form of the disease. Antibodies to titin, a major protein in striated muscles, are found in up to 40% of patients with MG and are associated with LOMG.

The thymus also appears to play a role in the autoimmune process of MG. Thymic hyperplasia is common in EOMG patients with AChR antibodies. The follicles in the thymus expand and contain ectopic germinal centers with autoantibody-producing B cells. In addition, about 10% to 15% of patients with LOMG have a *thymoma,* a tumor of the thymus that may contain autoreactive T cells. It is thought that inflammation of the thymus gland may be triggered by persistent activation of TLRs by viruses such as EBV. The autoreactive response is thought to be perpetuated by defective immunoregulatory mechanisms involving an imbalance between Th17 cells and Tregs, resulting in increased production of proinflammatory cytokines and B-cell growth factors.

Genetic factors have been implicated in susceptibility to MG. The HLA haplotype, A1, B8, DR3, has a strong association with EOMG, whereas the HLA antigens B7, DR2, and DRB1 are more likely to appear in LOMG, and HLA-DR14-DQ5 may increase susceptibility to MuSK antibody production in MG.

Treatment

Most patients with MG can have a good quality of life with appropriate treatment. Anti-cholinesterase agents to prevent destruction of the neurotransmitter ACh, are used as the main therapy. Thymectomy should be performed on patients who have a thymoma but may also have some benefit in patients who do not have a thymoma. If these treatments are not effective, immunosuppression is recommended. Treatment generally begins with high doses of glucocorticoid drugs followed by other immunosuppressive drugs, such as azathioprine or mycophenolate mofetil, to maintain the response. Plasmapheresis to remove the autoantibodies or intravenous immunoglobulin (whose mechanism of action is unknown) can be administered to patients in crisis. Biological agents such as monoclonal antibodies or fusion proteins targeted to specific components of the immune system involved in the pathogenesis of MG (e.g., the anti-CD20 agent, rituximab) may be given to MG patients who are unresponsive to conventional therapies. All of these treatments have allowed MG patients to maintain a quality of life that is nearly normal.

Laboratory Diagnosis of Myasthenia Gravis

Diagnostic testing for MG is based on a combination of clinical and laboratory testing. Clinical testing involves demonstration of decreased muscle response to repetitive stimulation of a motor nerve and increased muscle strength following inhibition of acetylcholinesterase, an enzyme that breaks down ACh.

The gold standard for detecting binding AChR antibodies is a quantitative radioimmunoassay based on the reaction of patient serum with AChRs isolated from human muscle that are radio-labeled with α-bungarotoxin, a snake venom that binds with high affinity to a different site on the receptors. This assay is highly sensitive and can be used to determine antibody titers. Blocking and modulating AChR antibodies can be detected by radioimmunoprecipitation with AChR isolated from human muscle or by a semiquantitative flow cytometry method in which patient serum is incubated with an AChR-expressing cell line, followed by addition of a fluorescent-labeled α-bungarotoxin.

Patients who are negative for AChR antibodies should be tested for MuSK antibodies; this can be done by a quantitative RIA. Testing for titin antibodies may also be useful in these patients and can be performed by a semiquantitative ELISA. IIF assays for LPR4 antibodies may also be done but are not widely used. The use of additional markers, such as antibodies to agrin, a protein involved in the development and maintenance of the neuromuscular junction, is being studied.

Anti-Glomerular Basement Membrane Disease (Goodpasture's Syndrome)

Anti-glomerular basement membrane (Anti-GBM) disease, formerly known as **Goodpasture's syndrome,** is a small-vessel vasculitis characterized by the presence of an autoantibody to a basement membrane antigen in the glomeruli of the kidneys, alveoli of the lungs, or both. The basement membranes are composed of a thin, fibrous matrix that separates the epithelial cell layer within these organs from underlying connective tissue. Originally identified by Ernest Goodpasture in 1919, Goodpasture's syndrome is a rare disorder that is found mainly in Caucasians of European origin. It primarily affects two age groups—men in their late 20s and men and women in their 60s and 70s.

The clinical presentation of patients varies, but most patients initially experience fatigue and malaise followed by clinical signs of kidney involvement, such as edema and hypertension, which can rapidly progress to acute renal failure if left untreated. Some patients develop chronic renal failure that requires lifetime hemodialysis or kidney transplantation. About 60% to 70% of patients with anti-GBM disease have pulmonary involvement and exhibit symptoms such as cough, shortness of breath, and hemoptysis (coughing up blood).

The standard treatment for anti-GBM disease involves the administration of high-dose corticosteroids to stop inflammation, followed by immunosuppressive drugs such as cyclophosphamide to inhibit further production of autoantibodies. In addition, plasmapheresis is performed to remove circulating autoantibodies. The monoclonal antibody rituximab (anti-CD20) has been used as a supplemental treatment in some patients. Prompt initiation of therapy is important because symptoms can be life threatening. If started early, therapy is successful in preventing acute renal failure in most patients. Long-term prognosis depends on the severity of symptoms at initial diagnosis and patient response to treatment.

Etiology and Immunopathology

Although little is known about the circumstances that trigger the autoimmune response in anti-GBM disease, there is a strong genetic association, with many patients carrying the HLA-DRB1-15 antigen. Exposure to cigarette smoke and other pulmonary irritants, organic solvents, or infection has been implicated in disease pathogenesis by causing tissue injury that exposes critical antigenic epitopes. The autoantibodies produced in anti-GBM disease are specifically directed against the noncollagenous domain of the alpha-3 chain of type IV collagen. This autoantibody reacts with collagen in the glomerular or alveolar basement membranes and is thought to cause damage by type II hypersensitivity. Complement binding to the immune deposits attracts neutrophils, which mediate injury to the membranes by releasing chemically reactive oxygen-containing molecules and proteolytic enzymes. These immune reactants progressively destroy the renal tubular, glomerular, and pulmonary alveolar basement membranes. T-cell–mediated mechanisms are also thought to contribute to destruction of the basement membranes. Loss of membrane integrity results in leakage of blood and proteins into the urine.

Laboratory Diagnosis

Laboratory evidence of renal involvement includes gross or microscopic hematuria, proteinuria, a decreased 24-hour creatinine clearance, and elevated blood urea and serum creatinine levels. Abnormally shaped RBCs and casts can be found in the urine sediment. In those patients with pulmonary involvement, decreased total lung capacity and increased uptake of carbon monoxide are evident. An iron-deficiency anemia with decreased hemoglobin and hematocrit can develop if pulmonary hemorrhage is severe. The ESR and CRP level may be normal or increased.

Circulating antibodies to the GBM can be detected in the majority of patients, and their detection plays an important role in disease diagnosis. An IIF assay was long held as the standard, using frozen kidney sections incubated with patient serum and then overlaid with a fluorescein-labeled anti-IgG. However, the results can be hard to interpret, and there is a high percentage of false positives and false negatives. Currently, GBM antibodies are routinely detected by commercially available ELISA or fluorescent microbead immunoassays that use purified or recombinant alpha-3(IV) antigen substrates. A sensitive and specific Western blot method can be used to confirm positive results or retest negative samples. High-antibody titers are usually associated with rapidly progressing disease. Some patients are also positive for ANCAs, which are usually specific for myeloperoxidase and exhibit the perinuclear staining pattern on IIF. ANCAs may be detectable months to years before anti-GBM and symptoms are evident.

Histological analysis is important for confirmation of the diagnosis and for assessment of tissue damage. Tissue-bound anti-GBM can be detected by performing direct immunofluorescence on biopsy sections from kidney or lung specimens. In patients with renal disease, these antibodies are indicated by formation of a smooth, linear, ribbonlike pattern of fluorescence along the GBM. In contrast, glomerulonephritis caused by other autoimmune diseases shows a granular pattern of immunofluorescence caused by nonspecific deposition of immune complexes in the glomeruli. Examination of renal biopsy tissue also reveals crescent formations of inflammatory macrophages in the glomeruli. In patients with pulmonary involvement, linear IgG staining of the alveolar cell walls can be seen on direct immunofluorescence of lung biopsy tissue or bronchial washings. Thus, laboratory testing plays a key role in differentiating anti-GBM disease from other diseases that can cause similar symptoms and in facilitating an early diagnosis that can lead to prompt treatment and better clinical outcomes.

SUMMARY

- Autoimmune diseases result from a loss of self-tolerance, a delicate balance set up in the body to restrict the activity of T and B lymphocytes. Immunologic tolerance is achieved at two levels. Central tolerance affects potentially reactive B cells and T cells as they mature in the bone marrow and thymus, respectively, whereas peripheral tolerance occurs in the secondary lymphoid organs.
- Autoimmune disease is thought to result from complex interactions between the genetic makeup of an individual, exposure to environmental factors, and defects in immune regulation. Associations between certain HLA types or polymorphisms in non-MHC genes involved in the immune response have been observed for several autoimmune diseases. Other factors, including sex hormones, tissue injury, and exposure to microbial infections, are thought to trigger the development of autoimmunity in genetically susceptible individuals.
- Infectious microorganisms are believed to trigger autoimmune responses in a variety of ways, including molecular mimicry (a resemblance to self-antigens), epitope spreading (induction of a local inflammatory response that affects immune reactivity to unrelated antigens), and the presence of superantigens that can bind to class II MHC molecules and several TCRs, regardless of their antigen specificity.
- Autoimmune diseases can be classified as organ specific or systemic, depending on whether tissue destruction is localized or affects multiple organs. SLE, RA, Sjögren's syndrome, SSc, polymyositis, dermatomyositis, and GPA are examples of systemic diseases, whereas Hashimoto's thyroiditis, Graves' disease, type 1 diabetes mellitus, celiac disease, autoimmune hepatitis, primary biliary cholangitis, multiple sclerosis, myasthenia gravis, and anti-GBM disease are considered organ-specific diseases.
- Specific autoantibodies are strongly associated with the presence of certain autoimmune diseases and are useful in their diagnosis. For example, anti-dsDNA antibodies are found in SLE, anti-CCP (cyclic citrullinated proteins) antibodies are seen in RA, and antibodies against the TSH receptor are specific for Graves' disease.
- Anti-nuclear antibodies (ANAs) are found in the majority of patients with SLE and in a significant number of patients with other systemic autoimmune rheumatic diseases. The most commonly used method in ANA testing is IIF using the human epithelial cell line HEp-2 as the substrate. Some of the main fluorescent patterns observed in this test are homogeneous, speckled, nucleolar, centromere, and discrete nuclear dots. Each pattern is correlated with the presence of certain ANAs and should be followed up by confirmatory tests to more specifically characterize the antibodies.
- Rheumatoid factor is an autoantibody directed against the Fc portion of IgG molecules. It is found in the majority of patients with rheumatoid arthritis but is not specific for the disease because it is also present in a significant number of patients with other autoimmune diseases involving the connective tissues.
- Anti-neutrophil cytoplasmic antibodies (ANCAs) are strongly associated with autoimmune syndromes involving vasculitis. ANCAs are routinely detected by IIF using ethanol- or formalin-fixed leukocytes as the substrate. Two patterns of fluorescence can result: c-ANCA, a diffuse, granular staining of the cytoplasm of the neutrophils, mainly caused by antibodies against PR3 and seen in the vast majority of patients with active systemic GPA; and p-ANCA, characterized by fluorescence surrounding the nuclear lobes of ethanol-fixed neutrophils, caused by antibodies to positively charged antigens such as MPO.

CASE STUDIES

1. A 25-year-old female consulted her physician because she had been experiencing symptoms of weight loss, joint pain in the hands, and extreme fatigue. Her laboratory results were as follows: RF rapid slide test positive at 1:80; ANA positive at 1:160; RBC 3.5×10^{12} per L (normal is 4.1 to 5.1×10^{12} per L); WBC count 5.8×10^{9} per L (normal is 4.5 to 11×10^{9} per L).

Questions

a. What is a possible explanation for positive results on both the RF test and the ANA test?
b. What is the most likely cause of the decreased RBC count?
c. What further testing would help the physician distinguish between RA and SLE?

2. A 40-year-old female went to her doctor because she was feeling tired all the time. She had gained about 10 pounds in the last few months and exhibited some facial puffiness. Her thyroid gland was enlarged and rubbery. Laboratory results indicated a normal RBC and WBC count, but her FT4 level was decreased, and an assay for anti-thyroglobulin antibody was positive.

Questions

a. What condition do these results likely indicate?
b. What effect do anti-thyroglobulin antibodies have on thyroid function?
c. How can this condition be differentiated from Graves' disease?

REVIEW QUESTIONS

1. All of the following may contribute to autoimmunity *except*
   a. clonal deletion of self-reactive T cells.
   b. molecular mimicry.
   c. increased expression of class II MHC antigens.
   d. polyclonal activation of B cells.

2. Which of the following would be considered an organ-specific autoimmune disease?
   a. SLE
   b. RA
   c. GPA
   d. Hashimoto's thyroiditis

3. SLE can be distinguished from RA on the basis of which of the following?
   a. Joint pain
   b. Presence of anti-nuclear antibodies
   c. Immune complex formation with activation of complement
   d. Presence of anti-dsDNA antibodies

4. Which of the following would support a diagnosis of drug-induced lupus?
   a. Anti-histone antibodies
   b. Antibodies to Smith antigen
   c. Presence of RF
   d. Antibodies to SS-A and SS-B antigens

5. A speckled pattern of staining of the nucleus on IIF may be caused by which of the following antibodies?
   a. Anti-dsDNA
   b. Antibody to histones
   c. Centromere antibody
   d. Anti–SS-A/Ro antibody

6. Which of the following would be considered a significant finding in Graves' disease?
   a. Increased TSH levels
   b. Antibody to TSH receptor
   c. Decreased T3 and T4
   d. Anti-thyroglobulin antibody

7. Destruction of the myelin sheath of axons caused by the presence of antibody is characteristic of which disease?
   a. Multiple sclerosis
   b. Myasthenia gravis
   c. Graves' disease
   d. Anti-glomerular basement membrane disease

8. Blood was drawn from a 25-year-old woman with suspected SLE. A FANA screen was performed, and a speckled pattern resulted. Which of the following actions should be taken next?
   a. Report out as diagnostic for SLE.
   b. Report out as drug-induced lupus.
   c. Perform an assay for specific ANAs.
   d. Repeat the test.

9. Which of the following is a mechanism used to achieve peripheral tolerance?
   a. Negative selection of autoreactive T cells in the thymus
   b. Apoptosis of autoreactive B cells in the bone marrow
   c. Editing of B-cell receptors that weakly recognize self-antigens in the bone marrow
   d. Lack of a costimulatory signal to autoreactive T cells in the lymph nodes

10. *Epitope spreading* refers to
    a. post-translational modifications to self-antigens.
    b. modifications in gene expression that are not caused by changes in DNA sequence.
    c. expansion of the immune response to unrelated antigens.
    d. cross-reaction of the immune response to a pathogen with a similar self-antigen.

11. Anti-CCP (cyclic citrullinated proteins) is specifically associated with which autoimmune disease?
    a. Rheumatoid arthritis
    b. Myasthenia gravis
    c. Autoimmune hepatitis
    d. Systemic sclerosis

12. Which autoantibodies are strongly associated with granulomatosis with polyangiitis (Wegener's granulomatosis)?
    a. ANA
    b. ANCA
    c. AMA
    d. SMA

13. A technologist performs an IIF test for ANCAs and observes that there is an intense fluorescent staining of the nuclear lobes of the neutrophils. How can this type of staining be differentiated from an ANA?
    a. Perform the test on formalin-fixed leukocytes.
    b. Perform IIF with HEp-2 cells.
    c. Perform an ELISA for ANCAs.
    d. All of the above

14. A 20-year-old woman made an appointment to see her physician because she was experiencing intermittent diarrhea. Laboratory testing revealed that she also had an iron-deficiency anemia. To determine if the patient has celiac disease, her doctor should order which of the following laboratory tests?
    a. Anti-tTG
    b. Anti-gliadin
    c. Anti-gluten
    d. All of the above

15. Anti-mitochondrial antibodies are strongly associated with which disease?
    a. Autoimmune hepatitis
    b. Celiac disease
    c. Primary biliary cholangitis
    d. Anti-glomerular basement membrane disease

16 Transplantation Immunology

John L. Schmitz, PhD, D(ABMLI, ABHI)

LEARNING OUTCOMES

After finishing this chapter, you should be able to:

1. List the histocompatibility systems relevant to clinical transplantation.
2. Compare the mechanisms of direct and indirect alloantigen recognition.
3. Distinguish between an allograft, autograft, xenograft, and syngeneic graft (isograft).
4. Compare the immunologic mechanisms involved in hyperacute, acute, and chronic graft rejection.
5. Identify risk factors for graft-versus-host disease (GVHD) and the types of grafts in which this mechanism of rejection could occur.
6. List the major classes of immunosuppressive agents and their effects on the immune system.
7. Explain the principles of laboratory methods for human leukocyte antigen (HLA) typing.
8. Describe laboratory methods for detecting and identifying HLA antibodies (i.e., antibody screening, identification, and crossmatching).
9. Identify common tests used to monitor patients post-transplant.
10. Deduce the suitability of a possible donor for a transplant recipient, based on results of HLA typing and antibody identification.
11. Describe the nomenclature used for HLA antigens and alleles.

CHAPTER OUTLINE

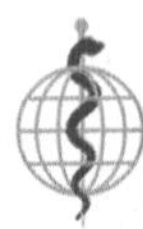

Go to FADavis.com for the laboratory exercises that accompany this text.

KEY TERMS

Acute rejection (AR)
Allograft
Autograft
Chronic rejection
Complement-dependent cytotoxicity (CDC)
Crossmatch
Direct allorecognition
Graft-versus-host disease (GVHD)
Haplotype
HLA antibody screen
HLA genotype
HLA matching
HLA phenotype
HLA typing
Human leukocyte antigen (HLA)
Hyperacute rejection
Immunosuppressive agents
Indirect allorecognition
Isograft
Major histocompatibility complex (MHC)
Minor histocompatibility antigen (mHA)
Mixed lymphocyte reaction (MLR)
Percent panel reactive antibody (%PRA)
Polymorphism
Syngeneic graft
Xenograft

Transplantation is a lifesaving treatment for end-stage organ failure, cancers, autoimmune diseases, immune deficiencies, and a variety of other diseases. In addition, vascular composite allograft (VCA) transplantation (craniofacial, uterus, and limb) is now a reality. In 2019, 39,719 organ and vascular composite allograft transplants were performed in the United States. More than 50,000 hematopoietic cell transplants (HCTs) are performed worldwide each year for a variety of indications, including cancer, autoimmune disease, immunodeficiencies, and other diseases. The number of transplants performed is a testament to the numerous developments during the past few decades in patient management pre- and post-transplant and in the technologies for organ or hematopoietic cell acquisition and sharing. Of critical importance has been the growing knowledge of the immunologic mechanisms of graft rejection and **graft-versus-host disease (GVHD)**, in particular the role of **human leukocyte antigens (HLAs)** and the development of pharmacological agents that promote graft survival by interfering with various components of the immune system.

The HLA system is the strongest immunologic barrier to successful allogeneic organ and HCT transplantation (see Chapter 3 for details). This system consists of cell surface proteins that play a central role in the thymic education of T lymphocytes, initiation of adaptive immune responses, and regulation of innate immune system components such as natural killer (NK) cells. HLA proteins are found on the surface of almost all nucleated cells and are antigenically very diverse, with thousands of unique variants in the human population. Because of this diversity and high level of immunogenicity, they elicit strong immune responses that aim to eliminate the foreign (non-self) antigens. Therefore, transplantation of a solid organ or hematopoietic stem cells (HSCs) into an allogeneic host is likely to result in graft rejection or GVHD in the absence of immunosuppressive therapy.

Histocompatibility Systems

Major Histocompatibility Complex (MHC) Antigens

The classical (transplant) antigens consist of the class I and class II proteins. Class I proteins include HLA-A, HLA-B, and HLA-C; class II proteins consist of HLA-DR, HLA-DQ, and HLA-DP. HLA proteins are encoded by a set of closely linked genes located on the short arm of chromosome 6 within the **major histocompatibility complex (MHC)**. HLA genes are inherited as **haplotypes** from parental chromosomes **(Fig. 16–1)**. A haplotype is a group of closely linked alleles on a single chromosome, for example, HLA-A1, HLA-Cw7, HLA-B8, HLA-DR3, and HLA-DQ2. Offspring receive one maternal and one paternal HLA haplotype. Based on Mendelian inheritance, there is a 25% chance that any two siblings will inherit the same two haplotypes (i.e., are HLA identical), a 50% chance of them being HLA haploidentical (i.e., share one of two HLA haplotypes), and a 25% chance of them being HLA nonidentical (i.e., share neither HLA haplotype). Recombination between maternal or paternal chromosomes can take place, resulting in the inheritance of unexpected haplotypic

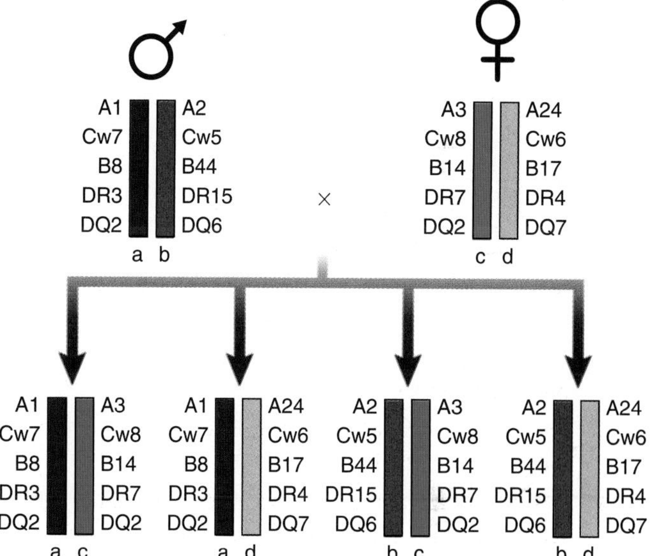

FIGURE 16–1 HLA genes are linked and inherited in Mendelian fashion as haplotypes. One paternal (a or b) and one maternal (c or d) haplotype is passed to each offspring. Four different combinations of haplotypes are possible in offspring. Elucidation of haplotype sharing between siblings is an important assessment in the search for a transplant donor. *(Figure courtesy of John Schmitz.)*

combinations; however, this occurs in less than 1% of families that are HLA typed.

HLA proteins are heterodimeric molecules consisting of two different polypeptide chains chemically bound to each other (see Chapter 3). They are also members of the immunoglobulin superfamily, which shares structural similarities with immunoglobulin molecules.

Class I proteins are the product of the HLA-A, HLA-B, and HLA-C genes and are expressed on the cell surface covalently bound to β2–microglobulin. Class I heterodimers are codominantly expressed on virtually all nucleated cells. Class II heterodimers are the products of the HLA-D region genes. Class II proteins are codominantly expressed, primarily on antigen-presenting cells (APCs; e.g., dendritic cells, monocytes, macrophages, B lymphocytes). For stable expression on the cell surface, both class I and II molecules also are complexed with a short peptide that can be derived from self-proteins or foreign proteins such as proteins from an infectious agent or other exogenous (non-self) protein.

As discussed in Chapter 3, HLA proteins have critical roles in the development and functioning of the innate and adaptive immune systems. They serve as recognition elements for antigen receptors on T lymphocytes, thus initiating adaptive immune responses. In addition, they serve as ligands for regulatory receptors on NK cells in the innate immune response. The CD8 molecule on cytotoxic T lymphocytes interacts with class I HLA proteins, whereas the CD4 molecule on T helper (Th) cells interacts with class II HLA proteins.

A cardinal feature of the genes encoding HLA proteins is the extensive degree of allelic **polymorphism.** Polymorphism refers to the presence of two or more different genetic compositions among individuals in a population. The HLA system is the most polymorphic genetic system in humans; many HLA genes exist in the population, and numerous combinations of these genes are possible in individuals (see **Tables 16–1 and 16–2**). This degree of polymorphism is believed to have resulted from the survival benefit of initiating an immune response to a broad array of peptides from an innumerable array of pathogenic microbes that populations encounter. Although this has successfully enabled populations to survive infectious challenges, it severely restricts the ability to transplant foreign tissues or cells between any two individuals because the HLA proteins are immunogenic and elicit robust allogeneic immune responses.

Table 16–1 Approximate Number of HLA Antigens and Alleles Defined at the Classical Transplant Loci*

HLA LOCUS	# ANTIGENS	# ALLELES
A	28	6,291
B	62	7,562
C	10	6,223
DRB1	24	2,838
DQB1	9	1,930

**Note: The number of HLA alleles identified has increased tremendously in recent years because of the availability of improved molecular techniques. The numbers in this table were current as of September, 2020. To view the most up-to-date information about the HLA alleles discovered, access the websites https://www.ebi.ac.uk/ipd/imgt/hla/stats.html and http://hla.alleles.org/antigens/recognised_serology.html*

Minor Histocompatibility Antigens (mHAs)

Researchers identified a second set of transplantation antigens based on studies in mice and humans. These studies demonstrated tissue rejection in MHC-identical transplants and the development of GVHD in HLA-identical sibling HSC transplants. The scientists conducting these studies also observed that a "slower" rejection pace was mediated by these transplantation antigens, thus their name—**minor histocompatibility antigens (mHAs).**

The mHAs are non-HLA proteins that demonstrate variation in the amino acid sequence between individuals. Both X-linked and autosomally encoded mHAs have been identified. Transplanting one individual's tissue or cells containing a polymorphic variant of one of these proteins into another individual possessing a different polymorphic variant can induce a recipient's immune response to the donor variant. CD4 and CD8 T cells recognize the variant protein in an MHC-restricted fashion and mediate the immune response. This response is analogous to the reaction to a microbial antigen. Several mHAs have been identified, including proteins encoded by the male Y chromosome, proteins for which the recipient has a homozygous gene deletion, proteins that are autosomally encoded, and proteins that are encoded by mitochondrial DNA.

MHC Class I–Related Chain A (MICA) Antigens

The MHC class I–related chain A (MICA) gene encodes a cell surface protein that is involved in gamma/delta T-cell responses. MICA is polymorphic, with more than 100 allelic variants. MICA proteins are expressed on endothelial cells, keratinocytes, fibroblasts, epithelial cells, dendritic cells, and monocytes, but they are not expressed on T or B lymphocytes. As such, MICA proteins could serve as targets for allograft immune responses. Antibodies to MICA antigens have been detected in as many as 11% of kidney-transplant patients and are associated with rejection episodes and decreased graft survival.

ABO Blood Group Antigens

The ABO system is the only blood group system that affects clinical transplantation. ABO blood group incompatibility is a barrier to solid-organ transplantation because these antibodies can bind to the corresponding antigens that are expressed on the vascular endothelium. Binding activates the complement cascade, which can lead to very rapid rejection of the transplanted organ. This phenomenon, known

Table 16–2 Listing of Individual HLA Antigens*

HLA-A		HLA-B			HLA-C	HLA-DR	HLA-DQ
1	68	5	42	65	1	1	1
2	69	7	44	67	2	103	2
203	74	703	45	70	3	2	3
210	80	8	46	71	4	3	4
3		12	47	72	5	4	5
9		13	48	73	6	5	6
10		14	49	75	7	6	7
11		15	50	76	8	7	8
19		16	51	77	9	8	9
23		17	5102	78	10	9	
24		18	5103	81		10	
2403		21	52	82		11	
25		22	53	Bw4		12	
26		27	54	Bw6		13	
28		2708	55			14	
29		35	56			1403	
30		37	57			1404	
31		38	58			15	
32		39	59			16	
33		3901	60			17	
34		3902	61			18	
36		40	62			51	
43		4005	63			52	
66		41	64			53	

**Note: HLA antigen names begin with the prefix "HLA-," followed by the gene locus (A, B, C, or D) and the antigen number (e.g., HLA-A2). A "w" was originally placed after newly identified antigens at International Histocompatibility Workshops. The "w" has been retained for HLA-C antigen names to differentiate them from complement proteins (e.g., HLA-Cw1).*

as **hyperacute rejection,** occurs within minutes to hours after the vascular supply to the transplanted organ is established (see *Transplant Rejection*). Anti-A or anti-B antibodies develop in individuals lacking the corresponding blood group antigens. As such, recipient–donor pairs must be ABO identical or compatible to avoid this adverse outcome. For example, an individual of blood Group A will possess anti-B antibodies and can thus receive an organ only from an ABO type A or type O donor. Likewise, a B-expressing individual has anti-A antibodies and can receive an organ only from an ABO type B or type O donor.

Transplantation approaches using plasma exchange and intravenous immunoglobulin administration have allowed successful transplantation of kidneys from ABO-incompatible donors. These treatments reduce the ABO antibody to levels that significantly lower the risk of hyperacute rejection.

Killer Immunoglobulin-Like Receptors (KIRs)

Another polymorphic genetic system that affects allogeneic transplantation is the killer immunoglobulin-like receptor (KIR) system. KIRs are one of several types of cell surface molecules that regulate the activity of NK lymphocytes. The KIRs contain activating and inhibitory receptors that vary in number and type on any individual NK cell. The balance of signals received by the activating and inhibitory receptors regulates the activity of the NK cell (see Fig. 2–7).

The ligands for the inhibitory KIRs have been defined as several of the class I MHC molecules, including specific HLA-A, HLA-B, and HLA-C proteins. Normally, an NK cell encounters self class I MHC proteins as it circulates in the body. This interaction between MHC protein and the inhibitory

KIR maintains the NK cells in a quiescent state. If an NK cell encounters a cell with absent or decreased HLA class I expression, inhibitory receptors are not engaged, and a loss of negative regulatory activity occurs, resulting in NK cell activation.

The regulatory role of KIRs has been exploited in haploidentical stem cell transplantation. Stem cell donors have been selected for recipients who lack a corresponding class I MHC protein for the donor's inhibitory KIR type. This results in alloreactivity by NK cells that repopulate the recipient after transplant. These alloreactive NK cells have been shown to mediate a graft-versus-leukemia (GVL) reaction and prevent relapse after transplantation for certain types of hematologic malignancies.

Self-Antigens

In addition to these well-described alloantigen systems, humoral immune responses to self-antigens in transplant recipients have been associated with poor transplant outcomes, although a direct causal relationship has yet to be firmly established. Among the several proteins to which antibody has been described post-transplantation are angiotensin II type 1 receptor, vimentin, K-alpha1 tubulin, collagen-V, and myosin.

Allorecognition

Transplantation of cells or tissues is classified by the genetic relatedness of the donor and the recipient. An **autograft** is the transfer of tissue from one area of the body to another of the same individual. A **syngeneic graft** (also known as an **isograft**) is the transfer of cells or tissues between individuals of the same species who are genetically identical, for example, identical twins. An **allograft** is the transfer of cells or tissue between two genetically disparate individuals of the same species. Finally, a **xenograft** is the transfer of tissue between two individuals of different species. Most transplants fall into the category of allografts. The HLA disparity between donor and recipient that occurs with allografts and xenografts will result in a vigorous cellular and humoral immune response to the foreign MHC antigens. This response is the primary stimulus of graft rejection.

The recipient's immune system recognizes foreign HLA proteins via two distinct mechanisms—direct and indirect allorecognition **(Fig. 16–2)**. In **direct allorecognition,** recipient T cells bind and respond directly to foreign (allo) HLA proteins on donor APCs. Although an individual T lymphocyte can recognize self-HLA + peptide, foreign HLA proteins may mimic a self-HLA + peptide complex because of similarities in the structure of the allo-HLA protein itself or to structural similarities of allo-HLA protein + peptide. Evidence suggests that virus-specific T cells may be an important source of alloreactive cells. Either way, direct allorecognition is characterized by a high frequency (up to 10%) of responding T cells compared with the responder frequency in a typical T-cell response to a foreign antigen.

The **mixed lymphocyte reaction (MLR)** is an in vitro correlate of direct allorecognition. In this assay, lymphocytes from an individual needing a transplant are incubated with lymphocytes from a potential donor that have been inactivated so they cannot proliferate. A disparity in the HLA-D antigens (class II antigens) found on the two populations of lymphocytes results in the proliferation of the recipient cells, which can be quantitated by incorporation of radio-labeled (^{3}H) thymidine into the DNA of the proliferating cells. The amount of radioactivity taken up by the cells increases in proportion to the amount of

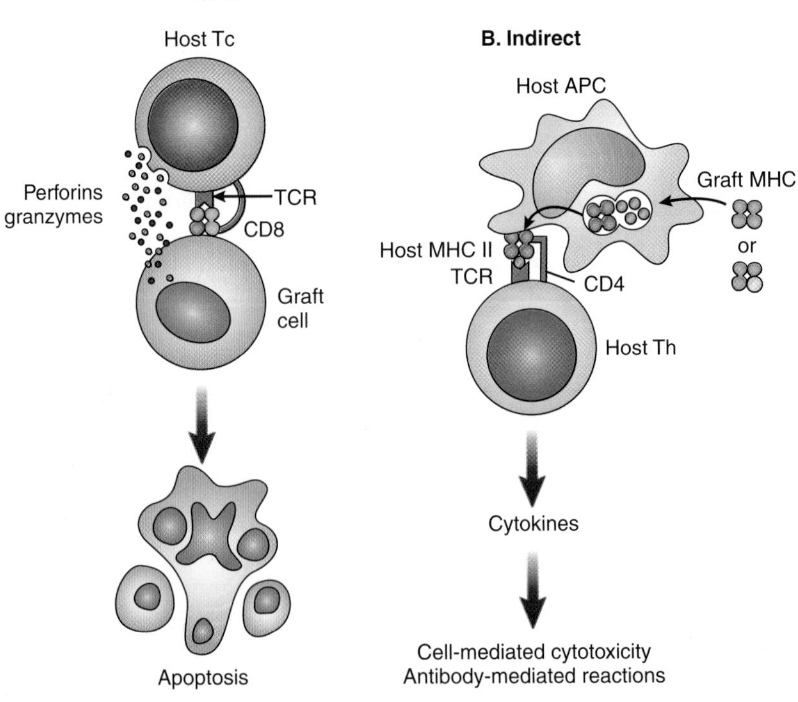

FIGURE 16–2 Direct versus indirect allorecognition. (A) In direct allorecognition, cytotoxic T cells from the host bind directly to foreign HLA (MHC I) proteins on graft cells. (B) In indirect allorecognition, APCs from the host present foreign MHC I or MHC II antigens to CD4+ Th cells, which produce cytokines that stimulate graft rejection.

cell proliferation. Thus, a high level of radioactivity indicates that the recipient's T cells have divided in response to different HLA-D antigens on a potential donor's cells and that such a donor would be more likely to stimulate graft rejection.

Indirect allorecognition is the second pathway by which the immune system recognizes foreign HLA proteins. Indirect allorecognition involves the uptake, processing, and presentation of foreign HLA proteins by recipient APCs to recipient T cells. It is analogous to the normal mechanism of recognition of foreign antigens. Indirect allorecognition may play a predominant role in induction of alloantibody and chronic rejection.

The effector responses against transplanted allogeneic tissue include direct cytotoxicity, delayed-type hypersensitivity (DTH) responses, and antibody-mediated mechanisms. Antibody can mediate antibody-dependent cellular cytotoxicity reactions and fix complement, resulting in cell death. Rejection episodes vary in the time of occurrence and the effector mechanism that is involved. The next section will cover three types of rejection: hyperacute, acute, and chronic.

Transplant Rejection

Hyperacute Rejection

As previously discussed, hyperacute rejection occurs within minutes to hours after the vascular supply to the transplanted organ is established (in some cases, rejection may occur in an accelerated fashion several days after transplant and has been referred to as *accelerated vascular rejection*). This type of rejection is mediated by preformed antibody that reacts with donor vascular endothelium. ABO, HLA, and certain endothelial antigens may elicit hyperacute rejection. Antibodies to these antigens may be present because of blood transfusion, prior transplantation, or exposure of a pregnant woman to fetal antigens of paternal origin. Binding of preformed antibodies to the alloantigens activates the complement cascade and clotting mechanisms and leads to thrombus formation. The result is ischemia and necrosis of the transplanted tissue.

Hyperacute rejection is seldom encountered in clinical transplantation. Donor–recipient pairs are chosen to be ABO identical or compatible, and patients awaiting transplantation are screened for the presence of preformed HLA antibodies. In addition, the absence of donor HLA-specific antibodies is confirmed before transplant by the performance of a **crossmatch** test (see *HLA Antibody Screening, Identification, and Crossmatching*). These approaches have virtually eliminated hyperacute rejection episodes.

Acute Rejection

Days to months after transplant, individuals may develop **acute rejection (AR).** AR can be mediated by a cellular alloresponse (ACR) or by donor-specific antibody (also known as *antibody-mediated response*; AMR).

ACR is characterized by parenchymal and vascular injury. Interstitial cellular infiltrates contain a predominance of CD8+ T cells as well as CD4+ T cells and macrophages. CD8 cells likely mediate cytotoxic reactions to foreign MHC-expressing cells, whereas CD4 cells likely produce cytokines and induce DTH reactions. Antibody may also be involved in acute graft rejection by binding to vessel walls and activating complement. The antibody induces transmural necrosis and inflammation as opposed to the thrombosis typical of hyperacute rejection. Diagnostic criteria include characteristic histological findings, deposition of the complement protein C4d in the peritubular capillaries, and detection of donor-specific HLA antibody. The development and application of potent immunosuppressive drugs that target multiple pathways in the immune response to alloantigens has improved early graft survival of solid-organ transplants by reducing the incidence of AR and by providing approaches for its effective treatment.

Chronic Rejection

Chronic rejection results from a process of graft arteriosclerosis characterized by progressive fibrosis and scarring with narrowing of the vessel lumen caused by proliferation of smooth muscle cells. Chronic rejection remains the most significant cause of graft loss after the first year post-transplant because it is not readily amenable to treatment. Several predisposing factors affect the development of chronic rejection, including prolonged cold ischemia, reperfusion injury, AR episodes, and toxicity from immunosuppressive drugs. Chronic rejection is also thought to have an immunologic component, presumably a DTH reaction to foreign HLA proteins. This is indicated in studies employing animal models of graft arteriosclerosis in which mice lacking interferon-gamma (IFN-γ) do not develop graft arteriosclerosis. In addition, similar studies support an important role for CD4 T cells and B cells in this process. Cytokines and growth factors—secreted by endothelial cells, smooth muscle cells, and macrophages activated by IFN gamma—stimulate smooth muscle cell accumulation in the graft vasculature. Alloantibody production likely contributes to the development of chronic rejection as well.

Graft-Versus-Host Disease (GVHD)

HCT transplants (and less commonly lung and liver transplants) are complicated by a unique allogeneic response—GVHD. In this condition, lymphoid cells in the graft mount an immune response against the host's histocompatibility antigens **(Fig. 16–3).** Recipients of HCT transplants for hematologic malignancies typically have depleted bone marrow before transplantation because of the chemotherapy used to treat the malignancy and make room for incoming stem cells to repopulate the marrow. The individual receives an infusion of donor bone marrow or, more commonly, peripheral blood stem cells. The infused products often contain some mature T cells. These cells have several beneficial effects, including promotion of engraftment, reconstitution of immunity, and mediation of a GVL effect. However, these mature T cells may also mediate GVHD.

Acute GVHD occurs during the first 100 days post-infusion and manifests in the skin, gastrointestinal tract, and liver. In

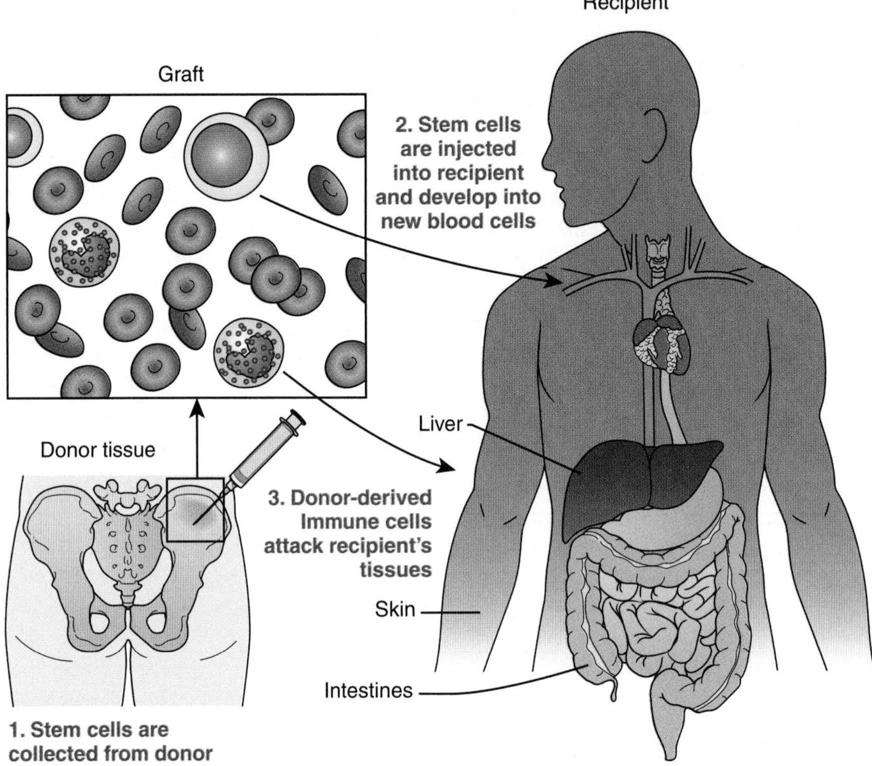
Recipient
Graft
2. Stem cells are injected into recipient and develop into new blood cells
Liver
Donor tissue
3. Donor-derived Immune cells attack recipient's tissues
Skin
Intestines
1. Stem cells are collected from donor

FIGURE 16-3 Graft-versus-host disease (GVHD). GVHD is caused by the reaction of T cells in the donor graft (e.g., bone marrow or peripheral blood stem cells) against mismatched HLA proteins in the recipient's tissues. This results in damage to the recipient's tissues, especially the skin, intestines, and liver.

mismatched allogeneic stem cell transplantation, the targets of GVHD are the mismatched HLA proteins, whereas in matched stem cell transplantation, mHAs are targeted. The infused T cells can mediate GVHD in several ways, including a massive release of cytokines because of large-scale activation of the donor cells by MHC-mismatched proteins and by infiltration and destruction of tissue.

The incidence and severity of GVHD is related to the match status of the donor and recipient as well as other factors. The recipient's medical team can take several approaches to reduce the incidence and severity of GVHD, including immunosuppressive therapy in the early post-transplant period and removal of T lymphocytes from the graft. T-cell reduction, achieved by purification of donor hematopoietic cells from the peripheral blood or bone marrow collection, is very effective in lowering the incidence of GVHD, but it can also reduce the GVL effect of the infused cells and increase the incidence of graft failure. The GVL effect is similar to the GVH response but targets the recipient's malignant cells as opposed to healthy tissues of the recipient, such as the skin and gastrointestinal tract.

Beyond 100 days post-transplant, patients may experience chronic GVHD. This condition resembles autoimmune disease, with fibrosis affecting the skin, eyes, mouth, and other mucosal surfaces.

Immunosuppressive Agents

The list of agents employed to suppress antigraft immune responses in solid-organ and HCT transplantation is growing. **Immunosuppressive agents** are used in several ways, including induction and maintenance of immune suppression and treatment of rejection. Combinations of different agents are frequently used to prevent graft rejection. However, the immunosuppressed state (and graft survival) induced by these agents comes at a price of increased susceptibility to infection, malignancies, and other associated toxic side effects. There are several classes of immunosuppressive agents:

Corticosteroids—Corticosteroids are potent anti-inflammatory and immunosuppressive agents used for immunosuppression maintenance. At higher doses, they are used to treat AR episodes. Steroids act by blocking the production and secretion of cytokines, inflammatory mediators, chemoattractants, and adhesion molecules. These activities decrease macrophage function and alter leukocyte-trafficking patterns. However, long-term use is associated with several complications, including hypertension and diabetes mellitus.

Antimetabolites—Antimetabolites interfere with the maturation of lymphocytes and kill proliferating cells. Azathioprine was the first such agent employed. It has been replaced in large part by mycophenolate mofetil, which has a more selective effect on lymphocytes compared with azathioprine and thus fewer side effects.

Calcineurin inhibitors—Cyclosporine and Tacrolimus are compounds that block signal transduction in T lymphocytes, resulting in impaired synthesis of cytokines such as interleukin (IL) 2, IL-3, IL-4, and INF-γ. Inhibition of cytokine synthesis blocks the growth and differentiation of T cells, impairing the antigraft response. Rapamycin (sirolimus) is an agent that inhibits T-cell proliferation by binding to specific intracellular proteins, including mammalian target of rapamycin (mTOR). mTOR is an intracellular molecule involved in cellular functions such as proliferation and motility.

Monoclonal antibodies—Several monoclonal antibodies that bind to cell surface molecules on lymphocytes are used at the time of organ transplant and to treat severe rejection episodes after transplantation. Basiliximab binds CD25 (IL-2 receptor) and thus interferes with IL-2–mediated T-cell activation. It may also deplete CD25-expressing cells. Another monoclonal antibody, alemtuzumab, targets the CD52 receptor found on T and B lymphocytes and may be used for induction therapy at the time of transplantation. A problem with some monoclonal antibody preparations is that patients can develop antibodies that may interfere with the effectiveness of these agents. The potential for this problem to occur is being reduced with increased use of humanized and fully human monoclonal antibodies (see Chapters 5 and 25).

Polyclonal antibodies—Two polyclonal anti–T-cell antibody preparations have been used as induction agents or to treat severe rejection. Thymoglobulin is an antithymocyte antibody prepared in rabbits, and ATGAM is a polyclonal antiserum prepared from the immunization of horses. Both are potent immunosuppressive agents that deplete lymphocytes from the circulation. A drawback associated with the administration of polyclonal antibody preparations is the development of serum sickness because of antibody responses to the foreign immunoglobulins (see Chapter 14).

Clinical Histocompatibility Testing

Appreciation of the beneficial role of **HLA matching** and the detrimental role of antibody to HLA proteins in graft survival provided the impetus for development and application of specialized testing to aid in the selection of the most appropriate donors for patients needing transplantation. Histocompatibility laboratories provide specialized testing for both solid-organ and stem cell transplantation programs. Two main activities are carried out by these laboratories in support of transplantation: HLA typing and HLA antibody screening and identification.

HLA Typing

HLA typing is the identification of the HLA antigens (phenotype) or genes in a transplant candidate or donor. For clinical HLA testing, phenotypes or genotypes of the classical transplant antigens or genes are determined (HLA-A, HLA-B, HLA-C, HLA-DR, HLA-DQ, HLA-DP). This information is used to find the most suitable donor–recipient combination from an immunologic standpoint. It must be stressed that other factors must also be considered when choosing a particular donor for any given patient, be it a solid-organ or stem cell transplant. For example, ABO compatibility and infectious disease status are important considerations in donor selection.

HLA Phenotyping

The classic procedure for determining the **HLA phenotype** is the **complement-dependent cytotoxicity (CDC)** test. Panels of antisera or monoclonal antibodies that bind to individual specific HLA proteins or groups of immunologically similar HLA antigens are incubated with lymphocytes from the person to be HLA typed in separate wells of a microtiter plate (Terasaki tray). Each well of the plate contains a different antibody preparation. It is important to note that multiple antisera are used for HLA typing. This requirement is based on the presence of both unique (private) epitopes on HLA molecules (those that define the phenotypic specificity of a specific HLA antigen) and public epitopes (epitopes that are present on more than one unique HLA protein). Because responses to public epitopes are common, multiple sera must be used to define a pattern of reactivity that correlates with a specific HLA antigen. T and B lymphocytes are used for HLA class I typing, whereas purified B lymphocytes are used for HLA class II typing because class II antigens are not found on most T cells. Binding of antibody occurs only if the lymphocytes express the HLA antigen targeted by the antisera. After incubation with the antisera, rabbit complement is added. If the cells possess the HLA antigen recognized by the antibody in that well, complement is activated, and the cells are killed. A vital dye such as eosin red or trypan blue is added to distinguish live cells from dead cells, and the well of the Terasaki tray is viewed microscopically. The dead cells, whose membranes have been made more permeable, are able to take up the dye and appear colored, whereas the live cells, whose membranes remain intact, cannot take up the dye and remain colorless. The proportion of dead cells is estimated by microscopic examination and scored according to the following scale, established by the American Society for Histocompatibility and Immunogenetics (ASHI):

- 1 = 0% to 10% cell death; negative
- 2 = 11% to 20% cell death; doubtful negative
- 4 = 21% to 50% cell death; weak positive
- 6 = 51% to 80% cell death; positive
- 8 = 81% to 100% cell death; strong positive
- 0 = unreadable

The principle of the CDC test is illustrated in **Figure 16–4.** Using this assay, an extensive array of HLA antigens can be defined (see Table 16–2).

The CDC method has several limitations for HLA typing. Viable lymphocytes must be used, which demands timely performance of the assay. Separation of T and B lymphocytes is required for differentiation of class I versus class II antigens. In addition, the source of antisera for HLA typing is not always consistent or reliable. Thus, reagents can vary in quality or quantity through time. Finally, the level of resolution (i.e., the ability to distinguish two closely related yet distinct HLA antigens) is limited. The limits of resolution don't significantly affect the role of this technology for matching solid-organ donors and recipients. However, for allogeneic stem cell transplantation, a higher level of resolution is required. DNA-based (molecular) HLA typing methods are now commonly

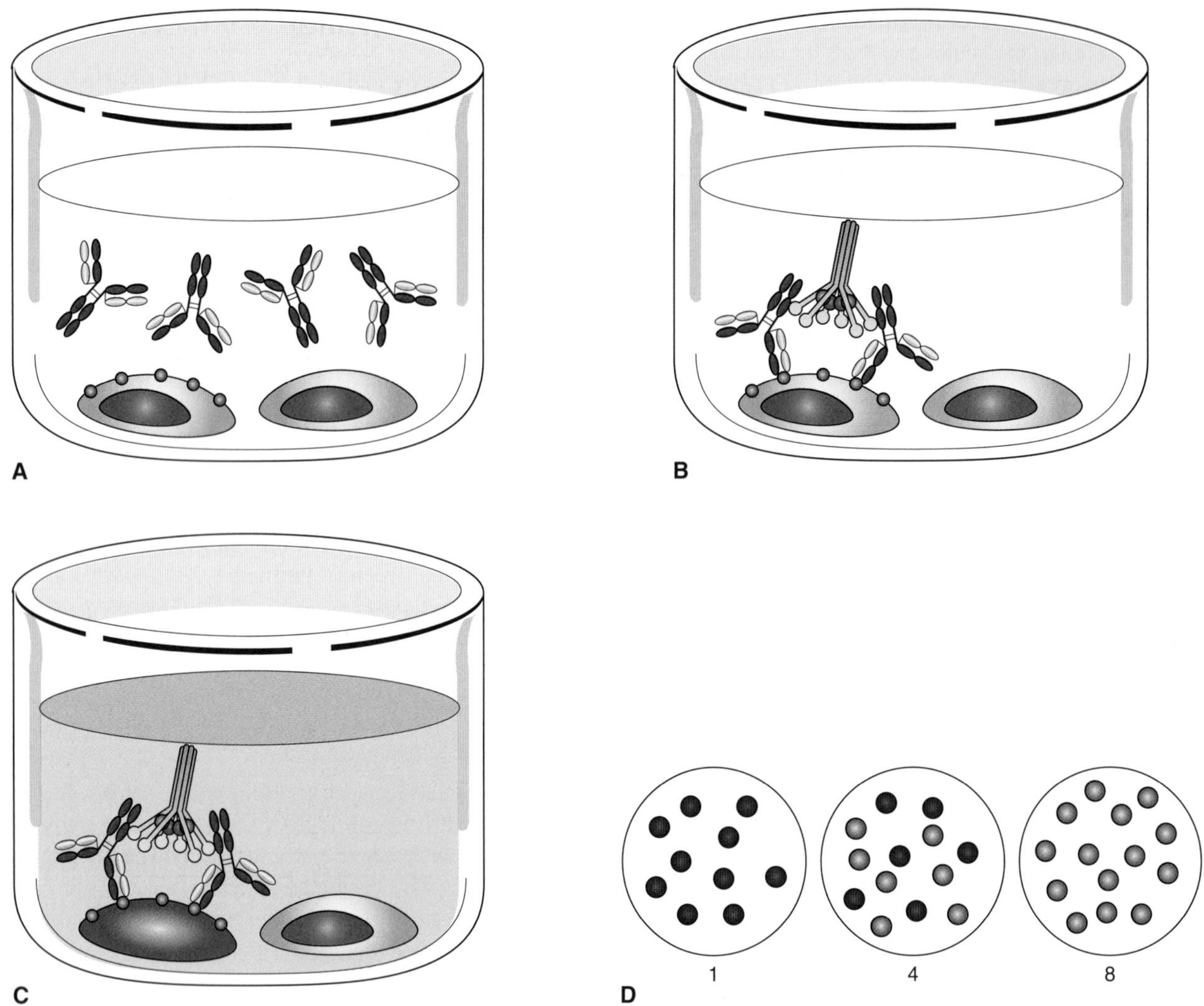

FIGURE 16–4 Principle of the complement-dependent cytotoxicity (CDC) test. A) Addition of patient lymphocytes to well containing specific HLA antisera; B) Addition of reagent complement; C) Addition of vital dye; D) Scoring of results.

employed in histocompatibility laboratories because their higher resolution, reagent quality and consistency, and amenability to higher throughput formats overcomes the limitations of CDC-based methods.

HLA Genotyping

Molecular HLA genotyping methods use polymerase chain reaction (PCR)-based amplification of HLA genes followed by analysis of the amplified DNA to identify the specific HLA allele or allele group (see Chapter 12). Three DNA-based HLA typing methods are in use: PCR with sequence-specific primers (PCR-SSP), PCR-sequence-specific oligonucleotide probe hybridization (PCR-SSOP), and sequence-based typing (SBT). One of the common approaches for analysis involves PCR amplification of HLA genes with panels of primer pairs, each of which amplifies specific alleles or related allele groups (PCR-SSP). Only those primer pairs that are perfectly base-pair matched to the target gene result in the generation of an amplification product **(Fig. 16–5).** Amplification is detected by agarose gel electrophoresis or using a fluorescent label in a real-time detection approach (qPCR). The **HLA genotype** is then identified by determining which primers resulted in amplification.

A second common approach for HLA genotyping is to perform PCR-SSOP. This involves a single PCR reaction that will amplify all HLA gene variants at a specific locus (referred to as a *generic amplification*). The amplified gene is then subjected to hybridization with a panel of DNA probes, each specific for a unique HLA allele or allele group. Only those probes that specifically hybridize to the amplified DNA will be detected. The HLA genotype is determined by assessing which probes are hybridized **(Fig. 16–6).**

A third common method for HLA genotyping is SBT, which involves sequencing of PCR-amplified HLA genes. SBT can be carried out using Sanger dideoxy chain terminator sequencing. A generic amplification of the HLA gene of interest is conducted, followed by a sequencing reaction using dideoxy nucleotides. The dideoxy terminators are fluorescently labeled. Incorporation into the synthesized DNA molecule is detected using automated DNA sequencers with fluorescent detectors. The sequence of the target gene is compared with an HLA sequence database to determine the specific HLA allele for the patient. SBT for HLA typing is considered the

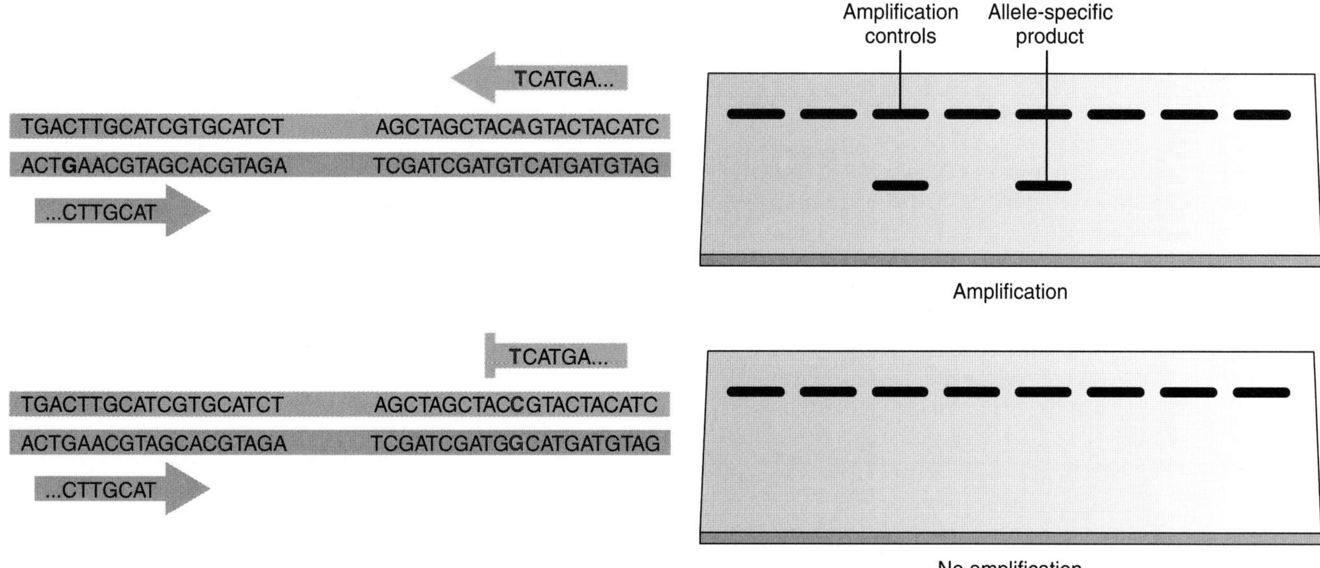

FIGURE 16–5 Principle of PCR-SSP. The sequence-specific primer ending in 3′ TCATGA . . . 5′ will be extended only from a template carrying the polymorphism shown.

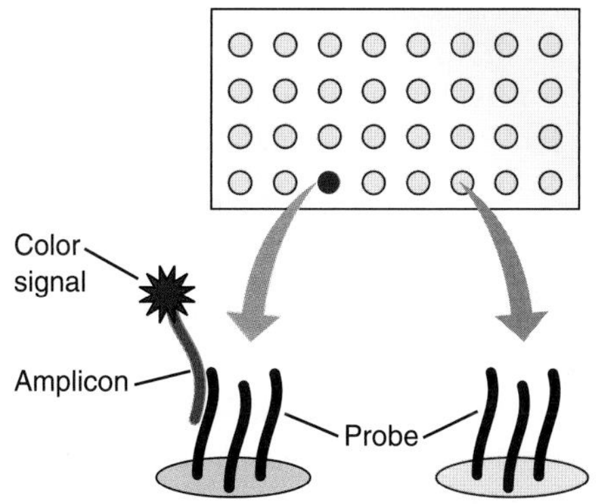

FIGURE 16–6 Principle of PCR-SSOP. Patient DNA is amplified using primers labeled with biotin or digoxigenin at the 5′ end. The amplicons are then hybridized to panels of probes immobilized on a membrane. If the sequence of the amplicon matches and hybridizes to that of the probe, a secondary reaction with enzyme-conjugated avidin or antidigoxigenin will produce a color or light signal when exposed to substrate (bottom left). If the sequence of the amplicon differs from that of the probe, no signal is generated (bottom right).

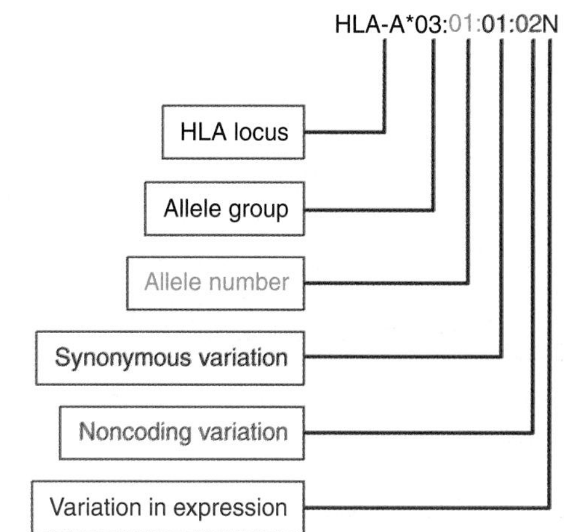

FIGURE 16–7 The nomenclature used for naming HLA alleles includes identification of the HLA locus, which is separated from the allele number by an asterisk (*). The first two digits of the allele number typically correspond to the phenotypic group. The next position after the ":" identifies the specific allele within the allele group. This position can accommodate up to three digits. The next position identifies allelic variants resulting from synonymous nucleotide substitutions (i.e., they do not result in a change in amino acid). The next position identifies allelic variants resulting from polymorphisms in noncoding regions of the gene (i.e., introns). Lastly, a letter may be added that indicates unique features of the allele, such as "N" indicating the allele is null (i.e., not expressed on the cell surface). *(Figure courtesy of John Schmitz.)*

gold standard and is able to detect new allelic variants because it interrogates all nucleotides in the amplified target region as opposed to PCR-SSP and PCR-SSOP, which target small stretches of previously defined nucleotides. More recently, next-generation sequencing technologies have been developed and used for HLA genotyping. This technology has the advantage over Sanger sequencing of providing unambiguous allele level typing more consistently.

HLA genotyping overcomes the limitations of CDC-based HLA phenotyping. Cells do not need to be viable to obtain DNA for HLA genotyping. Typing reagents are chemically synthesized; thus, there is no reliance on human donors of antisera. HLA genotyping can provide varying levels of resolution that can be tailored to the specific clinical need. DNA-based typing can provide results at a level of resolution comparable with CDC-based typing (low-resolution-antigen equivalent) or can provide results at the allele level, which are required for matching of unrelated HSC donors and recipients. Allele-level HLA typing has demonstrated the incredible extent of polymorphism within the HLA loci (see Table 16–1). The nomenclature used for HLA typing is explained in **Figure 16–7.**

Connections

Polymerase Chain Reaction

Recall from Chapter 12 that the PCR is a molecular method that is used to produce millions of copies of a DNA segment. It is commonly used to amplify a piece of DNA to levels that can be detected in the laboratory. Amplification is achieved by a three-step cycle: (1) heat denaturation of the target DNA (in this case, DNA coding for a specific HLA allele) to form single strands; (2) cooling the reaction and binding of short, complementary nucleotide sequences called *primers* to the 3′ ends of the target strands to initiate replication; and (3) heating the reaction in the presence of DNA polymerase and the four deoxynucleotide triphosphates (i.e., the DNA building blocks) to extend the strands. These heating–cooling cycles are performed by an automated thermocycler.

HLA Antibody Screening, Identification, and Crossmatching

Antibodies to HLA antigens can be detected in candidates and recipients of solid-organ transplants. These antibodies can develop in response to multiple blood transfusions or to prior HLA-mismatched transplants. They can also be produced by women who have had multiple pregnancies in response to paternally derived fetal antigens. Because of the potential adverse impact HLA antibodies can have on graft survival, patients awaiting solid-organ transplantation are screened periodically for their presence through an **HLA antibody screen.** If detected, the HLA specificity of the antibodies is then determined so that donors possessing those HLA antigens can be eliminated from consideration for donation to that patient. Patients are tested periodically for the presence of HLA antibodies while they are waiting for an organ offer. Antibody screening and identification is also performed post-transplantation to aid in the diagnosis of antibody-mediated rejection or to assess the effectiveness of therapy for antibody-mediated rejection. Crossmatching is performed just before transplant to confirm the absence of donor-specific antibody.

The methods used for antibody detection, identification, and crossmatching have changed significantly in recent years. The CDC method used for HLA typing is also used for HLA antibody detection and identification. In this case, panels of lymphocytes with defined HLA phenotypes are incubated with the patient's serum. If the serum contains HLA antibodies, they will bind to those lymphocytes in the panel that express the corresponding HLA antigen. Binding is detected by addition of rabbit complement and a vital dye to assess cell death microscopically (see Fig. 16–4). Usually 30 to 60 unique lymphocyte preparations are included in the panel; the proportion of lymphocytes in the panel that are killed by the patient's serum is referred to as the **percent panel reactive antibody (%PRA).** In addition, the specificity of the antibodies can be determined by evaluating the phenotype of the panel cells.

In some scenarios, the level of antibody in a serum sample may be below the level detectable by the CDC assay. In these cases, anti-human globulin (AHG) can be added to the CDC assay to increase the test's sensitivity. The AHG-CDC assay can detect lower levels of antibody as well as isotypes of bound antibody that don't activate complement and thus wouldn't normally be detected in the standard CDC assay. More recently, the determination of PRA for solid-organ allocation has been modified. Currently, a calculated PRA (cPRA) is determined for organ allocation. In this approach, the HLA antigens to which a candidate has HLA antibody are determined using solid-phase immunoassays. These antigens are then classified as unacceptable antigens for that candidate. Accordingly, donors expressing those antigens are excluded from donation for that candidate. The proportion of potential donors in the donor pool possessing one or more of the unacceptable antigens is determined and reported as the cPRA value. For example, a recipient with an HLA-A2 antibody would have a cPRA value of 47% because 47% of potential donors are projected to be HLA-A2 expressing, based on historic HLA typing data.

Another approach for antibody detection and identification is flow cytometry. Antibody in patient serum can be captured by incubation with beads that are coated with purified HLA antigens, either from a pool of donors, an individual donor, or a single purified or recombinant HLA protein. Beads coated with pooled HLA proteins are a sensitive qualitative screen for the presence of HLA antibody because they will detect antibodies to the majority of common HLA antigens. Beads coated with purified HLA proteins from individual donors or with a single HLA antigen type (referred to as single-antigen beads) are used to determine the specificity of the HLA antibodies in a patient's serum; this information is used to determine the cPRA. Patient serum is incubated with the beads, and bound antibody is detected by adding a fluorochrome-labeled anti-immunoglobulin G (IgG) reagent **(Fig. 16–8).** A more recent version of flow cytometry–based antibody detection is the multiplex bead array system that can classify patient antibodies to up to 100 different HLA antigens in a single tube using a dedicated flow-based detection system such as a Luminex bead array. Solid-phase methods are the most sensitive technology for detecting HLA antibodies. In addition, they can provide the best determination of the specificity of HLA antibodies when beads coated with a single HLA antigenic type are used.

Once a suitable donor has been identified for a particular patient, a donor–recipient crossmatch test is performed to confirm the absence of donor-specific antibody. Donor T and B lymphocytes are incubated with recipient serum in a CDC assay. Microscopic analysis is used to verify a lack of binding after the addition of complement and a vital dye to differentiate live cells from dead cells. Cell death is an indication of recipient antibody binding to donor HLA antigen(s). Alternatively, binding of antibody can be detected by flow cytometry using a fluorochrome-labeled anti-IgG reagent. As for antibody screening and identification, the flow cytometric crossmatch is the most sensitive method for detecting donor-specific antibody.

Post-Transplant Testing

Patients who have received solid-organ transplants or HCT are intensely monitored after transplantation. Two types of histocompatibility tests are commonly performed after these transplants: HLA antibody testing for solid-organ transplants and chimerism after HCT.

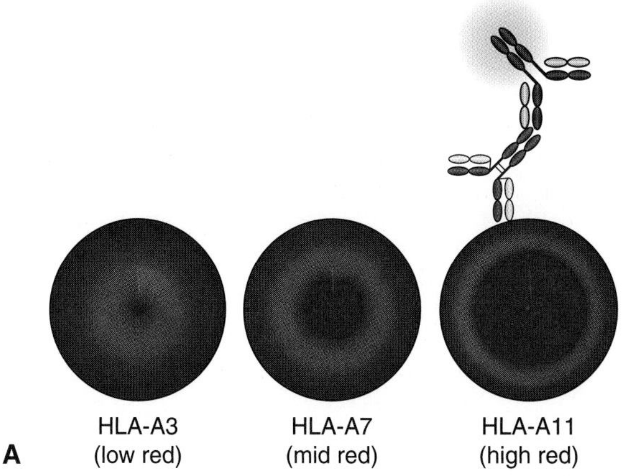

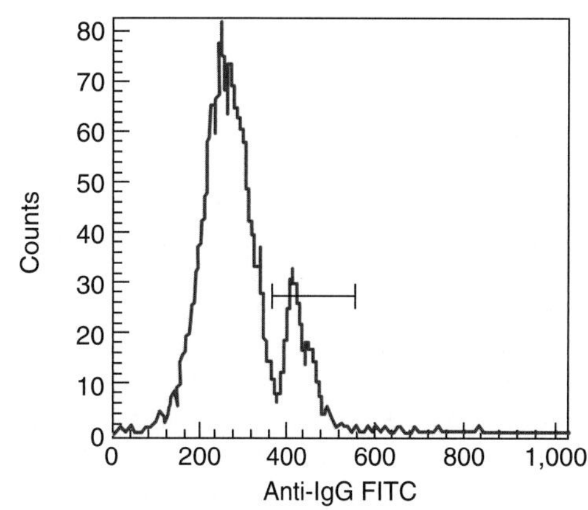

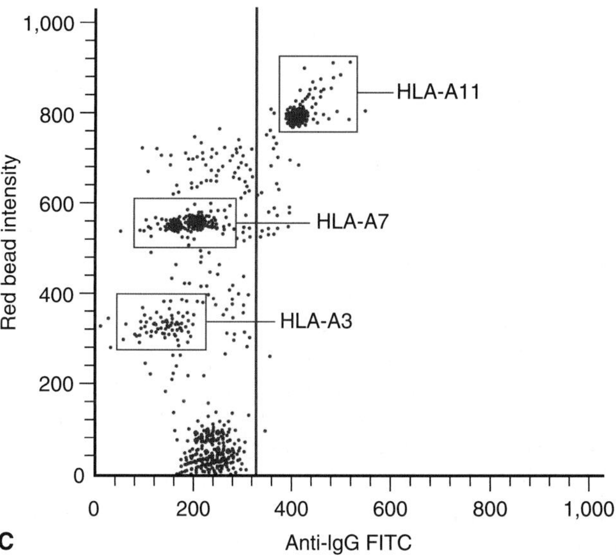

FIGURE 16–8 Flow cytometric detection and identification of antibodies. (A) Patient serum is incubated with a mixture of polystyrene beads coated with different HLA proteins (e.g., HLA-A3, HLA-A7, HLA-A11). The beads have been labeled with various amounts of a red dye for identification. Any HLA antibodies present in the serum will bind to the corresponding beads. After washing, patient antibodies bound to the beads are detected by the addition of a fluorescein isothiocyanate (FITC)-labeled anti-IgG reagent. After a second wash, the beads are analyzed for fluorescence on a flow cytometer. (B) Single-parameter histogram display of an HLA class I antibody screen using the three types of HLA-coated beads. The large peak represents beads with no bound antibody, whereas the smaller peak to the right indicates the presence of HLA antibody bound to approximately 29% of the HLA class I coated beads. This represents a positive HLA class I antibody screen. (C) The individual bead populations are identified in the dual-parameter dot plot. The beads coated with HLA-A11 have shifted to the right relative to the other beads, indicating that the HLA antibodies in this patient's serum are specific for the A11 antigen.

Solid-organ transplant recipients are at risk of developing HLA antibodies to donor-specific antigens (DSAs) after transplant. The development of DSAs after transplant has been associated with several outcomes. Some individuals have DSA but suffer no apparent clinical consequences. Others may suffer from antibody-mediated rejection or be at risk for acute cellular rejection. In the long term, post-transplant DSA development has been associated with lower graft survival compared with recipients who don't develop DSAs. The most common method to assess DSA involves the use of multiplex single-antigen bead arrays, as already described.

The intent of HCT is to repopulate the recipient's immune system with donor-derived white blood cells and eliminate malignant cells if transplanted for cancer. To monitor the patient for engraftment of donor cells, a blood sample can be assessed for the presence of donor-specific genetic markers. The relative quantity of donor cells versus recipient cells can be determined. A common method to accomplish this is the use of short tandem repeat (STR) testing. STRs are short segments (2 to 6 base pairs) of a specific, repeated DNA sequence. The number of repeats at a locus can vary from individual to individual; thus, determination of repeat number can be used to distinguish donor from recipient DNA in the blood. To determine the relative STR length in a sample, PCR is used to amplify several different STR loci in the pre-transplant recipient and donor DNA as well as in post-transplant DNA. PCR amplicons are separated according to the size of the repeats by capillary electrophoresis. Post-transplant electropherograms are compared with individual donor and recipient electropherograms. The peak heights or areas are determined for donor and recipient loci and reflect the relative proportions in the post-transplant blood sample. In this fashion, donor engraftment, or lack thereof, can be determined.

SUMMARY

- The immune system's ability to recognize and respond to the myriad of infectious agents that humans encounter has obvious benefits. However, the mechanisms that impart this ability make the transplantation of organs and cells between allogeneic individuals difficult.
- The targets of the response to transplanted tissues are HLA proteins and, to a lesser extent, minor histocompatibility

antigens. These proteins play critical roles as antigen-presenting molecules for CD4 and CD8 T cells, resulting in the phenomenon of MHC restriction.

- Although an individual's immune system develops to respond to the foreign proteins presented on its own MHC antigens, it responds intensely to foreign MHC proteins. Both the humoral and cellular branches of the immune system contribute to this allogeneic immune response and mediate graft rejection.
- The likelihood of developing an immune response to a graft depends on the genetic relatedness of the transplant donor and recipient. Autografts involve transfer of tissue from one area of the body to another in the same individual. Syngeneic grafts (isografts) involve the transfer of tissue between two genetically identical members of the same species. In allografts, tissue is transplanted between genetically nonidentical members of the same species, whereas in xenografts, tissue is transplanted between members of different species.
- Because of the disparity in HLA antigens, allografts and xenografts have the potential to induce strong immune responses in the transplant recipient.
- Hyperacute rejection occurs within minutes to hours after transplantation and is mediated by preformed HLA antibodies that react with donor vascular epithelium, resulting in activation of the complement cascade and clotting mechanisms. Preformed antibodies can also cause accelerated rejection, which occurs during a span of several days.
- Acute rejection develops days to months after transplantation and is mediated by a cellular or humoral response to foreign HLA antigens, involving cytokine production by CD4+ T cells, cytotoxic activity of CD8+ T cells, and/or antibody-mediated effector mechanisms.
- Chronic rejection can occur after the first year of transplantation through cellular and humoral responses to foreign HLA proteins, resulting in graft arteriosclerosis, fibrosis, and scarring.
- Graft-versus-host disease (GVHD) can occur in HLA-mismatched recipients of HSC transplants or, less commonly, via other transplants that contain lymphoid cells. In this condition, the donor's T lymphocytes destroy the recipient's cells, primarily in the skin, gastrointestinal tract, and liver.
- Even in the face of intense immune responses, transplantation has become an effective treatment for a variety of diseases because of the development of immunosuppressive agents that, in various ways, inhibit the immune system from responding to the allogeneic MHC proteins in the transplanted tissue. The classes of immunosuppressive agents include corticosteroids, antimetabolites, calcineurin inhibitors, monoclonal antibodies, and polyclonal antibodies. Unfortunately, these agents also interfere with immune responses to infectious organisms and tumors.
- Identifying the MHC antigens of donors and recipients and monitoring the allospecific immune response are critical components of clinical transplantation. Greatly improved outcomes of transplantation are seen when donor and recipient are matched for HLA types as much as possible and when the recipient does not have preformed antibodies to the donor's HLA antigens.
- The classic method of HLA phenotyping is the complement-dependent cytotoxicity test (CDC), in which HLA antigens are typed by incubating the individual's lymphocytes with a panel of antisera and reagent complement. Positive cells are identified by their ability to bind specific antisera and complement, resulting in membrane permeabilization and uptake of vital stains.
- Molecular methods such as PCR-SSP, PCR-SSOP, and SBT provide greater resolution than HLA antigen typing by determining the HLA genotype at the allele level.
- Screening and identification of preformed HLA antibodies in transplant recipients can be performed by the CDC method through incubation of patient serum with panels of lymphocytes with known HLA antigens, flow cytometry, or Luminex technology.
- Crossmatching is performed by incubation of recipient serum with donor lymphocytes in a CDC assay to confirm the absence of donor-specific antibody.
- Engraftment of donor-derived white blood cells in an HCT recipient can be determined by testing for donor-specific genetic markers known as *STRs*.

Study Guide: Classification of Grafts

TYPE OF GRAFT	DEFINITION	EXAMPLES
Autograft	Transfer of tissue within the same individual	Skin graft from a leg to the face of a burn patient Transfer of a saphenous vein from the leg of a cardiac bypass patient to his or her heart
Syngeneic (Iso) graft	Transfer of cells or tissues to a genetically identical individual	Transplant between identical human twins Grafts between genetically identical strains of mice
Allograft	Transfer of cells or tissues to a genetically nonidentical member of the same species	Human transplant from a deceased or living donor other than an identical twin Grafts between genetically nonidentical strains of mice
Xenograft	Transfer of cells or tissues to a member of a different species	Transplant of a pig valve into a human heart

Study Guide: Types of Graft Rejection

TYPE	TIMING (AFTER TRANSPLANT)	IMMUNOLOGIC MECHANISM
Hyperacute	Minutes to hours	Preformed antibodies to ABO, HLA, and certain endothelial antigens bind to donor vascular endothelium, activating complement and clotting factors. This leads to thrombus formation, ischemia, and necrosis of transplanted tissue.
Accelerated	Days	Same as for hyperacute rejection.
Acute	Days to months	Cell-mediated response to foreign MHC-expressing cells. CD4+ T cells produce cytokines and induce delayed-type hypersensitivity. CD8+ T cells mediate cytotoxic reactions. Antibodies produced against HLA antigens bind to vessel walls, activate complement, and induce transmural necrosis and inflammation.
Chronic	1 year or more	Delayed type hypersensitivity response, and possibly antibodies, to foreign HLA antigens on graft. Graft arteriosclerosis and smooth muscle proliferation occur, resulting in fibrosis, scarring, and narrowing of vessel lumen.
Graft-versus-host disease (GVHD)	100 days or more	T cells in HSC, lung, or liver transplants react against foreign HLA proteins in the recipient's cells, causing massive cytokine release, inflammation, and tissue destruction in various locations throughout the body.

CASE STUDIES

1. A 40-year-old mother of three needs to have a second kidney transplant. Her first transplant was lost because of chronic rejection. The mother's HLA type, HLA antibodies, and ABO blood group status were determined. The patient was found to have antibodies to HLA-B35 by flow cytometric testing with HLA-B35–coated beads. The HLA type and blood group were also determined for two of her siblings and two close friends who are interested in donating a kidney to the patient.

Question

a. From the available donors, who would likely be the most compatible with this patient?

Identification	Blood Group	A	B	C	DR	DQ
Recipient	O					
		1,2	8,44	7,5	17,4	2,7
Sibling 1	O	1,11	8,35	7,4	17,1	2,5
Sibling 2	A	3,11	7,35	7,4	15,1	6,5
Friend 1	B	2,24	57,7	6,7	7,15	2,6
Friend 2	O	2,24	57,7	6,7	7,15	2,6

2. A 59-year-old male with leukemia needed an HCT for his disease. Clinicians were hopeful that the patient's single sibling might be a suitable donor. However, the sibling was determined to be medically unsuitable for donation. As such, the transplant center conducted an unrelated donor search for this patient, and a potential donor was identified. The transplant registry provided the HLA type for the donor, which was determined using CDC-based testing (phenotyping). The patient's HLA type was determined at high resolution by SBT.

ID	HLA-A*	HLA- B*	HLA- C*	HLA-DRB1*	HLA-DQB1*
Patient	01:01	08:01	07:02	03:01	02:01
	02:01	44:02	02:01	15:01	06:02
Donor	1	8	7	3	2
	2	44	2	15	6

Questions

a. Is this donor–recipient pair HLA identical? Yes / No / Maybe
b. The transplant physician requested high-resolution HLA typing for the donor. Why?

3. A 56-year-old female with end-stage renal disease is seen by a transplant nephrologist, and the determination is made to list the patient for a deceased donor renal transplant. A histocompatibility workup is ordered for the patient, including HLA typing and HLA antibody testing. The patient's initial HLA antibody screen was positive for class I HLA antibodies. A single-antigen multiplex bead array assay was then performed to determine which specific HLA antigens the patient's serum reacted with. This test determined that the patient had antibodies to HLA-A1, B8, and DR17. Using the cPRA calculator that can be accessed at https://optn.transplant.hrsa.gov/resources/allocation-calculators/cpra-calculator/, place a checkmark in the box next to each HLA antigen that the patient has made antibody to. Next, click the "Calculate" button to determine the cPRA.

Questions

a. What is the resultant cPRA of this patient?
b. What does this value mean?

REVIEW QUESTIONS

1. Which of the following responses is the type of allograft rejection associated with vascular and parenchymal injury with lymphocyte infiltrates?
   a. Hyperacute rejection
   b. Acute cellular rejection
   c. Acute humoral rejection
   d. Chronic rejection
2. Antigen receptors on T lymphocytes bind HLA class II + peptide complexes with the help of which accessory molecule?
   a. CD2
   b. CD3
   c. CD4
   d. CD8
3. Patients who have received the following types of grafts are at risk for graft-versus-host disease (GVHD) *except* for recipients of
   a. bone marrow transplants.
   b. lung transplants.
   c. liver transplants.
   d. irradiated leukocytes.
4. Which of the following properties is *not* exhibited by HLA molecules?
   a. They belong to the immunoglobulin superfamily.
   b. They are heterodimeric.
   c. They are integral cell membrane glycoproteins.
   d. They are monomorphic.
5. Kidney allograft loss from intravascular thrombosis without cellular infiltration 5 days post-transplant may indicate which primary rejection mechanism?
   a. Hyperacute rejection
   b. Accelerated humoral rejection
   c. Acute humoral rejection
   d. Acute cellular rejection
6. Which reagents would be used in a donor–recipient crossmatch test?
   a. Donor serum and recipient lymphocytes + rabbit serum complement
   b. Recipient serum and donor lymphocytes + rabbit serum complement
   c. Donor stimulator cells + recipient responder cells + complete culture medium
   d. Recipient stimulator cells + donor responder cells + complete culture medium
7. The indirect allorecognition pathway involves which one of the following mechanisms?
   a. Processed peptides from polymorphic donor proteins restricted by recipient HLA class II molecules
   b. Processed peptides from polymorphic recipient proteins restricted by donor HLA class I molecules
   c. Intact polymorphic donor protein molecules recognized by recipient HLA class I molecules
   d. Intact polymorphic donor protein molecules recognized by recipient HLA class II molecules
8. Which immunosuppressive agent selectively inhibits IL-2 receptor-mediated activation of T cells?
   a. Mycophenolate mofetil
   b. Cyclosporine mofetil
   c. Corticosteroids
   d. Basiliximab
9. Phenotyping for HLA class II antigens requires B lymphocytes because
   a. B lymphocytes express HLA class II antigens.
   b. B lymphocytes do not express HLA class I antigens.
   c. B lymphocytes are exquisitely sensitive to complement-mediated lysis.
   d. B lymphocytes represent the majority of lymphocytes in the peripheral blood.
10. A renal transplant candidate was crossmatched with a donor who was mismatched for only the HLA-B35 antigen. The candidate was known to have an antibody specific for HLA-B35. Which of the following combinations of T- and B-cell flow cytometric crossmatch results would be expected?
    a. T-cell negative, B-cell negative
    b. T-cell positive, B-cell positive
    c. T-cell negative, B-cell positive
    d. T-cell positive, B-cell negative
11. Which of the following HLA alleles differs from A*02:01:02 by a synonymous nucleotide substitution?
    a. A*01:01:01:01
    b. A*02:01:03
    c. A*02:02
    d. A*02:03:01

12. Which one of the following donors would be expected to elicit a positive mixed lymphocyte response in lymphocytes from a patient who has the HLA-DRB1*01:01, 01:03 alleles?

a. DRB1*01:01, 01:03
b. DRB1*01:01, 01:01
c. DRB1*01:03, 01:03
d. DRB1*01:01, 01:05

13. Which of the following donors would be the most appropriate, based on ABO compatibility, for a renal transplant candidate with the ABO type = O?

a. O
b. A
c. B
d. AB

14. Which of the following HLA antigens would be expected to elicit an HLA antibody response in a kidney transplant recipient with the following HLA type: HLA-A*01,03; B*07,14; C*01,04N; DRB1*16,07?

a. HLA-A*01
b. HLA-B*14
c. HLA-C*04
d. HLA-DRB1*16

15. Suppose a 30-year-old man was found to be a suitable donor for a kidney transplant to his younger sister. This transplant would be an example of a(an)

a. autograft.
b. allograft.
c. isograft.
d. xenograft.

17 Tumor Immunology

Linda E. Miller, PhD, MB^{CM}(ASCP)SI

LEARNING OUTCOMES

After finishing this chapter, you should be able to:

1. Describe the characteristics that differentiate cancer cells from normal cells and the process by which malignant cells are thought to develop.
2. Differentiate between various types of tumor antigens and recognize examples of each.
3. Summarize the uses of tumor markers in screening for cancer, diagnosing malignancy, detecting prognosis, and monitoring patient responses to treatment.
4. Identify the characteristics that should be possessed by an ideal tumor marker and explain how nonideal features can affect the clinical utility of a marker.
5. Explain the principles of immunohistochemistry as they apply to tumor marker detection.
6. Distinguish the clinical applications of each of the following tumor markers: alpha-fetoprotein (AFP), cancer antigen 125 (CA 125), carcinoembryonic antigen (CEA), human chorionic gonadotropin (hCG), and prostate-specific antigen (PSA).
7. Contrast the advantages and limitations of immunoassays for tumor markers.
8. Summarize key principles of molecular and proteomic testing for tumor markers.
9. Describe the innate and adaptive immune responses that play a role in defense against tumors and how they contribute to immunosurveillance.
10. Discuss the process of immunoediting and how this relates to mechanisms of tumor escape from the immune system.
11. Cite the overall goal of immunotherapy and provide specific examples of active, passive, and adoptive immunotherapy for cancer.
12. Discuss principles and applications of molecular tests for cancer diagnosis.

CHAPTER OUTLINE

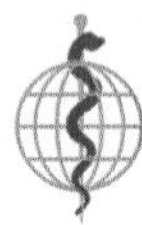

Go to FADavis.com for the laboratory exercises that accompany this text.

KEY TERMS

Adoptive immunotherapy
Alpha-fetoprotein (AFP)
Antibody arrays
Antibody–drug conjugates
Apoptosis
Benign
Biomarker profiling
Cancer
Cancer antigen 125 (CA 125)
Cancer vaccines
Carcinoembryonic antigen (CEA)
Carcinogenesis
Carcinomas
CAR-T cell therapy
CD45
Colony-stimulating factors (CSFs)
Cytogenetics
Fluorescence in situ hybridization (FISH)
Hematopoietic growth factors
High-dose hook effect
Human chorionic gonadotropin (hCG)
Human epidermal growth factor receptor 2 (HER2)
Immune-checkpoint inhibitors
Immunoediting
Immunohistochemistry
Immunosurveillance
Immunotherapy
Immunotoxins
Karyotype analysis
Malignant
Metastasis
Microarray
Mutations
Neoplasm
Oncofetal antigen
Passive immunotherapy
Prostate-specific antigen (PSA)
Proteomics
Proto-oncogenes
Sarcomas
Tumor
Tumor-infiltrating lymphocytes (TILs)
Tumor markers
Tumor suppressor genes

Introduction to Tumor Biology

Tumor immunology is the study of the relationship between the immune system and cancer cells. The field encompasses several areas, including the antigens associated with tumor cells, the host's immune responses to tumors, mechanisms by which tumors are thought to escape these responses, and therapeutic use of the immune system in an attempt to eradicate tumors. Tumor immunology is a major area of interest to immunologists because cancer is a leading cause of mortality, responsible for more than 9 million deaths each year and accounting for one out of every six deaths worldwide.

Tumor immunology is best understood with a background on the origin of cancer cells and their differences from normal cells. Normally, cell growth and division are carefully regulated processes that allow the body to rapidly produce new cells when necessary. At the same time, cell division is inhibited when enough cells are present, and the life span of cells is limited through a normal physiological process of cell death called **apoptosis.** These activities make it possible for the human body to carry out functions necessary for life, such as generation of new skin cells to replace those that are dying, proliferation of lymphocytes in immune responses, and regeneration of tissue during wound healing and repair. However, if these processes are allowed to continue unchecked, they can lead to excessive cell growth and division, resulting in the development of an abnormal cell mass called a **tumor** (from the Latin, meaning "to swell") or **neoplasm** (from the Greek, meaning "new growth"). See **Figure 17–1.**

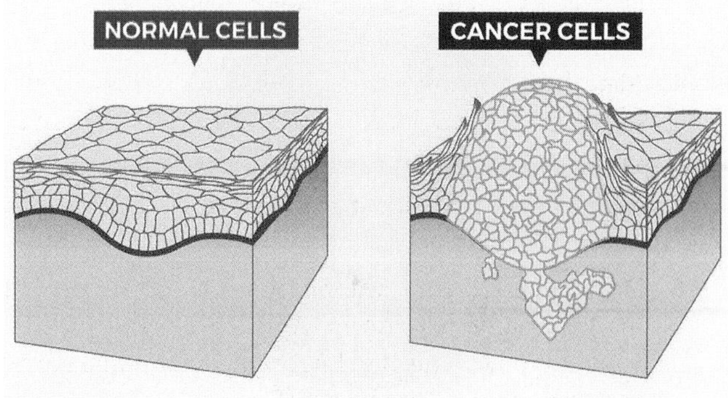

FIGURE 17–1 Cancer is a disease caused by cells dividing uncontrollably and spreading into surrounding tissues. *(Source: National Cancer Institute [NCI]).*

Tumors can be classified as **benign** or **malignant.** Benign tumors are composed of slowly growing cells that are well differentiated and organized, similar to the normal tissue from which they originated. These tumors are surrounded by a capsule, which secures them in place and prevents them from circulating to other parts of the body. In contrast, malignant tumors, or cancer cells, are disorganized masses that are rarely encapsulated, allowing them to invade nearby organs and destroy their normal architecture. **Cancer,** named after the Latin word for "crab," derives its name from this property of invasiveness, which can resemble the legs of a crab when viewed in microscopic tissue sections. In addition, malignant tumors commonly exhibit **metastasis,** or the ability of cells to break away from the original tumor mass and spread through the blood to nearby or distant sites in the body (**Fig. 17–2**). Malignant tumors can vary in their degree of differentiation, from completely differentiated, or mature, to completely undifferentiated tumors that tend to grow more aggressively and have a poorer prognosis.

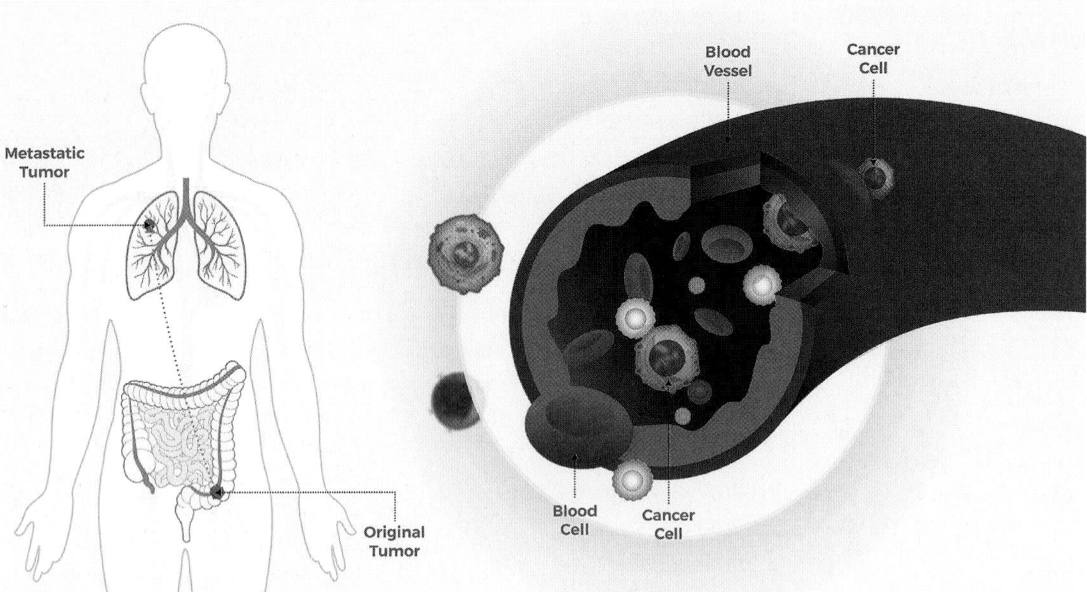

FIGURE 17–2 The process of metastasis. Cancer cells can break away from the original tumor and travel through the blood or lymphatic system to distant locations in the body, where they exit the vessels to form additional tumors. *(Source: National Cancer Institute [NCI]).*

Connections

Apoptosis

Recall that apoptosis is a normal homeostatic mechanism that is necessary for maintaining normal cell numbers. This process occurs through a series of biochemical reactions within a cell that lead to chromatin condensation, DNA fragmentation, cell shrinkage, and membrane blebbing. Cell death occurs in the absence of cell lysis and does not provoke an inflammatory reaction that could damage neighboring cells. Genetic changes within a cell that cause it to become resistant to apoptosis are important in the development of cancer.

Malignant tumors are classified according to their tissue of origin. Approximately 80% of cancers are **carcinomas,** derived from the skin or epithelial linings of internal organs or glands; about 9% are *leukemias or lymphomas,* malignant white blood cells (WBCs) present in the circulation or lymphatic system; and about 1% are **sarcomas,** derived from bone or soft tissues such as fat, muscles, tendons, cartilage, nerves, and blood vessels. Other types of tumors include melanoma (a malignancy of the cells that make the pigment of skin), brain and spinal cord tumors, germ cell tumors (arising from cells involved in the production of sperm and eggs), and neuroendocrine tumors (derived from cells that produce hormones after receiving signals from the nervous system). To make a specific diagnosis and guide treatment decisions, physicians use staging systems based on the site and type of the primary tumor, tumor size, involvement of regional lymph nodes, presence or absence of metastasis, and degree of resemblance to normal tissue. The most widely used staging scheme is the TNM system of the American Joint Committee on Cancer (AJCC).

Clinical Correlations

The TNM System

In the TNM system, tumors are classified according to the size and extent of the primary tumor (T0 to T4), the degree of spread to adjacent lymph nodes (N0 to N3), and the presence or absence of distant metastases (M0 or M1). For example, breast cancer that is classified as T2N1M0 would involve a tumor between 2 to 5 cm in diameter that has spread to one to three regional lymph nodes but has not spread to distant sites. For many types of cancer, the TNM criteria also correspond to one of five stages (stage 0, I, II, III, or IV). Although the specific criteria vary according to the type of cancer, in general, stage 0 represents noninvasive (in situ) carcinoma; stages I, II, and III are tumors that are larger or that have spread beyond the organ in which they first developed to nearby lymph nodes or tissues; and stage IV tumors are those that have metastasized to distant sites.

The transformation of a normal cell into a malignant tumor is thought to be a multistep process involving a series of genetic mutations that cause the phenotype of a cell to be changed over time. This process, called **carcinogenesis,** is thought to be initiated by exposure of the host to factors in the environment that induce genetic changes in the cell. These factors include chemical carcinogens, such as asbestos and cigarette smoke; radiation, such as ultraviolet rays from the sun and ionizing radiation from x-rays; and certain pathogenic viruses that have been linked to specific types of cancer. These agents are all believed to create genetic changes, or **mutations,** in the DNA of our cells that affect the body's mechanisms that normally control cell growth.

Two major types of genes are involved in malignant transformation: proto-oncogenes and tumor suppressor genes. **Proto-oncogenes** are normal genes that stimulate cell proliferation and growth. Sometimes mutations in proto-oncogenes can convert them to oncogene-like genes, which have DNA sequences similar to those found in the *oncogenes* of transforming viruses. These genetic alterations—which include point mutations, chromosomal translocations, and gene amplifications—cause continual activation of the proto-oncogenes, resulting in changes that allow cells to divide uncontrollably.

Excessive cell division is normally inhibited by the action of **tumor suppressor genes.** These genes exert their effects by controlling the entry of cells into the cell cycle and preventing cells from completing the cell cycle if they contain damaged DNA or other abnormalities. If a mutation occurs in which the function of a tumor suppressor gene is lost, normal growth-inhibitory signals are removed. Tumor suppressor genes also play an important role in recognizing damaged DNA in a cell and repairing it. If repair is not possible, the cell is induced to undergo apoptosis. Thus, mutations in tumor suppressor genes can result in genetic instability and allow abnormal cells to survive.

In their classic papers, Hanahan and Weinberg defined eight characteristics that differentiate a cancerous cell from a normal cell:

1. Sustained signaling of proliferation
2. Resistance to cell death
3. Ability to induce angiogenesis (development of new blood vessels to provide oxygen and nutrients to the tumor)
4. Immortality in terms of cell division
5. Invasion and metastasis
6. Ability to avoid suppressors of cell growth
7. Reprogramming of energy metabolism to support malignant proliferation
8. Ability to evade destruction by the immune system

These characteristics are made possible by genetic mutations that occur in the proto-oncogenes and tumor suppressor genes as well as a state of chronic inflammation in the tumor microenvironment that promotes excessive cell growth. In most cases, the development of a cancerous tumor is believed to result from a series of mutations in proto-oncogenes and tumor suppressor genes that accumulate in the same cell over a lifetime **(Fig. 17–3).**

Today, it is recognized that cancer is not a single disease but, rather, a diverse group of diseases that show variability in the characteristics mentioned. In fact, heterogeneity is commonly found among different cancer cells in the same patient. The extent to which a tumor exhibits these characteristics will determine its ability to survive, grow, and metastasize. This, in turn, has important implications that influence disease aggressiveness, patient prognosis, and choice of therapy. The immune system is thought to have important effects on tumor growth. In this chapter, we will discuss the interactions between tumors and the immune system in more detail, as well as tumor antigens that can be used as markers for various types of cancer.

Tumor Antigens

The concept of tumor immunology is based on the premise that tumors possess antigens that are recognized as foreign by the immune system. Some of these antigens are unique to tumor cells, whereas others are also found on normal cells. The discussion that follows describes various types of tumor antigens, which can be grouped in terms of their molecular basis and source. **Table 17–1** summarizes the features of the various types of tumor antigens and provides examples of each.

Advances in next-generation sequencing (NGS; see Chapter 12) have led to the discovery of *mutation-derived tumor antigens* (MTAs), also known as *neoantigens,* or *tumor-specific antigens.* These antigens are created because of various mutations that occur as the cell progresses through the cell cycle and can occur in proto-oncogenes, tumor suppressor genes, or unrelated genes. The new antigens can then bind to MHC molecules and be presented to T lymphocytes and stimulate anti-tumor responses (see *Adaptive Immune Responses*).

A well-known example of an MTA is a fusion protein that is produced in chronic myelogenous leukemia (CML) cells. This protein is a result of a reciprocal chromosome translocation commonly known as the *Philadelphia chromosome,* which involves the *BCR* (breakage cluster region) gene on chromosome 9 and the c-*ABL* gene on chromosome 22. c-*ABL* is a cellular proto-oncogene that codes for tyrosine kinase, a key enzyme in cell-signaling pathways that promote cell division. During the translocation, the two chromosomes break and exchange parts so that the c-*ABL* gene is combined with part of the *BCR* to produce a hybrid gene that is constantly expressed **(Fig. 17–4).** The *BCR/ABL* gene rearrangements result in uncontrolled cell proliferation and are found in the majority of CML patients.

Other MTAs originate from point mutations (i.e., genetic changes involving a single base pair) in key genes involved in cell proliferation, such as the tumor suppressor gene *p53* and the gene coding for caspase 8, an enzyme important for apoptosis (both of which are associated with head and neck tumors and squamous cell carcinoma). MTAs can also be produced by mutations induced by carcinogenic chemicals and radiation.

Another group of tumor antigens consists of proteins encoded by cancer-causing viruses **(Table 17–2).** For example, antigens coded for by genes of the Epstein-Barr virus (EBV) can be found in cells from B-cell lymphomas that are associated with the virus. These antigens have been observed in the nucleus, cytoplasm, or plasma membrane of the associated tumor cells. The antigens are produced inside of the cells infected with an oncogenic virus and can be processed by class I MHC molecules and displayed on the tumor cell surface, where they are presented to T cells.

Other types of tumor antigens are present in some types of normal cells but are overexpressed or abnormally expressed by cancer cells. These types include the cancer/testis antigens, differentiation antigens, and overexpressed antigens.

Cancer/testis antigens are present in testicular germ cells (i.e., spermatogonia and spermatocytes), placental trophoblasts,

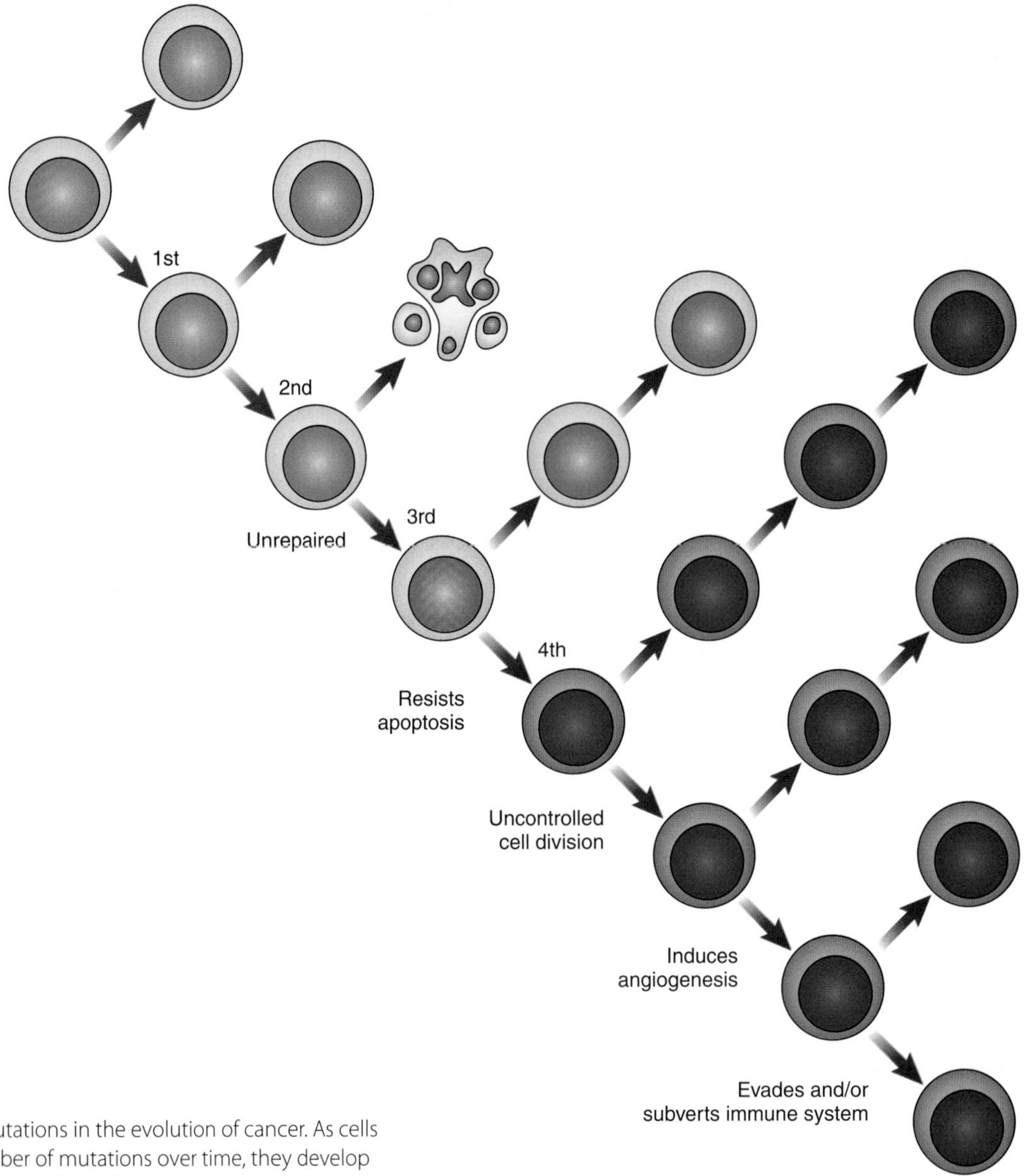

FIGURE 17–3 Genetic mutations in the evolution of cancer. As cells acquire an increasing number of mutations over time, they develop more of the characteristics that allow them to evolve into invasive cancer cells (numbers indicate mutations).

and ovaries but not in normal somatic cells. They become tumor antigens when the transformation process causes them to be expressed on tumors originating from other cell types. These antigens have been identified on many tumors of epithelial or mesenchymal origin. The best-known examples of tumor-associated antigens (TAAs) in this category are the melanoma antigen gene (MAGE) proteins that are expressed by melanoma tumors.

Differentiation antigens are expressed on immature cells of a particular lineage. An example of a tumor antigen in this group is the CD10 antigen (previously known as the *CALLA*, or common acute lymphoblastic leukemia antigen), which is normally found on pre-B cells but not on mature B cells. This group of antigens also includes the *oncofetal* or embryonic antigens that are normally expressed on developing cells of the fetus but not on cells in the adult. It is thought that the genes coding for these antigens are silenced during development of the embryo but that the process of malignant transformation allows them to be re-expressed. Examples of oncofetal antigens include carcinoembryonic protein (CEA), alpha-fetoprotein (AFP), and prostate-specific antigen (PSA). Many of these antigens are tumor markers that can be detected in the clinical laboratory (see the next section).

The *overexpressed antigens* are found in higher levels on malignant cells than on normal cells. Genetic mutations that occur during transformation are thought to deregulate expression of these proteins, resulting in levels up to 100 times greater than normal. A well-known example of a tumor antigen in this category is the **human epidermal growth factor receptor 2 (HER2)** protein, a transmembrane receptor that

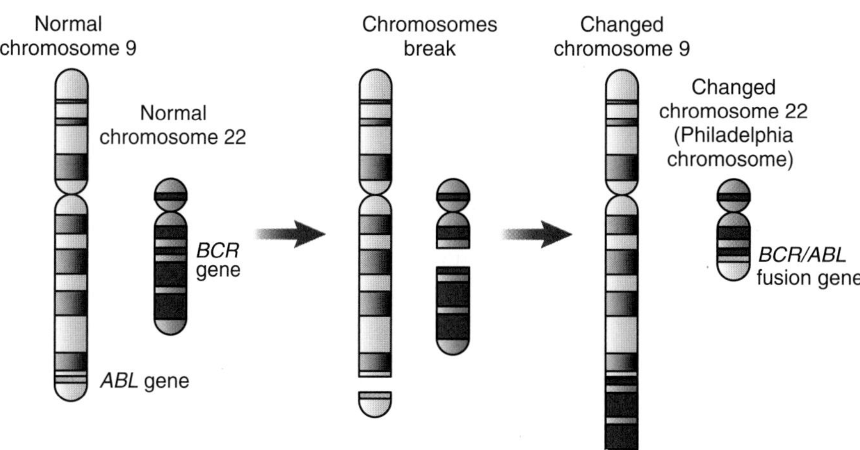

FIGURE 17–4 The *BCR/ABL* gene rearrangement characteristic of CML.

Table 17–1 Types of Tumor Antigens*

CATEGORY	DESCRIPTION	EXAMPLES*
Mutation-derived tumor antigens (neoantigens)	Antigens that are created because of mutations; these are unique to a tumor or shared by tumors of the same type	*BCR/ABL* fusion protein (CML) p53 CASP-8
Antigens from oncogenic viruses	Antigens that are expressed because of infection with a cancer-causing virus	Epstein-Barr virus (EBV) antigens in EBV-associated B-cell lymphomas
Cancer/testis antigens	Expressed in gametes and in many tumors but not in somatic cells	MAGE (melanoma)
Differentiation antigens	Expressed on immature cells of a particular lineage	CD10 (ALL) CEA (mainly in colorectal cancer) AFP (HCC) PSA (prostate cancer)
Overexpressed antigens	Found in higher levels on malignant cells than on normal cells	HER2 (mainly in some breast cancers)

**Primary cancer associations are shown in parentheses.*

AFP = alpha-fetoprotein; ALL = acute lymphoblastic leukemia; CD10 = cluster of differentiation 10; Casp = caspase; CEA = carcinoembryonic antigen; CML = chronic myelogenous leukemia; HCC = hepatocellular carcinoma; HER2 = human epidermal growth factor 2; MAGE = melanoma antigen gene; PSA = prostate-specific antigen.

Table 17–2 Human Viruses Associated With Cancer

VIRUS	CANCER ASSOCIATIONS
Epstein-Barr virus (EBV)	Burkitt lymphoma Hodgkin lymphoma Leiomyosarcomas Post-transplant lymphoproliferative disease Nasopharyngeal carcinoma
Hepatitis B virus (HBV)	Hepatocellular carcinoma
Hepatitis C virus (HCV)	Hepatocellular carcinoma
Human herpes virus 8 (HHV-8)	Kaposi sarcoma
Human papilloma virus (HPV)	Cervical cancer Other genital and anal cancers Oral cancers
Human T-lymphotropic virus I (HTLV-1)	Adult T-cell leukemia or lymphoma
Merkel cell polyomavirus	Merkel cell carcinoma (a type of skin cancer)

binds human epidermal growth factor. Gene amplification in a certain type of breast cancer can result in increased production of this protein, which serves as a marker for detection and therapy (see *Immunotherapy* later).

An updated list of tumor antigen peptides that have undergone comprehensive scientific study is maintained in an online database promoted by the Cancer Research Institute. Researchers are continually discovering new tumor antigens by using molecular techniques. Some of these antigens can serve as targets for specifically directed therapies (see *Immunotherapy* later).

In addition to peptide TAAs, glycolipid and glycoprotein antigens may also be overexpressed in some tumors. Examples of these antigens include cancer antigen 125 (CA 125), which is associated with ovarian cancer, and cancer antigen 19-9 (CA 19-9), which is associated with pancreatic cancer. In the next section, we will discuss clinical applications of some of these markers.

Clinically Relevant Tumor Markers

Tumor markers can be defined as biological substances that are found in increased amounts in the blood, body fluids, or tissues of patients with a specific type of cancer. These substances can be produced by the tumor itself or by the patient's body in response to the tumor or related benign conditions. The concentration of a tumor marker in the serum depends on the degree of tumor proliferation, the size of the tumor mass, the proteolytic activities of the tumor, or release of the marker from dying tumor cells. An elevated level of a tumor marker suggests that a significant amount of a particular type of tumor is present.

Tumor markers can be proteins, carbohydrates, oncofetal antigens, hormones, metabolites, receptors, or enzymes. **Table 17–3** lists some examples of clinically relevant tumor markers in each category, along with their disease associations.

An ideal tumor marker should have the following characteristics. A marker should:

- Be produced by the tumor itself or by the patient's body in response to the tumor.
- Be secreted into a biological fluid, where it can be inexpensively and easily quantified.
- Have a circulating half-life long enough to permit its concentration to rise with increasing tumor load.
- Increase to clinically significant levels above the reference level while the disease is still treatable.
- Have a high sensitivity; in other words, it should easily detect the majority of individuals in the population who have a particular cancer.
- Have a high specificity; in other words, the marker should be absent from, or present at background levels in, all individuals without the malignant disease in question to minimize false-positive test results.

Unfortunately, many of the tumor markers in clinical use are not tumor specific. This limitation affects the performance of tumor markers in each of the four applications introduced in the next section.

Clinical Uses of Tumor Markers: Benefits and Limitations

In general, tumor markers have four major clinical applications: screening, diagnosis, prognosis, and monitoring. It is a well-established fact that patient survival rates are usually higher when cancer is diagnosed in its earliest stages. Detecting cancer early, before it begins to invade normal tissues

Table 17–3 Categories of Clinically Relevant Tumor Markers

TUMOR MARKER CLASS	EXAMPLES	DISEASE ASSOCIATIONS
Cell surface markers	Estrogen or progesterone receptors	Prognosis for hormone therapy in breast cancer
	Cluster of differentiation (CD) markers on white blood cells (WBCs)	Clonality and lineage of WBC neoplasms
Proteins	Thyroglobulin (TG)	Well-differentiated papillary or follicular thyroid carcinoma
	Immunoglobulins (Ig) and Ig light chains (Bence Jones proteins)	Multiple myeloma and lymphoid malignancies
Oncofetal antigens	Alpha-fetoprotein (AFP)	Germ cell carcinomas, hepatocellular carcinoma
	Carcinoembryonic antigen (CEA)	Colorectal, breast, or lung cancer
Carbohydrate antigens	CA 125	Ovarian cancer
	CA 15-3	Breast cancer
	CA 19-9	Pancreatic and gastrointestinal cancers
Enzymes and isoenzymes	Prostate-specific antigen (PSA)	Prostate cancer
	Alkaline phosphatase (ALKP)	Bone and liver cancer
	Neuron-specific enolase	Neural tissue neoplasms
Hormones	Human chorionic gonadotropin (hCG)	Germ cell carcinoma, trophoblastic tumors
	Calcitonin	Medullary thyroid cancer
	Gastrin	Pancreatic gastrinoma

and is difficult to target, requires good screening methods. Tumor markers can be used to screen asymptomatic individuals in a population for the presence of cancer. The individuals screened may belong to a healthy population or to a high-risk population. For example, PSA has been routinely used to screen men aged 50 or older for the presence of prostate cancer.

Secondly, tumor markers can be helpful in making an initial diagnosis of cancer. For example, an elevated level of PSA might suggest the presence of prostate cancer. A third use of tumor markers is in predicting the prognosis of a cancer patient. In general, an initial high concentration of a tumor marker or an increasing level of a tumor marker over time points to a poorer prognosis. A fourth use of tumor markers is to monitor known cancer patients to determine whether their treatment is working and to check for recurrence of the tumor. Decreasing levels of a marker indicate that the treatment is effective in reducing the amount of tumor harbored by the patient, whereas increasing levels indicate that the treatment is ineffective and that the number of tumor cells in the patient is increasing. Each of these applications will be discussed in more detail in the text that follows.

The second half of this section will focus on traditional tumor markers that are commonly detected in the serum. This section will also introduce the role of molecular and proteomic methods in detecting newer tumor markers that are being increasingly evaluated in the clinical laboratory.

Screening for Tumor Markers

The detection of tumor markers provides an ideal way to screen for tumors because the markers can be detected by a simple blood test. However, the benefits and limitations of using a particular marker to screen a population must be considered before testing is implemented. On the positive side, screening asymptomatic individuals can lead to earlier detection of tumors with a need for less aggressive treatment. In addition, many people who have been screened can receive reassurance from true-negative results. However, there are also significant disadvantages associated with screening. Besides the actual dollar costs of the screening test, harm to the individuals tested may also occur. For example, misleading reassurance can be experienced by individuals with false-negative results. In contrast, false-positive results can lead to patient anxiety; possible harm from more invasive, unnecessary follow-up testing; and overtreatment of questionable diagnoses. For example, PSA, a marker elevated in prostate cancer, can also be increased in men with a harmless enlargement of the prostate known as *benign prostatic hypertrophy* (BPH) (see *PSA* section). In these cases, the finding of an elevated PSA value can lead to unnecessary testing and potentially harmful treatments, such as a prostate biopsy.

The effectiveness of a tumor marker in screening for cancer depends on the sensitivity and specificity of the marker, as well as the cancer's prevalence in the population. Screening is most effective when it is conducted in populations at a high risk for developing the disease, such as certain ethnic groups or those with a family history of a particular type of cancer. For example, AFP, a tumor marker for hepatocellular carcinoma (HCC), is not used for screening in the United States but is used to screen people in China, where the incidence of liver cancer is high. In high-risk populations, the predictive value of the tumor marker will be highest. In other words, a positive test result is most likely to be found in a person who truly has the disease, whereas a negative result is most likely to occur in a person who truly does not have the disease.

Using Tumor Markers to Aid in Diagnosis

A second application of tumor markers is to help physicians distinguish between different diseases with similar symptoms, a process called *differential diagnosis*. For example, if a computerized tomography (CT) scan revealed the presence of a lung nodule, histological examination of a lung biopsy could help differentiate whether the nodule was caused by cancer or another disease process, such as an infection. Follow-up staining of the biopsy for tumor markers could help determine the neoplasm's tissue origin. To improve the sensitivity and specificity of the testing, multiple tumor markers could be examined, or testing for tumor markers could be combined with other laboratory tests. It is important to recognize that tumor markers can serve as a valuable aid in making a cancer diagnosis when they are used in conjunction with clinical findings and other tests, but they are not diagnostic by themselves.

Using Tumor Markers to Determine Prognosis

A third application of tumor markers is to assess prognosis in a known cancer patient. A high concentration of a tumor marker at the time of diagnosis or increasing levels of a tumor marker over time can indicate the presence of an aggressive tumor that has metastasized and requires rigorous treatment. Tumor markers can also be used to determine the type of therapy that would be most effective for a patient. For example, in breast cancer, anti-HER2 agents such as trastuzumab work best in patients whose tumors overexpress the HER2 protein or gene; anti-endocrine therapies such as tamoxifen are suitable for patients whose tumors overexpress the estrogen receptor.

Connections

Specificity

A problem with many tumor markers is that they lack specificity for the disease they are intended to detect. Recall from Chapter 9 that specificity is the ability of a test to be negative for a person who does not have a particular disease. For example, suppose a tumor marker has a specificity of 90%. Although this may seem to be a good attribute because the test will give a true negative result in every 90 out of 100 people tested, 10% of those tested will have a false-positive result. If 100,000 people in a population were tested, 10,000 would have a positive result even though they did not have the intended disease and would likely be recommended to have additional unnecessary testing or invasive procedures.

Using Tumor Markers to Monitor Patient Response to Treatment and Determine Tumor Recurrence

One of the most important uses of tumor markers is to monitor known cancer patients to determine whether their treatment is effective and to check for recurrence of the tumor. This can be done because the level of a serum tumor marker often correlates with the amount of tumor in the patient's body. The laboratory typically determines a baseline concentration of the marker before treatment begins, followed by serial measurements over time. A significant decrease in the concentration of a tumor marker after surgery, chemotherapy, or other treatment indicates that the therapy has been effective in reducing the tumor mass. In contrast, an increasing level of the marker after a return to normal indicates that the tumor has recurred and that more aggressive treatment may be needed. Elevation in a tumor marker can become evident several months before the cancer is detected by other methods.

The clinical significance of monitoring a tumor marker is illustrated in **Figure 17–5.** This figure shows tumor marker levels from a hypothetical cancer patient who has been treated with surgery and two chemotherapy drugs. As expected, the level of the tumor marker in the patient's serum declined after the initial tumor mass was removed by surgery. However, after a few months, the concentration of the tumor marker began to increase, indicating that the tumor had recurred. The tumor was unresponsive to Chemotherapy #1, as reflected by the sustained elevation in the marker after treatment with that drug. This prompted a change in treatment to Chemotherapy #2, which was successful in decreasing the amount of tumor present in the patient, as indicated by the decline in the tumor marker to an undetectable level.

Serum Tumor Markers

The number of tumor markers in clinical use has increased over the years. The next few sections will discuss some of the more commonly used tumor markers that can be detected in patient serum. The major characteristics of these and other selected markers are listed in **Table 17–4,** along with their clinical applications and important noncancerous conditions that can cause elevations.

Alpha-Fetoprotein (AFP)

Alpha-fetoprotein (AFP) is a 70,000-MW glycoprotein that is similar to albumin in its physical and chemical properties. It is classified as an **oncofetal antigen** because it is synthesized by the fetal liver and yolk sac and is abundant in fetal serum, but it declines to low levels (10 to 20 ug/L) by 12 months of age. AFP is frequently elevated in patients with primary HCC and nonseminomatous testicular cancer but can also be elevated in other types of cancers and in nonmalignant conditions such as pregnancy and hepatitis.

AFP is the most widely used tumor marker for HCC, serving as a tool in diagnosis, staging, prognosis, and monitoring patients undergoing therapy. The sensitivity of AFP for HCC is 41% to 65%, and its specificity ranges between 80% and 94%. Therefore, the utility of AFP in screening for HCC has been a matter of debate. However, screening for HCC with AFP is routinely performed in high-prevalence areas of the world such as China and Southeast Asia. In the United States, AFP screening is usually conducted in patients with a high risk for HCC, along with liver ultrasound. Many of these patients have liver cirrhosis because of hepatitis B or hepatitis C infection. The diagnostic utility of AFP may be improved by testing specifically for the isoform AFP-L3, which has a stronger

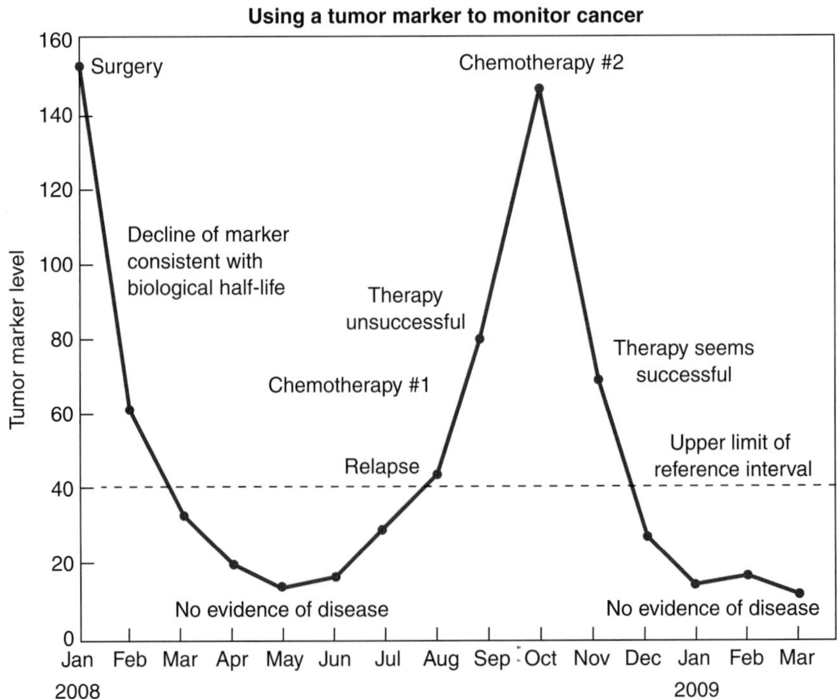

FIGURE 17–5 Tumor marker analysis. A curve showing a sample scenario monitoring a cancer patient for tumor recurrence and for therapy efficacy using levels of a circulating tumor antigen.

Table 17–4 Common Tumor Markers

MARKER	CANCER(S)	USES	NORMAL SOURCES	NONCANCEROUS CONDITIONS WITH ELEVATIONS	COMMENTS
AFP	Nonseminomatous testicular germ cell Liver	Screening Diagnosis and staging Prognosis Monitoring	Fetal liver and yolk sac, adult liver	Pregnancy, nonneoplastic liver disease	Screening conducted in high-risk populations for liver cancer, such as those with liver cirrhosis and chronic hepatitis. In germ cell tumors, both AFP and hCG are elevated.
β2–microglobulin	B-lymphocyte malignancies	Prognosis Monitoring	Part of class I MHC molecule	Inflammatory and high cell turnover conditions	High levels imply poor prognosis in multiple myeloma.
Calcitonin and Ca++	Familial medullary thyroid carcinoma	Diagnosis Monitoring	Thyroid	In hypercalcemia, increased calcitonin is expected. Serum Ca++ may be low when calcitonin is elevated in medullary carcinoma.	Can be elevated in other forms of cancer.
CD markers	WBC	Diagnosis Monitoring	All WBCs	WBC increase caused by other conditions such as infections	Different CD markers are associated with specific WBC malignancies.
CEA	Colorectal Breast Lung	Prognosis Monitoring	Tissues of endodermal origin	Renal failure, nonneoplastic liver and intestinal disease, age	Values increased with age and in cigarette smokers.
CA 125	Ovarian adenocarcinoma	Screening Diagnosis Prognosis Monitoring	Ovaries and various other tissues	Endometriosis, pelvic inflammatory disease, uterine fibroids, and pregnancy	Increases can occur during menstruation. Screening is only recommended for women with a family history of ovarian cancer.
CA 15-3	Breast cancer Can also be increased in pancreatic, lung, colorectal, ovarian, and liver cancers	Prognosis Monitoring	Mammary tissue	Benign breast disease, benign liver disease	Anti-CA 15-3 is a monoclonal antibody directed against an epitope of episialin.
CA 19-9	Pancreatic	Diagnosis Prognosis Monitoring	Sialylated Lewis[a] blood group antigen	Benign hepatobiliary and pancreatic conditions	Can be elevated in some nonpancreatic malignancies. Lewis[a] and [b]-negative persons cannot synthesize CA 19-9.
ER/PR	Breast adenocarcinoma	Prognosis	Breast	N/A	ER+/PR+ breast cancers benefit from estrogen or progesterone reduction therapy.

(continued)

Table 17–4 Common Tumor Markers—cont'd

MARKER	CANCER(S)	USES	NORMAL SOURCES	NONCANCEROUS CONDITIONS WITH ELEVATIONS	COMMENTS
hCG	Nonseminomatous testicular cancer germ cell trophoblastic (hydatidiform mole, choriocarcinoma)	Diagnosis Prognosis Monitoring	Placenta	Pregnancy	hCG has a high homology with luteinizing hormone (LH). Malignancies can produce free α and β chains as well as intact α and β dimers. Immunoassays that detect only intact hCG should not be used for tumor marker detection. In germ cell tumors, both AFP and hCG are elevated.
HER2 (neu)	Breast	Prognosis	Growth factor gene in all cells	N/A	Cancers associated with overexpression of HER2 (neu) have a good response to monoclonal antibody therapy (trastuzumab).
Monoclonal free Ig light chains	Plasma cell, B lymphocytes	Diagnosis Monitoring Prognosis	Normal Igs are polyclonal. Few free light chains exist.	Monoclonal gammopathy of undetermined significance (MGUS), amyloidosis, nonsecretory myeloma	Bence Jones proteins are free Ig light chains in urine detected by urine immunofixation electrophoresis or serum free light-chain assays.
Monoclonal Igs	Plasma cell, B lymphocytes	Diagnosis Monitoring Prognosis	Normal Igs are polyclonal	Monoclonal gammopathy of undetermined significance	Monoclonal IgG/IgA—multiple myeloma Monoclonal IgM—Waldenström macroglobulinemia
PSA	Prostate	Screening Diagnosis Monitoring Prognosis	No tissues other than prostate	UTI or prostatitis, benign prostatic hypertrophy	Levels directly proportional to prostate size. Many elevations are benign or not clinically significant. Screening may be conducted in men aged 50 and older, based on patient decision. Decreased percent of free PSA and a PSA velocity greater than 0.75 ng/mL/year are more strongly associated with prostate cancer. Collect specimen before ejaculation, digital rectal examination, or prostate manipulation.

Table 17-4 Common Tumor Markers—cont'd

MARKER	CANCER(S)	USES	NORMAL SOURCES	NONCANCEROUS CONDITIONS WITH ELEVATIONS	COMMENTS
PTH and Ca++	Parathyroid carcinoma	Diagnosis Prognosis Monitoring	Parathyroid glands	In hypocalcemia, increased PTH is expected. Serum Ca++ may be high when PTH is elevated in parathyroid carcinoma.	PTH has a short half-life, so levels are commonly measured minutes after surgery to ensure complete parathyroid tumor removal.
TG	Thyroid	Monitoring	Thyroid	TG reflects thyroid mass, injury, and TSH levels. Thyroid markers (T4, TSH) are generally normal in thyroid cancer.	Assays must simultaneously test for thyroglobulin antibodies because these can cause falsely decreased results. Often tested after TSH stimulation (or less often, by withholding thyroid medication) to see if TG production by residual tumor cells occurs.

AFP = alpha-fetoprotein; CA = carbohydrate antigen; Ca++ = serum calcium; CD = clusters of differentiation in WBC; CEA = carcinoembryonic antigen; ER or PR = estrogen or progesterone receptors;
hCG = human chorionic gonadotropin; Ig = immunoglobulis; PTH = parathyroid hormone; PSA = prostate-specific antigen; TG = thyroglobulin; TSH = thyroid-stimulating hormone; UTI = urinary tract infection; WBC = white blood cell.

correlation with HCC, and by combining AFP with other laboratory markers, such as des-γ-carboxy-prothrombin (DCP), the liver enzyme alanine aminotransferase (ALT), and platelet count. In addition, high levels of AFP are associated with a poor prognosis in patients with HCC, whereas decreasing levels over time indicate a good response to therapy.

AFP is also an established tumor marker for nonseminomatous germ cell cancers of the testes (NSGCTs). This marker, along with other markers such as human chorionic gonadotropin (hCG; see section later in this chapter) and lactate dehydrogenase (LDH), plays an important role in patient diagnosis, tumor staging, therapeutic monitoring, and detection of relapse. AFP is elevated in 10% to 20% of patients with stage I NSGCT and in nearly all patients in later stages of the disease. As in HCC, increased concentrations are associated with a poor prognosis, whereas declining levels reflect responsiveness to therapy.

In addition to its applications as a tumor marker, AFP is widely used as a marker to detect abnormalities in the fetus. An increased level of AFP in the serum or amniotic fluid of a pregnant woman is seen with open neural tube defects such as spina bifida, whereas low levels of AFP are associated with Down syndrome.

Cancer Antigen 125 (CA 125)

Cancer antigen 125 (CA 125) is a large, heavily glycosylated, mucin-like protein that is a marker for ovarian cancer. This marker is not unique to ovarian tumors because it is also found in the normal ovary as well as other tissues, including the endocervix, endometrium, fallopian tubes, pleura, pericardium, and peritoneum and the epithelial tissues of the colon, pancreas, lung, kidney, prostate, breast, stomach, and gallbladder.

CA 125 has been the standard marker for ovarian cancer. It has multiple applications to the disease, ranging from screening and diagnosis to prognosis and monitoring response to therapy. Serum CA 125 levels greater than 35 kU/L are considered to be above normal. Although 90% or more of women with ovarian cancer in stages II to IV have elevated CA 125, the marker is not recommended for screening of the general population because it lacks sensitivity and specificity. Elevated CA 125 levels are only seen in 50% to 60% of women with stage I ovarian cancer; therefore, generalized screening would miss about half of the women during the period when the disease is most treatable. In addition, CA 125 is not specific because it can increase during pregnancy or menstruation or because of benign gynecological conditions such as endometriosis, nongynecological conditions involving inflammation, and other malignancies. However, annual CA 125 testing, together with transvaginal ultrasound, is recommended for women with a family history of ovarian cancer because early detection and intervention are likely to be beneficial in this population. In addition, the sensitivity and specificity of testing can be increased when CA 125 is combined with testing for human epididymis protein 4 (HE4), a glycosylated protein that is elevated in about 80% of patients with the epithelial subtype of ovarian cancer.

The value of CA 125 can also be seen in clinical applications other than screening. For example, an elevated CA 125 concentration combined with imaging has been shown to be highly sensitive and specific for a differential diagnosis of ovarian cancer from benign pelvic masses, especially in postmenopausal women. Serial CA 125 testing is beneficial in monitoring a patient's response to chemotherapy and is recommended before treatment is initiated, during treatment, and during patient follow-up. Rising concentrations of CA 125 over time can predict recurrence of the disease. Persistent elevations of CA 125 or an initial CA 125 value greater than 65 kU/L point to a poor prognosis.

Carcinoembryonic Antigen (CEA)

Carcinoembryonic antigen (CEA) is a glycoprotein with a molecular weight of 180,000 to 200,000, depending on the exact structure of its carbohydrate side chains. CEA was the first oncofetal antigen to be discovered. In 1965, Gold and Freedman described its presence in tissues from the fetal colon and colon adenocarcinoma, as well as its absence in colon tissues from healthy adults.

Increased serum concentrations of CEA are associated with colorectal cancer, and CEA is the most widely used marker for that cancer. The main application of CEA is in monitoring patients undergoing therapy for colorectal cancer. It is recommended that the medical team obtain a baseline CEA value from the laboratory just before therapy, followed by CEA testing every 1 to 3 months during active treatment. Increasing CEA levels are a highly sensitive indicator of liver metastasis and can detect recurrent colorectal cancer by an average of 5 months before clinical symptoms appear. CEA measurement should be used in conjunction with clinical examination, radiological testing, and histological confirmation to maximize its sensitivity in detecting disease recurrence. CEA levels can also be used in determining the most appropriate treatment for colorectal cancer patients because those with higher baseline levels before surgery tend to have a poorer prognosis.

However, CEA is not recommended for colon cancer screening because of its low sensitivity and specificity in this situation. CEA is not increased in all patients with colorectal cancer, and elevated CEA levels can be present because of other conditions, including colitis, diverticulitis, irritable bowel syndrome, and nonmalignant liver disease. Cigarette smoking can cause an increase in CEA level to nearly twice that of nonsmokers. CEA levels can also be elevated in other cancers, notably those of the breast, gastrointestinal tract, pancreas, and lung.

Human Chorionic Gonadotropin (hCG)

Human chorionic gonadotropin (hCG) is best known as the "pregnancy hormone" because it is synthesized by trophoblasts, cells that contribute to the development of the placenta and promote implantation of the embryo. Accordingly, it rises during the first few weeks of gestation, when it can be detected in the blood and urine of pregnant women. In addition, hCG can be produced by certain malignant tumors; elevations are associated with germ cell tumors of the ovary and testes as well as choriocarcinoma, a rare type of cancer that is caused by malignant transformation of the trophoblast cells. In these tumors, testing for hCG is recommended as an aid in diagnosis, prognosis, monitoring response to therapy, and detection of recurrence.

hCG is a 45,000-MW glycoprotein that is composed of an α subunit, which is shared by luteinizing hormone (LH), follicle-stimulating hormone (FSH), and thyroid-stimulating hormone (TSH), and a β subunit that is unique to hCG. Most serological tests for hCG measure multiple forms of hCG—intact hCG, the hCG β subunit, and hCG fragments—because some patients with testicular cancer may only produce a single form in elevated amounts. This reduces the chance of obtaining false-negative results. Patients should be monitored using the same test because assays can have variability in the hCG forms detected. Because hCG levels can also increase in men as the result of malfunction of the testes, it is important to observe rising values in sequential tests before making a diagnosis of testicular cancer. Elevations of hCG can also occur because of gonadal suppression caused by chemotherapy and do not necessarily indicate tumor recurrence.

Prostate-Specific Antigen (PSA)

Prostate-specific antigen (PSA) is the most widely used marker for prostate cancer. It is a 28,000-MW glycoprotein that is produced specifically by epithelial cells in the prostate gland. PSA was first discovered in semen, where its function is to regulate the viscosity of the seminal fluid to facilitate mobility of the sperm cells. Its presence was subsequently noted in serum, where it is frequently elevated in patients with prostate cancer.

The specificity of PSA for the prostate gland led to its routine use as a screening test for prostate cancer. Since its approval by the U.S. Food and Drug Administration (FDA) in 1994, PSA testing has resulted in a dramatic increase in the detection rate of early-stage prostate cancer and in the rate of 5-year patient survival. Despite these successes, general screening for prostate cancer has been a controversial issue because it may potentially lead to unnecessary testing and treatment. There are several reasons for this concern. Although PSA is specific for prostate tissue, it is *not* specific for prostate cancer. PSA can also be elevated in other conditions affecting the prostate gland, such as *benign prostatic hyperplasia (BPH)*, an enlargement of the prostate gland that commonly occurs as men age, or prostatitis, an inflammation of the gland occurring because of infection or irritation. Transient increases in PSA levels can also occur if samples are collected shortly after ejaculation, digital rectal examination (DRE), or prostate manipulation. As such, there is concern that general PSA screening can lead to the performance of unnecessary prostate biopsies and risk of infection and other complications. In addition, many prostate cancers are slow growing and would be unlikely to cause death during an older man's remaining life span. Furthermore, the conventional treatments for prostate cancer, radical prostatectomy, and radiotherapy can be associated with significant side effects, most notably urinary incontinence, erectile dysfunction, and problems with bowel function. Therefore, some clinicians believe that it may be better to carefully monitor the condition over time, by active surveillance and observation ("watchful waiting"), than to initiate treatment for early-stage prostate cancer that could decrease quality of life.

Large clinical trials that tested thousands of men to determine the benefits and harms of PSA screening have produced conflicting results. Therefore, the American Cancer Society, the American Urological Association, and the U.S. Preventative Services Task Force recommend that the decision to receive PSA testing should be up to individual patients following a discussion with their physician about the benefits and harms of testing. Testing should be performed along with a DRE. The largest benefit is thought to be for men aged 55 to 69. A total PSA value of 0 to 4.0 ng/mL is generally considered to be normal. Prostate biopsy is recommended for men with a total PSA value greater than 4.0 ng/mL to determine whether the elevation is caused by malignancy.

Another application of PSA testing is to assist in the differential diagnosis of prostate cancer. It is important to distinguish between BPH, weakly aggressive prostate cancers, and highly aggressive cancers using PSA. Modifications in PSA testing may be helpful in making this differentiation. One modification involves testing for free PSA and the naturally occurring PSA-α-1-anti-chymotrypsin complex, in addition to total serum PSA. This combination increases the specificity of testing because the proportion of free PSA is higher in benign conditions, whereas the proportion of complexed PSA is greater in prostate cancer. Because free PSA quickly degrades at temperatures above 4°C, it is important to perform testing within 3 hours of sample collection or to store the sample at –70°C if a longer time interval is required.

Another approach is to calculate the PSA velocity (PSAV), or the rate of increase in PSA values over time. PSAV is calculated as the difference in PSA concentration divided by the number of years spanning the interval between sequential tests (reported as ng/mL/year). The rationale for this approach is that PSA will increase more rapidly if a growing tumor is present. A PSAV greater than 0.75 ng/mL/year has been shown to be strongly associated with the presence of prostate cancer. To rule out the possibility that an increase in PSAV is because of an infection of the prostate gland, a repeat measurement of PSAV can be conducted after a course of antibiotics is administered.

Calculation of the PSA density (PSAD), or the ratio of total PSA to the prostate gland volume, may also be performed to increase the specificity of the PSA measurement. The rationale behind this test is that an increase in serum PSA is more likely to be caused by cancer in a man with a small prostate gland versus a large prostate gland. PSAD is calculated as the total serum PSA concentration divided by the volume of the prostate gland, which is determined by transrectal ultrasonography.

In addition, molecular testing for PCA3, a noncoding ribonucleic acid (RNA) specific to prostate tissue, may be performed on urine samples. PCA3 is overexpressed in men with prostate cancer and may provide additional information in determining whether a prostate biopsy is needed.

PSA testing also plays an important role in the management of patients known to have prostate cancer. PSA values, in conjunction with histological observation of prostate biopsy tissue, can be used to predict the stage of prostate cancer and to guide physicians in determining optimal treatment. In addition, a rapid rise in PSAV or in the amount of time it takes for the PSA level to double are indicators of more aggressive disease. A persistently high level of PSA after radical prostatectomy indicates that residual disease is present. When surgery is successful in removing the tumor, PSA will decrease to undetectable levels. Rising PSA levels after surgery are a sign that the malignancy is recurring and can precede other indicators of disease recurrence by many years. PSA testing is a sensitive indicator of disease recurrence in men who have undergone hormonal therapy but is less sensitive in detecting recurrence after radiation therapy because circulating PSA levels decline more slowly after that type of treatment.

Laboratory Detection of Tumors

Three types of laboratory methods are routinely used for cancer screening and diagnosis: gross and microscopic morphology of tumors, detection of tumor markers by immunohistochemistry or automated immunoassays, and molecular diagnostics to detect genetic mutations in the malignant cells. These techniques are complementary in that many of the changes in DNA and subsequent mRNA expression result in altered protein antigens or morphology.

Tumor Morphology

Pathologists and histology laboratories process suspected tumor tissue with gross dissection and preparation of slides for microscopic analysis. Tumor marker antibodies, special stains, and nucleic acid probes can be applied to the slides to enhance visible features. Even so, evaluation of morphology and staining patterns can be very subjective, and classification categories can be rather broad. Considerable skill is required to accurately diagnose cancer on the basis of morphology; the final diagnosis is generally made with supplemental clinical information and additional testing.

Immunohistochemistry

Immunohistochemistry detection uses labeled antibodies to detect tumor antigens in formalin-fixed or frozen tissue sections of tumor biopsy material. Before testing, formalin-fixed sections must be treated with heat to make the antigen epitopes accessible. The indirect staining method is used because larger immune complexes are formed, providing more sensitive amplification of the signal than is achieved through direct staining. An unlabeled primary antibody specific for the antigen to be detected is applied to the tissue section on a slide. Following an incubation and wash, a labeled secondary antibody directed against the Fc portion of the primary antibody is applied. The label can be an enzyme such as peroxidase, alkaline phosphatase, or glucose oxidase; or a fluorescent dye such as fluorescein isothiocyanate (FITC), rhodamine, or Texas red. Immunofluorescence provides a greater dynamic range than immunochromatographic staining and is particularly useful for the identification and quantification of co-localized proteins. Binding is visualized by light microscopy after the addition of the appropriate chromogen in the case of enzyme labels and by fluorescent microscopy when fluorescent labels are used.

The use of positive and negative control tissues is essential for accurate results. Negative controls are necessary to ensure that the staining observed is because of antibody binding and not the background (i.e., nonspecific reactivity), whereas positive controls confirm that the antibody reagents are working properly. Normal tissue on the same slide can serve as an excellent internal control. The accuracy of the results is also increased when a broad panel of antibodies is used.

Clinically, immunohistochemistry is used as an effective technique of classifying tumors of uncertain origin because many tumors can have a similar appearance histologically. To be helpful in pathological diagnosis, the marker must be differentially expressed in the tumor of origin as compared with other tumors. The first step in immunohistochemistry is to broadly classify the tumor into one of three major lineages: *epithelial, mesenchymal,* or *hematopoietic*. This can be accomplished through the use of stains for specific markers that are characteristic of each type of tissue. Routinely, *cytokeratins,* which are intermediate filaments found in all types of epithelial cells, are used as markers for tumors of epithelial lineage. There are 20 different cytokeratin subtypes, whose expression is often organ and tissue specific and dependent on the stage of differentiation of the cells. *Vimentin,* an intermediate filament that is found in most mesenchymal cells, is used as a marker to indicate the presence of a sarcoma or melanoma, but its specificity is low because it is expressed in some other tumor types as well. **CD45**, a WBC marker (see Chapter 1), can be used to identify hematopoietic malignancies.

Once these broad differentiations are made in terms of cell lineage, antibodies for more specific markers can be used for more precise classification of the neoplasm. For example, antibodies to numerous CD antigens can be used to identify the various lymphoid and myeloid cell types (see Chapter 18). In addition, antibodies to estrogen receptors, progesterone receptors, and the HER2 antigen can be used to classify breast cancer and guide decisions about appropriate therapy. Automated immunohistochemistry assays have been developed that allow for quantitation of the proteins expressed by different cell populations.

Connections

Detecting Immune Complexes With Streptavidin-Biotin

Immune complexes can be more easily detected if an additional layer is added to the reaction. A common way to add this layer is to take advantage of streptavidin-biotin binding. Streptavidin, a bacterial protein similar to the avidin protein found in egg whites, has a strong affinity for the B vitamin, biotin. Therefore, in some enzyme-labeling assays, the secondary antibody is labeled with biotin, and a streptavidin-labeled enzyme is added in the next step. This forms a larger complex that contains more enzyme molecules, increasing the signal intensity and making the assay more sensitive (see Chapter 11).

Immunoassays for Circulating Tumor Markers

Serum tumor markers are most commonly measured by immunoassays because they are highly sensitive, lend themselves to automation, and are relatively easy to use. Despite their advantages, immunoassays can be affected by several factors that need to be considered when the results are interpreted. These factors are related to the use of antibodies as reagents.

First, antibody reagents from different manufacturers can vary greatly in terms of what they detect, particularly if monoclonal antibodies are used. Thus, it is important to use the same method for monitoring patients through time because the results can be affected if patients change clinics or laboratories. It also means that if laboratories switch methods, they must provide a transition period during which samples are measured by both methods and specimens are archived until new data are established for each patient.

Second, although antibodies are employed for their specificity, it is not absolute. Antibodies will cross-react with similar structures, which is particularly problematic when the cross-reacting substances are present in excessive amounts, as can occur with cancer. For example, the α subunit of hCG is virtually identical to the α subunit of LH, and the β subunits of the two hormones are 80% homologous, so epitope choice is quite important. Furthermore, assay configuration influences what is measured. For example, some tumors may produce free α and free β chains in addition to intact hCG, so an immunochemical method that detects only β chain epitopes to minimize LH interference will measure something completely different than a method that measures intact hCG.

A third factor that can affect immunoassay results is antigen excess. By virtue of their unchecked growth and aggressive metabolism, some neoplasms may produce massive amounts of tumor marker molecules. When the measurements exceed the linear range of reportable results, a **high-dose hook effect** can be created, which can result in a falsely decreased measurement in the area of antigen excess. In such cases, the sample must be diluted to determine its value within the reportable range. It is critical that criteria be developed to identify situations in which the hook effect may be present so that specimens can be systematically diluted and accurate results obtained. A related problem of antigen excess in automated systems is sample carryover, so testing of the sample adjacent to the specimen with excessive antigen may also need to be repeated.

Connections

Postzone and High-Dose Hook Effect

Recall from Chapter 10 that equivalent amounts of antigen and antibody are required for the formation of large lattice-like complexes that can be detected in a laboratory test. If a tumor antigen is present in extreme excess as compared with the reagent antibody, a *postzone* is created in which saturation of the antibody binding sites with antigen inhibits the cross-linking required to form the lattices. The curve that shows the relationship of the tumor marker concentration and the intensity of the reaction signal takes on the shape of a hook (see Fig. 11–6). Samples in the downward slope of the hook have a large amount of antigen but give a decreased reaction signal. Sandwich-type immunoassays are most susceptible to this effect.

A final problem with immunoassays is that interference can be caused by the presence of endogenous heterophile, anti-animal, or autoantibodies in the patient sample. Significant interferences can result from human anti-mouse antibodies (HAMAs), which are high-avidity antibodies produced by some patients who have received passive immunotherapy with mouse monoclonal immunoglobulins (see Chapter 25). Because many immunoassays use mouse monoclonal antibodies as reagents, endogenous HAMAs in the patient sample can interfere profoundly with the reaction, causing either falsely elevated (most commonly) or falsely decreased test results. The principle of interference resulting in a false-positive result is illustrated in Figure 11–7.

Connections

Autoantibodies and Heterophile Antibodies

Autoantibodies are produced in response to self-antigens (see Chapter 15). An example of an autoantibody that can cause interference is rheumatoid factor, an anti-immunoglobulin G (IgG) that could potentially bind to IgG antibodies in an immunoassay reaction. Heterophile antibodies may be produced in a variety of conditions and are capable of reacting with similar antigens from unrelated species. These antibodies generally have low avidity but can bind to a broad range of antigens, which may include reagents used in immunoassays, to produce aberrant results.

To confirm the presence of interfering antibodies, the sample can be diluted, and the linearity of the results can be analyzed. Specimens with interfering antibodies tend to exhibit nonlinear behavior. The laboratory can also test directly for the antibodies themselves. The likelihood of interference by endogenous antibodies can be reduced by pretreatment of the sample with commercial blocking reagents. These reagents are typically mouse or rabbit immunoglobulins that bind to the interfering antibodies and neutralize them. Interference with tumor marker tests can also be caused by factors that can affect other immunoassays, such as icterus, lipemia, and hemolysis. In any case, patient results should not be reported until the interference issue is resolved.

Some additional recommendations should be considered in the performance of tumor marker tests. Cutoff values for screening tests are typically selected under the presumption that a relatively low number of people being screened actually have cancer and that it would be worse to miss a cancer than to do further testing on a normal person to exclude cancer. Thus, a very high number of false positives is expected because of low disease prevalence. Establishment of a baseline level at initial diagnosis followed by serial testing over time can provide valuable information when a patient is being monitored for response to treatment or tumor recurrence. In this case, it is not a single absolute value of the tumor marker that is important but, rather, the upward or downward trend when the marker's biological half-life is considered. When performing serial testing, each test should be performed by the same laboratory with the same test kit to minimize variations in results. Testing for multiple markers, if possible, will increase sensitivity and specificity. The limitations of immunoassays have prompted a search for more specific and sensitive markers using molecular and proteomic technologies. The National Academy of Clinical Biochemistry (NACB) has published consensus guidelines regarding the clinical use of tumor markers.

Molecular Methods in Cancer Diagnosis

Because cancer is a disease process that involves many genetic alterations, scientists have searched for changes in the genome that characterize the various types and subtypes of cancer. Identification of genetic mutations has become an important tool in cancer diagnosis and the determination of prognosis.

Genetic Biomarkers

Molecular characterization is an essential component of testing for hematologic malignancies (see Chapter 18). For example, as we previously mentioned, the chromosome 9/22 (*BCR/ABL*) gene rearrangement is a well-established biomarker for CML. Rearrangements in immunoglobulin genes and T-cell receptor (TCR) genes are used to identify malignant clones of B cells or T cells, respectively, in leukemias and lymphomas. Genetic analysis is also helpful in the diagnosis of solid tumors. For example, mutations in the *MSH* genes of the DNA mismatch-repair system are helpful in the diagnosis of hereditary colorectal cancer; these alterations create microsatellite instability, an alteration in the length of repetitive DNA sequences that can be visualized by molecular testing. Molecular analysis of gene expression for the estrogen receptor (ER), progesterone receptor (PR), and HER2 can create a genetic profile that is used to classify breast cancer patients into subtypes that provide prognostic information and guide physicians in choosing therapeutic plans that have the best chances of success.

Genetic biomarkers can also be used for prospective and postdiagnostic evaluation of malignancies. Prospective markers can provide valuable information regarding the risk of an asymptomatic person of developing a particular type of cancer, the growth rate of the cancer, or the development of metastatic disease. For example, women with hereditary mutations in the *BRCA1* or *BRCA2* genes carry a 40% to 80% lifetime risk for developing breast cancer, as well as an 11% to 40% lifetime risk for ovarian cancer.

Postdiagnostic genetic markers are used to guide clinicians in making appropriate treatment decisions for known cancer patients. The FDA has approved a growing list of targeted drugs for administration in cancer patients with the appropriate genetic biomarkers. The list of approved therapies includes drugs that target tumors with alterations in the *BRAF* gene (metastatic melanoma), *KRAS* gene (colorectal cancer), *EGFR* gene (non–small cell lung cancer; NSCLC), *ALK* gene

(NSCLC), *HER2* gene (breast cancer), and *ESR1* and *PGR* genes (breast cancer). Testing for these and other genetic markers is incorporated into the clinical practice guidelines published by the National Comprehensive Cancer Network and the College of American Pathologists. Molecular testing plays an important role in identifying responders and nonresponders to the targeted medications so that the drugs can be given to patients who would most likely benefit from them.

Testing for biomarkers has been made possible through scientific advances in molecular techniques, including nucleic acid amplification techniques (NAATs), *fluorescence in situ hybridization (FISH),* microarray, and DNA sequencing. In NAATs, such as the *polymerase chain reaction (PCR),* millions of identical copies of a specific target sequence within a nucleic acid are synthesized in the laboratory from an original DNA template derived from the cancer cell population (see Chapter 12). These methods are used to amplify the sequence that potentially contains the genetic mutation of interest, allowing tiny changes in the sequence to be detected by the differences in fragment sizes that can be visualized by gel electrophoresis or binding of fluorescent probes.

Cytogenetics

Cytogenetics studies play a large role in the diagnosis and management of cancer. **Karyotype analysis** involves a visual arrangement of a person's chromosomes by their size, banding pattern, and position of the centromere (**Fig. 17–6**). This technique has been used for many years to detect the chromosomal abnormalities associated with many cancers. The number of these aberrations can increase as the disease advances. One type of abnormality that can be detected by karyotyping is *aneuploidy,* a condition in which individual chromosomes are gained or lost. Another type of abnormality that can be present in cancer cells is a *deletion,* in which a portion of a chromosome has been lost. A third type of abnormality is a *rearrangement,* involving breakage of two different chromosomes and translocation of the fragments onto the opposite chromosomes (as discussed in Chapter 18).

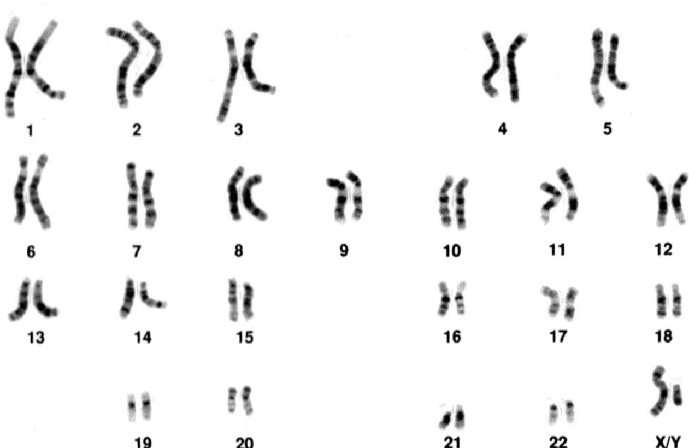

FIGURE 17–6 A normal male karyotype, containing 22 pairs of autosomal chromosomes and one pair of sex chromosomes. Karyotype analysis of tumor cells often reveals abnormalities in the number or structure of the chromosomes. *(Source: National Cancer Institute [NCI]).*

The development of **fluorescence in situ hybridization (FISH)** has allowed chromosomal abnormalities to be characterized more precisely at a molecular level. In FISH, interphase cells from the patient's tumor are incubated with fluorescent-labeled nucleic acid probes that are complementary to the sequence of interest. Cells containing the sequence will bind the probes and can be visualized with a fluorescent microscope. In oncology, FISH is most often used to detect chromosome rearrangements and gene amplification. To detect a chromosome translocation, such as the one seen in the *BCR/ABL* rearrangement characteristic of CML, two single probes are used, each specific for one of the two chromosomes involved and each labeled with a different fluorochrome (commonly, red and green). Normally, each cell should have two red signals and two green signals. If a translocation has occurred, a fusion probe signal is generated, in which the red signal is adjacent to the green signal, producing a yellow color (see Fig. 18–12B). To detect gene amplification, the probe hybridizes to the gene of interest. If that gene is overexpressed, multiple copies of the fluorescent signal representing the probe will be observed (see Fig. 12–13). This application of FISH is commonly used to detect the *HER2* gene amplification seen in some cases of breast cancer. Although FISH is a highly specific method to detect molecular abnormalities in tumor cells, it can only detect gene sequences that are complementary to the probes used; as such, it may not detect rare, tiny deletions.

Microarrays

As more clinically significant genetic abnormalities associated with cancer have been identified, **microarray** technology has been developed to test for panels of markers, rather than individual mutations. In this method, single-stranded DNA or RNA from the tumor is tagged with a fluorescent label and incubated with known nucleic acid sequences that have been spotted onto different areas of a membrane. The sample will hybridize to any complementary sequences on the tiny spots, allowing for simultaneous testing of the specimen for multiple genes. Microarrays can also be used to compare the levels of gene expression in cancer cells with those of normal cells by using two different colors of fluorescence to tag nucleic acid from each cell type (see Fig. 12–11). The microarray is interpreted with a fluorescent reader and analysis software. Microarrays can screen tens of thousands of gene sequences at the same time for their ability to bind to the sample nucleic acid, thus generating an enormous volume of information.

Sophisticated mathematics and computer software are necessary to analyze the vast amount of biological data. The collection and analysis of such data is referred to as *bioinformatics.* This approach is uncovering molecular signatures that can characterize specific tumor types and subtypes to provide better information regarding patient diagnosis and prognosis. Gene-expression arrays, such as the MammaPrint and Oncotype Dx for breast cancer, are being used to aid in predicting the likelihood of cancer recurrence and guiding treatment decisions in cancer patients.

Next-Generation Sequencing

Another molecular method that provides a large amount of data is *next-generation sequencing (NGS).* With NGS, thousands of genes within the tumor can be sequenced simultaneously in just a few hours to identify genetic variations (see Chapter 12). NGS can also be used to detect metastases by analyzing DNA from tumor cells circulating in the peripheral blood.

NGS has played a major role in generating an enormous volume of data for The Cancer Genome Atlas (TCGA). TCGA was established through a large-scale collaborative project funded by the National Cancer Institute and the National Human Genome Research Institute to catalogue and characterize the genomic changes that occur in cancer. The project has identified thousands of pertinent genomic alterations in several tumor types. This information is helping scientists to better understand the molecular aspects of cancer and has led to the development of drugs targeted to specific genetic mutations associated with malignancy. Because of the ongoing studies, molecular techniques have evolved from esoteric research tools into routine laboratory assays that have revolutionized cancer diagnosis and therapy.

Proteomics

Researchers are also analyzing the proteins produced by cancer cells. Analysis of the entire protein complement of a cell population is referred to as **proteomics.** This analysis is being done through the use of two-dimensional electrophoresis coupled with tandem mass spectrometry (MS/MS), surface-enhanced laser desorption/ionization mass spectrometry (SELDI-TOF), and **antibody arrays.** The latter is typically based on a principle of a double sandwich enzyme-linked immunoassay and is available in several different multiplex formats. The most common format uses beads that are coated with specific capture antibodies to bind the target proteins and streptavidin- or fluorescent-labeled detection antibodies that can be detected by flow cytometry. Although mass spectrometry can detect more proteins, antibody arrays do not require fractionation or depletion of high-abundance proteins to detect proteins that are present in lower concentrations; thus, the different types of methods complement each other. Proteomic methods may allow laboratories to identify unique patterns of proteins and their metabolites that are characteristic of particular types of cancer. This process is called **biomarker profiling.** In the future, data generated from proteomic methods may help clinicians diagnose cancer earlier and lead to the development of personalized therapies that can effectively target the underlying biology of this highly complex disease entity.

Interactions Between the Immune System and Tumors

Paul Ehrlich proposed the idea over 100 years ago that the immune system plays an important role in eliminating tumor cells. Ehrlich reasoned that if this were not the case, we would see cancer much more frequently in animals of advanced age. In the 1950s, after scientists learned more about how the immune system works, F. MacFarlane Burnet and Lewis Thomas independently proposed the theory of **immunosurveillance** to address this issue. This theory states that the immune system continually patrols the body for the presence of cancerous or precancerous cells and eliminates them before they become clinically evident. Burnet and Thomas based their hypotheses on early studies that involved transplantation of tumor cells in genetically inbred mice. Cells of the immune system isolated from these laboratory animals as well as from humans have been shown to kill tumor cells in the laboratory. The protective role of the immune system against tumors has also been supported by clinical evidence in humans. Notably, a significantly higher incidence of cancer has been observed in transplant patients who received immunosuppressive therapy and patients with immunodeficiency diseases than in the general population. In addition, the incidence of cancer rises greatly after the age of 60, at which point there is a decline in immune function. Although the validity of the immunosurveillance theory was challenged in the 1970s and 1980s, technical advances in genetics and monoclonal antibody technology have increased our knowledge in this area, and there is renewed enthusiasm among scientists that the immune system indeed plays an important role in defense against tumors. Ironically, some aspects of the immune response may actually promote tumor growth, and these will be discussed in the section *Immunoediting and Tumor Escape.*

Immune Defenses Against Tumor Cells

Both innate and adaptive immune responses are thought to contribute to protection of the host from cancer. The main components of the immune system that are thought to participate in defense against tumor cells are natural killer (NK) cells, macrophages, cytotoxic T lymphocytes (CTLs), cytokines, and possibly T helper (Th) cells and antibodies. The mechanisms by which each of these components function are the same as those that are involved in the elimination of pathogenic organisms **(Fig. 17–7).**

Innate Immune Responses

The key cells involved in innate immune responses to tumors are thought to be NK cells and possibly macrophages. People or laboratory animals with genetic defects in NK cells have been observed to be more susceptible to developing tumors. As we discussed in Chapter 2, NK cells act in a manner that is similar to CTLs (see the text that follows) but can kill tumor cells without prior sensitization to tumor antigens. In addition, they are activated to kill cells that lack class I MHC molecules, a property that is often seen in transformed cells (see the *Immunoediting and Tumor Escape* section later in this chapter). Activating receptors on NK cells bind to tumor antigens or substances released from stressed tumor cells, initiating intracellular signals that promote degranulation and the release of perforin and granzymes, which ultimately kill the cells by inducing apoptosis. The activity of NK cells can be increased by incubation with interleukin (IL)-2. NK cells may also participate in antibody-dependent cellular cytotoxicity (ADCC) in the presence of tumor-specific antibodies (see the text that follows). NK cells are thought to be most effective against malignant cells circulating in the bloodstream during the early stages of tumor development. Their effectiveness in eliminating well-established solid tumors is questionable, however, and requires further study.

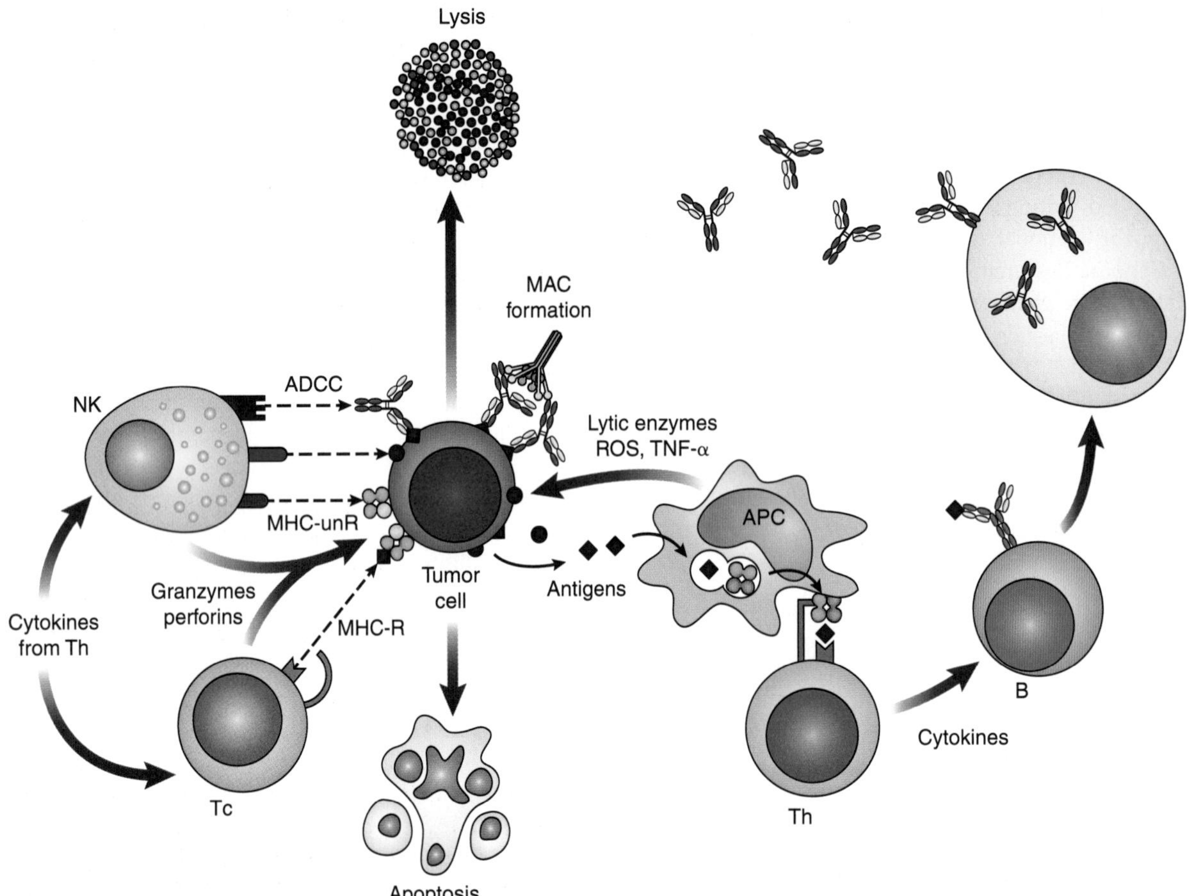

FIGURE 17–7 Immune defenses against tumor cells (MHC-R = MHC-restricted killing; MHC-unR =MHC unrestricted killing).

A subset of macrophages (called *M1*) may also play a role in innate immunity against tumors. Macrophages activated in vitro by interferon-gamma (IFN-γ) have been shown to possess tumoricidal capabilities. They appear to kill tumor cells by the same mechanisms they use to kill infectious organisms, including release of lysosomal enzymes, reactive oxygen species, and nitric oxide. In addition, they produce tumor necrosis factor alpha (TNF-α), a cytokine that is thought to cause necrosis of tumors by inducing local inflammation and thrombosis in the blood vessels within the cancerous mass. However, the significance of macrophages in anti-tumor responses in the body is unclear.

Adaptive Immune Responses

The primary mechanism of adaptive immunity against tumors is mediated by CTLs. CTL responses are thought to be initiated by dendritic cells, which act as antigen-presenting cells (APCs) by processing tumor antigens and displaying the peptides derived from these antigens on their surface in conjunction with class I MHC molecules. This mechanism is known as *cross-presentation* because the exogenous tumor antigens are presented in context with class I MHC molecules rather than class II MHC molecules. The APCs present the tumor peptide–antigen complexes to specific TCRs on the surface of the CTLs and provide costimulatory signals that promote maturation of the CTLs. The mature CTLs use their antigen-specific TCRs to bind class I MHC-associated tumor antigens on the surface of the tumor cell. Within minutes, their granules migrate toward the plasma membrane and release cytotoxic proteins within the synapse formed between the CTL and the tumor cell. Among these proteins are perforin, which creates pores in the membrane of the tumor cell, and granzymes, which enter through the pores and cause apoptosis of the tumor target (**Fig. 17–8**). NKT cells, which express surface antigens of both NK cells and T cells, are able to destroy tumor cells in a mechanism that is similar to the CTLs, but they have a unique type of TCR that recognizes glycolipid antigens instead of peptide antigens.

Dendritic cells are thought to activate CD4+ Th1 cells through presentation of tumor antigens in conjunction with class II MHC molecules. The activated Th1 cells may play a role in tumor immunity by secreting cytokines such as IL-2, which can promote CTL development and enhance NK cell activity, and IFN-γ, which activates macrophages and increases class I MHC expression on the tumor cell surface.

Tumor-bearing individuals can also produce antibodies against tumor antigens. In vitro studies have demonstrated that these antibodies can kill tumor cells by inducing complement-mediated lysis or ADCC. The latter mechanism occurs when the antibodies coat the tumor cells and bind to Fc receptors on the surface of macrophages, NK cells, or neutrophils, stimulating them to release enzymes that can destroy the tumor targets. However, the relevance of these antibodies in vivo is unclear.

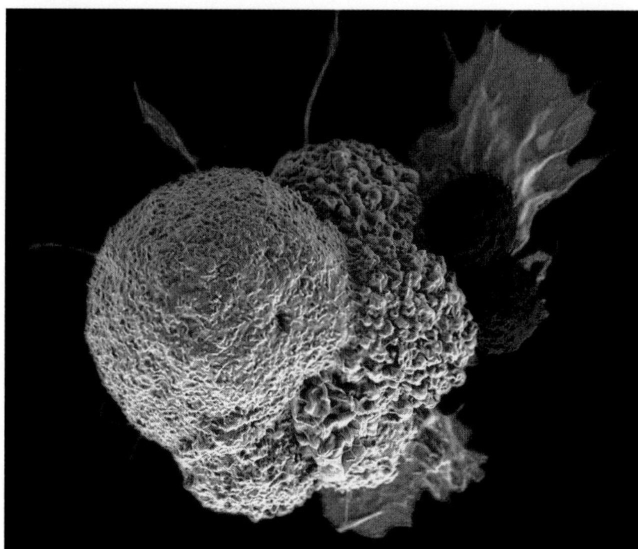

FIGURE 17–8 Tumor cell attack by cytotoxic T cells. Shown here is a pseudo-colored scanning electron micrograph of an oral squamous cancer cell (white) being attacked by two cytotoxic T cells (red). *(Source: National Cancer Institute [NCI]).*

Immunoediting and Tumor Escape

Despite evidence for innate and adaptive immune responses capable of attacking tumors, cancer occurs at a high frequency in individuals who appear to be immunocompetent. Medical scientists have long been trying to find the answer to this intriguing puzzle. As the field of tumor immunology advances, scientists are recognizing that immunosurveillance is only part of a broader process that explains the complex relationship between the immune system and cancer. This process is thought to consist of three phases: *elimination, equilibrium,* and *escape*. It involves changes in the genetics and characteristics of the tumor cells, termed **immunoediting,** that allow them to survive despite the host's immune responses **(Fig. 17–9).**

Elimination

The elimination phase of the cancer immunoediting process is essentially the same as the immunosurveillance concept that we previously discussed. If the immunologic mechanisms involved in immunosurveillance, such as destruction of cancerous cells by the host's NK cells and cytotoxic T cells, are highly effective, they will likely result in complete elimination of the tumor. If the immune responses are not completely effective, some of the tumor cells will remain in the body. These cells are then thought to enter the equilibrium phase.

Equilibrium

In this phase, tumor cells are thought to enter a state of dynamic equilibrium with the immune system, which keeps the altered cells under control so that they are not clinically evident. During this period, tumor cells may remain dormant or evolve slowly over time. The dynamic interactions between the tumor and the immune system are thought to shape the phenotype of the tumor and its ultimate outcome, hence the term *immunoediting*. Therefore, the tumor may eventually be eliminated by the body, establish permanent residence in the equilibrium phase, or evolve into a phenotype that can escape the immune system and cause disease.

During the equilibrium phase, mutations can occur in the genetically unstable transformed cells. Under selective pressure from immunologic forces of attack by cells in the tumor microenvironment (**Fig. 17–10**), some of the tumor cells may develop into genetic variants that are resistant to immune defenses, similar to the development of antibiotic resistance by bacteria. These cells move past the equilibrium phase and enter the escape phase.

Escape

During this phase, the balance between immunologic control and tumor development is tipped in favor of the neoplasm, and tumor growth progresses, even in the presence of anti-tumor immune responses. Cancer is a heterogeneous disease, and tumors have developed a variety of strategies for evading the immune system (see Fig. 17–9). Some of the escape mechanisms employed by tumors are a result of changes in the edited tumors themselves, which lead to reduced immunogenicity. For example, some tumors downregulate the expression of tumor antigens or MHC molecules on the cell surface, making them less likely to be recognized by T cells. Other modifications may involve defects in components of the antigen-processing machinery associated with class I MHC molecules. Tumor antigens may also be masked by glycoproteins and glycolipids on the cell surface, making them inaccessible to the immune system. Other alterations in surface molecules can result in tumor resistance to immune defenses. For example, impaired cell surface binding to perforin or defective apoptosis-inducing receptors, such as Fas, have been noted in some tumors.

Another way that tumors can escape the immune system is by suppressing anti-tumor immune responses. Tumors can do this directly by secreting immunosuppressive substances, or indirectly by recruiting T regulatory (Treg) cells, myeloid-derived suppressor cells, or a subset of macrophages that produce cytokines such as transforming growth factor-β and IL-10, which can inhibit protective immune responses.

Suppression of anti-tumor responses may also occur if the tumor is able to upregulate the expression of inhibitory receptors on T cells. Normally, T-cell responses are regulated by an appropriate balance of stimulatory receptors such as CD28, which activate the immune response (see Chapter 4), and inhibitory receptors called *immune checkpoint molecules*, which suppress T-cell activity. This balance maintains the necessary level of T-cell function in order to avoid autoimmune responses and damage to surrounding tissues. Two immune-checkpoint molecules that have been thoroughly studied are cytotoxic T lymphocyte antigen-4 (CTLA-4), which competes with CD28 for binding to molecules on APCs called CD80 (B7-1) and CD86 (B7-2), and programmed death-1 (PD-1), which binds to programmed death-ligand 1 (PDL-1) and programmed death-ligand 2 (PDL-2) on APCs. Increased expression of these immune-checkpoint molecules on some tumor cells may inhibit T-cell killing of those tumors.

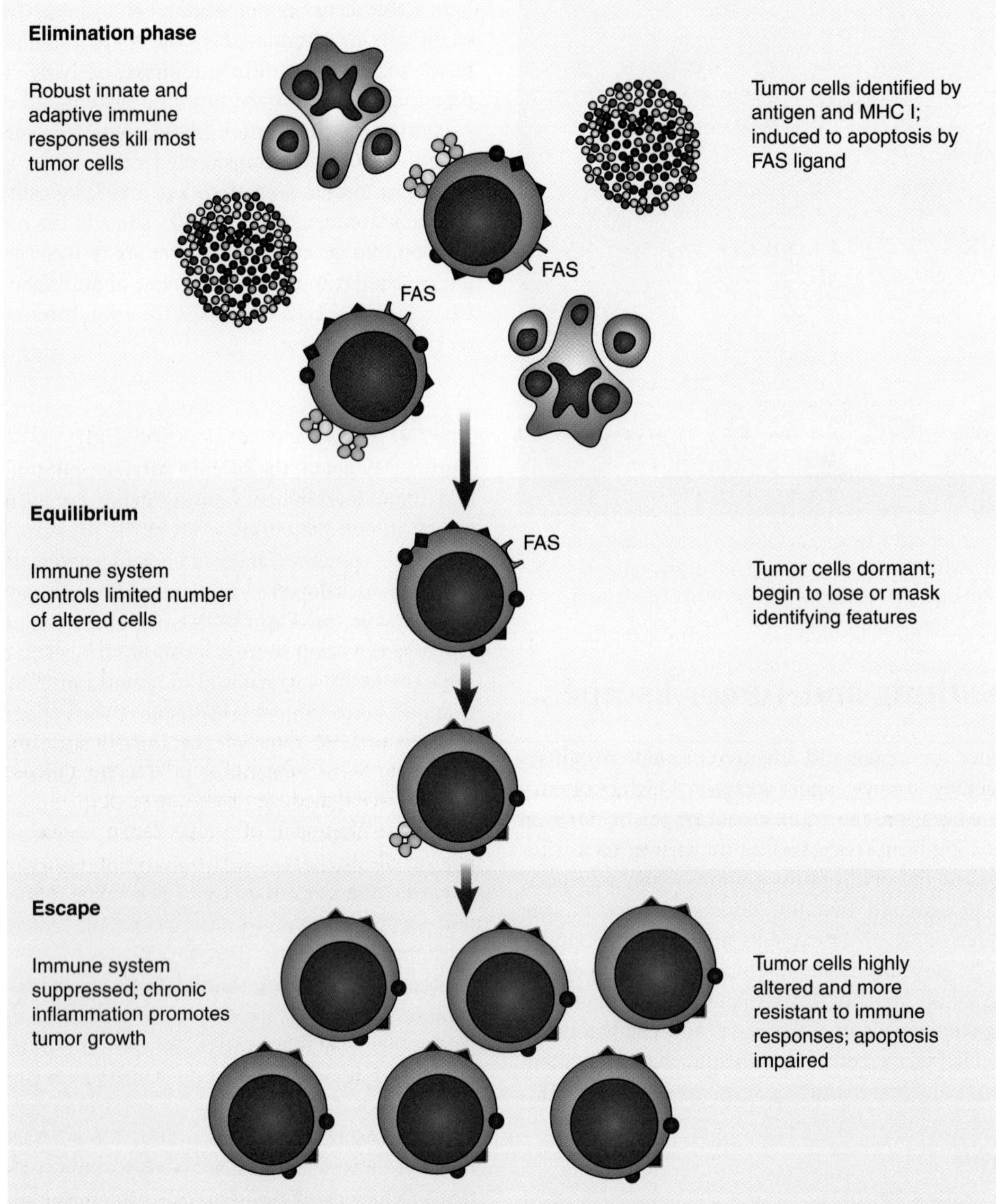
Elimination phase
Robust innate and adaptive immune responses kill most tumor cells
Tumor cells identified by antigen and MHC I; induced to apoptosis by FAS ligand
FAS
FAS
Equilibrium
Immune system controls limited number of altered cells
FAS
Tumor cells dormant; begin to lose or mask identifying features
Escape
Immune system suppressed; chronic inflammation promotes tumor growth
Tumor cells highly altered and more resistant to immune responses; apoptosis impaired

FIGURE 17–9 Relationship between the immune system and cancer: Immunoediting and mechanisms of tumor escape.

Another factor that likely contributes to tumor progression is inflammation. Although acute inflammation may be protective to the host, chronic inflammation is believed to modify the cellular microenvironment in ways that promote the development of tumors. Chronic inflammation and its associated proinflammatory cytokines may contribute to tumorigenesis in a number of ways, including generation of cellular stress and free radicals, production of growth factors that induce cell proliferation, enhancement of angiogenesis and tissue invasion, and suppression of adaptive immune responses.

The various defenses and escape mechanisms discussed in the previous paragraphs are summarized in a study guide at the end of this chapter. A clear understanding of the evasion mechanisms used by tumors and of the immune responses they suppress is critical in developing rational approaches to targeted immunotherapy. The section that follows presents specific approaches that have been taken in an attempt to influence interactions between tumors and the immune system in order to promote tumor rejection.

Immunotherapy

Many different types of treatments can be used for cancer patients. The type of therapy used for a particular patient depends on the type of tumor present and the stage of disease. Traditional therapies include surgery to remove solid tumors, radiation therapy to reduce tumor size, and chemotherapy and hormone therapy to target residual tumor cells and metastases. Advances in medical science have allowed immunotherapy to gain a position among these conventional types of

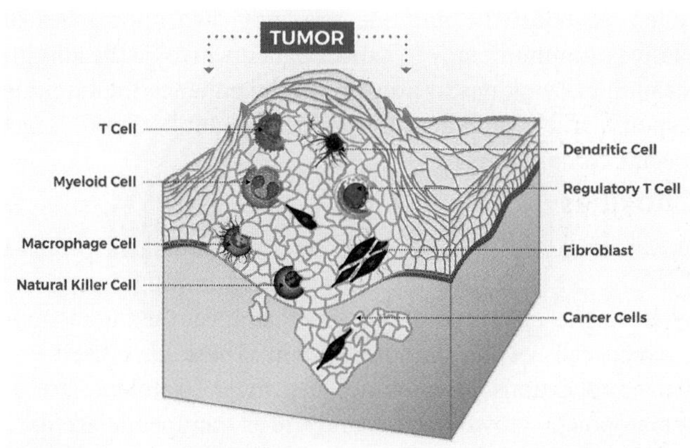

FIGURE 17–10 What is the tumor microenvironment? Within a tumor, cancer cells are surrounded by a variety of immune cells, fibroblasts, molecules, and blood vessels—what's known as the *tumor microenvironment.* Cancer cells can change the microenvironment, which in turn can affect how cancer grows and spreads. *(Source: National Cancer Institute [NCI]).*

treatment in the management of cancer. The goal of **immunotherapy,** which is also known as *biological therapy* or *biological response modifier therapy,* is to harness the ability of the immune system to destroy tumor cells.

Immunotherapeutic methods can be classified into three major types: active, passive, and adoptive. With active immunotherapy, patients are treated in a manner that stimulates them to mount an immune response against their tumors. Passive immunotherapy involves administration of tumor-specific antibodies or cytokines to patients who may not be able to develop an adequate immune response. In adoptive immunotherapy, cells from the immune system are provided to patients. Some treatments may combine different types of immunotherapy. Although it is well beyond the scope of this chapter to cover all the different protocols, the following sections present the major types of immunotherapy that have been developed and their applications to specific kinds of cancer.

Active Immunotherapy and Cancer Vaccines

The possibility of stimulating a patient's own immune system to respond to tumor antigens has long intrigued scientists. In 1891, the bone sarcoma surgeon William Coley began the first systematic study of immunotherapy. In his review of the literature, he noted that cancer patients who developed an infection after surgery experienced tumor regression and had a better prognosis than patients who did not acquire an infection. Inspired by this knowledge, he decided to inject one of his cancer patients with *Streptococcus pyogenes* bacteria. To his amazement, the patient's tumor shrank, and the patient became cancer-free. He went on to treat additional patients and observed shrinkage of their malignant tumors, although some of the patients died from infection because the bacteria were alive and virulent. Coley then developed a less dangerous version of his treatment, which consisted of a mixture of killed *S. pyogenes* and killed *Serratia marcescens* bacteria. This formulation later became known as "Coley's toxins" and was widely used by Dr. Coley and other physicians for the next 30 years to treat patients with inoperable bone and soft-tissue sarcomas.

However, Coley's treatment was controversial, and many doctors who used the toxins did not get good results, particularly with other types of cancer. In 1962, the FDA refused to recognize the formulation as an effective cancer therapy, and it became illegal to use Coley's toxins to treat cancer. Despite the criticism of Coley's work, the medical community later recognized that his premise of stimulating the immune system to effectively treat cancer bore some merit. Today we acknowledge Coley as the "Father of Immunotherapy."

Although Coley's toxins are no longer in use today, other agents have been used to nonspecifically boost the immune system. For example, Bacillus Calmette Guerin (BCG), a live but weakened strain of *Mycobacterium bovis* bacteria, is the most common immunotherapy for noninvasive bladder cancer. Serial treatments in which BCG is directly delivered into the urinary bladder through a catheter have been shown to be effective in reducing the progression of tumor growth and in delaying recurrence of the cancer in these patients. The exact mechanism by which BCG works is unknown, but it is believed to stimulate cytokine production by macrophages and activated lymphocytes, increase the anti-tumor effects of macrophages and other cells of the innate defense system, and increase T-cell–mediated immune responses.

The development of prophylactic **cancer vaccines** offers an effective approach to active immunotherapy. These vaccines have been generated for the purpose of preventing virus-associated cancers (see Chapter 25). Notably, the human papilloma virus (HPV) vaccine is effective in preventing cervical cancer, and the hepatitis B virus (HBV) vaccine has been successful in reducing the incidence of HBV infection of the liver and its associated complications, including HCC. These vaccines are routinely used and are incorporated into standard vaccination schedules.

Other cancer vaccines are being administered to patients who have already developed cancer. These vaccines are designed to induce an immune response against tumor antigens, with the hope of eliminating existing tumor cells and producing long-lasting immunity. Early cancer vaccines used tumor cell lysates or whole tumor cells that were inactivated by treatments such as irradiation. The advantages of this approach were that no knowledge was required about the tumor antigens themselves; the vaccine could theoretically contain all the antigenic components of the tumor. Unfortunately, clinical trials found that most killed tumor cell vaccines did not have a significant effect on patient survival; therefore, this approach is generally not used today.

The focus of more recent research has been on the development of antigen-specific vaccines for cancer. Some examples of common tumor antigens studied in vaccine trials include the HER2 antigen to treat a subset of breast cancer patients, the MAGE antigens for some patients with melanoma, and the p53 antigen, which is overexpressed by many tumors. A newer approach involves the use of DNA sequencing techniques to identify neoantigens that can be specifically recognized by CTLs from individual patients in a personalized form of treatment. Clinical trials are investigating ways to effectively deliver these antigens, including administration of synthetic peptides, viral vectors containing DNA that codes for the peptide antigens, mRNA packaged in carrier molecules, antigen-loaded nanoparticles, and antigen-primed dendritic cells to immunize patients against their own tumors. In some cases, the antigens are delivered along with other substances called *adjuvants* (see Chapter 25) to enhance the immune response.

Clinical Correlations

Dendritic Cell Vaccines and Provenge

To make dendritic cell (DC) vaccines, the DCs are isolated from the cancer patient and incubated with the pertinent tumor antigen or transfected with the gene that codes for the antigen. The antigen-loaded DCs are then re-administered to the patient, where they are believed to function as potent APCs. Sipuleucel-T (Provenge), the first FDA-approved cancer vaccine, is based on this technology. The vaccine is designed to treat patients with advanced prostate cancer. It is produced by incubating the patient's own peripheral blood cells with a fusion protein composed of the antigen, prostatic acid phosphatase (PAP), and the cytokine GM-CSF, which is thought to promote DC activation and induce a PAP-specific T-cell response. Clinical use of Provenge has shown a modest improvement in median overall patient survival.

Although cancer vaccines show much promise for the future, they have some important limitations. As previously mentioned, tumor cells can evade the immune response by creating an immunosuppressive microenvironment in which T cells are unable to fully exert their tumoricidal potential. It may therefore be necessary to return the tumor microenvironment to an immunosupportive tissue before a cancer vaccine can be fully effective. Scientists are attempting to do this by promoting local production of certain cytokines (e.g., IL-12 and IFN-α) and using antibodies to eliminate Treg cells or block molecules that inhibit immune responses (see *Passive Immunotherapy* later).

Unlike vaccines for infectious diseases, which are used to *prevent* infection, most cancer vaccines are immunotherapeutic, being administered *after* the disease has occurred. They are frequently given to patients in the advanced stages of disease when other treatment options have been exhausted. In this situation, the patient's immune system has often been compromised because of the disease process or the effects of chemotherapy; therefore, the response to the vaccine may be suboptimal. In these cases, it may be more beneficial to provide the patient with components of the immune system through passive or adoptive immunotherapy to more effectively target destruction of the tumor. These approaches to cancer immunotherapy will be discussed in the sections that follow.

Passive Immunotherapy

Passive immunotherapy, as previously mentioned, involves the administration of soluble components of the immune system to boost the immune response. Two approaches to passive immunotherapy in cancer patients involve the administration of cytokines to nonspecifically enhance the immune response and treatment with monoclonal antibodies to target specific tumor antigens.

Cytokines

As we discussed in Chapter 6, cytokines are small proteins that play an important role in regulating immune responses by serving as chemical messengers that affect the interactions between cells of the immune system. There have been two main applications of cytokines in cancer treatment: use as hematopoietic growth factors and use as therapeutic agents.

Because chemotherapy drugs inhibit cell division, they often adversely affect the development of hematopoietic stem cells in the bone marrow, resulting in decreased production of WBCs, red blood cells (RBCs), and platelets. **Hematopoietic growth factors,** also known as **colony-stimulating factors (CSFs),** can be administered to patients to help them recover from or prevent these toxicities. Some of the main CSFs that have been used to treat cancer patients are granulocyte colony-stimulating factor (G-CSF), granulocyte-macrophage colony-stimulating factor (GM-CSF), erythropoietin, and IL-11 (see Chapter 6). G-CSF stimulates hematopoietic stem cells to develop into granulocytes, whereas GM-CSF stimulates hematopoietic stem cells to develop into granulocytes and monocytes, thus reducing the patient's risk for severe infections. Erythropoietin stimulates production of RBCs from the bone marrow and can be used to treat patients with severe anemia. IL-11 stimulates the maturation of megakaryocytes, helping patients to recover from chemotherapy-induced thrombocytopenia.

The therapeutic application of cytokines is aimed at enhancing patients' immune responses to their tumors. Preclinical and clinical investigations have been conducted for the interferons (IFNs), tumor necrosis factors (TNFs), and several interleukins. Two examples of cytokines that have been widely studied are IFN-α and IL-2.

IFNs were the first cytokines that were used as biological response modifiers. IFN-α has been the most commonly used IFN in cancer therapy and has been approved by the FDA for the treatment of several types of cancer, including malignant melanoma, hairy cell leukemia, chronic myeloid leukemia, and Kaposi's sarcoma. IFN-α is thought to promote anti-tumor effects by increasing tumor immunogenicity, enhancing dendritic cell responses to the tumor, enhancing Th1 responses and cell-mediated cytotoxicity, promoting tumor apoptosis, and inhibiting angiogenesis. Although high doses of IFN-α are associated with better clinical responses than low doses of the cytokine, they also generate strong adverse effects, including fever, asthenia (loss of muscle strength), neutropenia, and nausea and vomiting.

Of all the interleukins, IL-2 has been the most extensively studied. IL-2 induces T-cell proliferation and enhancement of CTL and NK cell function (see Chapter 6). However, clinical trials revealed that systemic administration of IL-2 as immunotherapy was limited because of its short half-life (fewer than 10 minutes) and serious adverse effects, including vascular leakage syndrome, marked fluid retention, and shock. Although this cytokine is still used to treat metastatic melanoma and advanced renal cancer, it is rapidly cleared from the body, and its most effective use may be to activate immunocompetent cells in vitro for adoptive immunotherapy (see *Adoptive Immunotherapy* later).

Although cytokines continue to be incorporated in immunotherapy, their use has been limited because of the serious and sometimes life-threatening side effects associated with high-dose systemic treatment, as previously discussed. The cytokine network is very complicated, and the administration of a cytokine can have multiple, and sometimes unwanted, effects. For example, in addition to its immunostimulatory effects, IL-2 is also thought to be necessary for the generation and maintenance of Treg cells, which can be involved in enhancing tumor growth. Studies are under way to see if some of these obstacles can be overcome through more localized administration of cytokines, use of cells that are genetically engineered to express specific cytokine genes, or therapies using small doses of cytokines combined with each other or with chemotherapy drugs.

Monoclonal Antibodies

Monoclonal antibodies take a more specific approach to immunotherapy and play an important role in the treatment of cancer patients. As we discussed in Chapter 5, these antibodies are derived from a single clone of cells, providing for an abundant source of highly specific antibodies directed toward one particular epitope of an antigen. Monoclonal antibodies in cancer immunotherapy have been directed against many different types of antigens: CD antigens, glycoproteins, glycolipids, carbohydrates, vascular targets, stromal and extracellular antigens, and growth factors. These antibodies have different mechanisms of action, depending on their targets. The major approaches to monoclonal antibody therapy are discussed in the text that follows and summarized in **Table 17–5.**

Table 17–5 Approaches to Cancer Immunotherapy Using Monoclonal Antibodies

TARGET OF THERAPY	MECHANISM OF ACTION	EXAMPLES
Surface antigens on tumor cells	Opsonization Complement-mediated cytotoxicity ADCC	*Rituximab,* an MAb directed against the CD20 antigen on B cells; used to treat B-cell neoplasms *Alemtuzumab,* an MAb directed against mature lymphocyte antigen, CD52; used to treat chronic lymphocytic leukemia and T-cell lymphomas
Cell surface receptors	Block signaling pathways involved in cell proliferation and survival	*Panitumumab,* an MAb directed against epidermal growth factor receptor (EGFR), used to treat colorectal cancer *Trastuzumab,* an MAb directed against HER2, used to treat breast and gastroesophageal tumors with overexpressed HER2
Antigens involved in angiogenesis	Inhibit formation of blood vessels necessary for delivery of oxygen and nutrients to the tumor	*Bevacizumab,* an MAb directed against vascular endothelial growth factor (VEGF); for treatment of colorectal, glioblastoma, lung, renal, cervical, and ovarian cancers
Immune-checkpoint molecules—block T-cell activation and proliferation by binding to molecules on antigen-presenting cells	Immune-checkpoint inhibitors—enhance anti-tumor-specific T-cell responses by preventing T-cell inhibition	*Ipilimumab,* an MAb directed against cytotoxic T-lymphocyte antigen 4 (CTLA-4); for treatment of metastatic melanoma *Pembrolizumab* and *Nivolumab,* MAbs directed against programmed death-1 (PD-1); used to treat melanoma, colon cancer, and other tumors
Antibody–drug conjugates (immunotoxins) directed against tumor antigens	Deliver potent toxic molecules directly to tumor cells	*Brentuximab vedotin,* an immunotoxin directed against the CD30 antigen; used to treat Hodgkin lymphoma and systemic anaplastic large-cell lymphoma *Trastuzumab emtansine,* an immunotoxin directed against the HER2 antigen; for treatment of HER2-positive metastatic breast cancer
Bi-specific monoclonal antibodies with two different variable regions, one that binds to the tumor antigen and the other, to a T-cell surface marker	Bring T cells close to tumor cells to facilitate direct contact and destruction of tumor cells	*Blinatumomab,* an MAb that binds to CD19 and CD3, approved for relapsed or refractory B-cell precursor ALL

ADCC = antibody-dependent cellular cytotoxicity; ALL = acute lymphoblastic leukemia; CD = clusters of differentiation; HER2 = human epidermal growth factor 2; MAb = monoclonal antibody.

Some monoclonal antibodies are directed against antigens found on the surface of the tumor cells. These antibodies are believed to destroy the tumor through the same mechanisms that are used to attack infectious organisms, namely, opsonization, complement-mediated cytotoxicity, and ADCC. A second group of immunotherapeutic monoclonal antibodies targets surface receptors involved in intracellular pathways that lead to the growth and immortality of cancer cells. These receptors are expressed at higher-than-normal levels on epithelial cancers of the colon, breast, lung, head, and neck. Therapeutic antibodies bind to these receptors and block cell signals that are necessary for activation of the molecular pathways involved in cell growth and survival.

A third group of monoclonal antibodies targets antigens involved in angiogenesis or the formation of blood vessels that are necessary to provide the oxygen and nutrients needed for tumor growth. Many of the antibodies in this category are directed against the vascular endothelial growth factor (VEGF) family of proteins or their receptors. A fourth group of monoclonal antibodies boosts the immune response to the tumor by blocking inhibitory pathways that inactivate T cells. This approach uses monoclonal antibodies to the inhibitory receptors CTLA-4 and PD-1 or its ligand PD-L1, which we discussed in a previous section. These antibodies, which are called **immune-checkpoint inhibitors**, have shown a high level of effectiveness in treating several different types of cancer. Their mechanism of action is illustrated in **Figure 17–11.**

One strategy to increase the effectiveness of monoclonal antibodies involves linking them to potent cytotoxic drugs that can be taken up by the tumor cells. These products are known as **antibody–drug conjugates** or **immunotoxins.** They reduce the systemic side effects of the toxins by localizing a small number of toxic molecules directly to the tumor cells using a tumor-specific antibody. After binding to an antigen on the tumor surface, the conjugate is quickly internalized by the cancer cell through receptor-mediated endocytosis and transported to the lysosomes. The cytotoxic drug is released from its antibody into the cytoplasm of the tumor cell, where it exerts potent toxic effects.

The first immunotoxins, derived from the plant toxin ricin, or from toxins of diphtheria-causing or *Pseudomonas* bacteria, had some effectiveness against tumors but produced toxic side effects. Improvements in linker technology and conjugate design have led to the development of products that are

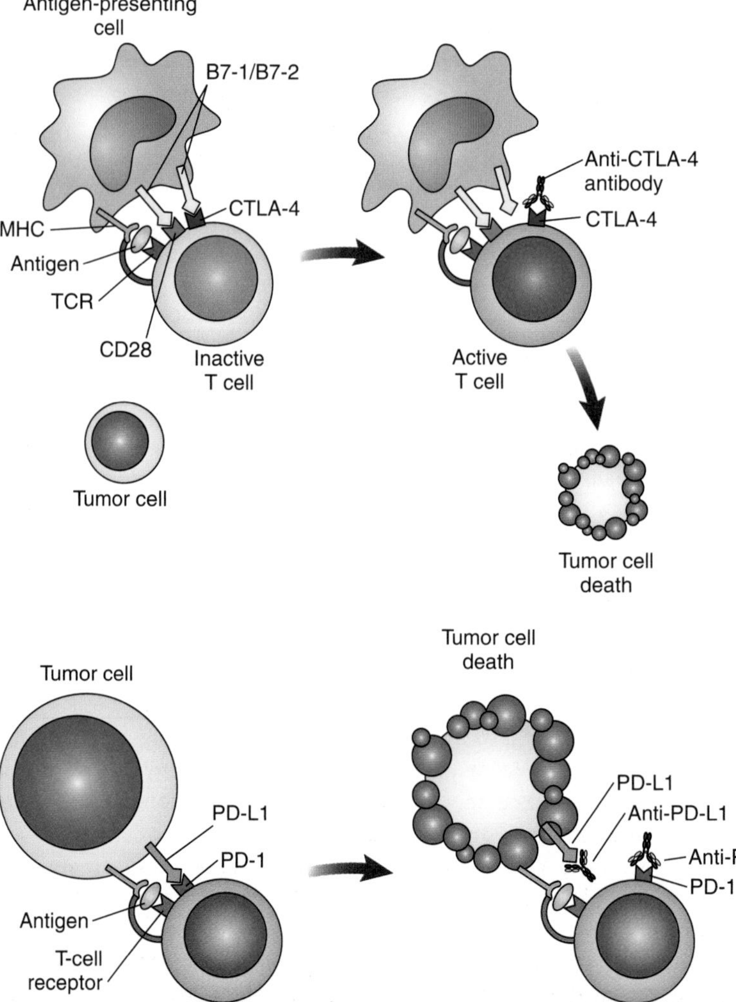

FIGURE 17–11 Immune-checkpoint molecules and inhibitors. (A) CTLA-4. The CTLA-4/B7 binding inhibits T-cell activation. Blocking CTLA-4 enables the T cell to kill the tumor cell. (B) PD-1. The PD-L1 binds to PD-1 and inhibits the T cell from killing the tumor cell. Blocking PD-L1 or PD-1 enables the T cell to kill the tumor cell.

more effective and have fewer side effects. Newer-generation antibody-drug conjugates are made from modified toxins that can be genetically engineered by cloning genes for antibody fragments with genes for the adapted toxin. Two FDA-approved preparations in clinical use are brentuximab vedotin, an immunotoxin directed against the CD30 antigen that is used to treat Hodgkin lymphoma (HL) and systemic anaplastic large cell lymphoma (sALCL), and trastuzumab emtansine, which has specificity for the HER2 antigen and is used to treat patients with HER2-positive metastatic breast cancer.

Another advance is the development of bi-specific monoclonal antibodies. These agents are produced by recombinant DNA technology and have two antigen binding sites, one that attaches to the tumor antigen and the other that binds to a T-cell marker such as CD3. Such antibodies are presumed to function by bringing T cells closer to the tumor cells of interest, so they can be more easily activated to attack the tumor cells. At the time of this writing, a bi-specific antibody that binds to CD19 has been approved for the treatment of B-cell acute lymphocytic leukemia, and several other agents are under development.

Monoclonal antibodies have been used to treat almost all major subtypes of cancer; therefore, this treatment modality has been established as one of the most successful therapeutic strategies for cancer. A listing of FDA-approved monoclonal antibodies and other drugs in oncology can be found at http://www.centerwatch.com/drug-information by searching in the FDA-approved-drugs category for the term *oncology.*

Although monoclonal antibodies have had a large impact in treating cancer, they have some limitations. Some patients develop hypersensitivity reactions to the antibody proteins. This problem has been substantially reduced as monoclonal antibody technology has evolved from making purely mouse antibody products to manufacturing fully human products (see Chapters 5 and 25). Monoclonal antibody treatment can also cause toxicity if the target antigen is expressed on normal cells. Therapy with monoclonal antibodies may be ineffective if the antibodies are unable to permeate through tumor tissues or bind their target antigen molecules with high affinity. Finally, cancer cells can develop resistance to monoclonal antibodies, analogous to the way that bacteria can develop resistance to antibiotics. Scientists are researching several new approaches to monoclonal antibody therapy that may overcome these limitations in the future.

Adoptive Immunotherapy

Scientists have reasoned that because cell-mediated immunity is so important in defense against tumors, the transfer of cells of the immune system to cancer patients may effectively assist them in eliminating tumor cells. This approach, known as **adoptive immunotherapy,** is discussed in detail in Chapter 25.

Early experiments conducted in mice in the 1960s showed that lymphoid cells from mice immunized with certain tumors were able to protect against tumor growth when they were transplanted into genetically identical mice; this response was enhanced in the presence of IL-2. In pioneering studies conducted in the late 1980s by Dr. Steven Rosenberg and his colleagues, it was discovered that adoptive immunotherapy could be applied to the treatment of human cancer. These scientists isolated lymphocytes from the surgically removed tumors of patients with metastatic melanoma and grew them in the laboratory in the presence of IL-2. They found that these cells, referred to as **tumor-infiltrating lymphocytes (TILs),** demonstrated potent cytolytic activity against autologous melanoma cells. Taking these findings a step further, they prepared expanded populations of TILs from melanoma patients in the laboratory and infused them back into the same patients in the presence or absence of IL-2. These early studies found only a slight improvement in patient response but demonstrated the potential value of adoptive immunotherapy for human cancer.

Subsequent modifications of technique resulted in significantly improved patient outcomes. Instead of administering the entire population of TILs, cells are subcultured and individually tested for their reactivity to the tumor **(Fig. 17–12).** Only the cultures that show potent anti-tumor activity are selected for further expansion and infusion into patients. In addition, the effectiveness of the therapy has been improved by pretreating patients with total body irradiation or high-dose chemotherapy before conducting the adoptive cell transfer. This pretreatment is thought to eliminate cells that could exert immunosuppressive effects before the treatment begins. Adoptive therapy with autologous TILs has shown good clinical response rates in patients with malignant melanoma but has not yet been successful with other types of cancer, which are probably less immunogenic.

An alternative type of treatment that has created much excitement among immunologists is **CAR-T cell therapy.** In this type of therapy, a patient's peripheral blood WBCs are collected and enriched for T cells, which are then genetically engineered to possess *chimeric antigen receptors (CARs)* and infused back into the patient. CARs are most often constructed by combining the antigen-binding variable fragment of a monoclonal antibody to a specific tumor antigen with intracellular domains of the TCR and costimulatory molecules to provide activating signals to the T cells (see Chapter 25 and Fig. 25–11 for more details). CAR-T cell therapy has generated much interest because CARs can target specific tumor antigens in an MHC-independent manner so that the product can be universally used instead of being restricted for patients with a particular HLA type. At the time of this writing, CD19-specific CAR-T cell therapies have been approved by the FDA for patients with B-cell ALL or large B-cell lymphoma for whom other treatments have not been effective.

Although adoptive immunotherapy holds much promise, some toxicities have been reported, notably an intense inflammatory response resulting from excessive release of cytokines. In addition; resistance to the therapy may develop in some patients because the targeted antigen may be lost by tumor cells that have not been depleted by the treatment. Finally, adoptive-based therapies are expensive, personalized treatments that are available in only a limited number of sites worldwide. Advances in technology are being explored that may make it possible to mass-produce tumor-specific T cells for use in adoptive immunotherapy in the future.

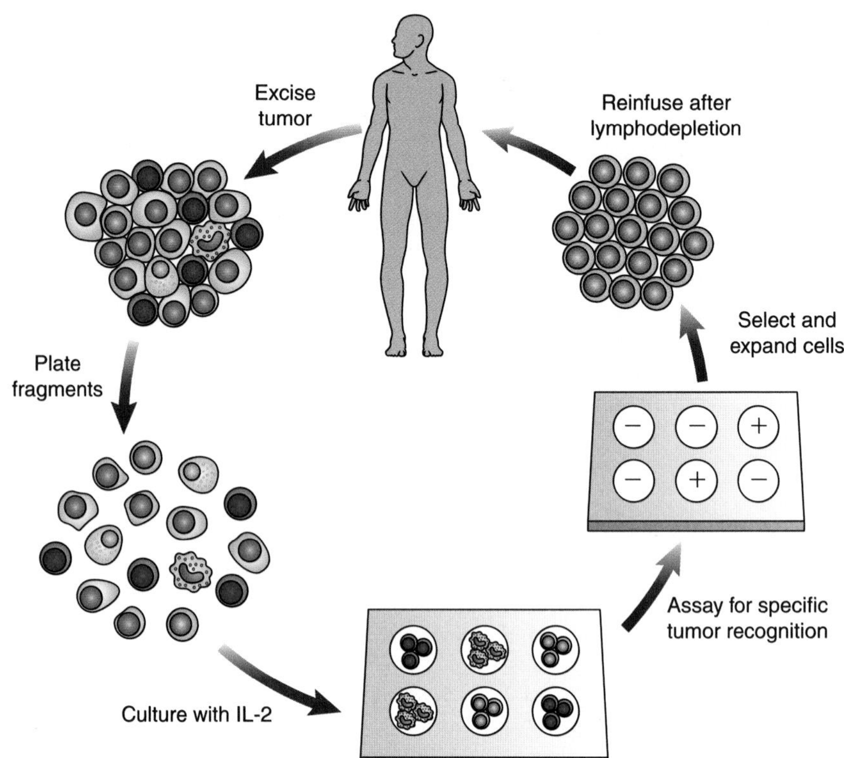

FIGURE 17–12 Adoptive immunotherapy with tumor-infiltrating lymphocytes (TILs). The patient's tumor is surgically removed and cut into fragments, which are cultured in vitro with IL-2. The cultures are screened for lymphocytes with potent anti-tumor activity. Positive cultures are expanded further in the presence of IL-2 and are infused into the cancer patient. Before infusion, the patient is treated with high-dose chemotherapy or radiation to deplete immunosuppressive cells.

SUMMARY

- Cancer arises from exposure of the host to environmental factors that induce mutations in proto-oncogenes and tumor suppressor genes. The former influence cell proliferation, and the latter regulate entry of cells into the cell cycle, maintain genetic stability, and repair damaged DNA.
- Malignant tumors consist of immortal cells that resist apoptosis and proliferate in an unregulated manner. They can also induce angiogenesis, invade nearby tissues, and spread to distant sites in the body. These characteristics are influenced by mutations, genomic instability, and inflammatory responses of the immune system.
- The concept of tumor immunology is based on the premise that tumor cells possess antigens that can be recognized as foreign by the immune system. Some antigens are tumor specific, or unique to a particular type of tumor cell, whereas others are also expressed by normal cells. The latter include the cancer/testis antigens, differentiation antigens, and overexpressed antigens.
- Tumor markers are biological substances that are increased in the blood, body fluids, or tissues of patients with a particular type of cancer. They can be detected by immunohistochemistry, automated immunoassays, or molecular methods and are used in cancer screening and diagnosis, determining patient prognosis, and monitoring patient response to therapy.
- The ideal tumor marker should be produced by the tumor or by the patient's body and be secreted into a biological fluid, where it can be easily and inexpensively quantified. It should rise with increasing tumor load and have a high sensitivity and specificity. Most tumor markers do not possess these characteristics and are therefore not suitable for screening the general population.
- Tumor markers are best used to monitor patient response to therapy by performing serial measurements over time. If therapy is effective, the amount of tumor marker will decrease. Ineffective therapy and recurrence of cancer are indicated by an increase in the tumor marker level.
- Some commonly used serum tumor markers and their primary cancer associations are presented in Table 17–4.
- Tests for circulating tumor markers are most commonly performed by highly sensitive, automated immunoassays. Their results can be affected by reagent variability among manufacturers, cross-reactivity with similar antigens, tumor antigen excess (producing a high-dose hook effect), or presence of heterophile, anti-animal, or autoantibodies in the patient sample.
- Molecular techniques such as PCR, FISH, and microarray are commonly used in clinical testing for tumor markers. DNA sequencing is being used increasingly to identify mutations associated with cancer.
- The hypothesis of immunosurveillance states that the immune system continually patrols the body for cancer cells and eliminates them before they become clinically evident.

- There are innate and adaptive immune responses against tumor cells. Innate responses are mediated by NK cells and macrophages. Adaptive immune responses are mediated by cytotoxic T cells and possibly by antibodies, activated Th cells, and cytokines.
- Tumor cells are thought to escape these responses through the process of immunoediting, which allows some of the tumor cells to develop into genetic variants that are resistant to immune defenses.
- Mechanisms by which tumor cells can escape immune defenses include avoiding immune recognition by downregulation of surface class I MHC molecules, resistance to apoptosis, suppression of anti-tumor immune responses, and chronic inflammation.
- The purpose of immunotherapy is to harness the ability of the immune system to destroy tumor cells. Immunotherapeutic approaches include stimulating the immune system with cancer vaccines, passive therapy with monoclonal antibodies, and adoptive immunotherapy with tumor-infiltrating lymphocytes or genetically engineered T cells.

Study Guide: Clinical Applications of Tumor Markers

CLINICAL APPLICATION	PURPOSE AND COMMENTS	BENEFITS	LIMITATIONS	EXAMPLE
Screening	To identify cancer in asymptomatic individuals in a population.	Detection of cancer at an early stage.	False-positive results can lead to patient anxiety, unnecessary testing, and overtreatment. False-negative results can give misleading reassurance.	PSA
Diagnosis	To identify cancer in a particular patient Presence of the marker or an elevation of the marker above normal levels suggests the presence of the cancer.	Helps distinguish between diseases with similar clinical manifestations.	Tests by themselves are not diagnostic and should be used in conjunction with other tests and clinical findings.	PSA
Prognosis	To predict the clinical outcome of a cancer patient and aid in therapeutic decision-making. An initial high concentration or an increasing level of the tumor marker over time indicates a worse prognosis.	Used to identify the level (minimal to aggressive) and type of therapy that is best for a particular patient.		HER2
Monitoring	To observe the response of a cancer patient to treatment. Effective treatment is indicated by decreasing levels of the marker over time. Increasing levels of the tumor marker indicate that the therapy is not effective.	Elevations can indicate tumor recurrence before other signs become evident.	The cancer must be positive for the marker before treatment begins.	CA 125

CA 125 = cancer antigen 125; HER2 = human epidermal growth factor 2; PSA = prostate-specific antigen.

(continued)

Study Guide: Immune Defenses to Tumors and Escape Mechanisms—cont'd

Defenses	
INNATE DEFENSES	**ADOPTIVE DEFENSES**
NK Cells	**Cytotoxic T cells**
• Kill tumor cells that lack class I MHC without prior sensitization to tumor antigens • Release perforins and granzymes, which destroy tumor cells	• Most important adaptive defense against tumors • Bind specifically to surface tumor antigens complexed with class I MHC • Release perforins and granzymes, which destroy tumor cells
Macrophages	**Th1 T helper cells**
• Some macrophages may kill tumor cells through release of lysosomal enzymes, reactive oxygen species, nitric oxide, and the cytokine TNF-α	• May bind to tumor antigens in complex with class II MHC and release cytokines that activate cytotoxic T cells and enhance NK cell activity
	Antibodies
	• Role in tumor defense is unclear • May cause tumor cell destruction through complement-mediated lysis or ADCC
ESCAPE MECHANISMS	
Antigen Modulation	**Suppression/Alteration of Immune Response**
• Altered or downregulated expression of tumor antigens because of genetic mutations • Downregulated expression of class I MHC on tumor cell surface • Defective antigen processing by APCs • Masking of tumor antigens by glycoproteins and glycolipids • Impaired surface binding to perforin or apoptosis-inducing receptors	• Tumor cells produce immunosuppressive substances • Recruitment of Tregs, myeloid suppressor cells, and macrophages that suppress immune responses against the tumor • Upregulation of inhibitory receptors such as CTLA-4 or PD-1, which block protective T-cell responses • Chronic inflammation with release of proinflammatory cytokines may promote tumor growth

ADCC = antibody-dependent cellular cytotoxicity; APC = antigen-presenting cell; MHC = major histocompatibility complex; NK = natural killer; TNF = tumor necrosis factor; Treg = T regulatory.

CASE STUDIES

1. A 45-year-old woman went to her physician's office after noticing a lump during her breast self-examination. She had a strong family history of breast cancer. The lump was detected on mammography and was found to be a 0.5-cm mass that was adherent to her skin. Analysis found her CA 15-3 levels to be 60 IU/mL, which is double the upper limit of the reference interval. After surgery, the levels of CA 15-3 dropped, but at a rate that was slower than the biological half-life. They remained above 30 IU/mL. The tumor morphology indicated malignancy, so it was tested for HER2 expression, which was elevated, and estrogen and progesterone receptors, which were negative.

Questions

a. Do you think that there is a residual tumor? If so, why?

b. In addition to chemotherapy, what other therapy would you recommend? Why?

c. What type of therapy is unlikely to be successful? Why?

2. A 66-year-old male went to his urologist complaining of frequent urination with only small volumes of urine, creating great urgency. During the DRE, the urologist felt an enlarged prostate with no distinct nodules or abnormal areas. The patient's serum level of PSA was

determined and compared with the level from the previous year. The physician also asked that the free-to-total PSA ratio be determined. The test results are shown in the data that follow.

Laboratory Results

Test	Patient Results	Reference Interval
PSA October 2020	4.2 ng/mL	0–4.0 ng/mL
PSA October 2019	3.9 ng/mL	0–4.0 ng/mL
PSA Velocity	0.30/ng/mL/year	<0.35 ng/mL/year
% free PSA/total PSA	26.2%	N/A*

Values greater than 25.0% are associated with the lowest probability of finding prostate cancer on prostate biopsy.
PSA = prostate-specific antigen.

Questions

a. Do any tissues other than the prostate produce PSA? Could there be another source of the PSA in this case?
b. What is PSA velocity?
c. Should this man have a biopsy? Do you think this man has cancer? Explain your answer.

REVIEW QUESTIONS

1. How can normal cells become malignant?
   a. Overexpression of oncogenes
   b. Mutations in tumor suppressor genes
   c. Viral infection
   d. All of the above

2. Which of the following best summarizes the concept of tumor development through immunoediting?
   a. Tumor cells produce cytokines that are toxic to T cells.
   b. Tumor cells that can escape the immune system have a growth advantage over tumor cells that are destroyed during immunosurveillance.
   c. T-cell activity causes an increase in MHC expression on tumor cells that allows them to escape the immune system.
   d. Secreted tumor antigens saturate T-cell receptors, making T cells incapable of binding to tumor cells.

3. Which of the following is an example of a tumor-specific antigen?
   a. *BCR/ABL* fusion protein
   b. CEA
   c. CA 125
   d. PSA

4. Most tumor markers are not used to screen the general population because they
   a. cannot be inexpensively quantified.
   b. do not rise to high enough levels in the presence of cancer.
   c. can also be elevated in conditions other than the cancer.
   d. vary too much between patients belonging to different ethnic populations.

5. Both AFP and hCG exhibit serum elevations in
   a. pregnancy.
   b. ovarian germ cell carcinoma.
   c. nonseminomatous testicular cancer.
   d. all of the above.

6. Suppose a patient with ovarian cancer had a serum CA 125 level of 50 kU/L at initial diagnosis. After her tumor was surgically removed, her CA 125 level declined to 25 kU/L. She received chemotherapy drug #1; after 1 year, her CA 125 level was 40 kU/L. She was then given chemotherapy drug #2, and her CA 125 level rose to 60 kU/L. These results indicate that
   a. surgery was effective in removing the patient's tumor.
   b. chemotherapy drug #1 was more effective than chemotherapy drug #2.
   c. both chemotherapy drug #1 and chemotherapy drug #2 were effective.
   d. neither chemotherapy drug #1 nor chemotherapy drug #2 was effective.

7. The hook effect that can occur in immunoassays for circulating tumor antigens is caused by which of the following in the patient sample?
   a. An excess of tumor antigen
   b. A very low concentration of tumor antigen
   c. Heterophile antibodies
   d. Autoantibodies

8. The best use of serum tumor markers is considered to be in
   a. screening for cancer.
   b. initial diagnosis of cancer.
   c. monitoring patients undergoing cancer treatment.
   d. determining patient prognosis.

9. In order to use a tumor marker to monitor the course of the disease, which of the following must be true?
   a. The laboratory measures the marker with the same method over the entire course of the patient's treatment.
   b. The marker must be released from the tumor or, because of the tumor, into a body fluid that can be obtained and tested.
   c. The marker's half-life is such that the marker persists long enough to reflect tumor burden but clears fast enough to identify successful therapy.
   d. All of the above

10. Which of the following markers could be elevated in nonmalignant liver disease?
    a. AFP
    b. CEA
    c. CA 15-3
    d. All of the above

11. Each of the following markers is correctly paired with a disease in which it can be used for patient monitoring *except*
    a. CEA/choriocarcinoma.
    b. CA 15-3/breast adenocarcinoma.
    c. CA 125/ovarian adenocarcinoma.
    d. CA 19-9/pancreatic adenocarcinoma.

12. Which of the following is a marker used in immunohistochemical staining to identify tumors of epithelial origin?
    a. Cytokeratin
    b. Vimentin
    c. CD45
    d. CD10

13. Which of the following assays would you recommend to test for chromosomal rearrangements such as the *BCR/ABL* translocation seen in CML?
    a. PCR
    b. FISH
    c. Microarray
    d. NGS

14. Innate immune responses thought to be involved in defense against tumors include
    a. NK cell-mediated apoptosis.
    b. MHC I–restricted T-cell–mediated destruction.
    c. ADCC.
    d. all of the above.

15. A woman with breast cancer is treated with a monoclonal antibody to HER2. This is an example of
    a. a cancer vaccine.
    b. an immunotoxin.
    c. passive immunotherapy.
    d. active immunotherapy.

18

Immunoproliferative Diseases

Linda E. Miller, PhD, MB^CM^(ASCP)SI

LEARNING OUTCOMES

After finishing this chapter, you should be able to:

1. Differentiate leukemias, lymphomas, and plasma-cell dyscrasias, and provide examples of each type of malignancy.
2. Describe some of the cellular properties and genetic changes that occur during malignant transformation of hematologic cells.
3. Cite the cellular characteristics used in the classification scheme recommended by the World Health Organization (WHO) for identification of the hematopoietic neoplasms.
4. Describe cell surface markers and cytogenetic abnormalities commonly associated with acute lymphoblastic leukemia, chronic lymphocytic leukemia, and hairy-cell leukemia.
5. Differentiate between Hodgkin lymphomas and various types of non-Hodgkin lymphomas in terms of their cellular origin and characteristic surface markers.
6. Associate specific CD markers with selected hematologic malignancies.
7. Describe the relationship between monoclonal gammopathy of undetermined significance (MGUS), smoldering multiple myeloma (SMM) and multiple myeloma, as well as the laboratory and clinical criteria that differentiate these conditions.
8. Correlate clinical manifestations and laboratory results with multiple myeloma or Waldenström macroglobulinemia.
9. Specify the ways in which laboratory tests can be used to diagnose and follow the progression of immunoproliferative disorders.
10. Explain the underlying principles of serum and urine protein electrophoresis (UPE), immunofixation electrophoresis (IFE), immunosubtraction (immunotyping), and serum free light-chain (sFLC) analysis.
11. Contrast the serum protein electrophoresis (SPE) and IFE results seen in monoclonal gammopathies with those observed in polyclonal increases in immunoglobulins.
12. Discuss the types of genetic abnormalities that are frequently seen in hematologic malignancies and the laboratory methods used to detect them.

CHAPTER OUTLINE

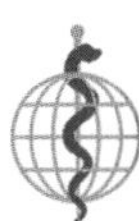

Go to FADavis.com for the laboratory exercises that accompany this text.

KEY TERMS

Bence Jones proteins
Cryoglobulins
Fluorescence in situ hybridization (FISH)
Hairy-cell leukemia
Heavy-chain diseases
Hodgkin lymphoma (HL)
Immunophenotyping
Immunosubtraction (immunotyping)
Leukemias
Lymphomas
Monoclonal
Monoclonal gammopathies
Monoclonal gammopathy of undetermined significance (MGUS)
Multiple myeloma
Non-Hodgkin lymphomas (NHLs)
Paraprotein (M protein)
Plasma-cell dyscrasias
Polyclonal
Postzone
Proto-oncogenes
Tumor suppressor genes
Waldenström macroglobulinemia

The immunoproliferative diseases refer to a diverse group of hematologic malignancies that arise from hematopoietic cells of a lymphoid or myeloid lineage. This chapter focuses on the lymphoid malignancies, which can be broadly classified as leukemias, lymphomas, and plasma-cell dyscrasias. **Leukemias** are malignancies that originate from hematopoietic cells in the bone marrow, which migrate to the peripheral blood. In contrast, **lymphomas** are solid tumors whose cells usually arise in the lymph nodes and other lymphoid tissues, such as the tonsils and spleen, and proliferate in those sites. There can be an overlap between the sites affected by leukemias and lymphomas, as leukemic cells can also be found in the lymphoid tissues and other organs in the body, and lymphoma cells may also be seen in the peripheral blood, especially when the malignancy is far advanced. However, it is generally most useful to classify the malignancy according to the site where it first arose, rather than the sites it can ultimately involve.

The **plasma-cell dyscrasias**, also known as *plasma-cell disorders* or *monoclonal gammopathies*, include malignancies of the plasma cells as well as associated premalignant conditions. These commonly involve the bone marrow, lymphoid organs, and other nonlymphoid sites. They are considered biologically distinct from the leukemias and lymphomas.

This chapter presents an introduction to some of the lymphoid malignancies that are commonly evaluated by the clinical laboratory. It is not intended to provide a comprehensive discussion of hematologic malignancies. The chapter will also cover key principles and applications of some of the laboratory tests that are essential to the diagnosis and monitoring of lymphoid malignancies.

Malignant Transformation of Hematologic Cells

Cell Properties

Hematologic malignancies are characterized by excessive accumulation of cells in the blood, bone marrow, or other lymphoid organs. This accumulation may occur because of rapid proliferation and excess production of the cells or failure of the cells to undergo apoptosis, a normal physiological process of cell death. Malignancy may reflect the result of an initially normal process in which regulatory steps to control the level of cell proliferation have failed. In addition to a failure of growth regulation, mutations can result in arrested maturation of a cell. Thus, some malignant hematopoietic cells may not develop into properly functioning mature cells but may remain at an earlier stage of differentiation and continue to replicate. Malignant and premalignant proliferation of cells can occur at any stage in the differentiation of the lymphoid lineages.

Cells of the immune system are at great risk for malignant transformation because the features that characterize the development of malignancy are also a normal part of the immune response. For example, as we discussed in Chapter 4, proliferation of T and B lymphocytes is an integral part of the immune response to an antigenic stimulus. In addition, gene rearrangements are a normal part of lymphocyte maturation, and somatic hypermutations occur in the immunoglobulin genes of the B cells during immunoglobulin class-switching and the generation of high-affinity antigen receptors. Despite being affected by abnormal regulation, malignant lymphoid cells generally retain some or all of the morphological and functional characteristics of their normal counterpart—for example, their characteristic cell surface antigens or secretion of immunoglobulin. These characteristics are often used to classify lymphoid malignancies.

Connections

Somatic Hypermutations

Recall from Chapter 5 that mutations occur in the immunoglobulin variable-region genes of the B cells as they are rapidly dividing in response to a foreign antigen. Some of these mutations code for a variable region within the B-cell receptor that can bind to antigen more strongly. This process is called *affinity maturation* and results in enhancement of the immune response.

The immune system is naturally diverse and heterogeneous in its response against a wide range of potential pathogens. Normal immune responses are **polyclonal,** meaning that cells with different features such as antigen specificity all proliferate in response to an immune stimulus. In contrast, hematologic malignancies are **monoclonal,** arising from excessive proliferation of a single mutant parent cell to form a clone of genetically identical cells that are similar in their appearance and surface markers. Suspicion of a hematologic malignancy is raised when there are elevated numbers of a specific population of lymphocytic cells in the bloodstream, bone marrow, or lymphoid tissues.

Genetic Changes

Malignancies are generally multifactorial in origin. As we discussed in Chapter 17, malignant transformation is thought to be a multistep process involving exposures to environmental agents such as chemical carcinogens and radiation, which induce a series of genetic mutations. Recall that the key genes involved are the **proto-oncogenes,** which promote cell growth and division, and the **tumor suppressor genes**, which control cell division by regulating the progression of cells through the cell cycle and maintain the genetic stability of the cells by repairing damaged DNA. Changes in these genes can result in uncontrolled cell proliferation.

The genetic alterations in malignant cells of hematopoietic origin include point mutations involving a change in a single nucleotide base, duplications or deletions of specific genes, and chromosome translocations in which two different chromosomes break apart and exchange genetic material. Additions or deletions of specific chromosomes may also occur, resulting in abnormal numbers of chromosomes, a condition referred to as *aneuploidy*. Although aneuploidy is thought to be caused by common secondary events that are not specific to a particular hematologic malignancy, its presence can provide valuable prognostic information.

The detection of translocations is of particular value in the diagnosis of several hematologic malignancies. Many of the translocations involve an exchange between the immunoglobulin or T-cell receptor (TCR) loci with various partner chromosomes, leading to abnormal proto-oncogene expression. For example, some of the hematologic malignancies are characterized by translocations involving the proto-oncogene *c-MYC,* which stimulates the transcription of several other genes involved in cell proliferation. Overexpression of the *c-MYC* gene can occur because of a rearrangement in which c-*MYC* is placed under the control of a different gene promoter sequence. For example, a translocation involving the *c-MYC* gene on chromosome 8 and the immunoglobulin μ gene on chromosome 14, denoted as [t(8;14)], is believed to be involved in the pathogenesis of some cases of Burkitt lymphoma (BL), a B-cell malignancy. Because of persistent *c-MYC* expression, several genes that are involved in cell proliferation are activated beyond normal levels. The resulting high levels of c-MYC protein drive the affected cells to continually proliferate.

Other hematologic malignancies are associated with genes that affect apoptosis. For example, most cases of follicular lymphoma have a t(14;18) gene translocation, in which portions of chromosome 14 (which contains the immunoglobulin [Ig] heavy-chain genes) and chromosome 18 (which contains an anti-apoptotic gene called *BCL*-2) are exchanged. This exchange results in the rearrangement and constitutive overexpression of *BCL-2*. The *BCL-2* gene induces the production of an inner mitochondrial membrane protein that blocks apoptosis. Therefore, the cells affected by this translocation do not die normally. Even though the altered cells do not proliferate at an increased rate, an excessive number of cells accumulates because their survival is enhanced compared with normal cells.

Other characteristic translocations result in the production of a novel fusion protein. For example, chronic myelogenous leukemia is characterized by a translocation between the *BCR* (breakage cluster region) on chromosome 9 and the c-*ABL* proto-oncogene on chromosome 22 (see Fig. 17–4). This results in a BCR/ABL fusion protein, which codes for a continuously activated tyrosine kinase enzyme, causing unregulated cell division. Scientists have developed anticancer drugs such as Gleevec to specifically target the abnormal protein produced by this gene translocation. These drugs slow cell growth by inhibiting the activity of the altered kinase.

Classification of Hematologic Malignancies

The classification of hematologic malignancies has undergone many changes over the years as new laboratory techniques have been developed and more knowledge has been gained about these diseases. In the 1950s and 1960s, the classification and diagnosis of hematologic malignancies were based primarily on abnormalities in the morphological features of the malignant cells, which were viewed on peripheral blood or bone marrow samples fixed onto microscope slides and treated with stains such as Wright-Giemsa. Advances in understanding basic lymphocyte biology led to a major rethinking of the use of classification schemes based solely on cell morphology. The discovery of surface markers on T and B lymphocytes in the 1970s and 1980s allowed this information to be incorporated into the diagnosis of hematologic malignancies. The 1990s and 2000s witnessed a tremendous expansion of knowledge about the genetic changes of the tumors. Therefore, investigators and clinicians today are using a combination of morphological, immunologic, cytogenetic, and molecular techniques to assist in the classification of hematologic malignancies.

Several schemes have been used over the years to classify the hematologic malignancies, including the French-American-British (FAB) Cooperative Group consensus criteria for leukemias and myelodysplastic syndromes and the Revised European American Lymphoma (REAL) classification for leukemias and lymphomas.

The REAL scheme, which was adopted in 2001 and updated in 2008 and 2016 by the World Health Organization (WHO), became the basis for the classification scheme for all types of hematologic malignancies. This widely accepted system is considered the "gold standard" in the classification of tumors for diagnosis and determination of appropriate therapy. The WHO system classifies hematologic malignancies into several major groups and numerous subgroups. The groupings are based on cell lineage, and specific cancers are further defined by their immunologic markers and genetic features, in addition to their morphological and cytochemical staining properties. The major groupings for the tumors of lymphoid origin are the precursor lymphoid neoplasms, the mature B-cell neoplasms, the mature T- and natural killer (NK)-cell neoplasms, Hodgkin lymphomas, and immunodeficiency-associated lymphoproliferative disorders.

Some of the recognized types of lymphomas, leukemias, and plasma-cell dyscrasias are discussed in more detail in this chapter. The WHO classification scheme continues to evolve as new knowledge is gained about the characteristics that typify the various disease entities.

Leukemias

Leukemias can be broadly divided into two groups based on the cell type from which they originated: myeloid and lymphoid. The myeloid leukemias are derived from the common myeloid precursor and encompass the granulocytic, monocytic, megakaryocytic, and erythrocytic leukemias. This section will not cover this group in detail but will briefly present a classic genetic change associated with chronic myeloid leukemia and how it is identified in the clinical laboratory. The focus of this section will be the lymphoid leukemias, which originate from mature lymphocytes or their precursors.

The lymphoid and myeloid leukemias can be further divided into acute and chronic types. In acute leukemias, the malignant cells multiply rapidly in the bone marrow and crowd out normal hematopoietic precursors, resulting in a decrease in red blood cells (RBCs) and fatigue; decreased neutrophils with subsequent infections and fever; and decreased platelets, causing bleeding abnormalities. The acute lymphoid leukemias involve immature/precursor cells called *lymphoblasts* (or *blasts*) that multiply rapidly in the bone marrow and are present in the peripheral blood. They are small to medium-sized cells that contain little cytoplasm, dense nuclear chromatin, and indistinct nucleoli **(Fig. 18–1)**. The acute leukemias progress rapidly and can become fatal in weeks or months if left untreated; however, they have a high response rate to therapy, so prompt diagnosis is important. In contrast, chronic leukemias generally involve mature cells. They usually present with variable nonspecific symptoms and are more slowly progressive. This section will discuss examples of acute and chronic lymphoid leukemias.

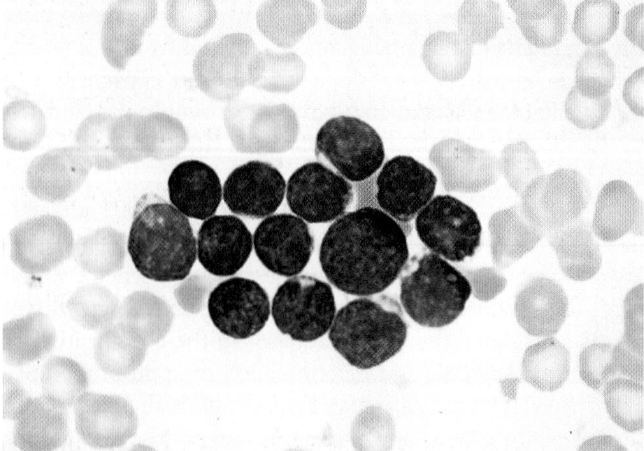

FIGURE 18–1 Lymphoblasts in the peripheral blood. *(From Harmening D.* Clinical Hematology and Fundamentals of Hemostasis. *5th ed. Philadelphia, PA: F.A. Davis; 2009.)*

Connections

Molecular and Cytogenetic Analysis

Compare the lymphoblasts in Figure 18–1 to the normal lymphocyte shown in Figure 1–8. Although differences can be seen in the morphology of the two cell types, not much else can be determined from simply observing the cells. Flow cytometry studies have added much detail to the traditional microscope-based laboratory evaluation of hematologic malignancies. Detection of cell surface markers provides insight into the lineage and maturation stage of the malignant cell type, which can be used to make a more accurate diagnosis. Molecular and cytogenetic analyses detect genetic mutations and chromosomal abnormalities in the cells, providing doctors with a more precise diagnosis and information about the patient's prognosis, which they can use to select the most effective therapy for the patient.

Acute Lymphoblastic Leukemias (ALLs)

Acute lymphoblastic leukemia (ALL) (also known as *acute lymphocytic leukemia*) is characterized by the presence of poorly differentiated precursor cells (blast cells) in the bone marrow and peripheral blood. These cells can also infiltrate soft tissues, leading to organ dysfunction. ALL is usually seen in children between 2 and 5 years of age and is the most common form of leukemia in this age group. ALL is a treatable disease with a high rate of remission and a cure rate of about 90% in children. Remission and cure rates are lower in adults with ALL. The main type of treatment is chemotherapy.

The majority of ALL cases are of B-cell origin, and these can be further characterized by their stage of maturation, as early-stage (pre-pro-B or pro-B) B-cell ALL, intermediate-stage (or common) B-cell ALL, and pre–B-cell ALL. The blasts are typically positive for terminal deoxynucleotidyl transferase (TdT), HLA-DR, CD79a, CD19, and CD22 and show variable expression of CD34. The CD10 marker, originally named "common acute lymphoblastic leukemia antigen" or "CALLA," is found in early stages of B-cell differentiation and is also commonly expressed. Slightly more mature B cells, at the pre–B-cell stage, express the cytoplasmic μ immunoglobulin heavy chain but are negative for surface immunoglobulin. Myeloid-associated antigens, such as CD13, CD15, and CD33, may also be expressed.

About 10% to 20% of ALL cases are of precursor T-cell origin and occur most commonly in teenaged males as a lymphoma or as leukemia/lymphoma combined. T-cell precursor ALL is characterized by presence of TdT, and the T-cell markers, CD7 and CD3. CD4 and CD8 are usually positive, and CD2 and CD5 have variable expression. Knowledge of the antigen expression pattern at the time of diagnosis is very important in monitoring patients for possible recurrence of the tumor (i.e., minimal residual disease) after treatment.

The WHO has classified ALL into several subtypes based on the genetic abnormalities associated with the cells, to precisely determine diagnosis. Cytogenetic analysis also provides information that aids in the prognosis of patients with ALL. For example, *hyperdiploidy*, in which the malignant cells contain more than 46 chromosomes, is associated with a good prognosis, whereas *hypodiploidy* is associated with a poorer prognosis. The most common translocation in ALL of B-cell origin, t(12:21)(p13;q22), also known as *ETV6/RUNX1* (or *TEL-AML-1*), is associated with an excellent prognosis in children.

Chronic Lymphocytic Leukemia (CLL)/ Small Lymphocytic Lymphoma (SLL)

The mature lymphoid neoplasms may involve B cells, T cells or NK cells. They include chronic lymphocytic leukemia (CLL) and small lymphocytic lymphoma (SLL). The WHO considers CLL and SLL a single disease with different clinical presentations. CLL is the most common leukemia in adults living in Western countries of the world. It primarily occurs in patients over 50 years of age and has a 2-to-1 male-to-female predominance.

The malignant clone in CLL/SLL is derived from small mature B lymphocytes. The cells appear to be cytologically normal but are dysfunctional, accumulating in the bone marrow and blood as well as in the spleen, lymph nodes, and other organs. Patients usually present with an increase in the peripheral blood lymphocyte count, which may be an incidental finding on a routine physical examination. Lymph node enlargement is prominent early in the disease. Anemia and thrombocytopenia are usually absent at the time of diagnosis. However, as the malignant lymphocytes continue to increase in number, replacement of normal elements in the bone marrow leads to anemia and thrombocytopenia. Treatment includes chemotherapy, monoclonal antibodies directed against the CD20 antigen, and targeted agents directed against various proteins involved in biological pathways that control cell proliferation. CLL is compatible with a long survival, as treatments can help control or reduce symptoms; however, they are not curative.

The malignant cells in CLL/SLL express the B-cell markers CD19, CD20 (weaker expression), CD23, and CD200 and are negative for CD10. Typically, the cells are dimly positive for surface immunoglobulin. In addition, they abnormally express the T-cell marker CD5. Cytogenetic analysis shows that patients whose malignant B cells have undergone somatic hypermutations in the variable immunoglobulin heavy-chain genes (see Chapter 5) have a better prognosis than those whose cells have not undergone such mutations. Another abnormality associated with an adverse patient outcome is a deletion in chromosome 17 that involves the TP53 tumor suppressor gene [del(17q)(TP53)].

Hairy-Cell Leukemia

Hairy-cell leukemia is a rare, slowly progressive disease characterized by infiltration of the bone marrow and spleen by leukemic cells without the involvement of lymph nodes. It has a male predominance and is most often seen in individuals over 50 years of age. Patients usually present with bone marrow disease and pancytopenia because of bone marrow infiltration; however, the blood lymphocyte count is usually not very high. Splenomegaly is striking, whereas lymphadenopathy is generally absent. The clinical presentation can resemble several other B-cell neoplasms, including CLL/SLL and splenic marginal-zone lymphoma.

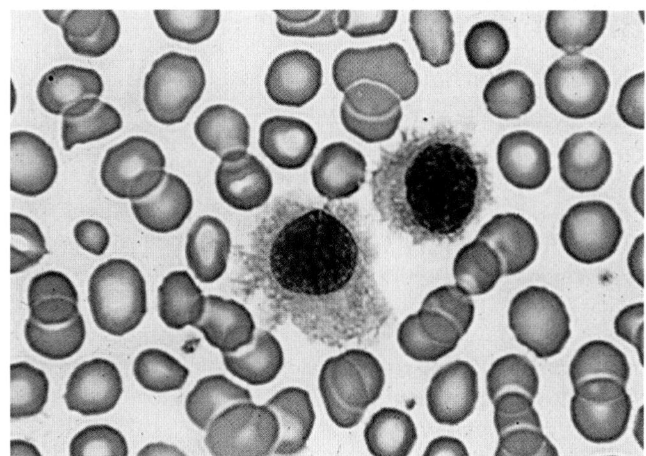

FIGURE 18–2 Hairy-cell leukemia. *(From Harmening D.* Clinical Hematology and Fundamentals of Hemostasis. *5th ed. Philadelphia, PA: F.A. Davis; 2009.)*

The malignant lymphocytes are medium-sized cells with round- to oval-shaped nuclei that occupy a large percentage of the cell volume. The cells often have irregular, "hairy" cytoplasmic projections from their surfaces **(Fig. 18–2).** They can be seen in the peripheral blood or bone marrow but are typically present in low numbers and may be difficult to find.

The malignant cells express the B-cell markers CD19, CD20, and CD22, and the interleukin (IL)-2 receptor CD25, which are not specific for the disease. The classic type of hairy-cell leukemia is also positive for CD103 and CD123, and these markers are helpful in making a specific diagnosis when used in combination with the other markers. Immunohistochemistry staining of bone marrow biopsy tissue with anti-CD20 can help identify the malignant B cells, and staining with antibody to Annexin A1 can help differentiate them from other mature B-cell neoplasms. An accurate diagnosis is made in most cases because of the cytomorphological and immunophenotypic characteristics. Polymerase chain reaction (PCR) for the detection of the mutated gene *BRAF-V600E* has been shown to be a sensitive and reliable test to aid in the diagnosis of hairy-cell leukemia. The mutation codes for an overly active kinase that enhances cell proliferation and is the target for a small molecule inhibitor that can be given to patients who do not respond to other therapies.

Lymphomas

The lymphomas have commonly been referred to as **Hodgkin lymphoma (HL)** and the **non-Hodgkin, or lymphocytic, lymphomas (NHLs).** Each of these entities will be discussed in more detail in the text that follows.

Hodgkin Lymphomas (HLs)

The HLs were first described by Thomas Hodgkin in 1832. The disease entity is common, with a reported incidence of about 3 cases per 100,000 people in the Western world. Studies suggest that HL has an infectious etiology, having possible association with the Epstein-Barr virus (EBV), which is known to preferentially infect B cells and immortalize them.

HL can occur in both young adults and the elderly and has a male predominance. The peripheral lymph nodes are primarily involved, although numerous organs, such as the liver, lung, and bone marrow, can be affected. Advances in chemotherapy and radiation therapy have made it possible to cure HL in the majority of cases. The WHO classification recognizes two major types of HL: classic HL, which comprises the majority of cases, and nodular lymphocytic-predominant HL (NLPHL). Classic HL is further divided into four subtypes: nodular sclerosis, mixed cellularity, lymphocyte-rich, and lymphocyte-depleted HL, based on the types of cells that comprise the background in which the tumor exists.

Classic HL is characterized by the presence of Reed-Sternberg (RS) cells in affected lymph nodes and lymphoid organs. RS cells are typically large, with one, two, or multiple nuclei containing a prominent nucleolus **(Fig. 18–3)**. These abnormal cells are not usually found in the peripheral bloodstream. RS cells are typically surrounded by a mixed population of lymphocytes, histiocytes, eosinophils, and plasma cells, which presumably have been attracted to the tumor in its immunoproliferative environment. The nontumor cells often account for the majority of the cells in the tumor biopsy.

Molecular studies have shown that the malignant RS cells are primarily of B-cell lineage, despite their lack of typical B-cell markers. RS cells in all subtypes of classic HL have a similar antigenic profile, being positive for CD30 and often for CD15. Expression of CD20 is typically weak or absent.

The malignant cells of NLPHL have a different morphology from those found in classic HL and are referred to as *lymphocytic and histiocytic (L&H) cells*. L&H cells are large, with a moderate amount of cytoplasm and a single, folded nucleus that resembles popcorn; thus, they are often referred to as "popcorn cells." These cells rarely express CD30 but instead express the mature B-cell antigens CD20 and CD22, as well as CD45. They are often surrounded by small lymphocytes.

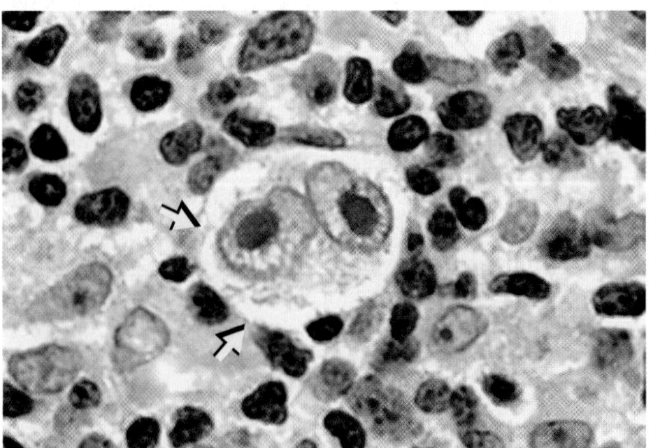

FIGURE 18–3 Hodgkin Reed-Sternberg cell with two nuclei, each containing prominent nucleoli, giving the cell an "owl's-eyes" appearance (arrows). *(From* Harmening D. Clinical Hematology and Fundamentals of Hemostasis. *5th ed. Philadelphia, PA: F.A. Davis; 2009.)*

Non-Hodgkin Lymphomas (NHLs)

NHLs include a wide range of neoplasms, and these may involve the B cells, T cells, or NK cells. B-cell lymphomas represent about 85% to 90% of all NHL cases, and the NK-cell malignancies are the most infrequent. Over two-thirds of the patients are older than 60 years of age, and the incidence is greater in men than in women. Immunosuppression seems to be the greatest risk factor for NHL; in fact, an increase in cases corresponded to the emergence of HIV. Other conditions associated with increased risk for NHL include certain autoimmune diseases, congenital immunodeficiency disorders, organ transplantation, and exposure to certain infectious agents.

B-cell lymphomas generally begin in the germinal centers of lymph nodes. Although these lymphomas can begin in any tissue, the gastrointestinal tract is the most common site for NHL outside of the lymph nodes. Three characteristics usually identify lymphomas as having a B-cell origin: (1) surface immunoglobulin, which is found on no other cell type; (2) other cell surface proteins, such as CD19 and CD20, that are sensitive and specific for B cells; and (3) rearranged immunoglobulin genes. In almost all cases, both the surface immunoglobulin and the rearranged immunoglobulin genes have features of clonality.

B-cell malignancies include diffuse large B-cell lymphoma (DLBCL), follicular lymphoma, mantle-cell lymphoma, and Burkitt lymphoma. The most common NHL is DLBCL, which accounts for 30% to 40% of NHL. DLBCL is a heterogeneous group of diseases characterized by diffuse growth of large atypical cells. The malignant cells display a mature B-cell phenotype, with surface immunoglobulin and B-cell markers such as CD19, CD20, and CD22. The cells are rapidly growing, but prompt, aggressive treatment with chemotherapy and monoclonal antibody to CD20 results in a high cure rate. CAR-T–cell therapy, involving the administration of genetically modified T cells directed toward the CD19 antigen, is approved for patients who don't respond to other treatments (see Chapters 17 and 25).

The next most common type of B-cell lymphoma is follicular lymphoma, which originates in the germinal centers within the follicles of the lymphoid organs. The cells have a mature B-cell phenotype and are positive for surface Ig, CD19, CD20, and CD22. The disease is associated with the chromosomal translocation t(14;18)(q32;q21), in which the Ig heavy-chain gene on chromosome 14 has been placed next to the *BCL-2* gene on chromosome 18. This results in overexpression of the Bcl-2 protein, which allows the malignant cells to survive by inhibiting apoptosis. Patients with the disease are typically asymptomatic at the time of diagnosis, except for painless lymphadenopathy. However, the disease has usually disseminated to the spleen, liver, and bone marrow and is incurable.

Mantle-cell lymphoma was so named because the malignant cells resemble lymphocytes in the mantle zone surrounding the germinal centers in terms of their morphology and immunophenotype. The classic form of this cancer is characterized by a diffuse infiltration of the lymph nodes with intermediate-sized cells that have irregular, cleaved nuclei. Small-cell and blastoid-cell variants also occur. The cells express B-cell antigens, such as CD19, CD20, CD22, CD79a+, and surface immunoglobulin as well as the T-cell marker CD5. The cells strongly express the anti-apoptotic protein Bcl-2 and are identified by their characteristic chromosome translocation, t(11;14)(q13;q32), between the Ig heavy-chain gene and the cyclin D1 gene. Most patients have an aggressive clinical course that is unresponsive to therapy, but some may have a slower disease progression that does not require therapy for several years.

Burkitt lymphoma (BL) is a malignancy of the mature B cells that can occur in three forms: endemic, sporadic, and immunodeficiency-associated. The endemic form, which was discovered by Dennis Burkitt, represents the prototype of the disease. It is the most common childhood tumor in equatorial Africa and other areas of the world where malaria is endemic. The tumor typically grows in the jaw or maxilla **(Fig. 18-4)** and is associated with EBV infection at an early age. The immunodeficiency-associated form is associated with EBV infection in patients with HIV/AIDS or other conditions involving profound immunosuppression. In contrast, the sporadic form is not associated with EBV infection and typically involves the abdomen. The malignant cells in BL have a characteristic morphology. They are medium-sized cells with finely clumped chromatin, numerous nucleoli, and a deeply basophilic cytoplasm containing several distinct vacuoles. Bone marrow and lymph node tissue may have a "starry sky" appearance, resulting from a mixture of the cells from the tumor with macrophages that have phagocytized apoptotic cells. The cells are typically positive for the B-cell antigens CD19, CD22, CD20, CD79a, and often CD10, as well as surface Ig. Most cases display the characteristic chromosome translocation, t(8;14)(q24;q32), involving the *c-MYC* oncogene on chromosome 8 and the Ig heavy-chain gene on chromosome 14, resulting in uncontrolled cell proliferation. Laboratory testing plays a critical role in diagnosis, as BL is a fast-growing tumor that is rapidly fatal if untreated but has a high cure rate if recognized early and treated with chemotherapy.

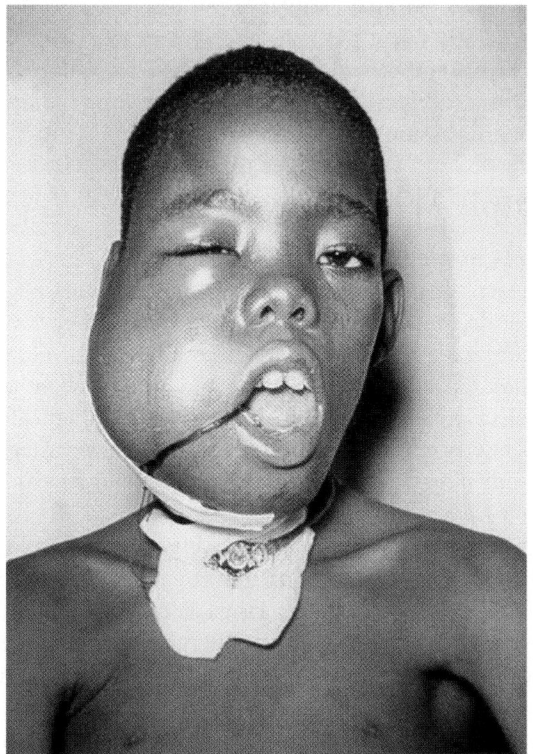

FIGURE 18-4 Child from Nigeria with a large facial tumor, caused by Burkitt lymphoma, a form of non-Hodgkin lymphoma. The solid tumor is composed predominantly of abnormal B cells. *(Courtesy of the CDC Public Health Image Library/Robert S. Craig.)*

T-cell lymphomas are a diverse group of more rare disorders that include mycosis fungoides (MFs), Sézary syndrome (SS), and adult T-cell leukemia/lymphoma. MF and SS are cutaneous T-cell lymphomas that involve the skin. Patients develop dermatitis lesions that form plaques, which develop into ulcerative tumors over time. Although MF is a slowly progressive disease that is mostly confined to the skin, it can disseminate to the lymph nodes, liver, spleen, and other organs in the later stages. SS is a systemic disorder in which the malignant cells are present in the peripheral blood; it has a worse prognosis than MF. The malignant cells in both MF and SS are mature CD4+ T cells that display TCR gene rearrangements. They appear abnormal, having irregular-shaped, folded (cerebriform) nuclei. Treatment in the early stages involves topical application of steroid creams or phototherapy. In the later stages, patients are treated with various chemotherapy agents and monoclonal antibodies in attempt to improve the clinical outcome.

Adult T-cell leukemia/lymphoma is a T-cell malignancy that is endemic in Japan and certain other areas of the world. It is associated with infection with the retrovirus HTLV-I, which is transmitted through the placenta or breast milk, intravenous drug use, blood transfusion, or sexual contact. The malignancy develops in a small percentage of infected persons after a long latency period. The acute form of the disease has an aggressive clinical course in which there is extensive involvement of the lymph nodes, blood, skin, and bones. The malignant cells are moderately large blasts that have convoluted or clover-leaf–shaped nuclei and condensed chromatin; because of their appearance, they have been referred to as "flower cells." The cells have the phenotype of mature T helper cells, being positive for CD3 and CD4 and TCR gene rearrangements. The acute form of the disease does not respond well to chemotherapy and has a low survival rate, but allogeneic stem cell transplant and targeted therapies show promise for the future. More details on HTLV-I and adult T-cell leukemia/lymphoma can be found in Chapter 23.

Plasma-Cell Dyscrasias

The plasma-cell dyscrasias are plasma-cell disorders that include several related syndromes: multiple myeloma, Waldenström macroglobulinemia, heavy-chain diseases, and the premalignant conditions **monoclonal gammopathy of undetermined significance (MGUS)** and smoldering multiple myeloma (SMM). These conditions are characterized by overproduction of a single immunoglobulin component called a *myeloma protein* **(M protein),** or **paraprotein,** by a clone of identical plasma cells. Therefore, these disorders are also known as the **monoclonal gammopathies.** Although monoclonal immunoglobulins may also be produced in other lymphoproliferative disorders of B-cell origin, laboratory detection and characterization of the M protein play an important role in the diagnosis, differentiation, and monitoring of the plasma-cell dyscrasias.

Monoclonal Gammopathy of Undetermined Significance (MGUS) and Smoldering Multiple Myeloma (SMM)

As with other types of cancer, multiple myeloma is thought to arise from a multi-step process in which plasma cells in the bone marrow undergo genetic changes that lead to their malignant transformation. As this process progresses, the cells are thought to evolve into the premalignant condition, MGUS, followed by an intermediate state, SMM, before they eventually develop into the cancer.

MGUS is a common condition that is present in about 3.5% of people aged 50 or older. People with MGUS produce a monoclonal immunoglobulin but do not have symptoms of organ damage or other laboratory findings that are associated with multiple myeloma or the other plasma-cell dyscrasias. MGUS is usually diagnosed incidentally when patients with various nonspecific symptoms undergo laboratory testing such as serum protein electrophoresis (SPE). The International Myeloma Working Group (IMWG) has identified three criteria that define the presence of MGUS:

1. a serum monoclonal protein (immunoglobulin G [IgG] or immunoglobulin A [IgA]) concentration less than 3 g/dL; and
2. a plasma-cell count of lower than 10% of the total cells in the bone marrow; and
3. the absence of signs or symptoms associated with multiple myeloma.

> **Clinical Correlations**
>
> **CRAB Features**
>
> The clinical findings associated with multiple myeloma are commonly referred to as "CRAB," with each letter in the acronym standing for one of the features—increased serum **c**alcium, **r**enal failure, **a**nemia, and lytic **b**one lesions.

Studies have found that people with MGUS have an average lifetime risk of developing multiple myeloma or other related disorders of about 1% per year. MGUS patients who produce an IgG or IgA monoclonal Ig typically progress to multiple myeloma, patients who produce an immunoglobulin M (IgM) monoclonal Ig can develop Waldenström macroglobulinemia or other lymphoproliferative disorders, and patients with monoclonal light chains can develop light-chain multiple myeloma, amyloidosis, or light-chain deposition diseases. Greater risk of disease progression has been associated with the production of an M protein that is not IgG, a monoclonal Ig concentration of 1.5 g/dL or greater, and an abnormal free light-chain (κ:λ) ratio (see section on *Serum Free Light-Chain [sFLC] Analysis*).

SMM is an intermediate stage in the malignant transformation process and has a higher risk of progression than MGUS: About 10% of people with SMM have been observed to progress to malignant disease within 5 years after diagnosis. The IMWG has identified the following criteria for SMM:

1. a serum monoclonal IgG or IgA concentration of greater than or equal to 3 g/dL; and/or
2. a plasma-cell count between 10% and 60% of the total cells in the bone marrow; and
3. the absence of signs or symptoms associated with multiple myeloma.

SMM has a higher risk for rapid progression to malignancy if the serum monoclonal protein levels are more than 30 g/L, the monoclonal antibody is IgA, there is a progressive increase in the monoclonal Ig concentration over 6 months, there is an abnormal free light-chain ratio (greater than 8), there are high numbers of bone marrow plasma cells (~50% to 60%), the plasma-cell phenotype is abnormal, or certain cytogenetic abnormalities are present.

Currently, there are no standardized treatments to prevent or delay the progression of MGUS or SMM. Lifelong follow-up of patients with medical examinations and pertinent laboratory testing (e.g., SPE, complete blood count [CBC], kidney function tests, serum calcium levels) is recommended to identify the development of malignancy before serious complications occur. SMM patients with high-risk factors can be offered clinical trials to receive treatment options with the hope that disease progression can be prevented.

Multiple Myeloma

Multiple myeloma, sometimes called *plasma-cell myeloma,* is a malignancy of mature plasma cells that accounts for about 10% of all hematologic cancers. It is the most serious and common of the plasma-cell dyscrasias. Multiple myeloma occurs most often after the age of 60, and men are slightly more likely than women to develop the disease. The American Cancer Society estimates that more than 32,000 newly diagnosed cases and more than 12,800 myeloma-related deaths occur annually in the United States.

Patients with multiple myeloma typically have excess plasma cells in the bone marrow, a monoclonal immunoglobulin component in the plasma and/or urine, and lytic bone lesions. Plasma cells infiltrating the bone marrow may be morphologically normal or may show atypical or bizarre cytological features. The malignant plasma cells phenotypically express CD38, CD56, and CD138. Approximately 20% of myeloma cells express CD20. Unlike normal plasma cells, myeloma cells have the ability to divide at a slow rate.

The immunoglobulin produced by the malignant clone can be of any type, with IgG being the most common (50% of cases),

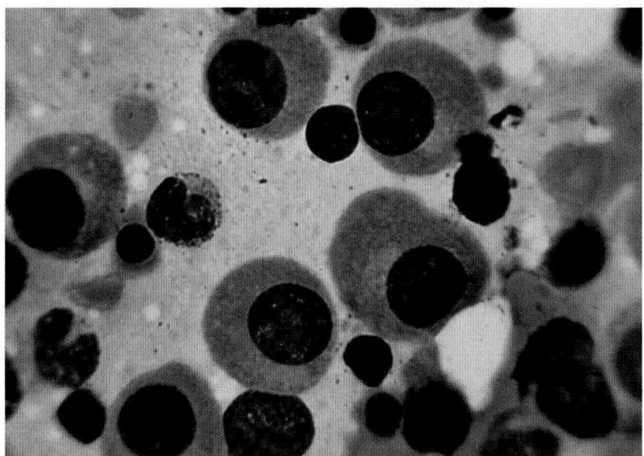

FIGURE 18–5 Bone marrow biopsy sample, showing replacement of marrow by plasma cells. *(From Harmening D.* Clinical Hematology and Fundamentals of Hemostasis. *5th ed. Philadelphia, PA: F.A. Davis; 2009.)*

followed by IgA and light chains only. Very often, the production of heavy and light chains by the malignant plasma cells is not well synchronized, and an excess of kappa or lambda light chains may be produced. In about 10% of cases, the myeloma cells exclusively produce light chains. These monoclonal light chains can be found in the blood, and about 60% to 70% of myeloma patients rapidly excrete them in the urine, where they are known as **Bence Jones proteins.** Rarely do myelomas produce IgM, immunoglobulin D (IgD), immunoglobulin E (IgE), or heavy chains only. Very rarely, two or more distinct M proteins are produced or a myeloma might not produce a detectable secretory product. The serum and urine M proteins are routinely detected and characterized by protein electrophoresis, immunofixation, and free light-chain assays (see sections that follow). The levels of normal immunoglobulins are often decreased in proportion to the amount of monoclonal immunoglobulin present in the serum because of the large number of myeloma cells.

The clinical manifestations of multiple myeloma are primarily skeletal, hematologic, and immunologic. Hematologic problems are often related to the failure of the bone marrow to produce a normal number of hematopoietic cells because myeloma cells progressively replace them **(Fig. 18–5).** The low number of hematopoietic precursors in the bone marrow leads to anemia, thrombocytopenia, and neutropenia. High levels of M protein can interfere with coagulation factors, leading to abnormal platelet aggregation and abnormal platelet function. These abnormalities, coupled with thrombocytopenia, make hemorrhaging, bruising, and purpura common complications of multiple myeloma.

Multiple myeloma preferentially involves bone, producing multiple lytic lesions that often lead to bone pain and pathological fractures **(Fig. 18–6).** Bone loss is caused by a complex interaction between the myeloma cells and normal cells in the bone. The myeloma cells trigger increased activity of the osteoclasts, whose function is to resorb bone tissue during the normal bone-remodeling process, and decreased activity of the osteoblasts, which help to replace the degraded bone with new bone tissue. Therefore, bone tissue is degraded faster than it can be replaced, and bone disease is a major contributing factor to disease morbidity. Bone pain, usually involving the spine or chest, is the most common presenting symptom of multiple myeloma. Hypercalcemia is very common because calcium is released as the bones degrade. In advanced disease, the hypercalcemia itself can reach life-threatening levels.

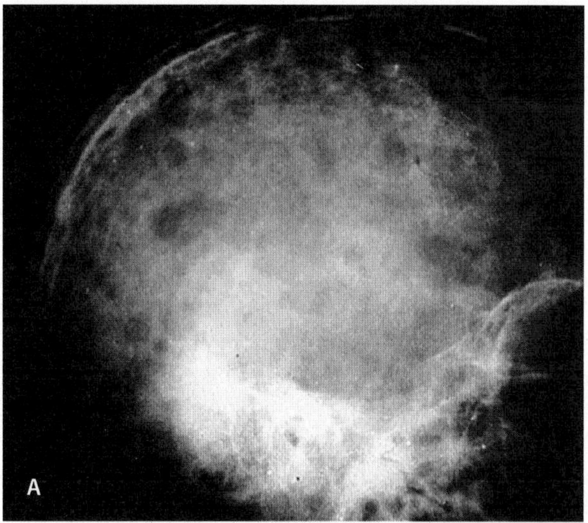

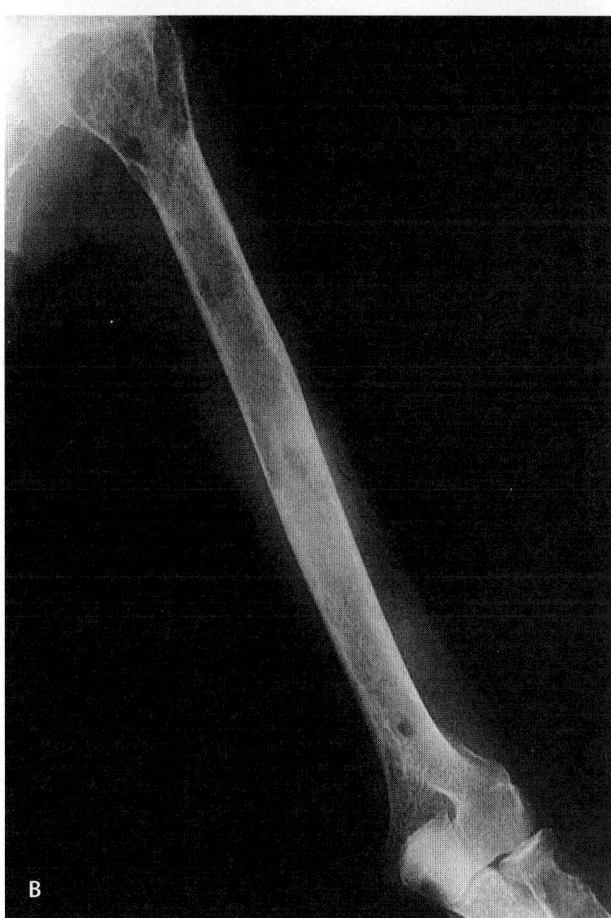

FIGURE 18–6 Bone lesions seen in a patient with multiple myeloma. (A) Lytic skull lesions. (B) Left humerus. *(From* Harmening D. Clinical Hematology and Fundamentals of Hemostasis. *5th ed. Philadelphia, PA: F.A. Davis; 2009.)*

Despite the dependence of multiple myeloma cells on the bone marrow, tumors may occasionally be found in the spleen and liver. These tumors are typically more aggressive.

When immunoglobulin levels in the blood are sufficiently high, they may cause the formation of rouleaux, stack-like formations of red blood cells (RBCs) that can be seen on examination of a peripheral blood smear. Excess production of the abnormal immunoglobulin is accompanied by a progressive decrease in the normal immunoglobulins. This leads to a deficiency of normal antibody responses and a higher incidence of infections. Hyperviscosity can develop when the level of M protein in the plasma is high. Because viscosity depends on the concentration and size of the molecule in solution and IgM is the largest of the immunoglobulins, hyperviscosity is most often seen with IgM-producing tumors. Hyperviscosity syndrome is also sometimes seen with an IgG3-producing myeloma because IgG3 is the largest of the IgG subclasses.

Up to 15% of patients with multiple myeloma develop light-chain deposition disease or amyloidosis. These are two related disorders in which free light chains or fragments of immunoglobulin are deposited in the tissues. Amyloid fibers stain with the dye Congo red and show apple-green birefringence when viewed with a polarizing microscope. Light chains can be identified in tissue sections by immunofluorescence or immunohistochemical staining with specific antibodies. The deposition of antibody-derived material results in organ dysfunction. The kidneys are most often affected, but every tissue in the body can develop amyloid deposits. Cardiomyopathy, peripheral neuropathy, hepatosplenomegaly, and ecchymoses (areas of skin discoloration caused by blood in the tissues) are the most common manifestations.

Patients with multiple myeloma can develop either acute or chronic renal failure. As many as two-thirds of patients with multiple myeloma exhibit some degree of renal insufficiency. Patients with myelomas that produce light chains or IgD are much more likely to develop renal failure than those with other types. Renal insufficiency caused by Bence Jones proteins is seen in about 50% of patients. After infection, this is the second-leading cause of death. Bence Jones proteins are thought to be directly toxic to tubular epithelial cells and can damage the kidneys by precipitating in the tubules, causing intrarenal obstruction.

The IMWG has identified the following criteria for the diagnosis of multiple myeloma:

1. Clonal bone marrow plasma cells present at greater than or equal to 10% or plasmacytoma observed in a biopsy within or outside of the bone marrow AND
2. One or more of the following:
   a. Presence of end-organ damage (CRAB features)
   b. Clonal bone marrow plasma-cell percentage greater than or equal to 60% in the absence of end-organ damage
   c. Serum free light-chain (sFLC) ratio greater than or equal to 100, with the monoclonal free light-chain concentration greater than or equal to 100 mg/L (see section on *Serum Free Light-Chain [sFLC] Analysis*)
   d. More than one focal lesion of at least 5 mm in size on magnetic resonance imaging (MRI) studies

The overall 5-year survival rate for patients with multiple myeloma is about 52%. The prognosis is generally worst in patients who are diagnosed in the later stages of disease or who show evidence of renal damage. Cytogenetics analysis of chromosomal abnormalities provides valuable information regarding patient prognosis. For example, the presence of trisomies (three copies of a single chromosome) or the translocations [t(11;14) or t(6;14)] are considered a standard risk for disease progression, whereas a deletion in the short arm of chromosome 17 or the translocations [t(14;16) or t(14;20)] indicate a high risk for more aggressive disease.

Different treatment options are available for multiple myeloma and are directed by the level of risk for disease progression. Various combinations of drugs are often used, along with supportive treatments, such as bone-strengthening and pain medications to manage patient symptoms. Therapies include immunomodulating agents such as thalidomide and lenalidomide; proteasome inhibitors such as bortezomib that stop enzyme complexes from degrading proteins that control cell division; and monoclonal antibodies, such as daratumumab, which is directed against the plasma-cell marker CD38, as well as chemotherapy and autologous stem cell transplantation. Measurements of M proteins are conducted along with other laboratory tests to monitor patients and determine the effectiveness of treatments. Successful treatment will result in a decrease in the M protein concentration, sometimes to undetectable levels. Although multiple myeloma is still an incurable disease, increased treatment options have improved the mortality rate.

Waldenström Macroglobulinemia

Waldenström macroglobulinemia, also known as a *lymphoplasmacytic lymphoma*, is a malignant proliferation of IgM-producing lymphocytes. It is a rare condition; only about 1,500 cases are reported annually in the United States. More cases occur in males than in females, and the median age at onset is about 70 years. The majority of patients have a genetic mutation in the *MYD88* gene, and about 30% of cases exhibit a mutation in the *CXCR4* gene. Both genes code for proteins that are involved in cell signaling pathways that regulate cell division and apoptosis, as well as overexpression of these proteins because the mutations result in increased cell proliferation and survival. The presence of MGUS increases the risk of Waldenström macroglobulinemia 200-fold over the general population.

The malignant cells in Waldenström macroglobulinemia possess the B-cell markers CD19, CD20, CD22, and CD79a and stain brightly for cytoplasmic IgM. They are also positive for CD38. They do not express CD3, CD5, CD10, and CD103. The tumor cells can have a variety of presentations, described as small lymphocytes, plasmacytoid lymphocytes, and cells resembling mature plasma cells. Typically one morphotype will predominate. The cells always infiltrate the bone marrow and are sometimes found in the spleen and lymph nodes. In bone marrow aspirates, the lymphocyte count can be within the reference range or severely elevated.

The clinical signs and symptoms of Waldenström macroglobulinemia are variable and are caused by infiltration of the malignant cells into the bone marrow, spleen, liver, and lymph nodes as well as the overproduction of monoclonal IgM. Accumulation of the cells in these organs can produce splenomegaly (enlargement of the spleen), hepatomegaly (enlargement of the liver), and lymphadenopathy (lymph node enlargement). Signs and symptoms often include weakness, fatigue, anemia, bleeding, and occasionally plasma hyperviscosity. Anemia is attributed to overgrowth of tumor cells in the bone marrow, displacing erythropoiesis. Thrombocytopenia and leukopenia are less commonly seen. Bleeding can be caused by a combination of thrombocytopenia and interference of platelet function by monoclonal IgM.

The monoclonal IgM can accumulate in any tissue, forming deposits that lead to inflammation and tissue damage. Because early diagnosis is possible, hyperviscosity is uncommon. Lytic bone lesions, hypercalcemia, and renal tubular abnormalities are rare, differentiating this disease from multiple myeloma. Approximately 20% of the patients with Waldenström macroglobulinemia present with peripheral neuropathy. It appears that the monoclonal IgM in these cases is directed against glycoproteins or glycolipids of the peripheral nerves, causing symptoms of neuropathology.

All individuals with Waldenström macroglobulinemia have an elevated serum monoclonal IgM that migrates in the gamma region during SPE. However, the concentration varies widely, and it is not possible to define a concentration that differentiates this disease from other B-cell lymphoproliferative disorders. IgM levels do not affect survival rate or correlate with symptoms. Patients with serum IgM concentrations over 5,000 mg/dL can be asymptomatic, whereas patients with levels of 500 mg/dL can have significant bone marrow infiltration and pancytopenia. The presence of IgM paraprotein is not specific for Waldenström macroglobulinemia. SPE should be used to evaluate the amount of the monoclonal protein, and the presence of IgM should be confirmed by immunofixation electrophoresis (IFE; see the section in the text that follows). In 70% to 80% of the patients, the light chain is κ. Bence Jones proteinuria is present in about 10% of the cases. Serum β_2–microglobulin levels are generally above 3.0 mg/dL, the upper limit of the reference range.

In 10% to 20% of patients, the IgM paraproteins behave as **cryoglobulins.** Cryoglobulins precipitate at cold temperatures and can occlude small vessels in the extremities in cold weather. Occlusion of small vessels can lead to hypoxia and the development of skin sores or even necrosis of portions of the fingers or toes. Cryoglobulins can also contribute to plasma hyperviscosity. Cryoglobulins can be detected when a blood or plasma sample is refrigerated in the clinical laboratory. The precipitate forms at low temperatures and dissolves upon warming.

Some of the clinical symptoms are caused by autoantibody activity of the monoclonal IgM antibody. Some IgM paraproteins have specificity for the *i* or *I* antigens and will agglutinate RBCs in the cold *(cold agglutinins)*. Antibodies can bind to RBCs, producing an autoimmune hemolytic anemia. Coating of the RBCs can produce rouleaux, which can be demonstrated on peripheral blood smears. A thrombocytopenic purpura-like syndrome can develop from binding of the paraprotein to thrombocytes. In addition, IgM can be demonstrated against polyclonal IgG. This results in immune complex disease characterized by vasculitis, affecting small vessels of the skin, kidneys, liver, and peripheral nerves.

Asymptomatic patients do not require treatment, but they should be monitored. Treatment includes anti-tumor chemotherapy, targeted therapies such as immunomodulating agents and proteosome inhibitors (see discussion on multiple myeloma), monoclonal antibodies directed against CD20, and plasmapheresis to reduce blood viscosity. With these treatments, the 5-year survival rate of patients with the disease is close to 80%.

Heavy-Chain Diseases

The **heavy-chain diseases** are rare B-cell lymphomas that are characterized by the production of a monoclonal Ig heavy chain. Genetic mutations in the affected B cells result in the production of abnormal heavy chains that have lost part of their CH1 or variable domain, so they are incapable of binding to Ig light chains. These diseases are classified according to the type of heavy chain produced, which can be alpha (α), gamma (γ), or mu (μ).

Alpha heavy-chain disease is the most common of the three types and is seen most often in young adults in their 20s or 30s who live in the Mediterranean region, including northern Africa and the Middle East. It has been associated with poor hygiene, poor nutrition, and chronic bacterial and parasitic infections. The disease is a lymphoma that involves the mucosal-associated lymphoid tissues (MALTs) and can occur as one of three forms: gastrointestinal, respiratory, or lymphomatous. Most patients have the gastrointestinal form, which is characterized by intestinal malabsorption with diarrhea, abdominal pain, and weight loss. The monoclonal α chains can be identified in patient serum through reaction with anti-IgA in IFE (see the text that follows). Because of their abnormal structure and tendency to polymerize, they may not be evident by SPE, which can appear normal or demonstrate a broad band that migrates to the α-2 or β region. Histological testing of biopsy tissue obtained from the small intestine or other affected areas demonstrates an infiltration of plasma cells and mature B cells. Early diagnosis is important because treatment with antibiotics in the early stage of the disease can improve prognosis. Patients unresponsive to antibiotics or those who have progressed to later stages of the disease are treated with chemotherapy.

Gamma chain disease is a very rare disorder that has been found in people around the world, usually appearing between the ages of 60 and 70. One-fourth of the patients also have an autoimmune disease such as rheumatoid arthritis (RA). The disease is heterogeneous and can present in one of three forms: disseminated lymphoma with lymphadenopathy and generalized symptoms such as fever and weight loss; localized disease with lymphoma limited to the bone marrow; or localized disease involving areas outside of the lymph nodes, such as the skin. The abnormal gamma chains tend to migrate to the β region on SPE, where they may be masked by other proteins. Serum IgG is elevated, and the abnormal protein can be seen by IFE, which demonstrates a monoclonal γ band in the absence of monoclonal light chains. Immunohistochemistry studies reveal the presence of malignant B cells and plasma cells in the bone marrow, spleen, lymph nodes, or other involved areas such as the skin. Patients are treated with chemotherapy, and the prognosis is highly variable, ranging from 1 month to many years.

Mu heavy-chain disease is an extremely rare disorder that has been diagnosed in a very small number of people throughout the world, mainly Caucasian males aged 50 to 60 years. The majority of patients also have a lymphoid malignancy that resembles CLL or SLL. Thus, patients have symptoms that are related to the associated lymphoma, such as splenomegaly, hepatomegaly, and anemia. More than half of patients have a normal SPE pattern, but IFE typically reveals μ polymers of various sizes that are not associated with κ or λ light chains. The urine does not usually contain μ heavy chains but demonstrates the presence of free monoclonal light chains (Bence Jones proteins) in more than half of patients. Bone marrow aspirates reveal a mixture of plasma cells containing prominent cytoplasmic vacuoles and small round lymphocytes resembling those of CLL. Patients are treated with chemotherapy, and overall survival is variable, ranging from under 1 month to many years.

Role of the Laboratory in Evaluating Immunoproliferative Diseases

The diagnosis of a hematologic malignancy is usually suggested by a patient's medical history and clinical symptoms and confirmed by laboratory testing. Laboratory evaluation of a patient suspected of having an immunoproliferative disorder begins with performance of a CBC and differential and examination of the cell populations on a peripheral blood smear. Blood samples from some patients with hematologic malignancies may show a decrease in RBCs (anemia) or platelets (thrombocytopenia) because of crowding out of normal hematopoietic precursors by the malignant-cell population. A decrease in normal white blood cells (WBCs) may also be evident and can result in increased susceptibility to infections. Microscopic examination of cell morphology in the peripheral blood smear can provide important clues about the lineage of the malignant-cell population. Differentiation between cells of monocytic or granulocytic origin and those of lymphoid origin can also be accomplished by the use of various cytochemical stains, such as peroxidase and Sudan Black B. Once abnormalities are detected in the CBC and differential, a bone marrow aspirate and biopsy are obtained to confirm the diagnosis. Although microscopic examination of the bone marrow cells can confirm the presence of a malignant population, specialized tests are required to more precisely identify the cells of interest.

This section will discuss three types of specialized tests that are used in the diagnosis and monitoring of patients with lymphoproliferative disorders: immunophenotyping by flow cytometry, evaluation of immunoglobulins, and genetic testing. The laboratory can assess the immunophenotype of hematopoietic cells in the blood, bone marrow, or lymphoid tissues by flow cytometry. This is done by detecting cell surface antigens that are characteristic of a specific lineage and stage of differentiation. This technology serves as an excellent complement to microscope-based traditional diagnostic methods and adds distinctive discriminatory capabilities that are unmatched by any other diagnostic technique. By performing immunophenotyping, the laboratory can determine whether the malignant cell population consists of B cells, T cells, NK cells, plasma cells, or cells of myeloid origin.

A second role of the laboratory is to evaluate the amount and characteristics of the immunoglobulins produced by malignant B cells or plasma cells. Because the B-cell lineage develops into plasma cells that produce antibody, malignancies of B cells are sometimes associated with excessive or abnormal antibody production. The concentrations and characteristics of the immunoglobulins in the patient's serum or urine can be used to diagnose and evaluate the plasma-cell dyscrasias.

Third, the laboratory is involved in the assessment of genetic and chromosomal abnormalities in hematologic malignancies. Genetic techniques play an important role in routine clinical practice. Cytogenetic analyses are used to detect chromosomal abnormalities such as translocations. Molecular techniques such as microarray and the PCR can be used to detect mutant sequences within genes that have been linked to particular diseases.

Immunophenotyping by Flow Cytometry

Immunophenotyping, or the analysis of cell surface marker expression, is commonly used in the diagnosis and classification of leukemias and lymphomas. Because the malignant cells express markers that often correspond to those of their normal precursors, insight into their lineage of origin and stage of maturation can often be determined by this technique.

The presence of cluster of differentiation (CD) antigens on the surface of hematopoietic cells is routinely detected by flow cytometry. **Table 18–1** lists some of the clinically relevant markers. In immunophenotyping, clinical samples containing cells that are potentially neoplastic are incubated with panels of antibodies that are specific for the relevant antigens. The clinical laboratory determines the specific antibodies used for testing on the basis of the suspected disease, the type of sample, and the amount of sample available. Each antibody in a single reaction tube is labeled with a different fluorescent dye. Thus, cells that express a specific antigen are bound by the corresponding antibody and emit fluorescence of a particular color. The fluorescence, along with cell size and other cell characteristics, is analyzed by flow cytometry (see Chapter 13). This allows the antigenic profile, or immunophenotype, of the cell population to be determined. **Table 18–2** lists the CD markers typically found on selected hematologic malignancies of lymphoid origin.

Flow cytometry is ideal for fluids such as blood, in which cells are naturally suspended, but it is also useful for lymphoid tissues, from which single-cell suspensions can be easily made. The advantages of flow cytometry are largely based on its ability

Table 18–1 Markers Commonly Detected by Flow Cytometry in the Analysis of Hematologic Malignancies*

CELL TYPE	ASSOCIATED MARKERS
T cells	CD1, CD2, CD3, CD4, CD5, CD7, CD8, TCR alpha-beta, TCR gamma-delta
B cells	CD10, CD19, CD20, CD22, CD23, CD79a, CD103, kappa (surface and cytoplasmic), lambda (surface and cytoplasmic)
Myeloid cells and monocytes	CD11b, CD13, CD14, CD15, CD33, CD64, CD117, myeloperoxidase
Miscellaneous	CD11c, CD16, CD25, CD26, CD30, CD34, CD38, CD41, CD42b, CD45, CD56, CD57, CD61, HLA-DR, glycophorin, TdT, CD123, CD138, CD200

**Modified from ARUP Laboratories. Laboratory Test Directory. Leukemia/Lymphoma Phenotyping by Flow Cytometry. https://ltd.aruplab.com/Tests/Pub/3001780. Accessed June 29, 2020.*

Table 18–2 Surface Markers Characteristic of Selected Leukemias and Lymphomas

HEMATOPOIETIC MALIGNANCY	CHARACTERISTIC SURFACE MARKERS*
Classic Hodgkin lymphoma	CD15+ (most), CD30+, CD3 +/–, CD20 – or weak, CD45–
Nodular lymphocytic predominant Hodgkin lymphoma (NLPHL)	CD20+, CD22+, CD45+, CD15–, CD30–
B-cell acute lymphocytic leukemia (B-ALL)	CD10+, CD19+, CD22+, CD34+/–, CD79a+, TdT+, HLA-DR+
T-cell acute lymphocytic leukemia (T-ALL)	CD2+/–, CD3+, CD4 (usually +), CD5+/–, CD7+, CD8 (usually +), TdT+
Chronic lymphocytic leukemia (CLL)	CD5+, CD19+, CD20 (weak+), CD23+, CD200+
Hairy-cell leukemia	CD19+, CD20+, CD22+, CD25+, CD103+, CD123+
Multiple myeloma	CD38+, CD56+, CD138+, ~20% are CD20+
Waldenström macroglobulinemia	CD19+, CD20+, CD22+, CD38+, CD79a+, CD3–, CD5–, CD10–, CD103–

**CD = cluster of differentiation; + = positive; – = negative; TdT = terminal deoxynucleotidyl transferase.*

to very rapidly and simultaneously analyze multiple cell properties, including size and granularity, as well as surface and intracellular antigens, even in small samples. The quantitative nature of the data produced, both with regard to cell population distributions and to expression of individual cell antigens, offers objective criteria for the interpretation of results.

However, laboratorians and clinicians must recognize that malignant cells can differ from their normal counterparts (e.g., B-cell ALL versus normal B cells) in terms of the antigens that they characteristically express. This difference can occur in any of the following ways:

1. There may be a gain of antigens not usually expressed by the normal cell type or lineage.
2. There may be abnormally increased or decreased levels of the antigens expressed by the malignant cells or, in some cases, a complete loss of normal antigens.
3. The malignant cells may express antigens at inappropriate times during the maturation process.
4. There may be a homogeneous expression of antigens that are typically heterogeneously expressed by the normal counterpart.

Because there is no single surface marker that is specific for a particular hematologic malignancy, the laboratory must use a panel of carefully selected antibodies to identify the markers necessary for making an accurate diagnosis. Examples of commonly used antibody panels are listed in Table 13-2, Chapter 13.

Evaluation of Immunoglobulins

As we discussed in Chapter 5, the basic immunoglobulin unit consists of two identical heavy chains and two identical light chains, covalently linked by disulfide bonds. The structure of the heavy chain defines the class, or isotype, of the antibody (e.g., γ heavy chain in IgG, μ heavy chain in IgM, etc.). The two types of light chains (κ and λ) can each occur in combination with any of the heavy-chain types. The heavy chains and light chains each contain constant and variable regions. The constant region contains the part of the immunoglobulin that binds to cell receptors and the part involved in complement fixation. The variable regions contain the *idiotypes*, which are responsible for the antigen specificity of the antibody. Normally, the pool of immunoglobulins in plasma is heterogeneous because it contains antibodies with different idiotypes that recognize a variety of different antigens. The variability in the isotype means that they also vary in their physical characteristics, such as molecular weight and charge.

B cells differentiate into antibody-producing plasma cells by maturation through several stages. Each B cell recognizes only a single antigenic site or epitope. An early B-cell precursor is stimulated to proliferate and mature when it encounters an immunogen that it recognizes. When a foreign molecule enters the body, the many different epitopes on it each stimulate a B-cell response, leading to the production of an array of different antibodies. However, in disorders such as multiple myeloma, the proliferation of one clone of transformed plasma cells leads to the overproduction of an immunoglobulin of a single class and antigen specificity. As we mentioned previously, these disorders are called *monoclonal gammopathies* because the diseases involve proteins that are produced by a single clone of plasma cells. These proteins are found mainly in the gamma region of an SPE analysis. The antibody produced by the malignant plasma cells is referred to as an *M* (monoclonal) *protein* or *paraprotein* (i.e., an abnormal protein). All of the antibody proteins produced by the clone of plasma cells are identical in terms of their heavy chains, light chains, and idiotypes.

The initial tests used to screen for the presence of a monoclonal gammopathy are serum immunoglobulin levels and SPE (see the text that follows). Quantitative measurement of immunoglobulin levels in the serum is routinely performed by automated nephelometric or immunoturbidimetric methods (see Chapter 10). Because each plasma cell produces only one type of immunoglobulin, the persistent presence of an elevated amount of a single immunoglobulin class suggests malignancy. In contrast, an increase in the amount of total immunoglobulin, without an increase in any one specific class, is characteristic of nonmalignant conditions such as infections or autoimmune diseases.

Serum Protein Electrophoresis (SPE)

SPE is a technique in which serum proteins are separated on the basis of their size and electrical charge, as we discussed in Chapter 5. SPE results in five regions: albumin, plus the alpha 1, alpha 2, beta, and gamma globulins. IgG, IgM, IgD, and IgE migrate in the gamma globulin region, whereas IgA migrates as a broad band in the beta and gamma regions. **Figure 18–7**, panel A, shows a stylized drawing of the protein distribution in normal serum. As you can see, immunoglobulins normally show a range of mobilities because they are derived from many clones of plasma cells (i.e., they are polyclonal) and have different variable-region sequences. The SPE pattern for a polyclonal increase in serum immunoglobulins is shown in panel B. Note the broad mobility but increased height of the gamma globulin peak. Polyclonal increases in serum immunoglobulins are seen in a variety of disorders, including infections, autoimmune diseases, liver diseases, and some immunodeficiency states (e.g., hyper-IgM syndrome). The SPE result in panel C depicts a monoclonal immunoglobulin,

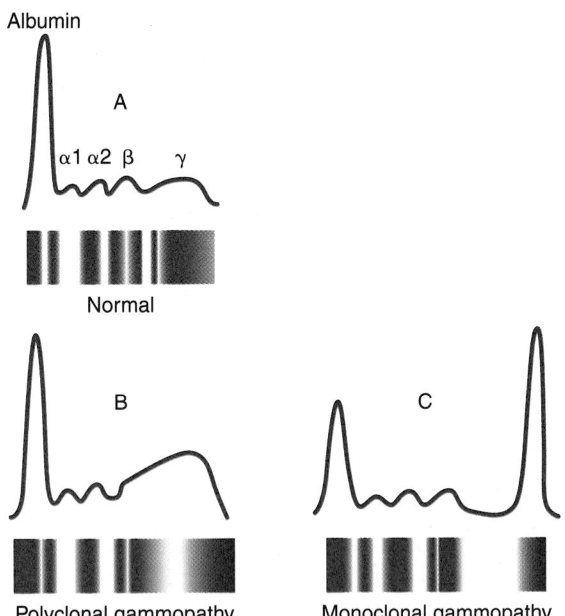

FIGURE 18–7 Serum protein electrophoresis of normal and abnormal samples. The lower portion of each panel is a representation of a stained agarose electrophoresis gel. The intensity of staining corresponds to the amount of protein in each region of the gel. In the upper portion of each panel is a densitometer tracing of a gel similar to the one beneath it. In the upper panel showing a normal serum sample, the largest peak is albumin. The globulin regions are as indicated.

which is increased in concentration and has limited mobility because it is produced by an identical clone of plasma cells. This is illustrated by the tall, narrow peak in the gamma region.

Additional evaluation of serum immunoglobulins by IFE is performed if the SPE shows a monoclonal component, if there is a significant quantitative abnormality of serum immunoglobulins, or if the clinical picture strongly suggests a plasma-cell dyscrasia. Myeloma cases in which only light chains are produced may not be detected on SPE because the light chains are rapidly cleared in the urine. Therefore, additional studies on a random or 24-hour urine sample may be indicated even in the presence of a normal SPE.

Immunofixation Electrophoresis (IFE)

Serum Immunofixation Electrophoresis

The performance of IFE is typically the next step in evaluating a monoclonal gammopathy. IFE is a highly sensitive and specific assay that is used to identify the type of monoclonal protein present in a sample. It can be performed by manual or automated capillary electrophoresis systems. In IFE, serum samples are electrophoresed in six separate lanes on an agarose gel, and specific antisera are applied directly to the lanes. The antisera used are selected to detect the most common M proteins and are directed against:

- Whole human serum (lane 1)
- Anti-γ (to detect IgG) (lane 2)
- Anti-α (to detect IgA) (lane 3)

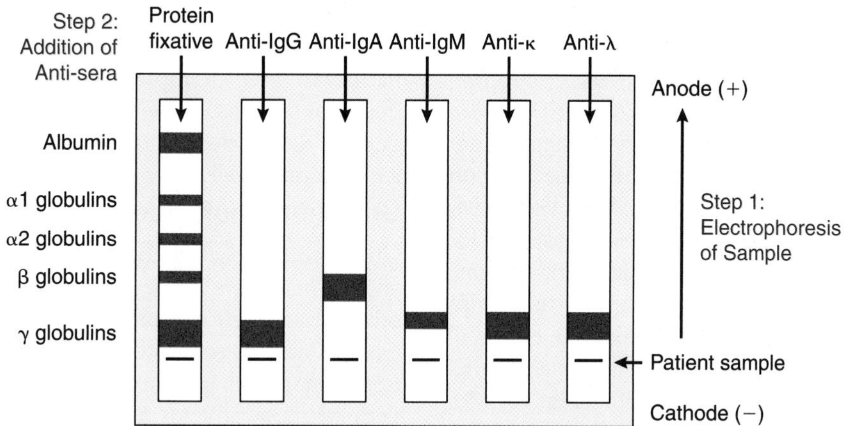

FIGURE 18–8 Principle of immunofixation electrophoresis (IFE). IFE involves two major steps. In step 1, proteins in the clinical sample (serum, urine, or cerebrospinal fluid) are applied to an agarose gel and separated according to their surface charge under the influence of an externally applied electrical field. At a pH of 8.6, the proteins acquire a negative charge and move toward the positively charged anode. Five major protein fractions result: γ globulins, β globulins, α1 globulins, α2 globulins, and albumin. Immunoglobulins are located primarily in the γ globulin fraction but can also migrate into the β-globulin fraction. In step 2, specific anti-sera are added to each one of the lanes and react with their corresponding protein to produce a precipitin band. A protein fixative is added to lane 1, which binds to all of the major protein fractions. The precipitin bands can be visualized after staining the gel with a protein stain and destaining with acetic acid to remove background color. *(Courtesy of Dr. Linda Miller.)*

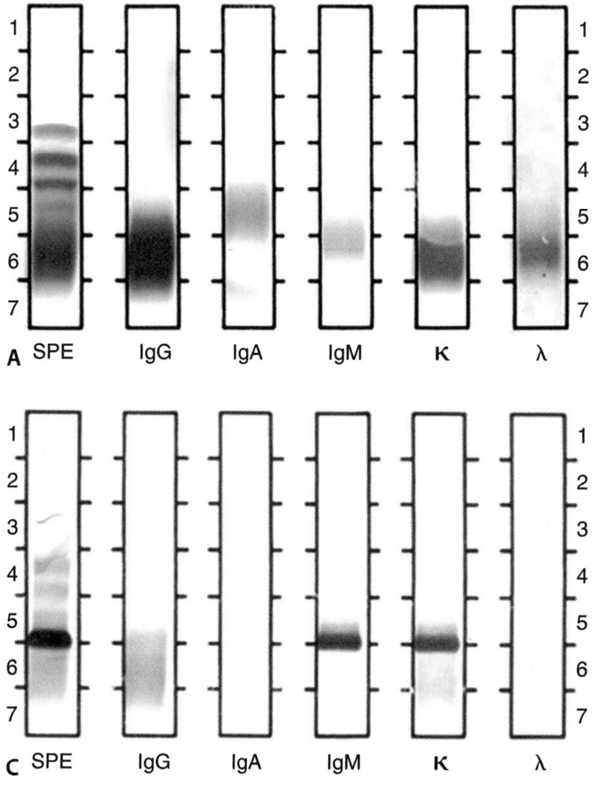

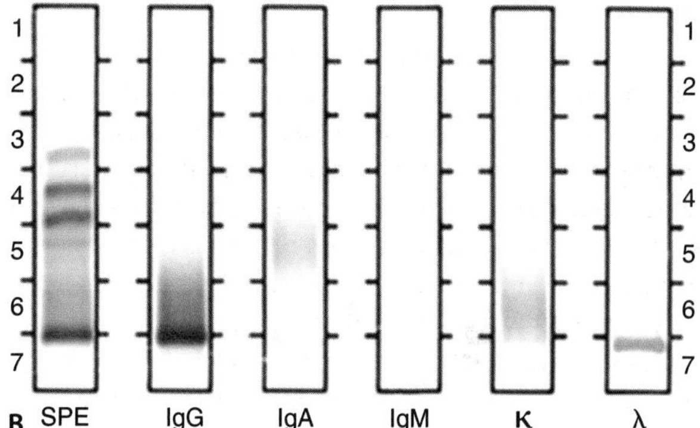

FIGURE 18–9 Sample IFEs from normal serum and sera from patients with monoclonal gammopathies. (A) Normal serum. Note the broad, diffuse bands in all the immunoglobulin lanes. These represent polyclonal antibodies that are heterogeneous in terms of their antigen specificity and structure and therefore migrate to slightly different positions on the gel. (B) Serum from a patient with a monoclonal IgG, λ antibody. Note the discrete, narrow bands in the IgG and λ lanes. The monoclonal antibody molecules produced by the patient are all identical and migrate to the same position on the gel. (C) Serum from a patient with monoclonal IgM, κ antibody. Note the discrete, narrow bands in the IgM and κ lanes. *(Courtesy of Dr. Linda Miller.)*

- Anti-μ (to detect IgM) (lane 4)
- Anti-κ (to detect kappa light chains) (lane 5)
- Anti- λ (to detect lambda light chains) (lane 6)

The antibodies combine with the immunoglobulin proteins in the sample to form complexes that are visualized by staining. **Figure 18–8** illustrates the principle of IFE. Areas of diffuse staining indicate polyclonal immunoglobulins, whereas monoclonal bands produce narrow, intensely stained bands **(Fig. 18–9)**.

Interpretation of IFE results requires a high level of expertise. When the monoclonal protein is in high concentration and the amount of polyclonal immunoglobulin of the same class is low, the bands produced in IFE gels are usually clear and easy to identify, as shown in Figure 18–9. However, the presence of higher levels of normal immunoglobulins can make it difficult to distinguish a minor monoclonal band against a background of normal proteins. These M proteins can sometimes be identified by a technique called *immunosubtraction* (see section that follows). Poorly resolved bands can also be caused by poor technique during the electrophoresis or anti-sera application steps. Other situations can also affect the quality of the results. For example, plasma is not recommended because fibrinogen can adhere to the β region of the gel and cause monoclonal proteins to stick nonspecifically, resulting in distinct bands in all of the anti-sera tracks. Samples with large amounts of rheumatoid factor or immune complexes can also produce unusual results, such as precipitin bands at the place of application. An extreme excess of monoclonal immunoglobulin can cause a *postzone* effect that produces a clear zone in the center of the band **(Fig. 18–10)**.

Connections

Postzone Effect in IFE

Recall from Chapter 10 that equivalent amounts of antigen and antibody are required for optimal formation of immune complexes and precipitation. Extreme antigen excess results in the formation of small immune complexes that cannot be visualized. This is called a **postzone** effect. When a sample with a very large concentration of an M protein is reacted with antisera on an IFE gel, precipitation will be visible on the outer edges of the band, where the reaction is in equivalence, but will not appear in the center of the band, where the reaction is in the postzone area. The problem can be corrected by diluting the sample and repeating the IFE procedure.

Immunosubtraction

A variation of immunofixation, called **immunosubtraction** or **immunotyping**, is a sensitive procedure that uses capillary electrophoresis to identify monoclonal immunoglobulin components. In this technique, antibodies to each heavy- or light-chain isotype are added to separate capillary runs of the patient's specimen. The binding of the antibody to its heavy- or light-chain antigenic target changes the electrophoretic mobility of the patient's immunoglobulin molecule. Monoclonal peaks thus "disappear" in the presence of antibodies to their components, allowing typing to occur by subtraction of peaks. **Figure 18–11** shows an example of a monoclonal IgG kappa protein detected by immunotyping.

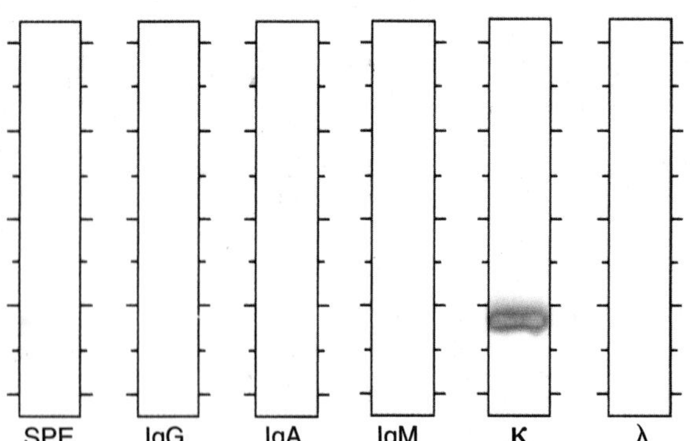

FIGURE 18–10 Postzone effect in immunofixation electrophoresis (IFE). IFE was performed on a 24-hour urine sample that was concentrated 50× by manual ultrafiltration (original protein concentration = 22 mg/dL). Note the clear area in the center of the κ band on the gel, reflecting decreased immunoprecipitation caused by an excess of κ chains relative to the amount of anti-κ reagent used in the κ lane. *(Courtesy of Dr. Linda Miller.)*

Urine Immunofixation Electrophoresis

Urine protein electrophoresis (UPE) and urine IFE also play an important role in the diagnosis of multiple myeloma and other plasma-cell dyscrasias. As previously discussed, some patients with these disorders produce an excessive amount of free monoclonal Ig light chains (i.e., Bence Jones proteins). Because these proteins are rapidly cleared from the circulation, they may not be detectable on serum IFE. However, the excess light chains are excreted into the urine and can be identified using UPE and urine IFE. The free light chains are believed to contribute to renal disease by depositing in the glomeruli and tubules of the kidneys and by their involvement in the development of renal casts. Therefore, UPE and urine IFE can be used to monitor patients with plasma-cell dyscrasias. These tests can also be used to assess the effect of therapy on the production of free monoclonal light chains and can indicate more extensive renal damage when large proteins such as intact immunoglobulins, which are normally retained in the blood, are demonstrated in the urine.

Urine samples for UPE and IFE are typically collected over a 24-hour period. The total protein concentration is determined and the sample is treated by filtration or centrifugation to remove any sediment that could interfere with performance of the tests. In addition, the samples must be concentrated so that enough protein is present to produce visible bands on the gel. Concentration can be accomplished by one of two ways. The first way involves the use of urine concentrators with ultrafiltration membranes that can retain large proteins (usually 10,000 daltons or more) but allow water, salts, and other small molecules to pass through, thus reducing the sample volume. In the process, the sample flows through a chamber containing the absorbent membranes and is collected when it reaches the desired volume and concentration. The second way involves the use of centrifugal concentrators that concentrate the sample by high-speed filtration. Centrifugal concentrators are faster than ultrafiltration membranes and can produce higher concentration factors. They are recommended for the preparation of urine samples in capillary electrophoresis systems.

In both systems, the desired concentration factor is based on the amount of protein in the urine sample and is determined by dividing the starting sample volume by the final volume. The concentrated sample is then applied to the electrophoresis gel, and the tests are completed as previously described for SPE and serum IFE.

Serum Free Light-Chain (sFLC) Analysis

Although UPE and urine IFE are sensitive methods for the detection of free monoclonal light chains, they have some limitations. For example, the requirement for a 24-hour urine collection can delay results. In addition, interpretation of the

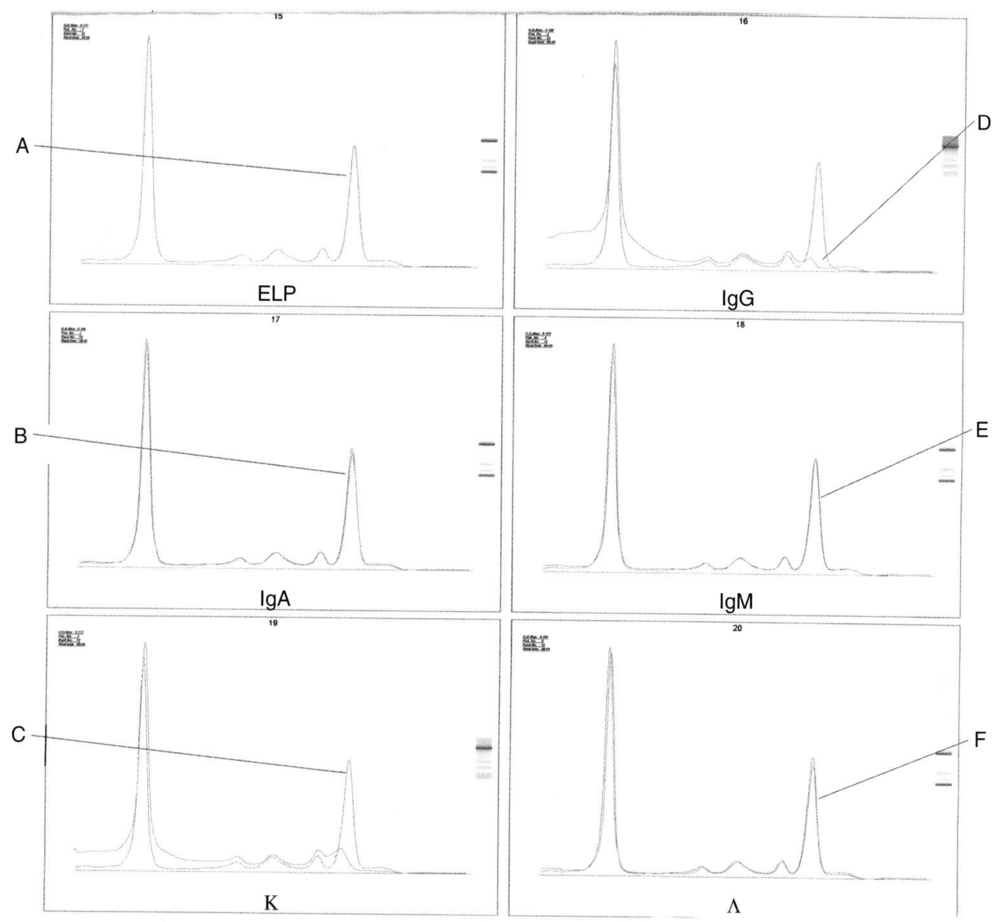

FIGURE 18–11 Immunotyping of a monoclonal IgG, κ protein. Panel A: Serum protein electrophoresis (SPE). The arrow points to the M-spike in the gamma region. Panel B: Electrophoresis with anti-alpha heavy chain. This pattern is overlaid with the original SPE. The patterns are identical. Panel C: Electrophoresis with anti-kappa light chain. The M-spike has disappeared, indicating the peak contains a kappa light chain (see arrow). Panel D: Electrophoresis with anti-gamma heavy chain. The M-spike has disappeared, indicating the peak contains IgG (see arrow). Panel E: Electrophoresis with anti-mu heavy chain. This pattern is overlaid with the original SPE. The patterns are identical. Panel F: Electrophoresis with anti-lambda light chain. This pattern is overlaid with the original SPE. The patterns are identical. *(Courtesy of Dr. Thomas Alexander.)*

results is subjective and can be difficult when a low level of free light chains is present with a high level of proteinuria, which can create a high degree of background staining. Automated tests for sFLC offer advantages over the traditional methods for urine testing described previously.

The sFLC assays are latex-enhanced immunoassays that measure free kappa and lambda light chains in the serum. The assays use polyclonal antibody reagents that recognize a diverse range of FLC epitopes that are normally hidden when the light chains are bound to heavy chains in intact immunoglobulins. This allows for quantitative measurement of free κ and free λ chain concentrations, as well as calculation of a κ/λ ratio, which is normally, between 0.26 and 1.65. An abnormal κ/λ ratio outside of the reference range, along with an increase of either κ or λ, is a sensitive indicator for the presence of a malignant plasma-cell clone, which is characteristic of a monoclonal gammopathy.

The sFLC assays are highly sensitive, being capable of detecting concentrations lower than 1 mg/L. This sensitivity allows them to detect monoclonal FLCs in patients previously thought to be negative for monoclonal Ig production by serum or urine IFE. Based on the quantitative nature and high level of sensitivity of sFLC testing and clinical studies, the IMWG developed consensus guidelines that recommend the use of the sFLC assay along with SPE and serum IFE to screen for multiple myeloma and related disorders. In addition, the group stated that the sFLC can replace the 24-h urine IFE to screen for most plasma dyscrasias (except for light-chain amyloidosis). The experts also concluded that sFLC measurements are valuable in monitoring patients with plasma-cell disorders and in helping to determine patient prognosis.

Evaluation of Genetic and Chromosomal Abnormalities

As we previously discussed, researchers have identified the specific mutations associated with malignant transformation for many of the hematologic malignancies. These genetic alterations are an integral part of the classification system outlined by the WHO. The detection of chromosome translocations is of particular value in diagnosis of hematologic malignancies. **Table 18–3** lists chromosome translocations that are characteristic of selected leukemias and lymphomas.

Often, these translocations can be detected by cytogenetic techniques. Malignant lymphoid cells can be made to proliferate in vitro, and their metaphase chromosomes can be examined for grossly visible abnormalities that correspond to characteristic translocations. Traditional cytogenetic evaluation by karyotyping has been supplemented by a technique known as **fluorescence in situ hybridization (FISH).** This technique is used to directly identify a specific region of DNA in a cell. It involves the preparation of short sequences of single-stranded DNA, called *probes,* which are complementary to the DNA sequences of interest. These probes bind to the complementary chromosomal DNA and, because they contain a fluorescent label, allow the location of those DNA sequences in the chromosomes to be visualized. **Figure 18–12** shows an example of a FISH result obtained from a patient with a hematologic malignancy. Probes can be used on chromosomes, interphase nuclei, or tissue biopsies. FISH on interphase chromosomes is quite sensitive and rapid because it does not require cell culture. However, it only provides information about the specific DNA sequence being detected by the probe used in the test.

Table 18–3 Cytogenetics Characteristic of Selected Leukemias and Lymphomas

HEMATOPOIETIC MALIGNANCY	CHARACTERISTIC CYTOGENETICS*
Burkitt lymphoma	Most commonly t(8;14) [IgH/*MYC*]; also t(2;8) and t(8;22)
Follicular lymphoma	t(14;18) [IgH/*BCL-2*]
Mantle cell lymphoma	t(11;14) [IgH/cyclin D1]
B-cell acute lymphoblastic leukemia (B-ALL)	t(12;21) [*ETV6/RUNX1*]
Chronic myelogenous leukemia (CML)	*t(9;22) [BCR/ABL]*

**t = translocation; IgH = immunoglobulin heavy-chain gene.*

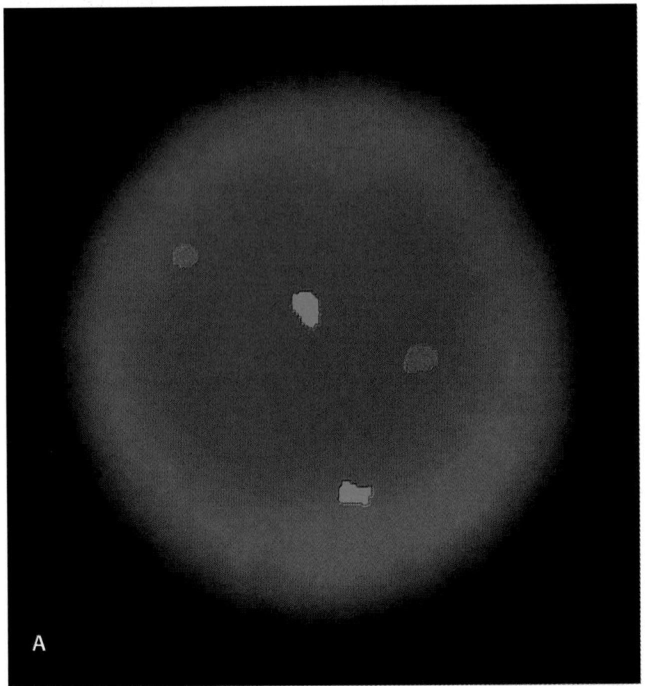

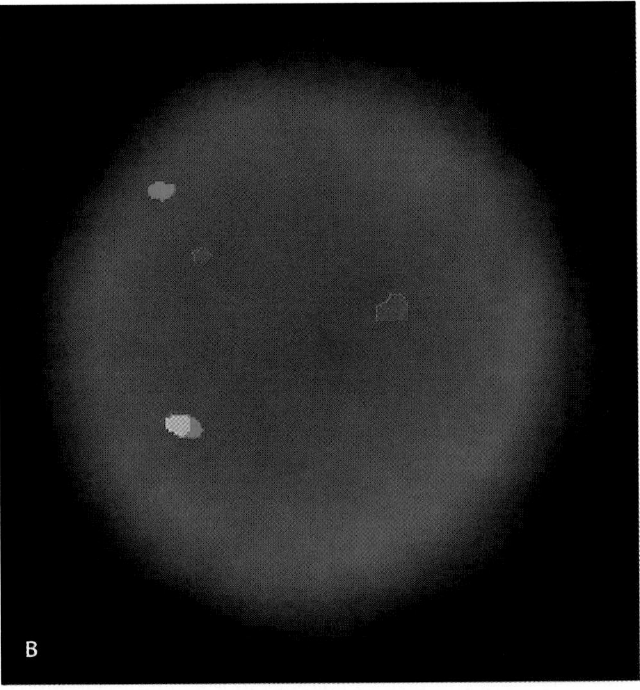

FIGURE 18–12 Fluorescence in situ hybridization (FISH) demonstrating a chromosomal translocation. In this assay, interphase cells were hybridized with molecular probes complementary to specific regions on chromosomes 9 and 22. The green signal represents the *BCR* (breakpoint cluster region) on chromosome 22, and the red signal represents the *ABL1* proto-oncogene on chromosome 9. A yellow signal represents the *BCR/ABL1* fusion caused by a 9;22 chromosome rearrangement. (A) A normal test result, showing two green signals representing two copies of chromosome 22 and two red signals representing two copies of chromosome 9. (B) Result from a patient with a translocation between chromosomes 9 and 22 [t(9;22)(q34.1;q11.2)]. The yellow signal indicates the fusion between the *BCR* and *ABL1* loci on the rearranged chromosome 22, which is also known as the *Philadelphia chromosome.* The smaller red signal detects the residual *ABL1* sequences present on the rearranged chromosome 9. This translocation is found in patients with chronic myelogenous leukemia (CML) as well as some individuals with acute myeloid leukemia (AML) and acute lymphoblastic leukemia (ALL). *(Courtesy of the Cytogenetics Laboratory, SUNY Upstate Medical University.)*

Lymphoid malignancies can also be evaluated by molecular techniques to identify abnormalities that are too subtle or diverse to be detected by karyotyping or FISH. Laboratorians can use molecular methods to find microdeletions or clonal rearrangements of the immunoglobulin genes in B-cell malignancies or of the TCR genes in T-cell malignancies. The PCR is a widely used technique to detect these gene rearrangements. To detect B-cell clonality, for example, the PCR amplifies the Ig heavy-chain gene sequence containing the variable and joining genes (see Chapter 5). The primers used in the assay are designed to detect conserved sequences so that most of the immunoglobulin genes in the sample will be amplified to detectable amounts, which can be seen on gel electrophoresis. If a malignant B-cell clone is present, a sharp band will migrate to a specific position on the gel, representing the unique V-D-J immunoglobulin heavy-chain gene (IgH) gene rearrangement contained in the cells of that clone (**Figure 18–13,** lanes 3, 6, 9, and 10). In contrast, normal polyclonal B cells produce a diverse array of V-D-J IgH gene rearrangements, which migrate to different positions on the gel, producing a smear (see Fig. 18–13, lanes 4, 8, and 11). Similarly, unique rearrangements in the TCR genes can be amplified by PCR to detect a malignant T-cell clone.

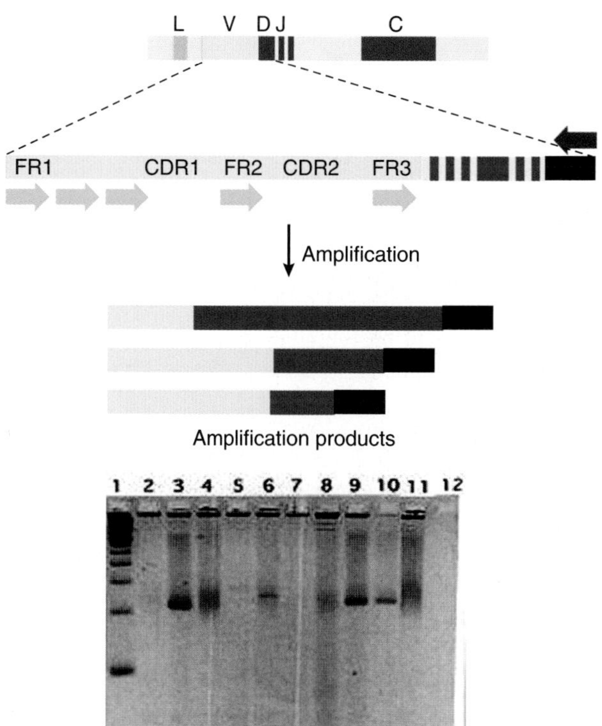

FIGURE 18–13 Immunoglobulin heavy-chain gene rearrangement by PCR with amplification from the variable region. Forward primers complementary to the variable region and reverse primers complementary to the joining region are used to amplify the diversity region (top). In a polyclonal specimen, amplification products in a range of sizes will result. These products produce a dispersed pattern on an ethidium bromide–stained agarose gel (lanes 4, 8, 11). If at least 1% of the sample is representative of a monoclonal gene rearrangement, that product will be amplified preferentially and revealed as a sharp band by gel electrophoresis (lanes 3, 6, 9, and 10). *(From Buckingham L.* Molecular Diagnostics. *2nd ed. Philadelphia, PA: F.A. Davis; 2012.)*

Connections

B-Cell Maturation and Rearrangements

Recall from Chapter 5 that rearrangements in the immunoglobulin heavy- and light-chain genes occur during B-cell maturation. The rearrangements occur randomly so that each B cell possesses a unique sequence of variable-heavy (V), diversity (D), and joining (J) gene segments. This unique sequence is retained as the B cell proliferates. Thus, the sequence can be used as a marker for the B-cell clonality that is characteristic of B-cell malignancies. It is visualized as a band of a distinct size when it is amplified by PCR and run on gel electrophoresis.

Although PCR and FISH are used to detect abnormalities in targeted genes, other molecular techniques can assay larger areas of the genome. DNA microarray technology enables efficient analysis of thousands of genes in the human genome in a single hybridization experiment by using a panel of molecular probes (see Chapter 12). The probes are complementary to portions of specific genes or chromosome regions and are spotted onto separate locations on a small glass slide or nylon membrane. Genomic DNA is isolated from a clinical sample, labeled with a fluorescent dye, and incubated with the microarray. Fluorescent spots will be visible in the locations where the sample DNA has bound. This technique is being used clinically to detect small genetic changes called *single-nucleotide polymorphisms* (SNPs), as well as larger chromosome deletions or additions that result in copy-number variations (CNVs) that may occur in hematologic malignancies. Next-generation sequencing (NGS) of tumor cells is also making its way into routine clinical practice. This technique is being used to analyze the nucleotide sequence of all of the genes (i.e., whole genome sequencing), the coding regions of the genome (referred to as *exome sequencing*), or the transcriptome (i.e., messenger RNA) in samples from cancer patients, including those with hematologic malignancies. The tremendous amount of data resulting from these analyses is allowing clinicians to identify genetic profiles associated with specific hematologic malignancies and is revealing new genetic alterations that are associated with the pathobiology of lymphoid neoplasms. Microarrays and NGS are enabling a more comprehensive analysis of the neoplastic genome, which is being translated into better patient diagnosis and more precise, targeted therapies for the hematologic malignancies.

SUMMARY

- The immunoproliferative diseases are a diverse group of malignancies that arise from hematopoietic cells of a lymphoid or myeloid lineage.
- Leukemias originate from hematopoietic cells in the bone marrow that migrate to the peripheral blood, whereas lymphomas are solid tumors that usually arise in the lymph nodes and affect other lymphoid tissues. However, there is often overlap in the sites affected by these malignancies.

- The WHO classification of hematologic malignancies is based on their morphological features, cytochemical staining, immunophenotype as determined by flow cytometry, and cytogenetics.
- The acute lymphocytic leukemias (ALLs) are characterized by the presence of poorly differentiated precursor cells called "blasts" that migrate rapidly in the bone marrow and are found in large numbers in the peripheral blood. They usually originate from immature precursors belonging to the B-cell lineage.
- Chronic lymphocytic leukemia (CLL)/small lymphocytic lymphoma (SLL) is a slowly progressive malignancy derived from mature B lymphocytes.
- Hairy-cell leukemia is a rare, slowly progressive disease that primarily affects the bone marrow and spleen. The malignant cells express mature B-cell markers and have irregular hairy cytoplasmic projections from their surface.
- Classic Hodgkin lymphoma is characterized by the presence of abnormal lymphocytes of B-cell origin called *Reed-Sternberg (RS) cells* in lymph nodes and other lymphoid organs. It can be divided into four subtypes based on the population of cells that surround the RS cells in the affected tissues.
- Nodular lymphocytic-predominant Hodgkin lymphoma (NLPHL) is characterized by the presence of large, lymphocytic and histiocytic (L&H) cells that express mature B-cell antigens and are surrounded by small lymphocytes. L&H cells have a single, folded nucleus that resembles popcorn and are often referred to as "popcorn cells."
- Non-Hodgkin lymphomas include a wide range of neoplasms involving the B cells, T cells, or NK cells. They are most commonly found in immunosuppressed patients and include the B-cell malignancies, diffuse large B-cell lymphoma, follicular lymphoma, mantle-cell lymphoma, and Burkitt lymphoma, and the T-cell malignancies, adult T-cell leukemia/lymphoma, mycosis fungoides, and Sézary syndrome.
- The plasma-cell dyscrasias, also known as *monoclonal gammopathies*, include plasma-cell malignancies as well as premalignant conditions of the plasma cells that are characterized by the production of a monoclonal immunoglobulin (M protein or paraprotein).
- Two premalignant conditions, monoclonal gammopathy of undetermined significance (MGUS) and smoldering multiple myeloma (SMM) are plasma-cell dyscrasias that are associated with an increased risk of progressing to multiple myeloma. They are defined by a specific concentration of monoclonal immunoglobulin and percentage of plasma cells in the bone marrow in the absence of clinical features associated with multiple myeloma.
- Multiple myeloma is a plasma-cell malignancy characterized by an increased number of plasma cells in the bone marrow that crowd out normal hematopoietic precursors. They produce an M protein, usually IgG, IgA, or free light chains. The clinical features of multiple myeloma are known as "CRAB" (increased serum <u>c</u>alcium, <u>r</u>enal failure, <u>a</u>nemia, and lytic <u>b</u>one lesions).
- Waldenström macroglobulinemia is a malignancy of plasmacytoid lymphocytes that produce an IgM paraprotein. The heavy-chain diseases are rare B-cell lymphomas that produce a monoclonal immunoglobulin heavy chain (alpha, gamma, or mu), which is incapable of binding to a light chain.
- Some patients with plasma-cell dyscrasias produce free monoclonal light chains (κ or λ) and excrete the excess in the urine, where they are known as *Bence Jones proteins*.
- Identification and quantification of the paraprotein are central to the diagnosis and monitoring of the monoclonal gammopathies. Serum protein electrophoresis (SPE) is used to detect the presence of an M protein, which is then characterized by immunofixation electrophoresis (IFE). The presence of a monoclonal immunoglobulin is indicated by a discrete, narrow band that migrates to a restricted position on the gel, whereas polyclonal immunoglobulins are diverse and produce broad, diffuse bands.
- Immunosubtraction, or immunotyping, is a procedure in which antibodies to heavy- and light-chain isotypes are added during capillary electrophoresis of the sample. The presence of an M protein is indicated by the disappearance of a monoclonal peak in the presence of its corresponding antibody.
- Analysis of urine by UPE and IFE is important in the detection of Bence Jones proteins, which can contribute to renal damage. Before testing, the urine must be concentrated by manual filtration or high-speed centrifugal filtration to yield enough protein to produce visible banding on the gel.
- Serum free light-chain assays are latex-enhanced automated immunoassays that measure free κ and λ light chains in patient serum. These are sensitive assays that can rapidly detect low levels of free light chains. An increase in κ or λ, along with an abnormal κ:λ ratio, indicates the presence of a malignant plasma-cell clone.
- The cellular origin of a lymphoid malignancy is determined in the laboratory by flow cytometry. Fluorescent-labeled antibodies are used to identify CD markers on the surface of the malignant cells to determine their lineage, their stage of maturation, and the presence of abnormal antigen expression. This procedure is called *immunophenotyping*.
- Evaluation of genetic and chromosomal abnormalities is a rapidly evolving area of laboratory practice. These alterations can be detected by a variety of cytogenetic and molecular techniques, including FISH, PCR, microarray, and NGS. These methods allow for the detection of abnormalities, such as chromosome translocations, nucleotide deletions, and unique V-D-J gene rearrangements that are characteristic of specific hematologic malignancies.

CASE STUDIES

1. A 73-year-old male visits his primary care physician complaining of fatigue and shortness of breath, upper back pain, and a cough that has become productive over the last 2 days. The patient was febrile and appeared acutely ill. A chest x-ray revealed pneumonia, and the following significant laboratory results were found:

   RBC count of 4.1×10^{12}/L (reference range 4.6 to 6.0×10^{12}/L), hemoglobin 13 g/dL (reference range 14.0 to 18.0 g/dL), WBC count of 4.8×10^9/L (reference range 4.5 to 11.0×10^9/L), and an erythrocyte sedimentation rate of 12 mm/hr (reference range 0 to 9 mm/hr).

   Based on these results, the physician ordered serum immunoglobulin levels. The following results were reported: IgG = 3,250 mg/dL (reference range 600 to 1,500 mg/dL), IgM = 48 mg/dL (reference range 75 to 150 mg/dL), and IgA = 102 mg/dL (reference range 150 to 250 mg/dL).

   Questions

   a. What disease(s) should you suspect? Why?
   b. What additional tests could help confirm the diagnosis, and what results would you expect to find?

2. A 47-year-old man presented with fever, pneumonia, and an enlarged spleen. His hemoglobin was 11.5 g/dL, the WBC count was 2,700/mm^3, and the platelet count was 70,000/mm^3. A bone marrow biopsy revealed, among the normal bone marrow cells, numerous diffuse cells 10 to 14 μm in diameter with abundant, clear to lightly basophilic or eosinophilic cytoplasm. The surface of the cells exhibited delicate broad projections. The nuclei were oval and indented with variable chromatin and no prominent nucleoli. Immunohistochemical analysis revealed that the leukemic cells were positive for CD20, DBA44 (a B-cell marker), CD68, and annexin A1. Expression of CD20, CD11c, CD25, and CD103 was demonstrated by flow cytometry.

   Questions

   a. What disease(s) should be considered in the differential diagnosis?
   b. What is the significance of the immunophenotyping results?

REVIEW QUESTIONS

1. Bence Jones proteins consist of
   a. monoclonal IgG.
   b. IgG–IgM complexes.
   c. free κ or λ light chains.
   d. free μ heavy chains.

2. Which of the following would be the best indicator of a malignant clone of cells?
   a. Overall increase in antibody production
   b. Increase in IgG and IgM only
   c. Increase in antibody directed against a specific epitope
   d. Decrease in overall antibody production

3. Which of the following laboratory techniques is routinely used to identify chromosome translocations associated with specific hematologic malignancies?
   a. FISH
   b. IFE
   c. Immunosubtraction
   d. PCR

4. All of the following features are commonly used to classify lymphoid neoplasms *except*
   a. cell of origin.
   b. presence of gene translocations.
   c. exposure of the patient to carcinogens.
   d. morphology or cytology of the malignant cells.

5. Hodgkin lymphoma is characterized by
   a. proliferation of T cells.
   b. excess immunoglobulin production.
   c. an incurable, rapidly progressive course.
   d. the presence of Reed-Sternberg cells in lymph nodes.

6. Chronic leukemias are characterized as
   a. usually being of B-cell origin.
   b. being curable with chemotherapy.
   c. usually occurring in children.
   d. following a rapidly progressive course.

7. Which of the following is characteristic of heavy-chain diseases?
   a. Usually of B-cell origin
   b. Rare lymphomas
   c. Production of abnormal Ig heavy chains
   d. All of the above

8. Flow cytometry results for a patient reveal a decrease of cells with CD2 and CD3. These results indicate a reduced number of what type of cells?
   a. B cells
   b. T cells
   c. Monocytes
   d. Natural killer cells

9. Which of the following is true of Waldenström macroglobulinemia?
   a. Monoclonal IgM production may be associated with hyperviscosity syndrome.
   b. Multiple Ig-producing clones are found.
   c. The malignant cells produce monoclonal free heavy chains.
   d. Bence Jones proteins are never produced.

10. The presence of anemia, bone pain, thrombocytopenia, and lytic bone lesions is suggestive of
    a. Hodgkin lymphoma.
    b. hairy-cell leukemia.
    c. chronic lymphocytic leukemia.
    d. multiple myeloma.

11. The presence of an M protein on immunofixation electrophoresis (IFE) is indicated by
    a. broad, diffuse banding.
    b. a narrow, discrete band.
    c. a few well-defined bands in the IgG lane.
    d. a single band at the point of application in all of the lanes.

12. Surface immunoglobulin on a leukemic cell indicates presence of a
    a. B cell.
    b. T cell.
    c. macrophage.
    d. plasma cell.

13. Which of the following is *not* a requirement for urine testing by IFE?
    a. Collection of a 24-hour sample
    b. Concentration of the sample
    c. Dilution of the sample
    d. Removal of sediment

14. Multiple myeloma is characteristically preceded by
    a. chronic hypogammaglobulinemia.
    b. EBV infection.
    c. non-Hodgkin lymphoma.
    d. monoclonal gammopathy of undetermined significance.

15. Which serum free light-chain (sFLC) assay result indicates the presence of a malignant plasma-cell clone?
    a. An abnormal κ:λ ratio
    b. A decrease in κ and λ concentrations
    c. A decrease in IgG, IgA, and IgM concentrations
    d. An increase in immunoglobulin concentrations over a 24-hour period

19 Immunodeficiency Diseases

Thomas S. Alexander, PhD, D(ABMLI)

LEARNING OUTCOMES

After finishing this chapter, you should be able to:

1. Differentiate between primary immunodeficiency diseases and secondary immunodeficiency diseases.
2. Indicate the general immunologic defects associated with each of the nine categories of primary immunodeficiency diseases.
3. Associate examples of specific immunodeficiencies with each category.
4. Describe the types of infections typically associated with defects in the B-cell, T-cell, myeloid, or complement systems.
5. Recognize the association between immunodeficiency states and the risk of developing malignancy.
6. Explain the immunologic defects and clinical manifestations associated with selected primary immunodeficiency diseases.
7. Select appropriate laboratory tests to screen for and confirm the presence of specific congenital immunodeficiencies.
8. Correlate laboratory results with the presence of different types of primary immunodeficiency diseases.

CHAPTER OUTLINE

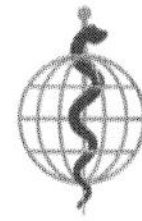

Go to FADavis.com for the laboratory exercises that accompany this text.

KEY TERMS

Agammaglobulinemias
Ataxia-telangiectasia (AT)
Bruton's tyrosine kinase (Btk) deficiency
Chronic granulomatous disease (CGD)
Common variable immunodeficiency (CVI)
DiGeorge syndrome
Immunodeficiencies
Immunofixation electrophoresis (IFE)
Inflammasome
Mitogen
Oxidative burst
Primary immunodeficiency diseases (PIDs)
Purine-nucleoside phosphorylase (PNP) deficiency
Secondary immunodeficiency
Severe combined immunodeficiency (SCID)
Transient hypogammaglobulinemia
22q11.2 deletion syndrome
Wiskott-Aldrich syndrome (WAS)

Immunodeficiencies are disorders in which a part of the body's immune system is missing or dysfunctional. People with these conditions have a decreased ability to defend themselves against infectious organisms and are more susceptible to developing certain types of cancer. The clinical symptoms associated with immunodeficiencies range from very mild or subclinical to severe, recurrent infections or failure to thrive. Immunodeficiencies can be inherited or acquired (secondary) because of other conditions, such as certain infections, malignancies, autoimmune disorders, and immunosuppressive therapies. An example of a **secondary immunodeficiency** is AIDS, which is caused by HIV. AIDS is discussed in detail in Chapter 24. This chapter focuses on the **primary immunodeficiency diseases (PIDs)**, which are *inherited* dysfunctions of the immune system. Several of the immunodeficiency syndromes show X-linked inheritance and, therefore, affect primarily males. Others show autosomal recessive or autosomal dominant inheritance.

The International Union of Immunological Societies has identified more than 350 different congenital forms of immunodeficiency. These phenotypes are the result of specific genetic defects, including defects in lymphoid cells, phagocytic cells, regulatory molecules, and complement proteins. With the exception of immunoglobulin A (IgA) deficiency, the PIDs are rare disorders with a combined incidence of about 1 in 1,200 live births. In spite of their rarity, it is important for physicians to consider the possibility of PID in children with recurrent infections because early detection and treatment can help prevent serious, long-term tissue damage or overwhelming sepsis. Early diagnosis can also provide the opportunity for appropriate genetic counseling, carrier detection, and prenatal diagnosis for other family members. The clinical laboratory plays an essential role in identifying these important diseases. This chapter serves as an introduction to the PIDs and the laboratory methods used to detect the presence of these disorders.

Clinical Effects of Primary Immunodeficiency Diseases

The PIDs can affect one or more parts of the immune system, depending on the specific disease. Some PIDs have their primary effect on B cells and humoral immunity, whereas others mainly affect the cell-mediated branch of the adaptive immune system. Other conditions involve components of the innate defense system, such as the phagocytic cells, complement, or natural killer (NK) cells. **Figure 19–1** illustrates points in the development of the immune system at which some PIDs exert their main effects.

The types of infection or symptoms displayed by a patient can give important clues regarding the specific immunodeficiency present. In general, defects in humoral immunity (antibody production) result in pyogenic (i.e., pus-forming) bacterial infections, particularly of the upper and lower respiratory tract. Recurrent sinusitis and otitis media (i.e., ear infections) are common. The clinical course of viral infections in patients with predominantly antibody deficiencies is not significantly different from that in normal hosts, with the exception of hepatitis B, which may have a fulminant course in patients with **agammaglobulinemias,** conditions in which antibody levels in the blood are significantly decreased.

Defects in T-cell–mediated immunity result in recurrent infections with intracellular pathogens such as viruses, fungi, and intracellular bacteria. Differentiating primary cellular deficiencies from HIV-induced immunodeficiency is essential for proper treatment. Patients with congenital T-cell deficiencies almost always develop mucocutaneous candidiasis, a yeast infection that involves the skin, nails, and mucous membranes. They are also prone to disseminated viral infections, especially with latent viruses such as herpes simplex, varicella zoster, and cytomegalovirus. Because T cells also play an important role in tumor immunity, patients with these conditions are more susceptible to developing certain types of cancer. Age-adjusted rates of malignancy in patients with immunodeficiency disease are much greater than those observed in immunocompetent individuals. Most of the malignancies are lymphoid and may be related to persistent stimulation of the remaining immune cells, coupled with defective immune regulation.

Defects in other components of the immune system also have significant consequences. For example, neutrophils are the first line of defense against invading organisms, and defects in neutrophil function are usually reflected in recurrent pyogenic bacterial infections or impaired wound healing. Abnormalities in macrophage function will have effects on both the innate and the adaptive defenses because macrophages are involved in the nonspecific phagocytosis of microorganisms during inflammation as well as in the processing of antigens and their

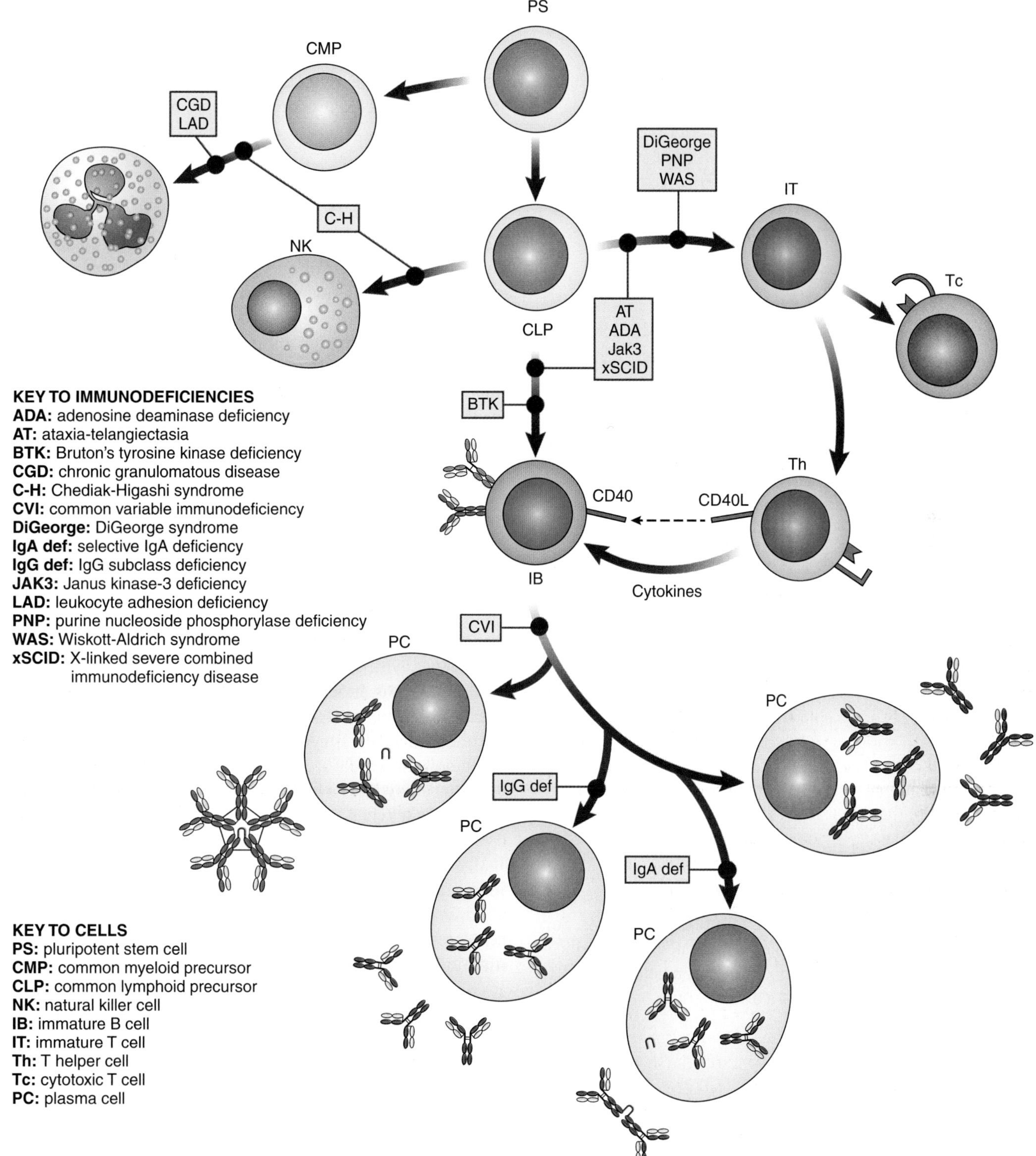

FIGURE 19–1 Examples of primary immunodeficiency diseases and their effects on the immune system.

presentation to T cells in humoral and cell-mediated immune responses. Reduction in the macrophage population by splenectomy is associated with an increased risk of overwhelming bacterial infection accompanied by septicemia. The complement system, as discussed in Chapter 7, is activated directly by antigens or by antigen–antibody complexes to produce biologically active molecules that enhance inflammation and promote lysis of microorganisms. Deficiencies of complement components result in recurrent bacterial infections and autoimmune-type manifestations. The severity of the conditions varies with the particular complement component that is deficient.

The components of the immune system play unique, but overlapping, roles in the host defense process. Therefore, defects in any one of the cellular or humoral components result in distinct clinical manifestations, as previously discussed. However, because the components of the immune system interact extensively through many regulatory and effector networks, a defect in one branch of the system may affect other aspects of immune function as well. In many cases, it appears that deficiency of one component of the immune system is accompanied by hyperactivity of other components. This may occur because persistent infections continuously stimulate the available immune cells or because a compensatory mechanism has been activated to correct for the deficient immune function.

In addition, the deficiency may involve a component that normally exerts regulatory control over other components of the immune system—control that is lacking in the deficiency state. For instance, T helper (Th2) cells secrete cytokines that regulate the development of B cells into plasma cells. A defect in Th2 cell function, such as a deficiency in CD154 (also known as the *CD40 ligand*, a molecule involved in binding to cell receptors during T-dependent immune responses), removes or creates an imbalance in the regulation of those immune responses. Whatever the mechanism, many partial immunodeficiency states are associated with allergic or autoimmune manifestations, currently referred to as *autoinflammatory disorders* (see discussion in the text that follows).

The Nine Categories of Primary Immunodeficiency Diseases

In the past, the immunodeficiencies were broadly classified as defects in T cells, B cells, phagocytes, complement proteins, and other components of the innate immune system. As scientific knowledge has been gained about the complexity of these disorders, experts have recognized that such a broad classification is overly simplistic. In 2014, the International Union of Immunologic Societies (IUIS) updated its classification of PIDs by grouping them into nine different categories based on their characteristic clinical features, immunologic defects, and genetic abnormalities. The IUIS again updated the classification system in 2017 and has published diagnostic flow charts to aid in classifying patients into a disease entity based on clinical symptoms and laboratory results. The nine categories are:

- Category 1: Immunodeficiencies Affecting Cellular and Humoral Immunity
- Category 2: Combined Immunodeficiencies With Associated or Syndromic Features
- Category 3: Predominantly Antibody Deficiencies
- Category 4: Diseases of Immune Dysregulation
- Category 5: Congenital Defects of Phagocyte Number, Function, or Both
- Category 6: Defects in Intrinsic and Innate Immunity
- Category 7: Autoinflammatory Disorders
- Category 8: Complement Deficiencies
- Category 9: Phenocopies of Primary Immunodeficiencies

Although the PIDs are separated into these categories, some diseases are listed in more than one category because they possess overlapping features. The following sections describe the main characteristics of each category and examples of specific PIDs that have been included in each category. Category 3, Predominantly Antibody Deficiencies, is discussed first because the conditions in this category are the most common immunodeficiencies, representing about one-half of all PIDs.

Category 3: Predominantly Antibody Deficiencies

This category encompasses conditions in which the main characteristic is low levels of serum immunoglobulins. Immunoglobulins migrate in the "gamma region" of the serum protein electrophoretic profile (discussed in Chapter 5). Therefore, deficiencies of immunoglobulins have been termed *agammaglobulinemias*. The mechanisms of the agammaglobulinemias include genetic defects in B-cell maturation or mutations leading to defective interactions between B cells and T cells. A wide range of immunoglobulin deficiency states have been reported and involve virtually all combinations of immunoglobulins and all degrees of severity. In some cases, only a single isotype of one immunoglobulin class is deficient, whereas all of the other isotypes are normal. Only the more common and well-characterized syndromes are described here. These are summarized in **Table 19–1.**

In evaluating immunoglobulin deficiency states, it is important to remember that blood levels of immunoglobulins change with age. The blood level of immunoglobulin G (IgG) at birth is about the same as the adult level, reflecting transfer of maternal IgG across the placenta. The IgG level declines during the first 6 months of life, as maternal antibody is catabolized. Levels of IgA and immunoglobulin M (IgM) are very low at birth. The concentrations of all immunoglobulins gradually rise when the infant begins to produce antibodies at a few months of age in response to environmental antigens. IgM reaches normal adult levels first, around 1 year of age, followed by IgG at about 5 to 6 years of age. In some normal children, IgA levels do not reach normal adult values until adolescence. Therefore, it is important to compare a child's immunoglobulin levels to age-matched reference ranges.

Transient Hypogammaglobulinemia of Infancy With Normal Numbers of B Cells

All infants experience low levels of immunoglobulins at approximately 5 to 6 months of age; however, in some babies, the low levels persist for a longer time. Because these children do not begin synthesizing immunoglobulins promptly, they can experience severe pyogenic sinopulmonary and skin infections as protective maternal IgG is cleared. Cell-mediated immunity is normal, and there may be normal levels of IgA and IgM. IgG appears to be the most affected, dropping to at least two standard deviations (SDs) below the age-adjusted mean with or without a depression of IgM and IgA. Immunoglobulin levels in infants with this condition usually normalize spontaneously, often by 9 to 15 months of age. The mechanism of this **transient hypogammaglobulinemia** is not known. These patients have normal numbers of circulating CD19+ B cells. This condition does not appear to be X-linked,

Table 19–1 Characteristics of Selected Predominantly Antibody Deficiencies (Category 3)

CONDITION	DEFICIENCY	LEVEL OF DEFECT	PRESENTATION
Transient hypogammaglobulinemia of infancy	All antibodies; especially IgG	Slow development of T helper function in some patients	2–6 months; resolves by 2 years
Selective IgA deficiency	IgA; some also with reduced IgG2	IgA-B cell differentiation	Often asymptomatic
Btk deficiency	All antibody isotypes reduced	Pre–B-cell differentiation	Infancy
Common variable immunodeficiency	Reduced antibody; many different combinations	B cell; excess T- cell suppression	Usually 20–30 years of age
Isolated IgG subclass deficiency	Reduced IgG1, IgG2, IgG3, or IgG4	Defect of isotype differentiation	Variable in the class and degree of deficiency
CD154 deficiency	Reduced IgG, IgA, IgE, with elevated IgM	Ig class switching in B cells	Variable

although it is more common in males. The cause may be related to a delayed maturation of one or more components of the immune system, possibly Th cells.

X-Linked Bruton's Tyrosine Kinase (Btk) Deficiency

Bruton's tyrosine kinase (Btk) deficiency, first described in 1952, is X-chromosome, so this syndrome affects males almost exclusively. Patients with X-linked agammaglobulinemia lack circulating mature CD19+ B cells and exhibit a deficiency or lack of immunoglobulins of all classes. Furthermore, they have no plasma cells in their lymphoid tissues. The patients do, however, have pre-B cells in their bone marrow. Because of the lack of B cells, the tonsils and adenoids are small or entirely absent, and lymph nodes lack normal germinal centers. T cells are normal in number and function. About half of the patients have a family history of the syndrome. They develop recurrent bacterial infections beginning in infancy as maternal antibody is cleared. The patients most commonly develop sinopulmonary infections caused by encapsulated organisms such as streptococci, meningococci, and *Haemophilus influenzae.* Other infections seen include bacterial otitis media, bronchitis, pneumonia, meningitis, and dermatitis. Some patients also have a susceptibility to certain types of viral infections, including vaccine-associated poliomyelitis. In general, live virus vaccines should not be administered to immunodeficient patients.

X-linked hypogammaglobulinemia results from arrested differentiation at the pre–B-cell stage, leading to a complete absence of B cells and plasma cells. The underlying genetic mechanism is a deficiency of an enzyme called the Btk in B-cell progenitor cells. Lack of the enzyme apparently causes a failure of immunoglobulin V_H gene rearrangement (see Chapter 5). The syndrome can be effectively treated by administration of intramuscular or intravenous immunoglobulin preparations and vigorous antimicrobial treatment of infections. Btk deficiency can be differentiated from transient hypogammaglobulinemia of infancy by the absence of CD19+ B cells in the peripheral blood, the abnormal histology of lymphoid tissues, and its persistence beyond 2 years of age. Immunologists have also described patients with a similar clinical presentation to Btk deficiency who have a genetic defect that is inherited in an autosomal recessive manner.

Selective IgA Deficiency

Selective IgA deficiency is the most common congenital immunodeficiency, occurring in about 1 in 500 persons of American or European descent. Most patients with a deficiency of IgA are asymptomatic. Those with symptoms usually have infections of the respiratory and gastrointestinal tract and an increased tendency to develop autoimmune diseases such as systemic lupus erythematosus (SLE), rheumatoid arthritis (RA), celiac disease, and thyroiditis. Allergic disorders and malignancy are also more common. About 20% of the IgA-deficient patients who develop infections also have an IgG2 subclass deficiency. If the serum IgA is lower than 5 mg/dL, the deficiency is considered severe. If the IgA level is two SDs below the age-adjusted mean but greater than 50 mg/dL, the deficiency is partial. Although the genetic defect has not been established, it is hypothesized that lack of IgA is caused by impaired differentiation of lymphocytes to become IgA-producing plasma cells.

IgE antibodies specifically directed against IgA are produced by 30% to 40% of patients with severe IgA deficiency. These antibodies can cause anaphylactic reactions when blood products containing IgA are transfused. Because many patients with severe IgA deficiency have no other symptoms, the IgA deficiency may not be detected until the patient experiences a transfusion reaction, resulting in the production of anti-IgA antibodies. Therefore, products for transfusion to known IgA-deficient patients should be collected from IgA-deficient donors, and cellular products should be washed to remove as much donor plasma as possible. IgA deficiency is also more common in patients with celiac disease (incidence of about 2%) than in the non-celiac population.

Most gamma globulin preparations contain significant amounts of IgA. However, replacement IgA therapy is not useful because the half-life of IgA is short (around 7 days) and intravenously or intramuscularly administered IgA is not transported to its normal site of secretion at mucosal surfaces. Furthermore, administration of IgA-containing products can

Connections

Anaphylaxis

Recall from Chapter 14 that anaphylaxis is a type I hypersensitivity reaction that is mediated by immunoglobulin E (IgE) antibodies. Blood transfusions or gamma globulin administration to IgA-deficient individuals can stimulate the production of IgE antibodies in response to the IgA contained in these products, which is recognized as a foreign antigen. The IgE antibodies sensitize mast cells in the IgA-deficient patients, and the surface IgE molecules are cross-linked upon repeated exposure to IgA. Therefore, the mast cells are triggered to release histamine and other chemical mediators, which cause increased vasodilation, vasopermeability, and smooth muscle contractions. These reactions result in a systemic response, including symptoms such as hypotension and respiratory distress, which can be rapidly fatal if it is not recognized and treated quickly.

induce the development of anti-IgA antibodies or provoke anaphylaxis in patients who already have antibodies.

Common Variable Immunodeficiency (CVI)

Common variable immunodeficiency (CVI) is a heterogeneous group of disorders with a prevalence of about 1 in 25,000. Although this is a low incidence, CVI is the most common PID with a severe clinical syndrome. Patients usually begin to have symptoms in their 20s and 30s, but children and the elderly can also develop the disease. The disorder can be congenital or acquired, or familial or sporadic, and it occurs with equal frequency in men and women. CVI is characterized by hypogammaglobulinemia that leads to recurrent bacterial infections, particularly sinusitis and pneumonia. In addition, up to 20% of CVI patients develop herpes zoster (shingles), a much higher incidence than in immunologically normal young adults. There is usually a deficiency of both IgA and IgG, but selective IgG deficiency may occur. CVI is often associated with a sprue-like syndrome characterized by malabsorption and diarrhea. CVI is also associated with an increased risk of lymphoproliferative disorders, gastric carcinomas, and autoimmune disorders. The most common autoimmune manifestations of CVI are immune thrombocytopenia and autoimmune hemolytic anemia. Other symptoms may include lymphadenopathy, splenomegaly, and intestinal hyperplasia.

CVI is diagnosed by demonstrating a low serum IgG level in patients with recurrent bacterial infections. Additionally, blood group isohemagglutinins, or the so-called naturally occurring antibodies, are typically absent or low. In contrast to X-linked agammaglobulinemia, most patients with CVI have normal numbers of mature B cells. However, these B cells do not differentiate normally into immunoglobulin-producing plasma cells. Three major types of cellular defects have been found in CVI patients. In some cases, T cells or their products appear to suppress differentiation of B cells into plasma cells. Secondly, T cells may fail to provide adequate help to support terminal differentiation of B cells. Finally, there appears to be a primary defect in the B-cell line in some patients. CVI is often a diagnosis of exclusion, where an immunodeficiency is present with no specific genetic defect defined.

CVI can usually be effectively treated with intramuscular or intravenous immunoglobulin preparations. However, because of their low levels of secretory IgA, patients are still susceptible to respiratory and gastrointestinal infections; clinicians should be vigilant for these infections and treat them vigorously with antibiotics.

Isolated IgG Subclass Deficiency

IgG subclass deficiencies are conditions in which the levels of one or more of the four IgG subclasses are more than two SDs below the mean age-appropriate level. Normally, about 66% of the total IgG is IgG1, 23% IgG2, 7% IgG3, and 4% IgG4. Therefore, a deficiency of a single subclass may not result in a total IgG level below the normal range. In patients with recurrent infections, levels of the different subclasses should be measured if the total IgG level is normal but the clinical picture suggests immunoglobulin deficiency.

Most IgG antibodies directed against protein antigens are of the IgG1 and IgG3 subclasses, whereas most IgG antibodies against carbohydrate antigens are IgG2 or IgG4. Thus, deficiencies involving IgG1 or IgG3 lead to a reduced capability of responding to protein antigens such as toxins, whereas selective deficiencies of IgG2 can result in impaired responses to polysaccharide antigens, which cause recurrent infections with polysaccharide-encapsulated bacteria such as *Streptococcus pneumoniae* and *H. influenzae*. A variety of genetic defects have been associated with IgG subclass deficiency. These include heavy-chain gene deletions and transcriptional defects. The most common subclass deficiency is IgG4, although IgG4 subclass deficiency may have the least clinical significance, and IgG1 deficiency is the least common.

Category 1: Immunodeficiencies Affecting Cellular and Humoral Immunity

This category contains diseases in which there are defects in both humoral (B-cell) and cell-mediated (T-cell) immunity. These deficiencies result from mutations that affect development of both types of lymphocytes or cause defective interaction between the two antigen-specific limbs of the adaptive immune system. Because helper T-cell functions are necessary for normal differentiation and antibody secretion by B cells, a severe defect of T-cell function will have effects on immunoglobulin levels as well. Combined deficiencies are referred to using a shorthand notation of $T^{+/-}B^{+/-}NK^{+/-}$ with the $^{+}$ or $^{-}$ superscript denoting whether or not each cell type is present in the deficiency.

Severe Combined Immunodeficiency (SCID)

The most serious of the congenital immunodeficiencies is **severe combined immunodeficiency (SCID).** SCID is actually a group of related diseases that all affect T- and B-cell function but with differing causes. A mutation in the interleukin-2 receptor gamma (IL2RG) gene located on the X-chromosome is the most common form of the disease, accounting for nearly half of the cases in the United States. The mutation occurs with a frequency of about 1 in 50,000 births. The IL2RG gene codes for a protein chain called the *common gamma chain* that is common to receptors for interleukins −2, −4, −7, −9, −15, and −21. Normal signaling cannot occur in cells with defective receptors, thus halting maturation of the lymphocytes. This may result in either a $T^-B^+NK^+$ or a $T^-B^+NK^-$ phenotype, depending on whether or not there is an additional defect in the *JAK3* gene. *JAK3* is required for processing an interleukin-binding signal from the cell membrane to the nucleus. No antibody production or lymphocyte proliferative response follows an antigen or mitogen challenge in such cases.

Several autosomal recessive forms of SCID, which affect both males and females, have also been discovered. For example, a *JAK3* deficiency may be found without the common gamma-chain deletion. The lack of the intracellular kinase *JAK3* means that lymphocytes are unable to transmit signals from IL-2 and IL-4. These patients have a $T^-B^+NK^-$ phenotype, and symptoms are similar to the X-linked form of the disease. The *JAK3* gene is located on chromosome 19, region p12. Other autosomal recessive forms of SCID are discussed in the paragraphs that follow.

About 15% to 20% of the patients with SCID have an adenosine deaminase (ADA) deficiency, leading to a $T^-B^-NK^-$ phenotype. The ADA gene is located on chromosome 1, region q21. ADA deficiency affects an enzyme involved in the metabolism of purines, similar to another form of PID, the PNP deficiency. In ADA deficiency, toxic metabolites of purines accumulate in lymphoid cells and impair proliferation of both B and T cells. In both ADA and PNP deficiencies, there is a progressive decrease in lymphocyte numbers. Several different mutations have been found to lead to ADA deficiency, and the degree of immunodeficiency correlates with the degree of ADA deficiency. Patients with only mildly reduced ADA activity may have only a slight impairment of immune function.

Other molecular defects have also been identified as causes of SCID. Infants with a lack of both T cells and B cells but with functioning NK cells were found to have a mutation in a recombinase-activating gene (RAG-1 or RAG-2). These mutations cause a profound lymphocytopenia because of the inability of T and B cells to rearrange DNA, a process that is necessary to produce functional immunoglobulins or T-cell receptors (TCRs). Patients with RAG-1 or RAG-2 deficiencies have decreased class II major histocompatibility complex (MHC) molecule expression. Human leukocyte antigen (HLA) class II molecules are intimately involved in antigen presentation; thus, this defect profoundly impairs the immune response. Another molecular defect that has been identified is a mutation in the gene encoding a common leukocyte protein called *CD45*. It is a transmembrane phosphatase that regulates signal transduction of T- and B-cell receptors.

Patients with SCID generally present early in infancy with infection by nearly any type of organism. Oral *Candida* yeast infections, pneumonia, and diarrhea are the most common manifestations. The administration of live vaccines can cause severe illness. Unless immune reconstitution can be achieved by bone marrow transplantation or by specifically replacing a deficient enzyme, patients with SCID typically die before they are 2 years old.

ADA deficiency is a special case because it presents a good opportunity for enzyme replacement therapy or somatic cell gene therapy. Although ADA is normally located within cells, its deficiency can be treated by maintaining high plasma levels of ADA. For some patients, red blood cell (RBC) transfusion can raise ADA to near-normal levels. However, bovine ADA conjugated with polyethylene glycol (PEG) has a longer half-life than native ADA and can raise the ADA level up to three times higher than normal. This treatment increases T-cell production and specific antibody responses. Side effects of ADA–PEG appear to be minimal. However, this therapy is very expensive and is primarily used in patients for whom a suitable hematopoietic stem cell donor cannot be found or for those patients who are too sick to undergo transplantation. Gene therapy for treatment of ADA deficiency has been accomplished by transfecting a normal ADA gene into patients' T cells or stem cells and reinfusing the gene-corrected cells into the patient. This type of therapy has resulted in sustained immune reconstitution and fewer infections in a significant number of patients.

Purine-Nucleoside Phosphorylase (PNP) Deficiency

Another immunodeficiency state for which a specific enzymatic basis has been defined is **purine-nucleoside phosphorylase (PNP) deficiency.** PNP deficiency is a rare autosomal recessive trait. The condition presents in infancy with recurrent or chronic pulmonary infections, oral or cutaneous candidiasis, diarrhea, skin infections, urinary tract infections, and failure to thrive. PNP deficiency affects an enzyme involved in the metabolism of purines. It produces a moderate to severe defect in cell-mediated immunity, with normal or only mildly impaired humoral immunity. The number of T cells progressively decreases because of the accumulation of deoxyguanosine triphosphate, a toxic purine metabolite. The levels of immunoglobulins are generally normal or increased. About two-thirds of PNP-deficient patients also have neurological disorders, but no characteristic physical abnormalities have been described. Because of the relatively selective defect in cell-mediated immunity, PNP deficiency can be confused with neonatal HIV infection. The two conditions can usually be distinguished by specific tests for HIV (see Chapter 24) and by assays for PNP activity.

Category 2: Combined Immunodeficiencies With Associated or Syndromic Features

This category differs from Category 1 in that the diseases in Category 2 are characterized by nonimmunologic features in addition to the combined immunodeficiency. Diseases in this category are typically caused by defects in cell-mediated immunity, which indirectly lead to problems with the other branches of the immune response. Often, these diseases can result from abnormalities at different stages of T-cell development. Many different molecular defects can result in a similar clinical picture (as in SCID). This is because T cells provide helper functions that are necessary for normal B-cell development and differentiation. Some of the more common defects of cellular and combined cellular and humoral immunity are summarized in **Table 19–2.**

In general, defects in cellular immunity are more difficult to manage than defects in humoral immunity. When immunoglobulin production is deficient, replacement therapy is often very effective. However, there is usually no soluble product that can be administered to treat a deficiency of cell-mediated immunity. Transplantation of immunologically intact cells, usually in the form of allogenic bone marrow or peripheral blood stem cells, is often required to reconstitute immune function.

Unlike patients with defects in humoral immunity only, those with severe defects in cell-mediated immunity may develop graft-versus-host disease (GVHD; see Chapter 16). Transfused lymphocytes are normally destroyed by the recipient's T-cell system. However, a severe defect in the T-cell system allows the donor lymphocytes to survive, proliferate, and attack the tissues of the recipient as foreign. GVHD can occur in any patient with a severe defect in cell-mediated immunity (e.g., in bone marrow transplant recipients) and can be fatal. Irradiation of cell-containing blood products (platelet concentrates, packed RBCs, and whole blood) before transfusion destroys the ability of the donor lymphocytes to proliferate and prevents the development of GVHD in immunodeficient recipients.

GVHD also occurs in patients who have received a bone marrow transplant as therapy for a congenital immunodeficiency. The closer the match between the genetic constitution of the patient and the graft donor, the less severe the GVHD is likely to be. Thus, although hematopoietic stem cell transplantation can potentially cure the immune defect, it can also have serious, lifelong complications of its own. Examples of specific immunodeficiencies in Category 2 are discussed in the text that follows.

Wiskott-Aldrich Syndrome (WAS)

Wiskott-Aldrich syndrome (WAS) is a rare X-linked recessive syndrome that is defined by the triad of immunodeficiency,

Table 19–2 Characteristics of Selected Immunodeficiencies Affecting Cellular and Humoral Immunity (Category 1) and Combined Immunodeficiencies With Associated or Syndromic Features (Category 2)

CONDITION	DEFICIENCY	LEVEL OF DEFECT	PRESENTATION
Category 1			
CD40 ligand deficiency	T cells with effects on antibody production	Defective isotype switching with increased or normal IgM but decreased concentrations of other isotypes	1–2 years of age
SCID	Both T cells and B cells	ADA, purine metabolism; RAG-1/RAG-2; *JAK3;* common gamma-chain receptor; others	Infancy
PNP deficiency	T cells; some secondary effects on antibody production	PNP synthesis, purine metabolism	Infancy
Category 2			
The 22q11.2 Deletion (DiGeorge) Syndrome	T cells; some secondary effects on antibody production	Chromosome 22 deletion, embryonic development of the thymus	Neonatal, with hypocalcemia or cardiac defects if severe; abnormal mental delay; defect in thymus development; incomplete forms may present later with infection
WAS	Reduced IgM and T-cell defect	CD43 expression	Usually infancy; with thrombocytopenia, small platelets, and eczema
AT	Reduced IgG2, IgA, IgE, and T lymphocytes	DNA instability	Infancy, with involuntary muscle movements and capillary swelling

ADA = adenosine deaminase; AT = ataxia-telangiectasia; PNP = purine-nucleoside phosphorylase; SCID = severe combined immunodeficiency; WAS = Wiskott-Aldrich syndrome.

Connections

Graft-Versus-Host Disease

As we discussed in Chapter 16, GVHD results from an immune response of donor T lymphocytes within the hematopoietic cell transplant to different HLA antigens on the recipient's cells. The immunocompetent cells within the graft can cause severe damage to the host's tissues, most notably the skin, gastrointestinal tract, and liver. GVHD may become chronic and is potentially lethal.

eczema, and thrombocytopenia. WAS is usually lethal in childhood because of infection, hemorrhage, or malignancy. Milder variants have also been described, such as an X-linked form of thrombocytopenia.

The laboratory features of WAS include a decrease in platelet number and size with a prolonged bleeding time. The bone marrow contains a normal or somewhat increased number of megakaryocytes. There are abnormalities in both the cellular and humoral branches of the immune system related to a general defect in antigen processing. Therefore, patients display a severe deficiency of isohemagglutinins (IgM antibodies to ABO blood group antigens). The absence of isohemagglutinins is the most consistent laboratory finding in WAS and is often used diagnostically. Patients with WAS can have a variety of different patterns of immunoglobulin levels, but they usually have low levels of IgM, normal levels of IgA and IgG, and increased levels of IgE. These patients also have persistently increased levels of serum alpha-fetoprotein, which can also be a useful diagnostic feature.

Clinical Correlations

Isohemagglutinins

Isohemagglutinins are antibodies, mainly of the IgM class, that are produced by individuals against antigens of the ABO system that they do not possess. Persons who are blood type A lack the B antigen on their RBCs and normally have anti-B antibodies in their serum. Likewise, type B individuals lack the A antigen and normally have anti-A in their serum. Type O persons lack both the A and B antigens and therefore produce both anti-A and anti-B. Isohemagglutinins are present in the serum of newborns and are commonly tested for when looking for a humoral immunodeficiency. Their origin is unclear, but they may be produced spontaneously by a subset of B lymphocytes (so-called "natural antibodies") and/or by adaptive immune responses to cross-reacting bacterial or food antigens.

The primary molecular defect in the syndrome appears to be an abnormality of the integral membrane protein CD43, which is involved in the regulation of protein glycosylation. The gene responsible for the defect, called the *WAS* gene, is located on the X chromosome, region p11. Abnormalities cause defective actin polymerization and affect its signal transduction in lymphocytes and platelets.

Platelets have a shortened half-life, and T lymphocytes are also affected, although B lymphocytes appear to function normally. Splenectomy can be very valuable in controlling the thrombocytopenia. Treatment for this immunodeficiency involves transplantation of hematopoietic stem cells from an HLA-identical sibling.

The 22q11.2 Deletion Syndrome (DiGeorge Syndrome)

The **22q11.2 deletion syndrome** is an autosomal dominant disorder that results from a deletion in chromosome 22, region q11. The deletion can be detected by fluorescence *in situ* hybridization (FISH). The syndrome has also been known by several other names, including **DiGeorge syndrome**, velocardiofacial syndrome, Shprintzen syndrome, and conotruncal anomaly face syndrome, because of the variations in the clinical features that may be seen.

The deleted genes result in abnormalities of the third and fourth pharyngeal pouches that affect thymus development in the embryo. All organs derived from these embryonic structures can be affected. Associated abnormalities include mental retardation, absence of ossification of the hyoid bone, cardiac anomalies, abnormal facial development, and thymic hypoplasia. The severity and extent of the developmental defect can be quite variable. Many patients with a partial deletion have only a minimal thymic defect and, thus, near-normal immune function. However, about 20% of children have a pronounced and persistent decrease in T-cell numbers. These children tend to have severe, recurrent viral and fungal infections. Severely affected children usually present in the neonatal period with tetany (caused by hypocalcemia resulting from hypoparathyroidism) or manifestations of cardiac defects.

The possibility of immunodeficiency can be overlooked if the association between the presenting abnormality and a possible thymic defect is not recognized. The immunodeficiency associated with the DiGeorge anomaly is a quantitative defect in thymocytes. Not enough mature T cells are made, but those that are present are functionally normal. The immunodeficiency associated with the syndrome can be treated with transplantation of hematopoietic stem cells or fetal thymus tissue.

Ataxia-Telangiectasia (AT)

Ataxia-telangiectasia (AT) is a complex, autosomal recessive syndrome that affects the nervous system and the immune system. It is characterized by cerebellar ataxia (involuntary muscle movements) and telangiectasias (capillary swelling, resulting in red blotches on the skin), especially on the earlobes and conjunctiva. Blood vessels in the sclera of the eyes may be dilated, and there may also be a reddish butterfly area on the face and ears. The majority of patients exhibit increased levels of serum alpha-fetoprotein. Patients have a combined defect of humoral and cellular immunity. Antibody response to antigens, especially polysaccharides, is blunted. The levels of IgG2, IgA, and IgE are often low or absent, although the pattern can be quite variable. In addition, the number of circulating T cells is often decreased.

Although the incidence of this disease is rare, as much as 1% of the population is heterozygous for the genetic mutation associated with the condition. Patients with AT have a defect in a gene that is apparently essential to the recombination process for genes in the immunoglobulin superfamily. The *AT* gene is located on chromosome 11, region q22. This abnormality results in a defective kinase involved in DNA repair and in cell cycle control. Rearrangement of TCR and immunoglobulin genes does not occur normally. Patients' lymphocytes often exhibit chromosomal breaks and other abnormalities involving the TCR genes in T cells and the immunoglobulin genes in B cells. These are sites of high levels of chromosomal recombination, and errors that occur during gene rearrangements may not be repaired properly.

The syndrome is associated with an even greater risk of lymphoid malignancy than other immunodeficiency syndromes, presumably because the failure to properly repair DNA damage leads to the accumulation of mutations. Immunoglobulin replacement therapy may be given to patients with low immunoglobulin levels, but treatments aimed at prolonged immune reconstitution have given inconclusive results. Death usually occurs in early adult life from either pulmonary disease or malignancy.

Category 4: Diseases of Immune Dysregulation

Category 4 includes many diseases with normal numbers of T or B cells but with reduced control over their functions. Many of the diseases in the category also have features of autoimmunity. The autoimmune lymphoproliferative syndrome (ALPS), for example, may involve mutations in genes coding for caspase enzymes involved in apoptosis. Defective apoptosis in the thymus may lead to autoreactive cells in the circulation. The CD25 deficiency is manifested by a lack of T regulatory (Treg) cells, which leads to lymphoproliferation and autoimmunity. Mutations in the *FoxP3* gene, which is required for Treg differentiation, may show a similar clinical presentation. Chediak-Higashi syndrome, an immunodeficiency with hypopigmentation (loss of skin color) caused by a mutation in the *LYST* gene, is characterized by a reduced number of NK cells and neutrophils, as well as an increased production of inflammatory proteins. Peripheral blood smears from patients with Chediak-Higashi syndrome show granulocytic inclusions attributed to enlarged lysosomes.

Category 5: Congenital Defects of Phagocyte Number, Function, or Both

Category 5 classifies the PIDs that are characterized by abnormalities in phagocytic cells. Recall from Chapter 1 that the majority of cells that perform phagocytosis are neutrophils. Neutrophils play a crucial role in the immediate and nonspecific response to invading organisms by responding before specific antibody and cell-mediated immune responses can be mounted. In addition, neutrophils are even more effective at ingesting and killing organisms coated with specific antibody, and they continue to play an important role in host defense even after an adaptive immune response is established. To destroy invading organisms, neutrophils must adhere to vascular endothelial lining cells, migrate through the capillary wall to a site of infection, and ingest and kill the microbes (see Chapter 2). Defects affecting each of these steps can lead to an increased susceptibility to pyogenic infections.

Chronic Granulomatous Disease (CGD)

Chronic granulomatous disease (CGD) is a group of disorders involving inheritance of either an X-linked recessive or autosomal recessive gene that affects neutrophil microbiocidal function. The X-linked disease accounts for 70% of the cases and tends to be more severe. Symptoms of CGD include recurrent suppurative infections, pneumonia, osteomyelitis, draining adenopathy, liver abscesses, dermatitis, and hypergammaglobulinemia. Typically, catalase-positive organisms such as *Staphylococcus aureus, Burkholderia cepacia,* and *Chromobacterium violaceum* are involved, in addition to fungi such as *Aspergillus* and *Nocardia*. Infections usually begin before 1 year of age, and the syndrome is often fatal in childhood.

CGD is the most common and best characterized of the neutrophil abnormalities. Several specific molecular defects have been described in this syndrome, all of which result in the inability of the patient's neutrophils to produce the reactive forms of oxygen necessary for normal bacterial killing. Three different autosomal recessive genes are involved, and all affect subunits of nicotinamide adenine dinucleotide phosphate (NADPH) oxidase. Normally, neutrophil stimulation leads to the production of reactive oxygen molecules, such as hydrogen peroxide (H_2O_2), by NADPH oxidase reactivity on the plasma membrane. The plasma membrane enfolds an organism as it is phagocytized, and hydrogen peroxide is generated in close proximity to the target microbe. Neutrophil granules fuse with and release the enzyme myeloperoxidase into the forming phagosome. The myeloperoxidase uses the hydrogen peroxide to generate the potent microbicidal agent hypochlorous acid (see Chapter 2). A genetic defect in any of the several components of the NADPH oxidase system can result in the CGD phenotype by making the neutrophil incapable of generating an **oxidative burst** (a process by which neutrophils generate partially reduced forms of oxygen).

CGD was historically diagnosed by measuring the ability of a patient's neutrophils to reduce the yellow dye nitroblue tetrazolium (NBT) to a deep blue product called formazan, which could be detected microscopically in a peripheral blood smear. More recently, a flow cytometric assay has been used. In this assay, neutrophils are labeled with dihydrorhodamine (DHR). DHR will fluoresce when it is reduced. The neutrophils are then activated using phorbol myristate acetate (PMA), which is mitogenic for neutrophils. The resultant oxidative burst will reduce the DHR, resulting in fluorescence that may be quantitated on a flow cytometer. Neutrophils from CGD patients are unable to undergo the oxidative burst and show less fluorescence than normal neutrophils. This technique is more objective and quantitative than the traditional NBT technique.

Although therapy with granulocyte transfusions may allow resolution of an acute infectious episode, it is impossible to provide enough granulocytes to treat the chronic condition. Administration of cytokines, such as interferon, may increase the oxidative burst activity in some patients. Continuous use of antibiotics can greatly reduce the occurrence of severe infections. Hematopoietic stem cell transplantation may result in a permanent cure.

Other Microbiocidal Defects

Several other recognized defects can result in impaired neutrophil microbiocidal activity. Neutrophil glucose-6-phosphate dehydrogenase deficiency leads to an inability to generate enough NADPH to supply reducing equivalents to the NADPH oxidase system. This shortfall leads to a defect in hydrogen peroxide production and a clinical picture similar to that of CGD. Myeloperoxidase deficiency is relatively common, occurring in about 1 in 3,000 persons in the United States. It is an autosomal recessive disorder, caused by several different mutations in the *MPO* gene. Deficient patients may have recurrent *Candida* infections, although severe infections are not common, probably because MPO-independent mechanisms may compensate for the defect. Abnormalities of neutrophil secondary granules have also been described.

Leukocyte Adhesion Deficiency (LAD)

Even if microbiocidal activity is normal, neutrophils cannot perform their functions properly if they fail to leave the vasculature and migrate to a site of incipient infection. Adhesion molecules on leukocytes and their receptors on endothelial cells and the extracellular matrix play important roles in these activities. In leukocyte adhesion deficiency (LAD), there is a deficiency in a protein called CD18, which is a component of adhesion molecules on neutrophils and monocytes (CD11b or CD11c) and on T cells (CD11a). The CD18 deficiency is transmitted through autosomal recessive inheritance and has variable expression. This defect leads to abnormal adhesion, motility, aggregation, chemotaxis, and endocytosis by the affected leukocytes. The defects are clinically manifested as delayed wound healing, chronic skin infections, intestinal and respiratory tract infections, and periodontitis. A defect in CD18 can be diagnosed by detecting a decreased amount of the CD11/18 antigen on patient leukocytes by flow cytometry.

Other types of adhesion molecule deficiencies have also been characterized (LAD II and LAD III). LAD II is caused by a deficiency in a carbohydrate molecule involved in adhesive interactions, called *CD15s* or *sialyl-Lewis X*. In LAD III, activation of the beta integrins is defective.

Category 6: Defects in Intrinsic and Innate Immunity

Category 6 was created because of the explosive increase in understanding of the innate immune system. At least one disease, chronic mucocutaneous candidiasis, which was previously classified as a T-cell defect, has been moved to this classification. Researchers identified two forms of this entity involving mutations in genes coding for IL-17. Other rare entities classified under this heading include mutations in Toll-like receptors (TLRs). For example, TLR3 deficiency results in herpes simplex encephalitis. Defects in TLR signaling pathways, such as IRAK4 deficiency, can also occur. Both types of defects can lead to bacterial infections. Few clinical laboratory assays are currently available for assessing innate immune system functional capabilities. Diagnosing these entities is based upon clinical presentation, which leads to molecular analyses to identify specific genetic mutations.

Category 7: Autoinflammatory Disorders

Autoinflammatory disorders are subdivided into two classifications: those involving the inflammasome and those that are noninflammasome conditions. The **inflammasome** is a protein oligomer that contains caspase enzymes and other proteins associated with apoptosis. The inflammasome is located primarily in myeloid cells and may be activated by various microbial substances. Once activated, the inflammasome stimulates the production of the proinflammatory cytokines IL-1 and IL-18.

Genetic defects involving the inflammasome include the hyper-immunoglobulin D (IgD) syndrome, also referred to as *periodic fever syndrome*, and Muckle-Wells syndrome. Hyper IgD is caused by a deficiency of mevalonate kinase, an enzyme involved in a sterol synthesis pathway. The syndrome has been seen primarily in northern European populations. Diagnosis includes clinical presentation of recurrent fevers, followed by IgD testing. Muckle-Wells syndrome is caused by a mutation in the *CIAS1* gene coding for cryopyrin, a component of the inflammasome. Patients may present with urticaria and amyloidosis. Molecular assays are necessary to confirm the diagnosis.

Defects not involving the inflammasome include tumor necrosis factor (TNF) receptor-associated periodic syndrome (TRAPS) and early-onset inflammatory bowel disease (IBD). TRAPS is caused by a mutation in the *TNFRSF1A* gene, which codes for a TNF receptor and may result in recurrent fevers, as well as ocular and joint inflammation. Early-onset IBD is caused by mutations in genes coding for IL-10 or its receptor.

Family history may be helpful in diagnosing diseases of Category 7. Muckle-Wells syndrome and TRAPS show autosomal dominant inheritance, whereas hyper IgD and early-onset IBD are autosomal recessive.

Category 8: Complement Deficiencies

Complement consists of a series of proteins that work in a cascade to assist antibody in the destruction of cells, as described in Chapter 7. The complement system is also part of the innate immune system and can work as part of the inflammatory process to directly eliminate a potential pathogen. Deficiencies in each of the major complement components have been described, leading to various clinical sequalae.

Deficiencies in the early complement components, C1q, C4, and C2, are usually associated with a lupus-like syndrome. Deficiency of C2 is believed to be the most common complement component deficiency. A C3 deficiency may also have a lupus-like clinical presentation, but it is more likely to involve recurrent infections with encapsulated organisms. Deficiencies of the later components of complement (C5–C9) are often associated with recurrent *Neisseria meningitidis* infections. A deficiency of C1 esterase inhibitor has been found in patients with hereditary neuroangioedema. Most complement deficiencies appear to be inherited in an autosomal recessive manner and are likely caused by random changes in the DNA nucleotide sequence.

Category 9: Phenocopies of Primary Immunodeficiencies

This category comprises the most recent classification of PIDs. Disorders that fall into this category have an inherited genetic component but also include an acquired component, such as somatic mutations or autoantibody production. New knowledge of these factors has led to reclassification of some PIDs. For example, chronic mucocutaneous candidiasis, a disease that was once classified as a cell-mediated deficiency, is now included in Category 9. This disease is induced by a genetic mutation in the *AIRE* gene (a gene that codes for the "autoimmune regulator" protein, which helps T cells to distinguish between self and non-self) but also involves production of an antibody to either (or both) IL-17 and IL-22. Mutations in the *nRAS* or *kRAS* genes are also associated with diseases that fall into this category.

Laboratory Evaluation of Immune Dysfunction

When performing diagnostic testing for immunodeficiency, it is important for laboratorians to compare the results for a patient with appropriate age-matched controls. In tests of cellular function, the patient's cells need to be tested in parallel with cells from a normal control. If an abnormal test result is obtained, it should be confirmed by repeat testing.

Screening Tests

Screening tests are used for the initial evaluation of a suspected immunodeficiency state. Most of these tests can be performed routinely in any hospital laboratory. The evaluation of possible immunodeficiency starts with a patient history, followed by a complete blood count (CBC) and white blood cell (WBC) differential, which may reveal a reduced lymphocyte count. Thrombocytopenia with small platelets can be detected in WAS.

Measurements of serum IgG, IgM, and IgA concentrations and levels of the IgG subclasses are used to screen for defects in antibody production. Testing for isohemagglutinins is easily performed by the transfusion service. By the age of 2, a child should have naturally occurring IgM antibodies against ABO blood group antigens. The absence of these antibodies suggests an abnormal IgM response.

An overall assessment of antibody-mediated immunity can be made by measuring antibody responses to antigens to which the population is exposed normally or following vaccination. This can be easily done by measuring the titer of the specific antibody produced in response to immunization with a commercial vaccine such as diphtheria/tetanus. In an unimmunized child, the development of tetanus or diphtheria antibodies is determined 2 weeks after immunization. In a previously immunized patient, the response to a booster injection can be evaluated, normally 4 to 6 weeks postvaccination. A wide range of other protein and polysaccharide antigens can also be used in these tests. This technique is often used to evaluate a possible IgG subclass deficiency. IgG1 and IgG3 isotypes normally respond to protein antigens, such as those found in tetanus and diphtheria vaccines. IgG2 normally responds to polysaccharide antigens, such as those in the *H. influenzae* and *S. pneumoniae* vaccines.

Delayed-type hypersensitivity skin reactions can be used to screen for defects in cell-mediated immunity (see Chapter 14). These tests are generally performed by clinicians and not by laboratory personnel. Delayed cutaneous hypersensitivity is a localized cell-mediated reaction to a specific antigen. The prototype is the tuberculin skin test. An antigen to which most of the population has been exposed, such as candida, mumps, or tetanus toxoid, is injected intradermally. The presence of induration 48 to 72 hours later indicates a cell-mediated immune response. A negative test is not always informative because the patient may not have been previously exposed to the test antigen. In vitro assays to measure cell-mediated immunity have also been developed, and these are detailed in the text that follows.

Screening for complement deficiencies usually begins with a CH50 assay. This procedure determines the level of functional complement in an individual. Undetectable CH50 levels may indicate a deficiency in a specific component of the classical pathway of complement. Based on the clinical history, individual component assays would be indicated. The laboratorian should be aware, however, that low CH50 levels may be caused by complement consumption and do not, by themselves, indicate a complement deficiency.

Defects in neutrophil oxidative burst activity may be detected by a flow cytometric assay, as previously mentioned. Neutrophils labeled with DHR are stimulated to undergo an oxidative burst by exposure to a mitogen. The oxidative burst will reduce the DHR, producing fluorescence, which can be measured objectively by flow cytometry. Flow cytometry can also be used to confirm a diagnosis of LAD type 1 by looking for the expression of the CD18 antigen.

Confirmatory Tests

If the screening tests detect an abnormality or the clinical suspicion is high, more specialized testing will probably be necessary to precisely identify an immune abnormality. Some of the tests used for confirming an immunodeficiency state are listed in **Table 19–3.**

Enumeration of classes of lymphocytes in the peripheral blood is performed by flow cytometry. Even though the different types of lymphocytes cannot be distinguished morphologically, they exhibit different patterns of antigen or surface immunoglobulin expression that correlate with functional characteristics. Before flow cytometric analysis, antibodies to antigens specific for different types of lymphocytes are labeled

Table 19–3 Specialized Confirmatory Tests for Immunodeficiencies

SUSPECTED DISORDER	SPECIALIZED TESTS
Humoral immunity	B-cell counts by flow cytometry B-cell proliferation in vitro (e.g., mitogen assays) Histology of lymphoid tissues
Cell-mediated immunity	T-cell counts by flow cytometry (total and T-cell subsets) T-cell function in vitro (e.g., mitogen assays) QuantiFERON-TB assay Cylex ImmuKnow assay Enzyme assays (ADA, PNP)
Phagocyte defects	Leukocyte adhesion molecule analysis (CD11a, CD11b, CD11c, CD18) Phagocytosis and bacterial killing assays Chemotaxis assay Enzyme assays (myeloperoxidase, glucose-6-phosphate dehydrogenase, components of NADPH oxidase)
Complement	Specific complement component assays

ADA = adenosine deaminase; NADPH = nicotinamide adenine dinucleotide phosphate; PNP = purine-nucleoside phosphorylase.

with a fluorescent probe. These antigens are generally referred to by a "cluster of differentiation" (CD) number (see Chapters 1 and 13). The antibodies are allowed to react with the patient's peripheral blood mononuclear cells in a direct immunofluorescence assay, and RBCs in the sample are lysed. The flow cytometer is used to count the WBCs that are labeled with each fluorescent antibody. Lymphocytes can then be assigned to specific types based on antigen expression: B cells (CD19+), T cells (CD3+), T helper (Th) cells (CD3+/CD4+), cytotoxic T cells (CD3+/CD8+), and NK cells (CD16+ or CD56+).

Flow cytometry is objective and quite reliable in detecting those defects that result in a decrease in one or more types of lymphocytes. For example, an absence of or profound decrease in the number of CD3+ cells would be consistent with DiGeorge syndrome. An absence of CD19+ B cells suggests Btk deficiency. One should remember, however, that in the actual clinical arena, secondary immunodeficiencies are more common than PIDs. For example, in the laboratory of the author (TA), the most common cause of absent B cells is not Btk deficiency but patients treated with rituximab, a monoclonal anti-CD20 antibody. This antibody, used to treat leukemic, transplant, and autoimmune patients, destroys B cells, resulting in no detectable CD19+ or CD20+ cells. **Figure 19–2** is a flow cytometry histogram from a patient treated with rituximab. Note that no CD19+ B cells are detectable.

Most of the genes associated with PIDs have been identified and localized. Thus, genetic testing is available for many conditions, including the 22q11.2 deletion syndrome, the Wiskott-Aldrich syndrome, and SCID. Although genetic testing is useful to understand the pathology of the disease, it is often not required for making a diagnosis. Genetic testing of family members of affected patients may be helpful in determining who may be at risk of developing the disease or passing it on to offspring.

T-cell function can be measured by assessing the ability of isolated T cells to proliferate in response to an antigenic stimulus or to T-cell mitogens in culture, such as phytohemagglutinin (PHA) or Concanavalin A (Con A). A **mitogen** is a substance that stimulates mitosis in all T cells or all B cells, regardless of antigen specificity. Classically, the T-cell response to a mitogen can be measured by quantitating the uptake of radioactive thymidine, a precursor of DNA. Increased thymidine uptake suggests cell division and activation. This assay requires experienced technologists, a radioactive materials license, and laboratory-determined reference ranges.

More recently, antigen- or mitogen-stimulated T-cell activation has been measured without the use of radioactive materials. The U.S. Food and Drug Administration (FDA) has cleared three such assays for diagnostic use. The QuantiFERON-TB assay and the T-SPOT assay measure an individual's response to *Mycobacterium tuberculosis* antigens. Following overnight incubation of whole blood (QuantiFERON gold plus) or isolated mononuclear cells (T-SPOT) with tuberculosis (TB) antigens, gamma interferon secreted by activated Th1 cells is quantitated by either an enzyme-linked immunosorbent assay (ELISA) or ELISPOT procedure. Either of these assays may be used as an in vitro assessment of exposure to *M. tuberculosis* (see Chapter 14).

The third assay, the Cylex ImmuKnow assay, measures total T-cell activity. This test uses the mitogen PHA to activate T cells. Following incubation, adenosine triphosphate (ATP) production is measured by a fluorescent immunoassay technique. This test is a general measurement of T-cell function and is often used to monitor individuals receiving immunosuppressive therapy. The assay may be used to determine overall T-cell functional capabilities in an individual suspected of a PID. PHA is also used as a positive control in the QuantiFERON and T-SPOT procedures.

Newborn Screening for Immunodeficiencies

All states in the United States include PID testing as part of their newborn screening programs. This testing is typically

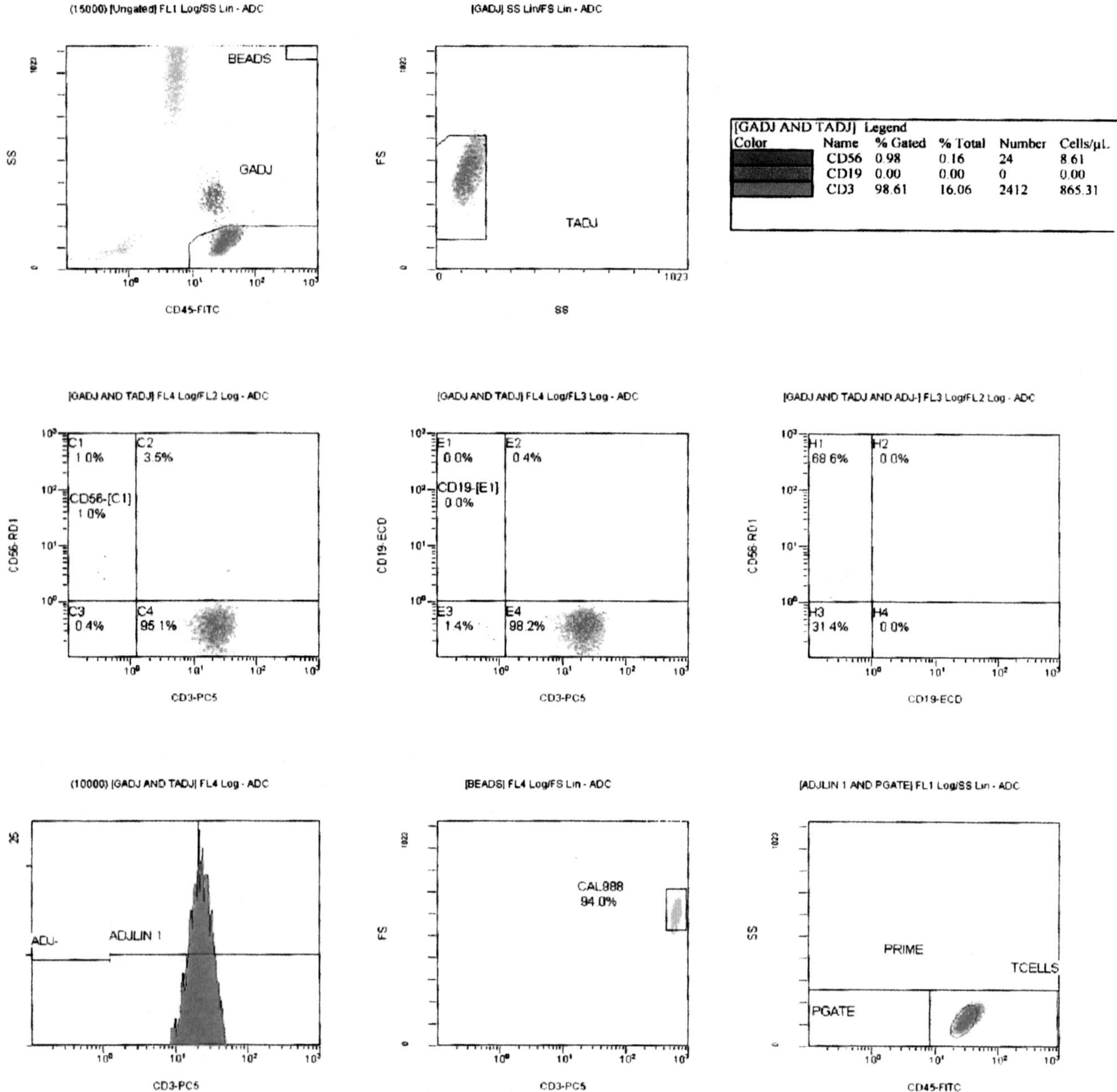

FIGURE 19–2 Flow cytometry histogram of peripheral blood stained with antibodies to CD3, CD19, and CD56. Note that no CD19+ cells are detected in this patient sample. *(Courtesy of Dr. Thomas Alexander.)*

performed to look for the presence of TCR excision circles (TRECs) in newborn blood. TRECs, identified by quantitative PCR (see Chapter 12), are present in T cells that have undergone alpha-beta receptor gene rearrangements. They are the genetic material that has been removed from the germline DNA during alpha V-J and beta V-D-J recombination **(Fig. 19–3)**. Their absence indicates a lack of functional T cells, allowing early identification of T-cell–related defects leading to SCID. The 22q11.2 deletion syndrome and other non-SCID diseases, such as Omenn syndrome, have also been detected using this method. Other molecular techniques not normally applied to newborn screening, such as whole exome sequencing and whole genome sequencing, have been used to identify genetic defects associated with PIDs and will likely see increased use in the future.

Evaluation of Immunoglobulins

Quantitative measurement of serum immunoglobulins is used in the workup of both immunodeficiency states and some lymphoproliferative disorders. This is usually performed by automated assays involving nephelometry or immunoturbidimetry but may also be performed by radial immunodiffusion (RID). In addition, serum protein electrophoresis (SPE) can be quantitative if the total serum protein is determined, and the results are read using a densitometer.

Connections

T-Cell Receptors (TCRs)

Recall from Chapter 12 that the TCR for antigen is composed of two different chains: an α chain and a β chain. During T-cell maturation, rearrangement of specific V and J genes that code for the variable region of the α chain and specific V, D, and J genes that code for the variable region of the β chain occur to produce a TCR that is specific for a particular antigen (see Fig. 4-3). In the process, the intervening sequences are cut out to form circles called *TRECs*.

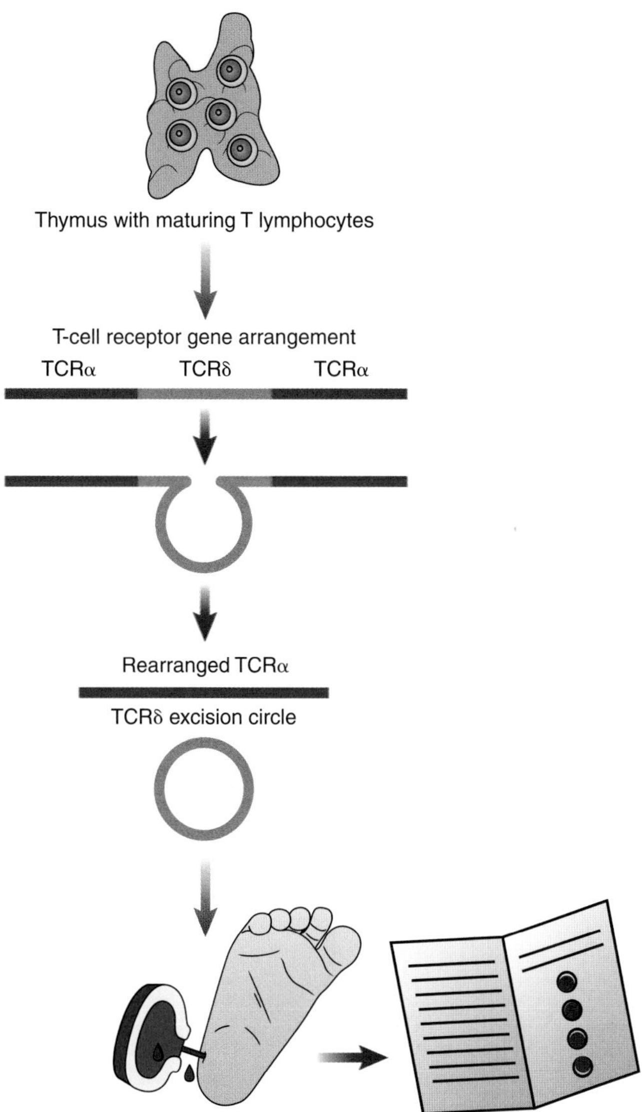

FIGURE 19–3 Newborn testing for T-cell receptor excision circles (TRECs) formed by normal T-cell receptor gene rearrangements.

Serum Protein Electrophoresis (SPE)

SPE is a technique in which molecules are separated on the basis of their size and electrical charge. SPE allows reproducible separation of the major plasma proteins. See Chapter 5 for details. The serum protein electrophoretic profile is traditionally divided into five regions: albumin, $alpha_1$ globulins, $alpha_2$ globulins, beta globulins, and gamma globulins. Some laboratories use six regions, dividing the beta region into the $beta_1$ (transferrin) and $beta_2$ (complement component C3) regions. IgG, IgD, and IgE migrate in the gamma globulin region, whereas IgM and IgA overlap the beta and gamma regions. Immunoglobulins normally show a range of mobilities. Additional evaluation of serum immunoglobulin is performed if the SPE shows a monoclonal component or if there is a significant quantitative abnormality of serum immunoglobulins. Classically, SPE has been performed using agarose gels. More recently, SPE may be performed using capillary electrophoresis (described in Chapter 12), which eliminates the need for gels and the drying and staining processes associated with the agarose-based technique.

Immunofixation Electrophoresis (IFE)

Another method of characterizing immunodeficiencies is **immunofixation electrophoresis (IFE)** (see Chapter 18). In IFE, serum samples are electrophoresed, just as for SPE, and then specific antibody is applied directly to the separating gel. The antibody–antigen complexes form and are visualized by staining. Polyclonal immunoglobulins are indicated by areas of diffuse staining, whereas monoclonal immunoglobulins produce narrow, intensely stained bands (see **Fig. 19–4** later in the Case Studies). Lack of bands indicates a deficiency of one or more immunoglobulin classes. The capillary electrophoresis version of immunofixation is referred to as *immunotyping, immune displacement*, or *immunosubtraction*. Recently, mass spectroscopy has been applied to detecting monoclonal gammopathies. This technique has several advantages over standard electrophoresis techniques, particularly when applied to low-level monoclonal proteins. For accurate interpretations, specific immunoglobulin isotype levels, determined by nephelometry or other immunoassay techniques, are necessary.

Bone Marrow Biopsy

A bone marrow aspirate and biopsy is indicated in any evaluation of a monoclonal gammopathy or immunodeficiency state. It is important in establishing the diagnosis of such disorders and for excluding other diseases. The bone marrow specimen will be analyzed microscopically and by flow cytometry. Cytogenetic analysis may also be performed to detect the specific genetic anomalies associated with the PID diseases.

Family History

The importance of obtaining a full family history as part of the PID diagnosis process cannot be overemphasized. The mode of inheritance, if known, can rule in or rule out many of the PIDs. The disease may be X-linked, such as in the common gamma-chain mutation, WAS, or the CD154 deficiency; autosomal dominant, such as in hyper-IgE or Muckle-Wells syndrome; or autosomal recessive, such as in AT or LAD. CGD may be either X-linked or autosomal recessive. Although obtaining a family history is not the responsibility of the clinical immunology laboratory, these diseases are not identified solely by laboratory testing. A team approach among the laboratory, clinicians, medical geneticists, and the family is required for a final diagnosis. Laboratory results are most useful when integrated into the entire clinical picture. Laboratories should not test in a vacuum!

Primary Immune Deficiencies in a Computer App

The phenotypic PID classification is now available as an app for both Android and Apple systems. These apps are based on the criteria published by the International Union of Immunological Societies. Although they provide useful information, especially for a quick review or study, they are not a substitute for a professional diagnosis.

SUMMARY

- Immunodeficiencies are disorders in which part of the body's immune system is missing or dysfunctional. There are two types of immunodeficiencies—primary (i.e., inherited) and secondary (acquired because of other factors, such as infections, malignancies, or immunosuppressive drugs).
- The International Union of Immunological Societies has classified the primary immunodeficiencies into nine categories based on their clinical features, immunologic defects, and genetic abnormalities.
- Defects in the development and regulation of individual parts of the immune system can affect the humoral or cell-mediated branches of the adaptive immune system or various components of the innate defense system, such as the phagocytic cells or the complement system.
- Defects in antibody-mediated immunity typically lead to recurrent infections with pyogenic bacteria, particularly of the respiratory and intestinal tracts.
- Defects in T-cell–mediated immunity generally lead to recurrent infections with intracellular pathogens, such as viruses, fungi, and intracellular bacteria.
- Defects in phagocyte function generally lead to pyogenic bacterial infections, often of the skin. Immunodeficiency states range from quite mild to lethal.
- Therapy to reconstitute the deficient immune component includes administration of immunoglobulin preparations and hematopoietic stem cell transplantation. Treatment must begin as soon as possible in an attempt to prevent permanent organ damage or death caused by infection.
- PIDs must be suspected clinically and are diagnosed with the help of screening tests to measure leukocyte counts and immunoglobulin levels, followed by specialized laboratory testing, such as flow cytometry, to determine numbers of specific lymphocyte subsets.
- Laboratory results correlate with the presence of a specific PID. For example, patients with Bruton's tyrosine kinase (Btk) deficiency typically have decreased serum concentrations of all the immunoglobulins and decreased numbers of CD19+ B cells, whereas patients with chronic granulomatous disease (CGD) would be expected to have decreased fluorescence in the DHR assay, which measures oxidative burst in neutrophils.
- Newborn screening is available to detect SCID, a combined immunodeficiency disease involving defective T-cell function. The screening assay looks for the absence of TRECs, T-cell receptor excision circles that have been removed during normal gene rearrangements that occur during T-cell development.

Study Guide: Classification of Primary Immunodeficiency Diseases

CATEGORY	DESCRIPTION	PROTOTYPIC DISEASES
1. Immunodeficiencies affecting cellular and humoral immunity	Low to absent humoral and cellular capabilities	SCID (common gamma chain deficiency, *JAK3* deficiency, ADA deficiency, MHC deficiencies) PNP deficiency
2. Combined immunodeficiencies with associated or syndromic features	Low to absent humoral and cellular capabilities with additional, nonimmunologic anomalies	Wiskott-Aldrich syndrome, ataxia-telangiectasia, 22q11.2 deletion (DiGeorge) syndrome
3. Predominantly antibody deficiencies	One or more immunoglobulin isotypes are decreased	Bruton's thymidine kinase (Btk) deficiency, transient hypogammaglobulinemia of infancy, common variable immunodeficiency, selective IgA deficiency, IgG subclass deficiencies
4. Diseases of immune dysregulation	Loss of T regulatory or other controlling mechanisms	Chediak-Higashi syndrome, autoimmune lymphoproliferative syndrome, CD25 deficiency
5. Congenital defects of phagocyte number, function, or both	Reduction in phagocytic function, number, or both	Chronic granulomatous disease, cyclic neutropenia, leukocyte adhesion deficiency
6. Defects in intrinsic and innate immunity	Interruption in signaling pathways of innate immune cells	Chronic mucocutaneous candidiasis, TLR3 deficiency, IRAK4 deficiency
7. Autoinflammatory disorders	Diseases usually associated with recurrent fevers with or without infections	Hyper IgD syndrome, familial Mediterranean fever, TNF-receptor–associated periodic syndrome

Study Guide: Classification of Primary Immunodeficiency Diseases—cont'd

CATEGORY	DESCRIPTION	PROTOTYPIC DISEASES
8. Complement deficiencies	Loss of individual complement components	C2 deficiency, C3 deficiency, C6 deficiency, hereditary angioedema
9. Phenocopies of PID	PID associated with an acquired mutation or autoantibody	Autoimmune lymphoproliferative syndrome, chronic mucocutaneous candidiasis associated with autoantibodies

ADA = adenosine deaminase; MHC = major histocompatibility complex; PID = primary immunodeficiency disease; PNP = purine-nucleoside phosphorylase; SCID = severe combined immunodeficiency.

Adapted from Picard C, Gaspar HB, Al-Herz W, et al. International Union of Immunological Societies: 2017 Primary immunodeficiency diseases committee report on inborn errors of immunity. J. Clin. Immunology. *2018;38:96–128.*

Study Guide: Screening Tests for Immunodeficiencies

SUSPECTED DISORDER	SCREENING TESTS
All immunodeficiencies	Complete blood cell count, white blood cell differential count
Humoral immunity	Serum IgG, IgA, IgM levels; IgG subclass levels; isohemagglutinin titers (IgM); IgG antibody response to protein and polysaccharide antigens
Cell-mediated immunity	Lymphocyte (T, B, NK) phenotyping Lymphocyte activation (mitogen; interferon gamma release) studies Delayed hypersensitivity skin tests (i.e., *Candida*, diphtheria, tetanus, PPD) Chest x-ray (thymus shadow) TREC screening
Phagocyte defect	DHR reduction test
Complement	CH50 (classical pathway) Serum complement levels (e.g., C3, C4)

DHR = dihydrorhodamine; PPD = purified protein derivative; TREC = T-cell receptor excision circles.

CASE STUDIES

1. A 7-month-old male child was diagnosed with bacterial meningitis. Previously he had been hospitalized with bacterial pneumonia. Laboratory testing results were as follows: RBC count: normal; WBC count: 22 × 10^9/L (normal is 5–24 × 10^9/L); differential: 70% neutrophils, 15% monocytes, 5% eosinophils, and 10% lymphocytes; SPE: no gamma band present.

Questions

a. What possible conditions do these results indicate?
b. How are these conditions inherited?
c. What type of further testing do you recommend?

2. A 37-year-old female presents with a history of recurrent upper respiratory infections. She states that she was always a sick child, usually with respiratory infections, but occasional diarrhea would also occur. She has received countless antibiotic regimens through the years. The physician orders an SPE and immunoglobulin levels. The SPE is read as a low gamma level with no monoclonal proteins detected. Levels of IgG, IgM, and IgA are below the reference ranges. The physician then orders an immunofixation assay.

Question

a. Figure 19–4 contains four patient immunofixations. Which pattern would be most representative of the expected pattern for this patient?
b. Explain why you chose this answer.

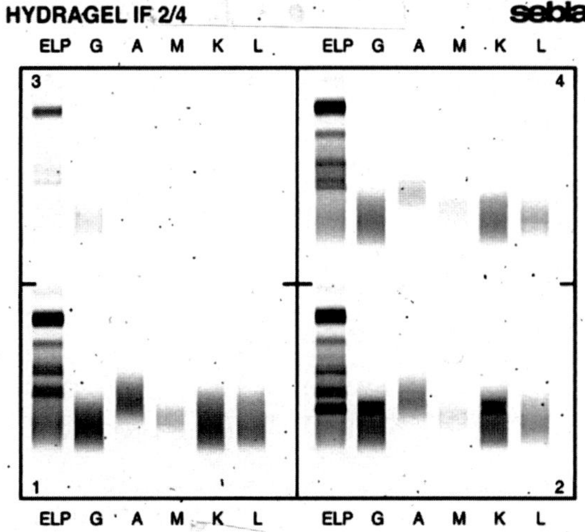

FIGURE 19–4 Case Study 2: Four different immunofixation patterns.

REVIEW QUESTIONS

1. Patients with which immunodeficiency syndrome should receive irradiated blood products to protect against the development of GVHD?
   a. Bruton's tyrosine kinase (Btk) deficiency
   b. Selective IgA deficiency
   c. SCID
   d. CGD

2. T-cell subset enumeration by flow cytometry would be most useful in making the diagnosis of which disorder?
   a. Bruton's tyrosine kinase (Btk) deficiency
   b. Selective IgA deficiency
   c. SCID
   d. Multiple myeloma

3. What clinical manifestation would be seen in a patient with myeloperoxidase deficiency?
   a. Defective T-cell function
   b. Inability to produce IgG
   c. Defective NK cell function
   d. Defective neutrophil function

4. Defects in which branch of the immune system are most commonly associated with severe illness after the administration of live virus vaccines?
   a. Cell-mediated immunity
   b. Humoral immunity
   c. Complement
   d. Phagocytic cells

5. Which of the following statements applies to Bruton's tyrosine kinase (Btk) deficiency?
   a. It typically appears in females.
   b. There is a lack of circulating CD19+ B cells.
   c. T cells are abnormal.
   d. There is a lack of pre-B cells in the bone marrow.

6. The 22q11.2 deletion syndrome is characterized by all of the following *except*
   a. autosomal recessive inheritance.
   b. cardiac abnormalities.
   c. parathyroid hypoplasia.
   d. decreased number of mature T cells.

7. A 3-year-old boy is hospitalized because of recurrent bouts of pneumonia. Laboratory tests are run, and the following findings are noted: prolonged bleeding time, decreased platelet count, increased level of serum alpha-fetoprotein, and a deficiency of naturally occurring isohemagglutinins. Based on these results, which is the most likely diagnosis?
   a. PNP deficiency
   b. Selective IgA deficiency
   c. SCID
   d. Wiskott-Aldrich syndrome

8. Which of the following is associated with ataxia-telangiectasia?
   a. Inherited as an autosomal recessive
   b. Defect in both cellular and humoral immunity
   c. Chromosomal breaks in lymphocytes
   d. All of the above

9. A 4-year-old boy presents with recurrent wound and soft tissue infections. Which of the following assays should be considered for diagnosing his presumed PID?
   a. DHR reduction
   b. CD4 quantitation
   c. CD19 quantitation
   d. CD56 quantitation

10. A patient with a deficiency in complement component C7 would likely present with
    a. recurrent *Staphylococcal* infections.
    b. recurrent *Neisserial* infections.
    c. recurrent *Escherichia coli* infections.
    d. recurrent *Nocardia* infections.

11. A *FoxP3* gene mutation may lead to a deficiency of what cell type?
    a. T helper cells
    b. T cytotoxic cells
    c. B cells
    d. T regulatory cells

12. The Cylex ImmuKnow assay is useful in determining the functional capabilities of which cell type?
    a. T cells
    b. B cells
    c. NK cells
    d. Neutrophils

13. Recurrent, periodic fevers may be associated with increased production of which immunoglobulin?
    a. IgG
    b. IgM
    c. IgD
    d. IgE

14. Chediak-Higashi syndrome is classified as which type of PID?
    a. Autoinflammatory disorder
    b. Intrinsic and innate immunity deficiency
    c. Predominantly antibody deficiency
    d. Disease of immune dysregulation

15. Prenatal screening for SCID involves detecting
    a. Tregs.
    b. TRECS.
    c. THELPS.
    d. TCYTOS.

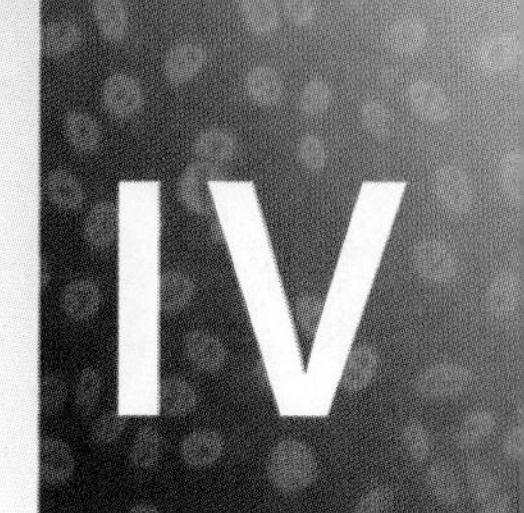

Serological and Molecular Diagnosis of Infectious Disease

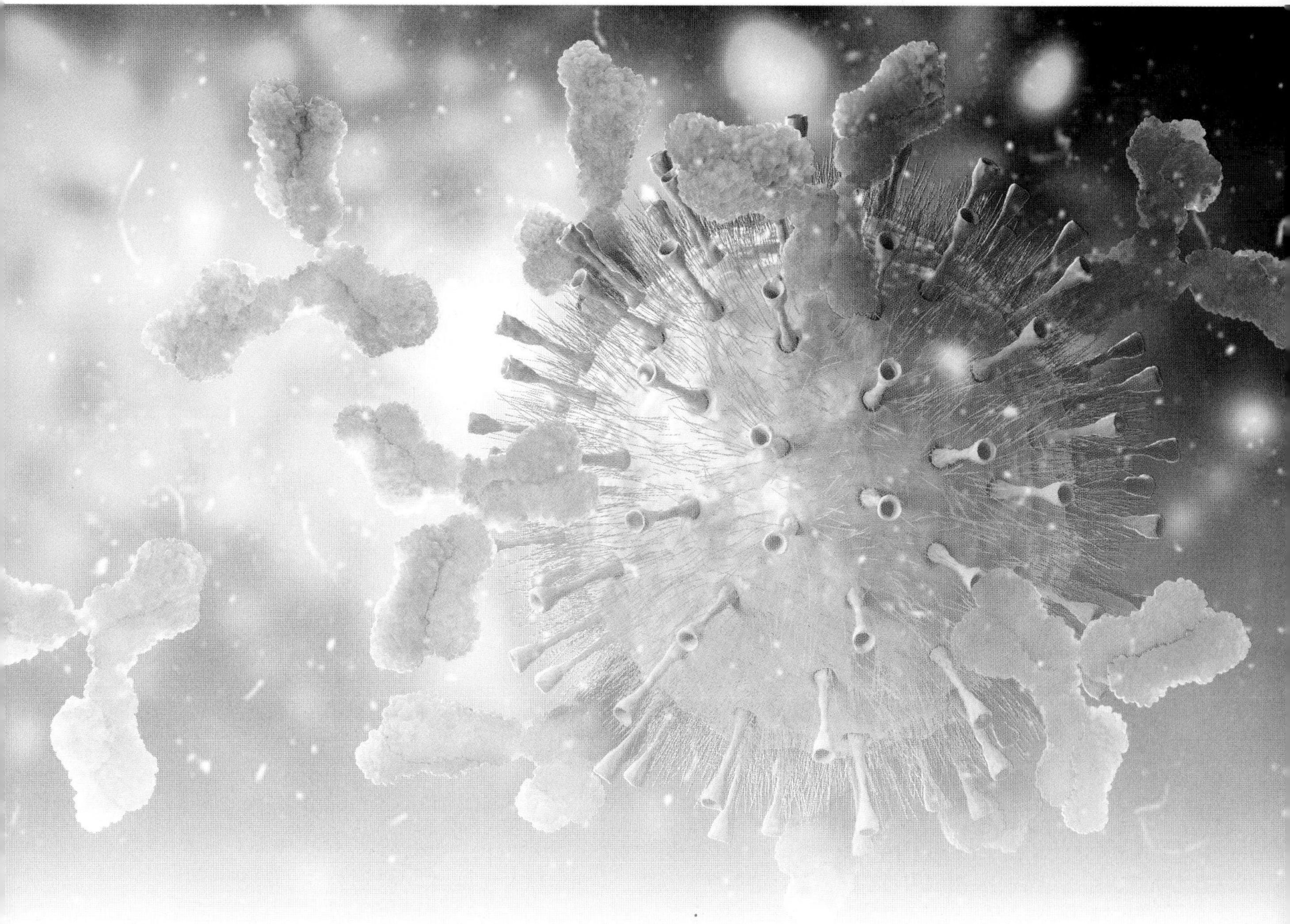

20 Serological and Molecular Detection of Bacterial Infections

James L. Vossler, MS, MLS^{CM}(ASCP) SM^{CM}

LEARNING OUTCOMES

After finishing this chapter, you should be able to:

1. Differentiate between commensalistic, mutualistic, and parasitic relationships.
2. Differentiate between pathogenicity, virulence, and infectivity.
3. Cite structural features of bacteria that contribute to increased virulence.
4. Describe host defenses against bacteria and the means by which bacteria can evade the immune system.
5. Compare and contrast endotoxins and exotoxins with respect to biological activity, immunogenicity, and the genetic encoding for the production of the two toxin categories.
6. Cite the five general laboratory means of detecting the causative agent of a bacterial infection.
7. Explain the principle of lateral flow immunochromatographic assays (LFA).
8. List the exotoxins produced by Group A streptococci and the roles they play in contributing to the virulence of *Streptococcus pyogenes.*
9. Describe the symptoms and pathogenesis of acute rheumatic fever and poststreptococcal glomerulonephritis.
10. Explain the principle, interpretation, and clinical significance of the anti-streptolysin O (ASO), anti-deoxyribonuclease B (anti-DNase B), and streptozyme tests.
11. Recognize the role *Helicobacter pylori* plays in gastrointestinal ulcers and the virulence factors that contribute to infection by this organism.

CHAPTER OUTLINE

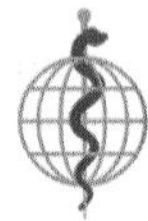

Go to FADavis.com for the laboratory exercises that accompany this text.

12. Discuss the various types of tests that may be performed to detect *H. pylori* infection.
13. Describe the respiratory and dermatological manifestations of *Mycoplasma pneumoniae* infections.
14. Discuss the use of serology for the diagnosis of *M. pneumoniae* infections, including the clinical value of detecting cold agglutinins.
15. Describe the epidemiology of Rocky Mountain spotted fever (RMSF) with respect to etiologic agent, transmission, and pathogenesis.
16. Select the appropriate serological and molecular techniques to diagnose Rocky Mountain spotted fever.

KEY TERMS

Acute rheumatic fever
Anti-DNase B
ASO titer
Commensalistic
Endotoxin
Exotoxin
Group A streptococcus (GAS)
Helicobacter pylori
Impetigo
Indigenous microbiota
Infectivity
Lancefield groups
Lateral flow immunochromatographic assay (LFA)
MALDI-TOF
Microbiome
Mutualistic
Mycoplasma pneumoniae
Parasitic
Pathogenicity
Plasmids
Poststreptococcal glomerulonephritis
Proteome
Proteomics
Rickettsiae
Rocky Mountain spotted fever (RMSF)
Scarlet fever
Streptococcus pyogenes
Streptolysin O
Streptozyme
Symbiotic
Typhus
Urease
Virulence
Virulence factors

The collection of microorganisms that exists on the body—bacteria, viruses, and single-celled prokaryotic organisms (e.g., yeast and fungi)—is referred to as the human **microbiome.** The bacteria comprising the human microbiome keep us healthy in many ways. They protect us against disease-causing bacteria, aid in digesting our food, produce certain vitamins, and stimulate both the innate and adaptive immune systems. The establishment of an organism that leads to host injury is referred to as an "infection." When a microbe causes damage to host cells or altered physiology that results in clinical signs and symptoms of disease, the phrase "infectious disease" applies. Traditional means of determining the cause of a bacterial infection have relied largely on growing the organism in culture and using stains to view the organism under the microscope. These infections can also be identified by immunoassays that detect bacterial antigens or antibodies and by molecular or proteomic techniques that detect nucleic acid or proteins from the organisms, respectively. This chapter will begin with an introduction to the human–microbe relationship and factors that influence the interactions between bacteria and the immune system. The chapter will then discuss laboratory methods that are commonly used to detect bacterial infections in the context of selected pathogenic bacteria.

Human–Microbe Relationships

When an individual is born, a dynamic relationship begins between the human host and the bacteria in the environment. Very quickly, various bacteria establish themselves on the surfaces of an individual, including the gastrointestinal tract, creating a **symbiotic** relationship. The bacteria and the host "live together," often maintaining a long-term interaction. Symbiotic bacteria that reside on and colonize these surfaces are referred to as the **indigenous microbiota** (previously known as "normal flora"). The bacterial populations that exist on the body are not homogenous; they vary in composition and numbers, depending on the area of the body.

The microbial populations outnumber human cells by 10 to 1. Collectively, they may account for 2 to 6 pounds of an individual's body weight. Although it was previously thought that a relatively limited number of bacteria make up the human microbiome, we now know that the microbial community is actually very diverse. Furthermore, greater than 90% of the bacteria that comprise the human microbiome cannot be cultured in vitro, most likely because their growth depends on specific conditions or substances that have not been duplicated in the laboratory.

Our relationship with our indigenous microbiota exists through co-evolution, co-adaptation, and co-dependency between the bacteria and the host. For a microorganism to survive, the organism needs to colonize the host and acquire nutrients. Importantly, it must not stimulate the host's immune response (in the case of the indigenous microbiota) or it must avoid or circumvent the immune responses. Once established, it needs to be able to replicate and disseminate to a preferred site in the body for survival and eventually be transmitted to a new susceptible host.

Three types of symbiotic relationships can exist between humans and bacteria. In **commensalistic** relationships, there is no apparent benefit or harm to either organism. The indigenous microbiota are often referred to as "commensals" or the "commensalistic bacteria," describing bacteria that are recovered in culture that do not represent a pathogen. An example of a commensalistic organism is *Staphylococcus epidermidis,* which colonizes and inhabits the human skin. In a **mutualistic** relationship, both humans and the bacteria benefit. One example is the *Lactobacillus* species that colonizes the epithelial surfaces of the vaginal canal. The human host provides conditions that allow the bacteria to grow and multiply, such as appropriate temperature, atmosphere, and nutrients. In exchange, the bacteria produce lactic acid, which prevents colonization of bacteria and yeast that may cause disease. Although the vast majority of the interactions between the host and members of the microbiome are harmless, the encounter with specific organisms or viruses occasionally results in harm to the host. In this case, a **parasitic** relationship exists between the other organisms and the host.

As previously mentioned, the establishment of an organism that leads to host injury is referred to as an *infection.* Although there is harm to the host, not all infections are symptomatic. In many instances, the infection may be *subclinical;* in other words, there are no signs or symptoms. An example is infection with *Chlamydia trachomatis,* a sexually transmitted organism. Only about 10% of infected males and 5% to 30% of infected females will show symptoms when infected with *C. trachomatis.* The organism may then be transmitted to other individuals or may result in complications such as pelvic inflammatory disease in women.

Several terms are used to describe the interaction between the infecting organisms and the host. The terms *infectivity, pathogenicity,* and *virulence* are often used interchangeably; however, each term has different meanings when discussing an organism's ability to cause an infection. **Infectivity** refers to an organism's ability to establish an infection. More specifically, infectivity describes the proportion of individuals exposed to a pathogen through horizontal transmission (i.e., person-to-person spread) who will become infected. Another term that is used with similar meaning is *contagious.* For example, the measles virus is extremely contagious and has a high degree of infectivity.

Pathogenicity refers to the inherent capacity of an organism to cause disease. This is a qualitative trait of the organism determined by its genetic makeup. Some organisms, such as the HIV virus, are considered to be primary or true pathogens that are capable of causing harm to a majority of individuals who have intact immune systems. Although an organism may be pathogenic in nature, it may not always cause disease. The outcome of the host–pathogen interaction is determined by several factors, including the host's immunologic status. Some microorganisms may only cause disease or infection in individuals who have compromised immune systems because of factors such as chemotherapy, radiation therapy, or various chronic diseases. These organisms are referred to as "opportunistic pathogens."

Virulence is a quantitative trait that refers to the extent of damage, or pathology, caused by the organism. For example, *Yersinia pestis,* the causative agent of bubonic and pneumonic plague, is considered to be extremely virulent and is likely to cause severe illness and death upon infection unless antibiotics are administered. If the bacterial strain is not capable of causing disease, the organism is said to be "avirulent." Not all members of a bacterial species are necessarily capable of causing disease. For example, *Escherichia coli* resides as commensal bacteria in the gastrointestinal tract, but only some strains of *E. coli* are capable of causing diarrheal disease.

The degree of damage is mediated by specific virulence factors. **Virulence factors** may increase an organism's pathogenicity by contributing to the organism's ability to establish itself on or in the host, invade or damage host tissue, or evade the host immune response.

Bacterial Virulence Factors

Bacterial properties or features that determine whether an organism is pathogenic and able to cause disease are referred to as "virulence factors." Factors that increase a bacterium's virulence may be classified as either structural components (e.g., endotoxin is a component of the cell walls of certain bacteria) or as extracellular substances produced by the bacteria, such as exotoxins. Various types of bacterial virulence factors are discussed in the sections that follow.

For an organism to be pathogenic, it needs to possess genetic determinants that allow for the production of either the structural components or the extracellular products that contribute to its virulence. Genetic determinants located on the bacterial chromosome are generally responsible for the production of structural or surface molecules, which help the organism to attach to and colonize the host. The genetic information needed to produce the extracellular substances that are virulence factors is most frequently located on independent genetic elements called *plasmids.* **Plasmids** are self-replicating extrachromosomal DNA molecules that are located in the bacteria's cytoplasm and contain a limited number of genes. In addition, plasmids are mobile genetic elements that can be transferred between bacteria through various mechanisms. Acquisition of exogenous DNA that codes for the production of virulence factors can convert an avirulent strain into a virulent strain.

Structural Virulence Features

Bacterial cells are classified as prokaryotic cells, whereas human cells are classified as eukaryotic cells. Although prokaryotic bacterial cells are relatively simple, they have a

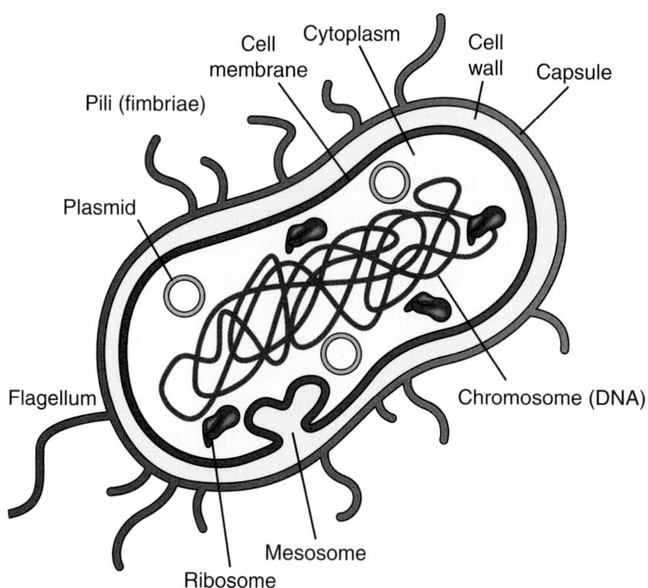

FIGURE 20–1 Cross section of a bacterial cell.

well-developed cell structure and contain several structural and genetic features that are not found in eukaryotic cells. One significant difference is that the bacterial chromosome is not enclosed inside of a membrane-bound nucleus but instead resides inside the bacterial cytoplasm. Also housed in the cytoplasm are internal cellular structures, such as ribosomes, mesosomes, and potentially plasmids, as well as other cytoplasmic inclusion bodies. Not present in bacterial cells are membrane-bound organelles such as the mitochondria found in eukaryotic cells **(Fig. 20–1).**

Other significant differences between eukaryotic and prokaryotic cells are features of the cell membrane and the presence of a cell wall in bacteria. Similar to the plasma membrane in eukaryotic cells, the bacterial plasma membrane plays a regulatory role in the transport of molecules in and out of the cell. The cell membrane in bacteria also contains various enzyme systems responsible for energy generation. In eukaryotic cells (except for plants and fungi) the plasma membrane is the outer surface of the cell. In contrast, bacteria have a cell wall as their outermost feature. The bacterial cell wall prevents osmotic lysis and confers shape and rigidity to the bacteria. Peptidoglycan is the primary component providing the shape and rigidity. The majority of antibiotics used to treat bacterial infections target the production of peptidoglycan in the cell wall.

The bacterial cell wall structure has two different variations, which are classified as either gram-positive or gram-negative, depending on their staining characteristics. Both gram-positive and gram-negative cell walls have features that increase an organism's virulence, as we will discuss later. One of the features found in the cell wall of gram-negative bacteria is the lipopolysaccharide (LPS) layer. There are three components that make up LPS—an outer core polysaccharide, an inner core polysaccharide, and lipid A. When released from a dead or dying cell, a portion of LPS called lipid A is exposed. Lipid A, also referred to as **endotoxin,** is a powerful stimulator of cytokine production that leads to a variety of systemic manifestations and potentially fatal endotoxic (gram-negative) shock (discussed later in this chapter).

To be successful in establishing an infection, bacteria must first adhere to and colonize the host tissue. Furthermore, to persist in the host, they must be capable of evading the immune system. Structural features are generally involved in the adherence of bacteria or the evasion of the immune system. Whip-like structures called *flagella* can facilitate adherence as well as movement of the bacteria toward a host cell.

Bacteria have surface structures or molecules that can bind specifically to complementary receptors on specific cells of host tissues. The most common surface structures involved in attachment are fimbriae, which are composed of protein. The fimbriae involved in specific attachment to prokaryotic surface ligands are referred to as the *common pili*. Other pili used to exchange genetic information, called the *F* or *sex pili*, are fewer in number than common pili. The sex pili may also function in the attachment of bacteria to host cells.

In addition to allowing the organism to attach to and colonize tissues, pili play a role in resisting phagocytosis by white blood cells (WBCs) and may undergo antigenic variation to evade the adaptive immune response. For example, the pili of *Neisseria gonorrhoeae* specifically adhere to human mucosal epithelial cells. *N. gonorrhoeae* can evade the immune response and resist phagocytosis by rearranging portions of its genome, thus changing the antigen makeup of the pili. Most strains of *E. coli* that colonize the gastrointestinal tract do not adhere to epithelial cells of the small intestine. The ability of certain strains of *E. coli* to cause gastrointestinal disease is associated with the expression of specific pili that allow for adherence to the epithelial cells of the small intestine. For example, enterotoxigenic *E. coli* (ETEC) strains have factor antigen I (CFA) pili that adhere to the cells in the small intestine; the organism then produces the toxins that cause diarrhea.

Attachment may also occur via adhesions or surface molecules on the bacterial cell. Attachment caused by the presence of surface molecules is referred to as *afimbrial* (non–pili dependent) attachment. Host-cell receptors recognized by bacterial surface molecules include proteoglycans, laminins, collagens, elastin, and hyaluronan. Glycoproteins such as fibrinogen, fibronectin, and vitronectin are also potential receptors for bacteria. The ability of ***Streptococcus pyogenes*** pili to attach to host cells is caused by the production of F protein, which attaches to fibronectin. In addition to aiding in attachment, surface M protein, the major virulence factor of *S. pyogenes,* allows the organism to resist phagocytosis.

A major structural feature that plays an important role in increasing an organism's virulence is the presence of a capsule, which is usually polysaccharide in nature. Capsules contribute to the organism's ability to resist innate and adaptive immune responses through a variety of means. They can block the attachment of antibodies, inhibit activation of complement, or act as a decoy when capsular material is released into the surrounding host environment. One of the most important features of a capsule is its role in blocking phagocytosis by WBCs. For example, *S. pneumoniae's* primary determinant of virulence is a polysaccharide capsule that prevents the ingestion of pneumococci by alveolar macrophages. In addition, extracellular capsular antigens are released and bind to immunoglobulins, thus reducing the effective immune response against the organism itself. Strains of bacteria that do not possess a capsule are, in most cases, avirulent and not able to produce disease.

Extracellular Virulence Factors

Extracellular substances produced by bacteria also contribute to an organism's virulence by breaking down primary or secondary defenses of the body, damaging the host tissues and cells, or facilitating the growth and spread of the organism. Substances that perform the latter function are called *invasins*. Several of the invasins include hyaluronidase, collagenase, phospholipases, lecithinases, coagulase, and various kinases.

Endotoxin and Exotoxins

Bacteria may also produce two types of toxins—endotoxin and exotoxins. Endotoxin (lipid A) is found in the LPS layer of the cell walls of all gram-negative bacteria. When the cell dies, the LPS layer is removed from the cell, releasing endotoxin in the host. The effects of endotoxin are complex. Endotoxin induces a variety of host responses, including the production of cytokines such as interleukin (IL)-1, IL-6, IL-8, tumor necrosis factor (TNF), and platelet-activating factor, which stimulate the production of prostaglandins and leukotrienes. This results in inflammation, increased heart rate, increased body temperature (fever), and a decrease in blood pressure. In addition, endotoxin activates the complement cascade, resulting in the formation of the anaphylatoxins C3a and C5a, which cause vasodilation and increase vascular permeability. The alternative coagulation cascade is also activated, producing coagulation, thrombosis, and acute disseminated intravascular coagulation (DIC), leading to hemorrhage and shock. A potential consequence of endotoxin release is septic shock, a life-threatening illness that is usually the result of a gram-negative *bacteremia,* or presence of bacteria in the blood. With septic shock, there is a large-scale release of inflammatory mediators that results in massive vasodilation and hypotension. Some refer to this as a "cytokine storm." If the condition worsens, there is widespread organ damage, including renal failure, liver dysfunction, heart damage, and eventual death. Although immunogenic, endotoxin does not elicit a protective immune response, so no vaccine is available against this bacterial component.

Clinical Correlations

Capsular Antigens and Vaccine Development

Most capsules evoke a strong humoral immune response and are used for the development of vaccines. For example, the vaccines for *Haemophilus influenzae* type b, *S. pneumoniae,* and certain types of *Neisseria meningitidis* consist of antigens derived from bacterial capsules (see Chapter 25).

Unlike endotoxin, which has multiple effects on the body, **exotoxins** have a very specific and targeted activity. They are protein molecules that are released from living bacteria (mostly gram-positive bacteria) and are considered to be some of the most potent molecules known to harm living organisms. Exotoxins may be classified as neurotoxins, cytotoxins, or enterotoxins, according to their effect on cells. Exotoxins bind to specific receptors on host cells. Most exotoxins have several subunits that bind to the receptor (B subunits) and a subunit that is actually responsible for the specific activity of the toxin (A subunit). An example of a cytotoxin is the diphtheria toxin, which interferes with protein synthesis in epithelial cells. Neurotoxins include the tetanus toxin, which prevents the release of inhibitory transmitters from the presynaptic membrane of neuromuscular cells, leading to continuous excitement of muscle cells and spasms. Botulism toxin works in a reverse manner—the toxin prevents the release of acetylcholine (ACh), resulting in paralysis of the motor system. Examples of enterotoxins are toxins A and B produced by *Clostridium difficile,* which cause fluid secretion (diarrhea), mucosal injury, and inflammation **(Fig. 20–2).** Exotoxins are extremely immunogenic and induce the production of protective antibodies. Inactivated exotoxins called "toxoids" are used for some vaccines. For example, the toxin of *Corynebacterium diphtheria* is used in the vaccine to prevent diphtheria.

Some exotoxins may act as "superantigens." Unlike other antigens, these superantigens are not processed by antigen-presenting cells (APCs). Instead, they bind directly to class II major histocompatibility complexes (MHC II) on APCs outside of the normal antigen-binding groove. The MHC II receptor binds to the T-cell receptor (TCR) with the whole antigen (toxin) attached. Normally, only 0.0001% of

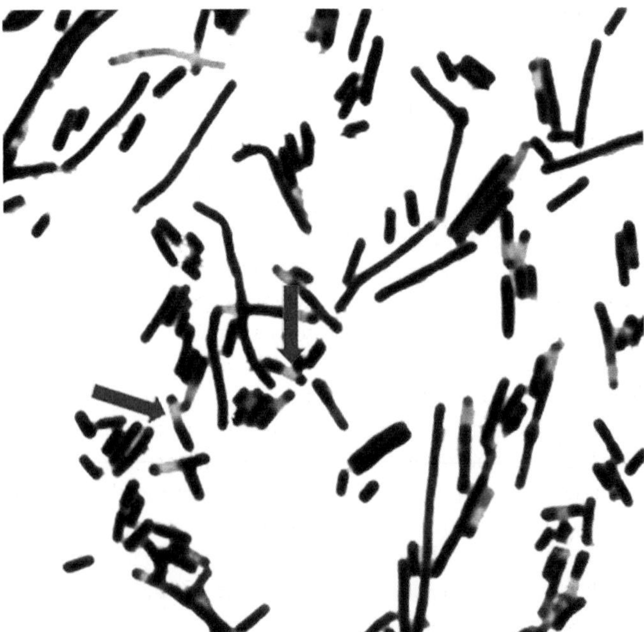

FIGURE 20–2 Gram stain of *Clostridium difficile* (a gram-positive rod). The clear areas in the cell represent a spore. Spores are resistant to disinfectants and contribute to the spread of the organism from person to person. *(Courtesy of James Vossler.)*

T cells are activated in an immune response. However, a superantigen induces activation of up to 20% of T cells, resulting in a massive release of cytokines. The systemic events brought on by the release of large amounts of cytokines leads to what is referred to as "toxic shock syndrome." Examples include the TSST-1 toxin produced by *Staphylococcus aureus* and the superantigens produced by *S. pyogenes,* the cause of streptococcal toxic shock syndrome (STSS).

Immune Defenses Against Bacterial Infections and Mechanisms of Evasion

Immune Defense Mechanisms

Although bacteria may possess various features that increase their virulence, they must be able to circumvent or overcome the host's defense mechanisms. As we discussed in previous chapters, both innate and adaptive responses may occur after an encounter with foreign antigens.

The first line of defense against potential pathogens involves intact skin and mucosal surfaces that serve as structural barriers. In addition, the epithelial surface may have enzymes and nonspecific antimicrobial defense peptides (ADPs), or defensins, and proteins that have antimicrobial activity. One example of an enzyme with specific antimicrobial activity is lysozyme, which is found in many secretions, including tears and saliva. Lysozyme destroys the peptidoglycan found in the cell wall of bacteria, especially gram-positive bacteria. Other enzymes include ribonucleases, which destroy RNA and have antimicrobial and antiviral activities. The body excretes a wide variety of ADPs and proteins that play a role in the innate defenses of the body. Some of the ADPs and proteins are only secreted by specific tissues or cells. One group of soluble peptides is the defensin peptides. *Defensins* are produced constitutively by the cells in the body.

The three main classes of defensins are alpha, beta, and theta. Alpha defensins are produced by neutrophils, certain macrophage populations, and Paneth cells of the small intestine. This class of defensins is believed to disrupt the microbial membrane. Beta defensins are produced by neutrophils as well as epithelial cells lining the various organs, including the bronchial tree and genitourinary system. They are believed to increase resistance of epithelial cells to colonization. Theta defensins are not found in humans.

Many antimicrobial proteins contribute to the innate immune response. For example, complement proteins can promote chemotaxis. Interleukins are involved in the regulation of immune responses and inflammatory reactions. Prostaglandins are involved in the dilation and constriction of blood vessels and modulation of inflammation. Leukotrienes are involved in inflammation and fever.

Acute-phase reactants also play important roles. For example, C-reactive protein (CRP) activates the complement system and promotes phagocytosis by macrophages. Haptoglobin binds free plasma hemoglobin, which deprives the bacteria of iron. Ceruloplasmin is a glycoprotein with bactericidal activities.

Bacteria, fungi, and viruses possess pathogen-associated molecular patterns (PAMPs), which are structural patterns consisting of carbohydrates, nucleic acids, or bacterial peptides. PAMPs are recognized by pattern recognition receptors (PRRs) expressed on the cells of the innate immune system. Engagement of the PRR with the appropriate PAMP triggers the release of immune mediators such as cytokines and chemokines, boosts production of various defensins and proteins, and initiates phagocytosis. The phagocytic process is enhanced by the activation of the alternative complement cascade, which is triggered by microbial cell walls or other products of microbial metabolism.

Adaptive immune responses include the production of antibodies directed against bacterial antigens or extracellular products produced by bacteria such as exotoxins. Antibody formation is the main defense against extracellular bacteria. The binding of antibodies to invading bacteria is referred to as *opsonization* (see Chapter 5).

Cell-mediated immunity (CMI), the other branch of the adaptive immune response, is helpful in attacking intracellular bacteria, such as *Mycobacterium tuberculosis, Legionella pneumophila, Listeria monocytogenes,* and *Rickettsia* species. Through the mechanism of delayed-type hypersensitivity, CD4 T cells produce cytokines, which activate macrophages to release enzymes that destroy the bacteria (see Chapter 14). The recruitment of inflammatory cells results in the formation of granulomas that surround the bacteria-infected cells to help prevent the spread of infection. Cytotoxic T cells are also recruited to the site of infection and mount an antigen-specific attack on the infected cells.

Bacterial Evasion Mechanisms

Bacteria have developed several ways to inhibit the immune system or make it more difficult for immune responses to occur. Three main mechanisms used by bacteria involve avoiding antibody, blocking phagocytosis, and inactivating the complement cascade **(Fig. 20–3).** Bacteria can evade antibodies by altering their bacterial antigens, a process called *antigenic variation.* They can also coat themselves with host proteins such as fibrin or immunoglobulin molecules *(S. aureus)* or fibronectin *(Treponema pallidum)* or hide their surface molecules through

Connections

Toll-Like Receptors (TLRs)

Recall from Chapter 2 that one of the main groups of PRRs are the Toll-like receptors (TLRs). TLRs are expressed on key cells of the innate immune system, such as macrophages and dendritic cells. They recognize molecules that are commonly found in microbial pathogens but not on host cells. Once TLRs have bound to their ligands, cell-signaling pathways are triggered that result in the production of cytokines that enhance the inflammatory response, resulting in more efficient pathogen destruction.

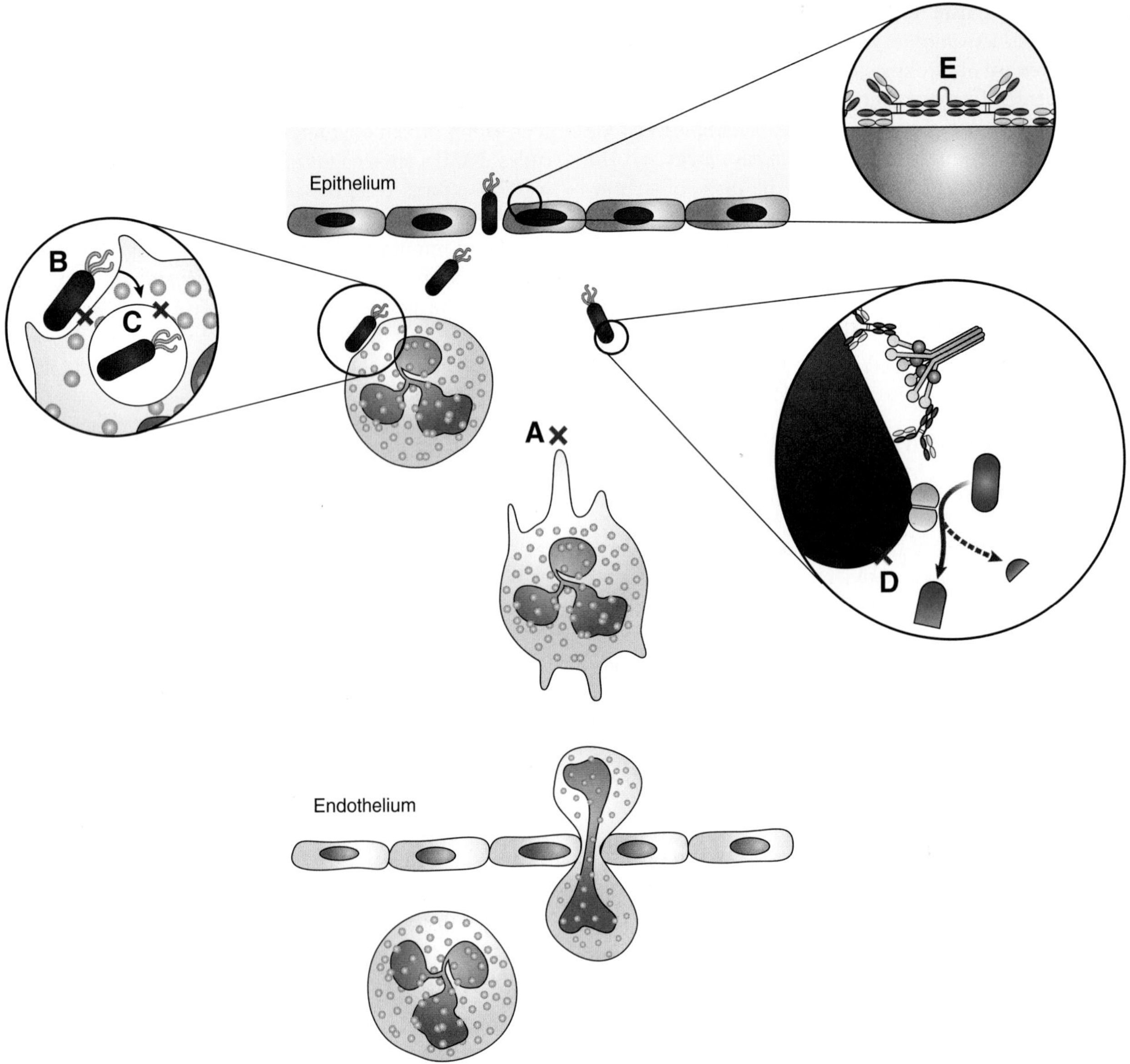

FIGURE 20–3 The strategies bacteria use to evade host defenses. (A) Inhibiting chemotaxis. (B) Blocking adherence of phagocytes to the bacterial cells. (C) Blocking digestion. (D) Inhibiting complement C3b binding. (E) Cleaving immunoglobulin A (IgA).

antigenic disguise (the hyaluronic acid capsule of *S. pyogenes*). Bacteria can also evade the specific immune response through downregulation of MHC molecules and production of proteases that degrade immunoglobulin A (IgA). *N. gonorrhoeae, H. influenzae,* and *Streptococcus sanguinis* are all examples of bacteria that can cleave IgA.

Most of the evasion mechanisms target the process of phagocytosis. Bacteria can mount a defense at several stages in the phagocytic process, including chemotaxis, adhesion, and digestion. Some pathogens such as *N. gonorrhoeae,* for example, inhibit the release of chemotactic factors that would bring phagocytic cells to the area. The cell walls of *S. pyogenes* produce an M protein that interferes with adhesion to the phagocytic cell. Additionally, the presence of a polysaccharide capsule found in such organisms as *N. meningitidis, S. pneumoniae, Y. pestis,* and *H. influenzae* inhibits the binding of neutrophils and macrophages needed to initiate phagocytosis.

Microorganisms use several different mechanisms to resist digestion. Some bacteria can block fusion of lysosomal granules with phagosomes after being engulfed by the phagocyte. *Salmonella* species are able to do this, as can *M. tuberculosis* and *Mycobacterium leprae.* In *M. tuberculosis* and *M. leprae* infections, each bacillus is contained in a membrane-enclosed fluid compartment called a *pristiophorus vacuole* (PV), which does not fuse with the lysosomes because of the complexity of the acid-fast cell walls.

An additional mechanism of resisting digestion involves the production of extracellular products after the bacteria are phagocytized. The primary effect is the release of lysosomal contents into the cytoplasm of the phagocytic cells, subsequently killing the WBC. Examples include leukocidin, produced by *S. aureus;* listeriolysin O, produced by *L. monocytogenes;* and streptolysin, produced by *S. pyogenes.*

The last major defense some bacteria use is to block the action of complement. Organisms mentioned previously that produce a capsule do not bind the complement component C3b, which is important in enhancing phagocytosis. Such organisms cannot easily be phagocytized unless coated by other opsonins (e.g., IgG). Additionally, some organisms express molecules that disrupt one or more of the complement pathways. Protein H, produced by *S. pyogenes,* binds to C1 but does not allow the complement cascade to proceed further. Another example is *Streptococcus agalactiae,* also known as *Group B streptococcus* or *GBS*. GBS has a capsule that is rich in sialic acid (a common component of host-cell glycoproteins), causing degradation of C3b and making the organism resistant to complement-mediated phagocytosis.

Laboratory Detection and Diagnosis of Bacterial Infections

Five general ways can be used to detect the causative agent of a bacterial infection: (1) culture or growth of the causative agent, (2) microscopy, (3) detection of bacterial antigens in the clinical sample, (4) molecular detection of bacterial DNA or RNA, and (5) serology to detect antibodies produced in response to the infection.

Bacterial Culture

Traditional means of determining the cause of a bacterial infection rely largely on growing the organism in culture. Various broth and solid media may be used to recover the organism. Some media may contain substances that enhance the growth of certain organisms and are referred to as *enriched media*. Selective media contain substances or antibiotics that suppress the growth of commensalistic bacteria and support the growth of other bacteria. Differential media contain substrates that allow for the differentiation of bacteria based on their ability to use the substrate. For example, MacConkey agar selects for gram-negative bacteria and differentiates between lactose- and non–lactose-fermenting bacteria. Some organisms, such as *Bordetella pertussis,* the causative agent of whooping cough, have very specific growth requirements for which specialized media must be used.

Although culture is the primary laboratory means of diagnosing bacterial infections, the culturing of bacterial pathogens has limitations. There are several bacterial pathogens for which clinically useful culture systems are not available. For other organisms, recovery in culture may take too long to be clinically useful. For example, although ***Mycoplasma pneumoniae,*** a leading cause of community acquired pneumonia, can be cultured, culturing is a challenge. The organism is extremely fastidious (difficult to grow) and may take weeks to recover in the laboratory. Other organisms present a danger to the laboratory technologist if they are not grown and handled using the most rigorous safety precautions (e.g., *Y. pestis*).

Microscopic Visualization

Visualization of the causative agents using microscopic techniques is most often done using differential or fluorescent stains. One example is the Gram stain for differentiating gram-positive bacteria, which stain purple with crystal violet **(Fig. 20–4)**, from gram-negative bacteria, which stain pink with safranin. Other examples are the acid-fast stain for the detection of *M. tuberculosis* **(Fig. 20–5)**, and the Giemsa stain for the detection of the causative agents of malaria. Direct fluorescent antibody assay, or DFA, involves the use of antibody conjugated with a fluorescent label to detect specific bacteria in a sample. Currently, many DFAs are being replaced by molecular tests because they lack sensitivity or because the reagents are not widely available. Although the various staining methods are not difficult to perform, a trained microscopist is necessary for proper interpretation. Another limitation

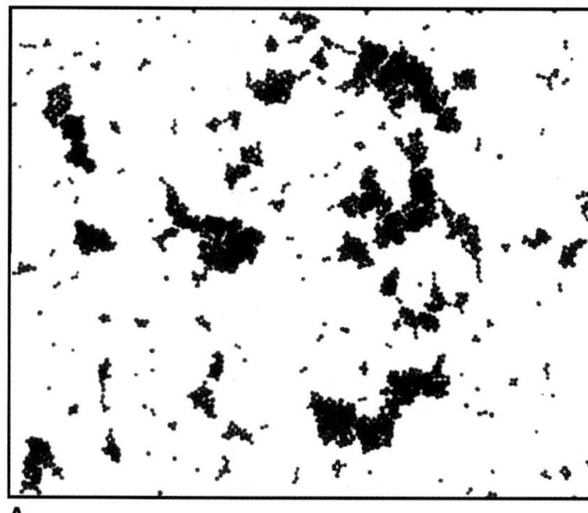

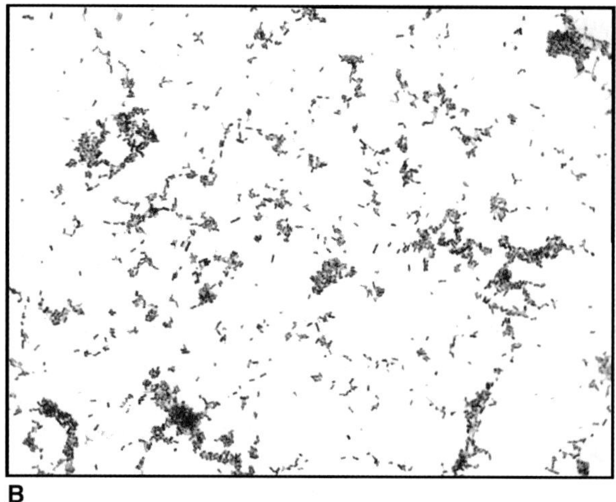

FIGURE 20–4 (A) Gram stain of Staphylococci showing gram-positive cocci in clusters. (B) Gram stain of *E. coli* showing gram-negative rods. *(Courtesy of James Vossler.)*

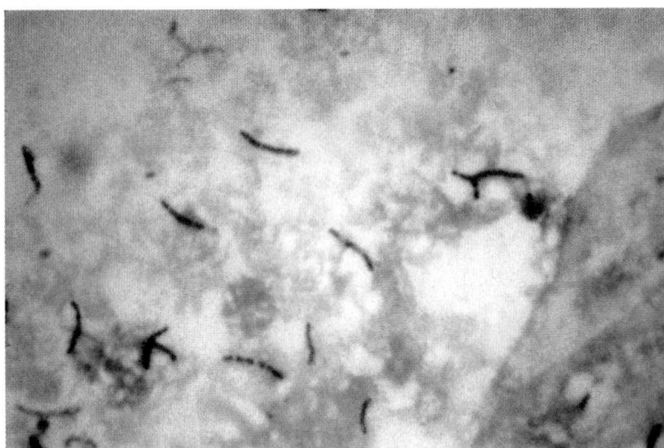

FIGURE 20-5 Photomicrograph of *Mycobacterium tuberculosis* bacteria using acid-fast Ziehl-Neelsen stain; magnified 1000×. The acid-fast stains depend on the ability of mycobacteria to retain the dye when treated with mineral acid or an acid–alcohol solution. *(Courtesy of the CDC/Dr. George P. Kubica, Public Health Image Library.)*

of microscopy is that not all organisms may be visualized through microscopic means.

Antigen Detection

Antigen detection assays are available for a wide variety of bacteria, viruses, parasites, and fungi in clinical samples. Testing methodologies include latex agglutination (LA), enzyme-linked immunosorbent assay (ELISA), and lateral flow immunochromatographic assays (LFA) that detect the presence of an analyte (e.g., bacterial antigen) in a sample. The LA and LFA assays are advantageous because of the relative ease by which the tests can be performed, their low cost, and the rapid turnaround time. Many of the LA and LFA assays are classified as "CLIA waived" tests. Under the Clinical Laboratory Improvement Amendments of 1988 (CLIA), simple, low-risk tests can be "waived" (i.e., laboratories performing the testing are not subject to routine inspection) and may be performed in physicians' offices and various other locations. Bacteria and viruses for which antigen detection is widely used include *S. pyogenes* (strep throat), *L. pneumophila* (Legionnaire disease), rotavirus (pediatric diarrheal disease), respiratory syncytial virus, and influenza A and B. Antigen detection assays are highly specific, and because of advances in technology, the sensitivities of the assays have improved dramatically. In many cases, antigen detection assays, particularly LFA, have replaced other methods used to detect infections with bacteria, viruses, and fungi.

Molecular Detection

Rapid developments in the field of molecular diagnostics have allowed for the increased availability and use of nucleic acid–based assays in the clinical laboratory to detect pathogenic microorganisms. Compact hybridization and gene amplification assays that are easy to perform have made their way into physicians' office laboratories. The most widely known molecular technology is the polymerase chain reaction (PCR), in which specific genetic sequences are amplified and detected. The development of real-time PCR or quantitative PCR (qPCR) has allowed for results to be obtained in a few hours, as compared with several days for traditional PCR. For some infectious agents, such as *N. gonorrhoeae* and *C. trachomatis,* nucleic acid–based assays are widely available and are more sensitive than traditional culture methods, making nucleic acid detection the method of choice for detection of these organisms.

Although nucleic acid–based assays are more sensitive than other methods, there are limitations associated with nucleic acid–based testing. At the time of this writing, there are relatively few U.S. Food and Drug Administration (FDA)-approved assays on the market for several infectious agents, and the cost of the instrumentation and disposables is prohibitive to many organizations. However, FDA-approved assays for the detection of agents causing infections are becoming available at a rapid rate. As more assays receive FDA approval and additional technological advances occur, the use of molecular-based assays for the detection of agents responsible for various infectious diseases will become even more widespread.

Serological Diagnosis

Serology has historically been used to detect and confirm infections from organisms that are difficult to grow or for which other laboratory methods of diagnosing the infection are not available. Serology may also be useful in determining the causative agent when the clinical symptoms are not specific enough to identify the cause of the infection. For certain organisms (e.g., *Anaplasma, Ehrlichia, Chlamydophila pneumoniae, Chlamydophila psittaci, Coxiella burnetii, Leptospira, Ricksettia* spp., and *T. pallidum*), serological testing remains useful and, in some cases, is the best means of detecting exposure to or infection with an organism. Detection of either immunoglobulin M (IgM) or immunoglobulin G (IgG) antibodies may indicate recent or previous exposure to an organism, and antibody titers may be used to assess reactivation or reexposure to an infectious agent (see Chapter 5).

Connections

Antibody Response Curve

A serological pattern of IgM+, IgG– generally indicates an early-stage, acute infection, whereas an IgM–, IgG+ pattern usually signifies a past exposure. The best indication of a current infection is a four-fold rise in antibody titer when comparing two serum samples collected from a patient during the beginning and later stages of the infection. This is a good time to review the typical antibody-response curve shown in Chapter 5.

The primary disadvantage of using serology in diagnosis is that there is usually a delay between the start of the infection and the production of antibodies to the infecting microorganism. Although IgM antibodies may appear relatively early (7 to 10 days after exposure), some infections have a rapid course; the need to initiate therapy limits the detection of IgM antibodies as a diagnostic tool in those instances. In some cases, demonstration of a high IgG antibody titer in the initial stage of infection is diagnostic; however, the high titer may be caused by a past infection, and the patient's symptoms may have an entirely different cause. When testing for the presence of IgG antibodies, it is ideal to collect serum samples during both the acute and convalescent phases of the illness so that a rising titer to the suspected pathogen can be observed. Another limitation of serology is that immunosuppressed patients may be unable to mount an antibody response.

Proteomics

The **proteome** is the total complement, or set, of proteins expressed by an organism or cell. **Proteomics** is the analysis and study of the proteins expressed by an organism's genome. Proteomics can be used to detect biomarkers—biological molecules found in blood, other body fluids, or tissues that are a sign of a normal or abnormal process, or of a condition or disease. The best-established clinical applications of proteomics so far are in the identification of markers for the early diagnosis of cancers.

Proteomics, which is still in its infancy, has the potential to be used to detect agents causing an infectious disease, monitor the effectiveness of treatment, or identify changes in a disease caused by a microorganism or virus. Advances in proteomic analysis are attributable largely to the introduction of mass spectrometry (MS) platforms capable of screening complex biological fluids for individual protein and peptide biomarkers. Proteomic-based approaches are being used to discover biomarkers that can be used in the detection and diagnosis of bacterial, viral, parasitic, or fungal infections. Specific protein biomarkers may also reveal the biological state of a particular organism (e.g., reproducing or dormant) or pathological changes within an infected host.

For example, the definitive diagnosis and monitoring of chronic hepatitis B virus (HBV) infection currently relies on liver biopsy. Research involving proteomic analysis of serum samples shows that the expression of at least seven serum proteins changes significantly in chronic HBV patients and that expression patterns correlate with fibrosis stage and inflammatory grade. Such markers could provide a non-invasive and definitive way to assess prognosis and guide treatment.

Proteomic analysis primarily relies on the use of MS platforms. Such platforms include matrix-associated laser desorption ionization time-of-flight MS (MALDI-TOF MS) and surface-enhanced laser desorption ionization time-of-flight MS (SELDI-TOF MS). Currently, the single most important application of **MALDI-TOF** is the identification of bacterial and fungal isolates growing from a culture.

To perform MALDI-TOF MS, the sample is placed on a solid surface matrix. The matrix is then placed in the instrument, where pulses of laser light vaporize the specimen, generating high-molecular-weight ions that absorb energy from the proteins and carbohydrates in the sample in a process known as *desorption*. The ions are then accelerated by an electrical field and a vacuum. Because the ions have the same energy, yet a different mass, they reach the detector at different times. The smaller ions reach the detector first because of their greater velocity, whereas the larger ions take longer owing to their larger mass. Hence, the analyzer is called "TOF" because the mass is determined from the ions' "time of flight" from being ionized and reaching the detector **(Fig. 20–6).** Identification of the microorganism in the sample is based on the generation of a characteristic "protein fingerprint" called a *profile* **(Fig. 20–7).**

SELDI-TOF is a variant of MALDI-TOF. SELDI-TOF has a higher sensitivity to low-molecular-weight proteins than MALDI-TOF and has been shown to detect various biomarkers associated with certain cancers better than MALDI-TOF. Research has shown that MALDI-TOF and SELDI-TOF can be used to detect certain parasitic and fungal infections in patients. The use of MALDI-TOF and SELDI-TOF to detect biomarkers associated with bacterial, viral, fungal, and parasitic agents shows promise in the detection and diagnosis of infections cause by these agents.

The remainder of this chapter reviews the infections caused by several bacteria and the clinical laboratory tests used to detect these infections.

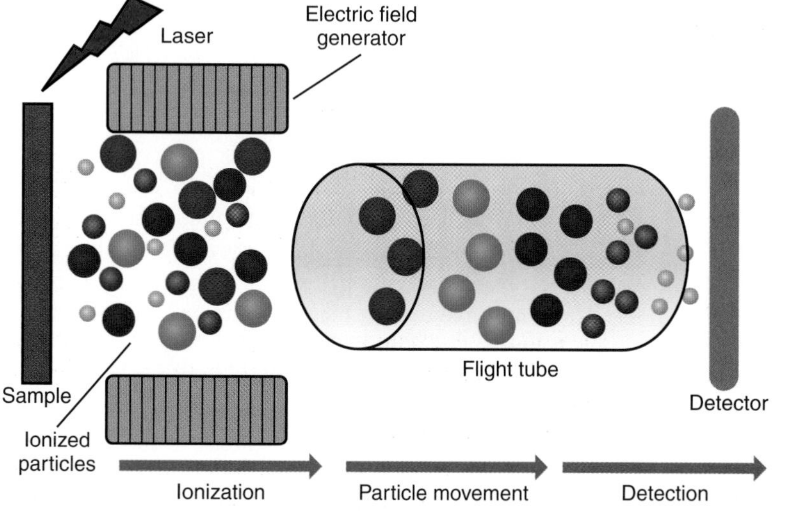

FIGURE 20-6 MALDI-TOF. The sample is ionized with a laser beam, breaking it into various-sized particles. The particles are accelerated into a tube with a magnetic field. Particles move through the tube via a vacuum. Smaller particles move faster through the tube (time of flight). The number of particles of each size is measured, creating a pattern unique to each organism and allowing for identification of the organism. (*Courtesy of James Vossler.*)

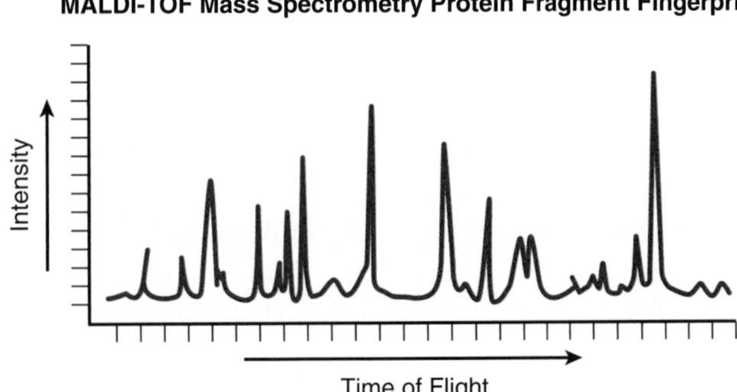

FIGURE 20-7 An example of a profile or pattern generated with MALDI-TOF. The pattern is compared with a database of known profiles, allowing for microorganism identification. (*Courtesy of James Vossler.*)

Group A Streptococci (*Streptococcus pyogenes*)

Classification and Structure

Streptococci are gram-positive cocci; these spherical, ovoid, or lancet-shaped organisms are often arranged in pairs or chains when observed on Gram stain **(Fig. 20–8)**. The streptococci are initially differentiated by their effect on sheep red blood cells (RBCs) when grown in culture. Those that completely lyse or hemolyze the blood cells are classified as being β-hemolytic. If the organisms only partially hemolyze the cells, causing them to appear green, they are classified as being α-hemolytic. If the organisms exhibit no effect on the cells, they are referred to as being γ-hemolytic. The β-hemolytic streptococci are further classified according to a group-specific carbohydrate composition that divides these bacteria into 20 groups designated A through H and K through V. These are known as the **Lancefield groups,** based on the pioneering work of Dr. Rebecca Lancefield.

A member of the β-hemolytic streptococci is *S. pyogenes*, a major cause of bacterial pharyngitis (a throat infection) and childhood impetigo (a skin infection). Because *S. pyogenes* has a Group A carbohydrate, the organism is also referred to as **Group A streptococcus (GAS)**. Additional cell wall components, the M and T proteins, allow for further classification and differentiation **(Fig. 20–9)**. The M protein is a filamentous molecule consisting of two alpha-helical chains twisted into a ropelike structure that extends out from the cell surface. Some strains possess a hyaluronic acid capsule outside the cell wall that contributes to the bacterium's antiphagocytic properties.

Serotyping and molecular techniques can be used to identify a particular strain of GAS. Serotyping involves identification of the M protein antigens by precipitation with type-specific anti-sera. More than 80 different serotypes have been identified by this method. However, serotyping has limitations, including limited availability of typing sera, new M protein types that do not react with the anti-sera, and difficulty in interpreting the results. Genotyping techniques involving PCR amplification of a portion of the *emm* gene, which codes for the M protein, followed by sequence analysis circumvents these problems. Pulsed-field gel electrophoresis (PFGE) has also been used for epidemiological studies. In PFGE, DNA from GAS is separated by using an alternating current to obtain a unique pattern or "fingerprint." The patterns from multiple sources may be compared when there is a Group A streptococcal outbreak.

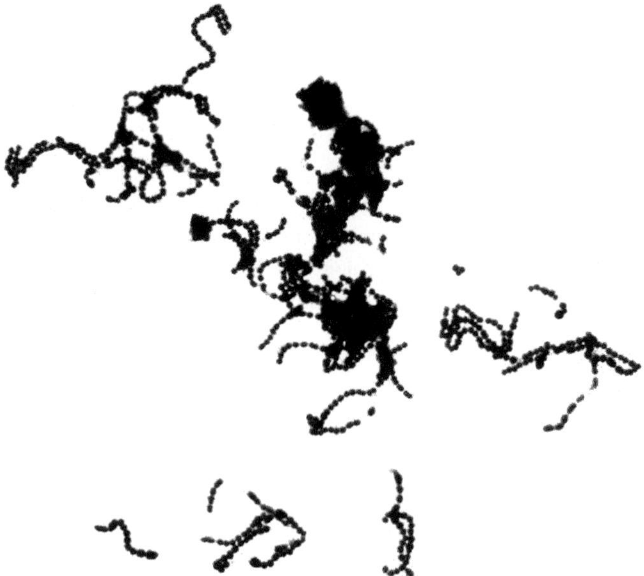

FIGURE 20–8 Gram stain of *Streptococcus pyogenes*, also known as Group A streptococci, which are gram-positive cocci that grow in pairs and chains. (*Courtesy of James Vossler.*)

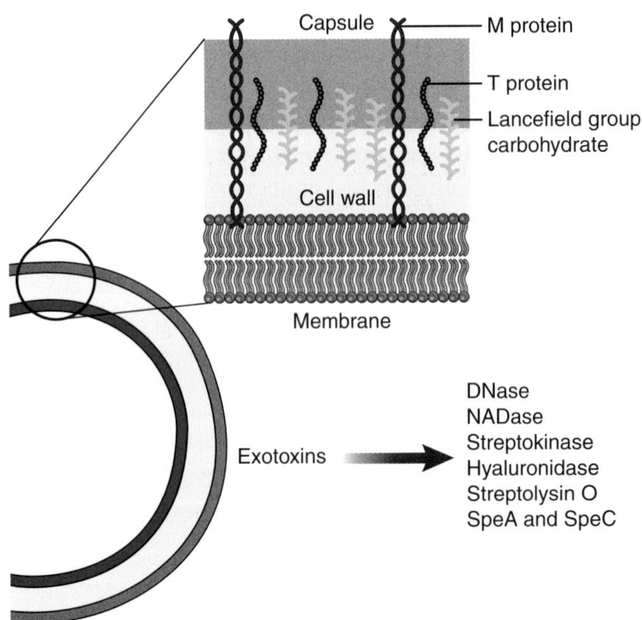

FIGURE 20–9 Diagram of antigenic components of *Streptococcus pyogenes.*

Virulence Factors

GAS is one of the most common and ubiquitous pathogenic bacteria and causes a variety of infections. The M protein is the major virulence factor of GAS and has a net-negative charge at the amino-terminal end that helps to inhibit phagocytosis. In addition, the presence of the M protein limits deposition of C3 on the bacterial surface, thereby diminishing complement activation. The M protein, along with lipoteichoic acid and protein F, help GAS attach to host cells. Immunity to GAS appears to be associated with antibodies to the M protein. There are more than 100 serotypes of this protein, and immunity is serotype-specific. Therefore, infections with one strain will not provide protection against another strain.

Additional virulence factors include various exotoxins that may be produced during the course of an infection. Pyrogenic exotoxins A, B, and C are responsible for the rash seen in scarlet fever and also appear to contribute to pathogenicity. Additional extracellular substances include the enzymes **streptolysin O**, deoxyribonuclease B (DNase B), hyaluronidase, nicotinamide adenine dinucleotide (NAD), and streptokinase. Antibodies produced against these substances are useful in the diagnosis of infection and for developing complications or sequelae associated with GAS infection (discussed later in the chapter).

Clinical Manifestations of Group A Streptococcal Infection

S. pyogenes can be responsible for infections ranging from pharyngitis (a throat infection) to life-threatening illnesses such as necrotizing fasciitis and streptococcal toxic shock syndrome. The two major sites of infections in humans are the upper respiratory tract and the skin, with pharyngitis ("strep throat") and streptococcal pyoderma (a skin infection) being the most common clinical manifestations. Symptoms of pharyngitis include fever, chills, severe sore throat, headache, tonsillar exudates, petechial rash on the soft palate, and anterior cervical lymphadenopathy **(Fig. 20–10)**. The most common skin infection is *streptococcal pyoderma* (also known as **impetigo**), characterized by vesicular lesions on the extremities that become pustular and crusted **(Fig. 20–11)**. Such infections tend to occur in young children. Other complications include otitis media, erysipelas, cellulitis, puerperal sepsis, and sinusitis. Septic arthritis, acute bacterial endocarditis, and meningitis also can result from a pharyngeal infection. Humans are the primary reservoir for GAS, and transmission of GAS is from person to person.

A small percentage of individuals develop **scarlet fever.** Although usually associated with pharyngeal infections, scarlet fever may occur with streptococcal infections at other sites. Symptoms include a fever of higher than 101°F, nausea, vomiting, headache, and abdominal pain. A distinct scarlet rash initially appears on the neck and chest and then spreads all over the body. Scarlet fever results from infection with a GAS that elaborates streptococcal pyrogenic exotoxins (erythrogenic toxins). Two of those toxins, streptococcal pyrogenic exotoxin A (SpeA) and streptococcal pyrogenic exotoxin C (SpeC), can act as superantigens that may induce toxic shock syndrome. Toxic shock syndrome is a life-threatening multisystem disease that often initiates as a skin or soft tissue infection and may proceed to shock and renal failure because of overproduction of cytokines.

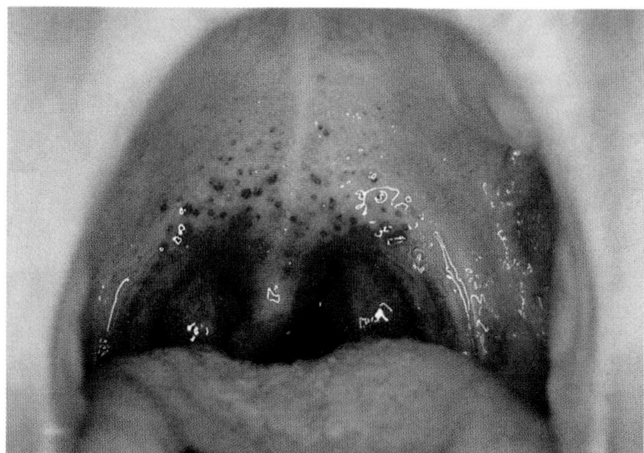

FIGURE 20–10 Pharyngitis, or sore throat, is characterized by swelling and reddening of the pharynx. Note the inflammation of the oropharynx and petechiae, or small red spots on the soft palate caused by *Streptococcal pharyngitis. (Courtesy of the CDC/Henry F. Eichenwald, Public Health Image Library.)*

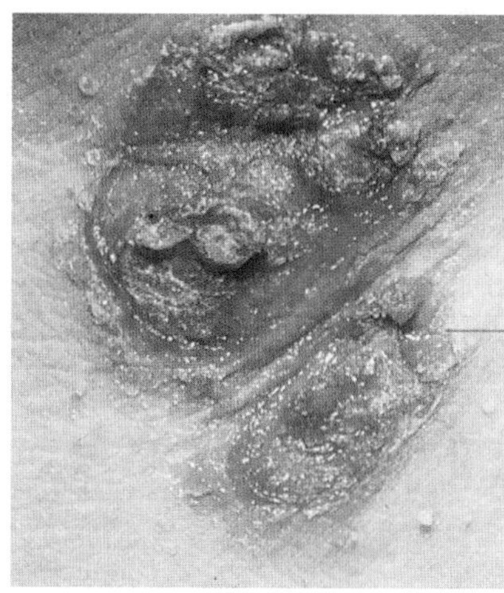

FIGURE 20–11 Impetigo is a dermatological streptococcal infection that is characterized by thick, golden-yellow discharge that dries, crusts, and sticks to the skin. It is also caused by the *S. aureus* bacteria.

Necrotizing fasciitis may occur when a GAS skin infection invades the muscles in the extremities or the trunk. The onset is quite acute and is a medical emergency. Exotoxins produced by *S. pyogenes* cause a rapidly spreading infection deep in the fascia, resulting in ischemia, tissue necrosis, and septicemia if not treated promptly. The disease may be associated with predisposing conditions such as chronic illness in the elderly or varicella in children, but healthy persons can be affected as well. Reporting of necrotizing fasciitis and toxic shock syndrome is part of a surveillance program conducted by the Centers for Disease Control and Prevention. Although the incidence of this syndrome has declined in the United States, a significant number of cases are still reported each year.

Group A Streptococcal Sequelae

The reason GAS receives so much attention is the potential for the development of two serious sequelae, **acute rheumatic fever** and **poststreptococcal glomerulonephritis** (*sequelae* are conditions that are the consequence of a previous disease or injury). The sequelae result from the host response to infection. Serological testing plays a major role in the diagnosis of these two diseases because the organism itself may no longer be present by the time symptoms appear.

Acute rheumatic fever develops as a sequela to pharyngitis or tonsillitis in 2% to 3% of infected individuals. It does not occur because of skin infection. The latency period is typically 1 to 3 weeks after onset of the sore throat. Characteristic features of acute rheumatic fever include fever, pain caused by inflammation in the joints, and inflammation of the heart. The disease is most likely caused by antibodies or cell-mediated immune responses originally produced against streptococcal antigens that cross-react with antigens present in human heart tissue.

Chief among the antibodies thought to be involved are those directed toward the M proteins, which have at least three epitopes that resemble antigens in heart tissue, permitting cross-reactivity to occur. Titers of some antibodies may remain high for several years following infection.

The second main complication following a streptococcal infection is acute glomerulonephritis, a condition characterized by damage to the glomeruli in the kidneys. This condition may follow infection of either the skin or the pharynx, whereas rheumatic fever follows only upper respiratory tract infections. Glomerulonephritis caused by a streptococcal infection is most common in children between the ages of 2 and 12 and is especially prevalent in the winter.

Symptoms of glomerulonephritis may include hematuria, proteinuria, edema, and hypertension. Patients may also experience malaise, backache, and abdominal discomfort. Renal function is usually impaired because the glomerular filtration rate is reduced, but renal failure is not typical. The most widely accepted theory for the pathogenesis of poststreptococcal glomerulonephritis is that it results from deposition of immune complexes containing streptococcal antigens in the glomeruli. These immune complexes stimulate an inflammatory response that damages the kidneys and impairs function because of release of the lysosomal contents of leukocytes and activation of complement.

Laboratory Diagnosis

Culture

Diagnosis of acute streptococcal infections typically is made by culture of the organism from the infected site. The specimen is plated on sheep blood agar and incubated. If GAS is present, small translucent colonies surrounded by a clear zone of β hemolysis will be visible **(Fig. 20–12)**. Identification is made on the basis of susceptibility to bacitracin, testing for L-pyrrolidonyl-β-naphthylamide (PYR) activity, or through Lancefield typing.

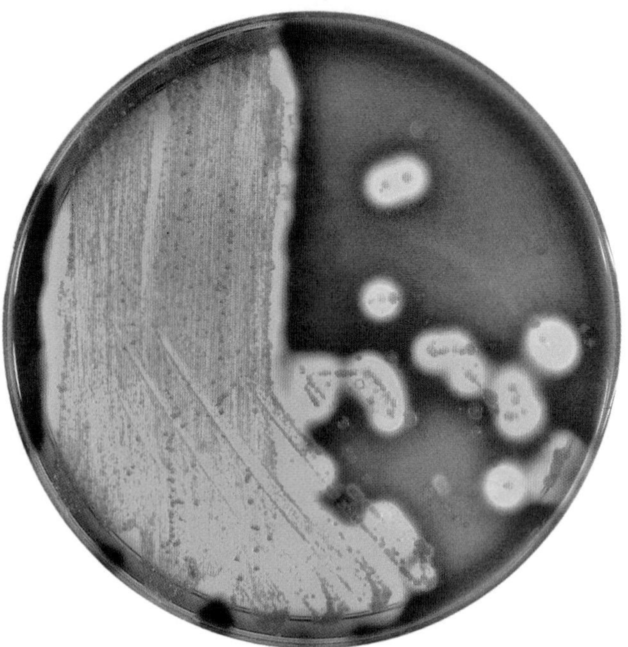

FIGURE 20–12 Throat culture plate showing a positive result for beta hemolytic Group A streptococci *(S. pyogenes)*. Bacterial colonies not producing beta hemolysis represent indigenous microbiota of the oropharynx. *(Courtesy of James Vossler.)*

Detection of Group A Streptococcal Antigens

As an alternative to culture, rapid assays have been commercially developed to detect Group A streptococcal antigens directly from throat swabs. The Group A antigens are extracted by either enzymatic or chemical means, and the process takes anywhere from 2 to 30 minutes, depending on the particular technique.

Lateral flow immunochromatographic assays (LFAs) are increasingly being used for the detection of bacterial, viral, fungal, and parasitic antigens in clinical samples. LFAs have largely replaced enzyme immunoassay (EIA) and LA assays to detect the antigens. LFAs are widely used in outpatient clinics, physician offices, and urgent care facilities for the rapid diagnosis of streptococcal pharyngitis.

The assays are technically easy to perform, allow for single-sample testing because of the incorporation of an internal control, and in many cases are more sensitive than traditional laboratory methods and other antigen detection methods (see Fig. 11–11). An example of an LFA used for the detection of GAS from a throat swab is shown in **Figure 20–13**.

Many of the assays require no more than 2 to 5 minutes of hands-on time. The specificity and sensitivity of the assays in many instances are higher than other methodologies. Although the assays have high sensitivities, cultures should be performed when rapid test results are negative. Molecular methods, including hybridization of specific rRNA sequences and real-time PCR, have also been developed as a means to rapidly detect Group A streptococcal infections.

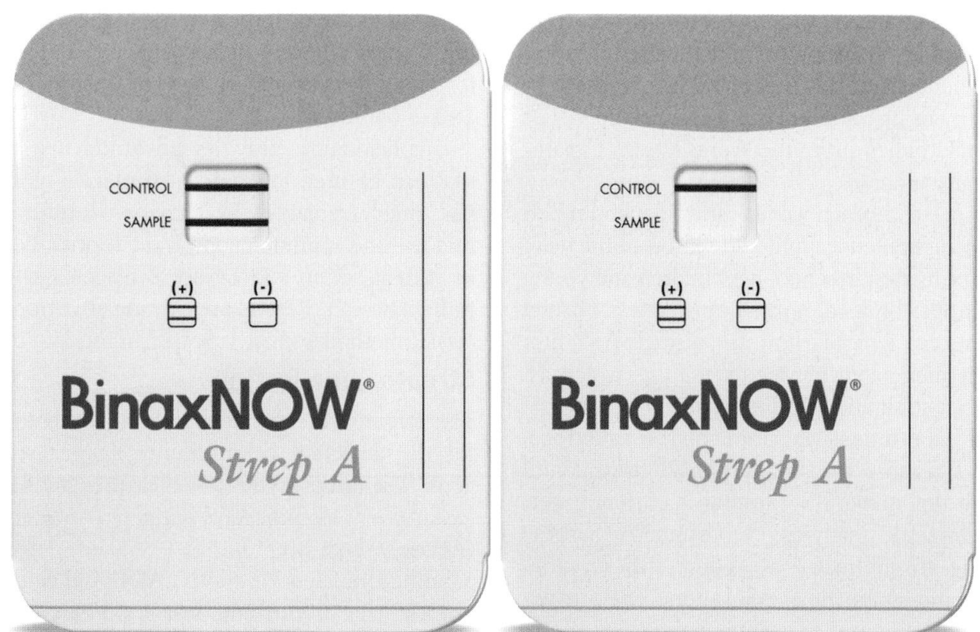

FIGURE 20–13 BinaxNOW lateral flow assay. The BinaxNOW Strep A Test immunochromatographic assay for the qualitative detection of *Streptococcus pyogenes* Group A antigen from throat swab specimens. To perform the test, a throat swab is inserted into the test card. Extraction reagents are added from dropper bottles. The test card is closed to bring the extracted sample in contact with the test strip. Strep A antigen captured by immobilized anti-strep A reacts to bind conjugated antibody. Immobilized species antibody captures the second visualizing conjugate. The test is interpreted by the presence or absence of visually detectable pink-to-purple colored lines. A positive result is indicated by production of both a sample line and a control line (shown on left), whereas a negative assay will produce only the control line (shown on right). *(BinaxNOW is a trademark of the Alere Scarborough, Inc. Used with permission.)*

Detection of Streptococcal Antibodies

Culture or rapid screening methods are extremely useful for diagnosis of acute pharyngitis. However, serological diagnosis must be used to identify acute rheumatic fever and post-streptococcal glomerulonephritis because the organism is unlikely to be present in the pharynx or on the skin at the time symptoms appear. Group A streptococci elaborate more than 20 exotoxins, and it is the antibody response to one or more of these that is used as documentation of nonsuppurative disease. Some of the exotoxin products include streptolysins O and S; deoxyribonucleases A, B, C, and D; streptokinase; NADase; hyaluronidase; diphosphopyridine nucleotidase; and pyrogenic exotoxins.

The antibody response to these streptococcal products is variable because of several factors, such as age of onset, site of infection, and timeliness of antibiotic treatment. The most diagnostically important antibodies are the following: anti-streptolysin O (ASO), anti-DNase B, anti-NADase, and anti-hyaluronidase (AHase). Assays for the detection of these antibodies can be performed individually or through use of the **streptozyme** test, which detects antibodies to all of these products (see *Streptozyme Testing* later). During Group A streptococcal infections, other antibodies are made to cellular antigens, such as the Group A carbohydrate and the M protein. Generally, detection of these antibodies is done in research or reference laboratories because commercial reagents are not available.

Serological evidence of disease is based on an elevated or rising titer of streptococcal antibodies. The onset of clinical symptoms of rheumatic fever or glomerulonephritis typically coincides with the peak of antibody response. If acute- and convalescent-phase sera are tested in parallel, a four-fold rise in titer is considered significant. The use of at least two tests for antibodies to different exotoxins is recommended because the production of detectable ASO does not occur in all patients. The most commonly used tests are those for ASO and anti-DNase B.

Antistreptolysin O (ASO) Testing

ASO tests detect antibodies to the streptolysin O enzyme produced by GAS. This enzyme is able to lyse RBCs. The presence of antibodies to streptolysin O indicates recent streptococcal infection in patients suspected of having acute rheumatic fever or poststreptococcal glomerulonephritis following a throat infection.

The classic hemolytic method for determining the **ASO titer** was the first test developed to measure streptococcal antibodies. This test was based on the ability of antibodies in the patient's serum to neutralize the hemolytic activity of streptolysin O. The traditional ASO titer involved preparing dilutions of patient serum to which a measured amount of streptolysin O reagent was added. These were allowed to combine during an incubation period, then reagent RBCs were added as an indicator. If enough antibodies were present, the streptolysin O was neutralized, and no hemolysis occurred. The titer was reported as the reciprocal of the highest dilution demonstrating no hemolysis. This titer could be expressed in either Todd units (by using a streptolysin reagent standard) or in international units (when using the World Health Organization international standard).

The range of expected normal values varies, depending on the patient's age, geographic location, and season of the year. ASO titers tend to be highest in school-age children and young adults. Thus, the upper limits of normal must be established for specific populations. Typically, however, a single ASO titer is considered to be moderately elevated if the titer is at least 240 Todd units in an adult and 320 Todd units in a child.

Because of the labor-intensive nature of the traditional ASO titer test and because the streptolysin O reagent and the RBCs used are not stable, ASO testing is currently performed by nephelometric methods. Nephelometry has the advantage of being an automated procedure that provides rapid, quantitative measurement of ASO titers. The antigen used in this technique is purified recombinant streptolysin. When antibody-positive patient serum combines with the antigen reagent, immune complexes are formed, resulting in an increase in light scatter that the instrument converts to a peak rate signal. All results are reported in international units, which are extrapolated from the classic hemolytic method described previously. When using the nephelometric method, individual laboratories must establish their own upper limits of normal for populations of different ages.

ASO titers typically increase within 1 to 2 weeks after infection and peak between 3 to 6 weeks following the initial symptoms (e.g., sore throat). However, an antibody response occurs in only about 85% of acute rheumatic fever patients within this period. Additionally, ASO titers usually do not increase in individuals with skin infections.

Anti-DNase B (Anti-Deoxyribonuclease B) Testing

Testing for the presence of **anti-DNase B** is clinically useful in patients suspected of having glomerulonephritis preceded by streptococcal skin infections because ASO antibodies often are not stimulated by this type of disease. In addition, antibodies to DNase B may be detected in patients with acute rheumatic fever who have a negative ASO test result.

DNase B is mainly produced by Group A streptococci, so testing for anti-DNase B is highly specific for Group A streptococcal sequelae. Macrotiter, microtiter, EIA, and nephelometric methods have been developed for anti-DNase testing. The classic test for the measurement of anti-DNase B activity is based on a neutralization method. If anti-DNase B antibodies are present, they will neutralize reagent DNase B, preventing it from depolymerizing DNA. The presence of DNase is measured by its effect on a DNA-methyl-green conjugate. This complex is green in its intact form; however, when hydrolyzed by DNase, the methyl green is reduced and becomes colorless. An overnight incubation at 37°C is required in some tests to permit antibodies to inactivate the enzyme. Tubes are graded for color, with a 4+ indicating that the intensity of color is unchanged and a 0 indicating a total loss of color. The result is reported as the reciprocal of the highest dilution demonstrating a color intensity of between 2+ and 4+. Normal titers for children between the ages of 2 and 12 years range from 240 to 640 units.

Nephelometry provides an automated means of testing that can be used for rapid quantitation of anti-DNase B and has largely replaced the enzyme-neutralization method. In this method, immune complexes formed between antibodies in patient serum and DNase B reagent generate an increase in light scatter. Results are extrapolated from values from the classic method and are reported in international units per mL.

Streptozyme Testing

The streptozyme test is a slide agglutination screening test for the detection of antibodies against streptococcal antigens. The streptozyme test measures antibodies against five extracellular streptococcal antigens: ASO, anti-hyaluronidase (AHase), anti-streptokinase (ASKase), anti-nicotinamide-adenine dinucleotide (anti-NAD), and anti-DNAase B antibodies. The streptozyme test is positive in 95% of patients with acute poststreptococcal glomerulonephritis because of GAS pharyngitis.

In this test, sheep RBCs are coated with streptolysin, streptokinase, hyaluronidase, DNase, and NADase so that antibodies to any of the streptococcal antigens can be detected. Reagent RBCs are mixed with a 1:100 dilution of patient serum. Hemagglutination represents a positive test, indicating that antibodies to one or more of these antigens are present. The test is rapid and simple to perform, but it appears to be less reproducible than other antibody tests. In addition, more false positives and false negatives have been reported for this test than for the ASO and anti-DNase B assays. Because a larger variety of antibodies are included in this test, the potential is higher for the detection of streptococcal antibodies. However, single-titer determinations are not as significant as several titrations performed at weekly or biweekly intervals following the onset of symptoms. The streptozyme test should be used in conjunction with the ASO or anti-DNase B tests when sequelae of Group A streptococcal infection are suspected and is especially useful when negative or borderline ASO results are obtained. (See the streptozyme test laboratory exercise online at Davis*Plus*.)

Helicobacter pylori

First isolated from humans in 1982, ***Helicobacter pylori*** is now recognized as a major cause of both gastric and duodenal ulcers. The organism resides in the mucus layer, the gastric epithelium, and occasionally the duodenal epithelium. This gram-negative, microaerophilic spiral bacterium is observed in 30% of the population in developed countries and more than 90% of the population in developing countries. In developing countries, more than 70% carry *H. pylori* by age 10, with carriage being nearly universal by the age of 20. Conversely, in the United States, there is little colonization during childhood. The rates gradually increase during adulthood, reaching a prevalence of 50% among persons older than 60 years. The high incidence of colonization in developing countries where living conditions are more crowded and sanitation conditions are suboptimal suggests that fecal–oral transmission is the most likely route. Since 1994, the National Institutes of Health has recommended that individuals with gastric or duodenal ulcers caused by *H. pylori* be given antibiotic treatment along with anti-ulcer medications. If untreated, *H. pylori* infection will last for the patient's life and may lead to gastric carcinoma.

Helicobacter pylori Virulence Factors

A major virulence factor of *H. pylori* is the production of the protein CagA, which is highly immunogenic. The organism has the ability to inject the CagA protein into the gastric epithelial cells. Once the CagA protein is in the epithelial cells, changes occur in the function of the cell's signal transduction pathways and in the structure of the cytoskeleton.

A second virulence factor is vacuolating cytotoxin, or VacA. The *VacA* gene codes for a toxin precursor. Epidemiological studies have shown that if the *CagA* and *VacA* genes are present in the strain of bacteria infecting the individual, there is a higher risk of developing gastric or peptic ulcers or gastric carcinoma.

Pathology and Pathogenesis

Unlike most other bacteria, *H. pylori* is able to survive and multiply in the gastric environment. This occurs because of several characteristics of the bacteria. Its spiral shape and flagella help the organism to be highly motile and to penetrate the viscous mucus layer in the stomach. The organism produces large amounts of **urease,** providing a buffering zone around the bacteria that protects it from the effects of the stomach acid. In addition, the acid-labile flagella are coated with a flagellar sheath, protecting them from the acidic environment of the stomach.

The pathology and mechanism of action leading to tissue damage are not clearly understood. Neutrophil-induced mucosal damage may be the result of the ammonia produced by urease. The ammonia has been shown to induce the release of chlorinated toxic oxidants from the neutrophils, which causes inflammation and damage to the mucosal cells. Once established below the mucosal layer, the organism does not invade the tissue. More likely, the pathology represents the host's response to extracellular products produced by the bacteria. Antibodies are formed against the signaling molecules CagA and VacA. Strains from individuals with stomach ulcers produce higher levels of VacA than strains from individuals without stomach ulcers.

The outcomes associated with *H. pylori* exposure vary. Not all individuals harboring the organism go on to develop disease, suggesting that there may be a genetic predisposition and that the interaction between the host and the bacteria plays a role. In some hosts, the organism is not able to establish itself. In others, asymptomatic colonization may persist, or hyperacidity may result in duodenal ulceration. Treatment of *H. pylori* consists of triple therapy with bismuth salts, metronidazole, and amoxicillin. Although highly effective, treatment will fail in some individuals because of poor patient compliance or resistance to metronidazole. An increased risk of developing gastric carcinoma and mucosa-associated lymphoid tumors (MALTomas) has also been shown.

Diagnosis of *H. pylori* Infection

Detection of *H. pylori* may be achieved by the invasive techniques of endoscopy or biopsy or through noninvasive techniques, including serological analysis, fecal antigen detection, and demonstration of urease production with urea breath tests. The most specific test to detect *H. pylori* infection is culture, but the sensitivity is usually lower than other methods because the organism is not evenly distributed throughout the gastric tissue.

Endoscopy and Biopsy

Endoscopy and biopsy are the most expensive and invasive methods for diagnosing an infection with *H. pylori*. However, histological examination of the tissue may reveal a great deal of information regarding the lesion. One method of testing for *H. pylori* involves the detection of urease from a biopsy taken from the antrum of the stomach. The antrum is the portion of the stomach before the pyloric sphincter or valve responsible for releasing stomach contents into the intestines. An example of a test that detects urease in a tissue biopsy is the CLOtest. The CLOtest (for *Campylobacter*-like organisms) detects urease activity in gastric mucosal biopsies. During the endoscopy, a small biopsy is taken (1 to 3 mm). The specimen is placed in the test cassette, resealed following the manufacturer's instructions, and sent to the laboratory. If urease is present, the yellow gel will turn a hot-pink color because of an increase in pH in the presence of urease. If urease is not present, the gel will remain yellow **(Fig. 20–14).** A majority of the tests will turn positive within 20 minutes; however, the test should be held and reexamined after 24 hours to allow time for the detection of a low-level infection. The test is easy to use, and results can be detected in a short period of time, making it ideal for rapid diagnosis of *H. pylori* infections.

Noninvasive Detection Methods

Procedures for detecting *H. pylori* that do not require the use of endoscopy include urea breath testing, enzyme or lateral flow immunoassays for the detection of bacterial antigens in the feces, molecular tests for *H. pylori* DNA, and serological testing. In the urea breath test, the patient ingests urea labeled with radioactive carbon (^{14}C) or, in newer tests, a nonradioactive ^{13}C urea is broken down by the urease enzyme of *H. pylori*, producing ammonia and bicarbonate. The bicarbonate is excreted in the breath, and the labeled carbon dioxide is measured by detection of radioactivity for ^{14}C or MS analysis for ^{13}C. The breath technique has excellent sensitivity and specificity and is helpful in determining if the bacteria have been eradicated by antimicrobial therapy.

Because of the potential for treatment failure, analysis of stool samples before and after antimicrobial therapy for

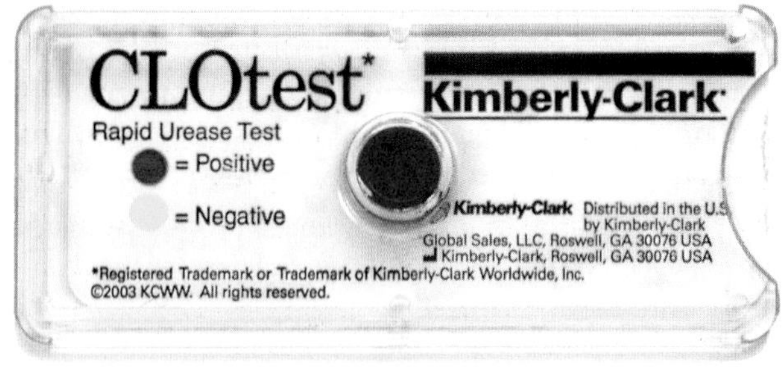

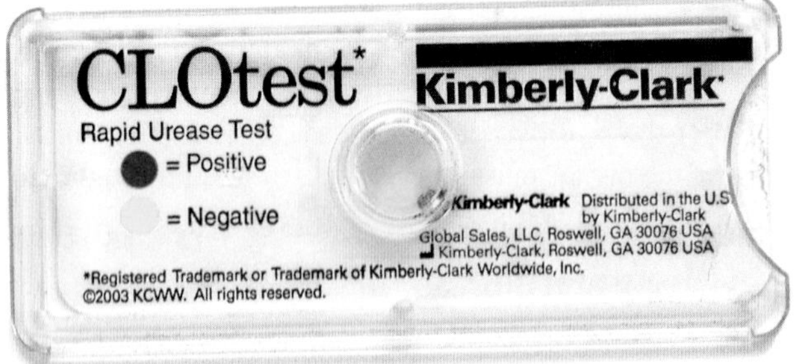

FIGURE 20–14 CLOtest. The CLOtest rapid urease method uses a tissue biopsy to detect *Helicobacter pylori*. The test consists of a well of indicator gel sealed inside a plastic cassette. The gel contains urea, phenol red, buffers, and a bacterial static agent to prevent the growth of contaminating urease-positive organisms. If the urease from *H. pylori* is present in the tissue sample, it changes the gel from yellow (bottom cassette) to bright magenta (top cassette). A majority of positive tests change color within 20 minutes. The test is reviewed after 24 hours because a low-level positive infection may not become detectable until then. *(Courtesy of Halyard Health, Inc., Irvine, CA. Used with permission.)*

H. pylori antigens is done to determine if the bacteria have been eliminated following treatment. ELISA tests as well as LFA methods are available. Because of the potential for asymptomatic carriage of the organism, stool antigen testing for initial diagnosis of *H. pylori* infection is not recommended.

Researchers also have developed molecular testing to detect *H. pylori* DNA. However, PCR-based methods, which detect the presence of the organism in fecal samples, cannot distinguish between living and dead *H. pylori*. Real-time PCR technology has been developed to determine the patient's bacterial load and has shown good correlation with the urea breath test. At the time of this writing, FDA-approved molecular assays for *H. pylori* are not available for clinical use.

Detection of *H. pylori* Antibodies

Serological testing is a primary screening method of determining infection with *H. pylori*. Infections from this organism result in production of IgG, IgA, and IgM antibodies. Most serological tests in clinical use detect *H. pylori*–specific antibodies of the IgG class. Although IgM antibody is produced in *H. pylori* infections, testing for its presence lacks clinical value because most infections have become chronic before diagnosis. Thus, IgG is the primary antibody found. IgA testing has a lower sensitivity and specificity than IgG testing, but it may increase the sensitivity of detection when used in conjunction with IgG testing.

The presence of antibodies in the blood of an untreated patient indicates an active infection because the bacterium does not spontaneously clear. Antibody levels in untreated individuals remain elevated for years. In treated individuals, the antibody concentrations decrease after about 6 months to approximately 50% of the level the patient had during the active infection. Therefore, convalescent testing should be performed 6 months to a year after treatment, which requires that the acute serum sample be stored for up to a year. A decrease in antibody titer of more than 25% must occur for treatment to be considered successful.

Measurement of the antibodies may be done with several techniques, including ELISA, immunoblot, and rapid tests using LA or LFA. Several LFAs are approved for CLIA-waived testing by physicians' office laboratories. The method of choice for the detection of *H. pylori* antibodies is the ELISA technique because it is reliable and accurate. Tests employing antigens from a pooled extract from multiple and genetically diverse strains yield the best sensitivity because *H. pylori* is so heterogeneous. Very few, if any, patients produce antibodies to all of the *H. pylori* antigens; most patients produce antibodies against the CagA and VacA proteins. Antibodies to these two proteins indicate a more severe case of gastritis or an increased risk of developing gastric carcinoma.

When compared with other techniques for antibody detection of *H. pylori*, ELISA tests are sensitive, specific, and cost effective for determining the organism's presence in untreated individuals. However, because antibodies are not rapidly cleared after treatment, antibody testing is not as well suited for determining eradication of infection as are other methods. Additionally, individuals who are immunocompromised (the elderly or immunosuppressed individuals) may have a false-negative result with antibody testing.

Rapid assays for the detection of *H. pylori* antibodies are also available. It is recommended that samples with positive rapid test results be tested by an ELISA method for confirmation.

Mycoplasma pneumoniae

Mycoplasma is a member of a unique group of organisms that belong to the class *Mollicutes*. Mycoplasmas represent the smallest known free-living life forms (150–250 nm) and have a small genome. Various members colonize plants, animals, and insects in addition to being human pathogens. These extracellular parasites attach to and exist on the surface of host cells using attachment organelles and adhesion molecules specific for their host cells. They absorb their nutrients from the host cells to which they are attached. The organisms lack cell walls (thus lacking peptidoglycan), have sterols in their cell membrane, and have complex growth requirements, making culture difficult and time consuming.

Mycoplasma pneumoniae Pathogenesis

The best-known *Mycoplasma* is *M. pneumoniae,* which is a leading cause of respiratory infections worldwide. *M. pneumoniae* infections are found in all age groups, with a majority of the infections involving the upper respiratory tract. *M. pneumoniae* is spread from one person to another by respiratory droplets. Relatively close association with an infected individual appears to be necessary for transmission of the organism. Unlike most respiratory infections, the incubation period is 1 to 3 weeks. The infection has an insidious onset, which differs from the acute onset observed with respiratory viruses such as influenza and adenovirus. Typically, there is development of a fever, along with headache, malaise, and a cough—the clinical hallmark of a *M. pneumoniae* infection. Depending on the age, approximately 5% to 10% of individuals progress to tracheobronchitis or pneumonia.

Originally, pneumonia caused by *M. pneumoniae* was referred to as "atypical pneumonia" because the infection could not be treated with penicillin. This is because the organism lacks the cell wall to which penicillin is directed against. In many cases, the pneumonia is mild, oftentimes appearing as a cold, and symptoms are generally mild enough that bedrest or hospitalization is not required. The infection has been referred to as "walking pneumonia" because individuals often do not stay home from work or school and still participate in their daily activities. Although many infections are mild, *M. pneumoniae* accounts for 20% of all hospitalizations for pneumonia in the United States. *M. pneumoniae* may remain in the respiratory tract for several months after resolution of the infection, causing chronic inflammation and a lingering cough. Based on nucleic acid detection of the organism, there is increasing evidence that *M. pneumoniae* may initiate or exacerbate asthma.

Dermatological Manifestations

Up to 7% of individuals with *M. pneumoniae* develop Stevens–Johnson syndrome, or erythema multiforme major, a condition in which the top layer of the skin dies and sheds. The syndrome is considered a medical emergency that usually requires hospitalization. The conjunctivae as well as the joints and various organs in the genitourinary and gastrointestinal tract may also be involved. The basis of Stevens–Johnson syndrome is not clearly known, but it may be caused by the immune response of the host or by augmented sensitivity to antibiotics while being treated for *M. pneumoniae*.

Another manifestation of *M. pneumoniae* infection is Raynaud syndrome, which is a transient vasospasm of the digits in which the fingers turn white when exposed to the cold. Although the exact cause is unclear, it may be related to the development and action of cold agglutinins in the body (see Chapter 14). Other extrapulmonary manifestations of Raynaud syndrome include arthritis, meningoencephalitis, pericarditis, and peripheral neuropathy.

Immunology of *Mycoplasma pneumoniae* Infection

In addition to stimulating the production of many proinflammatory and anti-inflammatory cytokines and chemokines, several classes of antibodies are produced in the course of a *M. pneumoniae* infection. As with any infection in which there is a humoral response, the body produces antibodies that neutralize the microorganism. *M. pneumoniae* also induces the production of autoantibodies, including agglutinins directed against the lungs, brain, cardiolipins, and smooth muscle.

The cold isoagglutinins observed with *M. pneumoniae* infection are among the most studied agglutinins by researchers. They are oligoclonal IgM antibodies directed against the altered I antigens found on the surface of human RBCs. These antibodies can agglutinate the RBCs at temperatures below 37°C. Development of the antibodies is thought to result from cross-reaction of antibodies formed against *M. pneumoniae* and the I antigen on human RBCs, or from alteration of the RBC antigen by the organism.

Laboratory Diagnosis of *Mycoplasma pneumoniae* Infection

Laboratory means of detecting *Mycoplasma* infection may involve culturing of the organism, detection of *M. pneumoniae*–specific antibodies in serum, and detection of *M. pneumoniae*–specific antigens or nucleotide sequences directly in patient specimens.

Detection of *Mycoplasma pneumoniae* by Culture

Although culturing has been considered the gold standard for diagnosis, culturing for the organism is rarely carried out in the clinical laboratory because of the fastidious nature of the organism. Collection and transport of the specimen differs from traditional methods used for culturing other microorganisms. The transport media may be trypticase soy broth with 0.5% albumin, SP4 medium, or a viral transport medium. If the sample cannot be plated immediately, it should be frozen at −70°C. Culturing requires the use of specialized media designed for the recovery of *Mycoplasma*. Growth of the organism takes several weeks in most cases. If the culture is successfully performed, the growth produces a "mulberry" colony with a typical "fried egg" appearance. Because of the difficulty in culturing for the organism and the time required for the organism to grow, culturing for the organism is rarely used except in research settings.

Detection of Antibodies to *Mycoplasma pneumoniae*

Detection of *M. pneumoniae*–specific IgM immunoglobulin is the most useful diagnostic test because it likely indicates a recent infection. Enzyme-linked immunoassays have been the most widely used methods for antibodies and can detect IgM or IgG directed against *M. pneumoniae*. Although IgM is the primary immunoglobulin response to infection, testing for the presence of IgG antibodies is necessary; the reason is that adults may only elicit an IgG response because of reinfection with the organism. ELISA methods have a specificity of more than 99% and a sensitivity of 98%.

Detection of Cold Agglutinins

For many years, before the development of antigen-specific serological tests, laboratory diagnosis of *M. pneumoniae* involved testing for cold agglutinins. The agglutinins are capable of clumping RBCs at 4°C. The reaction is reversible when the samples are warmed to 37°C. Cold agglutinins develop in about 50% of patients with *M. pneumoniae* infection. These antibodies are produced early in the disease (7–10 days) and can typically be detected at the time the patient seeks medical attention. The titer peaks at 2 to 3 weeks, and antibodies are present for 2 to 3 months after infection.

Although once considered the primary means of diagnosing *Mycoplasma* infection, the assay is not very specific (50% to 70%) nor is it very sensitive. Testing for cold agglutinins is no longer recommended because the development of cold agglutinins occurs in other circumstances, including some viral infections and collagen vascular diseases. However, a titer of 1:64 or greater, along with the clinical presentation of the patient, is suggestive of infection with *M. pneumoniae.* It should be noted that cold agglutinins may be found in patients with infections whose clinical presentations resemble *M. pneumoniae* infection, such as mononucleosis caused by Epstein-Barr virus (anti-i) and cytomegalovirus (anti-I).

Molecular Diagnosis of Mycoplasma Infections

Molecular methods will, in all likelihood, become the gold standard for the diagnosis of *Mycoplasma* infections. Before 2012, there were no FDA-approved assays available for the detection of *M. pneumoniae.* BioFire Diagnostics, Inc. (Salt Lake City, UT), now part of the BioMerieux corporation, received FDA approval in 2012 for its BioFire FilmArray Respiratory Panel. Using nested multiplex PCR, the assay is able to detect 20 respiratory viruses and bacteria, including *B. pertussis, C. pneumoniae,* and *M. pneumoniae.* The illumigene Mycoplasma Direct by Meridian Bioscience (Cincinnati, OH) detects *M. pneumonia* in throat swab specimens and became available in 2014. The illumigene uses Loop-Mediated Isothermal Amplification (LAMP) technology. As additional assays are developed and receive FDA approval, molecular testing will become more widespread and will likely replace serology as the primary means for the diagnosis of *M. pneumoniae* infections.

Rickettsial Infections

Members of the *Rickettsiaceae* family cause a variety of infections in man and animals. Because of advances in molecular technology, various members originally belonging to the genus ***Rickettsiae*** have been reclassified. These obligate intracellular, gram-negative bacteria now include the genera *Rickettsia* (rickettsiosis) and *Orientia* (*Orientia tsutsugamushi* causing scrub typhus). Additional members are the *Ehrlichia* group including *Ehrlichia* (ehrlichiosis), *Anaplasma* (anaplasmosis), *Neorickettsia* (associated with helminths), and *Neoehrlichia.*

Agents of *Rickettsia*-Related Disease

The genus *Rickettsia* is made up of two distinct groups: the spotted fever group (SFG) and the **typhus** group (TG). Each is responsible for a different set of diseases **(Table 20–1)**. In the United States, the main *Rickettsial* disease is **Rocky Mountain spotted fever (RMSF),** caused by *R. rickettsia* (SFG), with approximately 2,500 cases reported each year. Epidemic typhus, caused by *Rickettsia prowazekii* (TG), is the most prevalent member of the TG globally. Typhus fever (also known as *epidemic typhus*) occurs in conditions of poor hygiene and overcrowding, such as in prisons and refugee camps. Epidemic typhus was responsible for more than 3 million deaths

Table 20–1 Classification of Selected *Rickettsiae* Known to Cause Disease in Humans

ANTIGENIC GROUP	DISEASE	SPECIES	VECTOR	ANIMAL RESERVOIR(S)	GEOGRAPHIC DISTRIBUTION
Anaplasma	Human granulocytic anaplasmosis	*Anaplasma phagocytophilum*	Tick	Small mammals, rodents, and deer	Primarily United States, worldwide
Ehrlichia	Human monocytic ehrlichiosis	*Ehrlichia chaffeensis*	Tick	Deer, wild and domestic dogs, domestic ruminants, and rodents	Common in United States, probably worldwide
	Ehrlichiosis	*E. muris*	Tick	Deer and rodents	North America, Europe, Asia
	Ehrlichiosis	*E. ewingii*	Tick	Deer, wild and domestic dogs, and rodents	North America, Cameroon, Korea
Neoehrlichia	Human neoehrlichiosis	*Neoehrlichia mikurensis*	Tick	Rodents	Europe, Asia
Neorickettsia	Sennetsu fever	*Neorickettsia sennetsu*	Trematode	Fish	Japan, Malaysia, possibly other parts of Asia

Table 20–1 Classification of Selected *Rickettsiae* Known to Cause Disease in Humans—cont'd

ANTIGENIC GROUP	DISEASE	SPECIES	VECTOR	ANIMAL RESERVOIR(S)	GEOGRAPHIC DISTRIBUTION
Scrub typhus	Scrub typhus	*Orientia tsutsugamushi*	Larval mite (chigger)	Rodents	Asia-Pacific region from maritime Russia and China to Indonesia and North Australia to Afghanistan
Spotted fever	Rocky Mountain spotted fever	*Rickettsia rickettsii*	Tick	Rodents	North, Central, and South America
	Rickettsiosis	*Rickettsia aeschlimannii*	Tick	Unknown	South Africa, Morocco, Mediterranean shore
	Queensland tick typhus	*Rickettsia australis*	Tick	Rodents	Australia, Tasmania
	Boutonneuse fever or Mediterranean spotted fever	*Rickettsia conorii*	Tick	Dogs, rodents	Southern Europe, southern and western Asia, Africa, India
Typhus fever	Epidemic typhus, sylvatic typhus	*Rickettsia prowazekii*	Human body louse, flying squirrel ectoparasites, *Amblyomma* ticks	Humans, flying squirrels	Central Africa, Asia, Central America, North America, and South America
	Murine typhus	*Rickettsia typhi*	Flea	Rodents	Tropical and subtropical areas worldwide

Adapted from Centers for Disease Control and Prevention. *2018 Yellow Book: Traveler's Health.* Nicholson WL and Paddock CD. *Chapter 3. Rickettsial (Spotted & Typhus Fevers) & Related Infections, including Anaplasmosis & Ehrlichiosis.* Online version at https://wwwnc.cdc.gov/travel/yellowbook/2018/infectious-diseases-related-to-travel/rickettsial-spotted-and-typhus-fevers-and-related-infections-including-anaplasmosis-and-ehrlichiosis#5251. Accessed May 31, 2019.

in World War I. Once prevalent throughout the globe in the first half of the 20th century, only a few foci of epidemic typhus still exist in the world today (Ethiopia, Burundi, Rwanda, part of Mexico). Individuals traveling to areas with large homeless populations and regions that have recently experienced war or natural disasters leading to poor hygiene and crowded conditions (such as refugee camps) are at risk of acquiring typhus fever.

Each of the species responsible for the various *Rickettsial* diseases has a variety of animal reservoirs. The vectors responsible for the transmission are arthropods (ticks, mites, lice, or fleas) that transmit the organism through its bite after feeding on an infected animal **(Fig. 20–15)**. The one exception is typhus fever (epidemic louse-borne typhus), which is transmitted when an infected human body louse excretes *R. prowazekii* onto the skin while feeding and the individual becomes infected by rubbing louse fecal matter or crushed lice into the bite wound. Except for *R. prowazekii* (epidemic

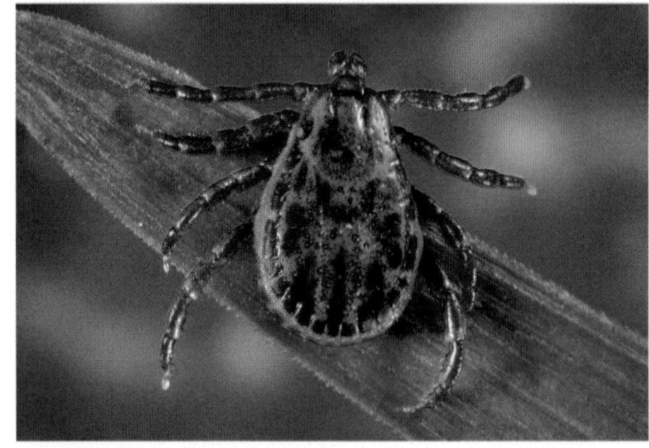

FIGURE 20–15 The Rocky Mountain wood tick, *Dermacentor andersoni*, is a known North American vector of *Rickettsia rickettsii*. *(Courtesy of the CDC/Dr. Christopher Paddock and James Gathany, Public Health Image Library.)*

typhus), humans are accidental hosts for *Rickettsia* and *Rickettsia*-related organisms. *Rickettsia* and *Rickettsia*-related organisms have worldwide distribution; however, certain members have a specific geographic distribution. For example, *Rickettsia japonica* is found only in Japan, whereas *R. rickettsii* is found in the Western hemisphere. Some species, such as *Rickettsia typhi,* are found everywhere in the world.

The members of the *Rickettsia* genus and *Anaplasma* and *Ehrlichia* cause several clinical diseases. Because of the prevalence of RMSF in North and South America, this chapter will focus on RMSF.

Rocky Mountain Spotted Fever

Epidemiology

RMSF is caused by *R. rickettsii.* The organism is transmitted to the human host by the bite of a tick. In the United States, the organism is transmitted by the American dog tick *(Dermacentor variabilis),* the Rocky Mountain wood tick *(Dermacentor andersoni),* and the brown dog tick *(Rhipicephalus sanguineus).* Although called *Rocky Mountain* spotted fever, five states—North Carolina, Oklahoma, Arkansas, Tennessee, and Missouri—account for more than 60% of RMSF cases in the continental United States. The occurrence of the disease has seasonal variation corresponding to tick activity, being most prevalent between May and September. The organism is transmitted transstadially in the tick (i.e., it remains present in the tick as the tick progresses from the nymph state to the adult) and is transmitted transovarially (from generation to generation through the eggs of the tick), allowing for maintenance of the organism in the tick population. Transmission occurs when the tick bites the host for a blood meal. When the tick has fed after 6 to 10 hours, the organism is injected into the host from the salivary glands.

Pathogenesis

Once introduced into the skin, the organisms spread via the lymphatic and circulatory system, where they attach to and invade their target cells, the vascular endothelium, by means of the OmpA and OmpB ligands. The organisms multiply by binary fission inside the endothelial cells, are released, and infect adjacent cells. This leads to hundreds of contiguous infected cells, producing the lesions and skin rash associated with the infection. The main pathophysiological event caused by the infection is endothelial cell damage, which leads to increased vascular permeability, resulting in edema, hypovolemia, hypotension, and hypoalbuminemia.

Clinical Manifestations

The symptoms observed with RMSF occur approximately 2 to 14 days (median 7 days) after a tick bite. Before the development of the hallmark rash, a large percentage of patients will experience a severe headache, nausea, vomiting, abdominal pain, diarrhea, and abdominal tenderness. The fever usually begins within the first 3 to 5 days after the onset of symptoms, and the rash usually appears 3 to 5 days after the onset of the fever. The rash typically starts on the hands and soles of the feet and proceeds to the trunk, although it may start on the trunk in some individuals **(Fig. 20–16).** With the classic form of RMSF, death occurs 7 to 15 days after the onset of symptoms if appropriate therapy is not provided. With the fulminant (i.e., severe and sudden onset) form of RMSF, death occurs within the first 5 days. The resolution or fatal outcome of the disease is largely related to the timeliness of initiating appropriate therapy. Immediate treatment with doxycycline reduces the severity of the infection.

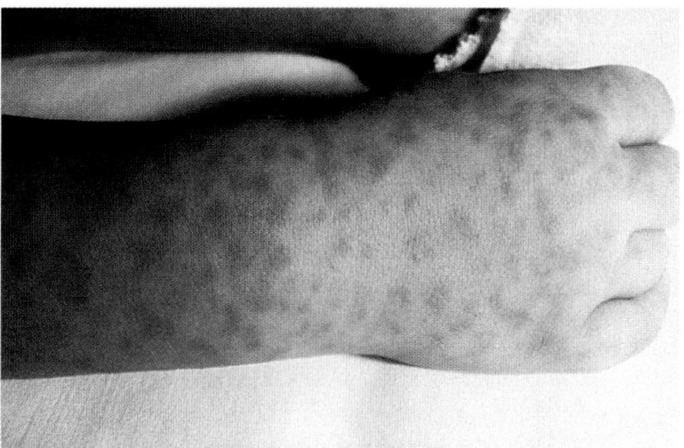

FIGURE 20–16 The characteristic spotted rash of Rocky Mountain spotted fever, the most severe and most frequently reported rickettsial illness in the United States. The disease is caused by *Rickettsia rickettsii.* *(Courtesy of the CDC, Public Health Image Library.)*

Diagnosis of RMSF

Initial diagnosis is often made clinically after ruling out a large variety of other conditions, including typhoid fever, measles, rubella, enteroviral infection, and respiratory tract infection. The overlapping symptoms, or clinical presentation, during the initial stages of the disease can make the diagnosis of RMSF extremely difficult. The diagnosis of fulminant RMSF is even more difficult because of its rapid course. The rash develops shortly before death, if at all; therefore, antibodies to *R. rickettsii* do not have time to develop.

Serological and Molecular Diagnosis

The organism infects the endothelial cells and does not circulate until the disease has severely progressed. Therefore, culturing for the organism and molecular methods are not always useful. If the patient has a rash, molecular diagnosis using DNA from the skin lesions is of value. Several assays using real-time PCR have been described in the literature, but at the time of this writing, there are no FDA-approved assays. Serology is the usual method for confirming the diagnosis of RMSF, but this is a retrospective diagnosis. Antibodies to *R. rickettsia* develop 7 to 10 days after the onset of symptoms, and a majority of patients do not have detectable antibodies during the first week of illness. For a successful outcome, therapy needs to be initiated before that time.

The gold standard for the serological diagnosis of RMSF is the indirect immunofluorescence assay (IFA) with *R. rickettsii* antigen, performed on two paired serum samples to demonstrate a significant (four-fold) rise in antibody titers. For many years, antibodies produced in patients with *Rickettsial* infections were detected by an agglutination test known as the *Weil-Felix test*, which was based on cross-reactivity of the patient's antibodies with polysaccharide antigens present on the OX-19 and OX-2 strains of *Proteus vulgaris* and the OX-K strain of *Proteus mirabilis*. This method lacks sensitivity and specificity and should not be relied on.

SUMMARY

- The indigenous microbiota varies at different sites of the body.
- The symbiotic relationship that exists between bacteria and humans is beneficial in protecting against infection, stimulating the immune system, aiding in digestion of food, and producing various vitamins.
- Humans exist in a commensalistic relationship with the bacteria that comprise the human microbiome. The encounter with some microbial organisms results in a parasitic relationship in which there is harm to the host that may result in an infection.
- *Pathogenicity* refers to the ability of an organism to cause disease, *virulence* refers to the extent that a pathogen causes damage to the host, and *infectivity* refers to the ability of an organism to spread from one host to another.
- To be virulent, an organism must possess structural features or produce extracellular substances that allow it to invade or cause damage to the host. These are referred to as *virulence factors*.
- Live bacteria may produce exotoxins that are generally specific to a particular bacterial organism and have specific modes of action on the host. Exotoxins are highly immunogenic, and antibodies formed against them are protective.
- Endotoxin, or lipid A, is part of the gram-negative bacterial cell wall that is released from dead bacteria. Endotoxin has a broad range of systemic effects on the body because it induces the release of cytokines that can lead to septic shock. Endotoxin, although immunogenic, does not result in the production of protective antibodies.
- Innate immune defenses (phagocytosis, production of antimicrobial defense peptides, various proteins) contribute heavily to the body's ability to overcome a bacterial infection.
- Humoral immunity plays a major role in defense against bacteria when the innate defenses are not sufficient in preventing infection. Antibodies attack bacteria by several mechanisms, including complement-mediated lysis, opsonization, and neutralization of bacterial toxins.
- Laboratory detection of the causative agent of a bacterial infection includes culturing of the organism, visualization of the bacteria in clinical specimens, detection of bacterial antigens in the clinical specimen, detection of the pathogen's DNA or RNA, proteomics, and demonstration of antibodies formed against the agent through serological tests.
- Highly sensitive, rapid lateral flow immunochromatographic assays (LFAs) are commonly used to detect bacterial, viral, fungal, and parasitic antigens. The principle behind LFAs involves movement of a liquid sample containing the analyte of interest along a strip that passes through various zones containing labeled antibodies specific to the analyte. If the antigen–antibody complex is present, it is captured by another antibody at the end of the strip, resulting in the development of a visible line.
- *Streptococcus pyogenes* (Group A streptococci or GAS) is the primary cause of bacterial pharyngitis. It is also a primary cause of a skin infection called *impetigo*. Untreated GAS infections may result in sequelae known as *acute glomerulonephritis* or *rheumatic heart disease*.
- The production of exotoxins contributes to the infections caused by GAS. Streptolysin O, hyaluronidase, deoxyribonuclease B (DNase B), and streptokinase all play a role in the infections associated with GAS.
- Scarlet fever occurs in a small percentage of individuals infected with GAS and is caused by the production of erythrogenic exotoxins that may also result in toxic shock syndrome.
- The laboratory diagnosis of GAS infection includes culture and antigen detection for acute infection, as well as anti-streptolysin O and anti-DNase B antibody detection for GAS sequelae.
- The streptozyme test measures antibodies against five extracellular streptococcal antigens—anti-streptolysin (ASO), anti-hyaluronidase (AHase), anti-streptokinase (ASKase), anti-nicotinamide-adenine dinucleotide (anti-NAD), and anti-DNAse B antibodies. The streptozyme test is positive in the majority of patients with acute poststreptococcal glomerulonephritis caused by GAS pharyngitis.
- *Helicobacter pylori* is the leading cause of gastric and duodenal ulcers and is associated with gastric carcinoma (stomach cancer). *H. pylori* produces a large amount of urease that protects the organism from the acidic environment in the stomach.
- Serological testing is a primary screening method of detecting *H. pylori* infection. Testing for urease is also used to detect and diagnose an infection with *H. pylori*. Detection of *H. pylori* antigen in stool samples can be used to monitor the effectiveness of treatment for *H. pylori* infections.
- *Mycoplasma pneumoniae* is a leading cause of community-acquired pneumonia. Infection with *M. pneumoniae* may not require bedrest or hospitalization and oftentimes is referred to as "walking pneumonia."
- Infection with *M. pneumoniae* may result in dermatological manifestations causing Stevens–Johnson syndrome. Raynaud syndrome, another manifestation that may be observed with *M. pneumoniae,* is a reversible variable vasospasm of the digits in which the fingers turn white when exposed to the cold.

- Production of cold agglutinins is observed in 50% of individuals with *M. pneumoniae*. Demonstration of cold agglutinins is neither specific nor sensitive when detecting infection by the organism. Detection of *M. pneumoniae*–specific IgM immunoglobulin is the most useful diagnostic assay because it likely indicates a recent infection.
- Rocky Mountain spotted fever (RMSF) is caused by *Rickettsia rickettsii* and is transmitted to the human host by the bite of a tick.
- The main pathophysiological event caused by RMSF is endothelial cell damage leading to increased vascular permeability, which then results in edema, hypovolemia, and hypotension. Various cytokines are released, and damage to the host may have a fatal outcome if therapy is not initiated in a timely fashion.
- The gold standard for the serological diagnosis of RMSF is the indirect immunofluorescence assay (IFA) with *R. rickettsii* antigen performed on two paired serum samples to demonstrate a significant (four-fold) rise in antibody titers.

Study Guide: Immune Defenses Against Bacterial Infection

INNATE DEFENSES	ADAPTIVE IMMUNE RESPONSES
Skin and mucosal surfaces	Antibodies produced against bacterial antigens promote opsonization and complement binding.
Antimicrobial defense peptides and proteins on epithelial surfaces (e.g., lysozyme, defensins)	Antibodies produced against bacterial exotoxins have neutralizing activity.
Other proteins (e.g., complement proteins, interleukins, prostaglandins, leukotrienes)	T-cell–mediated immune responses attack intracellular bacteria.
Acute-phase reactants (e.g., CRP, haptoglobin)	
Pattern recognition receptors (e.g., TLRs on macrophages and dendritic cells)	
Phagocytosis by neutrophils and macrophages	

Study Guide: Bacterial Virulence Factors

VIRULENCE FACTOR	DESCRIPTION	MECHANISM OF PATHOGENESIS	EXAMPLE(S)
Pili	Hair-like structures on the surface of bacteria	Adherence to and colonization of host tissue Resistance to phagocytosis Transfer of genetic material	Enterotoxigenic *E. coli* pili adhere to cells in small intestine.
Adhesion molecules	Molecules on surface of bacteria	Attach to a variety of host cell receptors, such as proteoglycans, collagen, fibrinogen	Fibronectin binding proteins of *S. pyogenes* facilitate attachment to host cells.
Capsule	A polysaccharide layer surrounding the cell wall of some bacteria	Blocks phagocytosis Blocks attachment of antibodies for opsonization Inhibits complement activation Acts as a decoy when released	Capsule of *S. pneumoniae* bacteria prevents phagocytosis by alveolar macrophages.
Endotoxin	Lipid A component of lipopolysaccharide on cell walls of gram-negative bacteria; released when bacteria die	Powerful stimulator of cytokine production	Gram-negative bacterial infection involving bacteremia can cause septic shock.
Exotoxins	Neurotoxins, cytotoxins, and enterotoxins released from live bacteria	Bind to specific receptors on host cells Some can act as superantigens that activate numerous T cells	Tetanus neurotoxin prevents transmitter release from neuromuscular cells, resulting in continuous muscle spasms. Exotoxins from *S. pyogenes* can cause toxic shock syndrome.

CASE STUDIES

1. A 6-year-old boy was brought to the pediatric clinic. His mother indicated he had been ill for several days with fever and general lethargy. The morning of the visit, the boy told his mother that his back hurt, and she had observed what appeared to be blood in his urine. History and physical examination indicated a well-nourished child with an unremarkable health history other than a severe sore throat with fever 3 weeks prior that was medicated with aspirin and throat lozenges. This child's temperature was 101.5°F, and the physician noted edema in the child's hands and feet. Blood and urine specimens were collected for a rapid GAS antigen test, streptozyme test, complete blood cell count, and urinalysis. Laboratory test results were as follows:

Complete Blood Count

RBC count: normal
Platelet count: normal
WBC count: 12.7×10^9/L (normal = 4.8 – 10.8×10^9/L)

Urinalysis

Color: red (normal = straw)
Clarity: cloudy (normal = clear)
Protein: 2+ (normal = negative/trace)
Blood: large (normal = none)

Rapid GAS Antigen Test

Negative

Streptozyme

Positive 1:600

Questions

a. What disorder is indicated by the child's history, physical examination, and laboratory test results?
b. What was the most likely causative agent of the sore throat preceding the current symptoms?
c. Discuss the most widely accepted theory explaining the physiological basis for this disease. Why didn't the physician order a throat culture?
d. What is the significance of the urinalysis results?
e. What is the significance of the streptozyme test results?

2. A 36-year-old female was seen by her physician because she had been experiencing flu-like symptoms along with a sore throat and chills for the past 3 days. She was also having difficulty breathing. The patient had a temperature of 100.2°F and was producing a moderate amount of sputum. Her physician decided that the probable diagnosis was some type of pneumonia and ordered the following laboratory tests to be performed: complete blood count, sputum culture, tests for influenza virus, and *M. pneumoniae* and cold agglutinin titers. The results were as follows:

Complete Blood Count

RBC: normal
WBC: 11.7×10^9/L (normal = 4.8 – 10.8×10^9/L) [somewhat elevated]

Sputum Culture

Negative

Mycoplasma Titers

IgM: none detected
IgG: 1:16

Cold Agglutinin Titer

Positive 1:128

Questions

a. What is the most probable cause of the pneumonia?
b. What is the significance of the *Mycoplasma* titer results?
c. Should additional *Mycoplasma* titers be ordered as a follow-up?
d. What is the significance of the cold agglutinin titer?

REVIEW QUESTIONS

1. All of the following are protective mechanisms against bacteria *except*
   a. production of antimicrobial defense peptides.
   b. phagocytosis.
   c. activation of complement.
   d. release of lipid A from the bacterial cell.

2. All of the following are characteristics of streptococcal M protein *except*
   a. It is the chief virulence factor of Group A streptococci.
   b. It provokes an immune response.
   c. Antibodies to one serotype protect against other serotypes.
   d. It limits phagocytosis of the organism.

3. An ASO titer and a streptozyme test are performed on a patient's serum. The ASO titer is negative, the streptozyme test is positive, and both the positive and negative controls react appropriately. What can you conclude from these test results?
   a. The ASO is falsely negative.
   b. The patient has an antibody to a streptococcal exoenzyme other than streptolysin O.
   c. The patient has not had a previous streptococcal infection.
   d. The patient has scarlet fever.

4. Which of the following applies to acute rheumatic fever?
   a. Symptoms begin after *S. pyogenes* infection of the throat or the skin.
   b. Antibodies to Group A streptococci are believed to cross-react with heart tissue.
   c. Diagnosis is usually made by culture of the organism.
   d. All patients suffer permanent disability.

5. Which of the following indicates the presence of anti-DNase B activity in serum?
   a. Reduction of methyl green from green to colorless
   b. Clot formation when acetic acid is added
   c. Inhibition of red blood cell hemolysis
   d. Lack of change in the color indicator

6. Which of the following is considered to be a nonsuppurative complication of streptococcal infection?
   a. Acute rheumatic fever
   b. Scarlet fever
   c. Impetigo
   d. Pharyngitis

7. All of the following are ways that bacteria can evade host defenses *except*
   a. presence of a capsule.
   b. stimulation of chemotaxis.
   c. production of toxins.
   d. lack of adhesion to phagocytic cells.

8. Antibody testing for Rocky Mountain spotted fever may not be helpful for which reason?
   a. It is not specific.
   b. It is too complicated to perform.
   c. It is difficult to obtain a blood specimen.
   d. Antibody production takes at least a week before detection.

9. Which of the following enzymes is used to detect the presence of *H. pylori* infections?
   a. DNase
   b. Hyaluronidase
   c. Urease
   d. Peptidase

10. Which of the following reasons make serological identification of a current infection with *Helicobacter pylori* difficult?
    a. No antibodies appear in the blood.
    b. Only IgM is produced.
    c. Antibodies remain after initial treatment.
    d. No ELISA tests have been developed.

11. *M. pneumoniae* infections are associated with the production of which antibodies?
    a. Cold agglutinins
    b. Antibodies to ATPase
    c. Antibodies to DNase
    d. Antibodies to *Proteus* bacteria

12. Which of the following *best* describes the principle of the IFA test for detection of antibodies produced in Rocky Mountain spotted fever?
    a. Patient serum is applied to a microtiter plate coated with a monoclonal antibody directed against the target antigen. A detection antibody labeled with biotin and directed against the target antigen is added. After addition of a substrate, a color reaction develops, indicating presence of the antigen.
    b. Specific antibodies in the serum sample attach to the antigens fixed to a microscope slide. In a second step, the attached antibodies are stained with fluorescein-labeled anti-human immunoglobulin and visualized with a fluorescence microscope.
    c. The serum sample is treated chemically to link the target antibodies to a fluorophore. The labeled sample is applied to a microscope slide to which the antigen has been attached. Following a wash step, the slide is examined for fluorescence.
    d. Patient serum is applied to a slide to which a specific antigen is bound. Following a wash step, a chromogenic dye is applied that binds to the Fc region of IgG and IgM antibodies. After a second wash step, the slide is examined for fluorescence.

13. Which of the following is true regarding exotoxins and endotoxins?
    a. Both endotoxins and exotoxins are highly immunogenic, allowing for the development of protective antibodies and vaccines.
    b. Endotoxins have targeted activity, whereas exotoxins have systemic effects when released.
    c. Endotoxins are released from the cell wall of dead bacteria, whereas exotoxins are released from live bacteria.
    d. Both endotoxins and exotoxins bind to specific receptors on a bacterial cell, leading to cell lysis.

14. Characteristics of a bacterial capsule include which of the following?
   a. It cannot be used for vaccine development.
   b. It is composed of peptidoglycan.
   c. It is an important mechanism for protecting a bacterium against ingestion by polymorphonuclear leukocytes PMNs.
   d. It is what causes bacteria to stain as gram-negative.

15. Which of the following statements regarding *Helicobacter pylori* is *not* true?
   a. It is associated with an increased risk of gastric carcinoma.
   b. It is the cause of most cases of acute food poisoning in the United States.
   c. It is a major cause of peptic ulcers in the United States.
   d. It is positive for urease.

21 Spirochete Diseases

Hamida Nusrat, PhD, PHM

LEARNING OUTCOMES

After finishing this chapter, you should be able to:

1. Describe identifying characteristics of *Treponema pallidum*, *Borrelia burgdorferi*, and *Leptospira* species.
2. Explain how syphilis, Lyme disease, and leptospirosis are transmitted.
3. Discuss the different stages of syphilis.
4. Discuss the advantages of direct fluorescent staining for *T. pallidum* over dark-field examination without staining.
5. Define *reagin*.
6. Distinguish treponemal tests from nontreponemal tests for syphilis.
7. Describe the principle of the following tests for syphilis: Venereal Disease Research Laboratory (VDRL), rapid plasma reagin (RPR), fluorescent treponemal antibody absorption (FTA-ABS), and *T. pallidum* particle agglutination (TP-PA).
8. Provide reasons for false-positive nontreponemal test results.
9. Compare and contrast typical results of treponemal and nontreponemal testing during the various stages of syphilis.
10. Discuss the advantages and limitations of polymerase chain reaction (PCR) and enzyme immunoassay (EIA) testing for syphilis.
11. Explain the traditional and reverse algorithms for syphilis and discuss their advantages and limitations.
12. Select appropriate laboratory methods for testing of cerebrospinal fluid (CSF) for neurosyphilis and testing for congenital syphilis.
13. Describe early and late clinical manifestations of Lyme disease.
14. Discuss the role of immunoglobulin M (IgM) and immunoglobulin G (IgG) antibody responses in the diagnosis of Lyme disease.
15. Discuss serological methods that play a key role in the laboratory evaluation of Lyme disease and describe recommended two-tier testing algorithms.
16. Discuss causes of false positives and false negatives in serological testing for Lyme disease.
17. Discuss the etiology, mode of transmission, clinical presentation, and laboratory diagnosis of leptospirosis.

CHAPTER OUTLINE

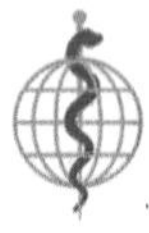

Go to FADavis.com for the laboratory exercises that accompany this text.

KEY TERMS

Borrelia burgdorferi
Chancre
Congenital syphilis
Flocculation
Fluorescent treponemal antibody absorption (FTA-ABS) test
Gummas
Immunoblotting
Leptospira
Leptospirosis
Lyme disease
Microscopic agglutination test (MAT)
Nontreponemal tests
Particle agglutination (PA) tests
Prozone
Rapid plasma reagin (RPR) test
Reagin
Spirochetes
Syphilis
T. pallidum particle agglutination (TP-PA) test
Treponema pallidum
Treponemal test
Venereal Disease Research Laboratory (VDRL) test
Weil's disease

Spirochetes are long, slender, helically coiled bacteria containing *axial filaments,* or periplasmic flagella, which wind around the bacterial cell wall and are enclosed by an outer sheath. These gram-negative, microaerophilic bacteria exhibit a characteristic corkscrew flexion or motility. Diseases caused by these organisms have many similarities, including a localized skin infection that disseminates to numerous organs as the disease progresses, a latent stage, and cardiac and neurological involvement if the disease remains untreated. This chapter discusses clinical manifestations and laboratory testing for the two major spirochete diseases, syphilis and Lyme disease, and provides an introduction to leptospirosis. Serological testing plays a key role in diagnosis of these diseases because isolation of the organisms themselves is difficult to accomplish in the laboratory and clinical symptoms are not always apparent.

Syphilis

Syphilis is a commonly acquired spirochete disease in the United States. It is typically spread through sexual transmission. Although the incidence of syphilis in the United States reached an all-time low in 2000, it slowly increased through 2017. According to the Centers for Disease Control and Prevention (CDC) surveillance report for sexually transmitted diseases, more than 30,600 cases of syphilis were reported in the United States in 2017, representing a 76% rise since 2013. Homosexual transmission between men was responsible for much of this increase. Despite the current emphasis on safe sexual practices, syphilis remains a major health problem in many areas of the world; more than 5 million new cases are reported worldwide each year. Early detection of syphilis is of major importance because treatment with antibiotics in the early stages of the disease can usually provide a cure. This section discusses characteristics of the organism that causes syphilis, its clinical manifestations, and laboratory methods essential to its diagnosis.

Characteristics of *Treponema pallidum*

The causative agent of syphilis is ***Treponema pallidum,*** subspecies *pallidum,* a member of the family *Spirochaetaceae.* Organisms in this family have no natural reservoir in the environment and must multiply within a living host. Three other pathogens in this group are so morphologically and antigenically similar to *T. pallidum* that all but one are classified as subspecies. These other organisms are *T. pallidum* subspecies *pertenue,* the agent of yaws; *T. pallidum* subspecies *endemicum,* the cause of nonvenereal endemic syphilis; and *Treponema carateum,* the agent of pinta. Yaws is found in the tropics, pinta is found in Central and South America, and endemic syphilis is found in desert regions.

T. pallidum (which will hereafter be used to refer to the subspecies *pallidum*) varies in length from 6 to 20 μm and in width from 0.1 to 0.2 μm, with 6 to 14 coils **(Fig. 21–1)**. The outer membrane of *T. pallidum* is a phospholipid bilayer with very few exposed proteins. Several identified membrane proteins, called *treponemal rare outer membrane proteins (TROMPs),* have been characterized. It appears that the scarcity of such proteins delays the host immune response.

Mode of Transmission

Pathogenic treponemes are rapidly destroyed by heat, cold, and drying, so they are almost always spread by direct contact. Sexual transmission is the primary mode of dissemination; this occurs through contact of abraded skin or mucous membranes with an open lesion. Approximately 30% to 50% of the

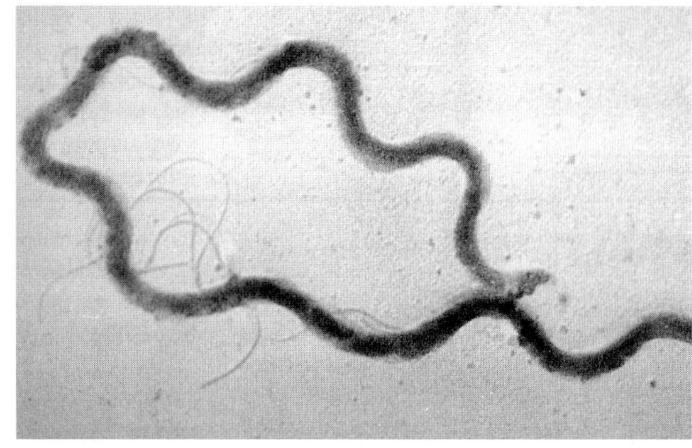

FIGURE 21–1 *Treponema pallidum.* Electron micrograph showing the coils and periplasmic flagella. (*Courtesy of CDC.*)

individuals who are exposed to a sexual partner with active lesions will acquire the disease. Congenital infections (transplacental) can also occur during pregnancy. In utero syphilis infection is generally severe and mutilating, affecting almost every tissue of the fetus. Infants born to mothers infected with early-stage syphilis tend to have symptoms resembling secondary syphilis in adults, characterized by cutaneous lesions, snuffles, hepatosplenomegaly, and central nervous system (CNS) involvement. The symptoms of early-onset syphilis generally manifest at younger than 2 years of age. Late-stage congenital syphilis occurs in infants older than 2 years when they are conceived by mothers having chronic and untreated infection. This type of manifestation corresponds to tertiary syphilis in adults, and symptoms include interstitial keratitis, bone and tooth deformities (Hutchinson's teeth), eighth-nerve deafness, and perforation of the hard palate. There may be a variety of manifestations in congenital syphilis, ranging from stillbirth and neonatal death to long-term physical and physiological deformities in the surviving infants.

Other potential means of transmission include parenteral exposure through contaminated needles or blood, but this is extremely rare. For the past 30 years, the lack of transfusion-transmitted syphilis in the United States has actually called into question the necessity of testing potential donors for the presence of the disease. However, current guidelines by the American Red Cross require that people wait 12 months after treatment for syphilis before donating blood. Because syphilis can only be transmitted by means of fresh blood products, the use of stored blood components has virtually eliminated the possibility of transfusion-associated syphilis.

Stages of the Disease

Untreated syphilis can progress through four stages: primary, secondary, latent, and tertiary.

Primary Stage

Once contact has been made with a susceptible skin site, endothelial cell thickening occurs with aggregation of lymphocytes, plasma cells, and macrophages. The initial lesion, called a **chancre,** develops between 10 and 90 days after infection, with an average of 21 days. A chancre is a painless, solitary lesion characterized by raised and well-defined borders **(Fig. 21–2).** In men, these usually occur on the outside of the penis, but in women they may appear in the vagina or on the cervix and, thus, may go undetected. This *primary stage* lasts from 1 to 6 weeks, during which time the lesion heals spontaneously.

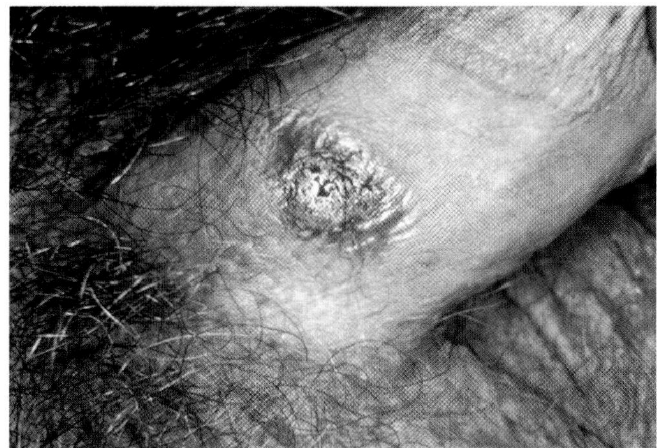

FIGURE 21–2 Primary chancre in the early stage of syphilis. *(Courtesy of the CDC/Dr. N. J. Fiumara, Public Health Image Library.)*

Secondary Stage

About 25% of patients who are untreated in the primary stage progress to the *secondary stage,* in which systemic dissemination of the organism occurs. This stage is usually observed about 1 to 2 months after the primary chancre disappears; however, in some cases, the primary lesion may still be present. Symptoms of the secondary stage include generalized lymphadenopathy, or enlargement of the lymph nodes; malaise; fever; pharyngitis; and a rash on the skin and mucous membranes. The rash may appear on the palms of the hands and the soles of the feet. Neurological signs, such as visual disturbances, hearing loss, tinnitus, and facial weakness, appear in nearly half of patients with secondary syphilis, indicating involvement of the CNS. Lesions persist from a few days up to 8 weeks, and spontaneous healing occurs, as in the primary stage.

> **Clinical Correlations**
>
> **The Great Imitator**
>
> Patients with syphilis can be difficult to diagnose because their clinical presentations can vary widely. Because the symptoms of syphilis can mimic those of many other diseases or conditions, the disease has often been referred to as "The Great Imitator."

Latent Stage

The *latent stage* follows the disappearance of secondary syphilis. This stage is characterized by a lack of clinical symptoms. It is arbitrarily divided into early latent (fewer than 1 year's duration) and late latent, in which the primary infection has occurred more than 1 year previously. Patients are not infectious at this time, with the exception of pregnant women, who can pass the disease on to the fetus even if they exhibit no symptoms.

Tertiary Stage

About one-third of the individuals who remain untreated develop *tertiary syphilis.* This stage occurs most often between 10 and 30 years following the secondary stage. Tertiary syphilis has three major manifestations: gummatous syphilis, cardiovascular disease, and neurosyphilis.

Gummas are localized areas of granulomatous inflammation that are most often found on bones, skin, or subcutaneous tissue. Such lesions contain lymphocytes, epithelioid cells, and fibroblasts. They may heal spontaneously with scarring, or they may remain destructive areas of chronic inflammation. It is likely that they represent the host response to infection.

Cardiovascular complications usually involve the ascending aorta, and symptoms are caused by destruction of elastic tissue in the aortic arch. The destruction may result in aortic aneurysm, thickening of the valve leaflets causing aortic regurgitation, or narrowing of the ostia, producing angina pectoris.

Neurosyphilis is the complication most often associated with the tertiary stage, but it actually can occur any time after the primary stage and can span all stages of the disease. Immunodeficient individuals such as HIV patients are susceptible to early neurosyphilis. During the first 2 years following infection, CNS involvement often takes the form of acute meningitis. Late manifestations of neurosyphilis include degeneration of the lower spinal cord with partial paralysis and chronic progressive dementia. It usually takes more than 10 years for these to occur; both are the result of structural CNS damage that cannot be reversed. Fortunately, symptoms of tertiary syphilis are now very rare because of early detection and effective treatment with antibiotics such as penicillin.

Connections

Gummas

A gumma is a form of granuloma characteristic of tertiary syphilis. As discussed in Chapter 14, granulomas are organized clusters of white blood cells (WBCs) and epithelial cells that are formed because of a type IV hypersensitivity reaction. This cell-mediated mechanism develops in response to chronic persistence of the antigen. Granulomas can form in patients with various infectious diseases, including leprosy, tuberculosis, cutaneous leishmaniasis, yaws, and syphilis.

Congenital Syphilis

Congenital syphilis occurs when a woman who has early syphilis or early latent syphilis transmits treponemes to the fetus. The occurrence of congenital syphilis rose from 362 cases in the year 2013 to 918 cases in 2017. Although the disease can be transmitted at any stage of pregnancy, typically the fetus is most affected during the second or third trimester. Fetal or perinatal death occurs in approximately 10% of the cases.

Infants who are born live often have no clinical signs of disease during the first few weeks of life. Some may remain asymptomatic, but the majority of these infants develop later symptoms if not treated at birth. Such infants may exhibit clear or hemorrhagic rhinitis (runny nose). Skin eruptions, in the form of a maculopapular rash that is especially prominent around the mouth, the palms of the hands, and the soles of the feet, are also common. Other symptoms include generalized lymphadenopathy, hepatosplenomegaly, jaundice, anemia, painful limbs, and bone abnormalities. Neurosyphilis may occur in up to 60% of infants with congenital disease.

Nature of the Immune Response

The primary body defenses against treponemal invasion are intact skin and mucous membranes. Once the skin is penetrated, T cells and macrophages play a key role in the immune response. Primary lesions show the presence of both CD4+ and CD8+ T cells. Cytokines produced by these cells activate macrophages, and it is ultimately macrophage phagocytosis that heals the primary chancre. The protective role of antibodies is uncertain, however, as coating the treponemes with antibodies does not necessarily bring about their destruction. *T. pallidum* is also capable of coating itself with host proteins, which delays the immune system's recognition of the pathogen. The rare treponemal proteins, or TROMPs, are important in triggering the activation of complement, which ultimately kills the organism. However, the chronic nature of the disease is an indicator that the organisms are able to evade the immune response. Treponemes may persist in the host for years if antibiotic therapy is not obtained.

Laboratory Diagnosis

Traditional laboratory tests for syphilis can be classified into three main types: direct detection of spirochetes, nontreponemal serological tests, and treponemal serological tests. These vary in their ability to detect syphilis at different stages of the disease. Principles and procedures of each type of testing are discussed in the text that follows. Special considerations in laboratory testing for neurosyphilis and congenital syphilis are also introduced.

Direct Detection

Direct detection of spirochetes can be accomplished by dark-field microscopy or fluorescent antibody testing. The performance of either test requires that the patient have active lesions.

Dark-Field Microscopy

Primary and secondary syphilis can be diagnosed by demonstrating the presence of *T. pallidum* in exudates from skin lesions. In dark-field microscopy, a dark-field condenser is used to keep all incidental light out of the field except for that captured by the organisms themselves. It is essential to have a good specimen in the form of serous fluid from a lesion. The serous fluid is usually obtained by cleaning the lesion with sterile saline and rubbing it with clean gauze. Pathogenic treponemes are identified on the basis of their characteristic corkscrew morphology and flexing motility.

Because observation of motility is the key to identification, specimens must be examined as quickly as possible before they dry out. False-negative results can occur when there is a delay in evaluating the slides, an insufficient specimen is obtained, or the patient is pretreated with antibiotics. Thus, a negative test does not exclude a diagnosis of syphilis. In addition, an experienced microscopist should perform testing. If a specimen is obtained from the mouth or the rectal area, morphologically identical nonpathogenic microbes can be found that must be differentiated from the true pathogens.

Fluorescent Antibody Testing

The use of a fluorescent-labeled antibody is a sensitive and highly specific alternative to dark-field microscopy. Testing can be performed by either a direct method, which uses a fluorescent-labeled antibody conjugate to *T. pallidum,* or an indirect method using antibody specific for *T. pallidum* and a second labeled anti-immunoglobulin antibody. An advantage of these methods is that live specimens are not required. A specimen can be brought to the laboratory in a capillary tube, and fixed slides can be prepared for later viewing. Treponemes can be washed off the slide even after fixing; therefore, each slide must be handled individually, and rinsing must be carefully performed. The use of monoclonal antibodies has made fluorescent antibody testing very sensitive and specific. However, monoclonal antibodies can still cross-react with other subspecies of *T. pallidum,* and this must be taken into account when making a diagnosis.

Serological Tests

If a patient does not have active lesions, as may be the case in secondary or tertiary syphilis, then serological testing for antibodies is the key to diagnosis. Serological tests can be classified as nontreponemal or treponemal, depending on the reactivity of the antibody that is detected. Nontreponemal tests have traditionally been used to screen for syphilis because of their high sensitivity and ease of performance. However, false-positive results are common because of the nonspecific nature of the antigen. Therefore, any positive results must be confirmed by a more specific **treponemal test,** which detects antibodies to *T. pallidum.*

Connections

Complement Fixation

The first nontreponemal serological test for syphilis was developed in 1906 by the bacteriologist August Paul von Wassermann. This test used a crude liver extract from a fetus that was infected with syphilis as the source of the lipid antigen. The Wasserman test was based on the principle of complement fixation. Patient serum was incubated with cardiolipin antigen in the presence of rabbit serum as the source of complement; this was followed by a detection system consisting of antibody-coated sheep red blood cells (RBCs). If the patient serum contained cardiolipin antibody, complexes were formed that bound the reagent complement, and the indicator RBCs were not lysed. In contrast, if cardiolipin antibody was not present in the patient serum, the reagent complement was free to react with the antibody-sensitized sheep RBCs to cause hemolysis.

Nontreponemal Tests

Nontreponemal tests determine the presence of an antibody that forms against cardiolipin, a lipid material released from damaged host cells. This antibody has sometimes been referred to as **reagin.** It is found in the sera of patients with syphilis and several other disease states. An antigen complex consisting of cardiolipin, lecithin, and cholesterol is used in the reaction to detect the nontreponemal reagin antibodies, which are either of the immunoglobulin G (IgG) or immunoglobulin M (IgM) class.

Connections

Reagin

The term *reagin* as it applies to syphilis should not be confused with the same word that was originally used to describe immunoglobulin E (IgE). They are not the same. Fortunately, the term *reagin* in reference to IgE is rarely used today.

The most widely used nontreponemal tests are the **Venereal Disease Research Laboratory (VDRL) test** and the **rapid plasma reagin (RPR) test.** These tests are based on flocculation reactions in which patient antibody complexes with the cardiolipin antigen. **Flocculation** is a specific type of precipitation that occurs over a narrow range of antigen concentrations. The antigen consists of very fine particles that clump together in a positive reaction.

Typical serological results for nontreponemal tests during the course of untreated and treated syphilis are shown in **Figure 21–3.** In general, nontreponemal tests become positive within 1 to 4 weeks after the appearance of the primary chancre. Titers usually peak during the secondary or early latent stages. In primary disease, up to about 40% of individuals appear nonreactive; however, by the secondary stage, almost all patients have reactive test results. However, testing of sera from patients in the secondary stage is subject to false negatives because of the **prozone** phenomenon (antibody excess). In this case, a nonreactive pattern that is typically granular or rough in appearance is seen. If a prozone is suspected, serial two-fold dilutions of the patient's serum should be made to obtain a titer.

Cardiolipin antibody titers tend to decline in the later stages of the disease, even if the patient remains untreated. After several years, about 25% of untreated syphilis cases become nonreactive for reagin. This decline occurs more rapidly in individuals who have received treatment. A first-time infection, if in the primary or secondary stage, should show a four-fold decrease in titer by the third month following treatment and an eight-fold decrease by 6 to 8 months. Following successful treatment, tests typically become completely nonreactive within 1 to 2 years.

VDRL Test

The VDRL test, which was designed by the Venereal Disease Research Laboratories, is both a qualitative and quantitative slide flocculation test for serum that includes a modification for use on spinal fluid. Antigen for all tests must be prepared fresh daily and in a highly regulated fashion. The antigen is an alcoholic solution of 0.03% cardiolipin, 0.9% cholesterol, and 0.21% lecithin. The antigen suspension is prepared by adding the VDRL antigen with a dropper to a buffered saline solution while continuously rotating the mixture on a flat surface; attention must be paid to required rotation speed and timing. A daily calibrated Hamilton syringe is used to deliver one drop of antigen for the slide test. If the delivery is off by more than 2 drops out of 60, the syringe must be cleaned with alcohol and recalibrated.

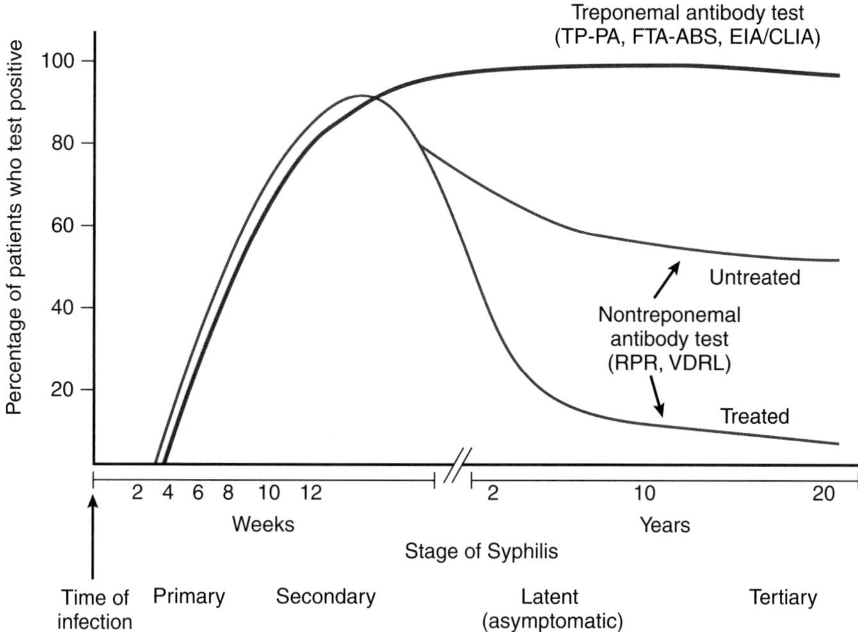

FIGURE 21–3 Typical nontreponemal and treponemal antibody patterns in syphilis. *(Adapted from Peeling RW, Ye H. Diagnostic tools for preventing and managing maternal and congenital syphilis: an overview.* Bull World Health Organ *2004;82(6):439–446.)*

The serum specimens to be tested are heated at 56°C for 30 minutes to inactivate complement, after which 0.05 mL is pipetted into a ceramic ring of a glass slide. Three control sera—nonreactive, minimally reactive, and reactive—are pipetted into separate rings on the glass slide in the same manner. Control sera and patient samples are spread out to fill the entire ring. One drop (1/60 mL) of the VDRL antigen is then added to each ring. The slide is rotated for 4 minutes on a rotator at 180 rpm. It is read microscopically to determine the presence of flocculation, or small clumps. The results are recorded as reactive (medium to large clumps), weakly reactive (small clumps), or nonreactive (no clumps or slight roughness). Tests must be performed at room temperature within the range of 23°C to 29°C (73°F to 85°F) because results may be affected by temperature changes. All sera with reactive or weakly reactive results must be tested using the quantitative slide test, in which two-fold dilutions of serum ranging from 1:2 to 1:32 are initially used. Sera yielding positive results at the 1:32 dilution are titered further.

RPR Test

The RPR test is a modified VDRL test involving macroscopic agglutination. The cardiolipin-containing antigen suspension is bound to charcoal particles, making the test easier to read. The suspension is contained in small glass vials, which are stable for up to 3 months after opening. The antigen is similar to the VDRL antigen, with the addition of ethylenediaminetetraacetic acid (EDTA), thimerosal, and choline chloride, which stabilize the antigen and inactivate complement so that serum does not have to be heat-inactivated before use. Patient serum (approximately 0.05 mL) is placed in an 18-mm circle on a plastic-coated disposable card using a micropipette or Dispenstir device. Cardiolipin antigen is dispensed from a small plastic dispensing bottle with a calibrated 20-gauge needle. One free-falling drop of antigen is placed onto each test area, and the card is mechanically rotated at 100 rpm for

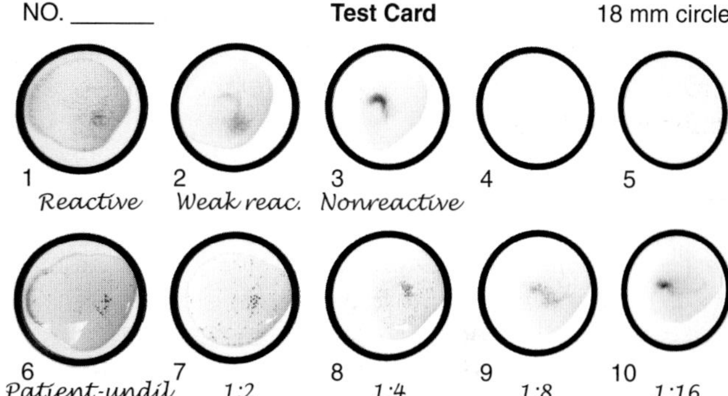

FIGURE 21–4 RPR test results. Well 1: reactive control, showing large clumps. Well 2: weakly reactive control, showing small clumps. Well 3: nonreactive control, showing slight roughness and a "tail" upon swirling. Wells 6 to 10 show results of a serially diluted sample of patient serum with a titer of 8. *(Courtesy of Linda Miller.)*

8 minutes under humid conditions. Cards are read under a high-intensity light source; if flocculation is evident, the test is positive **(Fig. 21–4).** All reactive tests should be confirmed by retesting using doubling dilutions in a quantitative procedure. The RPR test appears to be more sensitive than the VDRL in primary syphilis.

Treponemal Tests

Treponemal tests detect antibody directed against the *T. pallidum* organism or against specific treponemal antigens. Typical treponemal antibody results during various stages of syphilis are shown in Figure 21–3. Treponemal tests usually become positive before nontreponemal tests, although patients with early primary syphilis may be nonreactive. In secondary and latent syphilis, tests are usually 100% reactive. Once a patient is reactive, that individual remains reactive for life. Although there are fewer false positives compared with reagin tests, reactivity is seen with other treponemal diseases, notably yaws and pinta.

Connections

Antibody Response

Recall from Chapter 5 that IgG antibody produced in the secondary immune response is of high titer and persists for a long period of time. This is the reason that treponemal tests, which mainly detect IgG, remain positive for life after they have become reactive.

Two main types of manual treponemal tests are the indirect **fluorescent treponemal antibody absorption (FTA-ABS) test** and agglutination tests. Because these tests are highly specific for syphilis, they have been used to confirm positive nontreponemal test results. More recently, automated immunoassays for treponemal antibodies have been developed. Their applications will be discussed later.

FTA-ABS test

The FTA-ABS test is one of the earliest confirmatory tests developed. In this test, a dilution of heat-inactivated patient serum is incubated with a *sorbent* consisting of an extract of nonpathogenic treponemes *(Reiter strain)*, which removes antibodies that cross-react with treponemes other than *T. pallidum*. Diluted patient samples and controls are applied to individual wells on a test slide fixed with the *Nichols strain* of *T. pallidum*. Following a 30-minute incubation at 37°C, the slides are washed, and air-dried and antibody conjugate (anti-human immunoglobulin conjugated with fluorescein) is added to each well. Slides are re-incubated as before and washed to remove excess conjugate. Mounting medium is applied, and coverslips are placed on the slides, which are then examined under a fluorescence microscope.

If specific patient antibody is present, it will bind to the *T. pallidum* antigens. The antibody conjugate will, in turn, only bind where patient immunoglobulin is present and bound to the spirochetes. When slides are read under a fluorescence microscope, the intensity of the green color is reported on a scale of 0 to 4+. No fluorescence indicates a negative test, whereas a result of 2+ or above is considered reactive. A result of 1+ means that the specimen was minimally reactive, and the test must be repeated with a second specimen drawn in 1 to 2 weeks. Experienced personnel are needed to read and interpret fluorescent test results. False-positive results may occur in patients with systemic lupus erythematosus (SLE) or other autoimmune diseases and can appear as an atypical, beaded pattern of fluorescence. The FTA-ABS is highly sensitive and specific, but it is time consuming to perform and has been replaced in many laboratories with particle agglutination methods.

TP-PA (MHA-TP)

The **particle agglutination (PA) tests** originally used sheep RBCs coated with *T. pallidum* antigen and were referred to as *MHA-TP* (microhemagglutination assay for *T. pallidum* antibody). Current PA tests for *T. pallidum*, such as the Serodia ***T. pallidum* particle agglutination (TP-PA) test,** use colored gelatin particles coated with treponemal antigens and are more sensitive in detecting primary syphilis. In the Serodia

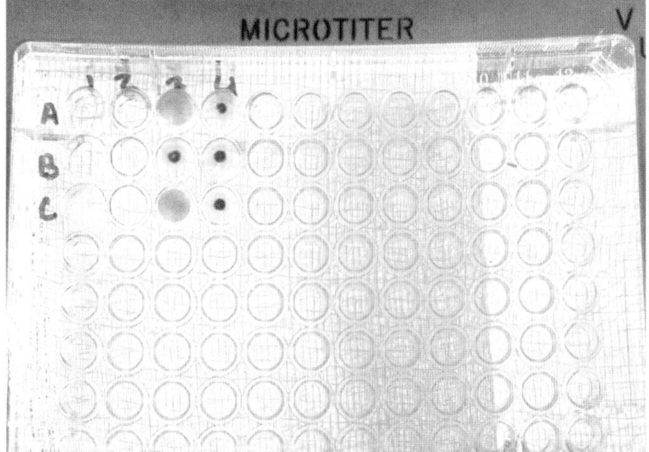

FIGURE 21–5 TP-PA test results. Row A: positive control. Row B: negative control. Row C: serum from a positive patient. *T. pallidum*–sensitized gel particles were placed in column 3 of each row, and unsensitized gel particles were pipetted into column 4 of each row. Positive wells (A3 and C3) are indicated by a diffuse mat of particles that spread over the surface of the well, whereas negative results are indicated by a compact button. *(Courtesy of Linda Miller.)*

TP-PA test, patient serum or plasma is diluted in microtiter plates and incubated with either *T. pallidum*–sensitized gel particles or unsensitized gel particles as a control. The presence of *T. pallidum* antibodies is indicated by agglutination of the sensitized gel particles, which bind to the antibodies to form a lattice-like structure that spreads to produce a smooth mat covering the surface of the well. If a sample is negative for the antibody, the gel particles settle to the bottom of the well and form a compact button **(Fig. 21–5)**.

Automated Immunoassays for *T. Pallidum* Antibodies

A variety of automated immunoassays have been developed for the detection of antibodies to *T. pallidum*. These include enzyme immunoassays (EIAs), chemiluminescent immunoassays (CLIAs), and multiplex flow immunoassays (MFIs). EIAs have been manufactured in a variety of formats, including one- or two-step sandwich assays, one-step competitive assays, and immune capture assays. In the sandwich assays, antibodies in the patient sample bind to recombinant *T. pallidum* antigens coated onto microtiter plate wells. An enzyme-labeled antibody or antigen conjugate and substrate are added to detect binding. In the immune capture format, microtiter wells are coated with antibody to IgM or IgG and are reacted with patient serum. Antigens that are labeled with an enzyme are then added **(Fig. 21–6)**. The capture EIA tests are especially useful in diagnosing congenital syphilis in infants because they look for the presence of IgM, which cannot cross the placenta. They can also be used to monitor response to therapy in the early stages of syphilis because many patients are negative for IgM treponemal antibodies 6 to 12 months after treatment. In competitive EIAs, treponemal antibody in the patient sample competes with an enzyme-labeled treponemal antibody conjugate for *T. pallidum* antigens bound to microtiter plate wells. Test sensitivities of the various EIAs range from about 95% to 99%, and test specificities are 100%.

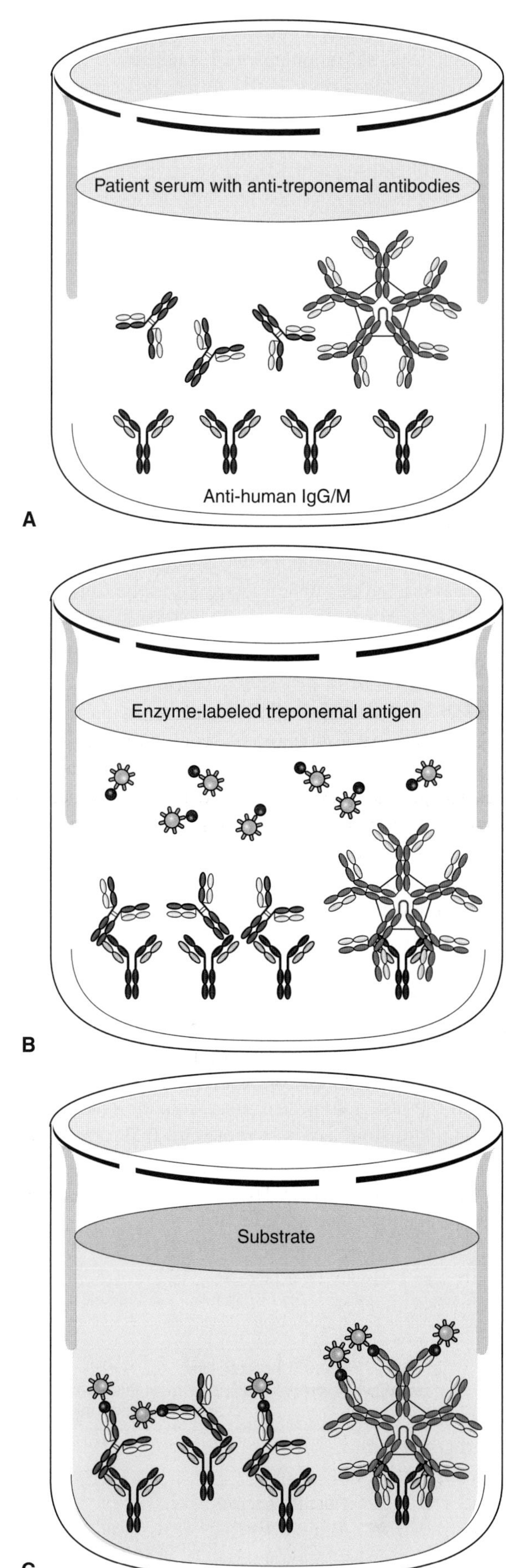

FIGURE 21–6 Antibody capture enzyme-linked immunosorbent assay (ELISA) test. Only specific anti-treponemal antibody will react with enzyme-labeled antigen.

CLIAs are available as a one-step sandwich technique in which the patient sample is incubated with paramagnetic microparticles that have been coated with *T. pallidum* antigens linked to a chemiluminescent derivative. After a wash step to remove unbound material, a catalyst is added and a chemical reaction occurs, producing emissions of light if the test sample is positive. The number of relative light units (RLUs) is proportional to the amount of treponemal antibody in the sample. CLIAs have many advantages as compared with EIAs, including a higher sensitivity in the early stages of syphilis, faster performance, and more stable reagents.

MFIs involve incubation of the patient sample with microspheres coated with recombinant *T. pallidum* antigens. Microspheres that have bound immune complexes are detected after addition of a phycoerythrin-labeled reporter antibody and are analyzed by flow cytometry. This method can simultaneously detect antibodies to multiple *T. pallidum* antigens in a small volume of sample and has a rapid turnaround time. Treponemal MFI, EIA, and CLIA yield comparable results to the FTA-ABS but have the advantage of automation.

Molecular Testing by Polymerase Chain Reaction (PCR)

PCR technology, which involves isolating and amplifying a specific sequence of DNA, has been used to test for the presence of treponemes in whole blood, spinal fluid, amniotic fluid, various tissues, and swab samples from syphilis lesions. Although there are many variations of this procedure, basically DNA is extracted from the sample and then replicated using a DNA polymerase enzyme and a primer pair to start the reaction (see Chapter 12). One variation is (real-time) quantitative PCR (qPCR), which is automated, faster, and more sensitive than traditional PCR.

PCR is an extremely sensitive technique capable of detecting as little as one treponeme in some clinical samples. Sensitivity is highest in patients with primary syphilis but is greatly reduced in detecting disease in secondary syphilis. The clinical availability of PCR is currently limited; however, in the future, PCR could be a useful tool for diagnosis when serological testing is inconclusive and may provide a viable alternative to dark-field microscopy in directly detecting the organism in ulcers from patients with primary disease. PCR may also be helpful in detecting treponemes in the blood of neonates with symptoms of congenital syphilis and in the cerebrospinal fluid (CSF) of patients suspected of having neurosyphilis. Better standardization of PCR may help the method to gain more widespread use in testing for syphilis in the future.

Clinical Applications

Nontreponemal tests are sensitive, inexpensive, and simple to perform. Thus, they have been very useful as a screening tool for syphilis. In addition, because antibody titers can be determined by testing serial dilutions of the patient sample, these methods have also been useful in monitoring the progress of the disease and in determining the outcome of treatment. As noted previously, nontreponemal titers will decrease if treatment is effective. Their main disadvantage is that they are subject to false positives. Transient false positives occur in diseases such as hepatitis, infectious mononucleosis, varicella, herpes, measles, malaria, and tuberculosis, as well as during pregnancy. Chronic conditions causing sustained false-positive results include SLE, leprosy, intravenous drug use, autoimmune arthritis, advanced age, and advanced malignancy.

A reactive nontreponemal test should be confirmed by a more specific treponemal test. In pregnancy, this is especially important because nontreponemal titers from a previous syphilis infection may increase nonspecifically. Titers can be considered to be nonspecifically increased if lesions are absent, the increase in titer is less than four-fold, and documentation of previous treatment is available.

Although treponemal tests are usually reactive before nontreponemal tests in primary syphilis, they suffer from a lack of sensitivity in congenital syphilis and neurosyphilis. Nontreponemal tests should be used for these purposes. Treponemal tests have been traditionally used as confirmatory tests to distinguish false-positive from true-positive nontreponemal results. They also help establish a diagnosis in late latent syphilis or late syphilis because they are more sensitive than nontreponemal tests in these stages.

Testing Algorithms

The traditional testing algorithm for syphilis involves screening the sample with a nontreponemal test and confirming any positive results with a more specific treponemal test **(Fig. 21–7)**. This testing strategy was used in most clinical laboratories for many years.

Because of the development of sensitive, automated methods for treponemal antibodies that can be easily performed in the clinical laboratory, a change in the testing strategy for syphilis has become increasingly popular, especially among large reference laboratories. Under this "reverse sequence algorithm," the testing order is reversed from the traditional algorithm, in that patient samples are screened by an automated treponemal immunoassay, and positive results are confirmed by a nontreponemal test. The reverse algorithm has several advantages over the traditional algorithm. The first advantage is cost. Automated testing can be performed on LIS-interfaced high-throughput analyzers as opposed to labor-intensive manual methods, saving time and reducing errors. Secondly, this algorithm can potentially detect more early, late, and treated syphilis cases because of the higher sensitivity of the specific treponemal tests. In the traditional algorithm, these cases may be missed because testing stops with a negative nontreponemal test result and the treponemal test is not run.

In the reverse algorithm, if the initial assay is negative, no further testing is done unless early syphilis is suspected (i.e., before seroconversion). If the automated assay result is positive and the subsequent RPR is positive, the results are considered positive for syphilis. However, discrepant results can be obtained in some cases, with the initial automated test result being positive and the RPR that follows giving a negative result. This combination of results can be problematic because it could be caused by a false-positive treponemal antibody test result, a past syphilis infection, or early primary syphilis, in which patients have not yet produced nontreponemal antibodies. To help distinguish between these possibilities, the CDC recommends that if laboratories choose to use the reverse algorithm, all discrepant results should be tested reflexively using the TP-PA test as a secondary confirmatory treponemal test. If the TP-PA is positive, then late or latent syphilis or previous history of syphilis would be considered. If the TP-PA is negative, the patient would be considered negative for syphilis at the time of testing. Careful evaluation of the patient's history should be considered, and the patient may be reevaluated for syphilis at a later date **(Fig. 21–8)**.

Testing for Congenital Syphilis

Nontreponemal tests for congenital syphilis performed on cord blood or neonatal serum detect the IgG class of antibody in addition to IgM. It is difficult to differentiate passively transferred IgG maternal antibodies from those produced by the neonate, so there are problems in establishing a definitive diagnosis. Late maternal infection may result in a nonreactive test because of low levels of fetal antibody. Additionally, testing the infant's spinal fluid for the presence of treponemes often lacks sensitivity. Nontreponemal titers in the infant that are higher than those in the mother may be a good indicator of congenital disease, but this does not always occur.

Several approaches have focused on detecting IgM antibodies in the infant. An FTA-ABS test for IgM alone lacks sensitivity, and the test is subject to interference because of the presence of rheumatoid factor. However, an IgM capture assay is more sensitive, and a Western blot assay (see Chapter 24 for details) using four major treponemal antigens has demonstrated high sensitivity and specificity.

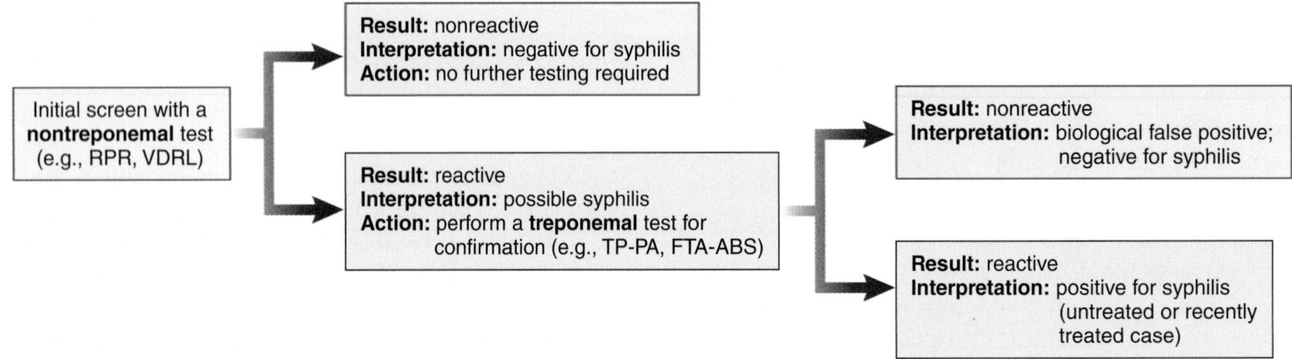

FIGURE 21–7 Traditional testing algorithm for syphilis.

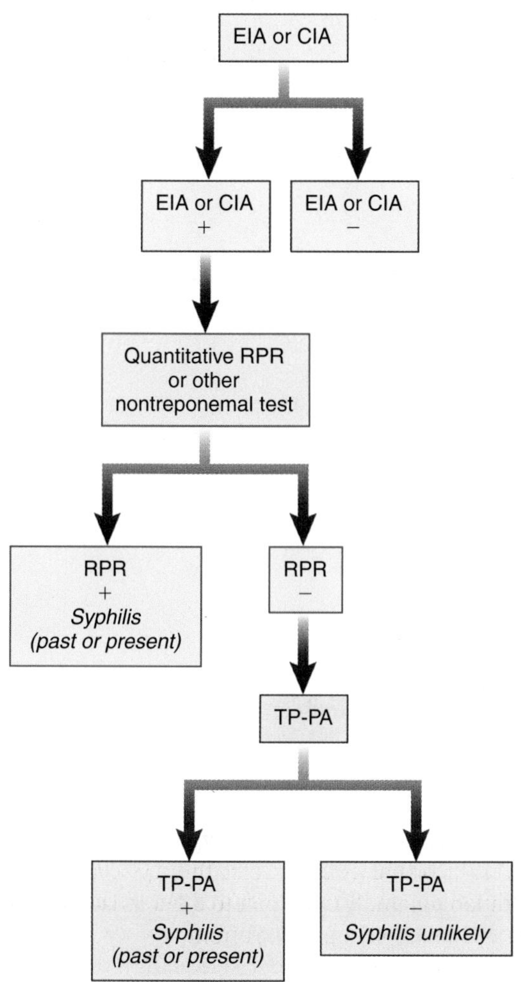

EIA = enzyme immunoassay; CIA = chemiluminescence immunoassay; TP-PA = *Treponema pallidum* particle agglutination.

FIGURE 21–8 The algorithm for reverse sequence syphilis screening involves treponemal test screening followed by nontreponemal test confirmation. The CDC recommends that discrepant results be followed by performance of the TP-PA test. *(Adapted from Centers for Disease Control and Prevention. Discordant results from reverse sequence syphilis screening: five laboratories, United States, 2006–2010.* MMWR. *2011;60*[05]*:133–137).*

Currently, it is recommended that in high-risk populations, nontreponemal tests be performed on both the mother and infant at birth, regardless of previously negative maternal tests. Because symptoms are not always present at birth, if congenital syphilis is suspected because of maternal history, tests should be repeated on infant serum within a few weeks. If infection is present in the infant, the titer will remain the same or will increase. The Western blot test is recommended to confirm congenital syphilis.

Clinical Applications

Testing of Cerebrospinal Fluid

CSF is typically tested to determine whether treponemes have invaded the CNS. Such testing is usually more reliable if CNS symptoms are present. The VDRL test and some of the newer enzyme-linked immunosorbent assay (ELISA) tests are the only ones routinely used for the testing of spinal fluid. For VDRL spinal fluid testing, the antigen volume used is less than the serum test and is at a different concentration. In addition, different slides are used (Boerner agglutination slides). The test is read microscopically as in the VDRL serum test. If a test is reactive, two-fold dilutions are made and retested following the same protocol to determine the titer.

A positive VDRL test on spinal fluid is diagnostic of neurosyphilis because false positives are extremely rare. However, sensitivity is lacking because samples from fewer than 70% of patients with active neurosyphilis give positive results. If a negative test is obtained, other indicators such as increased lymphocyte count and elevated total protein (45 mg/dL) are used as signs of active disease. PCR has been advocated in diagnosing neurosyphilis and may play an important role in CSF testing in the future.

Treatment

Penicillin has been the treatment of choice for syphilis since its availability in the late 1940s. Infection can be easily cured by administering a single dose of intramuscular long-acting benzathine penicillin G. Doxycycline and tetracycline are other alternatives for patients who are allergic to penicillin and are not pregnant.

Lyme Disease

Lyme disease was first described in the United States in 1975 when an unusually large number of cases of juvenile arthritis appeared in a geographically clustered rural area around Old Lyme, Connecticut (hence the disease name), in the summer and fall. Two mothers recognized this and brought it to the attention of health officials. Because of the epidemiological features of this newly described "Lyme arthritis," transmission by an arthropod vector was suggested. In 1982, the agent was isolated and identified as a new spirochete. It was given the name ***Borrelia burgdorferi*** after Willy Burgdorfer (first author in the original description). The clinical features of Lyme disease were soon recognized to extend beyond arthritis; it is now known to be a multisystem illness involving the skin, nervous system, heart, and joints. Lyme disease is the most common vector-borne disease in the United States; more than 42,743 confirmed and probable cases were reported in 2017, almost 9% more than in 2016. According to the CDC, the number of cases in high-incidence states has remained stable but has increased in neighboring states with previously low incidence.

Characteristics of *Borrelia* Species

Several species of *Borrelia* are known to be the causative agents of Lyme disease. In North America, it is exclusively *B. burgdorferi sensu stricto,* whereas in Europe, several species are known to cause Lyme disease (*Borrelia afzelii, Borrelia garinii, Borrelia sensu stricto,* and occasionally other *Borrelia* species). All share similar characteristics; for simplicity, they will be referred to as *B. burgdorferi*. The organism is a loosely coiled spirochete,

5 to 25 μm long and 0.2 to 0.5 μm in diameter. The outer membrane, which consists of glycolipid and protein, is extremely fluid and only loosely associated with the organism. Several important lipoprotein antigens, outer surface proteins (OSPs) OSP-A through OSP-F, are located within this structure and are actually encoded by plasmids. Surface proteins allow the spirochetes to attach to mammalian cells.

Just underneath the outer envelope are 7 to 11 *endoflagella* or *periplasmic flagella*. These run parallel to the long axis of the organism and are made up of 41-kDa subunits that elicit a strong antibody response. This immunodominant characteristic is of diagnostic importance because the response is not only strong but is also very early. Unfortunately, the flagellin subunit has homology to that of other nonpathogenic and pathogenic spirochetes, notably *B. recurrentis* and *T. pallidum*, causing cross-reactivity in serological testing. Because of this, a large number of uninfected people have low levels of antibodies to the 41-kDa protein. Although this is usually not a problem in the current diagnostic scheme of testing, it can become an issue when these individuals become ill with certain viruses that are known polyclonal B-cell activators (such as Epstein-Barr virus). In these cases, this normally low-level antibody becomes high enough to cause biological false positivity.

The organism divides by binary fission approximately every 12 hours. It can be cultured in the laboratory in a complex liquid medium (Barbour-Stoenner-Kelly) at 33°C, but it is difficult to isolate from patients. The spirochetemia (presence of spirochetes in the blood) is short-lived and is generally only found early in the illness. Cultures often must be incubated for 6 weeks or longer to detect growth and are therefore of little diagnostic utility.

Mode of Transmission

The main reservoir host is the white-footed mouse (*Peromyscus leucopus*), although in California and Oregon the spirochete is also harbored by the dusky-footed woodrat. Several types of *Ixodes* ticks serve as vectors of transmission: *Ixodes scapularis* in the Northeast and Midwest United States **(Fig. 21–9)**, *Ixodes pacificus* in the West, *Ixodes ricinus* in Europe, and *Ixodes persulcatus* in Asia. White-tailed deer are the main host for the tick's adult stage. Nymphs and adult stages of the tick can transmit the disease. The peak feeding is in the late spring, early summer, and fall, which corresponds to the peak biphasic occurrence of Lyme disease. The tick must feed for a period of time before the spirochete can be transmitted, typically more than 36 hours; one study found that transmission is still low at 72 hours.

Stages of the Disease

Lyme disease resembles syphilis in that manifestations occur in several stages. These have been characterized as (1) localized rash, (2) early dissemination to multiple organ systems, and (3) a late disseminated stage that often includes arthritic symptoms. These stages are not always sharply delineated; therefore, it may be easier to view Lyme disease as a progressive infectious disease that involves diverse organ systems.

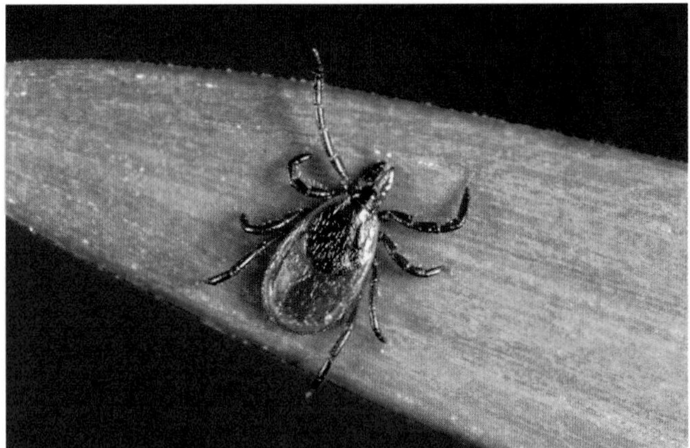

FIGURE 21–9 Adult tick *I. scapularis*, which transmits Lyme disease. *(Courtesy of the CDC/Michael L. Levin, PhD, and Jim Gathany, Public Health Image Library.)*

Localized Rash Stage

The clinical hallmark of early infection is the rash known as *erythema migrans* (EM), which appears between 2 days and 2 weeks after a tick bite. EM begins as a small red papule where the bite occurred, then rapidly expands to form a large ring-like erythema and often a central area that exhibits partial clearing **(Fig. 21–10)**. The clinical diagnosis of early Lyme disease relies on the recognition of this characteristic rash, which should be at least 5 cm in diameter. At this stage, the patient may be asymptomatic or have nonspecific flu-like symptoms. The EM usually continues to expand for more than a week; even if untreated, it gradually fades within 3 to 4 weeks. Unfortunately, approximately 20% of patients do not develop the rash. At this early stage, the antibody response is minimal, and most serology results are negative.

Early Dissemination Stage

Early dissemination occurs via the bloodstream in the days to weeks following the EM rash. The skin, nervous system, heart, or joints may be affected. Some patients display multiple skin lesions. Migratory pain often occurs in the joints, tendons, muscles, and bones. If treatment is not obtained, neurological or cardiac involvement develops in about 15% of patients within 4 to 6 weeks after the onset of infection. The most prevalent neurological sign is facial palsy, a peripheral neuritis that usually involves one side of the face. Pain and weakness can occur in the limb that was bitten. Some patients develop sleep disturbances, mild chronic confusion, or difficulty with memory and intellectual functioning. An aseptic meningitis can also be seen.

Late Dissemination Stage

Late Lyme disease may develop in some untreated patients months to years after acquiring the infection. The major manifestations of late Lyme disease are arthritis, peripheral neuropathy, and encephalomyelitis. These symptoms usually respond well to conventional antibiotic treatment, but treatment-resistant arthritis has been associated with particular

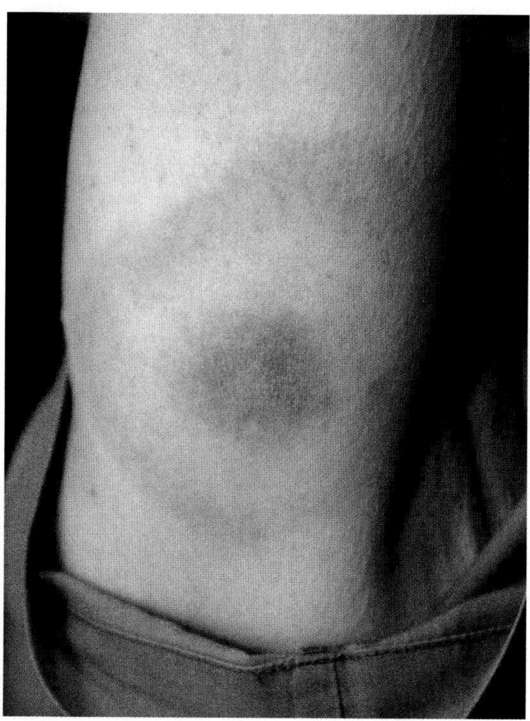

FIGURE 21–10 Erythema chronicum migrans rash, which appears after a tick bite in Lyme disease. *(Courtesy of the CDC/Jim Gathany, Public Health Image Library.)*

HLA–DRB alleles. Despite resolution of objective manifestations of *Borrelia* infection after antibiotic treatment, a small percentage of patients develop chronic fatigue, concentration and short-term memory problems, and musculoskeletal pain. These symptoms can last longer than 6 months in some cases.

Nature of the Immune Response

The immune response in Lyme disease is highly variable and complex. A well-documented humoral and cellular response is known to exist. Spirochete lipoproteins also trigger the production of macrophage-derived cytokines, which further enhance the immune response. However, the clinical effectiveness of these responses is questionable and not necessarily protective because late Lyme disease occurs despite high levels of circulating antibody and cellular responses.

Laboratory Diagnosis

The diagnosis of Lyme disease is a clinical one, with laboratory testing used as supporting evidence. Unfortunately, the clinical diagnosis is often difficult. If the characteristic rash is present, this can be used as a presumptive finding, but as many as 20% of patients do not develop or do not recognize the rash. Direct isolation of the organism from skin scrapings, spinal fluid, or blood is possible, but the yield of positive cultures is extremely low. Therefore, culture is not used as a routine diagnostic tool.

The antibody response is variable and may not be detectable until 3 to 6 weeks after the tick bite. The IgM response occurs first, followed by the IgG response. The IgG response does not peak until the third and fourth weeks of infection. These antibody responses are also not mutually exclusive and can be variable (e.g., an IgM response can occur in late Lyme disease). In most cases of acute early Lyme disease (first 2 weeks), serological testing is too insensitive to be diagnostically helpful. If patients with symptoms are tested in fewer than 7 days after infection, seropositivity is only about 30%. Therefore, the decision to start treatment for early Lyme disease must be made before seroconversion, similar to many acute infectious diseases. However, untreated seronegative patients having symptoms for 6 to 8 weeks are unlikely to have Lyme disease, and other possible diagnoses should be pursued. Antibiotic therapy begun shortly after the appearance of EM may delay or abrogate the antibody response.

The CDC recommends a two-tiered approach to providing laboratory support for the diagnosis of Lyme disease (**Fig. 21–11**). The standard approach has been in use since 1995. Using the standard testing algorithm, patients with clinical evidence of Lyme disease are screened with a sensitive ELISA or, alternatively, with an IFA. If the first serology test is positive or borderline, a Western blot test is performed on that specimen to confirm the result. Some important limitations to this approach are the cost and complexity of performing and interpreting the Western blot, which must be done in reference laboratories. The standard testing algorithm is highly specific but has low sensitivity in detecting early Lyme disease.

The limitations of the standard algorithm have led to the development of alternative testing strategies, referred to as a *modified two-tiered algorithm* (see Fig. 21–11). In this approach, symptomatic patients are first tested with a sensitive ELISA that uses purified *Borrelia* peptide antigens. Samples with positive or borderline results are retested with a different ELISA method for confirmation. The modified algorithm was approved by the U.S. Food and Drug Administration (FDA). In addition to being easier to perform and interpret, this approach demonstrates comparable specificity to the standard algorithm and increased sensitivity in detecting early Lyme disease.

Lyme testing should not be performed in the absence of supporting clinical evidence. A positive test performed under these circumstances has a low positive predictive value, even when done in an endemic area, whereas it rises to nearly 100% when clinical symptoms and history are present and consistent with Lyme disease. Some of the current testing procedures are discussed next.

Immunofluorescence Assay (IFA)

The IFA was the first test used to evaluate the antibody response in Lyme disease, followed by various forms of EIAs shortly thereafter. Basically, doubling dilutions of patient serum are incubated with commercially prepared microscope slides coated with antigen from whole or processed *Borrelia* spirochetes. Following a wash step to remove unbound material, an anti-human globulin with a fluorescent tag attached is added and reacts with any specific antibody bound to the spirochetes on the slide. After a second wash step, the slide is viewed under a fluorescent microscope.

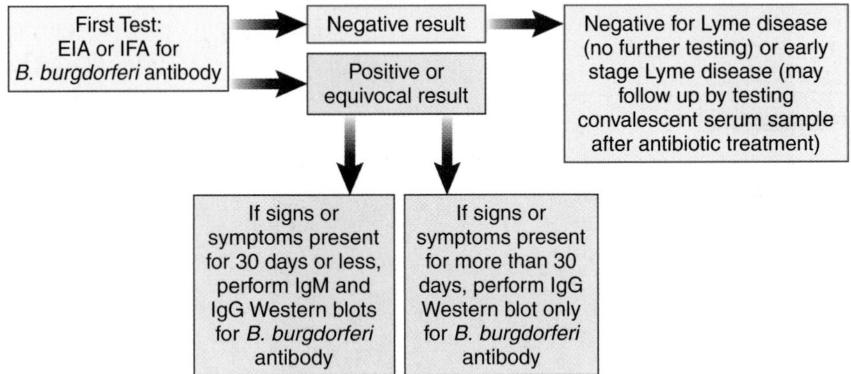

Modified Algorithm

Perform EIA #1 for *B. burgdorferi* antibody

Negative result

Positive or equivocal result

Negative for Lyme disease (no further testing) or early stage Lyme disease (may follow up by testing convalescent serum sample after antibiotic treatment)

Perform EIA #2 for IgM and IgG *B. burgdorferi* antibody

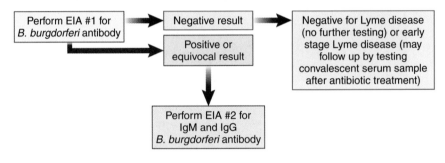

FIGURE 21–11 Two-tiered testing for Lyme disease *(Adapted from Centers for Disease Control and Prevention [https://www.cdc.gov/lyme/healthcare/clinician_twotier.html] and Branda JA, Strle K, Nigrovic LE, Lantos PM, Lepore TJ, et al. Evaluation of modified 2-tiered serodiagnostic testing algorithms for early Lyme disease.* Clin Infec Dis. *2017;64:1074–1080.)*

Typically, a test result is only considered positive if a titer of 1:256 or higher is obtained, although this varies between manufacturers. As previously mentioned, specimens obtained in the first few weeks are usually negative because the level of antibody present is below the detection limit of this (and other) assays. As might be expected, other closely related organisms, such as *B. recurrentis* (relapsing fever), *T. denticola* and others associated with periodontal disease, and *T. pallidum* (syphilis), may cross-react and cause biological false-positive results. Autoimmune connective tissue diseases such as rheumatoid arthritis (RA) and SLE can also produce false positives in the IFA for Lyme disease. An astute technologist can recognize a false positive by the beaded fluorescent pattern it produces. Reading of fluorescent patterns tends to be very subjective and requires highly trained individuals. However, if performed correctly by experienced personnel, the test can provide sensitive and accurate results. This test is best suited for low-volume testing.

Enzyme Immunoassay (EIA)

EIA testing has used ELISAs that are relatively inexpensive to perform and yield timely results. The test is reproducible because the results are objective, and the method lends itself well to automation and high-volume testing. For these reasons, EIAs are widely used in the initial evaluation of patients for Lyme disease. In addition, EIAs have recently been recommended by the CDC as an alternative to the Western blot test in the two-tier testing algorithm for Lyme disease, as we discussed previously.

Antigen preparations used in various forms of the assay include crude sonicates of the organism, purified proteins, synthetic proteins, and recombinant proteins such as the VIsE C6 peptide and pepC10 (peptide derived from OSP-C). The manufacturer's selected antigen is then coated onto 96-well microtiter plates or strips by various proprietary methods. Patient sera is added; during incubation, if antibodies to the *B. burgdorferi* antigens are present, they will bind to the solid phase. After a washing step, anti-human immunoglobulin conjugated with an enzyme tag such as alkaline phosphatase is added to each well. The conjugate can also be adapted to test for IgM and IgG, IgM only, or IgG only. Adding specific substrate produces a color change. Plates are read in a spectrophotometer, and the antibody is quantitated based on color intensity. EIAs provide objective results, and the titer is based on a continuum range rather than serial dilutions of patient sera. Thus, a more accurate measurement of the specific antibody is possible.

Similar to the IFA, EIAs have decreased sensitivity during the early stages of Lyme disease when patients may not have mounted a sufficient antibody response. In addition, as with IFAs, false positives can occur due to syphilis or other treponemal diseases such as yaws and periodontal disease, as well as relapsing fever and leptospirosis. Patients with infectious mononucleosis, Rocky Mountain spotted fever, and other autoimmune diseases may also be positive with an EIA. Lyme disease patients do not test positive with RPR, so this may be helpful if syphilis is in the differential diagnosis.

Western Blot

Immunoblotting, or Western blotting, has been used as a confirmatory test for samples that initially test positive or equivocal by EIA or IFA. It has been employed as the second test in the CDC-recommended two-tier testing scheme for Lyme disease. The CDC does not recommend testing seropositive or borderline patients for IgM antibodies if they have had symptoms for more than 4 weeks. Serological evidence of Lyme disease in these patients is indicated by a positive result in the IgG immunoblot.

The Lyme disease immunoblot is very complex **(Fig. 21–12)**. The technique consists of electrophoresis of *Borrelia* antigens in an acrylamide gel followed by transfer of the resulting pattern to nitrocellulose paper. This step is performed by the manufacturer, and nitrocellulose antigen strips are provided in the test kit. These strips are reacted with patient serum and developed with an anti-human immunoglobulin (either anti-IgG or anti-IgM) to which an enzyme label is attached. Further incubation with the enzyme's substrate allows for visualization of any antibody that has bound to a particular antigen. The reactivity is then scored and interpreted.

Ten proteins are used in the CDC-recommended interpretation of this test. They are designated by their molecular weights: 18, 23, 28, 30, 39, 41, 45, 58, 66, and 93 kDa. For a result to be considered positive for the presence of specific IgM antibody, two of the following bands must be present: 23 (OSP-C), 39, and 41 (flagellin) kDa. An IgG immunoblot is considered positive if any 5 of the 10 bands previously listed are positive. Because of the complexity of the Lyme immunoblots, testing and interpretation of blots should be done only in qualified laboratories that follow CDC-recommended evidence-based guidelines on immunoblot interpretations.

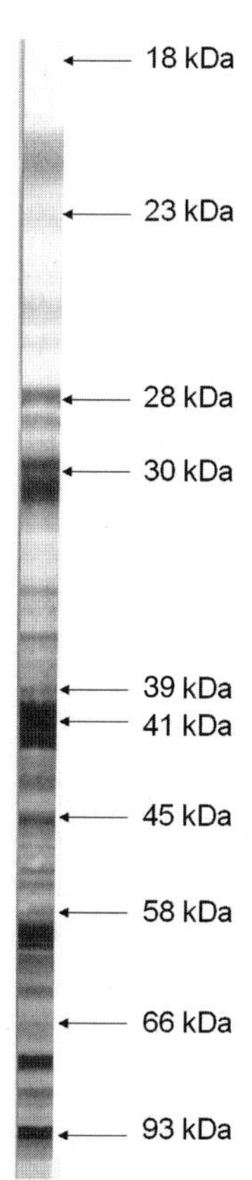

FIGURE 21–12 Immunoblot for Lyme disease.

Polymerase Chain Reaction (PCR)

In testing for Lyme disease, the PCR has found a niche in certain scenarios. Although only a few organisms need to be present for detection under optimal conditions, the number of spirochetes in infected tissues and body fluids is low, making specimen collection, transport, and preparation of DNA critical to the accuracy of the test results.

Several probes for target DNA that is present only in strains of *B. burgdorferi* are used in PCR testing. The procedure involves extracting DNA from the patient sample, followed by amplification using specific primers, DNA polymerase, and nucleotides. The patient DNA is combined with a known DNA probe to see if hybridization takes place. The single-stranded *Borrelia* DNA probe will bind only to an exact complementary strand, thus positively identifying the presence of the organism's DNA in the patient sample. This is much more specific than testing for antibody because there is little cross-reactivity. The specificity of PCR ranges from 93% to 100%. However, sensitivity remains problematic. In a series of studies, the median sensitivity of PCR on skin biopsies was 69%; of blood components, 14%; of CSF, 38%; and of synovial fluid, 78%. However, the range of sensitivities in any one type of specimen is quite large, suggesting that testing remains to be standardized. Furthermore, it would be hard to clinically justify a skin biopsy for PCR as a diagnostic method for an EM rash in most cases. However, PCR on CSF and synovial fluid is often used in difficult diagnostic neurological and arthritic cases. PCR for *Borrelia* is typically performed in reference laboratories. Modifications of the PCR, as well as proteomic assays, are being developed and tested for their potential utility in Lyme disease diagnosis as well.

Treatment

Borrelia is sensitive to several orally administered antibiotics, including penicillins, tetracyclines, and macrolides. Oral doxycycline is the first treatment of choice for patients with early Lyme disease who are not pregnant. Intravenous antibiotic therapy is required for patients with neurological symptoms, cardiac involvement, or arthritis that does not respond to oral therapy. Prophylaxis, full-course treatment, or serological testing of all patients with tick bites is not recommended. A single dose of doxycycline may be offered to adults and children older than 8 years of age when the tick can be reliably identified, and treatment can begin within 72 hours of tick removal.

Currently, there are no effective vaccines for humans. A human vaccine made with the OSP-A surface antigen has had limited usefulness; it has been associated with side effects and has been recalled from the market. There are renewed efforts to create a new vaccine, but as of this writing, no vaccines have been approved for clinical use.

Leptospirosis

Leptospirosis is caused by bacteria of the genus ***Leptospira***. It is more prevalent in temperate zones of the world with a warm climate. The incidence is higher in livestock and dairy farming communities. It is primarily a zoonotic infection commonly associated with occupational and recreational activities. Coming into contact with infected animals, especially rat-infested surroundings, poses increased exposure for veterinarians, dairy farmers, slaughterhouse workers, sewer cleaners, and miners. In the United States, most of the leptospirosis cases are associated with exposure to recreational water activities. Leptospirosis was a nationally reportable disease up until 1995, at which time it was dropped from the list of notifiable diseases. However, it was reinstated as a reportable infection in 2013. According to the CDC, an estimated 100 to 150 cases are reported annually in the United States; 50% of cases are from Puerto Rico, and Hawaii has the second highest incidence.

Characteristics of *Leptospira* Species

Organisms belonging to the genus *Leptospira* ("leptospires") are thin, flexible, and tightly coiled spirochetes. They are 0.1 µm wide and 6 to 20 µm long with pointed ends bent into a typical hook-like shape. Unlike *Treponema* and *Borrelia* organisms, the spirals of *Leptospira* are so close together that they tend to appear similar to a chain of cocci **(Fig. 21–13)**.

The genus *Leptospira* was originally divided into two main species, namely, pathogenic saprophytes, *L. interrogans*, and environmental saprophytes, *L. biflexa*. However, more characteristic distinction can be achieved by serotyping. There are more than 200 serovars of *L. interrogans* and more than 60 for *L. biflexa*. Leptospires are obligate aerobes that can grow optimally at a temperature range of 28°C to 30°C. They can be grown in artificial culture media such as Fletcher semisolid medium, Ellinghausen-McCullough-Johnson-Harris (EMJH) semisolid medium, or Stuart liquid medium.

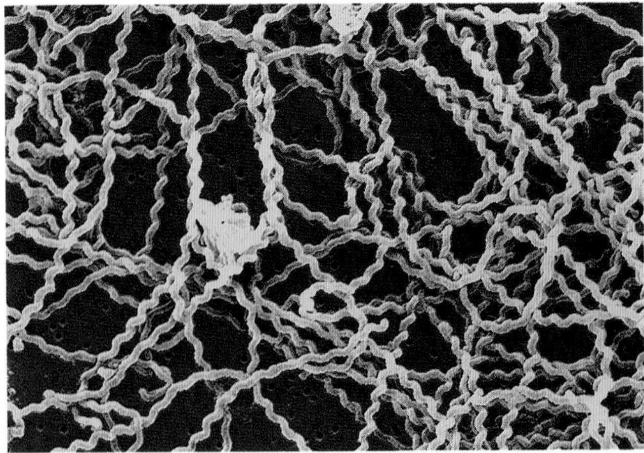

FIGURE 21–13 Scanning electron microscope (SEM) image shows many corkscrew-shaped *Leptospira* spirochetes atop a 0.1-µm polycarbonate filter. *(Courtesy of the CDC/Rob Weyant and Janice H. Carr, Public Health Image Library.)*

Mode of Transmission

Leptospires are naturally found inhabiting the renal tubules of infected animals such as rodents, dogs, pigs, horses, and livestock and, thus, are shed in the urine of these animals. The organisms can survive for weeks to months in urine-contaminated water and mud. Humans are exposed through mucous membranes, conjunctiva, skin abrasions, or ingestion when they come into contact with urine-contaminated water of rivers, streams, sewage, or floodwater. The risk of transmission increases by wading, swimming, or boating in floodwater or fresh water that may be contaminated with animal urine. Exposure to leptospirosis can be avoided by not wading or swimming in potentially contaminated water bodies, especially after heavy rainfall or flooding. Protective clothing such as rubber boots, gloves, and waterproof coveralls should be worn in situations involving occupational exposure.

Stages of the Disease

The incubation period in leptospirosis varies between 2 to 30 days, but most cases manifest 5 to 14 days after exposure. The clinical presentation of the illness is generally abrupt, starting with a nonspecific febrile episode of headache, myalgia, nausea, vomiting, diarrhea, and a characteristic conjunctival suffusion. Illness may be biphasic, with the patient briefly recovering from mild illness but then developing more severe disease with renal, hepatic, pulmonary, and CNS involvement. Severe systemic disease involving renal failure and jaundice caused by hepatic failure is referred to as **Weil's disease.** Patients with severe illness have a fatality rate of 5% to 15%. In pregnant women, leptospirosis can cause fetal abnormalities, death, or abortion.

Laboratory Diagnosis

Leptospires can be demonstrated in blood or serum samples in the first week of illness by dark-field, immunofluorescent, or phase contrast microscopy, but these techniques are not recommended because of lower sensitivity of microscopic examination. Serology is the most common method to diagnose leptospirosis, followed by molecular techniques. During the first week of illness, whole blood and serum are the preferred samples, and afterward, a serum and/or urine sample should be submitted for testing. IgM screening assays are available in the form of ELISA, ImmunoDOT, and lateral flow tests. Positive screening tests should be confirmed by a **microscopic agglutination test (MAT)**, which is the gold standard for diagnosing leptospirosis. Ideally, acute and convalescent serum samples collected 7 to 14 days apart are tested by MAT. This test is available only at regional or national reference laboratories. PCR assays are also available at the CDC and some commercial laboratories. The key advantage of PCR is quick turnaround time and prompt treatment of positive cases.

Treatment

Penicillin and doxycycline are the drugs of choice for treatment of leptospirosis. Early treatment leads to reducing the severity and duration of the illness. Studies have shown that prophylaxis with a weekly dose of oral doxycycline is considered effective for people in high-risk environments.

SUMMARY

- Syphilis and Lyme disease are two major diseases caused by spirochetes.
- Spirochetes are distinguished by the presence of axial filaments that wrap around the cell wall inside a sheath and give the organisms their characteristic motility.
- Syphilis is caused by the organism *Treponema pallidum,* subspecies *pallidum.* The disease is acquired by direct contact, usually through sexual transmission.
- Syphilis can be separated into four main clinical stages:
  - The *primary stage* is characterized by the presence of a painless ulcer called a *chancre* at the site of initial contact.
  - An untreated patient may progress from the primary stage to the *secondary stage,* in which systemic dissemination of the organism occurs and symptoms such as generalized lymphadenopathy, malaise, sore throat, and skin rash appear.
  - Disappearance of the secondary stage is followed by a lengthy *latent stage* in which patients are usually free of clinical symptoms.
  - About one-third of the individuals who remain untreated develop *tertiary syphilis.* This late-stage disease is characterized by three major clinical manifestations: granulomatous inflammation (gummas), cardiovascular disease, and neurosyphilis. Early diagnosis and treatment help to prevent later complications.
- Direct laboratory diagnosis of syphilis involves detecting the organism from a lesion and using dark-field microscopy, fluorescence microscopy, or PCR. If an active lesion is not present, diagnosis must be made on the basis of serological tests.
- Nontreponemal serological tests (i.e., the VDRL and RPR) determine the presence of antibody to cardiolipin, also known as *reagin.* These tests are fairly sensitive and simple to perform; however, they lack specificity, so specimens with positive results must be confirmed with a more specific treponemal antibody test.
- Traditional treponemal antibody tests include the FTA-ABS and particle agglutination (TP-PA). These tests detect antibody formed against *T. pallidum* itself. Treponemal tests are more specific and sensitive in early stages of the disease.
- Titers of treponemal antibodies remain detectable for life, whereas nontreponemal titers decline after successful treatment.
- More recent developments in testing include EIA and CLIA technology and PCR. EIA and CLIA tests for antibody to specific treponemal antigens, and separation of antibodies by class is possible. For large-volume testing, an EIA or CLIA is commonly used as a screening test, followed by confirmation with an RPR test. This testing sequence is known as the *reverse screening algorithm.*
- Lyme disease is the most common vector-borne infection in the United States. The organism responsible is the spirochete *Borrelia burgdorferi,* which is transmitted by the deer tick.
- Although an expanding red rash is often the first symptom noted in Lyme disease, the disease can be characterized as a progressive infectious syndrome involving diverse organ systems. Despite antibiotic treatment, a small percentage of patients continue to have fatigue; concentration and short-term memory problems; and musculoskeletal pain, which may last 6 months or longer. These symptoms may be caused by persistence of the infection.
- The presence of IgM and IgG to *B. burgdorferi* cannot usually be detected until 3 to 6 weeks after symptoms initially appear. A two-tier testing protocol is used that involves screening with an IFA or EIA and follow-up of equivocal or positive tests with immunoblotting or a different EIA. All serological findings must be interpreted carefully and in conjunction with clinical findings.
- Leptospirosis is a zoonosis associated with exposure to water contaminated with animal urine. It is caused by spirochetes of the genus *Leptospira* and has its highest incidence in tropical and subtropical regions of the world.
- Symptoms of severe *Leptospira* infection include fever, headache, myalgia, conjunctivitis, jaundice, and combined liver and renal failure, a condition usually referred to as *Weil's disease.*
- The microscopic agglutination test (MAT) is the gold-standard confirmatory method in the laboratory diagnosis of leptospirosis.

Study Guide: Comparison of Tests Used for the Diagnosis of Syphilis

TEST	ANTIGEN	ANTIBODY	COMMENTS
Direct Microscopic			
Dark-field	*T. pallidum* from patient	None	Requires active lesion; must have good specimen, experienced technologist; inexpensive
Fluorescent antibody	*T. pallidum* from patient	Anti-treponemal antibody with fluorescent tag	Requires active lesion; more specific than dark-field; specimen does not have to contain live organisms

(continued)

Study Guide: Comparison of Tests Used for the Diagnosis of Syphilis—cont'd

TEST	ANTIGEN	ANTIBODY	COMMENTS
Nontreponemal			
VDRL	Cardiolipin	Anti-cardiolipin (Reagin)	Microscopic flocculation; may be used for screening, treatment monitoring, spinal fluid testing; false positives are common
RPR	Cardiolipin	Anti-cardiolipin (Reagin)	Macroscopic flocculation with charcoal particles; more sensitive than VDRL in primary syphilis; false positives are common
Treponemal			
FTA-ABS	Nichols strain of *T. pallidum*	Anti-treponemal	Confirmatory; specific, sensitive; may be negative in primary stage
Serodia TP-PA (formerly, MHA-TP)	Gel particles sensitized with *T. pallidum* sonicate (formerly sensitized sheep RBCs)	Anti-treponemal	Not as sensitive as FTA-ABS
EIA, CLIA, MFI	Treponemal antigen	Anti-treponemal	Sensitive, automated testing provides objective results; used to screen for syphilis in many large laboratories; EIAs have been developed as competitive, sandwich, or capture immunoassays that can detect IgM or IgG antibodies
PCR	*T. pallidum* DNA in patient sample is amplified	None	Highest sensitivity is in primary-stage syphilis; availability is limited

CLIA = chemiluminescent immunoassay; EIA = enzyme immunoassay; FTA-ABS = fluorescent treponemal antibody absorption; MFI = multiplex flow immunoassay; MHA-TP = microhemagglutination assay for antibodies to Treponema pallidum*; PCR = polymerase chain reaction; RPR = rapid plasma reagin; TP-PA =* T. pallidum *particle agglutination; VDRL = Venereal Disease Research Laboratory.*

Study Guide: Comparison of Tests for the Diagnosis of Lyme Disease

TEST	ANTIGEN	ANTIBODY	COMMENTS
IFA	Whole or processed *B. burgdorferi*	Anti-*Borrelia* antibody from patient, anti-human globulin with fluorescent tag	Initial test for Lyme disease; labor intensive to perform; false positives; subjective
EIA	Sonicated *B. burgdorferi*	Anti-*Borrelia* antibody from patient, anti-human globulin with enzyme tag	Initial test for Lyme disease; easy to perform; false positives; more sensitive than IFA
	Purified flagellin protein	Anti-flagellin antibody from patient, anti-human globulin with enzyme tag	Initial test for Lyme disease; easy to perform; highly specific; sensitive in early Lyme disease
	C6 peptide	Conserved region of surface lipoprotein (VlsE)	Easy to perform; highly specific; sensitive in early and late Lyme disease; may be used as a confirmatory test for Lyme disease
Western blot or immunoblot	Antigens of *B. burgdorferi* separated by molecular weight	Detects antibodies (IgG or IgM) to individual *B. burgdorferi* antigens	Technically difficult to perform; scoring the blot can be challenging; used as a confirmatory test for Lyme disease
PCR	None. *B. burgdorferi* DNA in patient sample is amplified	None	Available in reference laboratories

EIA = enzyme immunoassay; IFA = immunofluorescence assay; PCR = polymerase chain reaction.

CASE STUDIES

1. A 30-year-old woman saw her physician to complain about repeated episodes of arthritis-like pain in the knees and hip joints. She recalled having seen a very small tick on her arm about 6 months before the development of symptoms. However, no rash was ever seen. Laboratory tests for rheumatoid arthritis and SLE were negative. An EIA test conducted on the patient's serum for Lyme disease was indeterminate.

Questions

a. Does the absence of a rash rule out the possibility of Lyme disease?
b. What might cause an indeterminate EIA test?
c. What confirmatory testing would help determine the cause of the patient's condition?

2. A mother who had no prenatal care appeared at the emergency department in labor. The physician safely delivered a baby boy who appeared to be normal. The physician obtained a blood sample from the mother for routine screening. An RPR test performed on the mother's serum was positive. The mother had no obvious signs of syphilis and denied any past history of the disease. She indicated that she had never received any treatment for a possible syphilis infection. Cord blood from the baby also exhibited a positive RPR result.

Questions

a. Is the baby at risk for congenital syphilis?
b. What is the significance of a positive RPR on a cord blood test?
c. How should the infant be managed, based on these results?
d. What is the significance of a positive RPR in pregnancy? How should it be confirmed for syphilis?

REVIEW QUESTIONS

1. False-positive nontreponemal tests for syphilis may occur because of which of the following?
   a. Infectious mononucleosis
   b. Systemic lupus
   c. Pregnancy
   d. All of the above

2. In the fluorescent treponemal antibody absorption (FTA-ABS) test, what is the purpose of absorption with Reiter treponemes?
   a. It removes reactivity with lupus antibody.
   b. It prevents cross-reactivity with antibody to other *T. pallidum* subspecies.
   c. It prevents cross-reactivity with antibody to nonpathogenic treponemes.
   d. All of the above.

3. Which test is recommended for testing cerebrospinal fluid for detection of neurosyphilis?
   a. RPR
   b. VDRL
   c. FTA-ABS
   d. Enzyme immunoassay

4. Advantages of direct fluorescent antibody testing to *T. pallidum* include all of the following *except*
   a. reading is less subjective than with dark-field testing.
   b. monoclonal antibody makes the reaction very specific.
   c. slides can be prepared for later reading.
   d. careful specimen collection is less important than in dark-field testing.

5. Which of the following is true of nontreponemal antibodies?
   a. They can be detected in all patients with primary syphilis.
   b. These antibodies are directed against cardiolipin.
   c. Nontreponemal tests remain positive after successful treatment.
   d. The antibodies are only found in patients with syphilis.

6. Which syphilis test detects specific treponemal antibodies?
   a. RPR
   b. VDRL
   c. FTA-ABS
   d. Dark-field exam

7. Which of the following is true of treponemal tests for syphilis?
   a. They are usually negative in the primary stage.
   b. Titers decrease with successful treatment.
   c. In large-volume testing, they are often used as screening tests.
   d. They are subject to a greater number of false positives than nontreponemal tests.

8. An RPR test done on a 19-year-old woman as part of a prenatal workup was negative but exhibited a rough appearance. What should the technologist do next?
   a. Report the result out as negative.
   b. Do a VDRL test.
   c. Send the sample for confirmatory testing.
   d. Make serial dilutions and do a titer.

9. Treponemal EIA tests for syphilis are characterized by all of the following *except*
   a. they are adaptable to automation.
   b. they are useful in monitoring antibody titers in syphilis patients undergoing therapy.
   c. subjectivity in reading is eliminated.
   d. they can be used to distinguish between IgG and IgM antibodies.

10. Which of the following tests is the most specific during the early phase of Lyme disease?
    a. IFA
    b. EIA
    c. Immunoblotting
    d. Detection of *B. burgdorferi* DNA by PCR

11. False-positive serological tests for Lyme disease may be caused by all of the following *except*
    a. shared antigens between *Borrelia* groups.
    b. cross-reactivity of antibodies.
    c. resemblance of flagellar antigen to that of *Treponema* organisms.
    d. a patient in the early stage of the disease.

12. A 24-year-old man who had just recovered from infectious mononucleosis had evidence of a genital lesion. His RPR test was positive. What should the technologist do next?
    a. Report out as false positive.
    b. Do a confirmatory treponemal test.
    c. Do a VDRL.
    d. Have the patient return in 2 weeks for a repeat test.

13. A 15-year-old girl returned from a camping trip. Approximately a week after her return, she discovered a small red area on her leg that had a larger red ring around it. Her physician had her tested for Lyme disease, but the serological test was negative. What is the best explanation for these results?
    a. She definitely does not have Lyme disease.
    b. The test was not performed correctly.
    c. Antibody response is often below the level of detection in early stages.
    d. Too much antibody was present, causing a false negative.

14. The reverse screening algorithm for syphilis testing
    a. is the CDC-preferred algorithm.
    b. is more labor intensive than the "traditional" method.
    c. has a significant number of false positives that must be resolved by doing a TP-PA test.
    d. is more prone to transcription errors in reporting.

15. All of the following statements are true for leptospirosis *except*
    a. It is caused by tightly coiled spirochetes under the genus *Leptospira.*
    b. Infection is zoonotic in nature.
    c. Leptospires cannot be cultured on artificial culture media.
    d. It is one of the nationally reportable diseases.

16. Which of the following specimens provides the most reliable means of detecting leptospires during the first week of infection?
    a. Urine
    b. Liver biopsy
    c. Blood
    d. Conjunctival swab

17. Which of the following statements regarding transmission of leptospirosis is *not* true?
    a. Infection can be acquired by coming into contact with urine-contaminated soil or water.
    b. People working in rat-infested areas run a high risk of contracting the infection.
    c. High-risk activities include swimming or wading in water bodies contaminated with animal urine.
    d. Person-to-person contact is a significant means of contracting the infection.

18. The gold standard method for diagnosis of leptospirosis is
    a. culturing the specimen on Fletcher semisolid or Stuart liquid media.
    b. enzyme-linked immunosorbent assay (ELISA).
    c. microscopic agglutination test (MAT).
    d. dark-field or phase contrast microscopy.

22

Serological and Molecular Diagnosis of Parasitic and Fungal Infections

James L. Vossler, MS, MLS^CM(ASCP)SM^CM

LEARNING OUTCOMES

After finishing this chapter, you should be able to:

1. Explain why a host has more difficulty overcoming parasitic diseases than those caused by bacteria or viruses.
2. Discuss potential outcomes of host and parasite interactions.
3. Cite strategies used by parasites to evade host defenses.
4. Discuss the role of immunoglobulin E (IgE) antibody and eosinophils in parasitic infections.
5. Discuss the roles of serological and molecular assays in the diagnosis of parasitic infections.
6. Discuss the role serology plays in the diagnosis of *Toxoplasma gondii* and cite the limitations of serological testing for toxoplasmosis in the newborn.
7. List possible limitations associated with parasitic serology.
8. Cite the role that rapid antigen detection systems (RDTS) play in the detection of parasitic diseases.
9. Briefly describe the principle of lateral flow assays.
10. List factors that have led to a notable increase in fungal infections in the past 25 years.
11. Describe the etiological and physiological factors to be examined when a mycosis is suspected.
12. Cite the four types of clinical manifestations that fungi can produce.
13. Describe the types of immune defenses mounted by the host in response to fungal infections and identify the immune response that plays the most important role in responding to a fungal infection.
14. Discuss the role of serological and molecular testing in the diagnosis of fungal infections.
15. Recognize the clinical diseases and epidemiology of aspergillosis, candidiasis, cryptococcosis, histoplasmosis, and coccidioidomycosis.

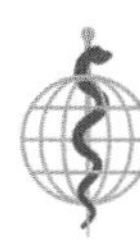

Go to FADavis.com for the laboratory exercises that accompany this text.

CHAPTER OUTLINE

KEY TERMS

Antigenic concealment	Conidia	Lateral flow assays
Antigenic mimicry	Cryptococcosis	Mycelial fungi
Antigenic shedding	Ectoparasites	Mycosis (mycoses)
Antigen switching	Fungi	Parasites
Antigenic variation	Helminths	Protozoa
Aspergillosis	Histoplasmosis	Rapid antigen detection systems (RDTS)
C-type lectin receptors (CLRs)	Hyphae	Toll-like receptors (TLRs)
Candidiasis	Immunologic diversion	Yeast
Coccidioidomycosis	Immunologic subversion	*Toxoplasma gondii*

The detection and diagnosis of fungal and parasitic infections rely on laboratory methods as well as the patient's clinical symptoms, medical history, geographic location, and travel history. The laboratory detection of fungal infections has relied on culture, direct microscopy, and histopathology for many decades. The laboratory identification of parasitic infections primarily relies on microscopy and has changed little since the development of the microscope in the 15th century. However, technological advancements have provided newer methodologies that are an improvement over conventional methods for the detection of both fungal and parasitic infections. Direct antigen detection, molecular assays, and newer serological assays have emerged. Although the sensitivity and specificity of serological assays for fungal and parasitic infections have improved over the years, the antigens used in parasitic and fungal assays are often cruder than those used in tests for viral and bacterial diagnosis, and antibodies raised against one parasite protein may cross-react with proteins from other species, thus decreasing their specificity.

Because of the advancements made in molecular technologies, there has been a focus on the development of molecular diagnostic techniques for detecting various parasitic and fungal agents responsible for human infections. A relatively new technology that shows promise in being able to diagnose fungal infections is the use of proteomics (see Chapter 20).

Despite the development of newer assays, the diagnosis of parasitic and fungal infections still remains a challenge. In many cases, the clinical presentations overlap or are nonspecific. Because of the shared antigenicity of several genera and species, the ability to distinguish a specific causative agent based on serology is sometimes not possible. Many fungal infections are opportunistic infections that occur in individuals who are immunocompromised. As such, those individuals may not mount a humoral antibody response, limiting the utility of serologically based assays. In addition, many of the parasitic diseases occur in impoverished countries. Because of the lack of resources and expertise in these countries, the development and use of serological assays has been hindered. Finally, for many of the agents, diagnostic serological or molecular assays are not available. This chapter provides information on the immunologic aspects of parasitic and fungal infections along with a discussion of available serological and molecular assays for the detection of the organisms that cause these infections.

Parasitic Immunology

Parasites are microorganisms that survive by living off of other organisms, referred to as *hosts*. Three types of organisms may cause parasitic infections: protozoa, helminths, and ectoparasites. **Protozoa** are a diverse group of single-celled organisms that can live and multiply inside of human hosts. Giardiasis is an example of a protozoal infection that can occur from drinking water infected with the parasites. **Helminths,** or parasitic worms, are multicelled organisms that can live either alone or in humans. They include flatworms, tapeworms, and roundworms. **Ectoparasites** are multicelled organisms that live on the skin. Common ectoparasites infecting humans include *Pediculus humanus capitis* (head lice), *Pthirus pubis* (pubic lice or crabs), and *Sarcoptes scabiei* (scabies). Other ectoparasites include fleas, ticks, and mites.

In many areas of the globe, parasitic diseases are on the rise, particularly in the tropic and subtropic regions, because of rapid and unplanned growth in the cities. The World Health Organization (WHO) reported that globally, one-third of all deaths are caused by infectious and parasitic diseases. In 2017, malaria alone was estimated to be the cause of 219 million infections and 435,000 deaths. Whereas malaria is well known for its impact in the developing world, there are several neglected tropical diseases (NTDs) that cause significant morbidity and mortality around the globe. A vast majority of the NTDs are caused by parasites. These diseases include leishmaniasis, schistosomiasis (snail fever), African trypanosomiasis (sleeping sickness), onchocerciasis (river blindness), and lymphatic filariasis (elephantiasis). In the United States, trichomoniasis, giardiasis, cryptosporidiosis, and toxoplasmosis are the most common parasitic infections.

Although effective vaccines have been developed for bacterial and viral agents, the development of vaccines for parasitic diseases has remained elusive. A variety of roadblocks have hindered the development of vaccines against parasitic agents. Parasites are complex organisms, many with elaborate life cycles; over time, they have developed well-honed mechanisms

Table 22–1 Potential Outcomes of Host and Parasite Interactions

LEVEL	HOST AND PARASITE INTERACTION	DESCRIPTION
1	Natural resistance	No invasion of host by parasite
2	Symbiosis	Colonization of host with parasite with benefit to both
3	Commensalism	Colonization of host with parasite with no benefit or harm
4	Sterilizing immunity	Parasite invades host and causes disease; host develops immunity and is cured
5	Concomitant immunity	Parasite invades host and causes disease; host develops an immune response and has some resistance to the parasite but is not cured
6	Ineffective immunity	Parasite invades host and causes disease; host does not develop resistance to the parasite and is not cured

Adapted from Playfair JHL. Effective and ineffective immune responses to parasites: evidence from experimental models. Curr Top Microbiol Immunol. *1978;80:37–64.*

for immune evasion. In addition, the immune responses to parasitic organisms are not fully understood, which also contributes to the lack of vaccine development in this area. This chapter covers the various strategies used by parasites to evade the immune response and survive in a host, as well as the use of serological and molecular techniques in the diagnosis of parasitic diseases.

The immune responses to bacterial infections are more clearly understood than the immune responses to parasitic infections. Bacteria are unicellular organisms with relatively simple life cycles. In addition, there is limited epitope variation in bacteria, allowing for the immune system to mount a response more easily. The immune response to parasitic infections differs from that associated with bacterial infections, mostly because of the multicellular nature of parasites. Chandra described general concepts that need to be considered in relation to host immune responses to parasites: (1) Heterogeneity with respect to life cycles and antigenic expression is a key feature of parasitic agents. (2) Many parasitic infections are chronic in nature. (3) The mechanisms of immune evasion are significantly different from those of bacterial infections. (4) Many parasites develop significant genetic and antigenic variation in a relatively short period. (5) The innate immunity in the natural hosts may be genetically determined. (6) Humans, as well as animals, differ widely in their ability to handle the complex antigens found in parasites.

Immune Responses to Parasites

When an organism encounters a host, the eventual outcome depends on a variety of factors. These include the number of organisms or size of the inoculum, the multiplication rate of the organism, and the virulence factors possessed by the organism. The degree to which the organism establishes an infection or is eradicated by the host depends on the organism's ability to mobilize sufficient host defenses for removal or the organism's ability to overcome those defense mechanisms.

If the parasite is able to establish itself, one of several possible outcomes may occur: death of the host, eradication of the parasite, or as is the case in the majority of parasitic infections, establishment of a persistent infection. The interaction and outcomes that parasites have within their hosts have been categorized into six different levels **(Table 22–1)**.

The most severe outcome is that the host is killed. Death of the host may be caused by a variety of reasons, ranging from the parasite overwhelming the host defenses to specific features of the parasite that contribute to the death of the host. One such example is *Plasmodium falciparum*. *P. falciparum* rapidly multiplies in the host and produces an erythrocyte membrane protein-1 (PfEMP1) that binds to the endothelium in the blood vessels, resulting in the small blood vessels becoming clogged. When this occurs in the brain, the result is cerebral malaria, which can be fatal.

Death of the host is not the best strategy for a parasite. If the parasite were to totally elude the host immune system and was sufficiently virulent, the parasite would kill the host on which its survival depends. If the host dies, then so does the parasite. Any parasite's survival depends on its ability to live in a peaceful manner with its host while living and feeding off the host.

Defenses to parasitic infection involve both innate and acquired (adaptive) immune mechanisms. The innate or nonspecific immune response may result in the destruction and removal of the parasite, thus preventing establishment of an infection. The nonspecific immune defenses can include activation of cells that may destroy the parasite by phagocytosis, release of cytokines that enhance the immune response (e.g., tumor necrosis factor alpha [TNF-α], interleukin-1 [IL]-1, type I interferons, and chemokines), or activation of the complement system, resulting in enhanced recognition by the immune system (see Chapters 2, 6, and 7). Similar to other organisms that may cause infection or disease, parasites have evolved strategies to evade natural nonadaptive host defenses. These include killing or avoiding being killed by phagocytes, interfering with complement's alternative pathway, producing iron-binding molecules, and blocking interferons.

If innate immunity is unsuccessful in eliminating the parasite, the parasite may be eliminated through activation of the adaptive immune responses. This results in either a humoral or a cell-mediated response to the parasite (see Chapter 4). In some parasites, complete immunity can be achieved through the humoral immune response. Specific antibodies can damage protozoa, neutralize parasites by blocking attachment to the host cell, prevent the spread of the parasite, promote complement lysis, enhance phagocytosis, and destroy the parasite through antibody-dependent cellular cytotoxicity (ADCC). Many parasitic infections are characterized by eosinophilia and high levels of immunoglobulin E (IgE). The IgE antibody binds to mast cells and basophils in the host (see Chapter 14). When specific antigen–antibody combinations occur, mast cells degranulate and release chemotactic factors, histamine, prostaglandins, and other mediators. One of the most important mediators released is eosinophil chemotactic factor, which attracts eosinophils to the infected area. Eosinophils can destroy some parasites by degranulation or through ADCC. Scientists believe that the ability to produce IgE evolved mainly to protect the host from parasitic infections. Studies indicate that high levels of anti-parasitic IgE correlate with resistance to reinfection by the parasite.

Connections

IgE Antibodies and Parasites

IgE antibodies are best known for their role in allergic reactions (see Chapter 14). However, they also play an important role in the defense against parasites such as helminths, which are too large to be phagocytized. Killing of the parasites is accomplished by ADCC. In this mechanism, parasite-specific IgE antibodies bind to the parasite, and the Fc portions of these antibodies bind to specific receptors on the surface of eosinophils, which are then stimulated to release enzymes from their granules that destroy the parasite. The concentration of IgE and the number of eosinophils in the peripheral blood are increased, indicating their importance in defense against parasitic infections.

Parasite Survival Strategies

In many host and parasite relationships, the host's adaptive defenses reduce the parasite load to low levels; however, they fail to eliminate the parasite completely, and transmission continues. For example, schistosomes (a type of helminth) have mechanisms that can downregulate the host's immune system. This immune modulation promotes the parasite's survival but also limits severe damage to the host. Therefore, adult schistosomes can live in the human host for up to 40 years before finally being eliminated.

Parasites have developed a variety of strategies to evade adaptive defenses that are more complicated than those for evading innate defenses. Survival strategies include antigenic concealment, antigenic variation, antigenic shedding, antigenic mimicry, immunologic diversion, and immunologic subversion.

In **antigenic concealment,** parasites hide their antigens from the host. One way in which parasites can conceal their antigens is by remaining inside of the host's cells without their antigens being displayed. If a parasite becomes sequestered within host cells, the parasite is hidden from the immune system and protected. Most parasites infect only a few cell types in their host. To infect a host, the parasite must reach its specific target cell. Once the parasite reaches its target cell, some parasites have developed strategies for entering and surviving within the host cell. The host cannot recognize the parasites while they reside inside cells. Examples of parasites that have an intracellular phase in their life cycle include *Plasmodium* species, *Trypanosoma cruzi, Leishmania,* and *Cryptosporidium parvum.*

Another process of evasion some parasites employ is **antigenic variation.** Evasion from the immune response depends on variation occurring in the parasite antigens that are recognized by the host's immune system. There are three main mechanisms for antigenic variation. The first mechanism involves the parasite's ability to generate novel antigens by random mutation. Some parasites have evolved mechanisms by which random mutations occur with a frequency sufficient to evade the immune system on an ongoing basis. An example of this is the antigenic variation of the malaria parasite through single-nucleotide replacement. The second mechanism of antigenic variation may occur through genetic recombination. Rearrangement of genes within an organism allows for the development and expression of new epitopes on the surface of the parasite for which a previous immune response has not taken place. The ability to rearrange genes and rapidly change surface molecules contributes to the virulence of *P. falciparum* and *T. cruzi.* The third mechanism is gene switching. Gene switching is the most dramatic form of antigenic variation observed in parasites. Organisms may carry upwards of one thousand different genes, allowing for the expression of distinct surface molecules. An organism employing this mechanism can switch from the use of one gene to another, thus persisting while the immune system is trying to catch up with it. Examples of parasites that use this mechanism are the trypanosomes *Trypanosoma gambiense* and *Trypanosoma rhodesiense.* These organisms are able to alter their surface glycoproteins to produce an unlimited group of variable antigen types. The process begins when the host produces antibody, mainly immunoglobulin M (IgM), to a parasite antigen, thereby reducing the infection. The parasite responds by swapping genes, thus changing its antigen and making the antibody ineffective. Gene switching may occur very rapidly, within 5 to 6 days. The host must then produce a new antibody. This process of **antigen switching** can continue for long periods of time.

A factor that must be considered with respect to antigenic variation is the parasite's life cycle. Parasites are large organisms compared with bacteria and viruses. Furthermore, they have complex life cycles and are antigenically diverse. The parasite's development and progression through its life cycle are adapted to the physiology and behavior of the host. Not all of the phases of a parasite's life cycle necessarily occur in one host. A particular host may be the *definitive host* that harbors the adult or sexual stage of the parasite (e.g., humans are the only definitive host for *Taenia saginata* and *Taenia solium*—the beef and pork tapeworms, respectively), an *intermediate host* in which the parasite lives during the larval or asexual stage (e.g., the malarial parasites in which humans are the intermediate host), or an *accidental* or *dead-end host* in which a relationship is not required for propagation or continuation of the parasite (e.g., *Echinococcus granulosus,* the causative agent of hydatid cysts, in which humans are the dead-end host).

Many parasites have complex life cycles that involve several hosts. Different antigens may be expressed, depending on the life-cycle stage in the different hosts. The parasite often undergoes complex growth cycles and differentiation in preparation for transmission to its next host. In doing so, an organism's surface antigens vary considerably while in a single host. For example, protozoa of the genus *Leishmania* can cause the development of skin sores or invade internal organs such as the spleen, liver, and bone marrow. The parasite is transmitted to humans by female sand flies that have been infected after sucking blood from an infected human or animal. In humans, the parasite is transformed from the promastigote stage in the blood to the amastigote stage when it invades the tissues. The presence of different antigens on the different developmental forms of the parasite can delay the effectiveness of the immune response and lead to severe illness.

In addition to variation of antigen expression, parasites may evade the immune system through antigen shedding. Similar to bacteria that shed capsular material into the host environment to evade the immune system, some parasites also exhibit **antigenic shedding**. *Entamoeba histolytica* is one example of a parasite that can shed antigens from its cell surface. Although antibody is formed against the parasite, the antibody attaches to the shed antigen rather than the parasite, allowing the parasite to escape the immune response.

Antigenic mimicry may occur when the parasite expresses epitopes that are similar, if not identical, to host molecules. The similarity between host and parasitic antigens may suppress the immune response and protect the invading parasite from being recognized and eliminated by the immune system. An example is the antigenic similarity between human host antigens and those of the *Schistosoma* species. The immune response may result in host and parasite cross-reactivity, which may lead to autoimmunity, manifested by the presence of autoantibodies or T cells capable of reacting with host antigens. An autoimmune response has been linked to the cardiac and intestinal symptoms that occur in the late stages of Chagas disease that may occur because of an infection with *T. cruzi,* a bloodborne parasite.

Some organisms enhance their survival by modulating the immune system. The ability to modulate the immune response is an important strategy employed by some parasites to enable their survival in the host. Some parasites can subvert the immune system. **Immunologic subversion** is achieved by avoiding the effector mechanisms of the immune response. Effector molecules include complement and cytokines. Effector cells include plasma cells, T helper (Th) cells, and cytotoxic T cells. For example, some parasites can subvert cytotoxic T cells by producing decoy human leukocyte antigen (HLA) molecules. Parasites may also subvert the Fc function of antibodies by making Fc receptor homologues, or they can subvert complement by making homologues of complement control proteins (CCPs). **Immunologic diversion** occurs when the parasite causes the immune system to produce proteins that divert the attention of the immune system. An example is the ability of some parasites to cause an increase in production of beta interferon (IFN-β), which allows for increased parasite survival. For example, IFN-β has been shown to decrease the ability of macrophages to kill *Leishmania* by significantly reducing the release of superoxide from these cells. Another example by which parasites can divert the immune system is seen with *P. falciparum*–infected erythrocytes (IEs), which have the potential to interact with B cells in different parts of the body, inducing them to divide and differentiate into antibody-secreting cells. The malaria parasite and some protozoa, viruses, and bacteria produce immunoglobulin-binding proteins (IBPs) that act as polyclonal B-cell activators. This results in the expansion of numerous B-cell clones and in antibody production not specific for the parasite. Thus, the IBPs may act as an evasion mechanism to divert specific antibody responses.

Serodiagnosis of Parasitic Diseases

In instances where demonstration of the parasite in biological or tissue samples is not possible, serological testing is the gold standard for diagnosis. Serological-based assays can be divided into those that detect parasitic *antigens* and those that detect *antibodies* against the parasite. These tests include enzyme-linked immunosorbent assays (ELISAs), indirect immunofluorescence, indirect hemagglutination, whole protozoan or antigen-coated particle agglutination, radioimmunoassays (now rarely used), and newer rapid diagnostic tests (RDTs). Previously, many of these assays used relatively crude antigens, making their sensitivity and specificity unpredictable. Advances in immunochemistry and molecular biology have allowed for the development of assays that have markedly improved sensitivity and specificity. However, assays utilizing these newer technologies are costly and not widely available in those countries that have the highest occurrence of parasitic diseases.

ELISA-based assays have been used to detect antigens of parasites that cause human and animal infections, such as amebiasis, babesiosis, fascioliasis, cutaneous and visceral leishmaniasis, cysticercosis, echinococcosis, malaria, schistosomiasis, toxocariasis, toxoplasmosis, trichinosis, and trypanosomiasis.

Whereas some parasitic diseases are readily diagnosed by demonstrating the causative agent in clinical material, such as infection with intestinal helminths, in which the worm's eggs are easily detected in fecal specimens, demonstration of other parasitic agents is difficult or not possible (e.g., toxoplasmosis). In those cases, serological assays can be very useful. **Table 22–2** indicates the usefulness of serological testing for the diagnosis of various parasitic diseases. Although serology may not be helpful in the diagnosis of some parasitic diseases, serology can play a role in epidemiological investigations.

Table 22–2 Usefulness of Antibody Detection for Parasitic Diseases

SEROLOGY INDICATED	SEROLOGY MAY BE USEFUL	SEROLOGY NOT INDICATED
Amebiasis (extraintestinal)	Amebiasis	Anisakiasis
Chagas disease	Amebic meningoencephalitis (caused by free-living amebae)	Ascariasis
Clonorchiasis	Anaplasmosis/Ehrlichiosis	Capillariasis
Cysticercosis	Babesiosis	Cryptosporidiosis
Hydatidosis	Malaria	Hookworm
Filariasis (lymphatic; suspect cases when microfilariae cannot be identified in blood)	Paragonimiasis (eggs not detectable in sputum or feces)	Trichuriasis
Leishmaniasis (cutaneous and visceral)		
Schistosomiasis (ectopic cases; chronic cases when eggs cannot be demonstrated in feces or urine)		
Toxocariasis (visceral and ocular)		
Toxoplasmosis		
Trichinellosis		

Adapted from Maddison SE. Serodiagnosis of parasitic diseases. Clin Microbiol Rev. *1991;4(4):457–469.*

Toxoplasmosis

Although advances have been made in the serological assays for some parasites, commercially available ELISAs still vary considerably in their sensitivity and specificity. One such example is the detection of antibodies against the protozoan ***Toxoplasma gondii.*** *T. gondii* has a high prevalence around the world and can infect all species of animals and birds. An estimated 11% of the U.S. population over the age of 6 is infected with this parasite, which usually remains dormant. Reactivation may occur if the individual becomes immunosuppressed. Members of the cat family *(Felidae)* serve as the definitive hosts for *T. gondii.*

The life cycle of *T. gondii* has three stages: the *tachyzoite,* which rapidly multiplies in the intermediate host (e.g., humans) and in nonintestinal epithelial cells of the definitive host (e.g., the cat); the *bradyzoite,* which forms the tissue cysts; and the *sporozoite,* which is found in the oocyst **(Fig. 22–1).** There are three routes by which *T. gondii* is potentially transmitted to humans. Humans can become infected with *T. gondii* by eating raw or insufficiently cooked infected meat (e.g., pork, mutton, or wild game) that contains the cysts or uncooked foods that have come into contact with the infected meat. Toxoplasmosis may also occur when humans ingest oocysts from cat feces present in a litter box or in the soil. Third, the tachyzoites, which are observed during the primary infection, can be transmitted transplacentally to the unborn fetus **(Fig. 22–2).** The incubation period for *T. gondii* in adults ranges from 10 to 23 days following ingestion of undercooked meat and from 5 to 20 days after ingestion of oocysts from cat feces. Following infection, the organism reproduces asexually and forms tissue cysts that remain for the life of the host. In the immunocompetent individual, a majority of initial *Toxoplasma* infections are asymptomatic or may only present with a mild lymphadenopathy. Immunity is usually sufficient to contain the latent infection. Toxoplasmosis can cause serious symptoms in the brain and other organs in immunocompromised patients, as well as in the developing fetus following congenital infection.

If the individual becomes immunosuppressed because of HIV infection, malignancy, or immunosuppressive drugs, reactivated toxoplasmosis can occur. The tissue cysts rupture and release the active bradyzoite, which results in clinical disease. *T. gondii* infection in the immunocompromised individual can be severe or even fatal. In immunosuppressed individuals, the organism can invade the central nervous system (CNS), leading to toxoplasma encephalitis. Over 95% of the cases are caused by reactivation of a latent infection.

Another concern is the organism's ability to be passed to the fetus during pregnancy. If a mother has been infected before pregnancy occurs, then the fetus is protected because of maternal antibodies. However, if the woman becomes infected just before or during pregnancy, congenital transmission of the organism can occur. Congenital toxoplasmosis may result in a miscarriage, a stillborn child, or mental deficits later on in life. Up to one-half of pregnant women who become infected can transmit *T. gondii* across the placenta. The trimester in which the infection was acquired influences the incidence and severity of congenital toxoplasmosis. The transmission risk during the first trimester of pregnancy is 10% to 25%, whereas the transmission risk is 60% to 90% during the third trimester. *Toxoplasma* infection can result from congenital infection or infection after birth.

Although the diagnosis of toxoplasmosis can be made by demonstrating the parasite in stained tissue samples or cerebrospinal fluid (CSF), diagnosis is usually made through serological means. A combination of tests needs to be performed to determine whether an individual has been recently infected or had a previous infection with *T. gondii.* The sensitivity and specificity of different commercial kits vary widely, and misinterpretation of the results, particularly in determining the presence and significance of IgM antibodies, may occur. This is concerning because serology results can influence decisions regarding continuation or termination of pregnancies. IgM antibodies may persist for up to 18 months after infection

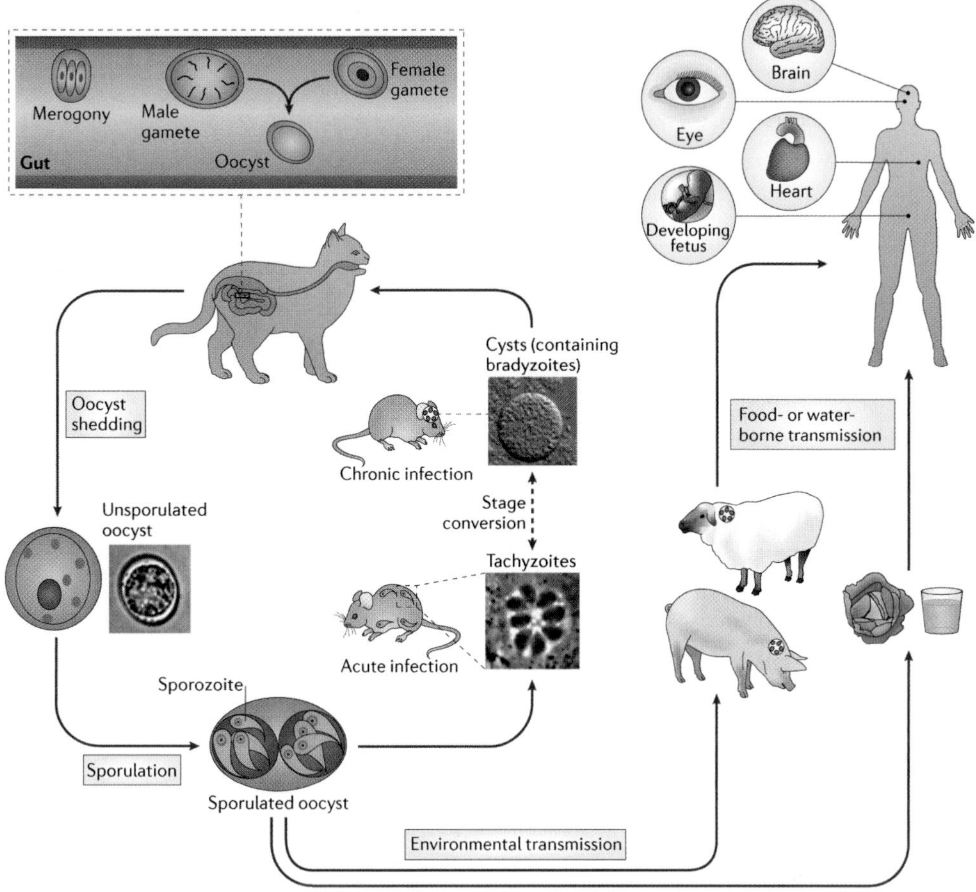

FIGURE 22–1 *Toxoplasma gondii* life cycle. Sexual replication of *T. gondii* occurs in cats, the definitive host for the parasite. *T. gondii* gametes are formed after merozoites replicate within enterocytes of the cat gut, a process known as *merogony*. The gametes fuse to form diploid oocysts, which are shed in cat feces and undergo meiosis in the environment to produce eight haploid progeny sporozoites. Asexual replication occurs in intermediate hosts such as rodents. Rapidly replicating forms called *tachyzoites* disseminate within the host during acute infection and can differentiate into slow-growing forms called *bradyzoites* inside tissue cysts. Other intermediate hosts or cats can acquire the infection by ingesting the tissue cysts, re-initiating the sexual phase of the life cycle. Oocysts can survive in the environment for a long time and develop into sporulated oocysts, which can be transmitted to intermediate hosts such as farm animals through contaminated food and water. Humans become infected by ingesting tissue cysts in undercooked meat or sporulated oocysts in contaminated water. *(Reprinted by permission from Macmillan Publishers Ltd: Nature Reviews Microbiology, 10:766–778, copyright 2012.)*

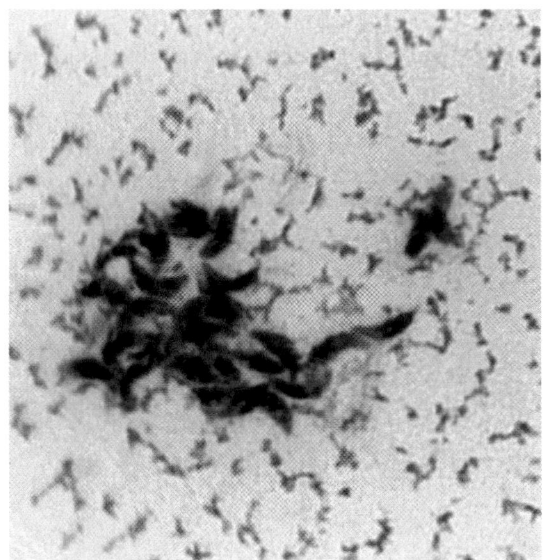

FIGURE 22–2 *Toxoplasma gondii* tachyzoites in mouse ascitic fluid stained with Giemsa stain. *(Courtesy of the CDC/Dr. L.L. Moore, Jr., Public Health Image Library.)*

with *T. gondii*. Therefore, the U.S. Food and Drug Administration (FDA) has recommended that anti-*Toxoplasma* IgM tests should be interpreted with caution and that the sole results of a single assay should not be used in determining a recent infection. The FDA has published guidelines for the interpretation of *T. gondii* serology results **(Table 22–3)**.

The greatest value of testing for IgM antibodies is in determining whether a woman has had a recent infection. If no IgM antibodies are detected and only immunoglobulin G (IgG) is detected, this excludes a recent infection before pregnancy. One of the problems when testing for *Toxoplasma*-specific IgM antibodies is that the current assays lack specificity. If only IgM antibodies are detected, additional testing should be performed. A second blood sample should be obtained from the patient 2 weeks after the first sample is collected and tested together with the first specimen. The second sample should demonstrate high levels of IgM and IgG antibodies if the first sample was collected early in the infection. If both specimens show the presence of IgM but absence of IgG, the IgM result should be considered to be a false positive.

Table 22-3 General Guidelines for Interpretation of *Toxoplasma gondii* Serology Results

IgG RESULT	IgM RESULT	REPORT AND INTERPRETATION (EXCEPT INFANTS)
Negative	Negative	No serological evidence of infection with *Toxoplasma*.
Negative	Equivocal	Possible early acute infection or false-positive IgM result. Obtain new specimen for IgM and IgG testing. If result for the second specimen remains the same, the patient is probably not infected with *Toxoplasma*.
Negative	Positive	Possible acute infection or possible false-positive IgM result. Obtain new specimen for IgM and IgG testing. If result for the second specimen remains the same, the IgM reaction is probably a false positive.
Equivocal	Negative	Indeterminate: obtain a new specimen for testing or retest this specimen for IgG using a different assay.
Equivocal	Equivocal	Indeterminate: obtain a new specimen for IgM and IgG testing.
Equivocal	Positive	Possible acute infection with *Toxoplasma*. Obtain new specimen for IgM and IgG testing. If the result for the second specimen remains the same or if the IgG becomes positive, both specimens should be sent to a reference laboratory with experience in diagnosing *Toxoplasma* infection.
Positive	Negative	Infected with *Toxoplasma* for 6 months or longer.
Positive	Equivocal	Infected with *Toxoplasma* for probably more than 1 year or false-positive IgM reaction. Obtain a new specimen for IgM testing. If results with the second specimen remain the same, both specimens should be sent to a reference laboratory with experience in diagnosing *Toxoplasma* infection.
Positive	Positive	Possible recent infection within the past 12 months or false-positive IgM result. Send the specimen to a reference laboratory with experience in diagnosing *Toxoplasma* infection.

Adapted from Centers for Disease Control and Prevention. DPDx—Laboratory identification of parasitic diseases of public health concern: toxoplasmosis. https://www.cdc.gov/dpdx/toxoplasmosis/index.html. Accessed July 9, 2019.

When both IgM and IgG antibodies are detected and the patient is pregnant, an IgG avidity test should be performed. Determination of the avidity of the antibody has proven useful in determining whether the IgG antibodies are from a recent infection or a previous infection. The presence of high-avidity IgG indicates an infection in the past, whereas IgG antibodies with a low avidity suggest a more recent infection. Although low avidity antibodies may persist for a prolonged period of time, their presence does not necessarily mean that the infection was recently acquired. However, the presence of high-avidity antibodies indicates an infection for at least 3 to 5 months and does not pose a risk to the fetus. The ELISA for IgG avidity utilizes a wash buffer containing urea to differentiate low-avidity from high-avidity antibodies. Antibodies with low avidity dissociate from the antigen in the presence of urea. The avidity is determined by running the assay in duplicate using buffer with and without urea. The avidity index (AI) is determined by dividing the *T. gondii*–specific IgG signal (optical density; O.D.) of the set washed with urea-containing buffer by the *T. gondii*–specific IgG O.D. of the set washed with non-urea buffer. AI values lower than 0.20 indicate the presence of low-avidity antibodies, values between 0.20 and 0.25 suggest intermediate avidity, and values greater than 0.25 are obtained with antibodies of high avidity.

Connections

High-Avidity Antibodies

The avidity of an antibody molecule represents the strength by which its antigen-binding sites can bind to an antigen. During the course of an immune response, somatic mutations occur in the immunoglobulin genes in the B cells, causing them to produce antibodies of higher avidity. This results in tight binding of the antibodies to the antigen, similar to a lock and key. The presence of high-avidity antibodies is a sign that the immune response has been going on for quite some time (see Chapter 5).

When using serology to detect congenital toxoplasmosis, several differences exist. Because of the passive transfer of IgG across the placenta, infants whose mothers are chronically infected will be born with toxoplasma IgG antibodies of maternal origin. Serological diagnosis can be made 5 or 10 days after birth by demonstration of positive *Toxoplasma* IgM or IgA antibody titers, respectively, in newborn sera. Detection of anti-*Toxoplasma* IgA antibodies is more sensitive than detection of IgM antibodies. It should be noted that commercial assays currently used in the United States have not been cleared by the FDA for diagnostic testing of infants. Therefore, samples from neonates suspected of having congenital toxoplasmosis should be sent to the Toxoplasma Serology Laboratory, Palo Alto, California, the site that has the most experience with infant testing.

Rapid Antigen Detection Systems (RDTS)

Rapid antigen detection systems (RDTS) (also called **lateral flow assays**) are based on immunochromatographic antigen detection and are widely used in many diagnostic laboratories. RDTS detect soluble proteins through their ability to bind to capture antibodies contained in a nitrocellulose strip (see Chapter 11). The clinical sample is placed on the strip and eluted by adding a few drops of buffer that contains a labeled antibody. A colored band representing the antigen–antibody complex can then be seen on the membrane. Many of the assays are stable at room temperature, easy to perform and interpret, and cost effective. Many clinical laboratories have discontinued the use of ELISAs in favor of immunochromatographic assays. For example, several years ago, ELISA-based assays were the predominant platform for the detection of *Giardia* and *Cryptosporidium*. Today, many clinical laboratories are using lateral flow assays. One example is the Xpect Giardia/Cryptosporidium assay from Remel (Lexena, Kansas) **(Fig. 22–3)**.

Because of their advantages, many RDTS can be used in rural regions. Assays have also been developed for the rapid diagnosis of malaria using this platform. The assays can be used in the field and allow for differentiation between *Plasmodium vivax* and the deadlier *P. falciparum*. At the time of this writing, the BinaxNOW Malaria Test (Abbott Rapid Diagnostics) is the only available RDTS for malaria in the United States. The test detects the histidine-rich protein II (HRPII) specific to *P. falciparum* (P.f.) and a pan-malarial antigen common to all four malaria species that can infect humans—*P. falciparum, P. vivax* (P.v.), *Plasmodium ovale* (P.o.), and *Plasmodium malariae* (P.m.) **(Fig. 22–4)**.

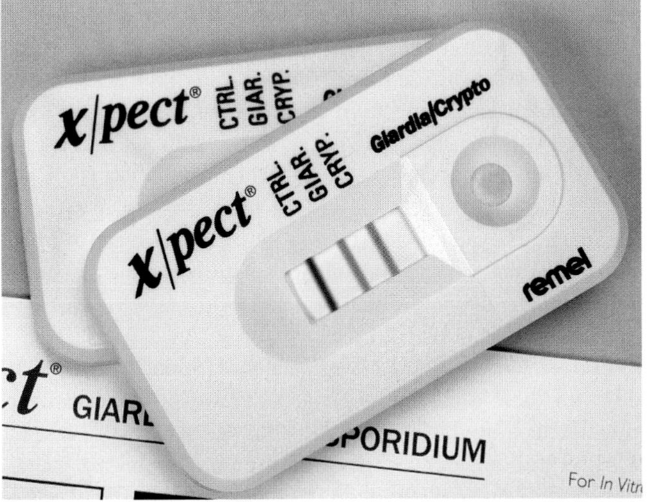

FIGURE 22–3 Remel Xpect® Giardia/Cryptosporidium immunochromatographic immunoassay. The test uses sample wicking to capture *Giardia* and *Cryptosporidium* antigens on discrete test lines containing antigen-specific antibodies for each organism. *(Reprinted by permission of Thermo Fisher Scientific, Lenexa, Kansas.)*

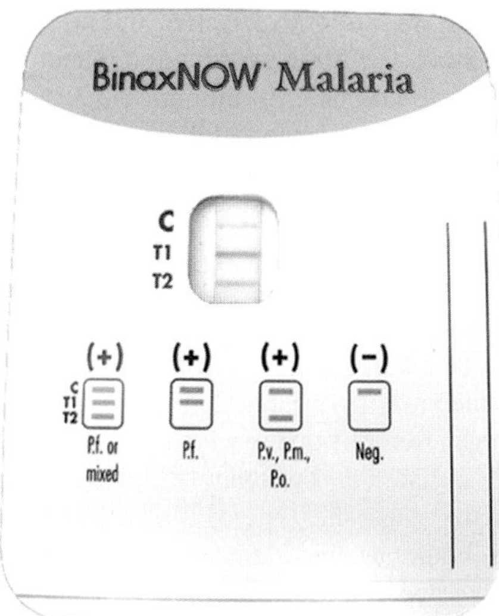

FIGURE 22–4 BinaxNOW Malaria Test. The immunochromatographic assay targets the histidine-rich protein II (HRPII) antigen specific to *Plasmodium falciparum* (P.f.) and a pan-malarial antigen common to all four malaria species capable of infecting humans—*P. falciparum, P. vivax* (P.v.), *P. ovale* (P.o.), and *P. malariae* (P.m.)—circulating in human venous and capillary ethylenediaminetetraacetic acid (EDTA) whole blood. *(Reprinted by permission of BioMed Central Ltd, Malaria Journal 14;10:300, copyright 2011.)*

Limitations of Parasitic Serology

As with all laboratory testing, it is important to use methods that are the most straightforward and cost effective for each test. However, it is also important to consider the specificity and sensitivity of the method when choosing a procedure. Currently, there is no external proficiency testing program offered in the area of parasitic serology except for the diagnosis of toxoplasmosis. Therefore, it is very difficult to evaluate the quality of commercial assays that are currently available. In the United States, commercial kit manufacturers must obtain FDA approval before selling their products. The FDA requires only that a new method be equivalent to a method that has already been approved. Researchers at the CDC have expressed concern that over time, the quality of new test kits may drift in a negative direction because a new kit may not be quite as good as the one used for comparison but may still receive approval.

In addition to the inability to evaluate an assay's performance using proficiency testing, a specific test may not detect a parasitic disease in an individual because of the inability of the assay to detect all species of the parasite causing the infection. For example, some serological tests, such as those for schistosomiasis, only detect antibodies that are species-specific. Therefore, the same sample can give a negative result in one test and a positive result in another. Also, the type of specimen submitted from a patient may give conflicting results. In one reported example, samples of serum, stool, and urine from a patient suspected of having schistosomiasis were submitted to a commercial laboratory for testing. Although the serum result was antibody negative and no parasites were found in the stool, the urine examination demonstrated eggs of *Schistosoma haematobium*. An immunoblot was positive for *S. haematobium* and negative for *Schistosoma mansoni* when the serum specimen was submitted to the CDC for blind retesting. In this example, the tests for schistosomiasis performed by the two laboratories were not equal in detecting the three *Schistosoma* species that infect humans. Situations such as these can lead to an inaccurate diagnosis.

Because of the antigenic complexity of parasites, the antibody formed may not be detected because the assay uses a different antigen from the one to which the patient has formed the antibodies. Also, the sensitivity of an assay may vary, depending on the stage and type of the patient's disease. For example, antibodies against *Plasmodium* species (malaria) rise rapidly in an acute infection but decline if the parasite becomes latent or dormant in the liver as a hypnozoite. Similarly, because of the potential for cross-reactivity of the antibodies formed in a parasitic infection, a positive result should be interpreted with caution.

Although there are commercially available tests for the serological diagnosis of several parasitic agents, only a few commercial kits are available in the United States, and they are not used by many clinical laboratories. In the United States, the majority of tests are performed by a few commercial laboratories, including Focus Technologies, Mayo Medical Laboratories, Parasitic Disease Consultants, Quest Diagnostics, and Specialty Laboratories. Most of the tests performed at the commercial laboratories and at the CDC are produced and evaluated in-house and use reagents that are not universally standardized. Because of the differences in the reagents used in the tests, discrepant results obtained by different laboratories are commonly observed.

Molecular-Based Diagnosis of Parasitic Disease

The microscopic detection and diagnosis of parasitic disease, although once considered to be the gold standard, is now recognized as having limitations in being able to detect agents responsible for parasitic infections. Decreased sensitivity associated with microscopic methods may be caused by intermittent shedding of the organism, as is seen with *Giardia lamblia,* or to low levels of the organism being present, as is observed with the bloodborne parasites such as the causative agents responsible for malaria or babesiosis. With the development of molecular-based assays, the diagnosis of parasitic infections using molecular-based technology is being used with increasing frequency. Although microscopy remains the means by which most blood and tissue parasites are detected, rapid real-time polymerase chain reaction (PCR) assays for babesiosis and malaria have recently been developed and are available from commercial reference laboratories (e.g., Mayo Medical Laboratories in Rochester, Minnesota, and Focus Diagnostics in Cypress, California) and from the CDC. At the time of this writing there are a limited number of FDA-approved molecular assays for the diagnosis and identification of gastrointestinal and blood and tissue parasites. Many laboratories have developed in-house assays for the identification and differentiation of parasites. Several new technologies, including nested multiplex PCR and loop-mediated isothermal amplification (LAMP), have the potential for the detection and identification of bloodborne and gastrointestinal parasites. Molecular tests are playing an increasingly important role as adjuncts to traditional diagnosis of parasitic infections and, in some cases, may even replace traditional methods as commercial companies develop molecular-based assays and seek FDA approval.

Fungal Immunology

Fungi represent a large heterogeneous group of eukaryotic organisms that are ubiquitous in the environment. Fungi can either be considered as parasites, deriving their nutrition from living matter, or more commonly as saprophytes, living off of dead and decaying matter. In the environment, fungi play an important role in maintaining the ecosystem with the decomposition of cellulose. At the time of this writing, there are an estimated 120,000 well-characterized fungal species. New organisms are being added as advances in molecular biology allow for the detection and differentiation of fungi. Despite the number and diversity of fungi, only about 300 fungal species are potentially pathogenic to humans and animals. Fewer than 50 of these species are responsible for approximately 90% of all fungal infections.

When a human or animal has an infection or disease caused by a fungus, it is referred to as a **mycosis** (plural: **mycoses**). Mycoses are classified into four groups—superficial, cutaneous, subcutaneous, or systemic—based on the type and amount of tissue involvement and the host response to the pathogen. Mycotic diseases are of growing importance for several reasons: (1) Fungi are widely distributed in nature and are able to maintain themselves in the environment, making them difficult to eradicate. (2) Many fungi are able to present with various clinical manifestations, ranging from invasive disease to localized infection, or allergic manifestations, as is observed with *Aspergillus*. (3) Diagnosis is difficult because of the varying clinical presentations. (4) Currently, vaccines are not available. (5) There are only a limited number of antifungal agents available for treating fungal infections. (6) Most fungal infections are opportunistic in nature, and increasingly, treatment of a primary disease puts individuals at risk for opportunistic infections.

Fungi do not possess a large array of virulence factors that allow for them to be true pathogens. However, opportunistic fungal infections have risen in recent years with the advent of AIDS and our increasing use of immunosuppressive therapies. Fungal diseases are often the first opportunistic diseases detected in patients with AIDS. One of the most common opportunistic diseases in AIDS patients is pneumonia caused by *Pneumocystis jirovecii* (previously *Pneumocystis carinii*). Although originally classified as a parasite, this organism now is designated a fungus in that it has a greater gene sequence homology with fungi than with parasites. Many saprophytic fungi formerly dismissed as cultural contaminants are now reported as opportunistic pathogens.

Characteristics of Fungi

Fungi are eukaryotic cells with nuclei and rigid cell walls composed primarily of chitin, glucans, mannans, and glycoproteins. Fungi can exist in two morphological states. They may exist as **yeast,** which are unicellular organisms, or as **mycelial fungi,** which are multicellular organisms. Yeast reproduce by budding, whereas the mycelial fungi reproduce through the production of spores or **conidia.** It should be noted that many individuals develop allergies to the spores and conidia produced by fungi. Although most fungi are *monomorphic* (existing in a single form), several fungi can exist as either yeast or mycelial fungi, depending on environmental conditions, and are referred to as *dimorphic* fungi.

Fungi grow more slowly than most bacteria (2 to 4 weeks versus 1 to 2 days) and have relatively simple nutritional requirements. Because most fungi are found in the environment, they prefer cooler temperatures to grow (25°C to 30°C).

Classification of Mycotic Infections (Mycoses)

Fungi can produce four types of clinical manifestations. Some individuals exhibit *hypersensitivity* to certain fungal agents. The hypersensitivity reaction generally occurs because of an allergic reaction to the spores. Hypersensitivity may occur only when an individual comes in contact with the specific spores he or she is allergic to, or it can occur as a chronic condition such as allergic bronchopulmonary aspergillosis (ABPA), which develops in response to the fungus *Aspergillus* (most commonly *Aspergillus fumigatus*). Fungi may also be responsible for *mycotoxicosis,* a poisoning of humans and animals by food products contaminated by fungi that produce toxins from a grain substrate. Major mycotoxins include aflatoxins, deoxynivalenol, fumonisins, zearalenone, T-2 toxin, ochratoxin, and certain ergot alkaloids. Mushrooms are classified as fungi. Thus, another type of disease that fungi can be responsible for is *mycetismus,* or mushroom poisoning, when the ingestion of toxin-producing mushrooms occurs. Potentially deadly mushrooms include *Amanita phalloides, Amanita verna, Amanita virosa,* and certain other species that contain neurotoxins.

The fourth type of mycotic disease is infection with clinical manifestations caused by the presence or growth of the fungi on or in the host tissue. Grouping the fungi according to their clinical manifestation is useful, both from a diagnostic standpoint and to facilitate identification of the agents in the laboratory. The *superficial* mycoses are fungal diseases that are restricted to the outer layers of the skin. These infections are cosmetic in nature and are not life threatening. *Cutaneous* mycoses are those infections that involve the keratinized body areas (skin, hair, nails) and rarely invade deeper tissue. Although not life threatening, these infections produce itchiness and cracking of the skin. Diseases of hair and nails are termed *dermatomycoses.* The fungi involved are called *dermatophytes* and can be transmitted through direct contact with an infected person or animal. The *subcutaneous* mycoses affect the subcutaneous tissue, where they usually form deep, ulcerated skin lesions. The causative agents are soil saprophytes, and acquisition of the fungal agent is generally caused by trauma to the skin, usually the feet or legs. The *systemic* mycoses can involve the deep viscera and spread throughout the body. These infections originate in the lungs and then disseminate to other locations. Although systemic mycoses are considered to be pathogenic to humans, many individuals infected with one of the causative agents are asymptomatic. Except for *Cryptococcus,* the causative agents in this group are dimorphic in nature. Several fungi previously not considered to be pathogenic in humans are responsible for opportunistic infections in the immunosuppressed patient. Several agents have been long known as causing infections in immunosuppressed individuals, including *Candida, Aspergillus,* and the fungi causing zygomycosis (*Rhizopus* species, *Mucor* species, *Cunninghamella bertholletiae,* and *Apophysomyces elegan*). **Table 22–4** lists the most frequent agents associated with the various classifications. Several fungi are considered to be commensalistic in nature, including *Candida albicans* and *Malassezia furfur;* however, these organisms may cause disease or clinical symptoms in some individuals.

Immune Responses to Fungi

As is the case with the immune responses to bacterial, viral, and parasitic agents, the immune defenses to fungal agents range from protective mechanisms that include the innate immunity present early in the infection to specific adaptive mechanisms that are induced later. The first line of innate defense includes skin and the mucous membranes of the respiratory, gastrointestinal, and genitourinary tracts that provide physical barriers that separate the host from the environment. Fungi possess very few factors that allow them to overcome those physical barriers; because of the nutrients and environmental conditions needed for many fungi, those mechanisms have not evolved. For example, among the most common fungal infections are those caused by the dermatophytes (*Trichophyton* species, *Microsporum* species, and *Epidermophyton floccosum*). These fungi cause infection of the skin, hair, and nails because they require dead keratin for growth. Infections caused by these fungi are also sometimes known as "ringworm" or "tinea." They do not possess any invasive factors, and the symptoms associated with these agents are caused by the inflammatory response of the host.

If the fungi penetrate the physical barriers, there are a variety of innate mechanisms for recognizing the organism. Innate immune cells express various pattern-recognition receptors (PRRs) that recognize specific structures and molecules present on bacteria and fungi called *pathogen-associated molecular patterns (PAMPs)*. There are several classes of PRRs that can be either transmembrane proteins located on the cell surface or cytoplasmic proteins contained within the cell. The four different classes are the **Toll-like receptors (TLRs)** and the

Table 22-4 Mycotic Infections Based on Site of Infection and Level of Tissue Involvement

CLASSIFICATION	REPRESENTATIVE AGENT	DISEASE
Superficial	*Malassezia furfur* *Phaeoannellomyces werneckii* *Piedraia hortae* *Trichosporon* species	Pityriasis versicolor (skin) Tinea nigra (skin) Black piedra (hair) White piedra (hair)
Cutaneous	*Trichophyton* species *Microsporum* species *Epidermophyton floccosum*	Tinea (e.g., ringworm, athlete's foot, jock itch)
Subcutaneous	*Sporothrix schenckii* *Fonsecaea pedrosoi* *Pseudallescheria boydii*	Sporotrichosis Chromoblastomycosis Eumycotic mycetoma
Systemic	*Histoplasma capsulatum*	Histoplasmosis (endemic in Ohio and Mississippi River valleys)
	Coccidioides immitis	Coccidioidomycosis (endemic in the southwestern United States)
	Paracoccidioides brasiliensis	Paracoccidioidomycosis (endemic in Central and South America, primarily Brazil)
	Blastomyces dermatitidis	Blastomycosis (predominantly a veterinary pathogen in Ohio and Mississippi River valleys)
	Talaromyces marneffei (previously *Penicillium marneffei)*	*Penicilliosis marneffei* (predominantly seen in AIDS patients in Southeast Asia)
	Cryptococcus neoformans	Cryptococcosis (causes meningitis in immunosuppressed patients [e.g., AIDS])
Opportunistic	*Candida albicans* *Aspergillus* species *Rhizopus* species	Candidiasis Aspergillosis Zygomycosis
Commensalistic	*Candida albicans* *Malassezia furfur*	Urinary tract infections, vaginal yeast infections Tinea versicolor (pityriasis versicolor), dandruff, and seborrheic dermatitis

C-type lectin receptors (CLRs), both of which are transmembrane proteins, and the retinoic acid-inducible gene (RIG)-I-like receptors (RLRs) and the NOD-like receptors (NLRs), which are cytoplasmic proteins (see Chapter 2). Of these, the TLRs play the most important role in defense against pathogenic microbial infection by stimulating the production of inflammatory cytokines and type I interferons. In addition to playing an important role in innate responses, TLRs are involved in shaping adaptive immunity. Several fungal components are recognized by TLRs, including phospholipomannans and β-glucans, which are recognized by TLR2, and glucuronoxylomannans, which are recognized by CD14 and TLR4.

Connections

Pathogen-Associated Molecular Patterns (PAMPs)

PAMPs are conserved among microbial species. As discussed in Chapter 2, PRRs on the innate immune cells—phagocytes, macrophages, and dendritic cells (DCs)—initiate the immune response by sensing and recognizing the presence of PAMPs on the bacteria, fungi, or viruses. The recognition of PAMPs by the PRRs stimulates the release of cytokines that upregulate the inflammatory response and influence adaptive immunity.

Although TLRs play a role in the immunologic response to fungi, CLRs are central for fungal recognition and for the induction of the innate and adaptive immune responses to fungi. Fungal cell walls consist mainly of multiple layers of carbohydrates, including mannans (cell wall polysaccharide), β-glucan, and chitins (the main component of fungal cell walls). The CLR transmembrane protein, dectin 1, recognizes β-glucans. Dectin 2 recognizes high-mannose structures that are common to many fungi and bind hyphal forms with higher affinity than yeast forms. Individuals with genetic deficiencies in CLRs are highly susceptible to fungal infections.

There has been a debate as to the roles of cell-mediated immunity versus humoral immunity in host defense to fungal infections. It is now accepted that the cell-mediated immune response plays the most important role in the adaptive response to fungal infections. Once the cells of the innate immune system have been activated, cytokines and chemokines are produced in response to the infection. Chemokines play a vital role in the recruitment of T cells to the site of the infection. Chemokines also aid in the formation of the adaptive immune response to fungi, specifically, those mediated by Th1 and Th2 cells. Th1 cells have been shown in mice to be vitally important to clearance of the organism in **cryptococcosis** and **histoplasmosis.** Once the T cells have committed themselves in response to the fungi, they express an effector function through the release of cytokines, primarily alpha interferon (IFN-α), TNF-α, and IL-17/22, contributing to protective immunity to pathogenic fungi.

Although there is a humoral response to fungal infections, the evidence that antibodies contribute to effective defense against fungal infections is not conclusive. One study has shown that humoral immunity can protect against experimental fungal infections if certain types of protective antibodies are present in sufficient quantities. The main functions of antibodies in fungal infections include opsonization, ADCC, prevention of adherence, and toxin neutralization. However, there is little evidence supporting the role of antibodies in host defenses in naturally acquired infections. The absence of an association between deficiencies in specific antibodies and susceptibility to fungal infections in patients with progressive fungal infections also provides evidence against a protective role of antibodies in fungal infections.

Laboratory Diagnosis of Fungal Infections

Because of the increased numbers of individuals who are immunosuppressed, the incidence of invasive fungal infections associated with significant morbidity and mortality has risen dramatically in the past several decades. The clinical diagnosis of fungal infections in many instances is difficult. The clinician must consider the patient's symptoms, history of other past or present infections, medical treatments, occupation, place of residence, and record of travel in evaluating the likely cause of a fungal infection. Available laboratory methods for diagnosing fungal infections include isolation of the organism in the laboratory, histopathological evidence of invasion, skin testing, and serological detection of antigens or antibodies. The traditional "gold standard" is the recovery of the organism in the laboratory. However, recovery is often difficult with uncommon fungi. In addition, once the organism is isolated, traditional identification methods may take several weeks because of the slow growth of fungi. Several nonculture laboratory methods, including antibody and antigen detection, are available for fungal pathogens that are commonly encountered in the clinical laboratory. These include *C. albicans*, *Aspergillus* species, *Cryptococcus neoformans*, and the dimorphic fungi *Histoplasma capsulatum* and *Coccidioides immitis*.

Although the humoral response to fungi is not the major defense against fungal infection, antibodies produced against the organisms may be readily detected and can be used to demonstrate current or past exposure to the agent. However, in that many fungal infections are opportunistic, serological diagnosis many times is of little value because of the fact that immunosuppressed individuals do not reliably produce antibodies during acute infections and serological assays are not available for the majority of the opportunistic fungi. In addition, in areas where a fungal agent is endemic to a geographic area, serological testing for antifungal antibodies is of little value because most people living in those areas will test positive for the antibodies.

Recently, molecular assays have been used in the detection and diagnosis of fungal infections. Examples include peptide nucleic acid fluorescence in situ hybridization (PNA-FISH) for identification of *Candida* species in blood cultures, real-time PCR assays for detection of *Aspergillus* species and *P. jirovecii* from bronchial lavage fluid, and multiplex PCR coupled with a bead probe fluid array for detection of numerous species of fungi in bronchial lavage fluid or blood. However, molecular-based diagnostic methods for fungal infections are in their infancy.

Fungal Pathogens

The following discussion provides information on five of the fungal infections for which serological testing is used.

Aspergillus Species

Aspergillus is a ubiquitous fungus that is found worldwide in nature **(Fig. 22–5)**. The genus has over 185 species and can be recovered from soil and plant material; its spores (conidia) may be recovered from the indoor air environment. *A. fumigatus* is the most commonly isolated species, with *Aspergillus flavus* and *Aspergillus niger* being the other frequently recovered species. Less commonly recovered isolates include *Aspergillus clavatus*, the *Aspergillus glaucus* group, *Aspergillus nidulans*, *Aspergillus oryzae*, *Aspergillus terreus*, and *Aspergillus versicolor*. In humans, *Aspergillus* is primarily an opportunistic pathogen causing a variety of infections. Infections in the immunocompetent individual include *Aspergillus otomycosis*, which is a superficial infection of the external auditory canal and auricle (otitis externa). Most of these infections are caused by *A. niger*. Another infection is caused by growth of *Aspergillus* in the lung cavity, forming a solid mass of **hyphae**, which can develop into a fungus ball referred to as an *aspergilloma*. Pulmonary aspergilloma usually occurs in

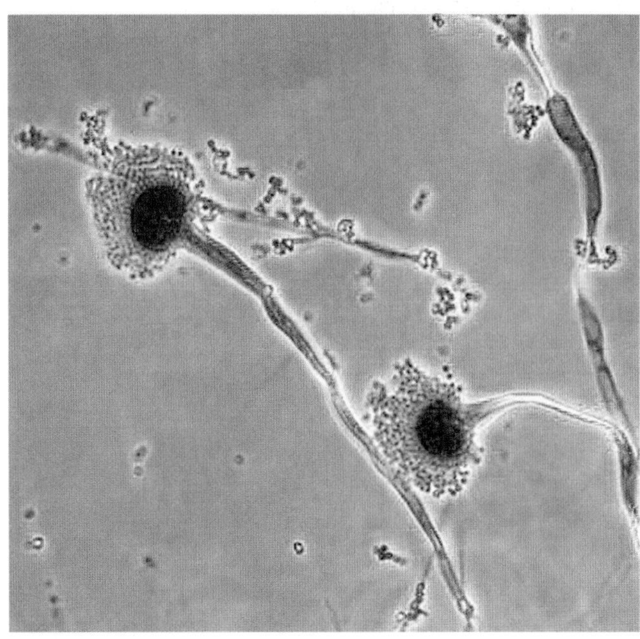

FIGURE 22–5 *Aspergillus fumigatus*, LPCB stain X 450. *(Courtesy of the CDC, Public Health Image Library.)*

scarred lung tissue or in a preexisting lung cavity resulting from a previous infection (e.g., tuberculosis, sarcoidosis). Some fungal antigens may elicit allergic responses to *Aspergillus,* causing ABPA, which results in a long-term allergic response. ABPA is thought to be present in 1% to 2% of patients with persistent asthma and in approximately 7% of patients with cystic fibrosis.

Invasive forms of *Aspergillus* most frequently begin in the lung, resulting from inhalation of the conidia. The organism grows and spreads in the lung tissue. Invasive pulmonary *Aspergillosis* (IPA) may occur in the neutropenic patient because of immunosuppression. Disseminated aspergillosis may occur through hematogenous spread to distant sites or by contiguous extension from the lung.

The diagnosis of **aspergillosis** generally requires a positive tissue biopsy demonstrating the hyphae or a positive culture for *Aspergillus.* Nonculture methods may also be used to diagnose invasive aspergillosis. Serological diagnosis is of limited utility because the immunosuppressed patient will fail to mount an antibody response, even with invasive disease. The detection of galactomannan in serum can be used to indicate a fungal infection and has increased the ability to diagnose invasive aspergillosis. At the time of this writing, there is one FDA-approved assay, the Platelia Aspergillus EIA (Bio-Rad Laboratories, Marne-La-Coquette, France). This assay is offered at larger or reference laboratories. Another assay to detect invasive fungal infections, including aspergillosis, measures β-D-glucan (BDG) in serum. BDG is a component of the cell wall of most fungi. Currently, there are five approved assays that can be used in the clinical diagnosis of invasive fungal infection. Scientists have developed molecular diagnostics, including PCR, for *Aspergillus,* which appear to be more sensitive than other methods, including galactomannan, and show promise in improving the diagnosis of invasive aspergillosis.

Candida Species

Candida ssp. are yeast (unicellular fungi) that may exist as commensalistic organisms in the human host. They are commonly found on the skin, in the gastrointestinal (GI) tract, and in the female genital tract. Of the more than 150 species of *Candida,* only a small percentage is regarded as frequently pathogenic for humans. *C. albicans* is the leading cause of human infections. Other members include *Candida guilliermondii, Candida krusei, Candida parapsilosis, Candida tropicalis, Candida pseudotropicalis, Candida lusitaniae, Candida dubliniensis,* and *Candida glabrata.* Following the introduction of antibiotics, *Candida* infections rose dramatically in the United States. In recent decades, *Candida* species have been the fourth most common organisms recovered from the blood of hospitalized patients in the United States. Invasive candidiasis is a major hospital-associated fungal disease in the United States and is associated with mortality rates of 30% to 40%. The incidence of candidemia-related hospitalizations has risen significantly in the past two decades. Increased use of immunosuppressive therapies, the use of advanced life-support therapies, and the incidence of HIV-1 infection have all contributed to the increased incidence of *Candida* infections. Infections in the immunocompetent host include diaper rash, vaginitis and urinary tract infections in the female, and thrush (oral candidiasis) caused by the use of broad-spectrum antibiotics. Individuals with thrush for no obvious reason should be evaluated for AIDS. The introduction of potent antiretroviral therapy has reduced the incidence of thrush in AIDS patients. *Candida* esophagitis, pneumonia, and septicemia may be observed in the neutropenic patient because of radiation and chemotherapy or use of broad-spectrum antibiotics.

The diagnosis of *Candida* infections generally involves the recovery of the causative agent. The organisms grow well in routine culture media. Direct examination of the clinical material through the use of 10% potassium hydroxide (KOH) preparation may also be used to detect *Candida* species. The serological diagnosis of **candidiasis** is limited because colonization by *Candida* species of the gastrointestinal tract or other body sites can stimulate antibody production in uninfected individuals. In addition, immunocompromised patients may not mount detectable antibody responses. Current recommendations include the combined detection of mannan and anti-mannan antibodies for the specific identification of *Candida* species in serum samples. These assays can be positive 6 days before blood cultures, on average. They also show a very high negative predictive value (greater than 85%).

Connections

Predictive Value

The predictive value of a laboratory test is the likelihood that the results it produces will lead to an accurate diagnosis. The predictive value depends on the sensitivity and specificity of the method, as well as the prevalence of the disease in the population undergoing testing (see Chapter 9). A negative predictive value is the likelihood that a negative test result is truly negative. Thus, an 85% negative predictive value means that there is an 85% chance that a patient with a negative test result does not have the disease in question. In general, negative predictive values are higher in populations with a low disease prevalence.

Over the years, tests for various serum antigens have been used to detect invasive *Candida* infections, including latex agglutination (LA), counterimmunoelectrophoresis, or ELISA-based assays; however, these have not proven to be useful. The use of molecular-based assays shows promise. Direct PCR of blood samples is a sensitive and specific method for the diagnosis of invasive candidiasis and may be used for early diagnosis of specific *Candida* species.

Cryptococcus neoformans

The genus *Cryptococcus* includes 19 species of encapsulated yeasts. *C. neoformans* evolved from being a rare cause of human disease to a significant opportunistic pathogen as the population of immunocompromised patients increased. *C. neoformans* is a *saprobe* in nature, obtaining its nutrition from dead or decaying organic matter. The organism lives in certain trees and rotting wood and has frequently been isolated from soil contaminated by guano from birds (e.g., pigeons). *C. neoformans* enters the host mainly through the lungs and has a predilection for invading the CNS of the susceptible host. Although pulmonary infections are common, *Cryptococcal* meningoencephalitis represents the primary life-threatening infection caused by *C. neoformans.* In the pre-AIDS era, cryptococcosis had an overall incidence of 0.8 cases per million persons per year. In 1992, during the peak of the AIDS epidemic, the rate in several large U.S. cities reached almost five cases per 100,000 persons per year. With the use of antiviral agents for the treatment of AIDS in developed countries, these numbers have declined.

The most important feature contributing to the organism's virulence and pathogenicity is its capsule. The capsule consists of polysaccharide containing an unbranched chain of alpha-1,3-linked mannose units substituted with xylosyl and β-glucuronyl groups. The capsule has many effects on the host's immune response. These include acting as a barrier to phagocytosis, depleting complement, producing antibody unresponsiveness, dysregulating cytokine secretion, interfering with antigen presentation, and enhancing HIV replication.

The two most common sites for infection with this encapsulated yeast are the lungs and CNS, with the respiratory tract being the most common portal of entry. The majority of cryptococcal infections are asymptomatic in individuals with a competent immune system, and most cases of cryptococcosis are diagnosed in individuals with compromised immune systems. Respiratory symptoms range from asymptomatic colonization of the airway to life-threatening pneumonia with evidence of an acute respiratory distress syndrome. Individuals with CNS involvement generally present with subacute meningitis or meningoencephalitis. Symptoms include headache, fever, lethargy, and memory loss over several weeks. Some patients may present with an acute onset of meningitis.

The laboratory diagnosis of *Cryptococcus* infections may be done using direct microscopic examination of the clinical material, culturing for the organism, or performing serological tests. Microscopic examination of the organism can be performed by mixing the biological fluid (usually CSF) with India ink. The encapsulated yeast displaces the India ink, creating a halo around the yeast cell **(Fig. 22–6).** Although the test is easy to perform and interpret and has high specificity, it shows poor sensitivity (50% to 80%).

Detection of cryptococcal polysaccharide antigen in serum and CSF can be performed by LA and enzyme immunoassays (EIAs). Both types of tests are more than 90% sensitive and specific. Although the LA test is a rapid and reliable serological method for the diagnosis of cryptococcosis, false-positive LA test results can occur. False-positive results are thought to be caused by rheumatoid factor or other interference factors. Pretreating the specimen with heat and pronase, or 2-Mercaptoethanol, destroys these factors and reduces the incidence of false positives.

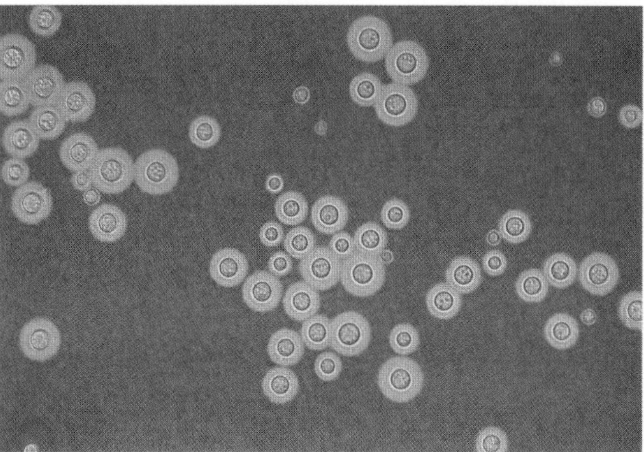

FIGURE 22–6 India ink prep showing *Cryptococcus neoformans* in CSF. The organism's large polysaccharide capsule displaces the India ink, allowing for visualization of the yeast. *(Courtesy of the CDC/ Dr. Leanor Haley, Public Health Image Library.)*

More recently, a lateral flow immunochromatographic assay (LFA) (Immy, Inc., Norman, OK) was approved by the FDA for the detection of cryptococcal antigen in CSF and serum **(Fig. 22–7).** The assay allows for the detection of cryptococcal antigen in fewer than 15 minutes. The assay has been shown to have a sensitivity of 100% and a specificity of 99.8% with serum samples, as well as a sensitivity of 99.3% and a specificity of 99.1% with CSF.

Measurement of cryptococcal antigen levels has been shown to have some clinical use. Serial polysaccharide antigen titers can be performed on serum or CSF. Initial high titers (1:1,024 or higher) indicate high levels of the yeast in the host and poor host immunity. These individuals have a greater chance of therapeutic failure. As is the case in many infectious diseases, increasing antigen titers are usually seen with worsening of the disease, whereas declining titers are usually associated with clinical improvement. Cryptococcal antigen may be detected even months after successful therapy, so cryptococcal antigen tests should not be used to indicate cure.

Histoplasma capsulatum

H. capsulatum is a common cause of infection in the Ohio and Mississippi River valleys. The organism is a dimorphic fungus, growing as a yeast at 35°C to 37°C and as a mycelial fungus at environmental temperatures. The organism is found and grows in soil under favorable conditions. The presence of bird and bat guano increases the likelihood of the organism being present in the soil. Whereas birds are not infected with the fungus, bats carry the fungus in their gastrointestinal tracts and shed it. Histoplasmosis is acquired by inhalation of mycelial fragments and microconidia. The majority of the infections are self-limiting and asymptomatic. The organism can cause a potentially lethal infection in patients with preexisting conditions. The organism causes opportunistic infection in patients with weakened immune systems (e.g., people with HIV infection). Of those who are symptomatic, pulmonary

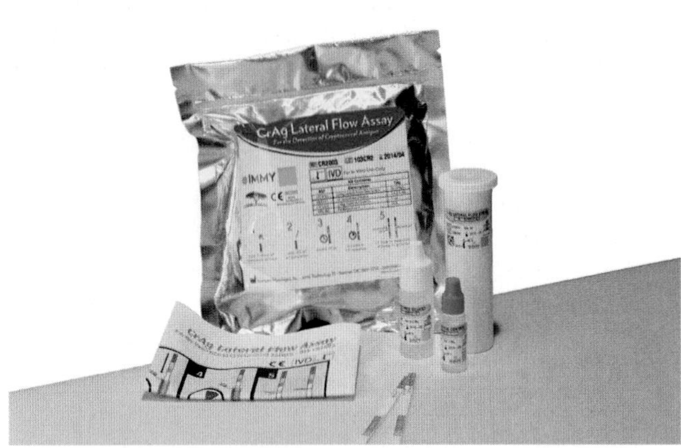

A

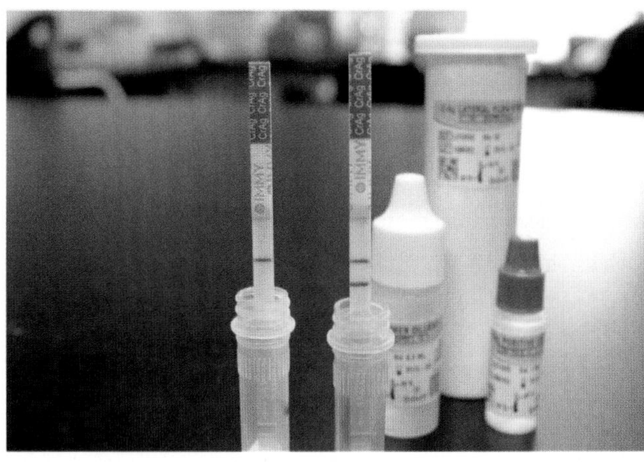

B

FIGURE 22–7 IMMY CrAg LFA (cryptococcal antigen lateral flow assay). (A) Kit components. The assay is a sandwich immunochromatographic dipstick assay for the qualitative and semiquantitative detection of cryptococcal antigen from CSF and serum. (B) Test results: The dipstick on the left shows one line for the control; the test sample is negative. The dipstick on the right shows two lines, indicating a valid control result and the presence of cryptococcal antigen in the test sample. *(Reprinted by permission of Immuno-Mycologics, Inc. [IMMY], Norman, Oklahoma.)*

histoplasmosis, either acute or chronic, is the most frequent clinical presentation. In a primary infection, the organism disseminates to organs rich in mononuclear phagocytes. Disseminated disease in the immunocompromised patient is 100% fatal if untreated. Survival rates of the acute episode exceed 80% when treated.

The diagnosis of histoplasmosis can be made by culture of the organism. The organism is generally recovered within 3 weeks of culture, with 90% of samples exhibiting growth within 7 days. The ability to recover the organism is affected by the number of specimens submitted for culture, the type of specimen submitted (e.g., respiratory secretions, blood, or CSF), and the severity of the infection.

Complement fixation (CF) and precipitation have been the most common tests used for detection of *Histoplasma* antibodies in the clinical laboratory. For CF antibodies, a titer of 1:8 to yeast or mycelial antigen is considered positive, and a titer of 1:32 may indicate histoplasmosis. Precipitin band testing looks for the presence of H and M antibodies in the serum of individuals. The H and M antigens are glycoproteins released by mycelial and yeast-phase cultures. H antibodies are detected in fewer than 10% of patients but, when present, signify active infection. Antibodies to the M antigen are detected in up to 80% of individuals who have been exposed to the fungus. These antibodies may be found in individuals who have previously been exposed to the organism or who have active disease; thus, their presence not useful in discriminating previous from current infection.

Skin testing, similar to the Mantoux tuberculin skin test, may also determine if an individual has been exposed to the organism. The *H. capsulatum* skin test becomes positive 2 to 4 weeks after infection, and the majority of infected people are asymptomatic. Repeat testing will usually give positive results for the rest of a person's life. Thus, in areas where the fungus is endemic, the skin test is of limited utility.

Connections

Skin Testing

Skin testing detects the cell-mediated immune response to antigens from a pathogen such as *H. capsulatum*. A commonly used skin test is the Mantoux test, which is used to detect exposure to the bacterium that causes tuberculosis (see Chapter 14). An antigen extract from the organism is injected under the skin, and the reaction is delayed, becoming visible 24 to 72 hours later. A positive test is indicated by the development of redness and firm swelling at the site of injection.

Laboratory diagnosis may be made by detecting the polysaccharide antigen in serum or urine by ELISA. Urinary antigen tests have been shown to have a high sensitivity and specificity for detecting *Histoplasma* infections. *Histoplasma* antigen was detected in the urine in 95% of AIDS patients with disseminated disease and in the serum of 86% of these patients. Ninety-two percent of patients without AIDS who have disseminated histoplasmosis demonstrate antigenuria, but only about 50% have *antigenemia*. Molecular assays appear to have promise in the diagnosis of histoplasmosis; however, at this point, no molecular assays for routine use are commercially available.

Clinical Correlations

"-emia" and "-uria"

The suffix "–emia" indicates the presence of a substance in the blood, whereas the suffix "–uria" indicates the presence of a substance in the urine. Thus, "antigenemia" means that a particular antigen (in this case, *Histoplasma* antigen) can be found in the blood, whereas "antigenuria" means that detectable antigen is present in the urine.

Coccidioides immitis

Similar to *H. capsulatum, C. immitis* is also a dimorphic fungus. For many years, **coccidioidomycosis** was thought to be a rare and nearly always fatal infection. In 1929, a medical student at Stanford University was accidentally exposed to the organism and experienced only a mild respiratory infection. His survival resulted in a reassessment of the coccidioidal infections. Coccidioidomycosis was initially recognized as a common respiratory condition in the San Joaquin Valley of California (valley fever). Although originally thought to be only found in the dry, arid regions of the southwestern United States, coccidioidomycosis has become more prevalent throughout both nonendemic and endemic regions of the world. The increased incidence of coccidioidomycosis can be mostly attributed to changes in demography. Populations at risk of exposure are greatly expanded. Regions in which *C. immitis* is endemic have major metropolitan centers, such as Phoenix, Arizona. These areas were previously sparsely populated. Along with increased population growth in the southwestern United States, there has been increased tourism, leading to movement of people into and out of endemic areas, increasing the numbers of people who are exposed to the organism and acquire coccidioidal infections.

In a vast majority of the cases, infections are the result of inhaling arthroconidia (a type of fungal spore). A single arthroconidium can be enough to produce a naturally acquired respiratory infection. Up to two-thirds of cases caused by *C. immitis* are either inapparent or so mild as to not prompt medical evaluation. In those individuals who do become symptomatic, the clinical presentation is similar to a community-acquired pneumonia. *Coccidioides* was estimated to be responsible for approximately one-third of all cases of community-acquired pneumonia in southern Arizona.

Once inhaled, there is an incubation period of 1 to 3 weeks before the development of respiratory symptoms. Thus, travel history is important if the person has traveled to an endemic area. Once coccidioidomycosis is suspected, diagnosis may be established by identifying the fungus in, or recovering *C. immitis* from, a clinical specimen or by detecting anticoccidioidal antibodies in serum, CSF, or other body fluid. The most frequent way in which coccidioidomycosis is diagnosed is through serology. Although the organism can be cultured, obtaining a sputum specimen in individuals is not often possible because of the lack of sputum production in infected individuals. In addition, fungal culturing in an outpatient setting is not available. The use and limitations of skin testing for *Coccidioides* infection are similar to those for *Histoplasma*. Once positive, the skin test generally remains positive for the rest of one's life; therefore, it is of limited utility in individuals living in endemic areas.

Complement fixation, immunodiffusion (ID), and LA have been the most commonly used serological methods for detecting infection. One of the original methods for detecting infection was the tube precipitin test (TPT). The detection of IgM antibodies by this test has been used to demonstrate infection. The test involves overnight incubation of the patient's serum with coccidioidal antigen. Formation of a precipitin button at the bottom of a test tube demonstrates the presence of IgM antibodies. A polysaccharide from the fungal cell wall is used as the antigen in the test. Tube precipitin antibodies are detected in 90% of patients within the first 3 weeks of symptoms. This test is often referred to as the "IgM test."

The other original test involved detection of coccidioidal antibodies using a CF assay. When mixed with a coccidioidal antigen, an immune complex is formed with the patient's antibodies, resulting in depletion of complement. When the complement is depleted, antibody-coated red blood cells (RBCs) added to the mixture fail to lyse. This test is often referred to as the "IgG test" because IgG is the immunoglobulin class usually involved in the formation of this type of immune complex. CF antibodies are detected later and for longer periods than tube precipitin-type antibodies. ID assays for detecting both IgG and IgM antibodies are available and have served as replacements for the earlier TPT and CF tests.

EIAs for coccidioidal antibodies are commercially available. The EIAs allow for the specific detection of IgM or IgG antibodies. A positive EIA result is a highly sensitive indicator for coccidioidal infection. Although the EIA tests for IgM and IgG are more sensitive than ID tests, false positives have been reported. At present, it is recommended that positive EIA results, particularly positive IgM results, should be confirmed with ID tube precipitin or CF test results. Similar to *H. capsulatum*, there are no commercially available molecular assays for the detection of *Coccidioides* infection.

SUMMARY

- Parasites are microorganisms that survive by living off of other organisms. The three major types of parasites are protozoa, helminths, and ectoparasites.
- Parasitic infections can result in eradication of the organism by the host's immune system, death of the host because of an ineffective immune response, or, in most cases, establishment of persistent infection because of the host's inability to completely eliminate the organism.
- Innate defenses (e.g., phagocytosis and cytokine release) and specific humoral and cell-mediated adaptive responses can be demonstrated against parasites. IgE antibodies and eosinophils can destroy some parasites by ADCC, and many patients with parasitic infections have increased levels of IgE and eosinophil numbers in the blood.
- Because of their complex, multistage life cycles, the immune responses to the agents responsible for parasitic diseases are often ineffective.
- Parasites have also developed several strategies to avoid the immune system—antigenic concealment, antigenic variation, antigenic shedding, antigenic mimicry, immunologic subversion, and immunologic diversion.
- Fungi are eukaryotic cells with nuclei and rigid cell walls. They can exist in two morphological states: unicellular yeasts or multicellular mycelia fungi.

- Fungal infections are known as *mycoses*. They can produce hypersensitivity, mycotoxicosis (a poisoning caused by fungal toxins), mycetismus (mushroom poisoning), skin infections, or systemic infections that disseminate from the lungs or skin to other sites of the body.
- Innate defenses, including physical barriers such as the skin and attachment of immune cells to pattern-recognition receptors (PRRs), are an important first line of defense against fungal infections. Cell-mediated immunity is the most important adaptive immune response to fungal infections.
- The diagnosis of many parasitic and fungal infections relies on traditional laboratory techniques either by the direct observation of the parasite in clinical material (feces, duodenal fluid, small intestine biopsy specimen, or blood) or by culture and growth of the fungal agent responsible for the infection.
- Serological testing for parasitic and fungal diseases is less routine than serology for other infectious diseases because test availability is limited and assays exhibit variable performance with respect to sensitivity and specificity. Many of these tests are only offered by reference laboratories.
- Serology results should be used in conjunction with the patient's symptoms, history, and other clinical findings to make a diagnosis of a fungal or parasitic infection.
- Toxoplasmosis is an example of a parasitic infection for which serological testing is useful. Detection of IgG, IgM, and IgA antibodies to *T. gondii* is helpful in determining whether the infection has been acquired recently or in the past and whether an infant has acquired a congenital infection with the organism.
- Fungal infections for which serological tests are useful include aspergillosis, candidiasis, cryptococcosis, histoplasmosis, and coccidioidomycosis. Serological testing can involve detection of fungal antibody or antigen, depending on the organism.
- To date, there are only a few commercial molecular tests that are available for the diagnosis of parasitic and invasive fungal infections, but advances in molecular technology will likely result in new diagnostic procedures in the future.

Study Guide: Escape Mechanisms of Parasites from Protective Host Responses

ESCAPE MECHANISM	NATURE OF RESPONSE	EXAMPLE(S)
Antigenic concealment	Intracellular survival within macrophages	*Leishmania donovani*
Antigenic variation	Random mutation Genetic recombination Gene switching Multistage parasitic life cycle	*Plasmodium* species *Plasmodium falciparum, Trypanosoma cruzi* *Trypanosoma gambiense, Trypanosoma rhodesiense* *Leishmania* species
Antigenic shedding	Shedding of surface antigens or components	*Entamoeba histolytica*
Antigenic mimicry	Incorporation of host "self" antigens into parasite surface	*Schistosoma* species
Immunologic subversion	Immunosuppression	*Schistosoma mansoni*
Immunologic diversion	Polyclonal B-cell activation	*Plasmodium* species

CASE STUDIES

1. An otherwise healthy infant developed a seizure 5 days following birth. The mother and baby returned to the hospital for evaluation. Upon examination of the infant, the physician found that the baby demonstrated chorioretinitis. Prescreening of the mother during the third trimester of pregnancy did not demonstrate the presence of antibodies against *T. gondii*. At that time, she was advised to refrain from cleaning the litter boxes of the family's two cats. Upon questioning, the mother stated that she had been cleaning the litter boxes when other family members failed to do so. The physician suspected that the child may have congenital toxoplasmosis. Serological testing of the mother and the fetus gave the following results:

	Anti–*T. gondii* IgM	Anti–*T. gondii* IgG
Mother	1:256	1:512
Baby	Not done	1:256

Questions

a. Evaluate the baby's status related to *T. gondii* infection.

b. What additional testing should be performed to confirm the baby's status?

2. A 60-year-old male with a medical history of chronic obstructive pulmonary disease (COPD), diabetes mellitus, and hepatitis C was seen in the emergency department. The patient admitted to using intravenous drugs in the past and has been receiving inhaled steroid therapy for his COPD. He complained of nausea and severe headaches, which interfered with his ability to carry out his normal activities. The patient also felt unbalanced and weak when standing. Head computed tomography (CT) and magnetic resonance imaging (MRI) revealed abnormalities in the cerebellum of the patient's brain. Cryptococcal meningitis was suspected. A lumbar puncture was performed, and a CSF sample was sent for laboratory testing to confirm the suspected diagnosis.

Questions

a. What clinical presentations of the patient point to a diagnosis of cryptococcosis?
b. What laboratory tests should be performed to confirm the patient's diagnosis?

REVIEW QUESTIONS

1. Compared with a host's response to a virus, overcoming a parasitic infection is more difficult for the host because of which of the following characteristics of parasites?
   a. Large size
   b. Complex antigenic structures
   c. Elaborate life cycle
   d. All of the above

2. Which of the following is indicative of a recent infection with *Toxoplasma gondii?*
   a. Anti-*Toxoplasma* IgM
   b. Anti-*Toxoplasma* IgE
   c. High-avidity anti-*Toxoplasma* IgG
   d. Low-avidity anti-*Toxoplasma* IgG

3. Parasites are able to evade host defenses by which of the following means?
   a. Production of antigens similar to host antigens
   b. Changing surface antigens
   c. Sequestering themselves within host cells
   d. All of the above

4. The chronic nature of parasitic infections is caused by the host's
   a. inability to eliminate the infective agent.
   b. type I hypersensitivity response to the infection.
   c. ability to form a granuloma around the parasite.
   d. tendency to form circulating immune complexes.

5. The presence of both IgM and IgG antibody in toxoplasmosis infections suggests that the infection
   a. occurred more than 2 years ago.
   b. occurred more recently than 18 months ago.
   c. is chronic.
   d. has resolved itself.

6. Which of the following is indicative of a parasitic infection?
   a. Increased IgA levels
   b. Increased IgE levels
   c. Increased IgG levels
   d. Increased IgM levels

7. In congenital toxoplasmosis, which class of antibodies is the most sensitive in detecting infection?
   a. IgA
   b. IgG
   c. IgM
   d. IgE

8. The most significant defense against fungal infections is
   a. cellular immunity.
   b. humoral immunity.
   c. phagocytosis.
   d. complement activation.

9. Clinical manifestations of fungal-related illness include
   a. hypersensitivity caused by fungal spores.
   b. poisoning caused by ingestion of mycotoxins.
   c. growth of fungi in or on tissue.
   d. all of the above.

10. Which of the following assay formats are increasingly being adopted by clinical laboratories for serological detection of fungal infections because of their ease of use?
    a. ELISA assays
    b. Lateral flow assays
    c. Radial immunodiffusion assays
    d. Indirect immunofluorescence assays

11. The presence of anti-H antibodies indicates which of the following?
    a. A previous infection with *Coccidioides immitis*
    b. A previous exposure to *Histoplasma capsulatum*
    c. An active infection with *Cryptococcus neoformans*
    d. An active infection with *Histoplasma capsulatum*

12. A limiting factor in reliably being able to detect antifungal antibodies in an acute infection is
    a. the lack of humoral response to fungal agents caused by immunosuppression.
    b. current assays lack specificity.
    c. antibodies are not normally formed against most fungi.
    d. antibodies tend to remain at low titer as a mycosis develops.

13. False positives may be observed in latex agglutination tests for the capsular antigen of *Cryptococcus neoformans* because of
    a. the use of serum instead of CSF.
    b. the presence of rheumatoid factor in the specimen.
    c. cross-reactivity with other fungal antigens.
    d. the low specificity of the assay.

14. A 27-year-old man from Ohio, diagnosed with AIDS, developed chest pains. After a short period of time, he also developed severe headaches with dizziness. In his free time, his hobby was exploring caves (a spelunker). His physician ordered a sputum culture and spinal tap, and both were positive for a yeast-like fungus. These findings are most consistent with infection by
    a. *Candida albicans.*
    b. *Coccidioides immitis.*
    c. *Cryptococcus neoformans.*
    d. *Histoplasma capsulatum.*

15. Which of the following serological tests detects the polysaccharide capsule antigen in serum and CSF of patients with suspected infection with *Cryptococcus neoformans?*
    a. Complement fixation (CF)
    b. India ink test
    c. Latex agglutination (LA)
    d. Hemagglutination test

16. Which of the following is a nondimorphic fungus that is found in concentrated bird droppings and can readily cause meningitis in immunocompromised individuals?
    a. *Coccidioides immitis*
    b. *Candida albicans*
    c. *Cryptococcus neoformans*
    d. *Histoplasma capsulatum*

23 Serological and Molecular Detection of Viral Infections

Linda E. Miller, PhD, MB^{CM}(ASCP)SI, and Deborah Josko, PhD, MLT(ASCP)M, SM

LEARNING OUTCOMES

After finishing this chapter, you should be able to:

1. Describe the immune defenses that are important in protecting humans from viral infections.
2. Discuss mechanisms by which viruses can escape host defenses.
3. Correlate the presence of viral immunoglobulin M (IgM) and immunoglobulin G (IgG) antibodies with their clinical significance in detecting current infections, congenital infections, or immunity to infections.
4. Discuss the role of molecular tests in diagnosing and monitoring patients with viral infections.
5. Differentiate between the different hepatitis viruses and their modes of transmission.
6. Correlate the various serological markers of hepatitis with their diagnostic significance.
7. Explain the laboratory methods that are most commonly used to screen for, confirm, or monitor hepatitis virus infections.
8. Associate the following viruses with the specific diseases they cause: Epstein-Barr virus (EBV), cytomegalovirus (CMV), varicella-zoster virus (VZV), rubella virus, rubeola virus, mumps virus, and the human T-cell lymphotropic virus type I.
9. Discuss the laboratory methods used to diagnose and monitor infections with the preceding viruses.
10. Correlate the heterophile antibody and EBV-specific antibodies with their clinical significance and describe the laboratory methods used to test for these antibodies.

CHAPTER OUTLINE

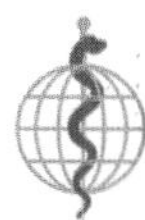

Go to FADavis.com for the laboratory exercises and a special online section on Coronavirus SARS CoV-2 that accompany this text.

KEY TERMS

Anti-HBe
Anti-HBs
Cytomegalovirus (CMV)
Epstein-Barr virus (EBV)
Hepatitis
Hepatitis A virus (HAV)
Hepatitis B surface antigen (HBsAg)
Hepatitis B virus (HBV)
Hepatitis Be antigen (HBeAg)
Hepatitis C virus (HCV)
Hepatitis D virus (HDV)
Hepatitis E virus (HEV)
Heterophile antibodies
Human T-cell lymphotropic virus type I (HTLV-I)
Human T-cell lymphotropic virus type II (HTLV-II)
IgM anti-HBc
Mumps virus
Parenteral
Rubella virus
Rubeola virus
Varicella-zoster virus (VZV)

Viruses are submicroscopic pathogens whose size is measured in nanometers. Their basic structure consists of a core of DNA or RNA packaged into a protein coat or capsid. In some viruses, the capsid is surrounded by an outer envelope of glycolipids and proteins derived from the host-cell membrane **(Fig. 23–1)**. It is remarkable that these tiny particles are capable of causing severe, and sometimes lethal, disease in humans, ranging from childhood infections to inflammatory diseases with a predilection for a specific organ, disseminated disease in immunocompromised patients, cancer, and congenital abnormalities.

Viruses are obligate intracellular pathogens that rely on the host cell for their replication and survival. They infect their host cells by attaching to specific receptors on the cell surface; penetrating the host cell membrane; and releasing their nucleic acid, which then directs the host cell's machinery to produce more viral nucleic acid and proteins. These components assemble to form intact viruses that are released by lysis of the cell or by budding off the cell's surface **(Fig. 23–2)**. Replication can occur quickly in cytolytic viruses that produce acute infections, or slowly in viruses that result in chronic infections. The free virions that are generated can then infect neighboring host cells and begin new replication cycles that promote dissemination of the infection. Thus, viruses can be present in the host as both freely circulating particles and intracellular particles.

This chapter briefly addresses the immunologic mechanisms required to attack the virus in its different states. Successful defense against viral infections requires a coordinated effort among innate, humoral, and cell-mediated immune responses **(Fig. 23–3)**. The remainder of the chapter discusses some of the most important viral infections detected by serology and molecular methods. These include the hepatitis viruses, herpes viruses, measles, mumps, rubella, and human T-cell lymphotropic viruses. Laboratory tests for the HIV virus are discussed separately in Chapter 24.

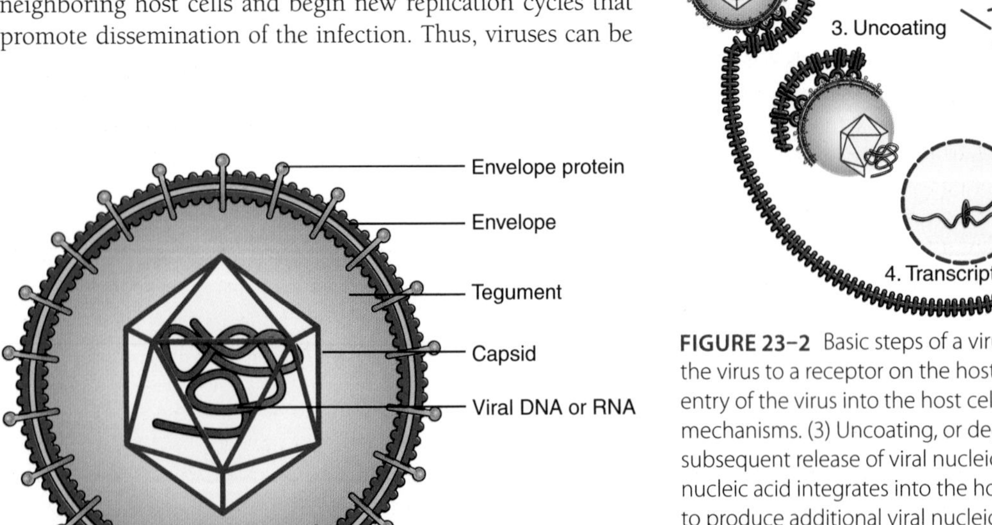

FIGURE 23–1 Basic structure of a virus.

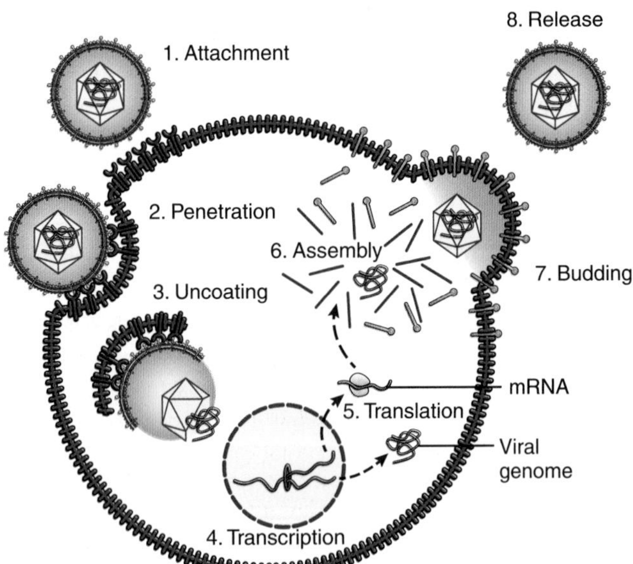

FIGURE 23–2 Basic steps of a virus life cycle. (1) Attachment of the virus to a receptor on the host cell surface. (2) Penetration, or entry of the virus into the host cell through endocytosis or other mechanisms. (3) Uncoating, or degradation of the viral capsid and subsequent release of viral nucleic acid. With some viruses, the nucleic acid integrates into the host-cell genome. (4) Transcription to produce additional viral nucleic acid. (5) Translation of viral nucleic acid to produce viral proteins. (6) Assembly of the viral components to produce intact virions. (7) Budding off the host-cell membrane or host-cell lysis results in (8) release of viral progeny. Modifications of these steps can occur with different viruses.

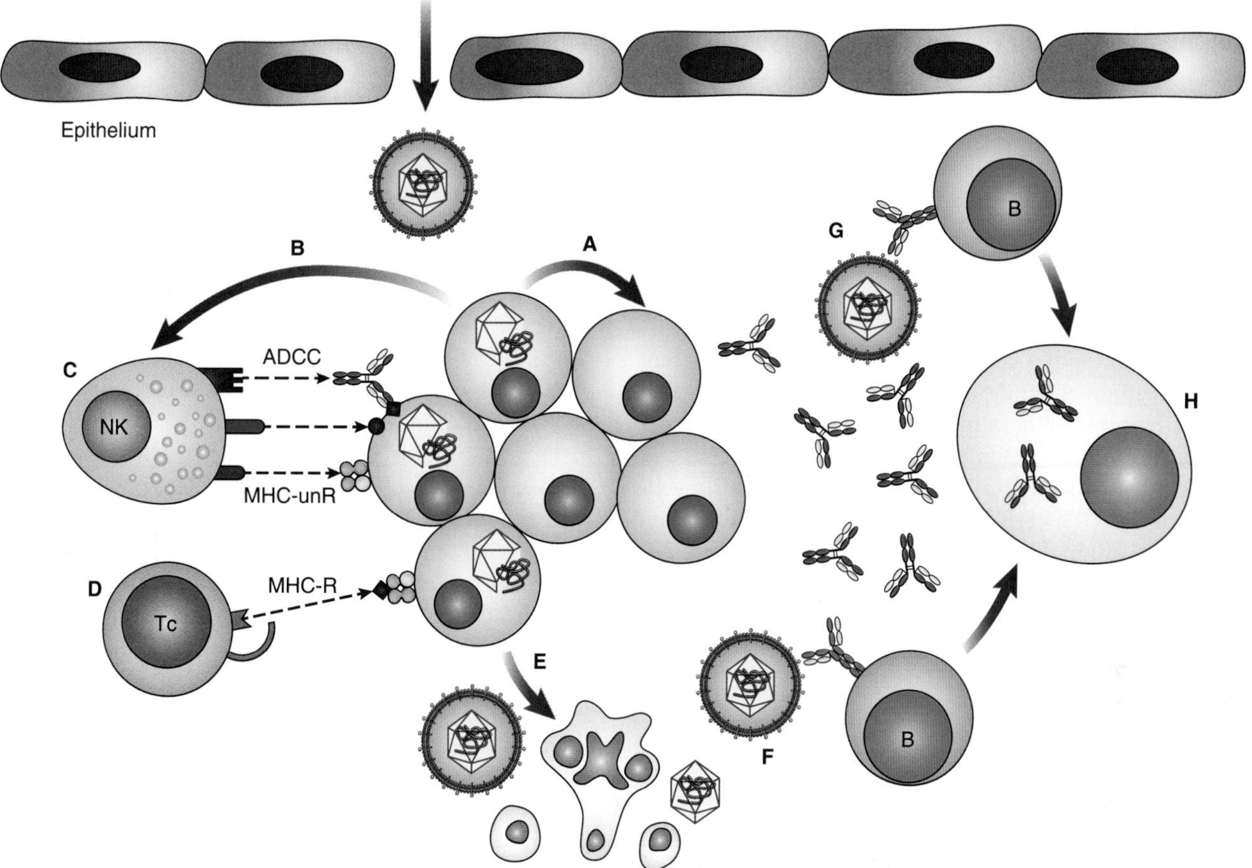

FIGURE 23–3 Innate defenses provide the initial barrier to viral infection. Infected cells release interferons (IFNs) α and β, which (A) inhibit viral replication in surrounding cells and (B) stimulate natural killer (NK) cells. Both NK and cytotoxic T (Tc) cells destroy virus-infected host cells (C, D), resulting in the release of free virions (E). Virus-specific B cells recognize these free virions (F), as well as virions that have penetrated the epithelium (G), leading to the production of antibodies (H) that bind free virions and mediate virus neutralization, opsonization, complement activation, and antibody-dependent cellular cytotoxicity (ADCC).

Immune Defenses Against Viral Infections

Innate immunity provides the first line of protection against viral pathogens. Viruses first encounter naturally occurring barriers in the body, such as the skin and mucous membranes. If they are able to invade these barriers, other innate defenses are activated when cells of the innate immune system recognize pathogen-associated molecular patterns (PAMPs) on the surface of, or within, virus-infected host cells. Two important nonspecific defenses against viruses involve type I interferons (IFNs) and natural killer (NK) cells. Virus-infected cells are stimulated to produce IFN-α and IFN-β following recognition of viral RNA by Toll-like receptors (TLRs). IFNs inhibit viral replication by inducing the transcription of several genes that code for proteins with antiviral activity—for example, a ribonuclease enzyme that degrades viral RNA. IFN-α and IFN-β also enhance the activity of NK cells, which bind to virus-infected cells and release cytotoxic proteins such as perforin and granzymes, causing the cells to die and release the viruses (see Fig. 2–7). These cell-free virions are now accessible to antibody molecules.

Connections

Interferons

IFNs "interfere" with the ability of viruses to replicate by stimulating infected host cells to produce proteins that degrade viral nucleic acid and proteins and induce an anti-viral state (see Chapter 6). IFNs exert their effects not only on the original infected cell but also on neighboring uninfected host cells.

When innate defenses are insufficient in preventing viral infection, specific humoral and cell-mediated defenses are activated. Virus-specific antibodies are produced by B cells and plasma cells and can attack free virus particles in several ways. Antibodies play a key role in preventing the spread of a viral infection through neutralization. This process involves the production of antibodies that are specific for a component of the virus that binds to a receptor on the host-cell membrane. When these neutralizing antibodies bind to the virus, they prevent it from attaching to and penetrating the host cell. Secretory immunoglobulin A (IgA) antibodies play an especially important role in this process because they neutralize viruses in the mucosal surfaces (e.g., respiratory and digestive tracts), which often serve as entryways for the pathogens. Meanwhile, immunoglobulin M (IgM) and immunoglobulin G (IgG) antibodies can bind to viruses in the bloodstream and inhibit dissemination of the infection. In addition, IgG antibodies promote phagocytosis of viruses through their opsonizing activity and promote destruction of viruses through antibody-dependent cellular cytotoxicity (ADCC). IgG and IgM antibodies also activate complement, which can mediate opsonization via C3b or lyse enveloped viruses by inducing formation of the membrane attack complex. IgM antibodies may also inactivate viral particles by agglutinating them.

Although antibodies can attack viruses in many different ways, they cannot reach viruses that have already penetrated host cells. Elimination of intracellular viruses requires the action of cell-mediated immunity. Type 1 helper (Th1) cells and cytotoxic T lymphocytes (CTLs) play a key role in this mechanism of defense. Th1 cells produce IFN-g, which induces an antiviral state within the virus-infected cells, and interleukin-2 (IL-2), which assists in the development of effector CTLs. In this process, CD8+ CTLs become programmed to expand in number and attack the virus-infected cells. To recognize the virus-infected host cell, the T-cell receptor (TCR) on the CTL must bind to a viral antigen complexed with class I major histocompatibility complex (MHC) on the surface of the infected cell (see Fig. 4-10 and Fig. 23–3). CD8 is a co-receptor in this interaction. These molecular interactions stimulate the granules in the CTL to release a pore-forming protein called *perforin*, which produces pores in the membrane of the infected host cell, and proteases called *granzymes*, which enter the pores. These enzymes activate apoptosis in the host cell, interrupting the viral-replication cycle and resulting in release of assembled infectious virions. The free virions can then be bound by antibodies. The CTL response is powerful and involves a series of cell divisions that can produce up to 50,000 times the original number of cells in a period of 1 to 3 weeks.

Viral Escape Mechanisms

Viruses can escape the host's defense mechanisms in several ways. First, viruses are rapidly dividing agents that undergo frequent genetic mutations. These mutations result in the production of new viral antigens, which are not recognized by the initial immune response to the virus. For example, continual antigenic variation in the influenza virus results in the emergence of novel infectious strains that require the development of new vaccines every year to protect the population. Antigenic variation is also seen in other viruses, including rhinoviruses, which cause the common cold, and HIV, which causes AIDS.

Second, some viruses can escape the action of components of the innate immune system such as IFNs, complement proteins, or the lysosomal enzymes in phagocytic cells. For example, the hepatitis C virus (HCV) can block IFN-mediated degradation of viral RNA, and herpes simplex viruses (HSV) produce a protein that binds to the complement component C3b, resulting in inhibition of the complement pathways.

Third, viruses can evade the host's defense by suppressing the adaptive immune system. Some viruses, such as the **cytomegalovirus (CMV)** and HIV, do this by reducing the expression of class I MHC molecules on the surface of virus-infected cells, making them less likely to be recognized by CTLs. Other viruses, such as rubeola, can cause decreased expression of class II MHC molecules, resulting in reduced Th cell activity. Some viruses can alter the function of certain cells of the immune system after directly infecting them. For example, the **Epstein-Barr virus (EBV)** causes polyclonal activation in B lymphocytes, whereas HIV suppresses the function of CD4 Th cells. EBV can also inhibit immune responses by producing a protein that can suppress Th1 cells because of its similarity to interleukin-10 (IL-10).

Finally, some viruses, such as CMV, **varicella-zoster virus (VZV)**, and HIV, can remain in a latent state by integrating their nucleic acid into the genome of the infected host cells. In this situation, the virus is only stimulated to replicate again if the host is exposed to other infectious agents or if the host's immune defenses decline. Latent viruses can remain silent within host cells for years because they are hidden from the immune system, although reactivation can occur later in life.

By using these evasion mechanisms, viruses have established themselves as successful human pathogens that can cause a range of mild to life-threatening diseases. Rapid, reliable laboratory detection of these pathogens is essential for early patient diagnosis and treatment. Laboratory identification also leads to prompt implementation of measures to prevent further spread of the virus to other members of the population.

Laboratory Testing for Viral Infections

As our knowledge of viruses has increased, so has the development of laboratory assays to detect viral infections. Serological and molecular tests can be easily and rapidly performed by the clinical laboratory. Therefore, they play an essential role in helping physicians establish a presumptive diagnosis so that treatment can be initiated promptly. Serological tests are also important in monitoring the course of infection, detecting past infections, and assessing immune status, whereas molecular tests have enhanced our ability to detect active infection and are essential in guiding antiviral therapy.

In general, the presence of virus-specific IgM antibodies in patient serum indicates a current or recent viral infection, whereas IgG antibodies to a virus signify either a current or past infection and, in many cases, immunity. Virus-specific IgM antibody in the newborn's serum indicates a congenital infection because IgM is actively made during fetal life. In contrast, IgG antibodies in the infant's serum are mainly maternal antibodies that have crossed the placenta. Current infections in the adult or newborn may also be detected by immunoassays for viral antigens in serum or other clinical samples or by the presence of viral nucleic acids that can be detected by molecular methods.

Hepatitis Viruses

Hepatitis is a general term that means inflammation of the liver. It can be caused by several viruses and by noninfectious agents, including ionizing radiation, chemicals, and autoimmune processes. The primary hepatitis viruses affect mainly the liver. Other viruses, such as CMV, EBV, and HSV, can also produce liver inflammation, but it is secondary to other disease processes. This section will focus on the primary hepatitis viruses. The **hepatitis A virus (HAV)** and the **hepatitis E virus (HEV)** are transmitted primarily by the fecal–oral route, whereas the **hepatitis B virus (HBV)**, the **hepatitis D virus (HDV)**, and the **hepatitis C virus (HCV)** are transmitted mainly by the **parenteral** route (i.e., through contact with blood and other body fluids). All of the hepatitis viruses may produce similar clinical manifestations. The early, or acute, stages of hepatitis are characterized by general flu-like symptoms and mild to moderate pain in the right upper quadrant (RUQ) of the abdomen. Progression of the disease leads to liver enlargement (hepatomegaly) and tenderness, jaundice, dark urine, and light feces.

Initial laboratory findings typically include elevations in bilirubin and in the liver enzymes, most notably alanine aminotransferase (ALT). These findings are nonspecific indicators of liver inflammation and must be followed by specific serological or molecular tests to identify the cause of hepatitis more definitively. The specific laboratory tests used to detect each type of hepatitis are listed in **Table 23–1.**

Hepatitis A

HAV is a nonenveloped, single-stranded ribonucleic acid (RNA) virus that belongs to the *Hepatovirus* genus of the *Picornaviridae* family. Two major genotypes of the virus are associated with human disease, and both can be detected by the same serological assays (see the text that follows). Hepatitis A is a common infection responsible for an estimated 1.4 million cases of hepatitis worldwide. HAV is transmitted primarily by the fecal–oral route, close person-to-person contact, or ingestion of contaminated food or water. Conditions of poor personal hygiene, poor sanitation, and overcrowding facilitate transmission. Rarely, transmission through transfusion of contaminated blood has been reported and may occur during a short period within the acute stage of infection when a high number of viral particles can be found in the source blood.

Following an average incubation period of 28 days, the virus produces symptoms of acute hepatitis in the majority of infected adults; however, most infections in children are asymptomatic. The infection does not progress to a chronic state and is usually self-limiting, with symptoms typically resolving within 2 months. Treatment is mainly supportive, involving bedrest, nutritional support, and medication for fever, nausea, and diarrhea. Massive hepatic necrosis resulting in fulminant hepatitis and death is rare and occurs mainly in those patients with underlying liver disease or advanced age.

HAV antigens are shed in the feces of infected individuals during the incubation period and the early acute stage of infection, but they usually decline to low levels shortly after symptoms appear and are not a clinically useful indicator of disease. Therefore, serological tests for antibody are critical in establishing diagnosis of the infection. Hepatitis A antibodies are most commonly detected by automated enzyme immunoassays (EIAs) and chemiluminescent microparticle immunoassays. Acute hepatitis A is routinely diagnosed in symptomatic patients by demonstrating the presence of IgM antibodies to HAV **(Fig. 23–4).** IgM anti-HAV is detectable at the onset of clinical symptoms and declines to undetectable levels within 6 months in the majority of infected individuals. Because false-positive results can occur, the test should be reserved for symptomatic individuals. Tests for total HAV antibodies also detect IgM but predominantly detect IgG, which persists for life. Thus, a positive total anti-HAV test result in combination with a negative IgM anti-HAV indicates that the patient has developed immunity to the virus, either through natural infection or vaccination. Negative total anti-HAV tests can be used to identify nonimmune individuals who may have been exposed to the virus.

Although IgM anti-HAV is the primary marker to detect acute hepatitis A, false-negative results can occur during the early phase of the infection. Molecular methods to detect HAV RNA have been shown to be more sensitive in this situation. The most common format of these methods is the reverse-transcriptase polymerase chain reaction (RT-PCR). Molecular methods can also be used to test samples of food or water suspected of transmitting the virus. Multiplex quantitative polymerase chain reaction (qPCR) methods that can simultaneously detect more than one type of hepatitis virus in clinical samples have also been developed.

A vaccine consisting of formalin-killed HAV was licensed in the mid-1990s to prevent hepatitis A. Currently, two inactivated single-antigen vaccines are licensed and available in the United States for hepatitis A prevention. Vaccination has resulted in a significant decrease in the number of HAV infections in the United States and other countries throughout the world. To prevent infection in unimmunized individuals who have been exposed to the virus, prophylactic administration of the hepatitis A vaccine or injections of immune globulin are recommended. The vaccine is the preferred treatment for persons aged 1 to 40 years, but intramuscular injection of immune globulin, a sterile preparation of pooled human plasma that contains antibodies to HAV, can be used to prevent infection in individuals of any age. To be effective, these treatments must be administered within 2 weeks of exposure.

Connections

Reverse-Transcriptase Polymerase Chain Reaction (RT-PCR)

In RT-PCR, viral RNA is treated with the enzyme reverse-transcriptase to generate a complementary DNA (cDNA) sequence. The cDNA is then amplified by the PCR to generate millions of copies that can be detected in the laboratory (see Chapter 12).

Table 23–1 The Hepatitis Viruses and Their Associated Serological and Molecular Markers

HEPATITIS VIRUS	TYPE AND FAMILY	TRANSMISSION	PROGRESSION TO CHRONIC STATE	COMPLICATIONS	SEROLOGICAL AND MOLECULAR MARKERS	CLINICAL SIGNIFICANCE
Hepatitis A (HAV)	RNA *Picornaviridae*	Fecal–oral, direct contact with infectious individual Blood transfusion (rare)	No	Low risk of fulminant liver disease	• IgM anti-HAV	• Acute hepatitis A
					• Total anti-HAV	• Immunity to hepatitis A
					• HAV RNA	• Detection of HAV in clinical, food, or water samples
Hepatitis B (HBV)	DNA *Hepadnaviridae*	Parenteral, sexual, perinatal	Yes	10% to 90% of cases may develop chronic hepatitis (depending on age), with increased risk for liver cirrhosis and hepatocellular carcinoma	• HBsAg	• Active hepatitis B infection
					• HBeAg	• Active hepatitis B with high degree of infectivity
					• IgM anti-HBc	• Current or recent acute hepatitis B
					• Total anti-HBc	• Current or past hepatitis B
					• Anti-HBe	• Recovery from hepatitis B
					• Anti-HBs	• Immunity to hepatitis B
					• HBV DNA	• Acute, atypical, or occult hepatitis B; viral load may be used to monitor effectiveness of therapy
Hepatitis C (HCV)	RNA *Flaviviridae*	Parenteral, sexual, perinatal	Yes	Eighty-five percent develop chronic infection, with increased risk of cirrhosis, hepatocellular carcinoma, or autoimmune manifestations	• Anti-HCV	• Current or past hepatitis C infection
					• HCV RNA	• Current hepatitis C infection; viral load may be used to monitor effectiveness of therapy; also used to determine HCV genotype
Hepatitis D (HDV)	RNA Genus *Deltavirus*	Mostly parenteral, but also sexual, perinatal; HBV infection required	Yes	Increased risk of developing fulminant hepatitis, cirrhosis, or hepatocellular carcinoma	• IgM-anti-HDV	• Acute or chronic hepatitis D
					• IgG-anti-HDV	• Recovery from hepatitis D or chronic hepatitis D
					• HDV RNA	• Active HDV infection; viral load may be used to monitor effectiveness of therapy
Hepatitis E (HEV)	RNA *Hepeviridae*	Fecal–oral Blood transfusion; vertical transmission	Yes, in immunocompromised individuals	Fulminant liver failure in pregnant women	• IgM anti-HEV	• Current hepatitis E infection
					• IgG anti-HEV	• Current or past hepatitis E infection
					• HEV RNA	• Current hepatitis E infection

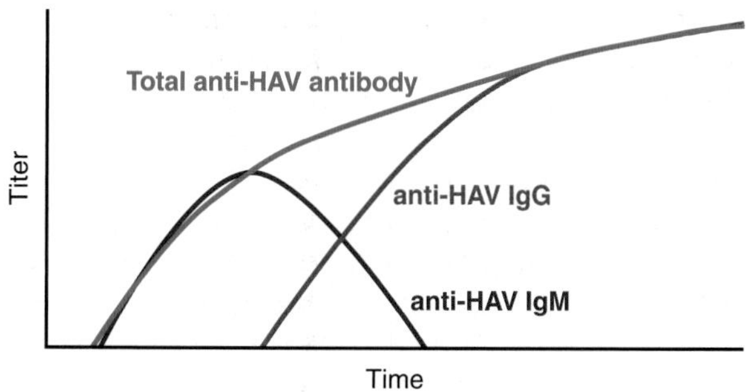

FIGURE 23–4 Hepatitis A Serology. Typical patterns of IgM and total (IgM plus IgG) anti-HAV.

Hepatitis E

HEV is a nonenveloped, single-stranded RNA virus that belongs to the genus *Hepevirus,* in the family *Hepeviridae.* HEV is a major cause of hepatitis worldwide. The World Health Organization (WHO) estimates that the virus causes 20 million infections, with over 3.3 million cases of acute hepatitis annually. In 2015, approximately 44,000 deaths were reported. Similar to the HAV, HEV is transmitted primarily by the fecal–oral route; however, person-to-person transmission is uncommon. The four genotypes of the virus differ in terms of their epidemiology and source of infection. Genotypes 1 and 2 are associated primarily with the consumption of fecally contaminated drinking water in developing regions of the world with poor sanitation, including parts of Africa, Asia, the Middle East, and Mexico. Outbreaks commonly occur in times of natural disasters such as flooding and earthquakes and can affect thousands of individuals. Genotypes 3 and 4 have been increasingly recognized in developed parts of the world, including Europe, North America, China, Taiwan, and Japan. HEV3 and HEV4 are zoonotic infections in which pigs are the primary host. Deer, wild boars, and other mammals are also known to harbor the virus. These infections are thought to be transmitted mainly by the consumption of infected pork and deer meat and possibly by direct contact with infected animals or fecally contaminated water. HEV has also been detected in the blood supply in several countries and can be transmitted through blood transfusions.

Although HEV infections are often silent, all genotypes are capable of causing acute hepatitis with symptoms that are indistinguishable from other types of hepatitis. Following an incubation period of 2 to 10 weeks, HEV infection in most people causes a self-limiting illness, with recovery occurring by 4 to 6 weeks. However, the infection can have severe consequences. Some patients may experience extrahepatic symptoms, including neurological syndromes, renal injury, pancreatitis, and hematologic abnormalities. Pregnant women infected with HEV1 or HEV2 have a mortality rate of 20% to 25% because of obstetric complications or development of fulminant hepatitis, which is associated with rapidly progressing liver disease and failure. The reason for this is unclear, but it may be caused by the hormonal and immunologic changes associated with pregnancy. HEV3 can result in chronic infection in immunocompromised individuals. Chronic infection can progress to liver fibrosis, cirrhosis, and liver failure, which may require liver transplantation.

Measures to prevent the infection include the provision of clean drinking water, improvement of sanitation conditions in developing countries, and in the case of HEV3, avoidance of eating undercooked meat, especially pork. A vaccine to prevent HEV1 infection has been licensed for use in the People's Republic of China. The vaccine consists of virus-like particles that have been genetically modified to express a gene that codes for a key HEV protein. To date, no U.S. Food and Drug Administration (FDA)-cleared vaccine is available in the United States.

Because HEV is not easily cultured, diagnosis relies on serology to detect antibodies to the virus and molecular methods to detect HEV nucleic acid. Antibodies to HEV are typically identified by sensitive EIAs that use recombinant and synthetic HEV antigens. Rapid immunochromatographic assays have also been developed. Antibody tests for HEV can detect all four genotypes of the virus because there is only one viral serotype. Acute infection is indicated by the presence of IgM anti-HEV, which is detectable at clinical onset, remains elevated for about 8 weeks, and becomes undetectable in most patients by 32 weeks. HEV-specific IgG antibodies appear soon after IgM, reach peak levels about 4 weeks after symptoms develop, and persist for several years. Immunoassays for IgG anti-HEV may be performed to detect patients in the later stages of infection, determine past exposure, and identify seroprevalence of the infection in a population.

Immunocompromised persons often yield negative antibody test results; molecular testing for HEV RNA is recommended in these patients. Quantitation of HEV nucleic acid can be performed by qPCR (the gold standard for diagnosis of acute HEV infections) or a loop-mediated isothermal amplification assay (LAMP), which is suitable for resource-limited settings because it is faster and does not require expensive equipment. These assays can be performed on blood or stool samples. HEV RNA can be detected just before clinical symptoms. It becomes undetectable in the blood about 3 weeks after symptom onset; in the stool, it becomes undetectable at about 5 weeks. Therefore, a negative result for HEV RNA does not exclude the possibility of a recent infection.

Hepatitis B

Hepatitis B is a major cause of morbidity and mortality throughout the world. The WHO estimates that HBV has infected 2 billion people worldwide, causing approximately 257 million chronic infections. In 2015, the WHO reported 887,000 deaths because of complications from the disease. The virus is highly endemic in the Far East, parts of the Middle East, sub-Saharan Africa, and the Amazon areas. In the United States, which is considered a low-prevalence area, approximately 2.2 million individuals are living with chronic HBV infections.

HBV is transmitted through the parenteral route by intimate contact with HBV-contaminated blood or other body fluids, most notably semen, vaginal secretions, and saliva.

Transmission has thus been associated with sexual contact, blood transfusions, sharing of needles and syringes by intravenous drug users, tattooing, and occupational needlestick injury. Inapparent transmission of HBV may occur through close personal contact of broken skin or mucous membranes with the virus. Transmission of HBV may also occur via the perinatal route, from infected mother to infant, most likely during delivery.

Several measures have been introduced to prevent HBV infection, including screening of blood donors, treating plasma-derived products to inactivate HBV, implementing infection-control measures, and most importantly, immunizing with a hepatitis B vaccine. The current vaccines, consisting of recombinant hepatitis B surface antigen (HBsAg) produced from genetically engineered yeast or mammalian cells, are some of the most widely used vaccines throughout the world. Immunization has been highly successful, resulting in a significant decline in the incidence of acute hepatitis B in the United States since routine immunization was implemented in 1991. Increasingly widespread use of the vaccine will likely continue to reduce the incidence of new HBV infections worldwide. The vaccine can also be administered to individuals thought to be exposed to the virus, along with hepatitis B immune globulin (HBIG), a preparation derived from donor plasma with high concentrations of antibodies to HBV that provides temporary protection.

Despite the preventative measures that have been implemented, a substantial number of HBV infections continue to occur, as we previously discussed. Infection with HBV results in an incubation period of 30 to 180 days, followed by a clinical course that varies in different age groups. Over 90% of newborns with perinatal HBV infection remain asymptomatic, whereas typical symptoms of acute hepatitis are observed in about 10% of children aged 1 to 5 years and in approximately one-third of adolescents and adults. Symptoms may last several weeks to several months and are usually managed through bedrest and other supportive treatment. Most HBV-infected adults recover within 6 months and develop immunity to the virus, but about 1% develop fulminant liver disease with hepatic necrosis. This highly fatal condition is treated with intensive life support, antiviral drugs, and in some patients, liver transplantation.

Development of chronic HBV infection, in which the virus persists in the body for 6 months or more, occurs in the majority of infected infants, about one-third of young children, and 10% of infected adults. Chronic infection is also more likely to develop in persons who are immunosuppressed and those who have HIV. Chronic infection with the virus results in inflammation and damage to the liver and places the patient at increased risk of developing cirrhosis or hepatocellular carcinoma. Patients with chronic infection can be treated with antiviral drugs to reduce liver inflammation and the risk of developing liver complications. Therapies consist of nucleoside analogues that inhibit the polymerase enzyme needed for viral replication and IFN-α, which enhances the immune response against the virus.

The virus responsible for hepatitis B, HBV, is a DNA virus belonging to the *Hepadnaviridae* family. Eight genotypes, designated A through H, have been identified based on nucleotide-sequence differences in their genomes. The genotypes vary in their geographic distribution, pathogenicity, and response to treatment but can be identified by the same serological assays. The intact HBV virion is a 42-nm sphere consisting of a nucleocapsid core surrounded by an outer envelope of lipoprotein. The core of the virus contains circular, partially double-stranded DNA; a DNA-dependent DNA polymerase enzyme; and two proteins, the hepatitis B core antigen and the **hepatitis Be antigen (HBeAg).** A protein called the **hepatitis B surface antigen (HBsAg)** is found in the outer envelope of the virus. HBsAg is produced in excess and is found in noninfectious spherical and tubular particles that lack viral DNA and circulate freely in the blood.

These antigens, and antibodies to them, serve as serological markers for hepatitis B and have been used in the differential diagnosis of HBV infection, monitoring the course of infection in patients, assessing immunity to the virus, and screening blood products for infectivity. The levels of these markers vary with the amount of viral replication and the host's immune response. They are useful in establishing the initial diagnosis of hepatitis B and monitoring the course of infection. Serological markers for hepatitis B are listed in Table 23–1 and are described in the text that follows. Typical patterns of the markers during acute and chronic hepatitis B are shown in **Figures 23–5** and **23–6.**

HBsAg is the first marker to appear, becoming detectable 2 to 10 weeks after exposure to HBV. Its levels peak during the acute stages of infection, then gradually decline as the patient develops antibodies to the antigen and recovers. Serum HBsAg usually becomes undetectable by 4 to 6 months after the onset of symptoms in patients with acute hepatitis B. In patients with chronic HBV infection, HBsAg remains elevated for 6 months or more. Thus, HBsAg is an indicator of active infection and is an important marker in detecting initial infection, monitoring the course of infection and progression to chronic disease, and screening of donor blood.

HBeAg appears shortly after HBsAg and disappears shortly before HBsAg in recovering patients. It may be elevated during chronic infection. This marker is present during periods of active replication of the virus and indicates a high degree of infectivity. The hepatitis B core antigen (HBc) is not detectable in serum because the viral envelope masks it.

As the host develops an immune response to the virus, antibodies appear. First to appear is IgM antibody to the core antigen, or **IgM anti-HBc.** This antibody indicates current or recent acute infection. It typically appears 1 to 2 weeks after HBsAg during acute infection and persists in high titers for 4 to 6 months and then gradually declines. IgM anti-HBc is useful in detecting infection in cases in which HBsAg is undetectable—for example, just before the appearance of antibodies to HBsAg (commonly referred to as the "core window" period), in neonatal infections, and in cases of fulminant hepatitis. Therefore, it is used in addition to HBsAg for the screening of donor blood. IgG antibodies to the core antigen are produced before IgM anti-HBc disappears and then persist for the individual's lifetime. They are the predominant antibodies detected in the test for total anti-HBc and can be used to indicate a past HBV infection.

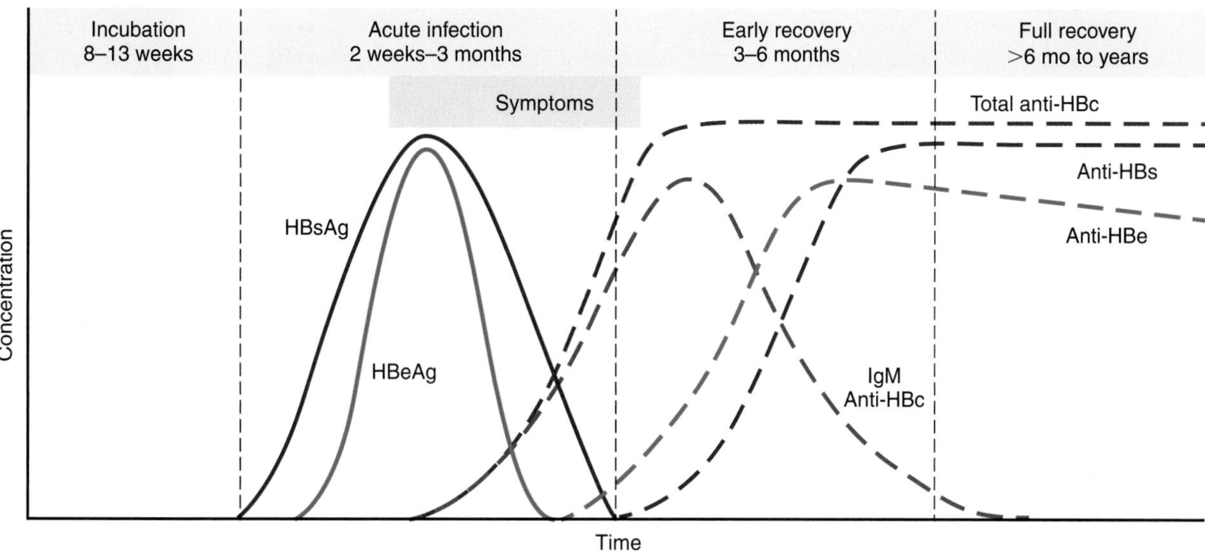

FIGURE 23–5 Typical serological markers in acute hepatitis B. Solid lines represent viral antigen concentrations, whereas dashed lines indicate antibody concentrations. Each antigen shares the same color with its associated antibody.

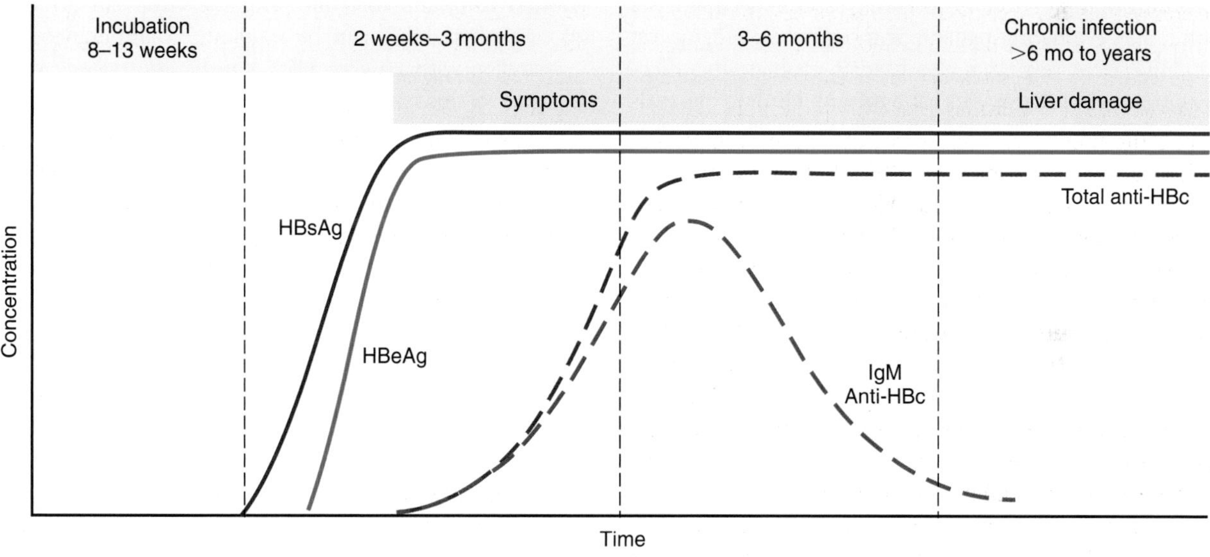

FIGURE 23–6 Typical serological markers in chronic hepatitis B.

The appearance of antibodies to the HBe antigen, or **anti-HBe**, occurs shortly after the disappearance of HBeAg and indicates that the patient is recovering from HBV infection.

Antibodies to HBsAg, or **anti-HBs**, also appear during the recovery period of acute hepatitis B, a few weeks after HBsAg disappears. These antibodies persist for years and provide protective immunity. Anti-HBs are also produced after immunization with the hepatitis B vaccine. Protective titers of the antibody in the serum are considered to be 10 mIU/mL or higher. Anti-HBs are not produced during chronic HBV infection, in which immunity fails to develop.

Serological markers for hepatitis B are most commonly detected by commercial immunoassays. These are available in a variety of formats, such as EIA and chemiluminescent immunoassay (CLIA). They are typically automated to ease batch testing in the clinical laboratory and have excellent sensitivity and specificity. An example of an immunoassay for detecting HBsAg is shown in **Figure 23–7.** Although these methods are highly sensitive and specific, false-positive and false-negative results can occur. Any initial positive results should be verified by repeated testing of the same specimen in duplicate, followed by confirmation with an additional assay, such as an HBsAg neutralization test or a molecular test that detects HBV DNA.

Several molecular methods have been developed to detect HBV DNA in serum or plasma and are mostly based on target amplification by traditional or qPCR (method of choice to quantify HBV DNA) or branched DNA (bDNA) signal amplification. HBV DNA can be detected in the serum about 21 days before HBsAg and may be a useful adjunct in detecting early acute HBV infection in certain situations, such as

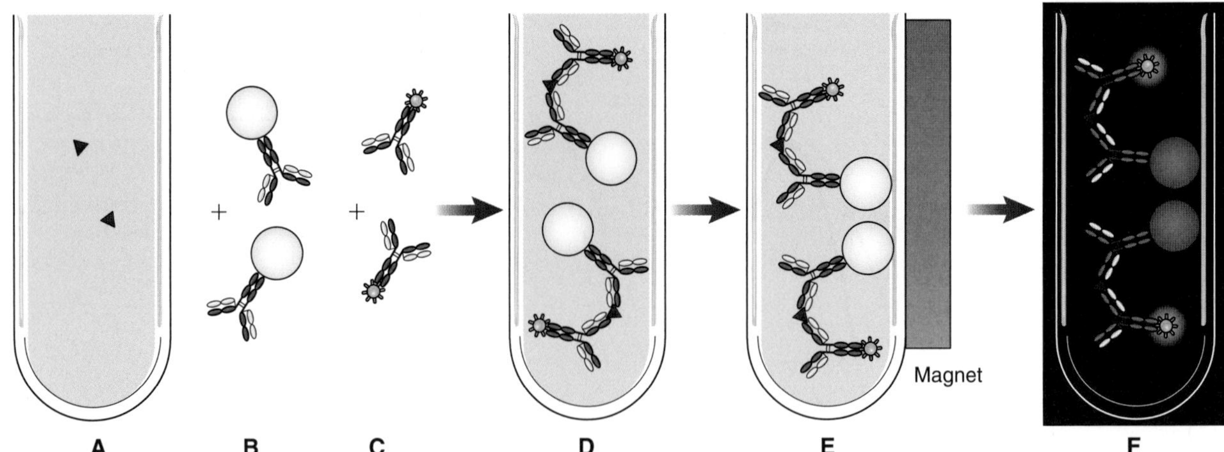

FIGURE 23–7 Detection of the HBs antigen by chemiluminescence microparticle immunoassay. Patient serum or plasma containing HBsAg (A) is mixed with magnetic microparticles coated with anti-HBs (B) and acridinium-labeled anti-HBs conjugate (C). During incubation, complexes form, with the antigen sandwiched in between the antibodies (D). Application of a magnetic field holds the microparticles and bound reagents in the tube while unbound materials are washed away and chemiluminescent reagents are added (E). The magnitude of light produced is measured in a luminometer (F) and is proportional to the concentration of HBsAg in the sample.

the screening of blood donors, assessing cases of occupational exposure, and evaluating patients with equivocal HBsAg test results. HBV DNA testing is also used to evaluate the effectiveness of antiviral therapy in patients with chronic hepatitis B. Successful treatment is indicated by a 1-$\log_{10}$ reduction in HBV DNA levels by 6 months, whereas persistently elevated HBV DNA levels indicate possible drug resistance and a need to change therapy. Molecular testing is also used to diagnose atypical cases of hepatitis B originating from mutations in the HBV genome that cause HBsAg tests to be negative. Molecular methods to detect HBV genotypes and HBV mutations associated with antiviral drug resistance have also been developed. These tests will likely be used more widely in the future to determine optimal patient therapy.

Hepatitis D

Hepatitis D, also known as *delta hepatitis,* is a parenterally transmitted infection that can occur only in the presence of hepatitis B. HDV is a defective virus that requires the help of HBV for its replication and expression. The only member within the *Deltavirus* genus, HDV consists of a circular RNA genome and a single structural protein called *hepatitis delta antigen* within its core, surrounded by a viral envelope that is of HBV origin and contains the HBsAg. Three genotypes have been identified: Genotype I (most common and found worldwide), Genotype II (Japan and Taiwan), and Genotype III (South America). Approximately 15 to 20 million people around the world are believed to be infected with HDV, which is highly prevalent in Mediterranean Europe, the Middle East, the Amazon basin, central Africa, and parts of Asia. The number of new infections appears to be increasing in certain parts of the world.

Similar to HBV, HDV is transmitted sexually in semen or vaginal secretions; through blood by intravenous drug use, needlestick injuries, or transfusions; or perinatally from mother to infant. Infection with the virus can occur in one of two ways: HDV can be transmitted simultaneously as a *co-infection* with HBV or HDV can be contracted as a *superinfection* of individuals who are already chronic HBV carriers. Clinically, most patients with co-infections experience an acute, self-limited hepatitis in which both viruses are cleared within a few months. Some patients may experience more severe symptoms of acute hepatitis than those infected with HBV alone, but only about 2% of cases progress to a chronic state. In contrast, more than 70% of patients with superinfections develop chronic liver disease with an accelerated progression to cirrhosis and liver failure. Combinations of IFN-α and antiviral drugs can be administered to patients with chronic or severe hepatitis D in an attempt to eradicate the virus.

Testing for hepatitis D should be performed in all patients who are HBsAg positive and involves the detection of HDV antibodies and HDV RNA. Antibodies are detected by immunoassays employing the hepatitis D antigen. The presence of IgG anti-HDV antibodies indicates exposure to the virus and can signify an acute, chronic, or past hepatitis D infection. Although IgM anti-HDV is produced during acute hepatitis D infections, its appearance may be delayed, it may persist for only a short period of time, and it may be missed. IgM antibodies to HDV can also persist during chronic infection. Serology testing for hepatitis B can be used to help distinguish HBV and HDV co-infections from HBV and HDV superinfections, which, as previously discussed, have different clinical outcomes. In addition to being positive for HDV antibodies, patients with co-infections are positive for IgM anti-HBc, whereas patients with superinfections are positive for IgG anti-HBc.

The detection of hepatitis D has been aided tremendously by the development of molecular methods to detect HDV RNA, a marker of active viral replication that is present in all types of active hepatitis D infections. HDV RNA testing is routinely used to confirm a positive HDV antibody screen. Molecular testing for serum HDV RNA is performed by sensitive, real-time RT-PCR assays. These assays also provide quantitative results that can be used to monitor the response of patients to antiviral therapy.

Hepatitis C

Hepatitis C is a major public health problem, with an estimated 71 million people infected worldwide. It is the most common bloodborne infection in the United States, with an estimated 2.4 million individuals living with chronic HCV. Hepatitis C is also the most frequent cause of chronic liver infection and the leading indicator for liver transplantation in the United States.

HCV, the virus that causes hepatitis C, is responsible for most of the infections previously classified as "nonA–nonB" before the discovery of the virus in 1989. It is an enveloped, single-stranded, positive-sense RNA virus belonging to the family *Flaviviridae* and the genus *Hepacivirus*. Scientists have discovered seven different genotypes of the virus, designated 1 through 7, and numerous subtypes for each, indicated by lowercase letters. The genotypes differ in their geographic distribution, pathogenicity, and response to antiviral treatment. Genotype 1, the most common, is responsible for 46% of hepatitis C infections worldwide and approximately 75% of HCV infections in the United States. Genotypes 1, 2, and 3 are predominant in North America, Europe, and Japan; genotypes 3 and 6 are found throughout south and southeast Asia; and genotypes 4, 5, and 7 are most common in parts of Africa. The variability of HCV, along with its ability to undergo rapid mutations within its hosts, has created difficulty in developing an effective vaccine.

Hepatitis C is transmitted mainly by exposure to contaminated blood, with intravenous drug use being the main source of infection. Blood transfusion was also a major vehicle of transmission before routine screening of blood donors for HCV antibody was implemented in 1992, but transmission by this means is rare today. Organ transplantation before 1992 was also a route of transmission. Other risk factors for acquiring hepatitis C include occupational exposures to contaminated blood, long-term hemodialysis, and unregulated body piercing or tattooing in environments such as correctional facilities where contaminated needles are likely to be used. Sexual transmission of HCV is thought to be less common but is higher in those who have had multiple sex partners or a history of sexually transmitted diseases. Perinatal transmission has been estimated to occur at a rate of about 6%.

HCV has an average incubation period of 7 weeks (range is 2 weeks to 6 months). The majority of infections are asymptomatic, with symptoms of acute hepatitis occurring in only about 20% of cases. Asymptomatic infection is problematic because chronic infection develops in about 70% of infected persons, and up to half of these individuals develop cirrhosis. Cirrhosis occurs slowly over a 25- to 30-year period, causing damage to the liver and posing an increased risk of developing hepatocellular carcinoma. Patients with chronic HCV infection may also develop extrahepatic manifestations, including rheumatological conditions; glomerulonephritis, vasculitis, or other autoimmune manifestations; neuropathy; ophthalmological symptoms; and dermatological symptoms. Early detection would help prevent these complications, but HCV is often missed in its early stages because of the asymptomatic nature of the infection in most individuals.

Clearance of the infection may occur spontaneously or may require treatment with antiviral drugs. The standard treatment involves a combination of pegylated IFN-α (PEG IFN-α) and ribavirin. Although this treatment has been successful in 80% of persons infected with genotypes 2 or 3, it is effective in only half of those with genotype 1 and is associated with numerous side effects. Increased understanding of the biology of HCV has led to the development of direct-acting antiviral drugs (DAAs) and host-targeted agents (HTAs) that inhibit specific steps of the viral replication cycle. Combination therapies employing these agents are being evaluated at a rapid pace and are revolutionizing the way hepatitis C is being treated.

The laboratory plays an essential role in screening for hepatitis C, monitoring patients known to have HCV infection, and guiding therapy. Between 1998 and 1999, the Centers for Disease Control and Prevention (CDC) issued recommendations that screening for HCV infection be conducted in high-risk individuals, including those who received blood or blood products. In 2012, the CDC extended these recommendations to include a one-time screening of all persons in the United States who were born between 1945 and 1965, regardless of risk factors. In 2013, the U.S. Preventative Task Force endorsed this recommendation. The rationale behind the latest recommendation was that about 75% of individuals living with HCV infection in the United States were born during this time period but are asymptomatic. Identification of these persons could lead to closer monitoring for disease progression and earlier administration of effective antiviral treatment.

Screening and diagnosis of hepatitis C begins with serological testing for HCV antibodies. Anti-HCV IgG is most commonly detected by sensitive EIAs or CLIAs that use recombinant and synthetic antigens developed from the conserved domains of the capsid core protein (C) and the nonstructural proteins NS3, NS4, and NS5. Alternatively, a rapid immunoblot assay can be used for point-of-care testing. Antibodies become detectable 8 to 10 weeks after HCV exposure and can remain positive for a lifetime. Thus, a reactive result can indicate the presence of a current HCV infection or a past HCV infection that has resolved. In addition, despite the excellent specificity of these methods, false-positive results may occur because of cross-reactivity in persons with other viral infections or autoimmune disorders. Therefore, any positive results from an anti-HCV screening test should be confirmed to distinguish between the various interpretations of these results. Current CDC guidelines recommend the use of nucleic acid testing (NAT) for HCV RNA for confirmation. If HCV RNA is detected, a current HCV infection is indicated. In contrast, if the NAT is nonreactive, this suggests a past HCV infection or false-positive antibody test result. To distinguish between a true-positive and false-positive result, HCV antibody testing can be repeated using a different assay from the initial test because a biological false-positive result is unlikely to occur in two different methods.

Molecular assays for HCV RNA can be classified as qualitative or quantitative. Qualitative tests distinguish between the presence or absence of HCV RNA in a clinical sample. These tests are used to confirm infection in HCV-antibody-positive patients (as previously mentioned), detect infection in antibody-negative patients who are suspected of having HCV, screen blood and organ donors for HCV, and detect perinatal infections in babies born to HCV-positive mothers. Qualitative RT-PCR and transcription-mediated amplification (TMA) methods are commercially available. These tests can detect as low as 5 International Units (IU) of HCV RNA per mL of serum (for TMA) or 50 IU/mL HCV RNA (for RT-PCR) and become positive within 1 to 3 weeks after infection. They are generally positive at the onset of symptoms but, in some patients, can transiently decrease to undetectable levels during the acute phase of the infection.

Quantitative tests are performed by RT-PCR, qPCR, or bDNA amplification. Commercial tests can detect a wide range of HCV concentrations, from about 10 IU/mL to 10 million IU/mL. They are used to monitor the amount of HCV RNA, or "viral load," carried by patients before, during, and after antiviral therapy in chronically infected individuals. The ultimate goal of such therapy is to achieve a sustained virological response (SVR) in which the patient continuously tests negative for HCV RNA 12 or 24 weeks after therapy is completed. The initial viral load level has also been used as a prognostic tool because those with a low initial viral load are most likely to achieve an SVR.

Genotyping, to determine the exact genotype and subtype of the virus responsible for the infection, should be performed on all HCV-infected patients before antiviral therapy. It is important to identify the patient's HCV genotype in order to determine the most effective treatment because HCV genotypes vary in their response to different antiviral drugs. For example, as we previously mentioned, PEG IFN-α/ribavirin treatment is more effective in patients with genotypes 2 or 3 than in patients with genotype 1. Genotyping is also useful in epidemiological studies to determine the source of HCV infection in specific populations.

Genotyping can be performed by PCR amplification and sequencing of the target gene, PCR followed by identification of the target gene with genotype-specific probes, or qPCR. PCR/direct sequencing (Sanger sequencing) is the reference method because it provides precise information regarding the genomic variability of the virus in patients during the course of the disease. However, sequencing is primarily performed in research laboratories because of the specialized equipment and analysis software required, whereas clinical laboratories typically use qPCR methods or PCR/probe hybridization.

Herpes Virus Infections

The herpes viruses are large, complex DNA viruses that are surrounded by a protein capsid, an amorphous tegument, and an outer envelope. These viruses are all capable of establishing a latent infection with lifelong persistence in the host. The *Herpesviridae* family includes eight viruses that can cause disease in humans: the herpes simplex viruses (HSV-1 and HSV-2); VZV; EBV; CMV; and the human herpes viruses HHV-6, HHV-7, and HHV-8, the latter being associated with Kaposi sarcoma. This section presents the clinical manifestations and laboratory diagnosis of some of these viruses.

Epstein-Barr Virus (EBV)

The EBV is ubiquitous in nature and causes a wide spectrum of diseases, including infectious mononucleosis (IM), lymphoproliferative disorders, and several malignancies. EBV infections most commonly result from intimate contact with salivary secretions from an infected individual. Although transmission of the virus can occur by other means, including blood transfusions, bone marrow and solid-organ transplants, sexual contact, and perinatal exposure, these routes appear to be much less frequent.

In developing nations of the world and lower socioeconomic groups living under poor sanitation, EBV infections usually occur during early childhood, whereas in industrialized nations with higher hygiene standards, infections are typically delayed until adolescence or adulthood. However, by adulthood (age 40), almost 100% of individuals have been infected, as evidenced by the presence of EBV antibodies in their serum.

Initial infection with EBV is believed to occur in the oropharynx, where the virus primarily infects epithelial cells and B lymphocytes. EBV binds to β1 integrins on the surface of the epithelial cells, which take up the virus by endocytosis. Inside the oropharyngeal epithelial cells, EBV enters a lytic cycle, characterized by viral replication, lysis of host cells, and release of infectious virions, until the acute infection is resolved. The virions spread to adjacent structures, including the salivary glands and tonsils. There, EBV infects B lymphocytes, which spread the virus throughout the lymphoreticular system. EBV enters the B cells by binding to surface CD21, which is also the receptor for the C3d component of complement. The virus-infected B cells become polyclonally activated, proliferating and secreting several antibodies, including EBV-specific antibodies; heterophile antibodies; and autoantibodies such as cold agglutinins, rheumatoid factor, and antinuclear antibodies. In healthy individuals, this process is kept in check by the immune response of NK cells and specific CTLs. However, EBV can persist in the body indefinitely in a small percentage of memory B cells, where it establishes a latent infection. In the latent state, EBV nucleic acid exists as episomal DNA outside of the chromosomes; in these cases, active viral replication does not occur. Periodic reactivation results in re-entry of the virus into the lytic cycle, with viral shedding into the saliva and genital secretions, even in healthy, asymptomatic individuals.

Several antigens have been identified in EBV-infected cells that are associated with different phases of the viral infection. Antibodies to these antigens have become an important diagnostic tool. Antigens produced during the initial stages of viral replication in the lytic cycle are known as the *early antigens (EAs)*. These antigens can be further classified into two groups based on their location within the cells: EA-D, which has a

Table 23–2 Epstein-Barr Virus Antigens

EARLY ACUTE PHASE	LATE PHASE	LATENT PHASE
EA-R (early antigen restricted) EA-D (early antigen diffuse)	VCA (viral capsid antigen) MA (membrane antigen)	EBNA (EBV nuclear antigens): EBNA-1, EBNA-2, EBNA-3 (3a), EBNA-4 (3b), EBNA-5 (LP), EBNA-6 (3c)
		Latent membrane proteins (LMP-1, LMP-2A, LMP-2B)

diffuse distribution in the nucleus and cytoplasm, and EA-R, which is *restricted* to the cytoplasm only. The late antigens of EBV are those that appear during the period of the lytic cycle following viral DNA synthesis. They include the viral capsid antigens (VCAs) in the protein capsid and the membrane antigens in the viral envelope. Antigens appearing during the latent phase include the EBV nuclear antigen (EBNA) proteins, EBNA-1, EBNA-2, EBNA-3 (or -3a), EBNA-4 (or -3b), EBNA-5 (or -LP), and EBNA-6 (or -3c), and the latent membrane proteins (LMPs), LMP-1, LMP-2A, and LMP-2B **(Table 23–2).**

The clinical manifestations of EBV vary with the host's age and immune status. Infections in infants and young children are generally asymptomatic or mild, whereas primary infections in healthy adolescents or adults commonly result in IM. More than half of patients with IM present with three classic symptoms: fever, lymphadenopathy, and sore throat. Symptoms usually last for 2 to 4 weeks, but fatigue, myalgias, and need for sleep can persist for months. Treatment is mainly directed at alleviating symptoms. Although the associated symptoms are essential in diagnosing IM, they can also be caused by many other infectious agents, so laboratory testing plays an important role in differentiating IM from other infections.

Characteristic laboratory findings in patients with IM include an absolute lymphocytosis of greater than 50% of the total leukocytes and at least 20% atypical lymphocytes **(Fig. 23–8)**. The atypical lymphocytes are predominantly activated cytotoxic T cells that are responding to the viral infection. Serological findings include the presence of a heterophile antibody and antibodies to certain EBV antigens.

By definition, **heterophile antibodies** are antibodies that are capable of reacting with similar antigens from two or more unrelated species. The heterophile antibodies associated with IM are IgM antibodies produced because of polyclonal B-cell activation and are capable of reacting with horse red blood cells (RBCs), sheep RBCs, and bovine RBCs. These antibodies are produced by 40% of patients with IM during the first week of clinical illness and by 80% to 90% of patients by the third week. They disappear in most patients by 3 months after the onset of symptoms but can be detected in some patients for 1 to 2 years. Because the heterophile antibody is present in most patients during the acute phase of illness, testing for this antibody has been typically performed to screen for IM in patients who present with symptoms of the disease.

For many years, the heterophile antibody of IM was detected by a rapid slide agglutination method called the "Monospot." In this test, serum premixed with guinea pig kidney antigen was still capable of agglutinating horse RBCs, whereas serum premixed with beef erythrocyte antigen could not agglutinate horse RBCs because the heterophile antibody

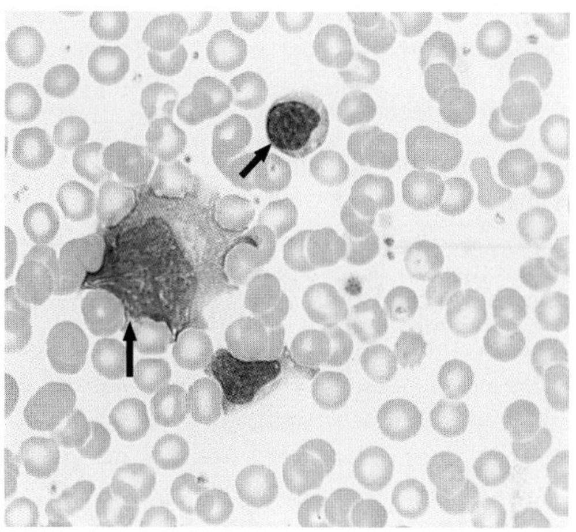

FIGURE 23–8 Atypical lymphocytes from a patient with infectious mononucleosis. Note the variation in size, nuclear:cytoplasmic ratio, and chromatin coarseness. *(From Harmening D. Clinical Hematology and Fundamentals of Hemostasis. 5th ed. Philadelphia, PA: F. A. Davis; 2009.)*

was absorbed during the first step. The test was used to distinguish the heterophile antibody of IM from heterophile antibodies produced in other conditions, which had different reactivity. The antibody could then be titered by incubating serial dilutions of the patient's serum with sheep RBCs in the Paul–Bunnell test (see the Lab Exercise on Davis*Plus*).

Today, these methods have been replaced by more sensitive, rapid agglutination tests or immunochromatographic assays using purified bovine RBC extract as the antigen. Although screening tests for the heterophile antibody are ideal for point-of-care testing, they are not as sensitive or specific as tests for antibodies to EBV, the direct cause of IM. Negative heterophile antibody results occur in about 10% of adult patients with IM and up to 50% of children younger than 4 years old. False-positive results, although uncommon, can occur in patients with lymphoma, viral hepatitis, malaria, and autoimmune disease or can be caused by errors in result interpretation.

Testing for EBV-specific antibodies can be performed to aid in the diagnosis of IM, especially in patients with a negative heterophile antibody screen, or to determine if individuals have had a past exposure to EBV. These antibodies can be detected by indirect immunofluorescence assays (IFAs) using EBV-infected cells, blot techniques, enzyme-linked immunosorbent assay (ELISA) or CLIA using recombinant or synthetic EBV proteins, or flow cytometric microbead immunoassays. Although all of these methods have a high level of sensitivity (95% to 99%), IFA tests have a higher level of specificity and

Table 23–3 Serological Responses of Patients With Epstein-Barr Virus-Associated Diseases

	ANTI-VCA			ANTI-EA			
CONDITION	IgM	IgG	IgA	EA-D	EA-R	ANTI-EBNA	HETEROPHILE ANTIBODY (IgM)
Uninfected	–	–	–	–	–	–	–
Acute IM	+	++	±	+	–	–	±
Convalescent IM	–	+	–	–	±	+	±
Past infection IM	–	+	–	–	–	+	–
Chronic active infection IM	–	+++	±	+	++	±	–
Post-transplant lymphoproliferative disease	–	++	±	+	+	±	–
Burkitt's lymphoma	–	+++	–	±	++	+	–
Nasopharyngeal carcinoma	–	+++	+	++	±	+	–

EA-D = early antigen—diffuse; EA-R = early antigen—restricted; EBNA = EBV nuclear antigen; IM = infectious mononucleosis; VCA = viral capsid antigen. Adapted from Straus SE, et al. Epstein-Barr virus infections: biology, pathogenesis, and management. Ann Intern Med. *1993;118:45, with permission.*

are considered the "gold standard" of EBV serology methods. However, many laboratories prefer ELISA or CLIA tests because they are automated and easier to interpret.

IgM antibody to the VCA is the most useful marker for acute IM because it usually appears at the onset of clinical symptoms and disappears by 3 months. IgG anti-VCA is also present at the onset of IM but persists for life and can thus indicate a past infection. Antibodies to EA-D are also seen during acute IM, whereas anti-EBNA appears during convalescence. Thus, acute primary infection is typically indicated by the presence of IgM anti-VCA and anti-EA-D, as well as the absence of anti-EBNA. A summary of serological responses during acute, convalescent, and post-IM is shown in **Table 23–3**.

Some individuals develop chronic active EBV infection, with severe, often life-threatening IM-associated symptoms that persist or recur for more than 6 months after the acute illness. In addition, EBV can sometimes integrate its DNA into the genome of the cells it infects and transform them into cancer cells. Therefore, EBV has been associated with several malignancies, both hematologic (e.g., Burkitt's lymphoma and Hodgkin disease) and nonhematologic (e.g., nasopharyngeal carcinoma and gastric carcinoma). EBV can also cause lymphoproliferative disorders in immunocompromised patients, including central nervous system (CNS) lymphomas in patients with AIDS, X-linked lymphoproliferative disease in males with a rare genetic mutation, and post-transplant lymphoproliferative disorders (PTLD) in patients who have received hematopoietic stem cell or solid-organ transplants. These disorders result from the inability of immunosuppressed patients to control primary EBV infection, leading to massive polyclonal expansion of the EBV-infected B cells and life-threatening illness with a high rate of mortality.

EBV-associated malignancies can be diagnosed with the help of serology tests for EBV antibodies and molecular methods to detect EBV DNA in blood and tissue samples. Typical patterns of EBV antibodies seen in some of these disorders are shown in Table 23–3. Molecular tests may be more reliable than serology in immunocompromised patients, who may not demonstrate a good humoral response. Quantitative real-time PCR is useful in monitoring viral load in transplant patients; a high or steadily increasing EBV viral load indicates the need to decrease immunosuppressive treatment and administer antiviral therapy. Detection of EBV-encoded RNA transcripts (EBERs) by in situ hybridization is the method of choice for detecting EBV in tumor tissue.

Cytomegalovirus (CMV)

CMV is a ubiquitous virus with worldwide distribution. The prevalence of CMV ranges from 40% to 100%, depending on the population, and increases with age; however, crowded living conditions and poor personal hygiene facilitate spread earlier in life. Transmission of the virus can occur in a variety of ways. CMV is spread through close, prolonged contact with infectious body secretions; intimate sexual contact; blood transfusions; solid-organ transplants; and perinatal exposure from infected mother to infant. The virus has been isolated in many body fluids, including saliva, urine, stool, vaginal and cervical secretions, semen, breast milk, and blood.

Primary, or initial, infections in healthy individuals are usually asymptomatic. However, some people experience a self-limiting, heterophile antibody-negative IM-like illness with fever, myalgias, and fatigue. A small number of immunocompetent individuals who have other underlying disorders may develop severe CMV disease, which most commonly involves the gastrointestinal tract, CNS, and hematologic abnormalities. An immune response against CMV is stimulated, but the virus persists in a latent state in monocytes, dendritic cells, myeloid progenitor cells, and peripheral blood leukocytes. It may be reactivated at a later time in the individual's life.

The clinical consequences of CMV infection are much more serious in the immunocompromised host, most notably organ-transplant recipients and patients with HIV/AIDS. CMV is the most important infectious agent associated with organ transplantation, with infections resulting from reactivation of CMV in the recipient or transmission of CMV from the donor organ. CMV infection of a previously unexposed recipient is associated with increased risk for allograft failure or graft-versus-host disease (GVHD) and poses a high risk for a variety of syndromes, such as fever and leukopenia, hepatitis, pneumonia, gastrointestinal complications, CNS dysfunction, and retinitis. Although combination antiretroviral therapy has reduced the incidence of CMV-related illness in patients with HIV infection, CMV remains a major opportunistic pathogen in patients with low CD4 T-cell counts.

Various measures can be undertaken to reduce the risk for CMV transmission and treat CMV infection in the immunocompromised host. Serological testing can be performed to identify CMV-positive donors so that transplantation of their organs into CMV-negative recipients can be avoided. If a CMV infection has been established in a transplant patient, immunosuppressive treatment should be reduced to the lowest dose possible. In addition, a variety of antiviral drugs are currently used to treat CMV infection and may, in some instances, be given prophylactically (i.e., before organ transplantation). Researchers are also investigating a vaccine design that involves the production of specific CMV antigens using genetic technologies.

CMV is also the most common cause of congenital infections, occurring in 0.3% to 2.3% of all neonates. Transmission of the virus may occur through the placenta, by passage of the infant through an infected birth canal, or by postnatal contact with breast milk or other maternal secretions. About 10% to 15% of infants with congenital CMV infection are symptomatic at birth. Mothers who acquire primary CMV infection during their pregnancy have a significantly higher risk of giving birth to a symptomatic or severely affected infant than do women in whom CMV was reactivated during pregnancy. Symptomatic infants present with a multitude of symptoms that reflect platelet dysfunction and CNS involvement. Ten percent of infants who are asymptomatic at birth progressively develop sensorineural hearing loss.

Several laboratory methods have been developed to detect CMV infection; the tests recommended for use depend on the clinical situation. Assays for direct detection of the virus, such as viral culture, identification of CMV antigens, and molecular tests for CMV DNA, are necessary to detect a current CMV infection in individuals who are immunocompromised or in neonates suspected of being congenitally infected with CMV. Serology is most beneficial in determining a past exposure to the virus, for example, in pregnant women or in patients in need of a transplant.

Isolation of the virus in culture is the traditional method of direct viral detection. In this method, human fibroblast cell lines are inoculated with CMV-infected specimens, most commonly urine, respiratory secretions, or anticoagulated whole blood. The presence of the virus is indicated by characteristic cytopathic effects (CPEs) that produce enlarged, rounded, refractile cells. Although conventional culture provides definitive results when positive, it is limited because CPEs do not appear until a few days to several weeks after inoculation, depending on the viral titer. Implementation of the rapid centrifugation-enhanced (shell vial) method has reduced the time of detection to within 24 hours after inoculation. In this assay, infected cells are grown on coverslips in shell vials and incubated with fluorescent-labeled monoclonal antibodies to CMV antigens produced early in the replication cycle. Fluorescent staining will appear in the nuclei of positive cells.

A widely used method for direct identification of CMV has been the CMV antigenemia assay, which uses immunocytochemical or immunofluorescent staining to detect the CMV lower-matrix protein pp65 in infected leukocytes from peripheral blood or cerebral spinal fluid. Following lysis of erythrocytes in the sample, the leukocytes are fixed onto a microscope slide, permeabilized, and stained with labeled monoclonal anti-pp65. Fluorescence appears in the nuclei of the infected cells, which can be counted to give quantitative results. The test can be completed in 2 to 4 hours, allowing for more rapid diagnosis and treatment of CMV infection in organ-transplant patients and individuals infected with HIV.

Although the antigenemia assay and shell vial culture methods are sensitive, specific, and rapid, they are labor-intensive and require personnel with expertise in performing and interpreting these tests. For these reasons, they are progressively being replaced with molecular methods that detect CMV DNA or mRNA. Real-time PCR is the most widely used molecular method because it is sensitive, simple to perform, and can provide quantitative results. PCR amplification of CMV DNA has been extremely useful for detecting CMV infections in HIV-infected hosts and establishing the diagnosis of CMV infection in transplant recipients. PCR also provides a more sensitive alternative to culture in diagnosing congenital CMV infections. Identification of CMV or CMV DNA in amniotic fluid after the 20th week of gestation is considered the gold standard for confirmation of fetal infection. Neonatal infection is established by detecting CMV or CMV DNA in the urine of the infant during the first 10 days of life. Quantitative PCR, which detects the CMV copy number in the peripheral blood, is used to monitor the effectiveness of antiviral treatment in immunocompromised hosts and to identify patients at risk for developing disseminated CMV disease. In addition, increasing CMV DNA levels over time can be helpful in distinguishing an active infection from asymptomatic or latent infections.

Although serology tests for CMV have been commercially available for many years, their clinical utility is limited. The serology methods performed most commonly are semi- or fully automated EIAs that use microtiter plates or microparticle systems. Assays for CMV IgG are most useful in documenting a past CMV infection and determining if an individual is at risk for future infection. For example, screening of blood and organ donors for CMV IgG is performed to identify those donors who are CMV-positive so that the risk of post-transfusion/post-transplant primary CMV infection in seronegative recipients can be reduced. In addition, screening of pregnant women for CMV IgG can determine if they have been exposed to the infection in the past or if they are susceptible to primary infection. In the latter case, the women could be educated on measures to reduce their chances of exposure while pregnant.

Although a single positive CMV IgG result indicates past exposure to the virus, conversion from a negative antibody result to a positive antibody result over time indicates a recent CMV infection. However, serial assays for CMV IgG are not routinely performed. Assays for IgM CMV antibodies have been developed but are limited in value because of the potential for false-negative results in newborns and immunocompromised patients and for false-positive results caused by other infections or the presence of rheumatoid factor. In addition, IgM antibodies may not necessarily indicate primary CMV infection because they can also be produced because of CMV reactivation and may persist for up to 18 months. Serological methods that distinguish CMV antibody avidity appear to be more useful in distinguishing a past exposure from a current primary infection. Low-avidity IgG antibodies indicate a recent infection, whereas high-avidity IgG antibodies reflect a past exposure because the avidity of the antibody increases during the course of the immune response. The presence of both IgM and low-avidity IgG antibodies can help identify pregnant women who have contracted a primary CMV infection. Because of the limitations of serology testing, direct methods of detecting CMV infection are essential.

Connections

Rheumatoid Factor

Recall that rheumatoid factor (RF) is an antibody (usually of the IgM class) that is directed against the Fc portion of IgG. RF can cause a false-positive result in some IgM assays because it binds to IgG antibodies in the patient serum that are directed against the viral antigen bound to the solid phase (see Chapter 11).

Varicella-Zoster Virus (VZV)

VZV is the cause of two distinct diseases: varicella, more commonly known as *chickenpox,* and herpes zoster, also known as *shingles.* The virus is transmitted primarily by inhalation of infected respiratory secretions or aerosols from skin lesions associated with the infection. Transplacental transmission to the fetus may also occur.

Primary infection with VZV results in varicella, a highly contagious illness characterized by a blister-like rash with intense itching and fever. Historically, the majority of varicella cases have occurred during childhood. In a typical infection, vesicular lesions first appear on the face and trunk and then spread to other areas of the body **(Fig. 23–9)**. The illness is usually mild and self-limiting in healthy children; however, in some cases, it may produce complications, the most common of which are secondary bacterial skin infections caused by scratching of the lesions. CNS involvement may occur in some cases but does not usually require hospitalization.

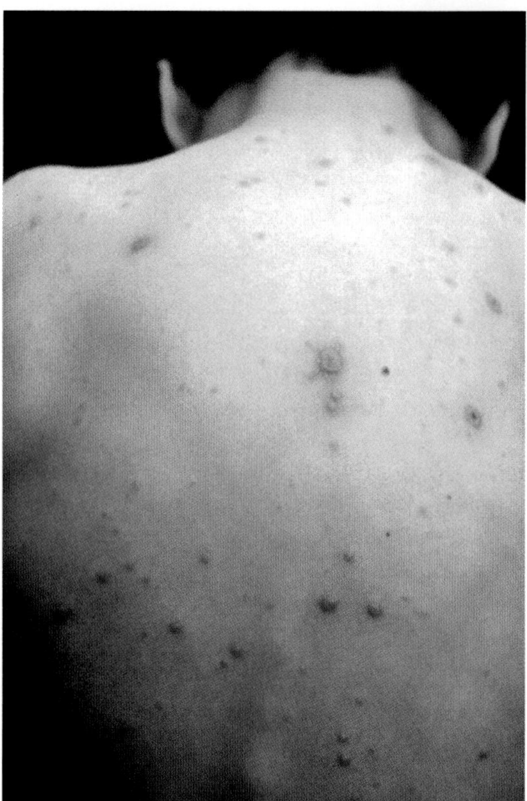

FIGURE 23–9 Vesicular lesions characteristic of chickenpox. These blisterlike lesions have a pus-filled center. *(Courtesy of the Centers for Disease Control and Prevention, Public Health Image Library.)*

Primary infections in adults, neonates, or pregnant women tend to be more severe, with a larger number of lesions and a greater chance of developing other complications such as pneumonia. Varicella infection in pregnant women may also cause premature labor or congenital malformations if the infection is acquired during the first trimester of pregnancy or may cause severe neonatal infection if transmission of the virus occurs around the time of delivery. Infections in immunocompromised patients are likely to result in disseminated disease, with extensive skin rash, neurological conditions (e.g., encephalitis), and other complications, including pneumonia, hepatitis, and nephritis.

During the course of primary infection, VZV is thought to travel from the skin lesions and the blood to sensory neurons, where it deposits its DNA and establishes a lifelong latent state in the dorsal root, autonomic, and cranial ganglia. The host's T-cell–mediated immune response is believed to keep the virus under control during this time.

Reactivation of VZV, with active viral replication, occurs in 15% to 30% of persons with a history of varicella infection. The number of cases increases with age or the development of an immunocompromised condition, probably because of decreased cell-mediated immunity. During reactivation, the virus moves down the sensory nerve to the dermatome supplied by that nerve, resulting in eruption of a painful vesicular rash known as *herpes zoster,* or *shingles,* in the affected area. The rash may persist for weeks to months and is more severe in immunocompromised and elderly individuals. A significant number of patients with herpes zoster develop complications, the most common being postherpetic neuralgia, characterized by debilitating pain that persists for weeks, months, or even years after resolution of the infection. Life-threatening complications, such as herpes ophthalmicus, that lead to blindness, pneumonia, and visceral involvement are more common in immunosuppressed persons.

Implementation of a vaccine consisting of a strain of live, attenuated varicella virus in 1995 has resulted in a significant decline in the incidence of chickenpox and its associated complications in the United States. In 2005, a vaccine was licensed for use in healthy children that combines the varicella vaccine with that for measles, mumps, and rubella. In addition, a single-agent live, attenuated VZV vaccine was licensed in 2006 for the prevention of herpes zoster in persons aged 60 or older, presumably by boosting T-cell immunity to the virus. Because these vaccines all contain a live agent, they are not recommended for use in immunocompromised persons.

GlaxoSmithKline developed a recombinant (genetically engineered) zoster vaccine for shingles, and the FDA licensed the vaccine in 2017. This vaccine is preferred over the live, attenuated vaccine. The CDC recommends healthy adults over the age of 50 receive two doses of the recombinant vaccine 2 to 6 months apart to protect against shingles.

Diagnosis of varicella and herpes zoster is usually based on identifying the characteristic vesicular lesions associated with the infection. Laboratory testing is most important in the diagnosis of atypical cases, such as those in which the rash is absent or delayed, and in immunocompromised patients with disseminated disease. Definitive diagnosis is based on identifying VSV or one of its products in skin lesions, vesicular fluids, or tissue. Older methods of identification involved cell culture and microscopy, but these have significant disadvantages. Culture of the virus and observation of characteristic CPE can be performed in several cell lines but is time consuming (4 days to 2 weeks) and may not yield productive results if clinical specimens do not contain sufficient amounts of the infectious virus. Microscopic detection of multinucleated giant cells called *Tzanck cells* in stained smears made from material from the vesicles allowed for rapid identification of the virus, but this procedure could not distinguish between VZV and HSV. Direct immunofluorescence staining of scrapings from vesicular lesions with monoclonal antibodies directed against VZV antigens provides a rapid, but more sensitive and specific means of detecting the virus. Today, qPCR for VZV DNA is the laboratory method of choice for diagnosing varicella zoster infection because it is highly accurate, sensitive, and rapid. Quantitative PCR is also useful in monitoring the response of immunocompromised patients to antiviral drugs. PCR can be performed on a variety of samples, including vesicular fluid or scabs, skin swabs, throat swabs, cerebrospinal fluid, blood, saliva, and tissues from biopsies or autopsies.

Serology testing is of limited use in detecting current infections because accurate detection requires demonstration of a four-fold rise in antibody titer between acute and convalescent samples, a process that takes 2 to 4 weeks to perform. In addition, testing for VZV IgM is not performed routinely for several reasons: IgM antibodies to VZV may not be detectable until the convalescent stage of illness, they cannot distinguish between primary and reactivated infection, and they may not be free of IgG antibodies when serum is processed for testing. In certain cases, IgG avidity assays may be used to differentiate between recent and past infection.

Serology is most useful in determining if immunity to VZV is present in certain individuals, such as health-care workers, pregnant women, and patients about to undergo organ transplantation. Therefore, most serology tests detect total VZV antibody, which consists primarily of IgG. Several methods have been developed for this purpose. The most sensitive and reliable method of detecting VZV antibody is a fluorescent test called *fluorescent antibody to membrane antigen* (FAMA) that detects antibody to the envelope glycoproteins of the virus. Although FAMA is considered to be the reference method for VZV antibody, it requires live, virus-infected cells and is not suitable for large-scale routine testing. The most commonly used method to detect VZV antibodies in the clinical laboratory is the ELISA because it is automated, provides objective results, and does not require viral culture. Although older ELISA methods that use a whole antigen extract are less sensitive than FAMA, a newer ELISA that detects antibody to a highly purified VZV envelope glycoprotein has been shown to have a high level of sensitivity. Despite this improvement, false-positive results can occur because the method can detect low levels of antibodies that do not confer long-term protection to varicella.

Other Viral Infections

Rubella

The **rubella virus** is a single-stranded, enveloped RNA virus of the genus *Rubivirus*, belonging to the family *Togaviridae*. It is transmitted through respiratory droplets or through transplacental infection of the fetus during pregnancy.

This virus is the cause of the typically benign, self-limited disease that is also known as *German measles* or *3-day measles*. Before widespread use of the rubella vaccine, this was mainly a disease of young children. However, today it occurs most often in young, unvaccinated adults. Following an incubation period of 12 to 23 days, the virus replicates in the upper respiratory tract and cervical lymph nodes, then travels to the bloodstream. It produces a characteristic erythematous, maculopapular rash, which appears first on the face, then spreads to the trunk and extremities, and usually resolves in 3 to 5 days. In adolescents and adults, this is usually preceded by a prodrome of low-grade fever, malaise, swollen glands, and upper respiratory infection lasting 1 to 5 days. However, up to 50% of rubella infections are asymptomatic. The infection usually resolves without complications, and no specific treatment is available. A significant number of infected adult women experience arthralgias and arthritis, but chronic arthritis is rare.

Rubella infection during pregnancy may have severe consequences, including miscarriage, stillbirth, or congenital rubella syndrome (CRS). The likelihood of severe consequences increases when infection occurs earlier in the pregnancy, especially during the first trimester. Infants born with CRS may present with several abnormalities, the most common of which are deafness; eye defects, including cataracts and glaucoma; cardiac abnormalities; mental retardation; liver and spleen damage; and motor disabilities. In mild cases, symptoms may not be recognized until months to years after birth.

Scientists developed a vaccine consisting of live, attenuated rubella virus with the primary goal of preventing infection of pregnant women by reducing dissemination of the virus in the population as a whole. The vaccine is part of the routine immunization schedule in infants and children and is usually given in combination with vaccines for measles and mumps (measles/mumps/rubella [MMR] vaccine) and sometimes with varicella (MMRV). Following licensure of the vaccine in 1969, the number of rubella infections and cases of CRS in the United States has dropped dramatically, with only limited outbreaks occurring, mostly among unvaccinated young immigrants to this country. However, rubella and CRS are still important health problems in parts of the world where routine immunization against the virus is not established.

Laboratory testing is helpful in confirming suspected cases of German measles because its symptoms may mimic those of other viral infections. It is essential in the diagnosis of CRS and in the determination of immune status in other individuals. Laboratory diagnosis of rubella infection can be accomplished through culture of the virus, demonstration of viral RNA, or detection of virus-specific antibodies. Rubella virus can be grown in a variety of cultured cells inoculated with throat swabs, nasopharyngeal secretions, or other clinical specimens and can be detected in almost all infected infants at the time of birth. However, viral growth is slow and may not produce characteristic CPE upon primary isolation, requiring at least two successive subpassages. In the absence of CPE, viral nucleic acid can be identified by RT-PCR, or viral proteins can be detected by IFA or EIA. Because culture is time consuming and labor intensive, it is increasingly being replaced by molecular methods that are more practical to perform in the clinical laboratory and provide more timely results. The most widely used molecular method is RT-PCR. RT-PCR is a highly sensitive and specific aid in prenatal or postnatal diagnosis and can be used to detect rubella RNA in a variety of clinical samples, including chorionic villi, placenta, amniotic fluid, fetal blood, lens tissue, products of conception, pharyngeal swabs, spinal fluid, or brain tissue.

Serology tests are the most common means of confirming a rubella diagnosis because they are rapid, cost effective, and practical in clinical laboratory settings. Several methods have been developed to detect rubella antibodies, including hemagglutination inhibition (HI), latex agglutination, and immunoassays. Although HI was once the standard technique for measuring rubella antibodies, the most commonly used method today is the ELISA because of its sensitivity, specificity, ease of performance, and adaptability to automation. More specific solid-phase capture ELISAs can be used to detect IgM rubella antibodies. Automated chemiluminescence assays and a multiplex bead immunoassay that can simultaneously detect measles, mumps, rubella, and varicella are also available and demonstrate comparable performance with ELISAs.

Primary rubella infection is indicated either by the presence of rubella-specific IgM antibodies or by a four-fold or greater rise in rubella-specific IgG antibody titers between acute and convalescent samples collected at least 10 to 14 days apart. The timing of serum collection is important because IgM antibodies to rubella do not appear in many patients until about 5 days after the onset of the rash, whereas IgG antibodies may not be detectable until 8 days after the rash. Only about 50% of patients are positive for IgM antibodies on the day that the rash appears; thus, a false-negative result can occur if the sample is obtained too early. False-positive results can also occur. Although IgM antibodies generally decline by 4 to 6 weeks, they may persist in low levels for a year or more in some cases. False-positive rubella IgM results have also been observed in individuals with parvovirus infections, enterovirus infections, heterophile antibodies, or rheumatoid factor. It is therefore recommended that positive IgM results, particularly in pregnant women, be confirmed by a more specific test, such as an EIA that measures the avidity of rubella IgG antibodies, to distinguish between recent and past rubella infections. In these assays, low antibody avidity indicates a recent infection (with a high risk for CRS), whereas high antibody avidity is seen in past infections, reflecting the normal change in avidity during the course of an immune response.

Laboratory diagnosis of congenital rubella infection begins with serological evaluation of the mother's antibodies and measurement of rubella-specific IgM antibodies in fetal blood, cord blood, or neonatal serum, depending on the age of the fetus or infant. To enhance the reliability of a CRS diagnosis, any positive IgM results should be confirmed by viral culture, RT-PCR–amplification of rubella nucleic acid, or demonstration of persistently high titers of rubella IgG antibodies after 3 to 6 months of age.

Serology tests are also used to screen for immunity to rubella in populations such as pregnant women or health-care workers. IgG antibodies provide immunity and persist for life. Rubella-specific IgG antibodies are produced because of natural infection or immunization. An antibody level of 10 to 15 IU/mL is considered to be protective.

Rubeola

The **rubeola virus** is a single-stranded RNA virus belonging to the genus *Morbillivirus* in the *Paramyxoviridae* family. It is a highly contagious infection that is spread by direct contact with aerosolized droplets from the respiratory secretions of infected individuals. After initial infection of the epithelial cells in the upper respiratory tract, rubeola virus is disseminated through the blood to multiple sites in the body, such as the skin, lymph nodes, and liver.

Rubeola virus infection is the cause of the disease commonly known as *measles*. Following an incubation period of

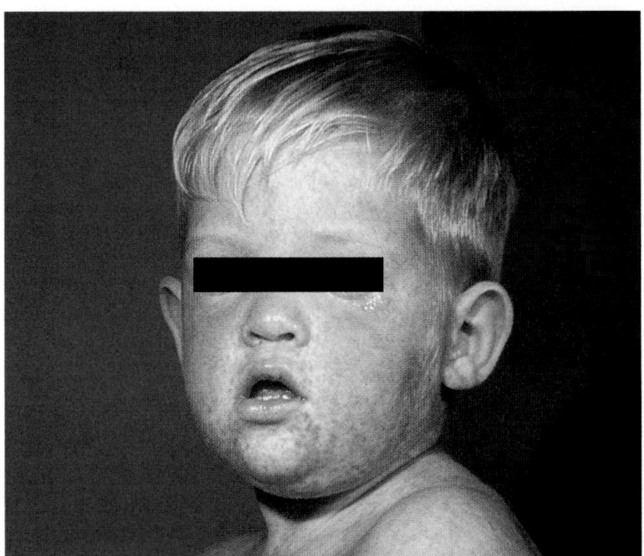

FIGURE 23–10 Characteristic rash of measles appearing on the face of a boy. *(Courtesy of the Centers for Disease Control and Prevention, Public Health Image Library.)*

about 10 to 12 days, the virus produces prodromal symptoms of fever, cough, coryza (runny nose), and conjunctivitis, which last 2 to 4 days. During the prodromal period, characteristic areas known as *Koplik spots* appear on the mucous membranes of the inner cheeks or lips; these appear as gray-to-white lesions against a bright red background and persist for several days. The typical rash of measles appears about 14 days after exposure to the virus and is characterized by an erythematous, maculopapular eruption that begins on the hairline, then spreads to the face and neck and gradually moves down the body to the trunk, arms, hands, legs, and feet **(Fig. 23–10).** The rash usually lasts 5 to 6 days.

Measles is a systemic infection that can result in complications, including diarrhea, otitis media, croup, bronchitis, pneumonia, and encephalitis. Rarely, a fatal degenerative disease of the CNS, called *subacute sclerosing panencephalitis (SSPE),* can result from persistent replication of measles virus in the brain. Measles infection during pregnancy can result in a higher risk of premature labor, spontaneous abortion, or low birth weight.

The incidence of measles has been greatly reduced in developed nations of the world since the introduction of a live, attenuated measles virus vaccine in 1968. A vaccine consisting of killed rubeola virus was originally licensed in 1963 but was ultimately ineffective because recipients developed a case of atypical measles if they were subsequently infected with the measles virus. The newer vaccine is used in the routine immunization schedule of infants and children, either in combination with rubella and mumps (MMR) or in combination with rubella, mumps, and varicella (MMRV). The recommended administration of the vaccine is in two doses, the first between the ages of 12 and 15 months and the second between ages 4 and 6. Administration of the first dose before the age of 12 months may result in vaccine failure because the presence of maternal antibodies can interfere with the infant's immune response. The vaccine was considered to be so successful that the CDC and WHO declared measles to be eliminated from the United States in the year 2000 and from the Americas in 2002. However, measles continues to be a global concern, and most cases in the United States and other industrialized nations are brought in by unvaccinated individuals from other countries. Measles outbreaks have occurred in recent years in the United States because some people in the population refuse to become vaccinated or have their children vaccinated on the basis of religious reasons or unfounded fears of vaccine associations with disorders such as autism. According to the CDC, in 2018, 349 individual cases of measles were reported in 26 states and in the District of Columbia. This was the second largest documented number of cases reported since 2000 (first largest number of cases was 667 in 2014). These cases are linked to unvaccinated individuals traveling to the United States, as well as communities of unvaccinated people living in close proximity in the United States.

The diagnosis of measles has typically been based on clinical presentation of the patient. However, the success of the U.S. immunization program in reducing the number of measles cases has decreased the ability of some physicians to recognize the clinical features of measles. In addition, atypical presentations of measles can occur in individuals who received the earlier form of the measles vaccine, who have low antibody titers, or who are immunocompromised. Laboratory tests are therefore of value in ensuring rapid, accurate diagnosis of sporadic cases; in addition, they are important for epidemiological surveillance and control of community outbreaks.

Isolation of rubeola virus in conventional cell cultures is technically difficult and slow and is not generally performed in the routine diagnosis of measles, but it may be useful in epidemiological surveillance of measles virus strains. The optimal time to recover measles virus from nasopharyngeal aspirates, throat swabs, or blood is from the prodrome period of 3 to 4 days after rash onset. The virus may be isolated from urine up to 1 week after the appearance of the rash.

Serological testing provides the most practical and reliable means of confirming a measles diagnosis. In conjunction with clinical symptoms, a diagnosis of measles is indicated by the presence of rubeola-specific IgM antibodies or by a fourfold rise in the rubeola-specific IgG antibody titer between serum samples collected soon after the onset of rash and 10 to 30 days later. SSPE is associated with extremely high titers of rubeola antibodies. IgM antibodies are preferentially detected by an IgM capture ELISA method, which is highly sensitive and has a low incidence of false-positive results. IgM antibodies are detectable by 3 to 4 days after appearance of symptoms and persist for 1 to 2 months. Samples collected before 72 hours may yield false-negative results, and repeat testing is recommended in that situation.

A variety of methods have been developed to detect IgG rubeola antibodies, but the most commonly used is ELISA. IgG antibodies become detectable 7 to 10 days after the onset of symptoms and persist for life. The presence of rubeola-specific IgG antibodies indicates immunity to measles because of past infection or immunization. Testing for IgG antibodies is therefore routinely performed on serum samples of individuals such as health-care workers to determine their immune status.

Molecular methods to detect rubeola RNA can be used in cases in which serological tests are inconclusive or inconsistent and can be used to genotype the virus in epidemiological studies. The preferred molecular technique is RT-PCR, performed by traditional or qPCR methodologies. These assays are sensitive, can be performed on a variety of clinical samples or on infected cell cultures, and can detect viral RNA within 3 days of rash appearance.

Mumps

The **mumps virus,** similar to rubeola, is a single-stranded RNA virus that belongs to the *Paramyxoviridae* family (genus *Rubulavirus*). It is transmitted from person to person by infected respiratory droplets, saliva, and fomites and replicates initially in the nasopharynx and regional lymph nodes. (Fomites are inanimate objects or substances that can transmit infectious organisms.) Following an average incubation period of 14 to 18 days, the virus spreads from the blood to various tissues, including the meninges of the brain, salivary glands, pancreas, testes, and ovaries, and produces inflammation at those sites. Inflammation of the parotid glands, or *parotitis,* is the most common clinical manifestation of mumps, occurring in 30% to 40% of cases **(Fig. 23–11).** The illness typically resolves in 7 to 10 days and does not require therapy other than supportive treatment to alleviate the symptoms. Mumps infection in pregnant women results in increased risk for fetal death when it occurs in the first trimester of pregnancy, but it is not associated with congenital abnormalities.

The number of mumps cases in the United States has declined significantly since the introduction of a live, attenuated mumps virus vaccine in 1967 and its routine use in childhood immunization schedules in 1977. The vaccine is most commonly combined with the vaccines for rubella and measles (MMR) or is used in combination with the rubella, measles, and varicella vaccines (MMRV). However, several outbreaks in the United States have been reported in close-knit communities and on college campuses. From January 1 to December 29, 2018, 47 states and the District of Columbia reported 2,251 cases of mumps to the CDC.

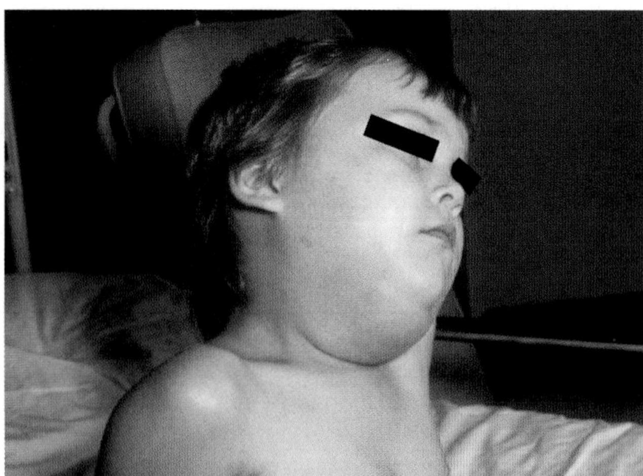

FIGURE 23–11 Parotitis characteristic of mumps. Note the swollen neck region caused by an enlargement of the boy's salivary glands. *(Courtesy of the Centers for Disease Control and Prevention, Public Health Image Library.)*

The diagnosis of mumps is usually made on the basis of clinical symptoms, especially parotitis, and does not require laboratory confirmation. However, laboratory testing is very useful in cases in which parotitis is absent or when differentiation from other causes of parotitis is required. Culture of the mumps virus from clinical specimens is considered to be the gold standard for laboratory confirmation of acute infection. Within the first few days of illness, the mumps virus can be isolated from saliva, urine, cerebrospinal fluid, or swabs from the area around the excretory duct of the parotid gland. The preferred specimens are a buccal swab or saliva from the buccal cavity collected within 3 to 5 days of symptom onset. The specimen can then be used to inoculate cell lines such as primary monkey kidney cells and Vero cells, which are grown in shell vial cultures and stained with fluorescein-labeled monoclonal antibodies to identify mumps antigens. However, culture methods require experienced personnel, and specialized reagents and are being increasingly replaced with molecular detection of viral nucleic acid.

Standard and real-time RT-PCR methods have been developed to detect mumps virus RNA in specimens collected from the buccal cavity, throat, cerebral spinal fluid, or urine of patients with a suspected mumps infection. In many laboratories, RT-PCR is recommended as the primary diagnostic test for mumps because it is more sensitive than serology. As with culture, buccal swabs collected early in the illness provide the best results, and false-negative results are frequent in clinical samples collected after 1 week of symptom onset. Genotyping may be performed to track transmission of the virus during mumps outbreaks.

When indicated, serological testing provides a simple means of confirming a mumps diagnosis, but it has some important limitations. EIA and IFA antibody kits are used; however, most only measure IgG mumps virus antibodies. ELISA is the most commonly used method to detect mumps antibodies because it is sensitive, specific, cost effective, and readily performed by the routine clinical laboratory. Use of solid-phase IgM capture assays reduces the incidence of false-positive results because of rheumatoid factor. Current or recent infection is indicated by the presence of mumps-specific IgM antibody in a single serum sample or by at least a four-fold rise in specific IgG antibody between two specimens collected during the acute and convalescent phases of illness. However, acute IgG titers are often high, and a four-fold increase in titer may not be evident in the convalescent sample. IgM antibodies can be detected within 3 to 4 days of illness and can persist for at least 8 to 12 weeks. However, a negative IgM test does not rule out mumps because negative results can occur if the serum was collected too early or too late. In addition, individuals who received any doses of the mumps vaccine tend to have lower or absent IgM antibody. IgG antibodies become detectable within 7 to 10 days and persist for years. However, the presence of mumps IgG antibodies does not necessarily correlate with the presence of neutralizing antibodies, which would confer immunity to the virus.

Human T-Cell Lymphotropic Viruses

Human T-cell lymphotropic virus type I (HTLV-I) and **human T-cell lymphotropic virus type II (HTLV-II)** are closely related retroviruses. Both viruses have three structural genes: *gag,* which codes for viral core proteins; *pol,* which codes for viral enzymes; and *env,* which encodes proteins in the viral envelope; as well as a region called *pX*, which encodes several regulatory proteins, including Tax and Rex. These viruses have RNA as their nucleic acid and the enzyme reverse transcriptase, whose function is to transcribe the viral RNA into DNA. The DNA then becomes integrated into the host cell's genome as a provirus. The provirus can remain in a latent state within infected cells for a prolonged period of time. Upon activation of the host cell, the provirus can proceed to complete its replication cycle to produce more virions. However, HTLV-I and HTLV-II exist predominantly in the proviral state and are spread directly to uninfected cells through a viral synapse. Additional copies of the viral nucleic acid are produced when the infected host cells replicate.

The human T-cell lymphotropic viruses preferentially infect CD4+ T lymphocytes but can also infect CD8+ T cells, dendritic cells, and macrophages. CD8+ CTLs effectively control the proliferation of virus-infected cells in most individuals. However, inflammatory cytokines released during the immune response may contribute to the pathogenesis of HTLV-associated diseases. In addition, researchers have reported that HTLV-I infection of CD4+ T cells can increase the production of proinflammatory cytokines, impair production of Th1 cytokines necessary for cell-mediated immunity, and induce differentiation of T regulatory (Treg) cells. The differentiated Treg cells can facilitate viral persistence by suppressing the host's immune response to the virus. HTLV-I also transforms CD4+ T lymphocytes into malignant cells in a small percentage of individuals through mechanisms mediated by the Tax protein, resulting in increased cell proliferation and accumulation of harmful genetic mutations.

HTLV-I and HTLV-II can be transmitted by three major routes: bloodborne (mainly through transfusions containing cellular components or through intravenous drug abuse), sexual contact (most commonly from men to women), and mother to child (mainly through breastfeeding). HTLV-I infection is endemic in southwestern Japan, the Caribbean islands, South and Central Africa, the Middle East, Romania, parts of South America, and Papua New Guinea. Between 5 million and 20 million people are thought to be infected with HTLV-I worldwide. Infections in the United States and Europe have resulted mainly from immigrants from endemic areas. HTLV-II infections are highest in various Native Indian populations in the Americas, a few Pygmy tribes in Central Africa, and intravenous drug abusers in North America and Europe.

HTLV-I is the cause of two diseases: adult T-cell leukemia/lymphoma (ATLL) and HTLV-associated myelopathy/tropical spastic paraparesis (HAM/TSP). ATLL can be classified into four different subtypes based on clinical manifestations: acute, T-cell non-Hodgkin's lymphoma, chronic, and smoldering. Over half of patients have the acute type, an aggressive variant with a median survival of 6 months. All four types of ATLL are characterized by a monoclonal proliferation of mature T cells that express the surface markers CD3, CD4, and CD25. The malignant cells have lobulated, "flower-shaped" nuclei that contain proviral HTLV-I nucleic acid. The lifetime risk of HTLV-I carriers for developing ATLL is 3% to 5% and is highest in those who acquired the infection perinatally. The disease typically appears after a latent period of 20 to 30 years following initial infection.

Individuals infected with HTLV-I also have a 4% lifetime risk of developing a progressive neurological disorder called *HTLV-I-associated myelopathy/tropical spastic paraparesis* (HAM/TSP). The risk is highest among those who contracted the infection through sexual transmission. The disease is characterized by slowly progressive weakness and stiffness of the legs, back pain, and urinary incontinence. HTLV-I has also been associated with a variety of autoimmune and inflammatory disorders, including uveitis (intraocular inflammation of the eyes), infective dermatitis, myositis (inflammation of the muscles), and arthropathy (inflammation of the joints); however, a causal relationship of the virus with these conditions has not been established. It is unclear what factors influence the development and types of clinical manifestations of HTLV-I infection, but differences in viral strains, viral load, mode of transmission, HLA haplotypes, and immune responses mounted by the host may all play a role.

The association of HTLV-II infection with disease is unclear, and most individuals infected with the virus are asymptomatic. However, there is evidence that HTLV-II may rarely be associated with a neurological disease that is similar to HAM/TSP, as well as certain hematologic and dermatological diseases and increased incidence of infections. In addition, a close link to cancer mortality in the United States has been identified. This evidence suggests that more research is needed to understand the pathogenicity of the virus.

Serological testing plays an important role in detecting HTLV-I and HTLV-II infections because culture of the viruses requires sophisticated techniques that cannot be performed in routine clinical laboratories. HTLV antibodies develop 30 to 90 days after exposure to the virus and persist for life. Tests for HTLV-I and HTLV-II antibodies are used to detect HTLV infections in individuals and to screen blood donors. The tests most commonly used for screening are EIA, CLIA, and IFA methods that incorporate recombinant antigens or synthetic peptides from both HTLV-I and HTLV-II. Particle agglutination tests have also been developed. Any sample producing a reactive result in the initial screen is retested by the same method and subsequently tested by a confirmatory method to reduce the incidence of false-positive results and to distinguish between HTLV-I and HTLV-II infection.

Commercially available Western blot assays are most commonly used for confirmation; line immunoassays (LIAs) and IFA tests have also been developed. Western blot and LIA identify antibodies to specific HTLV antigens. Specimens are considered positive if a particular band pattern representing antibodies to the gag and env proteins of HTLV-I or HTLV-II is obtained. According to criteria published by the WHO, for example, a sample is considered positive for HTLV-I antibodies if visible bands are produced for one of the env proteins (either gp46 or gp62/68) *and* one of the gag proteins (either p19, p24, or p53). A major problem with the Western blot and LIA methods is that indeterminate results can be obtained when a single band is observed or when multiple bands that do not meet the criteria for positivity are seen. PCR can be performed to detect HTLV-I or HTLV-II DNA in provirus-carrying peripheral blood mononuclear cells to clarify repeatedly indeterminate results. PCR methods can also be used to monitor the proviral load in patients with HTLV-associated diseases during therapy and to demonstrate the presence of the virus in cells from patients who are suspected of having HTLV-associated disease.

SUMMARY

- Viruses are obligate intracellular pathogens that can produce a wide range of diseases in humans.
- Viruses can exist as either free infectious virions or intracellular particles in infected host cells. These different states require a combined effort of innate, humoral, and cell-mediated immune responses to successfully defend the host against viral infections.
- Innate defenses against viruses include the skin and mucous membranes; IFNs to inhibit viral replication; and NK cells, which release cytotoxic proteins that destroy virus-infected host cells.
- Antibodies directed against specific viral antigens can prevent the spread of viral infection by neutralizing a virus and preventing it from binding to host cells, opsonizing a virus to make it more likely to be phagocytized, activating complement-mediated mechanisms of destruction, and agglutinating viruses.
- Cell-mediated immunity is needed to eliminate intracellular viruses. Virus-specific CTLs bind to viral antigen complexed with class I MHC on the surface of infected host cells and release cytotoxic proteins that cause the cells to undergo apoptosis.
- Viruses have evolved in several ways to escape the host's defenses. These include frequent genetic mutations to produce new viral antigens; evading the action of IFNs, complement, or other components of the immune system; or suppressing the immune system. Some viruses can establish a latent state by integrating their nucleic acid into the host's genome.
- Serological tests for viral antibodies can be used to indicate exposure to a viral pathogen. In general, the presence of IgM indicates a current or recent infection or a congenital infection, if present in infant serum. The presence of IgG antibodies indicates previous exposure to a virus or immunity because of vaccination.
- Culture, antigen detection, and molecular methods for viral nucleic acid can be used to directly identify viruses in clinical samples. Molecular methods have become increasingly important in the diagnosis of viral infections and can also be used to quantitate viral load to determine the effectiveness of antiviral therapy.
- The hepatitis viruses are those whose primary effect is inflammation of the liver. Hepatitis A and E are transmitted mainly by the fecal–oral route, whereas hepatitis B, C, and D are transmitted primarily by the parenteral route. Hepatitis B, C, and D can lead to chronic infections. Vaccines have been developed to prevent hepatitis A, hepatitis B, and hepatitis E.
- Serological markers of hepatitis infections consist of virus-specific antibodies and antigens that are commonly detected by automated immunoassays.
- IgM anti-HAV antibodies indicate current or recent hepatitis A infection, whereas IgG anti-HAV antibodies are developed later in the infection and indicate immunity to hepatitis A. Likewise, IgM anti-HEV antibodies are present during current or recent hepatitis E infection, and IgG anti-HEV antibodies indicate later infection and immunity.
- Hepatitis B infection is indicated by the presence of the antigen HBsAg; HBeAg indicates high infectivity. IgM antibodies to hepatitis B core antigen are present in acute hepatitis B, whereas IgG anti-HBc is present during past or chronic hepatitis B infection. Antibodies to HBsAg (anti-HBs) indicate immunity and can be produced because of past hepatitis B infection or immunization with the hepatitis B vaccine.
- The presence of anti-HCV indicates exposure to the hepatitis C virus but cannot distinguish between a current and a past infection. Molecular tests for HCV RNA are used to confirm antibody-positive results; if positive, they indicate a current infection. Molecular tests for hepatitis C are also used to quantitate viral load to determine the effectiveness of antiviral therapy. A third application of molecular testing is genotyping of the virus to guide decisions about therapy.
- Hepatitis D occurs as a super- or co-infection with hepatitis B and is indicated by antibodies to hepatitis D or molecular tests to detect HDV RNA. Patients with co-infections are also positive for IgM-anti-HBc, whereas patients with superinfections are positive for IgG-anti-HBc.
- The Epstein-Barr virus (EBV) is the cause of infectious mononucleosis (IM), Burkitt's lymphoma, Hodgkin disease, nasopharyngeal and gastric carcinomas, and lymphoproliferative disorders in immunosuppressed individuals.
- Most patients with IM produce heterophile antibodies, which can react with antigens from bovine, horse, or sheep RBCs. These antibodies are routinely screened for by the "Monospot" test, which is performed by rapid immunochromatographic or agglutination methods to detect antibodies to bovine or horse erythrocyte antigens.

- ELISA or IFA tests for EBV-specific antibodies are used to confirm a diagnosis of IM, detect heterophile-negative cases of IM, and diagnose other EBV-associated diseases. Acute IM is indicated by the presence of IgM anti-VCA and anti-EA-D, as well as the absence of anti-EBNA. Molecular tests are useful in detecting EBV DNA in immunocompromised patients, who may not develop a good antibody response, and in monitoring viral load in patients with EBV-related malignancies during therapy.
- Cytomegalovirus (CMV) infection is asymptomatic in most healthy individuals but may cause a mononucleosis-like syndrome, disseminated infection in organ-transplant recipients and patients with HIV/AIDS, and congenital abnormalities in infants born to infected mothers.
- CMV infection is best detected by molecular assays for CMV DNA, CMV antigenemia assays for pp65 antigen, or shell vial culture. Quantitative PCR is useful in determining the CMV DNA copy number in immunocompromised hosts undergoing antiviral treatment. Serological assays for CMV antibody are most helpful in documenting a past infection in potential blood and organ donors.
- Primary infection with varicella virus causes chickenpox (varicella), whereas reactivation of the virus in nerve cells supplying the skin causes shingles (zoster). Diagnosis of current varicella virus infection is usually based on clinical findings, but the detection of varicella virus DNA by PCR may be helpful in some clinical settings. Serological methods, most commonly ELISA and CLIA, are used mainly to document immunity to varicella virus.
- Vaccines have greatly reduced the incidence of three childhood infections: rubella, rubeola, and mumps. Rubella infection is the cause of German measles and can result in severe congenital abnormalities if it occurs during pregnancy. Rubeola viruses cause measles, a systemic infection that can cause complications in some individuals. Mumps virus is the cause of mumps, whose classic feature is swelling of the parotid glands.
- Although the diagnosis of rubella, measles, and mumps is usually based on clinical findings, laboratory testing may be helpful in confirmation. Current infections are indicated by the presence of IgM antibodies specific for the appropriate virus or by a four-fold rise in virus-specific IgG antibodies in two separate specimens collected during the acute and convalescent phases of disease. Testing for IgG antibodies is most commonly performed to screen for immunity to these viruses. RT-PCR is a useful adjunct to serology in detecting viral RNA in patients with inconclusive serology results, in epidemiological studies, and in the detection of congenital rubella infections.
- The human T-cell lymphotropic viruses, HTLV-I and HTLV-II, are retroviruses that infect CD4 T lymphocytes. HTLV-I is the cause of adult T-cell leukemia and lymphoma, HTLV-I-associated myelopathy/tropical spastic paraparesis (HAM/TSP), and other inflammatory disorders. HTLV-II may be associated with a HAM/TSP-like neurological disease as well as hematologic and skin disorders, but the disease associations of this virus are unclear. EIA and CLIA tests are used routinely to screen blood donors for antibodies to HTLV-I and HTLV-II and to detect exposure to HTLV in other individuals. Positive results are confirmed by Western blot or line immunoassays. PCR for proviral DNA can be used to clarify indeterminate results and monitor viral load in patients undergoing therapy.

Study Guide: Immune Defenses Against Viruses

IMMUNE DEFENSE	MECHANISM OF ACTION
Innate Defenses	First line of protection against viruses Skin and mucous membranes serve as barriers to prevent viruses from invading the body Type I IFNs inhibit viral replication NK cells bind to virus-infected host cells in a manner that is not antigen-specific and destroy the cells by releasing perforin and granzymes
Humoral Immunity	Antibodies bind to cell-free viruses and prevent them from infecting host cells by neutralizing their ability to bind to host cell receptors Antibodies also play a key role in opsonization, ADCC, and complement-mediated lysis of viruses
Cell-Mediated Immunity	T lymphocytes attack viruses in their intracellular state Th1 T helper cells produce cytokines that induce an anti-viral state and stimulate the development of CTLs CTLs bind specifically to viral antigens complexed with MHC class I on the surface of virus-infected host cells and destroy the cells by releasing perforin and granzymes

ADCC = antibody-dependent cellular cytotoxicity; CTL = cytotoxic T lymphocytes; IFN = interferon; NK = natural killer.

Study Guide: Immune Escape Mechanisms Commonly Used by Viruses

VIRAL ESCAPE MECHANISM	EXAMPLES
Acquisition of genetic mutations that result in new viral antigens	Influenza viruses, rhinoviruses, HIV
Inhibition of immunologic components	HCV blocks actions of IFNs; HSV inhibits C3b
Suppression of the immune system	CMV and HIV reduce expression of class I MHC on the surface of virus-infected cells, reducing their recognition by CTLs HIV destroys infected CD4 Th cells
Establishment of a latent state	CMV, VZV, and HIV integrate their nucleic acid into the host cell genome

CMV = cytomegalovirus; CTLs = cytotoxic T lymphocytes; HCV = hepatitis C virus; HIV = human immunodeficiency virus; HSV = herpes simplex viruses; MHC = major histocompatibility complex; VZV = varicella zoster virus.

CASE STUDIES

1. A 25-year-old male had been experiencing flu-like symptoms, loss of appetite, nausea, and constipation for 2 weeks. His abdomen was tender, and his urine was dark in color. Initial testing revealed elevations in his serum alanine aminotransferase (ALT) and aspartate aminotransferase (AST) levels.

Questions

a. What laboratory tests should be used to screen this patient for viral hepatitis?
b. If the patient tested positive for hepatitis B, which tests should be used to monitor his condition?
c. If the patient were to develop chronic hepatitis B, which markers would be present in his serum?

2. A 5-pound infant was born with microcephaly, purpuric rash, low platelet count, cardiovascular defects, and a cataract in the left eye. The infant's mother recalled experiencing flu-like symptoms and a mild skin rash early in her pregnancy. She had not sought medical attention at the time. The infant's physician ordered tests to investigate the cause of the newborn's symptoms.

Questions

a. What virus is the most likely cause of the infant's symptoms?
b. What laboratory tests would you suggest the doctor order for the mother to support your suggested diagnosis?
c. What tests should be performed on the infant's serum to support this diagnosis?

REVIEW QUESTIONS

1. The role of CTLs in immune responses against viruses is to

a. neutralize viral activity.
b. promote destruction of viruses by ADCC.
c. destroy virus-infected host cells.
d. attack free virions.

2. Viruses can escape immune defenses by

a. undergoing frequent genetic mutations.
b. suppressing the immune system.
c. integrating their nucleic acid into the host genome.
d. all of the above.

3. A patient who has developed immunity to a viral infection would be expected to have which of the following serology results?

a. IgM+, IgG–
b. IgM–, IgG+
c. IgM+, IgG+
d. IgM–, IgG–

4. A newborn suspected of having a congenital viral infection should be tested for virus-specific antibodies of which class?

a. IgM
b. IgG
c. IgA
d. IgE

5. Which of the following hepatitis viruses is transmitted by the fecal–oral route?
   a. Hepatitis B
   b. Hepatitis C
   c. Hepatitis D
   d. Hepatitis E

6. An individual with hepatomegaly, jaundice, and elevated liver enzymes has the following laboratory results: IgM anti-HAV (negative), HBsAg (positive), IgM anti-HBc (positive), and anti-HCV (negative). These findings support a diagnosis of
   a. hepatitis A.
   b. acute hepatitis B.
   c. chronic hepatitis B.
   d. hepatitis C.

7. The serum of an individual who received all doses of the hepatitis B vaccine should contain
   a. anti-HBs.
   b. anti-HBe.
   c. anti-HBc.
   d. anti-HDV.

8. Quantitative tests for HCV RNA are used to
   a. screen for hepatitis C.
   b. determine the HCV genotype.
   c. differentiate acute HCV infection from chronic HCV infection.
   d. monitor hepatitis C patients on antiviral therapy.

9. In the laboratory, heterophile antibodies are routinely detected by their reaction with
   a. B lymphocytes.
   b. bovine erythrocyte antigens.
   c. sheep erythrocyte antigens.
   d. Epstein-Barr virus antigens.

10. The presence of IgM anti-rubella antibodies in the serum from an infant born with a rash suggests
    a. a diagnosis of measles.
    b. a diagnosis of German measles.
    c. congenital infection with the rubella virus.
    d. passive transfer of maternal antibodies to the infant's serum.

11. A pregnant woman is exposed to a child with a rubella infection. She had no clinical symptoms but had a rubella titer performed. Her antibody titer was 1:4. Three weeks later, the test was repeated, and her titer was 1:128. She still had no clinical symptoms. Was the laboratory finding indicative of rubella infection?
    a. No, the titer must be greater than 256 to be significant.
    b. No, the change in titer is not significant if no clinical signs are present.
    c. Yes, a greater-than-four-fold rise in titer indicates early infection.
    d. Yes, but clinical symptoms must also correlate with laboratory findings.

12. The cause of shingles is
    a. cytomegalovirus.
    b. rubella virus.
    c. varicella-zoster virus.
    d. HTLV-I.

13. The method of choice for detecting VZV infection in immunocompromised hosts is
    a. serology to detect virus-specific IgM antibodies.
    b. serology to detect virus-specific IgG antibodies.
    c. viral culture.
    d. (real-time) qPCR.

14. Which of the following is true regarding laboratory testing for mumps?
    a. RT-PCR is recommended as the primary diagnostic test.
    b. Serology is necessary for confirmation of a suspected clinical case.
    c. IgM tests for mumps are highly specific.
    d. An acute infection must be confirmed by a four-fold rise in IgG titer.

15. A positive result on a screening test for HTLV-I antibody should be
    a. considered highly specific for HTLV-I infection.
    b. followed by PCR.
    c. confirmed by Western blot.
    d. validated by viral culture.

24 Laboratory Diagnosis of HIV Infection

Linda E. Miller, PhD, I, MB^{CM}(ASCP)SI

LEARNING OUTCOMES

After finishing this chapter, you should be able to:

1. Describe the classification system used to identify HIV isolates.
2. Explain the conditions under which transmission of HIV can occur.
3. Describe the structure of the HIV particle, including pertinent antigens and the genes that encode them.
4. Depict the replication cycle of HIV, beginning with entry of the virus into host cells.
5. Describe the host's immune responses to HIV and the effects of HIV on the immune system.
6. Describe the clinical manifestations of HIV infection.
7. Explain the Centers for Disease Control and Prevention (CDC) classification system for HIV infection.
8. Discuss antiretroviral treatments and the impact they have had on HIV infection.
9. Discuss the current CDC-recommended algorithm for screening for HIV infection, as well as its advantages and limitations as compared with the previous algorithm.
10. Discuss the principles and clinical uses of conventional immunoassays and rapid tests for HIV infection.
11. Describe the principle of the Western blot test for HIV antibody, interpretation of the results, and limitations of the test.
12. Discuss reasons for false-positive and false-negative results in HIV antibody testing.
13. Explain the principle and clinical utility of flow cytometric methods for CD4 T-cell enumeration.
14. Discuss the role of qualitative nucleic acid tests in the detection and diagnosis of HIV.
15. Describe the molecular techniques performed for HIV viral load testing and drug-resistance testing and their clinical utility.
16. Select appropriate methods for HIV testing of infants and children younger than 18 months of age.

CHAPTER OUTLINE

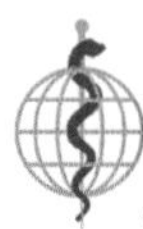

Go to FADavis.com for the laboratory exercises that accompany this text.

KEY TERMS

Acquired immunodeficiency syndrome (AIDS)
Antiretroviral therapy (ART)
Branched-chain DNA (bDNA)
CD4 T cells
Flow cytometry
Human immunodeficiency virus (HIV)
Opportunistic illnesses
p24 antigen
Reverse transcriptase
Seroconversion
Viral load tests
Viremia
Western blot test

Human immunodeficiency virus (HIV) is the etiologic agent of the **acquired immunodeficiency syndrome**, or **AIDS**, a disease that has posed one of the greatest medical challenges worldwide. According to the World Health Organization (WHO), at the end of 2019, about 38 million people were living with HIV infection, and 1.7 million people became newly infected. Since its discovery, the virus has claimed the lives of more than 32 million people worldwide. Although the majority of infected persons reside in developing countries, HIV infection has also created a significant problem in developed nations. For example, it was estimated that in the United States, there were 1.2 million cases of HIV infection at the end of 2018 (the most recent year for which these data were available).

The virus that is responsible for causing AIDS, HIV-1, was identified independently by the laboratories of Drs. Luc Montagnier of France and Robert Gallo and Jay Levy of the United States in 1983 and 1984, respectively. Isolates of HIV-1 have been classified into four groups: Group M (the main or major group), Group O (the outlier group), and two more recently named groups, N and P. Group M viruses are responsible for the majority of HIV-1 infections worldwide. This group contains nine subtypes or clades, designated A, B, C, D, F, G, H, J, and K. Subtype C is the predominant subtype worldwide, whereas subtype B is the most prevalent subtype in the United States, Europe, and Australia. Groups N, O, and P occur much less frequently and are largely confined to West Africa. A large number of circulating recombinant forms (CRFs) exist, which are produced because of genetic recombination between two subtypes that have infected a single individual.

A related but genetically distinct virus, HIV-2, was discovered in 1986. The majority of HIV-2 infections have occurred in West Africa, although the virus has also been identified in patients in other parts of the world. HIV-2 is transmitted in the same manner as HIV-1 and may also cause AIDS, but it is less pathogenic and has a lower rate of transmission. Although this chapter discusses the differences between the two viruses, our focus is on HIV-1 because it is much more prevalent throughout the world. In this chapter, the term *HIV* is used to refer to HIV-1, and HIV-2 is so named.

Accurate diagnosis is essential for early intervention and halting the spread of HIV. This chapter will discuss characteristics of the virus, immunologic and clinical manifestations of the disease, treatment and prevention, and laboratory techniques used to diagnose and monitor HIV infection.

HIV Transmission

Transmission of HIV occurs through one of three major routes: intimate sexual contact, contact with blood or other body fluids, or perinatally (from infected mother to infant). The majority of cases of HIV infection have occurred through sexual transmission involving either vaginal or anal intercourse. Worldwide, about 85% of cases of HIV infection can be attributed to heterosexual contact, whereas in the United States, the largest number of cases has resulted from male-to-male sexual contact. The presence of other sexually transmitted diseases, such as syphilis, gonorrhea, or genital herpes, increases the likelihood of transmission by disrupting protective mucous membranes and activating immunologic cells in the genital areas.

The second route of transmission is through parenteral exposure to infected blood or body fluids, which occurs mainly through the sharing of contaminated needles by intravenous drug users. Less frequently, transmission has taken place through blood transfusions, the use of clotting factors by hemophiliacs, occupational injuries with needlesticks or other sharp objects, or mucous-membrane contact in health-care workers exposed to infectious fluids. The virus has also been acquired by transplantation of infected tissue. The incidence of infection in recipients of blood transfusions, clotting factors, and organ transplants is rare in the United States because of screening of blood and organ donors for HIV.

Studies by the Centers for Disease Control and Prevention (CDC) have estimated the average risk of transmission to health-care workers to be approximately 0.3% after a percutaneous exposure to HIV-infected blood and about 0.09% after a mucous-membrane exposure. Body fluids considered to be potentially infectious include blood, semen, vaginal secretions, cerebral spinal fluid, synovial fluid, pleural fluid, peritoneal fluid, pericardial fluid, amniotic fluid, saliva from dental procedures, other fluids containing visible blood, and any body fluid that cannot be differentiated. The risk of transmission is increased in exposures involving a large quantity of blood, hollow-bore needles placed directly into an artery or vein, or deep tissue injury. The risk of infection is also increased if the source patient is in the acute or advanced stages of HIV infection, when the amount of virus circulating in the bloodstream is high.

The third route of transmission is perinatal, from an infected mother to her fetus or infant. Transmission can occur across the placenta during pregnancy, by transfer of blood at the time of delivery, or through breastfeeding. Perinatal transmission has been markedly reduced by HIV screening during pregnancy, administration of antiretroviral drugs to HIV-positive pregnant women and their newborn babies, and the use of infant formula by mothers who are infected with the virus. The WHO states that these measures have decreased the rate of perinatal transmission to less than 5%, as compared with rates of 15% to 45% in untreated mothers.

Characteristics of HIV

Composition of the Virus

HIV belongs to the genus *Lentivirinae* of the virus family *Retroviridae*. It is classified as a retrovirus because it contains ribonucleic acid (RNA) as its nucleic acid and a unique enzyme, called **reverse transcriptase,** which transcribes the viral RNA into DNA, a necessary step in the virus's life cycle. HIV is a spherical particle, 100 to 120 nm in diameter, which contains an inner core with two copies of single-stranded RNA surrounded by a protein coat or capsid and an outer envelope of glycoproteins embedded in a lipid bilayer. The glycoproteins are knob-like structures that are involved in binding the virus to host cells during the infection. **Figure 24–1** shows the structure of the HIV virion.

Structural Genes

The genome of HIV includes three main structural genes—*gag, env,* and *pol*—and several regulatory genes. **Figure 24–2** shows the relative locations of the major HIV genes and indicates their gene products. The *gag* gene codes for p55, a precursor protein with a molecular weight of 55 kd, from which four core structural proteins are formed: p6, p9, p17, and p24. All four are located in the nucleocapsid of the virus. The capsid that surrounds the internal nucleic acids contains p24, p6, and p9, whereas p17 lies in a layer between the protein core and the envelope, called the *matrix,* and is actually embedded in the internal portion of the envelope.

The *env* gene codes for the glycoproteins gp160, gp120, and gp41, which are found in the viral envelope. Gp160 is a precursor protein that is cleaved to form gp120 and gp41. Gp120 forms the numerous knobs or spikes that protrude from the outer envelope, whereas gp41 is a transmembrane glycoprotein that spans the inner and outer membrane and attaches to gp120. Both gp120 and gp41 are involved in fusion and attachment of HIV to receptors on host cells.

The third structural gene, *pol,* codes for enzymes necessary for HIV replication. These include reverse transcriptase (p51); ribonuclease (RNase H; p66), an enzyme involved in the degradation of the original HIV RNA; integrase (p31), an enzyme that mediates the integration of viral DNA into the genome of infected host cells; and a protease (p10) that cleaves precursor proteins into smaller active units used to make the mature virions. These proteins are located in the core of the virus in association with HIV RNA.

Several other genes in the HIV genome code for products that have regulatory or accessory functions. These genes include *tat* (transactivator), *rev* (regulator of expression of virion proteins), *nef* (negative effector), *vpu* (viral protein "U"), *vpr* (viral protein "R"), and *vif* (viral infectivity factor). Although the products of these genes are not an integral part of the viral structure, they serve important functions in controlling viral replication and infectivity. The HIV gene sequence is surrounded by 5′ and 3′ long terminal repeat (LTR) regions, which also play a role in regulating the expression of the genes. **Table 24–1** summarizes the major HIV-1 genes, their products, and their functions.

HIV-2 has *gag, env, pol,* and regulatory or accessory genes that have similar functions to those seen in HIV-1. The homology between the genomes of the two viruses is approximately 50%. The *gag* and *pol* regions are most similar, whereas the *env* region differs greatly. Thus, the viruses can most easily be distinguished on the basis of antigenic differences in their *env* proteins.

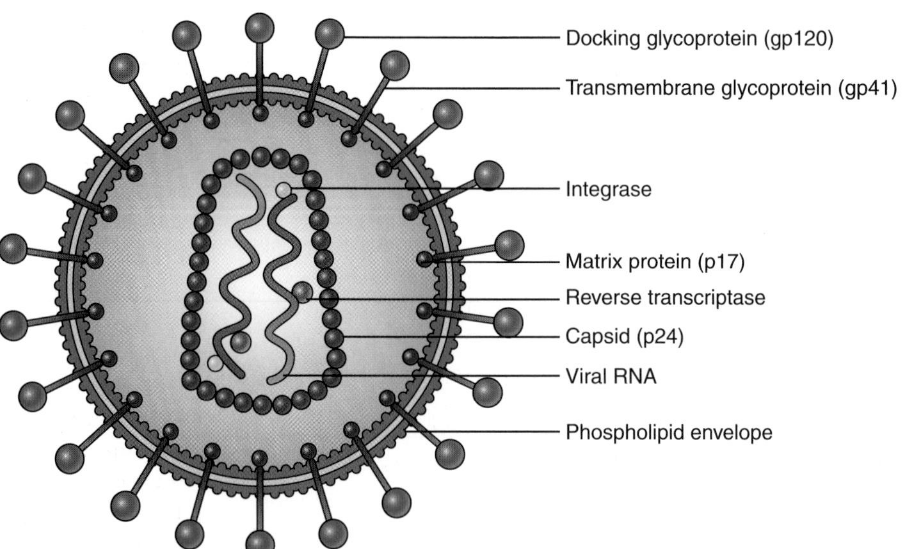

FIGURE 24–1 Structure of HIV virion, showing some of the major components. p = protein; gp = glycoprotein; the numbers refer to the molecular weights of the proteins in kilodaltons.

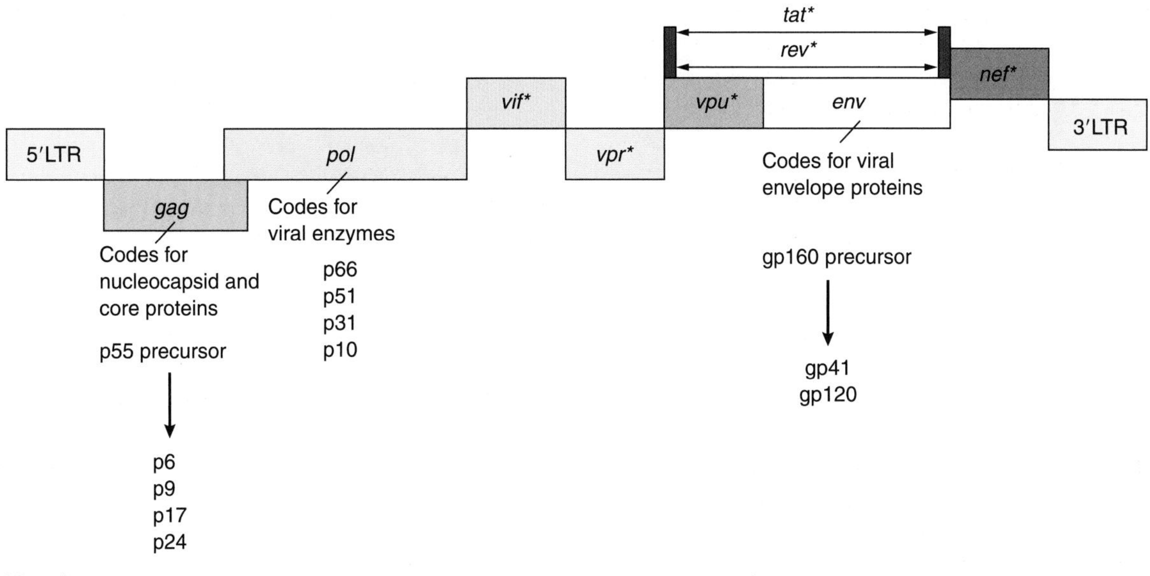

FIGURE 24–2 The HIV-1 genome. The relative locations of the major genes in the HIV-1 genome are indicated, as well as their gene products. * = regulatory genes.

Table 24–1 Major HIV Genes and Their Products

GENE	PROTEIN PRODUCT	FUNCTION
gag	p17	Inner surface of envelope
	p24	Core coat for nucleic acids
	p9	Core-binding protein
	p6	Binds to genomic RNA
env	gp120	Binds to CD4 on T cell
	gp41	Transmembrane protein associated with gp120
pol	p66	Subunit of reverse transcriptase; degrades original HIV RNA
	p51	Subunit of reverse transcriptase
	p31	Integrase; mediates integration of HIV DNA into host genome
	p10	Protease that cleaves *gag* precursor
tat	p14	Activates transcription of HIV provirus
rev	p19	Transports viral mRNA to the cytoplasm of the host cell
nef	p27	Enhances HIV replication
vpu	p16	Viral assembly and budding
vpr	p15	Integration of HIV DNA into host genome
vif	p23	Infectivity factor

Viral Replication

The first step in the reproductive cycle of HIV occurs when the virus attaches to a susceptible host cell. This interaction is mediated through the host-cell CD4 antigen, which serves as a receptor for the virus by binding the gp120 glycoprotein on the outer envelope of HIV. T helper (Th) cells are the main target for HIV infection because they express high numbers of CD4 molecules on their surface and bind the virus with high affinity. Other cells, such as macrophages, monocytes, dendritic cells, Langerhans cells, and microglial brain cells, can also be infected with HIV because they have some surface CD4. HIV viruses that preferentially infect T cells are known as *T-tropic* or *X4* strains, whereas those strains that can infect both macrophages and T cells are called *M-tropic* or *R5* strains.

Entry of HIV into the host cells to which it has attached requires an additional binding step, involving co-receptors that promote fusion of the HIV envelope with the plasma-cell membrane. These co-receptors belong to a family of proteins known as *chemokine receptors*, whose main function is to direct white blood cells (WBCs) to sites of inflammation. The chemokine receptor CXCR4 is required for HIV to enter T lymphocytes, whereas the chemokine receptor CCR5 is required for entry into macrophages. In fact, individuals who have a genetic mutation in the *CCR5* gene have been found to be resistant to HIV infection. Binding of the co-receptors allows for HIV entry by inducing a conformational change in the gp41 glycoprotein, which mediates fusion of the virus to the cell membrane.

After fusion occurs, the viral particle is taken into the cell, and uncoating of the particle exposes the viral genome. Action of the enzyme reverse transcriptase produces complementary

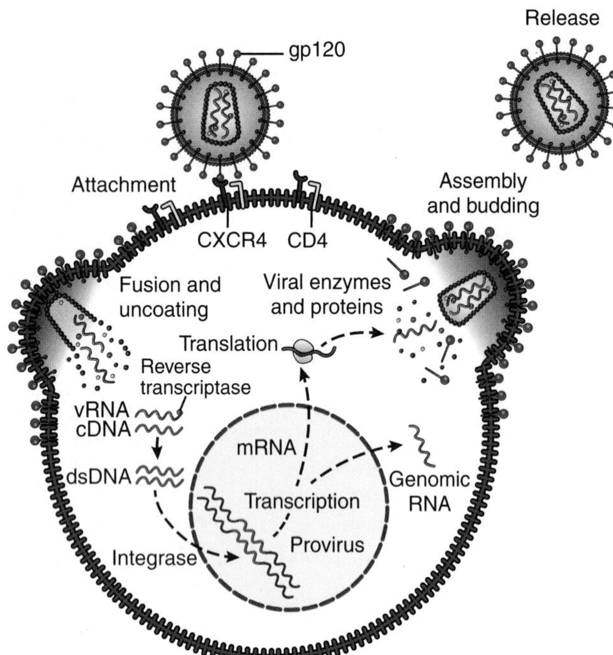

FIGURE 24–3 Replication cycle of HIV in a CD4+ T cell.

DNA from the viral RNA. Double-stranded DNA is synthesized and, with the help of the HIV integrase enzyme, becomes integrated into the host cell's genome as a provirus **(Fig. 24–3).** The provirus can remain in a latent state for a long time, during which viral replication does not occur. Eventually, expression of the viral genes is induced when the infected host cell is activated by binding to an antigen or by exposure to cytokines. Viral DNA within the cell nucleus is then transcribed into genomic RNA and messenger RNA (mRNA), which are transported to the cytoplasm. Translation of mRNA occurs, with production of viral precursor proteins and assembly of viral particles. The intact virions bud out from the host-cell membrane and acquire their envelope during the process. The precursor proteins are cleaved by the viral protease enzyme in the mature virus particles. These viruses can proceed to infect additional host cells. Viral replication occurs to the greatest extent in antigen-activated Th cells.

Because viral replication occurs very rapidly and the reverse transcriptase enzyme lacks proofreading activity, genetic mutations occur at a high rate, producing distinct isolates that exhibit an extraordinary level of antigenic variation. In fact, the level of HIV diversity in a single individual is greater than the diversity of all the influenza virus isolates throughout the world in a given year! This tremendous genetic diversity of HIV hinders the ability of the host to mount an effective immune response.

Immunologic Manifestations

Immune Responses to HIV

When HIV infects a healthy individual, there is typically an initial burst of viral replication followed by a slowing down of virus production as the host's immune response develops and keeps the virus in check. This initial viral replication can be detected in the laboratory by the presence of increased levels of **p24 antigen** and viral RNA in the host's bloodstream (see discussion in the text that follows). As the virus replicates, some of the viral proteins produced within host cells form complexes with class I major histocompatibility complex (MHC) antigens and are transported to the cell surface, where they stimulate lymphocyte responses. HIV-specific CD4+ Th cells are generated and assist both humoral and cell-mediated immune responses against the virus. However, the interactions between HIV and the immune system are complex, and these responses are unable to eliminate HIV from the body, as we will discuss in the text that follows.

B lymphocytes are stimulated to produce antibodies to HIV, which can usually be detected in the host's serum by 6 weeks after primary infection. The first antibodies to be detected are directed against the gp41 transmembrane glycoprotein, followed by production of antibodies to the *gag* proteins such as p24, and, finally, production of antibodies to the *env, pol,* and regulatory proteins. The most immunogenic proteins are in the viral envelope and elicit the production of neutralizing antibodies. These antibodies usually appear 2 to 3 months after infection and prevent the virus from infecting neighboring cells. Antibodies to the envelope proteins have also been shown to bind to Fc receptors on natural killer (NK) cells and participate in antibody-dependent cellular cytotoxicity (ADCC)-mediated killing of HIV-infected cells. However, these antibodies may also participate in the pathogenesis of HIV infection by facilitating Fc-receptor-mediated endocytosis of opsonized virus by uninfected cells. Furthermore, dense glycosylation of the *env* proteins can mask important epitopes, and the enormous diversity of the virus poses challenges to the host in producing a protective antibody response.

T-cell–mediated immunity is thought to play an important role in the immune response to HIV, as it does in other viral infections. CD8+ cytotoxic T lymphocytes, also known as *cytolytic T cells* (CTLs), appear within weeks of HIV infection and are associated with a decline in the amount of HIV in the blood during acute infection. CTLs attack HIV-infected host cells by binding to HIV proteins associated with class I MHC molecules on the surface of infected cells. HIV-specific CTLs are stimulated to develop into mature, activated clones through the effects of cytokines released by activated CD4 Th cells, a process that is common to immune responses against other viruses (see Chapter 4 for details). After the CTLs bind to HIV-infected host cells, cytolytic enzymes are released from their granules and destroy the target cells. Free virions are released from the damaged cells and can be bound by antibodies. CTLs can also suppress replication and spreading of HIV by producing cytokines such as interferon (IFN)-γ, which have antiviral activity.

Connections

CTL Versus Antibody Responses to HIV

Recall from Chapter 23 that antibodies can attach only to virions circulating freely outside of host cells. In contrast, CTLs can attack host cells harboring viruses internally.

Innate immune defenses may play a role in responding to HIV in the early stages of the infection. In particular, NK cells become activated during acute HIV infection and can mediate cytolysis of host cells infected with the virus. In addition, dendritic cells recognize viral components through pattern-recognition receptors, resulting in the release of proinflammatory cytokines that have antiviral effects and can activate other cells of the immune system.

Effects of HIV Infection on the Immune System

HIV has developed several mechanisms by which it can escape immune responses. Although the humoral and cell-mediated immune responses of the host usually reduce the level of HIV replication, they are generally not sufficient to completely eliminate the virus. CTL and antibody responses to HIV are hindered by the virus's ability to undergo rapid genetic mutations, generating escape mutants with altered antigens toward which the host's initial immune responses are ineffective. In addition, HIV can downregulate the production of class I MHC molecules on the surface of the host cells it infects, protecting them from CTL recognition. Numerous cells in the body can also harbor HIV as a silent provirus for long periods, including resting CD4 T cells, dendritic cells, cells of the monocyte and macrophage lineage, and microglial cells in the brain. In this proviral state, HIV is protected from attack by the immune system until cell activation stimulates the virus to multiply and display its viral antigens.

The ability of HIV to evade the immune response results in a persistent infection that can destroy the immune system. Because the virus's prime targets are the CD4 Th cells, these cells are most severely affected. Thus, a decrease in this cell population is the hallmark feature of HIV infection. The gastrointestinal immune system (GALT), which is the largest immune organ in the body, is the most profoundly affected. Early in the infection, HIV causes a rapid depletion of CCR5+ CD4+ memory T cells in the GALT. Th17 helper cells, which play an important role in the homeostasis of the epithelial cells lining the intestinal mucosa (enterocytes) as well as in the secretion of antimicrobial defensins, are also preferentially affected. This depletion results in damage to the intestinal epithelial barrier, with leakage of microbial products such as lipopolysaccharide (LPS) into the plasma and a general state of immune activation.

CD4 Th cells are thought to be killed or rendered nonfunctional by HIV through a variety of mechanisms, including loss of plasma-membrane integrity because of viral budding, destruction by HIV-specific CTL, and viral induction of apoptosis. Infected T cells turn over much more rapidly than they can be replaced, resulting in a progressive decrease in CD4 T cells during the natural course of untreated infections. In addition to reducing T-cell numbers, HIV also causes abnormalities in Th-cell function and impairment of memory Th-cell responses.

Because **CD4 T cells** play a central role in the immune system by regulating the activities of B and T lymphocytes (see Chapter 4), destruction of these cells results in decreased effectiveness of both antibody- and cell-mediated immune responses. These effects apply not only to the immune responses directed against HIV but also to the broad range of antigens that are encountered by the host. Dysregulated immune responses are also evident. HIV proteins actually stimulate polyclonal activation of B cells, resulting in maturational and functional defects with increased circulating immunoglobulin levels, immune complexes, and autoantibodies. However, B cells in HIV-infected individuals have a reduced ability to mount antibody responses after exposure to specific antigens, caused by the decrease in T-cell help.

Cell-mediated immunity is also affected by the reduction in Th activity, resulting in a decline in CTL activity and delayed-type hypersensitivity responses to specific antigens. Altered production of cytokines and chemokines has also been seen, including increases in the levels of some cytokines during the early stages of disease, followed by declining levels of interleukin-2 (IL-2) and antibody-dependent cellular cytotoxicity IFN-γ and a shift in the cytokine profile from Th1 to Th2 as the infection progresses toward development of AIDS. Extensive damage to the lymphoid tissues is evident late in the infection, with loss of germinal centers and follicular dendritic cells, resulting in an inability to activate T and B lymphocytes. Other immunologic abnormalities, including defective antigen presentation and oxidative burst by monocytes and macrophages and decreased NK-cell activity, have also been observed in AIDS patients.

Clinical Symptoms of HIV Infection

HIV causes a chronic infection that is characterized by a progressive decline in the immune system. Although the manifestations of the disease vary in individual patients, the infection progresses through a clinical course that begins with primary, or acute, infection, followed by a period of clinical latency that eventually culminates in AIDS. The acute, or early, stage of infection is characterized by a rapid burst of viral replication before the development of HIV-specific immune responses. In this stage, high levels of circulating virus, or **viremia,** can be seen in the blood of infected individuals; therefore, HIV begins to disseminate to the lymphoid organs. There is a reduction in the peripheral blood CD4 T-cell count, but this usually returns to slightly decreased or, sometimes, normal levels. As the immune system becomes activated, an acute retroviral syndrome may develop. This syndrome, which has been noted in 50% to 70% of patients with primary HIV infection, is characterized by flu-like or infectious-mononucleosis-like symptoms. Symptoms of the primary stage usually appear 3 to 6 weeks after the initial infection and resolve within 7 days to a few weeks. Many patients, however, are asymptomatic during this stage.

As HIV-specific immune responses develop, they begin to curtail replication of the virus, and patients enter a period of clinical latency. This stage is characterized by a decrease in viremia as the virus is cleared from the circulationand, and clinical symptoms are subtle or absent. However, studies have demonstrated that the virus is still present in the plasma, albeit at lower levels, and more so in the lymphoid tissues. The CD4 T-cell count remains stable for a variable period of time and then begins to progressively decline. A small proportion of HIV-infected individuals, termed *elite controllers*, have normal or mildly depressed CD4 T-cell counts and low viral loads and remain asymptomatic for many years in the absence of antiretroviral therapy. The presence of certain genetic factors, including HLA-B57-01 and HLA-B27-05, is thought to play a role in the ability of these individuals to mount vigorous immune responses that more effectively control replication of the virus.

Untreated individuals will ultimately progress to AIDS, the final stage of HIV infection, which is characterized by profound immunosuppression with very low numbers of CD4 T cells, a resurgence of viremia, and life-threatening infections and malignancies. The rate at which people progress to the development of AIDS varies, but progression typically occurs in untreated individuals within a median time of 10 years after the initial infection. The rate of progression has dramatically decreased with the use of antiretroviral therapies (see *Treatment and Prevention* in the text that follows).

A list of the **opportunistic illnesses** considered to be indicative of AIDS is found in the Clinical Correlations box. These conditions appear in immunocompromised individuals but do not usually affect people with a healthy immune system. In addition to infections and malignancies, HIV-infected individuals often demonstrate neurological symptoms resulting from the ability of HIV to infect cells in the brain. In early HIV infection, these symptoms may manifest as forgetfulness, poor concentration, apathy, psychomotor retardation, and withdrawal, whereas progression to late disease may result in confusion, disorientation, seizures, dementia, gait disturbances, ataxia, or paraparesis.

Clinical Correlations

Opportunistic Illnesses Indicative of AIDS (Stage 3 HIV Infection)

Bacterial infections, multiple or recurrent*
Candidiasis of bronchi, trachea, or lungs
Candidiasis of esophagus
Cervical cancer, invasive†
Coccidioidomycosis, disseminated or extrapulmonary
Cryptococcosis, extrapulmonary
Cryptosporidiosis, chronic intestinal (longer than 1 month's duration)
Cytomegalovirus disease (other than liver, spleen, or nodes), onset older than 1 month of age
Cytomegalovirus retinitis (with loss of vision)
Encephalopathy attributed to HIV
Herpes simplex: chronic ulcers (longer than 1 month's duration) or bronchitis, pneumonitis, or esophagitis (onset older than 1 month of age)
Histoplasmosis, disseminated or extrapulmonary
Isosporiasis, chronic intestinal (longer than 1 month's duration)
Kaposi sarcoma
Lymphoma, Burkitt (or equivalent term)
Lymphoma, immunoblastic (or equivalent term)
Lymphoma, primary, of brain
Mycobacterium avium complex or *Mycobacterium kansasii*, disseminated or extrapulmonary
Mycobacterium tuberculosis of any site, pulmonary†, disseminated, or extrapulmonary
Mycobacterium, other species or unidentified species, disseminated or extrapulmonary
Pneumocystis jirovecii (previously known as "*Pneumocystis carinii*") pneumonia
Pneumonia, recurrent†
Progressive multifocal leukoencephalopathy
Salmonella septicemia, recurrent
Toxoplasmosis of brain, onset older than 1 month of age
Wasting syndrome attributed to HIV

*Only among children aged younger than 6 years.
†Only among adults, adolescents, and children aged 6 years or older.
Courtesy of Centers for Disease Control and Prevention. Revised surveillance case definition for HIV infection—United States, 2014. *MMWR* 2014;63(3):1–10.

Symptoms of AIDS in infants include failure to thrive, persistent oral candidiasis, hepatosplenomegaly, lymphadenopathy, recurrent diarrhea, or recurrent bacterial infections. Abnormal neurological findings may be present. The rate by which HIV infection progresses in children varies and may be influenced by factors such as the maturity of the immune system at the time of infection, the dose of virus to which the child was exposed, and the route of infection.

The CDC first defined AIDS as "a disease, at least moderately predictive of a defect in cell mediated immunity, occurring in a person with no known cause for diminished resistance to that disease." The definition has been revised several times over the years as more information has been acquired about HIV and additional laboratory tests for HIV have been developed. The CDC also published a separate case definition for HIV infection in children. The latest definition at the time of this writing was published in 2014. It combines the case definitions for persons of all ages into a single definition that is intended to be used for surveillance of the disease. The 2014 definition bases a confirmed case of HIV infection on either laboratory criteria or clinical evidence, with laboratory results being the preferred criteria. Laboratory criteria consist of positive test results in multitest algorithms for HIV antibody or combination HIV antigen/antibody, whereas clinical evidence refers to physician documentation of HIV infection in the patient's medical record (see *Laboratory Testing for HIV Infection* in the text that follows).

HIV-positive patients are further classified into one of five stages (0, 1, 2, 3, or unknown). The stage can change for an individual patient in either direction over time. Stage 0 includes those individuals with early HIV infection who had an initial confirmed HIV-positive laboratory result followed by a negative or indeterminate HIV test result within a 6-month period. These patients can be reclassified in one of the other categories 180 days or more after initial diagnosis. Patients are classified as being in stages 1, 2, or 3 based on their peripheral blood CD4 T-cell count or percentage; if this information is

Table 24–2 CD4 T-Cell Parameters Used in HIV Staging

	AGE ON DATE OF CD4+ T-LYMPHOCYTE TEST					
	YOUNGER THAN 1 YEAR		1 TO 5 YEARS		6 YEARS OR OLDER	
STAGE	CELLS/μL	PERCENT	CELLS/μL	PERCENT	CELLS/μL	PERCENT
1	1,500	≥34	≥1,000	≥30	≥500	≥26
2	750–1,499	26–33	500–999	22–29	200–499	14–25
3	<750	<26	<500	<22	<200	<14

The stage is based primarily on the CD4+ T-lymphocyte count; the percentage is considered only if the count is missing.
Adapted from Centers for Disease Control and Prevention. Revised surveillance case definition for HIV infection—United States, 2014. MMWR *2014;63(3):1–10.*

missing, they are classified in the "unknown" category. The CD4 T-cell parameters used in this classification system are shown in **Table 24–2.** Stage 3 is also indicated if any of the opportunistic illnesses listed in the Clinical Correlations box are present.

Treatment and Prevention

Treatment of HIV infection involves supportive care of the associated infections and malignancies as well as administration of **antiretroviral therapy (ART)** to suppress the virus's replication. Several classes of antiretroviral drugs have been developed to treat HIV infection: nucleoside analogue reverse-transcriptase inhibitors (NRTIs), nonnucleoside reverse-transcriptase inhibitors (NNRTIs), protease inhibitors (PIs), integrase strand transfer inhibitors (INSTIs), fusion inhibitors, a CCR5 antagonist, and a CD4 post-attachment inhibitor. These drugs block various steps of the HIV replication cycle. Their mechanisms of action are summarized in **Table 24–3.** New drugs continue to be developed as advances in this area are made. Updated guidelines on the use of these drugs are available from the U.S. Department of Health and Human Services and the WHO.

Studies have shown that treatment with multiple drugs is more effective in killing the virus and preventing viral resistance than treatment with a single drug. Therefore, potent regimens involving a combination of drugs from different antiretroviral drug classes are the standard of treatment. The preferred initial treatment protocols at the time of this writing consist of two NRTIs plus an INSTI, an NNRTI, or a PI. The goal of this therapy is to reduce the patient's HIV viral load to a level that is below the detectable limit of quantitative plasma viral load assays (see *Quantitative Viral Load Assays* in the text that follows). This is most likely to be achieved if treatment is started early in the course of infection and the patient can adhere to the treatment as prescribed.

ART has had a dramatic effect on the clinical course of HIV infection, as evidenced by a significant decline in the incidence of opportunistic infections, a delay in progression to AIDS, and decreased mortality in patients who have received this multidrug treatment. Before the development of ART, the median survival time of AIDS patients was only 26 weeks from the time of diagnosis; today, HIV-infected patients who are treated appropriately with ART can be expected to live 50 years or longer. Because of this success, ART is recommended for all HIV-infected persons at the time of diagnosis. In addition, antiretroviral drugs given to pregnant women and newborns have had a significant impact in reducing perinatal transmission of HIV, as we discussed previously in this chapter. ART and avoidance of breastfeeding by HIV-positive women have reduced the rate of perinatal transmission to less than 1% in developed countries of the world.

Although antiretroviral drugs and ART have significantly improved morbidity and mortality in HIV-infected patients, they cannot be considered a cure for AIDS. Although blood levels of the virus are greatly reduced in patients treated with antiretroviral drugs, HIV is still harbored in lymphoid organs throughout the body and progressively destroys the immune system. Research is ongoing to develop additional drugs to target HIV that remains latent within infected cells.

Several other approaches for dealing with HIV have been directed toward preventing initial infection. Community-based education aimed at high-risk groups such as homosexual males and intravenous drug users has provided beneficial information on reducing transmission of the virus. The CDC has published guidelines for the use of antiretroviral drugs for pre-exposure prophylaxis (PrEP) to prevent transmission to individuals who are HIV-negative but at a high risk of contracting the infection, such as those who inject illicit drugs or are sexually active with an HIV-infected partner. In addition, the CDC and the Occupational Safety and Health Administration (OSHA) have published precautions to prevent the transmission of HIV and other bloodborne pathogens in health-care workers. Prophylactic therapy with antiretroviral drugs is also offered to health-care workers who may have been exposed to HIV through percutaneous or mucous-membrane contact with potentially infected blood or body fluids, in hope that early treatment will prevent infection. Because of these measures, fewer than 60 documented cases of occupational HIV transmission to health-care workers have been recorded by the CDC.

The ultimate means of preventing HIV infection would be the development of an effective vaccine. Much research has been directed in this area, but the task has been very difficult for many reasons. For example, HIV can rapidly mutate

Table 24–3 Antiretroviral Drugs for HIV Therapy

ANTIRETROVIRAL DRUG CLASSIFICATION	MECHANISM OF ACTION	EXAMPLES
Nucleoside analogue reverse-transcriptase inhibitors (NRTIs)	Similar in structure to nucleosides; incorporate into HIV nucleic acid and block synthesis of viral RNA	Zidovudine, lamivudine, emtricitabine, abacavir, tenofovir
Nonnucleoside reverse-transcriptase inhibitors (NNRTIs)	Bind to and inactivate reverse transcriptase	Nevirapine, doravirine, efavirenz, etravirine
Protease inhibitors (PIs)	Prevent cleavage of precursor proteins needed for assembly of HIV virions	Saquinavir, ritonavir, fosamprenavir
Integrase strand transfer inhibitors (INSTIs)	Prevent integration of HIV DNA into the host genome	Raltegravir, dolutegravir
Fusion inhibitors	Block viral infection by preventing fusion of HIV with target cells	Enfuvirtide
CCR5 Antagonists	Block binding of HIV to the chemokine co-receptor CCR5	Maraviroc
Post-attachment inhibitors	Block binding of HIV to the CD4 surface receptor	Ibalizumab-uiyk

and escape immune recognition, and there is no ideal animal model in which to study vaccine effects. In addition, an effective vaccine would need to induce mucosal immunity because HIV is usually transmitted through mucosal surfaces. An effective vaccine should also stimulate potent CTL and broad neutralizing antibody responses that could detect many variants of the virus. If a vaccine that can prevent HIV infection in the traditional sense cannot be developed, it is possible that a therapeutic vaccine given to already-diagnosed individuals may provide some benefits by stimulating a more effective immune response and lowering the level of viremia, thus reducing the risk of transmission to others.

Laboratory Testing for HIV Infection

The laboratory plays a key role in establishing the initial diagnosis of HIV infection and in monitoring known patients for their response to ART. In addition, recommendations published by the U.S. Preventative Task Force and the CDC for HIV screening, especially for those at high risk for HIV infection, have increased the number of infected individuals who are aware of their status.

Several types of laboratory tests have been used to diagnose and monitor HIV infection, including HIV antibody detection, HIV antigen detection, viral nucleic acid testing (NAT), and CD4 T-cell enumeration. The principles of each of these methods are discussed in the text that follows, along with their applications to the detection and monitoring of HIV infection. Although culturing the virus from patient samples is a definitive method of demonstrating HIV infection, it is not used in clinical settings because it is laborious, time consuming, costly, and potentially hazardous to laboratory personnel.

Screening and Diagnosis

Serological tests for HIV antibody have been used in the initial diagnosis of HIV infection because most individuals develop antibody to the virus within 1 to 2 months after exposure. Since 1985, these tests have played a critical role in screening the donor blood supply to prevent transmission of the virus through blood transfusions or administration of blood products. Serological tests are also used in epidemiology studies to provide health officials with information about the extent of the infection in high-risk populations. These groups can then be targeted for counseling, treatment, and vaccine trials, and their medical or social concerns can be addressed.

Different serological methods have been used to test for HIV. Standard screening methods for HIV antibody have involved automated immunoassays such as the enzyme-linked immunosorbent assay (ELISA) and chemiluminescent immunoassay (CLIA) (see Chapter 11). In addition, rapid tests have been developed that can detect HIV antibody within minutes, making them an attractive alternative to standard screening methods in certain situations. Confirmatory tests are performed on samples that test positive on a screening test, in order to differentiate true-positive from false-positive results. The Western blot test (see section in the text that follows) was the standard confirmatory test for HIV for several years, but it has been replaced by newer methods for routine testing. Serological testing for p24 antigen and NAT for HIV RNA have been incorporated into the initial HIV testing scheme, providing for earlier and more accurate detection. The principles of these methods are discussed in the text that follows, along with their use in HIV testing algorithms.

Testing Algorithms

Over the years, the CDC and the Association of Public Health Laboratories have developed algorithms that use a combination of laboratory tests performed in sequence to screen for the presence of HIV infection and resolve any discrepant results. These algorithms have been revised as improvements in laboratory tests have been made. In 1989, for example, the standard diagnostic algorithm recommended that testing begin with a sensitive ELISA for HIV-1 antibody, with positive samples being retested and then confirmed with a more specific Western blot test for HIV-1 antibody (or less frequently, an HIV-specific indirect immunofluorescence assay [IFA]). In 1992, the algorithm was modified so that initial testing was performed with an HIV-1/HIV-2 antibody test in cases where HIV-2 was likely to be present. In 2004, it was recommended that rapid HIV antibody tests could also be used for initial screening and that positive results should be confirmed by an HIV-1 Western blot or IFA.

In 2014, the CDC recommended that initial screening be performed with a combination immunoassay that detects antibodies to HIV-1 and HIV-2 as well as the HIV-1 p24 antigen. These recommendations apply to adults and children who are older than 24 months. There are separate recommendations for children younger than 2 years, as maternal antibodies may be present that are likely to confuse the interpretation of the test results (see the text that follows). All positive specimens should then undergo additional testing with a rapid immunoassay that discriminates between HIV-1 and HIV-2 antibodies. Any samples that are reactive in the initial test and nonreactive in the second test should then undergo NAT to resolve the discrepancy.

The 2014 algorithm is summarized in **Figure 24–4.** This testing scheme provides significant advantages over previous algorithms. First, it allows for earlier detection of infections, as the time between exposure and detectable results on the HIV-1/2/p24 combination assay is typically between 15 and 17 days. Secondly, it overcomes the limitations associated with use of the Western blot test. The Western blot is a lengthy procedure that is typically performed only by specialized reference laboratories. In addition, Western blot testing is less sensitive than the initial ELISA used for screening; therefore, indeterminate results can occur, which can take as long as 3 to 6 months to resolve. The 2014 testing algorithm allows for more rapid and accurate identification of HIV infection. This makes it possible to begin appropriate medical care and ART sooner in infected individuals. The 2014 testing protocol also helps to prevent additional infections by encouraging prompt initiation of counseling to reduce risky behaviors and earlier notification of sexual partners of diagnosed individuals.

Although the 2014 algorithm (the most current at the time of this writing) is highly sensitive in the detection of HIV infection, it has some limitations, which will be discussed in the

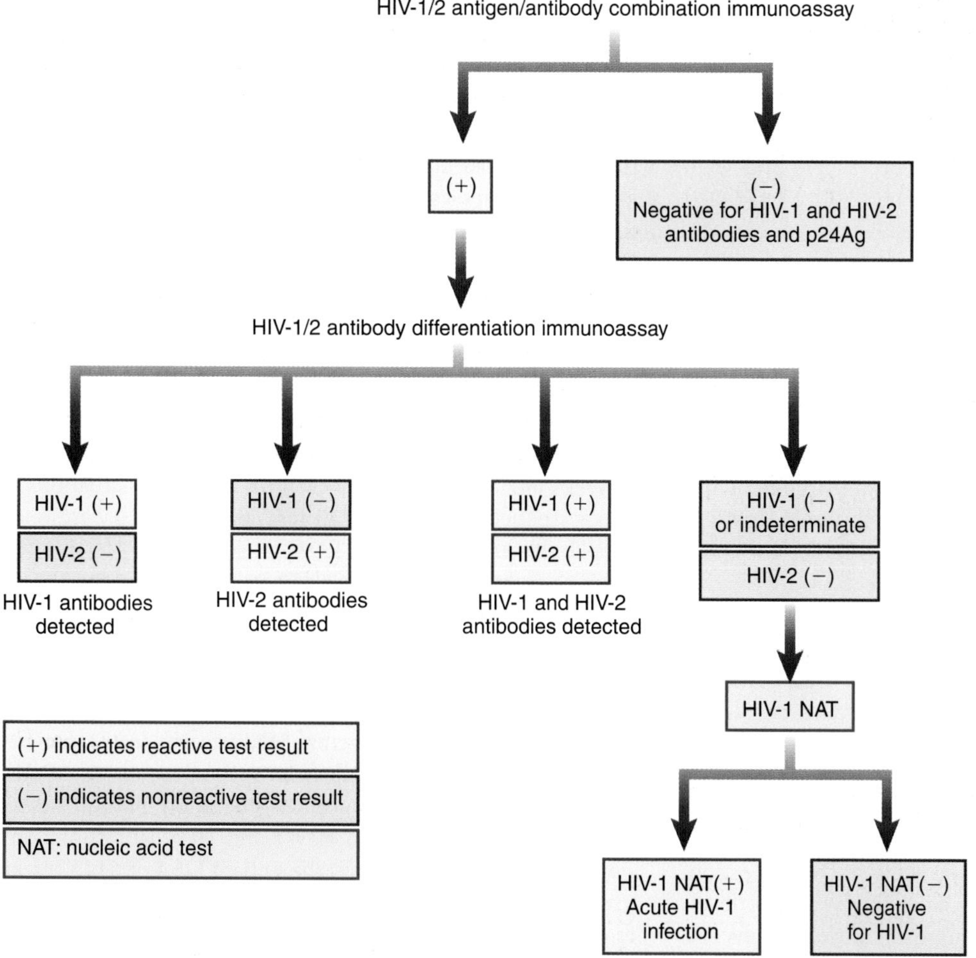

FIGURE 24–4 2014 Laboratory HIV testing algorithm recommended by the CDC. *(Adapted from Branson BM, Owen SM, Wesolowski LG, et al. Laboratory testing for the diagnosis of HIV infection: Updated recommendations. CDC Stacks. Web site. http://stacks.cdc.gov/view/cdc/23447. Updated 2014. Accessed December 18, 2014.)*

next section. The CDC continues to evaluate its algorithm as additional tests become available for clinical use. The principles of the major laboratory tests used in testing for HIV infection are discussed in the text that follows.

Serological Test Principles

Conventional Immunoassays

Conventional immunoassays have been the cornerstone of screening procedures for HIV because they are easy to perform, they can be adapted to test a large number of samples, and they are highly sensitive and specific. They were first used to detect HIV antibody in the United States in 1985 in response to the need to screen donated blood. Several manufacturers have developed commercial kits that are useful in screening blood products and in diagnosing patients. An updated list of kits approved for use in the United States is published by the FDA. Over the years, five generations of immunoassays have been developed, resulting in improved sensitivity and specificity.

The first generation of immunoassays were ELISAs that were based on a solid-phase, indirect technique that used viral lysate antigens from cultured cells to detect antibodies to only HIV-1. (See Chapter 11 for general principles of ELISA.) These first-generation assays were prone to false-positive results caused by reactions with HLA antigens or other components from the cells used to culture the virus, and they were unable to detect antibodies to HIV-2.

The second-generation ELISAs, introduced in the late 1980s, were indirect binding assays that used highly purified recombinant or synthetic antigens from both HIV-1 and HIV-2, rather than crude cell lysates. These assays demonstrated improved specificity and sensitivity overall and were able to detect antibodies to both HIV-1 and HIV-2 but failed to detect certain subtypes of HIV.

Third-generation tests were developed as sandwich ELISA and CLIAs. In these methods, antibodies in patient serum or plasma bind to recombinant HIV-1 and HIV-2 proteins coated onto a solid phase. After washing, bound antibody is detected by the addition of enzyme- or chemiluminescent-labeled HIV-1 and HIV-2 antigens and substrate or trigger solution. This test format was highly specific and improved sensitivity by simultaneously detecting HIV antibodies of different immunoglobulin classes, including immunoglobulin M (IgM), as well as antibodies to Group O HIV in addition to the more common Group M.

Currently, the most widely used assays are fully automated fourth-generation methods that can simultaneously detect HIV-1 antibodies, HIV-2 antibodies, and p24 antigen. Previously, separate immunoassays were used to detect the p24 antigen from the core of the HIV-1 virion as a marker of early infection. Levels of p24 in the circulation are high in the initial weeks of infection during the early burst of viral replication, providing a marker that can be detected before the appearance of HIV antibody during the acute stage of infection. The antigen becomes undetectable as antibody to p24 develops and binds the antigen in immune complexes; levels rise again during the later stages of infection when impairment of the immune system allows the virus to replicate.

The basic principle of the fourth-generation HIV-1 antibody/HIV-2 antibody/p24 antigen combination tests is illustrated in **Figure 24–5.** These tests employ a sandwich ELISA or CLIA in which patient serum is incubated with a solid phase onto which synthetic or recombinant HIV-1 antigens, HIV-2 antigens, and a monoclonal antibody to HIV-1 p24 have been attached. If antibody to HIV is in the sample, it will bind to the HIV-1 or HIV-2 antigens (or both, if both infections are present); if p24 antigen is in the sample, it will bind to the anti-p24 on the solid phase. Following a wash step to remove excess sample, a conjugate containing chemiluminescent- or enzyme-labeled anti-p24 and HIV-1/HIV-2 antigens is added. After a second incubation and wash step, the appropriate trigger solution or substrate/stop solution is added, and the relative light units released or optical absorbance is measured. As previously mentioned, these combination assays are used in the initial step of the 2014 laboratory testing algorithm recommended by the CDC.

A fifth-generation multiplex bead immunoassay has also been FDA-approved for screening for HIV infection. This assay can also detect both HIV antibodies and antigens, but in addition, it can differentiate between HIV-1 antibody, HIV-2 antibody, and p24 antigen.

Although the immunoassays used in HIV testing have a high level of sensitivity and specificity, they may sometimes give erroneous results. False-negative results for HIV antibody occur infrequently but may be caused by the collection of the test serum before the patient develops HIV antibodies (i.e., before **seroconversion**), administration of immunosuppressive therapy or replacement transfusion, conditions of defective antibody synthesis such as hypogammaglobulinemia, or technical errors attributed to improper handling of kit reagents. False-negative results may also occur if the patient harbors a genetically diverse, recombinant strain of HIV. The likelihood of false negatives occurring has been reduced by implementation of fourth-generation tests that can identify HIV infection several days earlier than third-generation tests because they detect p24 antigen in addition to HIV antibodies. This makes it possible for the infection to be diagnosed within 2 to 3 weeks after exposure. However, there are rare situations in which a patient can persistently test negative for HIV antibody despite the presence of HIV RNA.

False-positive results may also occur in these assays. These can result from several factors, including heat inactivation of the sample before testing, repeated freezing and thawing of specimens, the presence of heterophile or human-anti-mouse antibodies, passive immunoglobulin administration, or administration of an experimental HIV vaccine to the patient. False positives can also result from specimen mix-up or mislabeling. In addition, the fourth-generation immunoassays cannot distinguish between HIV-1 and HIV-2 infection. Any positive results obtained from the initial ELISA or CLIA screen must therefore be confirmed by additional testing that can differentiate the two viruses.

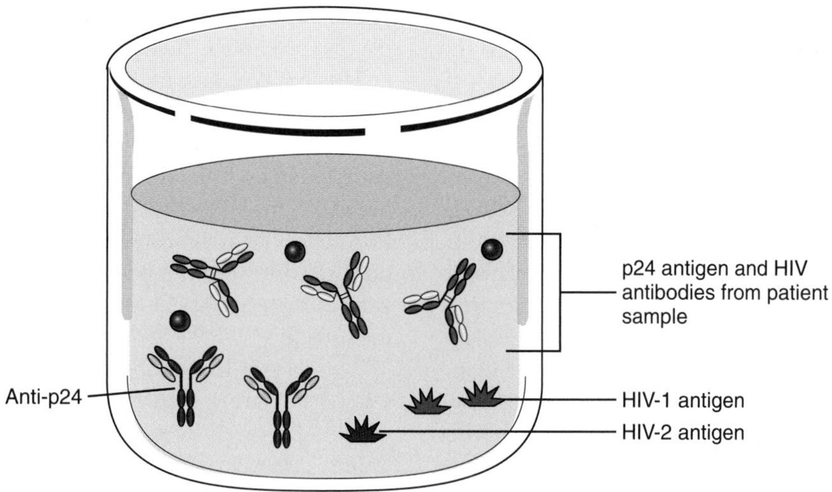

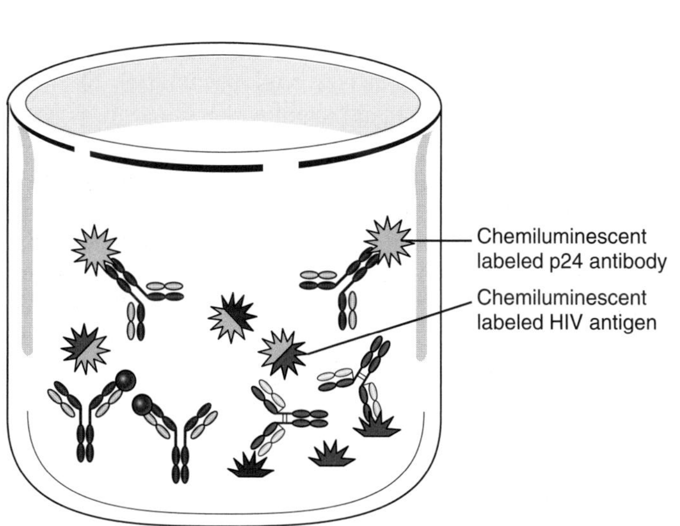

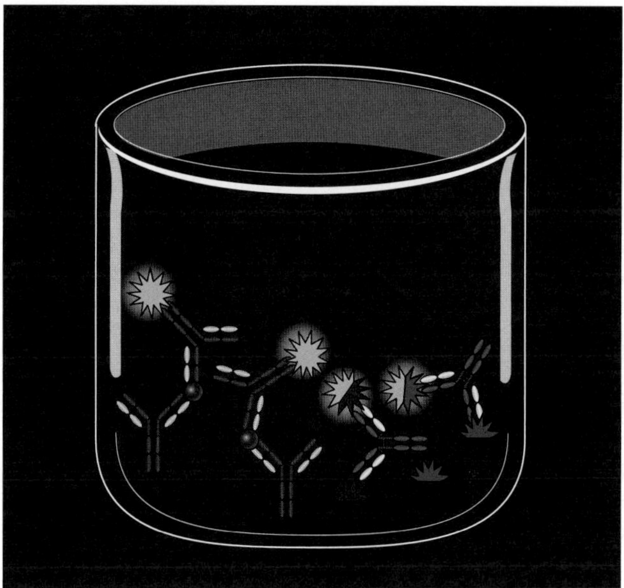

FIGURE 24–5 Principle of fourth-generation CLIA test for HIV. This test detects the HIV-1 p24 antigen as well as HIV-1 antibodies and HIV-2 antibodies.

Clinical Correlations

Seroconversion

By definition, seroconversion is the change of a serological test result from antibody negative to antibody positive. This occurs over time when the immune system is responding to HIV infection. Seroconversion can be detected by comparing the test results from two samples collected from the patient, the first soon after exposure to the virus and the second a few weeks later.

Rapid Tests for HIV Antibodies

Although conventional immunoassays are ideal tests for the detection of HIV antibodies in clinical laboratories that perform large-volume batch testing, they require expensive instrumentation and skilled personnel with technical expertise and may have a turnaround time of a few days. To overcome these limitations and to encourage more patients to be tested, simple, rapid methods to screen for HIV antibody have been developed. These tests are available for use around the world and provide results within 30 minutes.

Several commercially available rapid tests have been approved by the FDA. These kits detect antibodies to HIV-1 alone or to both HIV-1 and HIV-2; they can be used on serum, plasma, whole blood samples obtained by venipuncture or fingerstick, or for some kits, oral fluid. Although each test has unique features, all are lateral flow or flow-through immunoassays that produce a colorimetric reaction in the case of a positive result. The flow-through assays require multiple steps in which the sample and reagents are added to a solid support encased in a plastic device, whereas the lateral flow assays involve a one-step procedure in which the patient sample migrates along the test strip by capillary action (see Chapter 11). With either procedure, the patient's sample is applied to a test strip or membrane containing HIV antigens. The antigen–antibody complexes bind to an enzyme-labeled conjugate or an antibody-binding (protein A) colloidal gold conjugate and are detected by a colorimetric reaction that produces a colored line or dot in the case of a positive result. Interpretation of the results is made through visual observation of the test device and does not require instrumentation.

A primary use for rapid tests has been to screen for HIV infection; these are especially suitable in certain circumstances. Rapid tests are ideal for use in resource-limited settings around the world that do not have access to expensive equipment and highly trained personnel. They are also beneficial in situations in which fast notification of test results is desired. For example, rapid results are important in guiding decisions to begin prophylactic therapy with antiretroviral drugs following occupational exposures because this therapy appears to be most effective when administered soon after exposure. Other situations in which rapid tests are advantageous include testing women whose HIV status is unknown during labor and delivery and testing patients in sexually transmitted disease clinics or emergency departments who are unlikely to return for their test results.

Although rapid tests are highly specific, false positives can occur. In addition, rapid tests conducted with whole blood obtained by fingerstick or oral fluid are less sensitive than those performed on plasma or serum, and a negative test result does not rule out early acute HIV infection. For these reasons, rapid testing should be followed by the current recommended testing algorithm whenever possible. A rapid test that detects p24 antigen as well as HIV-1 and HIV-2 antibodies has also been approved for use in HIV screening.

Some rapid HIV kits are available through the Internet or over the counter for home testing; the FDA has approved two such kits, one for a blood sample obtained by fingerstick and the other for oral fluid. These tests offer the advantages of convenience, privacy, and anonymity and have the potential of encouraging more widespread screening among high-risk individuals. However, false-negative results can occur because home tests are not as sensitive as conventional testing, and there is concern that some people who test positive might not seek confirmatory testing and the appropriate medical care.

As we previously discussed, a rapid immunoassay that differentiates between HIV-1 and HIV-2 has also been recommended by the CDC for confirmation of results from samples that test positive in the HIV-1 antibody/HIV-2 antibody/p24 antigen combo screen. Rapid testing has several advantages over the previously recommended Western blot test (see the text that follows). Specifically, HIV antibodies are detected earlier, the incidence of indeterminate results is reduced, there is a shorter result-turnaround time, testing is less costly, and HIV-2 infections are detected as well as those caused by HIV-1.

Western Blot

Recall that because of the possibility of obtaining false-positive results, all positive samples from HIV screening tests must be referred for testing with a more specific confirmatory method. The **Western blot test**, or immunoblot, for HIV antibodies was introduced in 1984 and was the most common method used for confirmation of positive ELISA results from 1985 to 2014. This technique is more technically demanding than ELISA but can provide an antibody profile of the patient sample that reveals the specificities to individual HIV antigens.

Western blot kits are prepared commercially as nitrocellulose or nylon strips containing individual HIV proteins that have been separated by polyacrylamide gel electrophoresis and blotted onto the test membrane. The protein antigens are derived from HIV virus grown in cell culture. Antigens with low molecular weight migrate most rapidly and are therefore positioned toward the bottom of the test strip, whereas antigens of high molecular weight remain toward the top of the membrane.

The testing laboratory then applies patient serum to the test strip. During incubation, HIV antibodies in the sample will bind to their corresponding antigens on the test membrane. Unbound antibody is removed by washing; then an anti-human immunoglobulin conjugated to an enzyme label is added to the test strip and binds to specific HIV antibodies from the patient sample. Following a wash step, bound conjugate is detected by adding the appropriate substrate, which produces a chromogenic reaction. Colored bands appear in the positions where antigen-specific HIV antibodies are present. Separate HIV-1- and HIV-2-specific Western blot tests must be used to test for antibodies to each virus.

The bands produced by the test sample are examined visually for the number and types of antibodies present. Densitometry can also be performed to quantitate the intensity of the bands, which would reflect the amount of each antibody produced. Patients can be followed over time to determine whether there is a change in the antibody pattern.

Because Western blot testing is highly dependent on the laboratorian's technical skill and subjective interpretation, it is generally performed only in specialized reference laboratories that have an adequate proficiency testing program. Positive and negative control sera must be included in the test run to provide quality control. For the test to be valid, the negative control should produce no bands, and the positive control should be reactive with p17, p24, p31, gp41, p51, p55, p66, and gp120/160. A negative test result for the patient sample is reported if either no bands are present or if none of the bands present correspond to the molecular weights of any of the known viral proteins.

Criteria for determining a positive test result have been published by the Association of State and Territorial Public Health Laboratory Directors and CDC, the Consortium for Retrovirus Serology Standardization, the American Red Cross, and the FDA. According to these criteria, a result is considered positive if at least two of the following three bands are present: p24, gp41, and gp120/gp160 **(Fig. 24–6)**.

Specimens that have some of the characteristic bands present but do not meet the criteria for a positive test result are considered to be *indeterminate*. This result may be produced if the test serum is collected in the early phase of seroconversion or if the serum contains antibodies that cross-react with some of the immunoblot antigens, producing false-positive results. False positives may be caused by antibodies to contaminants from the cells used to culture HIV to prepare the antigens for the test; to autoantibodies, including those directed against

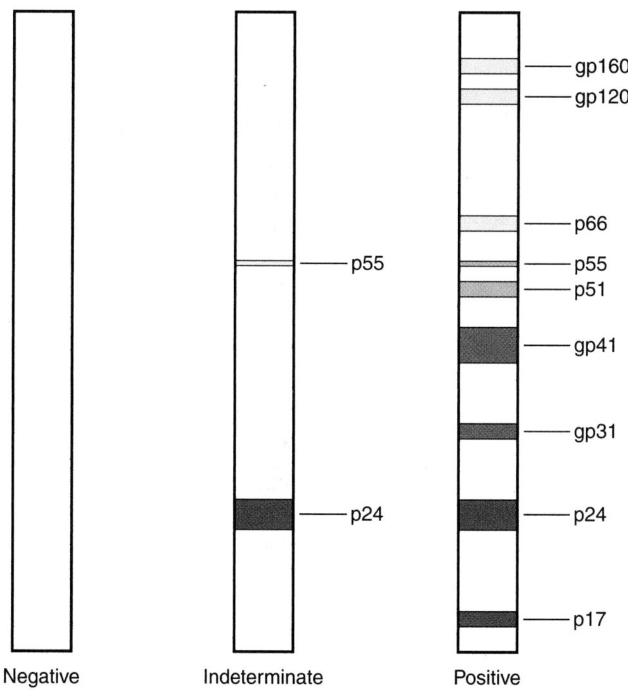

FIGURE 24–6 Western blot, showing results from a negative sample, an indeterminate sample, and a positive sample.

human leukocyte antigen (HLA), nuclear, mitochondrial, or T-cell antigens; or to antibodies produced after vaccinations.

The use of recombinant antigens instead of viral lysates has reduced the incidence of false-positive results. If an indeterminate test result is obtained, it is recommended that the test be repeated with the same or a fresh specimen; if the test is still indeterminate, testing may be performed with a new specimen obtained 4 to 6 weeks later. If the pattern converts to positive, it can be concluded that the first specimen was obtained during the early phase of seroconversion. Failure of an indeterminate test pattern to convert to positive after a few weeks strongly suggests that the pattern is caused by a false-positive test rather than HIV infection. During this period, HIV NAT can be performed to provide more conclusive results (see the text that follows).

Because of its relative insensitivity, level of technical difficulty, and long turnaround time to obtain results, the Western blot test was deemed inappropriate for use as an initial screen for HIV infection. For these same reasons, as we previously discussed, the CDC guidelines replaced the Western blot with a rapid HIV-1/HIV-2 antibody test as the standard method for confirming positive screening results. Rapid tests are more suitable for confirmation because they can be performed more quickly, detect infection earlier, reduce the incidence of indeterminate results, and detect HIV-1 and HIV-2 infections simultaneously. However, HIV-1 Western blot testing still available in some reference laboratories and may be used as a confirmatory method in special situations, such as the testing of dried blood or urine or of samples that have indeterminate antibody screening results and test negative for HIV-1 RNA.

Qualitative Nucleic Acid Tests (NATs)

Qualitative nucleic acid tests (NATs) are used to determine whether or not a detectable level of HIV nucleic acid is present in human plasma. These tests can be used to screen for infection or make an initial patient diagnosis. They are particularly beneficial in cases where serological results are inconclusive, such as in very early infection or in the diagnosis of infants, where the presence of maternal antibodies can confuse test results.

As previously mentioned, NAT is an integral part of the 2014 CDC recommendations for laboratory testing for HIV. The test is used to resolve discrepancies between a positive result in the initial antigen–antibody combo assay and the follow-up HIV-1/HIV-2 antibody differentiation assay. If the HIV-1 antibody/HIV-2 antibody/p24 antigen test is reactive, and the HIV-1/HIV-2 antibody test is also reactive, the result is considered positive for HIV-1 or HIV-2, and the qualitative NAT need not be performed. If the HIV-1 antibody/HIV-2 antibody/p24 antigen test is reactive, but the HIV-1/HIV-2 antibody test is indeterminate or negative, then NAT is performed. In this situation, if the NAT is reactive, this result is considered evidence for acute HIV-1 infection; in contrast, if the NAT is nonreactive, a false-positive result on the initial HIV antigen–antibody combo assay is indicated, and the result is considered negative for HIV-1. Performance of NAT may also be helpful if the HIV-1 antibody/HIV-2 antibody/p24 antigen test is nonreactive and a recent HIV exposure is suspected.

HIV NAT is highly sensitive; it is able to detect HIV RNA about 10 to 12 days after infection. Methods approved by the FDA include a qualitative polymerase chain reaction (PCR)-based assay to screen donors of whole blood, blood components, or organs and a transcription-mediated amplification (TMA) assay for diagnosis.

Disease Monitoring

Once a diagnosis of HIV infection has been established, it is essential to monitor patients over time to evaluate the effectiveness of their ART. This way, signs of disease progression can be detected early and guide decisions about further treatments. Two laboratory markers are routinely used to monitor patients with HIV infection for disease progression and guide their treatments: (1) the peripheral blood CD4 T-cell count, which is considered to be the best indicator of immune function in HIV-infected individuals, and (2) the HIV-1 RNA level, or "viral load," which reflects patient responses to ART. Each of these laboratory markers will be discussed in detail in the text that follows.

CD4 T-Cell Enumeration

Destruction of the CD4 T lymphocytes is central to the immunopathogenesis of HIV infection, and CD4 lymphopenia has long been recognized as the hallmark feature of AIDS. Therefore, enumeration of CD4 T cells in the peripheral blood has played a central role in evaluating the degree of

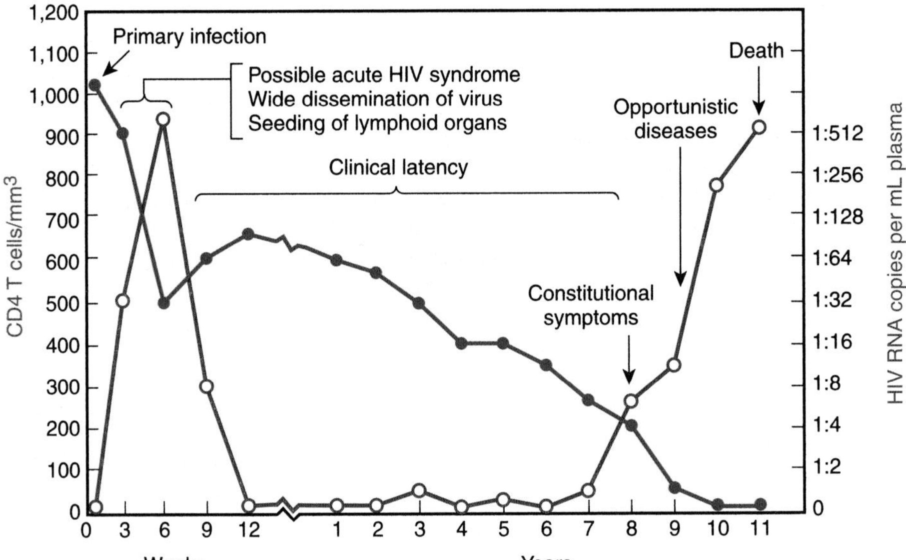

FIGURE 24–7 Typical CD4 T-cell numbers and plasma viremia during the natural course of HIV infection. *(Adapted from Pantaleo G, Graziosi C, Fauci AS. The immunopathogenesis of human immunodeficiency virus infection.* N Engl J Med. *1993;328:327–335.)*

immune suppression in HIV-infected patients for many years. Normally, the peripheral blood CD4 T-cell count ranges from 450 to 1,500 cells/μL (average, 1,000 cells/μL). In untreated patients, there is a progressive decline in the number of CD4 T cells during the course of infection **(Fig. 24–7)**. The rate of decline varies among patients and can be rapid or gradual. As we previously discussed, the CDC classification system uses CD4 T-cell counts to place patients into various stages of HIV infection, with those whose counts are below 200/μL being categorized as having stage 3 infection.

Another important clinical application of CD4 T-cell counts is to monitor the effectiveness of ART. Physicians use CD4 T-cell values to help determine whether a change in ART is necessary and if prophylactic drugs for certain opportunistic infections should be administered. According to guidelines published by the U.S. Department of Health and Human Services, a baseline CD4 T-cell measurement should be performed before the initiation of ART, then every 3 to 6 months for the first 2 years. Thereafter, annual measurements can be performed in patients whose CD4 T-cell counts have consistently remained between 300 and 500 cells/μL. More frequent testing should be performed if there is a change in the patient's clinical status. If there is a decline in the CD4 T-cell count of greater than 25%, the physician may change the ART. Patients with a CD4 T-cell count below 200/μL are placed on prophylactic therapy for *Pneumocystis jiroveci* pneumonia, whereas those with a count of lower than 50/μL are given prophylactic treatment for *Mycobacterium avium* complex.

The gold standard for enumerating CD4 T cells is immunophenotyping with data analysis by **flow cytometry** (see Chapter 13). The CDC has published guidelines to standardize the performance of CD4 T-cell determinations by flow cytometry. Early guidelines referred to a dual-platform technology in which both a flow cytometer and a hematology analyzer were required to make CD4 T-cell measurements. According to this protocol, the percentage of CD4 T cells in a sample was determined by dividing the number of lymphocytes positive for the CD4 marker by the total number of lymphocytes counted by the flow cytometer, according to the following equation:

$$\%\ \text{CD4 T Cells} = \frac{\#\text{CD4 Lymphocytes}}{\text{Total}\ \#\ \text{Lymphocytes}} \times 100$$

The percentage of CD4 T cells obtained for the patient sample was compared with a reference range established by the laboratory performing the test.

In the dual-platform approach, absolute numbers of CD4 T cells were calculated by multiplying the absolute number of lymphocytes (determined by the complete blood cell [CBC] count and differential from a hematology analyzer) by the percentage of CD4 T cells in the sample, according to the following equation:

$$\text{Absolute}\ \#\ \text{CD4 T Cells} = \text{WBC Count} \times \%\ \text{Lymphocytes} \times \text{CD4 T Cells}$$

The absolute CD4 T-cell count was then compared with the reference range, which is typically from 450 to 1,500 cells/μL peripheral blood.

Current technologies employ multicolor monoclonal antibody panels in a single-platform approach, which allows CD4 T-cell percentages and absolute numbers to be obtained from one tube using a single instrument, the flow cytometer. This is made possible by counting CD4+ T cells in a precisely measured blood volume or by incubating the sample with a known number of commercially available fluorescent microbeads, which function as an internal calibrator. The counts can then be determined by specific flow cytometry software, according to the following equation:

$$\frac{\#\ \text{of Events in the Bright CD45 Region}}{\#\ \text{of Events in the Microfluorosphere Region}} \times \frac{\text{Total}\ \#\ \text{Microspheres Added}}{\text{Volume of Blood Added}}$$

As with the dual-platform technology, lymphocytes are selected for analysis (or "gated") on the basis of their low-side scatter and ability to stain brightly with CD45 antibody.

Connections

Flow Cytometry

In flow cytometry, histograms display the patterns of light scatter and fluorescence emitted by individual cell populations. Multicolor IFAs are used in which the lymphocytes are differentiated from other cell types in the sample on the basis of their low-side scatter and their ability to stain brightly with fluorescent-labeled antibody to the CD45 marker, which is present on all WBCs. The side scatter represents the amount of cell complexity as determined by properties such as granularity and membrane irregularity. Because lymphocytes are more round and less granular than other types of WBCs, they reflect the laser light to a smaller degree and can be characterized by their low light scatter.

In addition to CD4+ T-cell percentages and absolute numbers, the ratio of CD4 T cells to CD8 T cells may be reported to assess the dynamics between the two T-cell populations. In HIV-infected patients, particularly those with AIDS, the large decrease in the number of CD4+ T cells, along with a possible increase in CD8+ cytotoxic T cells, results in an inverted ratio, or a ratio that is lower than 1:1.

Although flow cytometry is the accepted gold standard for enumeration of CD4 T cells, it is a costly method that requires the need for highly skilled personnel, a stable electricity supply, refrigeration of reagents, and regular instrument maintenance. These conditions are not available in many areas of the world. Therefore, there has been much interest in developing simpler, less expensive methods to determine CD4 T-cell measurements. This need has led to the manufacture of miniaturized flow cytometers that can be easily operated by smaller laboratories. These instruments are dedicated for CD3/CD4 measurements and use simple procedures that require a small volume of reagents.

Another major advance has been development of point-of-care devices that can be easily transported to remote regions. These devices can use blood obtained by fingerstick or venipuncture and contain stable, dried reagents that can withstand hot, humid temperatures. Disposable test cassettes are used to capture CD4+ cells with labeled antibodies, and the results are analyzed by small, portable instruments that can be powered by a rechargeable battery. Lateral flow devices that do not require instrumentation have also been developed for CD4+ T-cell enumeration. These methods are particularly suitable for resource-limited settings in developing countries where the incidence of HIV infection is high.

Quantitative Viral Load Assays

Quantitative **viral load tests** measure the amount of circulating HIV nucleic acid and play an essential role in helping physicians predict disease progression, monitor patient response to ART, and guide treatment decisions. The amount of HIV RNA in a patient's plasma is referred to as the "viral load" and reflects the natural history of HIV infection in that individual. HIV RNA levels become detectable about 11 days after infection and rise to very high levels shortly thereafter, during the initial burst of viral replication. Typically, over a period of a few months, the viral load drops as the individual's immune system clears viral particles from the circulation, and a stable level of plasma HIV RNA, known as the "set point," is achieved (see Fig. 24–7). In untreated individuals, this level can persist for a long time and then rise again later as the immune system deteriorates and the patient progresses to AIDS. In contrast, successful therapy with antiretroviral drugs will result in a drop in the viral load to an undetectable level within a few weeks to a few months after the initiation of ART.

Information obtained from viral load tests has prognostic value. Baseline plasma viral load values obtained in patients before the start of ART are an important predictor of disease progression because higher numbers of HIV RNA copies/mL of plasma are associated with more rapid development of an AIDS-defining illness or AIDS-related death.

Viral load tests are used routinely to monitor the effectiveness of ART in HIV-infected patients and play an essential role in the clinical management of these individuals. The U.S. Department of Health and Human Services recommends that plasma HIV RNA testing be performed before ART begins to obtain a baseline value; testing should be performed periodically thereafter to determine the effectiveness of the therapy. To obtain an accurate assessment of viral load dynamics in a single patient, it is recommended that the same assay be used for sequential viral load measurements because values may differ between different molecular tests. Patients who attain a lower number of HIV-RNA copies/mL of plasma are more likely to achieve a longer treatment response. The optimal goal of therapy is to reach an undetectable level of HIV RNA, below the lower limit of detection of a currently approved viral load assay. Patients who have a persistently elevated viral load should undergo resistance testing to determine if an alternative drug regimen is needed (see *Drug Resistance and Tropism Testing* in the text that follows).

Methods

Viral load assays are based on amplification methods that increase the number of HIV RNA copies (or their derivatives) in test samples to detectable levels. Several amplification methods have been developed for this purpose, the most common being PCR and the **branched-chain DNA** assay (**bDNA**). The basic principles of PCR and bDNA are discussed briefly in the section that follows and are covered in more detail in Chapter 12.

Another method that was developed for viral load determination is nucleic acid sequence-based amplification (NASBA). NASBA, which is based on the amplification of HIV RNA, is a technically complex method that is no longer suitable for clinical laboratory settings. In addition, simpler technologies have been developed to determine HIV viral load for use in areas of the world that lack skilled laboratory personnel as well as the resources to purchase costly instrumentation, refrigeration, and a continuous power supply. These include point-of-care devices such as closed cartridges that can provide semi-quantitative analysis with simpler instrumentation in a shorter period of time. Many of these technologies, including loop-mediated and helicase-dependent amplification, are based on isothermal reactions in which the temperature remains constant.

Polymerase Chain Reaction (PCR). Two kinds of PCR methods have been developed to detect HIV nucleic acid: the RT-PCR and, more recently, quantitative (real-time) PCR, also known as qPCR. A commercial RT-PCR was the first assay to be licensed by the FDA for the quantitative measurement of circulating HIV nucleic acid. The basic principle of this test is to amplify a DNA sequence that is complementary to a portion of the HIV RNA genome. In this assay, HIV RNA is isolated from patient plasma by lysis of the virions and precipitation with alcohol. The RNA is treated with a thermostable DNA polymerase enzyme that has both reverse-transcriptase activity and the ability to initiate DNA synthesis in the presence of the appropriate reagents. The reverse-transcriptase activity of the enzyme transcribes the HIV RNA into complementary DNA (cDNA). The cDNA is then amplified by standard PCR methodology (see Chapter 12).

Although the development of standard RT-PCR methods was a revolution in molecular testing for HIV infection, they have several disadvantages, including a limited dynamic range (i.e., the range of HIV RNA copies per mL that can be detected). In addition, they are highly susceptible to cross-contamination with extraneous nucleic acid. For these reasons, these assays have largely been replaced with qPCR assays that can detect and quantify the PCR products as they are being produced (see Chapter 12). This is accomplished by adding a fluorescent probe that binds to the amplicon during the reaction. The PCR amplification primers target highly conserved regions of the HIV-1 *gag* or *pol* genes. An internal control consisting of a different nucleic acid sequence is simultaneously amplified with each sample to compensate for the effects of inhibition and allow for more accurate quantitation. qPCR is highly sensitive and can detect a broad range of RNA copies, from 20 copies/mL to 10 million copies/mL.

Branched-Chain DNA Assay (bDNA). In contrast to RT-PCR, which involves amplification of the HIV target sequence, the bDNA method is based on amplifying the detection signal generated in the reaction. This is accomplished by using a solid-phase sandwich hybridization assay that incorporates multiple sets of oligonucleotide probes and hybridization steps to create a series of "branched" molecules. First, RNA isolated from lysed virions in patient plasma is captured on the wells of a microtiter plate coated with several probes. The captured RNA is then hybridized with branched amplifier probes and incubated with an enzyme-labeled probe that will bind to the DNA branches. Finally, a chemiluminescent substrate is added, and color change is measured with a luminometer. Quantitative results are generated from a standard curve.

The bDNA test can detect 75 to 500,000 copies of HIV RNA/mL of plasma. As compared with qPCR, the bDNA has higher reproducibility and higher throughput (rate of producing results). However, it requires a larger sample volume, lacks an internal control, and has a lower specificity. This method is most conducive for laboratories with high testing volumes.

Drug-Resistance and Tropism Testing

As we previously discussed, HIV is a rapidly replicating virus that has an intrinsically high rate of mutation. Because of these properties, it is possible for drug-resistant subpopulations of the virus to emerge during the course of ART. Drug resistance has been a major reason for the failure of ART in many people. Therefore, laboratory tests have been developed to assess drug-resistance patterns; these tests have had a major impact on guiding the selection of optimal ART for individual patients.

Two types of laboratory methods can be used to test for drug resistance: *genotype resistance assays* and *phenotype resistance assays*. Genotype resistance assays are performed more frequently than phenotype resistance assays because they are less expensive, more widely available, and have a shorter turnaround time.

Genotype resistance assays detect mutations in the reverse-transcriptase, protease, and integrase genes of HIV, as well as genes coding for envelope proteins that interact with entry and fusion inhibitors. These tests are available commercially and can be performed in clinical laboratory settings. In these tests, RNA is isolated from patient plasma, the desired genes are amplified by RT-PCR, and the products are analyzed for mutations associated with drug resistance by automated DNA sequencing. The nucleotide sequences of the genes of interest are identified and entered into a database, where they are compared with the corresponding sequences in wild-type HIV. The results are analyzed by commercially available software and reported qualitatively as "resistance," "possible resistance," or "no evidence of resistance" for each drug tested. Although genotyping tests have many advantages as compared with phenotypic methods, they can identify only known mutations and cannot assess the effects of combinations of individual mutations on drug resistance.

Phenotype resistance assays determine the ability of clinical isolates of HIV to grow in the presence of antiretroviral drugs. In these assays, recombinant viruses are created by inserting the reverse-transcriptase, protease, integrase, or *env* gene sequences from HIV RNA in the patient's plasma into a laboratory reference strain of HIV and transfecting the recombinant virus into mammalian cells. Varying concentrations of antiviral drugs are incubated with the transfected cells, and the IC_{50} or IC_{90} values, or drug concentrations needed to suppress the replication of the patient's viral isolate by 50% or 90%, respectively, are calculated. These values are then compared with the IC_{50} or IC_{90} values of cells transfected with a reference strain of HIV in order to determine drug resistance. The major advantage of phenotypic assays is that they measure drug susceptibility directly, on the basis of all mutations present in the patient's isolate. However, these assays are expensive and have a longer turnaround time than genotypic assays. In addition, phenotypic assays involve sophisticated technologies and are only performed by a few highly specialized reference laboratories.

Both genotypic and phenotypic assays require that a viral load of at least 500 to 1,000 copies of HIV RNA/mL be present in the test sample and for the resistant virus to constitute more than 25% of the total viral population in the patient to produce detectable results. Despite these limitations, studies have shown that patients undergoing drug-resistance testing, particularly by genotyping methods, have a better chance of receiving ART regimens that are more likely to result in greater reductions in viral load. Therefore, the U.S. Department of Health and Human Services recommends that drug-resistance testing be performed in individuals before initiating ART, in patients in whom ART has failed as evidenced by viral load values that have not been optimally reduced, and in all HIV-positive pregnant women. Genotypic testing is recommended for patients upon entry into medical care for HIV or after one to two unsuccessful treatment regimens because of its lower cost, faster turnaround time, and greater sensitivity for detecting wild-type/resistant virus mixtures. The addition of phenotypic testing is recommended when patients are thought to harbor HIV mutants with complex drug-resistance patterns.

Additional molecular tests are used to determine viral tropism and the suitability of a particular ART drug based on HLA type. Analysis of the co-receptor tropism is used to determine whether a patient is eligible for treatment with CCR5 antagonists such as maraviroc, which inhibits entry of HIV strains that use the CCR5 co-receptor to bind to host cells (the R5-tropic viruses). These drugs are only effective in patients who harbor these strains of HIV. Both genotypic and phenotypic tests are available for this purpose. Pharmacogenetic screening for the *HLA-B*5701* allele is helpful for patients who are being considered for treatment with the nucleoside reverse-transcriptase inhibitor abacavir because this allele has been associated with development of hypersensitivity to the drug. The test is typically performed by PCR amplification of the allele, followed by hybridization with sequence-specific oligonucleotide probes.

Testing of Infants Younger Than 18 Months

Serological tests are not reliable in detecting HIV infection in children younger than 18 months of age because of placental passage of immunoglobulin G (IgG) antibodies from an infected mother to her child. Maternal antibodies persist in the bloodstream of the infant during the first year of life (or longer in a small proportion of infants) and can confuse the interpretation of serological results from infant samples. Thus, a child born to an HIV-positive mother may test positive for HIV antibody during the first 18 months of life even though the child is not infected.

Because of the difficulties with serological testing, HIV infection in infants is best diagnosed using molecular methods. A qualitative HIV-1 RNA (discussed earlier) or an HIV-1 DNA PCR test may be used for this purpose. The latter test detects proviral DNA within the infants' peripheral blood mononuclear cells. Alternatively, quantitative HIV RNA assays may be used to diagnose HIV infection in infants. Although they are less sensitive than DNA assays, RNA tests can be used to provide a baseline viral load measurement and are more likely to detect infections with strains other than subtype B. They can also be used as a confirmatory test for infants who initially had a positive HIV DNA test.

It is recommended that nucleic acid tests for HIV be performed in infants with known perinatal exposure at the ages of 14 to 21 days, 1 to 2 months, and 4 to 6 months and possibly at birth for infants at high risk for HIV infection. A positive test result should be confirmed by repeat testing on a second specimen because false positives can occur. Two or more negative test results (the first at greater than 1 month and the second at greater than 4 months, or two separate tests conducted after 6 months) provide evidence for the absence of HIV infection and may be confirmed by serological tests at 12 to 18 months of age. The HIV status of breastfed infants, who are continually exposed to the virus, cannot be determined accurately until breastfeeding is stopped.

The CDC and the U.S. Department of Health and Human Services recommend that all pregnant women be tested for HIV infection so that those who are positive can be treated with ART and their infants can be evaluated for HIV infection after birth. Prompt detection of HIV infection in newborns is important because infected infants have a better prognosis when ART is started early and can benefit from treatment with prophylactic drugs for opportunistic infections.

SUMMARY

- Human immunodeficiency virus type 1 (HIV-1) is responsible for the majority of AIDS cases throughout the world. A related virus, HIV-2, may also cause AIDS but is generally less pathogenic.
- Transmission of HIV occurs by three major routes: (1) intimate sexual contact, (2) contact with contaminated blood or body fluids, or (3) vertical transmission from infected mother to her fetus or infant.
- HIV belongs to the retrovirus family, which contains RNA as the genetic material from which DNA is transcribed. HIV has three main structural genes: *gag*, which codes for the core proteins of the virus such as p24; *pol*, which codes for the enzymes reverse transcriptase, integrase, and protease; and *env*, which encodes the envelope proteins gp120 and gp41.
- The primary target cells for HIV are CD4 T lymphocytes and macrophages, which possess some surface CD4. The CD4 molecule acts as a receptor for attachment of the virus by binding to the gp120 envelope protein. Following attachment, entry of the virus into the host cells is mediated by the chemokine co-receptors, CXCR4 and CCR5.
- A burst of viral replication occurs after initial infection, followed by a period of latency during which viral DNA becomes integrated into the host genome as a provirus.
- Viral production slows down as the host's immune response develops and keeps the virus in check. The host

produces neutralizing antibodies, which prevent the virus from infecting neighboring cells, and develops HIV-specific CTLs that lyse virus-infected target cells. Innate defenses are also activated.

- Although the immune responses of the host reduce the level of HIV replication, they are usually not sufficient to completely eliminate the virus. HIV can escape these responses by undergoing rapid genetic mutations that generate altered antigens, downregulating production of class I MHC molecules on the surface of the infected target cells, and existing in a latent proviral state.
- The hallmark feature of HIV infection is a decline in the number of CD4 Th cells during the natural course of infection. This decline results in an immunodeficiency that affects both cell-mediated and humoral antibody responses to a variety of antigens.
- The clinical course of untreated HIV infection begins with an acute phase in which patients may experience flu-like symptoms. This is followed by a latent, asymptomatic period that lasts an average of 10 years. The infection culminates in AIDS, which is characterized by profound immunosuppression with life-threatening opportunistic infections and malignancies.
- The 2014 CDC case definition of HIV infection is based on laboratory criteria or clinical evidence and classifies patients into one of five stages based on CD4 T-cell measurements and the presence of opportunistic illnesses.
- Treatment with antiretroviral therapy (ART) is recommended for all HIV-infected persons and has resulted in a significant delay in disease progression, decreased mortality, and reduction in perinatal transmission.
- Several classes of antiretroviral drugs have been developed to block various steps of the HIV replication cycle: nucleoside analogue reverse-transcriptase inhibitors, nonnucleoside reverse-transcriptase inhibitors, protease inhibitors, integrase strand transfer inhibitors (INSTIs), fusion inhibitors, a CCR5 antagonist, and a CD4 post-attachment inhibitor. These drugs are most effective when administered in combination to reduce the development of drug resistance.
- The algorithm recommended by the CDC and the Association of Public Health Laboratories in 2014 to screen for HIV infection consists of a sequence of laboratory tests. The initial test is a fourth-generation immunoassay that simultaneously detects HIV-1 antibody, HIV-2 antibody, and p24 antigen. Positive test results must be confirmed by a rapid test that discriminates between HIV-1 antibody and HIV-2 antibody. Any samples that give discrepant results should undergo qualitative nucleic acid testing.
- Rapid screening tests for HIV antibodies are typically sensitive, lateral flow or flow-through assays that can provide results in fewer than 30 minutes. These tests are especially suitable for use in certain situations, including resource-limited settings, occupational exposures, labor and delivery, and clinics or emergency departments where patients are unlikely to make a return visit.
- The Western blot, which was used for many years to confirm positive HIV antibody screening test results, detects antibody specificities to individual HIV antigens. It is no longer recommended for routine diagnosis of HIV because it is labor intensive, relatively insensitive, and has a long result turnaround time, but it may be used for confirmation in special situations.
- HIV-infected patients are routinely monitored using two laboratory measurements: CD4 T-cell enumeration and HIV viral load.
- Peripheral blood CD4 T-cell counts and percentages are an excellent indicator of immune function and are routinely measured by multicolor immunofluorescence staining followed by analysis with flow cytometry. These measurements are used to stage HIV-infected patients and to monitor patients undergoing ART. Declining numbers can indicate if there is a need to change antiretroviral therapy or initiate prophylactic therapy for opportunistic infections.
- Qualitative nucleic acid tests can be used to screen for HIV infection or make an initial patient diagnosis. PCR and TMA are the approved methods for these purposes, respectively.
- Quantitative tests, which measure the amount of HIV nucleic acid circulating in patient plasma, are known as *viral load tests*. These tests have had an important impact on the clinical management of HIV-infected patients by allowing physicians to predict disease progression, monitor patient response to antiretroviral therapy, and guide treatment decisions.
- Viral load tests are performed by one of three molecular methods: reverse-transcriptase polymerase chain reaction (RT-PCR), a method that converts HIV RNA into cDNA and then amplifies the cDNA generated; qPCR, a quantitative real-time RT-PCR method; and the branched-chain DNA assay (bDNA), which amplifies a labeled signal bound to a test plate.
- Drug-resistance testing can be performed by genotypic assays that use molecular methods or by phenotypic assays in which HIV replication in clinical isolates is assessed in the presence of varying concentrations of antiretroviral drugs.
- Diagnosis of HIV in neonates is more complex than testing in adults. The presence of maternally acquired antibody in newborns makes tests for HIV antibody unreliable until a child is over 18 months old.
- Nucleic acid testing is recommended for the diagnosis of HIV infection in infants younger than 18 months. Testing can be performed with a qualitative PCR that detects HIV proviral DNA in the infant's peripheral blood mononuclear cells or a qualitative test for HIV RNA. Careful monitoring of HIV-infected mothers and early testing of infants at risk are recommended to facilitate prompt medical intervention.

CASE STUDIES

1. A young woman recently discovered that her boyfriend tested HIV-positive. She was concerned that she may have also contracted the infection because she had experienced flu-like symptoms 1 month ago. She decided to visit her physician for a medical evaluation.

Questions

a. What initial laboratory test should be performed on the young woman to determine if she has been exposed to HIV?
b. If the woman tests positive in the initial evaluation, what follow-up testing should be performed to confirm the results?
c. If the woman's test results are confirmed to be positive, what tests should be done to monitor her over time?

2. A pregnant woman had used intravenous drugs in the past and recently discovered that she was HIV-positive. She was concerned that her baby would also contract HIV infection and discussed this with her physician.

Questions

a. How is HIV infection transmitted from mother to infant, and what measures should be taken to reduce the risk of HIV infection to the infant?
b. Should testing for HIV antibody be performed to determine if the infant is HIV-positive after birth? Explain your answer.
c. What type of laboratory testing would be best to evaluate the infant for HIV infection after birth?

REVIEW QUESTIONS

1. All of the following describe HIV *except*
   a. it possesses an outer envelope.
   b. it contains an inner core with p24 antigen.
   c. it contains DNA as its nucleic acid.
   d. it is a member of the retrovirus family.

2. HIV virions bind to host T cells through which receptors?
   a. CD4 and CD8
   b. CD4 and the IL-2 receptor
   c. CD4 and CCR5
   d. CD8 and CCR2

3. Suppose a combination immunoassay to screen for HIV infection was positive, but the confirmatory test was negative. Which of the following tests should be performed?
   a. p24 antibody
   b. Western blot
   c. PCR for HIV-1 RNA
   d. No further testing is needed, and the screening test should be interpreted as a false positive.

4. Which of the following is typical of the latent stage of HIV infection?
   a. Proviral DNA is attached to cellular DNA.
   b. Large numbers of viral particles are synthesized.
   c. A large amount of viral RNA is synthesized.
   d. Viral particles with no envelope are produced.

5. The decrease in T-cell numbers in HIV-infected individuals is caused by
   a. lysis of host T cells by replicating virus.
   b. fusion of the T cells to form syncytia.
   c. killing of the T cells by HIV-specific cytotoxic T cells.
   d. all of the above.

6. The most common means of HIV transmission worldwide is through
   a. blood transfusions.
   b. intimate sexual contact.
   c. sharing of needles in intravenous drug use.
   d. transplacental passage of the virus.

7. The drug zidovudine is an example of a
   a. nucleoside analogue reverse-transcriptase inhibitor.
   b. nonnucleoside reverse-transcriptase inhibitor.
   c. protease inhibitor.
   d. fusion inhibitor.

8. False-negative test results in a laboratory test for HIV antibody may occur because of
   a. heat inactivation of the serum before testing.
   b. collection of the test sample before seroconversion.
   c. interference by autoantibodies.
   d. recent exposure to certain vaccines.

9. Which of the following combinations of bands would represent a positive Western blot for HIV antibody?
   a. p24 and p55
   b. p24 and p31
   c. gp41 and gp120
   d. p31 and p55

10. The fourth-generation combination immunoassays for HIV detect
    a. HIV-1 and HIV-2 antigens.
    b. HIV-1 and HIV-2 antibodies.
    c. p24 antigen.
    d. HIV-1 antibodies, HIV-2 antibodies, and p24 antigen.

11. The conjugate used in fourth-generation immunoassays for HIV consists of labeled
    a. anti-human immunoglobulin.
    b. HIV-1- and HIV-2-specific antibodies.
    c. HIV-1- and HIV-2-specific antigens.
    d. HIV-1- and HIV-2-specific antigens plus antibody to p24.

12. The characteristic laboratory finding in HIV infection is decreased
    a. numbers of CD4 T cells.
    b. numbers of CD8 T cells.
    c. numbers of CD20 B cells.
    d. immunoglobulins.

13. Which of the following tests is currently recommended by the CDC to confirm a positive screening test result for HIV infection?
    a. Rapid test for HIV-1 and HIV-2 antibodies
    b. Western blot
    c. Molecular testing for HIV RNA
    d. HIV viral culture

14. Which of the following tests would give the *least* reliable results in a 2-month-old infant?
    a. CD4 T-cell count
    b. ELISA for HIV antibody
    c. PCR for HIV proviral DNA
    d. p24 antigen

15. Which of the following measurements is/are routinely used to monitor patients with HIV infection who are undergoing antiretroviral therapy?
    a. HIV antibody titer
    b. p24 antigen levels
    c. CD4 T-cell and CD8 T-cell counts
    d. CD4 T-cell count and HIV RNA copy number

Immunization and Vaccines

25

Linda E. Miller, PhD, MB^CM(ASCP)SI

LEARNING OUTCOMES

After finishing this chapter, you should be able to:

1. Explain the underlying principles of active immunity, passive immunity, and adoptive immunity.
2. Provide examples of active immunity, passive immunity, and adoptive immunity.
3. Discuss the historical evolution of vaccines, from the early contributions of Edward Jenner through modern approaches to producing vaccines.
4. Define *vaccine, toxoid, attenuation, adjuvant,* and *recombinant protein vaccine.*
5. Describe the composition of live, attenuated vaccines; inactivated vaccines; and subunit vaccines. Contrast their advantages and limitations, and provide examples of each type of vaccine.
6. Explain how factors that influence the immune response to vaccines determine the ways in which vaccines are administered.
7. Recognize examples of adjuvants and explain the mechanisms by which they enhance the immune response to vaccines.
8. Contrast the benefits and adverse effects associated with vaccines.
9. Differentiate between standard human immune serum globulin (HISG) and specific HISG and their clinical applications.
10. Differentiate between monoclonal antibodies, chimeric antibodies, humanized antibodies, and fully human antibodies in terms of their structure and nomenclature.
11. Discuss some of the clinical applications of monoclonal antibody therapy and immunosuppressive therapy with gamma globulins.
12. Discuss clinical applications of adoptive immunotherapy.
13. Describe the structure of chimeric antigen receptors and the clinical utility of CAR-T cells.

CHAPTER OUTLINE

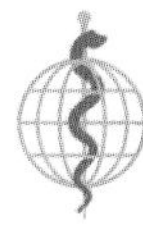

Go to FADavis.com for the laboratory exercises that accompany this text.

KEY TERMS

Active immunity
Adjuvant
Adoptive immunity
Adoptive immunotherapy
Antitoxin
Attenuation
CAR-T cells
Community immunity
Cross-reactivity
Herd immunity
Human immune serum globulin (HISG)
Immunization
Immunoprophylaxis
Immunotherapy
Passive immunity
Passive immunotherapy
Recombinant protein vaccine
Serotype
Toxoids
Tumor-infiltrating lymphocytes (TILs)
Vaccine
Virus-like particles (VLPs)

As we discussed in Chapter 1, *immunity* can be defined as the condition of being resistant to disease, most notably to infections. The process by which this state of protection is acquired is called **immunization.** There are three types of immunity that can be acquired through immunization: active, passive, and adoptive.

Active immunity results from immunization with a specific antigen by natural exposure to infection or administration of a vaccine. Adaptive, or antigen-specific, immune responses to bacteria, viruses, fungi, and parasites can all result in active immunity. For example, production of antibodies to a specific strain of Group A streptococci bacteria following a streptococcal sore throat protects the individual from future infection with that strain of bacteria. Active immunity is also stimulated through the administration of vaccines (see sections that follow). For example, after receiving all doses of the measles vaccine, most people develop immunity to the measles virus. In active immunity, the individual's own immune system is stimulated to mount an adaptive immune response to an antigen. The advantage of active immunization over other types of immunization is that it results in long-term memory to an antigen, providing potentially lifelong protection against the harmful effects of a pathogenic organism.

Passive immunity results from the transfer of antibodies from immunized hosts to a nonimmune individual. This state of immunity can occur naturally, from transfer of a mother's antibodies to her fetus or infant, or artificially, through passive immunization of an individual with commercial preparations of antibodies formed by other hosts to prevent or treat a disease. The latter application is also known as **passive immunotherapy.** The use of pooled human antibodies to protect a person who has an immunodeficiency disease is an example of passive immunotherapy. The main advantage of passive immunization is that it provides immediate protection to an individual who has not developed immunity to a particular antigen.

Adoptive immunity results from the transfer of cells of the immune system, usually lymphocytes, from an immunized host to a nonimmune individual. **Adoptive immunotherapy** involves the administration of these cells to treat patients with conditions such as immunodeficiency diseases or cancer. This type of therapy can be beneficial if the cells transferred are able to successfully establish themselves in the recipient. An example of adoptive immunotherapy is the transplantation of hematopoietic stem cells into leukemia patients who have undergone treatment with high doses of irradiation and chemotherapy to destroy the malignant cell population.

The primary difference between the immunity gained by active, passive, and adoptive immunization is that in active immunity, an individual's own immune system is responding to an antigen. In passive and adoptive immunity, immunity is provided to an individual through the transfer of antibodies or cells from another source to provide immediate protection.

This chapter discusses the mechanisms by which active, passive, and adoptive immunity occur in the context of their advantages and limitations. Clinical examples under each category are described so that the student can develop a better understanding of how knowledge of the basic principles of the immune system can be translated into therapies that can benefit humankind. A special focus is placed on the topic of vaccines because their use has significantly improved the health of populations throughout the world.

Vaccines

A **vaccine** is an antigen suspension derived from a pathogen. Vaccines are routinely administered to healthy individuals to stimulate an immune response to an infectious disease. Vaccination therefore is a form of **immunoprophylaxis,** or the prevention of disease through immunization. Vaccines have had a tremendous impact on public health by significantly reducing the incidence of illness and death from numerous diseases that had devastating effects on civilization. In addition, experimental "vaccines" for cancer have been developed as **immunotherapy** for patients who already have the disease (see Chapter 17). In this section, we will discuss the historical evolution of vaccines, the different forms of vaccines available, how they are routinely administered, factors that affect their efficacy, and vaccine design for the future.

Historical Evolution of Vaccines

As we discussed previously in Chapter 1, the science of immunology was born out of early observations of immunity and studies involving vaccination. The motivation behind these studies was the desire to eliminate the death and suffering caused by infectious diseases. Advances in science and technology during the 20th century and beyond have led to the creation of safer, more effective vaccines and remarkable success toward that goal.

Early Discoveries

One of the most feared diseases in ancient times was smallpox, a highly fatal illness characterized by a high fever and pustular rash. Those who survived the disease were usually left with disfiguring scars or blindness. However, it was noted in Greece as early as 430 BC that people who were fortunate enough to survive this infection became immune to the deadly disease. These observations led to the procedure of *variolation,* in which fresh material taken from a skin lesion of a person recovering from smallpox was subcutaneously injected with a lancet into the arm or leg of a nonimmune person. Recall from Chapter 1 that in an older form of the procedure practiced in ancient China, the material was dried into a powder and inhaled by the nonimmune person. The practice of variolation usually resulted in milder disease and recovery and was performed for centuries in Africa, India, and China. The practice was introduced to Europe in the 18th century. At that time, over 400,000 people in Europe died each year from smallpox, so the procedure became popular very quickly. However, variolation was not without risks; 1% to 2% of the recipients developed smallpox and died, whereas others contracted infectious diseases such as syphilis or tuberculosis (TB) from the injected material.

These observations led to the search for a safer procedure. Farmers observed that milkmaids who had a similar but milder disease called *cowpox* were protected from contracting the deadlier smallpox. The farmers, therefore, used cellular material from the cowpox lesions of milkmaids to variolate others and observed the same protective effects without the danger of contracting smallpox **(Fig. 25–1)**. The English physician Edward Jenner brought fame to this procedure when, in 1796, he injected fluid from the cowpox lesions of a milkmaid into an 8-year-old boy. When Jenner subsequently inoculated the boy with smallpox, he did not develop the disease, showing that the method was a success. Jenner called this procedure "vaccination" after the Latin word *vacca,* which means "cow." The protective effects induced by the vaccination were caused by the phenomenon of **cross-reactivity,** or antigenic similarity between the viruses that caused cowpox and smallpox. This early vaccine for smallpox led to the development of the modern smallpox vaccine, which is still derived from the *vaccinia* virus that causes cowpox **(Fig. 25–2)**. The vaccine was so successful that smallpox has been eradicated from the world, and the vaccine is no longer routinely administered.

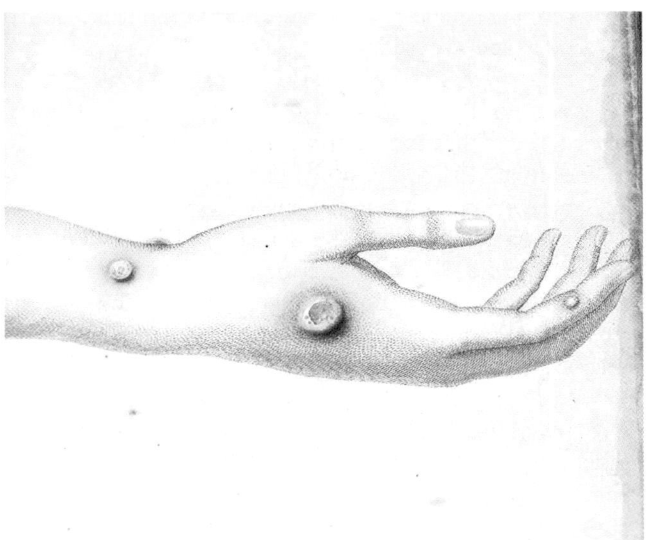

FIGURE 25–1 Color etching of a hand and wrist with cowpox lesions, from Edward Jenner's "Inquiry Into the Causes and Effects of the *Variolae Vaccinae.*" The etching shows several stages of cowpox, from early blistering to its later dimpled rupture. *(Courtesy of the National Library of Medicine, National Institutes of Health & Human Services. Bethesda, MD.)*

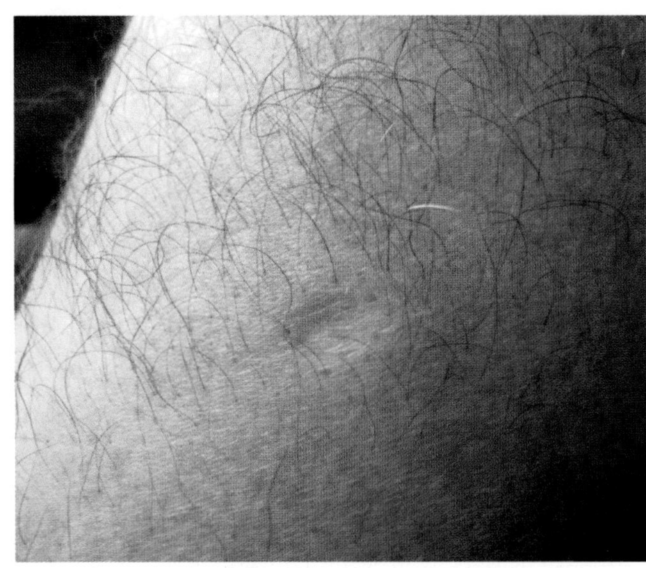

FIGURE 25–2 Evidence of smallpox vaccination. Individuals who have received the smallpox vaccine develop a blister, which dries up and forms a scab within the first 2 weeks. They can be easily identified by the scar that forms at the site of injection once the scab falls off. *(Courtesy of Linda Miller.)*

Despite the early development of the smallpox vaccine, many years passed before scientists understood that microbes were the underlying cause of infectious diseases and that components of these pathogens could be used to produce protective vaccines. Thus, it was not until 80 years later that the next vaccine was developed by Louis Pasteur against chicken cholera. Pasteur later went on to develop vaccines against anthrax and rabies. These vaccines were all based on the principle of attenuation. **Attenuation** involves the use of bacteria or viruses that have been weakened through exposure to modifying conditions such as chemical treatment, elevated or cold temperatures, or repeated *in vitro passage* in cell culture (a technique in which some of the cells are periodically transferred to a flask containing fresh nutrient medium). These weakened microorganisms do not cause disease in healthy individuals but are able to stimulate the immune response because they contain many of the same antigens as their pathogenic counterpart.

Connections

Pasteur's Discovery of Attenuation

It is thought that Pasteur discovered the effect of attenuation by accident during his studies of chicken cholera. After returning from a summer vacation in 1881, he noticed that he had left a culture of the bacteria that cause chicken cholera, now known as *Pasteurella multocida,* on his laboratory bench. Instead of disposing of the aged culture, he decided to use it to inoculate chickens. The chickens did not develop the disease; furthermore, when Pasteur later inoculated them with a fresh culture of the bacteria, they proved to be resistant to cholera. This series of events exemplified Pasteur's philosophy for science, that "success favors the prepared mind."

The rabies vaccine, for which Pasteur is most famous, was developed in 1885. Pasteur did not know the causative agent of rabies, but he recognized that it affected the central nervous system (CNS). He prepared an attenuated vaccine by repeatedly infecting rabbits with material contaminated with rabies, recovering the rabbits' spinal cords, and exposing them to dry air. In 1885, after testing the vaccine on dogs, he was convinced to administer his vaccine preparation to a 9-year-old boy who had been severely bitten by a rabid dog. The boy received a series of subcutaneous injections of the material over a period of 10 days and never developed rabies **(Fig. 25–3).** Pasteur received worldwide honors for this treatment and used the proceeds to build the famous Pasteur Institute in Paris, where vaccine studies and other biomedical research are conducted today. He was the first person to use the word *vaccination* in reference to all immunization procedures.

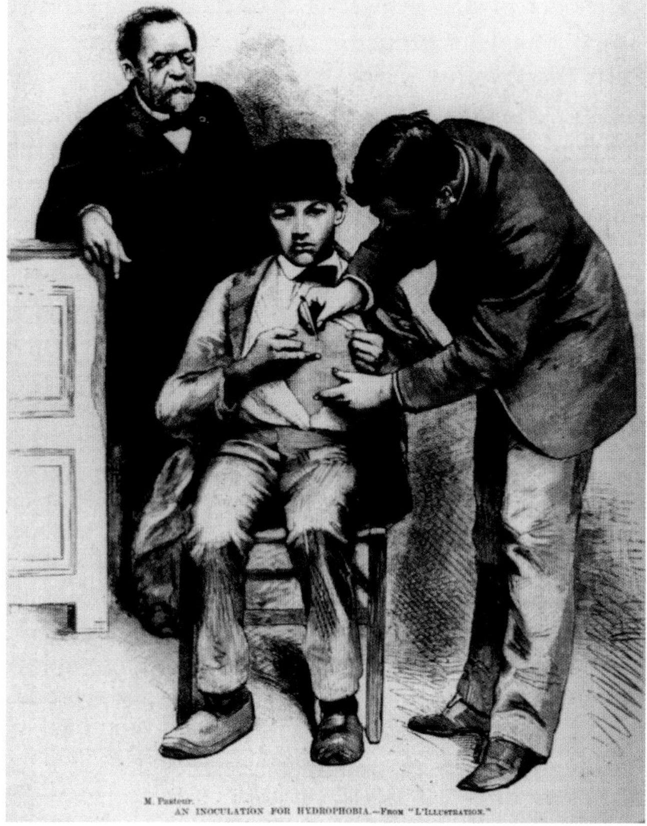

FIGURE 25–3 Louis Pasteur observes as a young boy receives an inoculation for hydrophobia (a symptom of rabies). *(Courtesy of the National Library of Medicine, National Institutes of Health & Human Services. Bethesda, MD.)*

Pasteur believed that only live, attenuated organisms could be used for effective immunization, and these remain the basis for many vaccines that are used today. However, in the late 1800s, Salomen and Smith showed that a killed suspension of *Vibrio cholerae* could provide pigeons with protection against cholera. A few years later, vaccines against human cholera, typhoid fever, and plague were developed using whole killed organisms.

20th-Century Vaccines

The 20th century witnessed a tremendous expansion in the development of vaccines because of advances in scientific research, techniques, and laboratory technology. New methods of attenuating microorganisms by repeated culture passage in special media resulted in the development of live, attenuated vaccines against TB and typhoid fever. Production of live, attenuated vaccines for yellow fever and influenza A was made possible in the 1930s, following Goodpasture's development of techniques that permitted viral growth in embryonic eggs.

Another major advance of the 20th century was the use of inactivated bacterial toxins in vaccine preparations. These preparations, referred to as **toxoids,** are made by chemically treating bacterially derived toxins known to cause pathogenesis so that they cannot cause harm to the host but retain their ability to stimulate an immune response. Using a formalin treatment, inactivated toxoid vaccines were developed against diphtheria by Glenny in 1923 and against tetanus by Ramon and Zoeller in 1926. Inactivated toxoids still serve as the basis for the diphtheria and tetanus vaccines in use today.

The second half of the 20th century has been referred to as the "golden age of vaccine development." During this period, researchers developed revolutionary techniques that enabled successful growth of viruses in cell culture. These important advances led to the development of numerous attenuated viral vaccines from 1950 to 1980, including those targeted against polio, measles, mumps, rubella, and varicella.

An important development in the last part of the 20th century was the use of purified polysaccharides to treat bacterial infections. These vaccine preparations were developed in the 1970s and 1980s to prevent meningococcal meningitis, pneumococcal pneumonia, and *Haemophilus influenzae* type b (Hib). In the late 1980s, these vaccines were made more effective by increasing the immunogenicity of the polysaccharides. This was accomplished by forming *glycoconjugates* consisting of polysaccharides linked to a protein that can be recognized by T cells.

The last part of the 20th century also saw the first applications of genetic technologies to vaccine development. The first **recombinant** (i.e., genetically engineered) **protein vaccine** was produced in 1986 against hepatitis B. This vaccine consists of purified hepatitis B surface antigen (HBsAg) made by genetically modified yeast cells that have incorporated the gene for HBsAg. It replaced an older form of the vaccine that

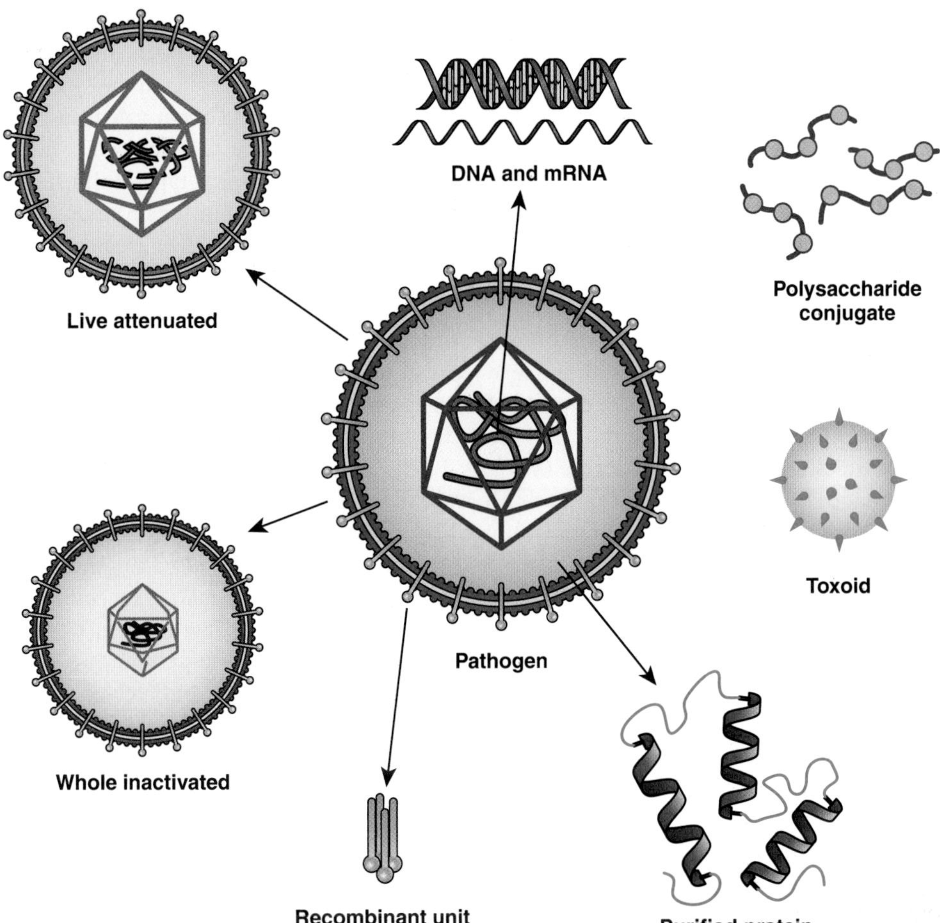

FIGURE 25–4 Major types of vaccines: attenuated, inactivated, toxoid, recombinant, DNA, mRNA, purified protein, and polysaccharide conjugate.

used a less purified preparation of HBsAg derived from the plasma of patients who were infected with hepatitis B. Genetic engineering was also used to develop recombinant vaccines to prevent other diseases, including pertussis and Lyme disease.

Beyond the 20th Century

The beginning of the 21st century has seen continued use and refinements in the vaccine technologies developed in the 1900s. The first decade of the 21st century witnessed the licensure of live, attenuated vaccines for influenza, rotavirus, and herpes zoster, as well as multivalent, glycoconjugate vaccines for pneumococcus and meningococcus. Vaccines composed of genetically recombinant antigens from the human papilloma virus (HPV; the cause of cervical and other genital cancers, as well as anal cancer) and the herpes zoster virus (the cause of shingles) were also introduced.

More than 25 infectious diseases are preventable by vaccines licensed in the United States. However, many diseases still present a challenge to the medical profession because they cannot be prevented through immunization. Future vaccines will likely be based on attempts to target these diseases through the application of advanced genetic technologies and the stimulation of innate defenses as well as humoral antibody production and cellular components of the adaptive immune system. Some of the challenges and strategies that are likely to be used in the future development of vaccines will be discussed later in this chapter.

Types of Vaccines

As we previously mentioned, vaccines are antigen preparations that are administered to prevent infectious diseases. Vaccines in routine use today consist of live, attenuated (nonpathogenic) microorganisms; inactivated (killed) microorganisms; or antigenic components of microorganisms, known as subunit vaccines. The main features of each of these vaccine forms are depicted in **Figure 25–4** and will be discussed in more detail in the sections that follow. Newer strategies for vaccine development, which incorporate modern genetic technologies and approaches to enhance immune responses, will also be introduced.

Live, Attenuated Vaccines

Live, attenuated vaccines have been in routine use since Jenner's discovery of the smallpox vaccine. As we previously discussed, this vaccine was based on the concept of cross-reactivity, in which material from the cowpox virus was used to develop immunity against the antigenically similar, but highly pathogenic, smallpox virus. However, most pathogens do not have an immunologically similar, but less pathogenic, counterpart.

Several laboratory techniques are currently used to modify bacteria or viruses so that they lose their pathogenic properties but are still capable of stimulating a good immune response. The techniques used to prepare conventional vaccines involve culture of the microorganism under conditions that are different from those present in the host and unfavorable to its growth. Pasteur used these principles to develop vaccines for chicken cholera and rabies. Another example of an attenuated preparation is the vaccine for tuberculosis developed by Albert Calmette and Camille Guerin at the Pasteur Institute in 1927. The vaccine, referred to as BCG *(Bacillus Calmette Guerin),* uses an attenuated strain of *Mycobacterium bovis* developed by growing the bacteria on culture media containing increasing concentrations of bile. After several years, the bacteria adapted to growing in media containing a high bile content and can be used in humans because the body's lower bile concentration is not conducive to pathogenic growth. A live, attenuated bacterial vaccine against typhoid fever, which consists of a mutated strain of *Salmonella typhi* packaged into capsules that are ingested orally, has also been developed. To produce this vaccine, the bacteria are chemically treated to induce genetic mutations that weaken them so that they are no longer pathogenic.

Attenuated vaccines are more easily prepared against viral infections than bacterial infections. A major viral disease for which an attenuated vaccine was developed is polio. Polio is a serious disease that causes aseptic meningitis and leaves its victims with disabling paralysis. In the early 1960s, Albert Sabin developed an oral polio vaccine from live, attenuated strains of poliovirus cultured in monkey kidney cells. The vaccine contained the three serotypes of poliovirus that are capable of causing the disease. Each **serotype** is a form of the virus that can be distinguished by the presence of specific antigens that can be identified by serological typing. Sabin's vaccine was the main poliovirus vaccine used in the United States from 1963 to 1997, before a potent inactivated polio vaccine was licensed. Although the oral polio vaccine is no longer available in the United States because of its potential for adverse effects (see *Benefits and Adverse Effects of Vaccines* in the text that follows), an oral vaccine is still used in some lower-income countries of the world because it is easier to administer than the attenuated vaccine, which requires injections.

The vaccines for measles, mumps, rubella, and varicella also consist of live strains of viruses that have been attenuated through repeated passage in cultured cells. The measles and mumps viral strains are produced in chick embryo cells, whereas the rubella strain is produced in human diploid cells. The vaccines to prevent chickenpox consist of live, attenuated Oka strains of varicella virus, which were originally isolated from a Japanese child with chickenpox and sequentially propagated in cultures of human or embryonic guinea pig cells. These strains are used to produce an individual varicella vaccine or a combination vaccine that also contains the vaccines for measles, mumps, and rubella (MMR or MMRV). A more potent formulation of the attenuated Oka varicella strain was used to prevent herpes zoster (shingles) in adults until a more recently developed recombinant vaccine was produced.

A live, attenuated vaccine has also been developed to prevent influenza. The vaccine is administered intranasally. The main antigens targeted by the vaccine are two surface glycoproteins of the influenza virus called *hemagglutinin* (H) and *neuraminidase* (N); these antigens are also used to classify the viruses on the basis of their serotype. Similar to the inactivated influenza vaccine discussed later, a new attenuated influenza vaccine must be prepared each year because of the high mutation rate of the influenza viruses, which results in the synthesis of new antigens. The vaccine consists of a quadrivalent suspension containing the most common circulating antigenic strains of influenza virus from four common virus types: influenza A (H3N2), influenza A (H1N1), and two influenza B strains. The viral strains have been cultivated in chicken eggs and attenuated for adaptation to colder temperatures so that they grow optimally at 25°C rather than body temperature (37°C).

The primary advantage of live, attenuated vaccines is that they are able to replicate at a low level in the host and are therefore capable of inducing both humoral and cell-mediated immune responses. This is especially important for viral infections because cytotoxic T cells are required to attack viruses during the intracellular phase of the viral life cycle. Because of the broad immunity induced by live, attenuated vaccines, they generally induce an effective immune response after just a single dose.

Despite these advantages, live, attenuated vaccines also have some significant limitations. It is important *not* to administer vaccines containing live organisms to immunocompromised individuals. Although the organisms are attenuated, they may cause severe, disseminated, and potentially fatal infections in patients with immunodeficiency diseases or patients receiving immunosuppressive treatments. Live vaccines may also not be recommended for use in pregnant women. On rare occasions, mutations may occur in the vaccine organism, causing it to lose its attenuation and revert to the pathogenic form. This unfortunately occurred during use of the live, attenuated (Sabin) vaccine for polio, which led to the vaccine's replacement with an inactivated polio vaccine in industrialized countries. The use of genomic techniques to design live, attenuated strains that lack the genes required for pathogenicity will hopefully prevent such an occurrence in the future.

Another limitation of live, attenuated vaccines is potential interference with replication of the organism in infants by maternal antibodies, necessitating a delay in the dosing schedule (see *Factors Influencing Immunogenicity* in the text that follows). Finally, careful handling and storage of attenuated vaccines is very important because exposure to heat and light may destroy the live organisms, causing the vaccines to be ineffective. This requirement can pose a major problem in developing countries of the world, where refrigeration is not readily available.

Inactivated Vaccines

Inactivated vaccines consist of intact, killed viruses or bacteria. The microorganisms are killed by heat or chemical treatment so that they are not pathogenic but retain their antigenic properties. Chemicals such as formaldehyde or β-propiolactone are used more frequently than heat treatment because they are less likely to alter the chemical structure of the surface epitopes. Examples of inactivated vaccines are the intramuscular vaccine for polio, the classic influenza vaccine, and the hepatitis A vaccine.

In the early 1950s, Dr. Jonas Salk developed the first effective inactivated vaccine for polio. The vaccine consisted of the three disease-related serotypes of polio virus killed by formaldehyde treatment. A more potent inactivated polio vaccine with greater antigenic content was developed in 1978. This form of the vaccine is used routinely today in developed countries of the world because of its effectiveness and safety.

Similar to the live, attenuated influenza vaccine, the inactivated influenza vaccines contain one influenza A (H3N2) virus strain, one influenza A (H1N1) virus strain, and one or two influenza B virus strains grown in embryonated hen eggs. However, these viruses have been killed by treatment with formaldehyde or β-propiolactone, and the vaccine is administered by intramuscular injection. More recently, influenza vaccines that use virus grown in cultured mammalian cells or recombinant hemagglutinin antigens have become available. These vaccines avoid or minimize the use of eggs, allowing for faster production and eliminating or reducing the likelihood of hypersensitivity to egg proteins.

The hepatitis A vaccine consists of purified hepatitis A virus (HAV) cultured in human fibroblasts and inactivated by formalin treatment. Although this vaccine was initially only given to individuals at high risk for contracting hepatitis A, it has been incorporated into routine childhood immunization programs to reduce the incidence of this common infection.

A major advantage of inactivated vaccines is that they can be safely given to immunocompromised people because the organisms have been killed and cannot replicate in the host. However, this property makes it necessary to provide a larger amount of antigen in order to stimulate an effective immune response. In addition, two or more booster doses administered over time may be required to produce protective immunity. Because the inactivated organisms do not infect host cells, these vaccines predominantly induce a humoral immune response, with little or no cell-mediated immunity.

Subunit Vaccines

Subunit vaccines consist of one or more purified components of a pathogen that are capable of stimulating an immune response. The forms of subunit vaccines that are routinely used are toxoids, capsular polysaccharides, purified proteins, and recombinant protein antigens.

Toxoid Vaccines. The pathology of some bacterial diseases, such as diphtheria and tetanus, is caused by a single exotoxin. Diphtheria is a contagious, life-threatening disease of the upper respiratory tract characterized by formation of a thick membrane that can cover the back of the pharynx, making it difficult to breathe. Tetanus is a serious bacterial infection that affects the nervous system, causing painful, prolonged muscle contractions and, sometimes, difficulty breathing.

As we previously mentioned, toxoids are bacterial exotoxins that have been chemically inactivated so that they cannot cause harm to the host but retain their ability to stimulate an immune response. Toxoids are used in vaccines to induce the production of antibodies that can bind to exotoxins and neutralize their effects. The first toxoid vaccine was developed in 1923 against diphtheria and consisted of a formalin-inactivated toxin from the causative organism, *Corynebacterium diphtheriae.* In 1926, scientists developed a toxoid vaccine against tetanus, which consisted of a formalin-inactivated toxin from the causative organism, *Clostridium tetani.* Toxoids are still used in the composition of today's vaccines for diphtheria and tetanus. Another commonly used toxoid, which consists of inactivated toxin from the bacterium *Bordetella pertussis,* is part of the acellular pertussis vaccine (see *Purified Protein Vaccines* in the text that follows). The vaccines for diphtheria, tetanus, and pertussis are available singly or in combinations known as *DTaP*, *TdaP*, *DT*, or *Td*, depending on the amounts of diphtheria, tetanus, and acellular pertussis components present.

Polysaccharide Vaccines. Another virulence factor possessed by some bacteria is the presence of a hydrophilic polysaccharide capsule, which covers the bacterial outer membrane. The capsule allows these bacteria to resist phagocytosis and other immune defenses by masking components of the membrane that might otherwise be targets of the immune response. However, if antibodies to the capsular polysaccharides are present, they can facilitate clearance of the bacteria by inducing opsonization or complement-mediated lysis. Therefore, vaccines against encapsulated bacteria contain purified capsular polysaccharides from specific bacterial strains that stimulate the production of antibodies. Because the structure of these capsular antigens varies with different bacterial serotypes, these vaccines contain multiple polysaccharide types to ensure an immune response that provides broad protection.

The first polysaccharide vaccine was developed against *Streptococcus pneumoniae,* the cause of pneumococcal pneumonia. The vaccines in use today contain polysaccharides from 13 or 23 different *S. pneumoniae* serotypes. Another polysaccharide vaccine has been developed against *H. influenzae* type b (Hib), which was a major cause of pneumonia and meningitis in infants and young children before the vaccine was implemented. The vaccine is composed of the polyribosylribitol phosphate component of the Hib capsule conjugated to a protein carrier. A polysaccharide vaccine has also been developed against *Neisseria meningitidis,* an important cause of bacterial meningitis, especially in young individuals living in close quarters such as dormitory buildings. The vaccine consists of four purified bacterial capsular polysaccharides (A, C, Y, W-135) from *N. meningitidis.*

A problem with polysaccharide antigens is that they do not induce a good immune response, especially in infants and the elderly, two populations that are at high risk for severe consequences of encapsulated bacterial infections. This is because polysaccharides are T-independent antigens that stimulate IgM production with no immunoglobulin class-switching or long-term memory response (see Chapter 4). This problem has been circumvented through vaccines composed of *glycoconjugates,* in which the polysaccharide antigens are linked to a carrier protein such as tetanus toxoid or diphtheria toxoid. These conjugates are able to induce a more effective immune response by activating T helper (Th) cells, resulting in immunoglobulin class-switching, with production of polysaccharide-specific IgG antibodies and generation of memory cells.

Purified Protein Vaccines. Vaccines can also be composed of proteins from a pathogen. One such vaccine protects against pertussis, a serious respiratory disease also known as "whooping cough" because of the characteristic whooping sound patients make while trying to breathe during violent coughing fits. The first vaccine against pertussis was composed of whole

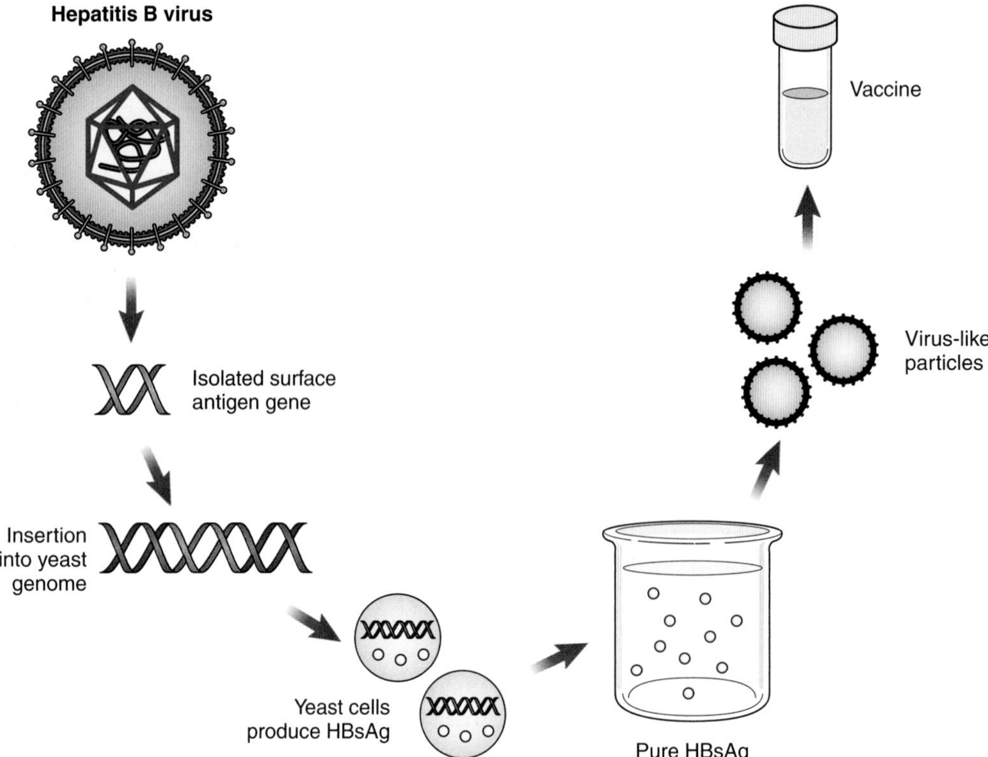

FIGURE 25–5 Production of the recombinant vaccine for hepatitis B.

killed *B. pertussis* bacteria and was thought to be associated with rare, but serious, neurological effects such as encephalitis or encephalopathy and convulsions, especially in children with neurological disorders. Today's pertussis vaccines are less frequently associated with side effects because they are composed of purified proteins from *B. pertussis* rather than whole bacterial cells. One of these proteins is a toxoid derived from the pertussis toxin (see *Toxoid Vaccines* in the previous text).

Recombinant Protein Vaccines and Virus-Like Particles. Recombinant DNA technology has made it possible to develop even more highly purified protein vaccines. In these methods, the gene coding for a specific protein antigen from a pathogenic microorganism is isolated and incorporated into the genome of nonpathogenic bacteria, yeast, or other cells. The genetically modified cells are cultured in large quantities and produce the desired antigen, which can then be purified by conventional biochemical methods. The first *recombinant protein vaccine* was developed in 1986 for hepatitis B and is widely used today. It is safer than the previous hepatitis B vaccine, which consisted of HBsAg isolated from pooled plasma of infected patients. The recombinant hepatitis B vaccine is produced by cloning the gene for HBsAg in yeast cells, then harvesting and purifying the HBsAg protein **(Fig. 25–5)**. The protein spontaneously assembles into **virus-like particles (VLPs)**. VLPs are formed when proteins from the viral capsid or envelope assemble to produce structures that are similar to the virus from which they were derived. VLPs do not replicate and are not infectious because they lack viral nucleic acid, but they induce an effective immune response because they display viral antigens in their native conformation.

Recombinant DNA technology is also the basis for vaccines developed against the HPV, which can cause cervical cancer, oropharyngeal cancer, anal cancer, and other genital cancers. These vaccines contain recombinant L1 major capsid proteins from nine HPV virus types (including types 16 and 18) that are highly associated with anal–genital cancers. The genes for the L1 proteins are cloned in yeast or insect cell lines infected with baculovirus, a type of virus that infects invertebrate cells. The isolated proteins then combine into VLPs that induce an effective immune response. HPV vaccination is recommended for adolescent girls and boys to confer protection before they become sexually active.

The production of recombinant DNA vaccines has become more common as technology has advanced, allowing for the manufacture of vaccines in a safer, more cost-effective manner that does not require the culture of highly pathogenic organisms and produces fewer side effects in recipients. Examples of more recently developed recombinant vaccines include those for shingles, influenza, and meningococcal meningitis serogroup B.

Factors Influencing Immunogenicity

There are many factors that affect the quality of the immune response to a vaccine antigen. Important factors include the age of the recipient, the individual's immune status, and the nature of the vaccine. All of these factors are considered by immunization experts when deciding how a vaccine should be administered to achieve an optimal immune response.

Age

Age is an important factor in determining how a vaccine should be provided to individuals in a population. Recommendations for the age at which a vaccine should be routinely administered are based on age-specific risks for contracting the disease and developing associated complications, as well as age-related ability to respond to the vaccine. Persons who are elderly or in early infancy typically exhibit reduced immune responses to traditional vaccines. Patients who are immunocompromised or have chronic diseases may also be less capable of mounting an effective immune response.

In general, it is recommended that vaccines be administered to the youngest individuals at risk for the vaccine's targeted disease, as long as the effectiveness and safety of the vaccine have been demonstrated in that age group. In the United States, vaccination schedules recommended by the Centers for Disease Control and Prevention's (CDC's) Advisory Committee on Immunization Practices (ACIP) are categorized according to age. Routine immunization against hepatitis B should begin soon after birth, for example, because the hepatitis B virus may have been transferred through the placenta, whereas vaccines for diphtheria, pertussis, tetanus, rotavirus, *H. influenza* type b, polio, and streptococcal pneumonia should begin at 2 months of age. Multiple inoculations of these vaccines, administered at specific time intervals through the first 18 months of life, are necessary to achieve optimal immunity because the young infant's immune system is immature. Additional doses of some of these vaccines are recommended during childhood, adolescence, or adulthood to maintain high antibody titers.

Some vaccines, such as the live, attenuated vaccine for measles, mumps, and rubella, are not started until 12 to 15 months of age because administration before that age does not result in an effective immune response. The response is less than optimal because passively acquired maternal antibodies present in the younger infant's serum limit replication of the attenuated viruses. Other vaccines, such as those for meningococcal meningitis (serogroups A, C, Y, W) and HPV, are routinely not administered until 11 to 12 years of age because the risk for contracting these infections is greater during adolescence. Still other vaccines, such as those for varicella zoster (the cause of shingles) and pneumococcal pneumonia, are not administered until later in adulthood because the natural decline of immune function in older individuals makes them more susceptible to developing these infections. A few vaccines, such as those for typhoid fever or yellow fever, are recommended only for individuals traveling to areas of the world where there is a high incidence of these diseases.

Vaccination schedules are revised annually by the ACIP in consultation with the American Academy of Pediatrics (AAP) and the American Academy of Family Physicians (AAFP). The 2020 immunization schedules for children, adolescents, and adults are shown in **Figures 25–6** and **25–7**. Up-to-date schedules can be accessed from the CDC at www.cdc.gov/vaccines.

These recommendations must be read with the notes that follow. For those who fall behind or start late, provide catch-up vaccination at the earliest opportunity as indicated by the green bars. To determine minimum intervals between doses, see the catch-up schedule (Table 2). School entry and adolescent vaccine age groups are shaded in gray.

Vaccine	Birth	1 mo	2 mos	4 mos	6 mos	9 mos	12 mos	15 mos	18 mos	19–23 mos	2–3 yrs	4–6 yrs	7–10 yrs	11–12 yrs	13–15 yrs	16 yrs	17–18 yrs
Hepatitis B (HepB)	1st dose	2nd dose					←3rd dose→										
Rotavirus (RV): RV1 (2-dose series), RV5 (3-dose series)			1st dose	2nd dose	See Notes												
Diphtheria, tetanus, acellular pertussis (DTaP <7 yrs)			1st dose	2nd dose	3rd dose			←4th dose→				5th dose					
Haemophilus influenzae type b (Hib)			1st dose	2nd dose	See Notes		←3rd or 4th dose, See Notes→										
Pneumococcal conjugate (PCV13)			1st dose	2nd dose	3rd dose		←4th dose→										
Inactivated poliovirus (IPV <18 yrs)			1st dose	2nd dose			←3rd dose→					4th dose					
Influenza (IIV)									Annual vaccination 1 or 2 doses						Annual vaccination 1 dose only		
or																	
Influenza (LAIV)												Annual vaccination 1 or 2 doses			Annual vaccination 1 dose only		
Measles, mumps, rubella (MMR)					See Notes		←1st dose→					2nd dose					
Varicella (VAR)							←1st dose→					2nd dose					
Hepatitis A (HepA)					See Notes			2-dose series, See Notes									
Tetanus, diphtheria, acellular pertussis (Tdap ≥7 yrs)														Tdap			
Human papillomavirus (HPV)													*	See Notes			
Meningococcal (MenACWY-D ≥9 mos, MenACWY-CRM ≥2 mos)								See Notes						1st dose		2nd dose	
Meningococcal B															See Notes		
Pneumococcal polysaccharide (PPSV23)														See Notes			

Range of recommended ages for all children

Range of recommended ages for catch-up immunization

Range of recommended ages for certain high-risk groups

Recommended based on shared clinical decision-making or *can be used in this age group

No recommendation/not applicable

FIGURE 25–6 Recommended immunization schedule for persons aged 0 through 18 years, 2020. *(Courtesy of Centers for Disease Control and Prevention.)*

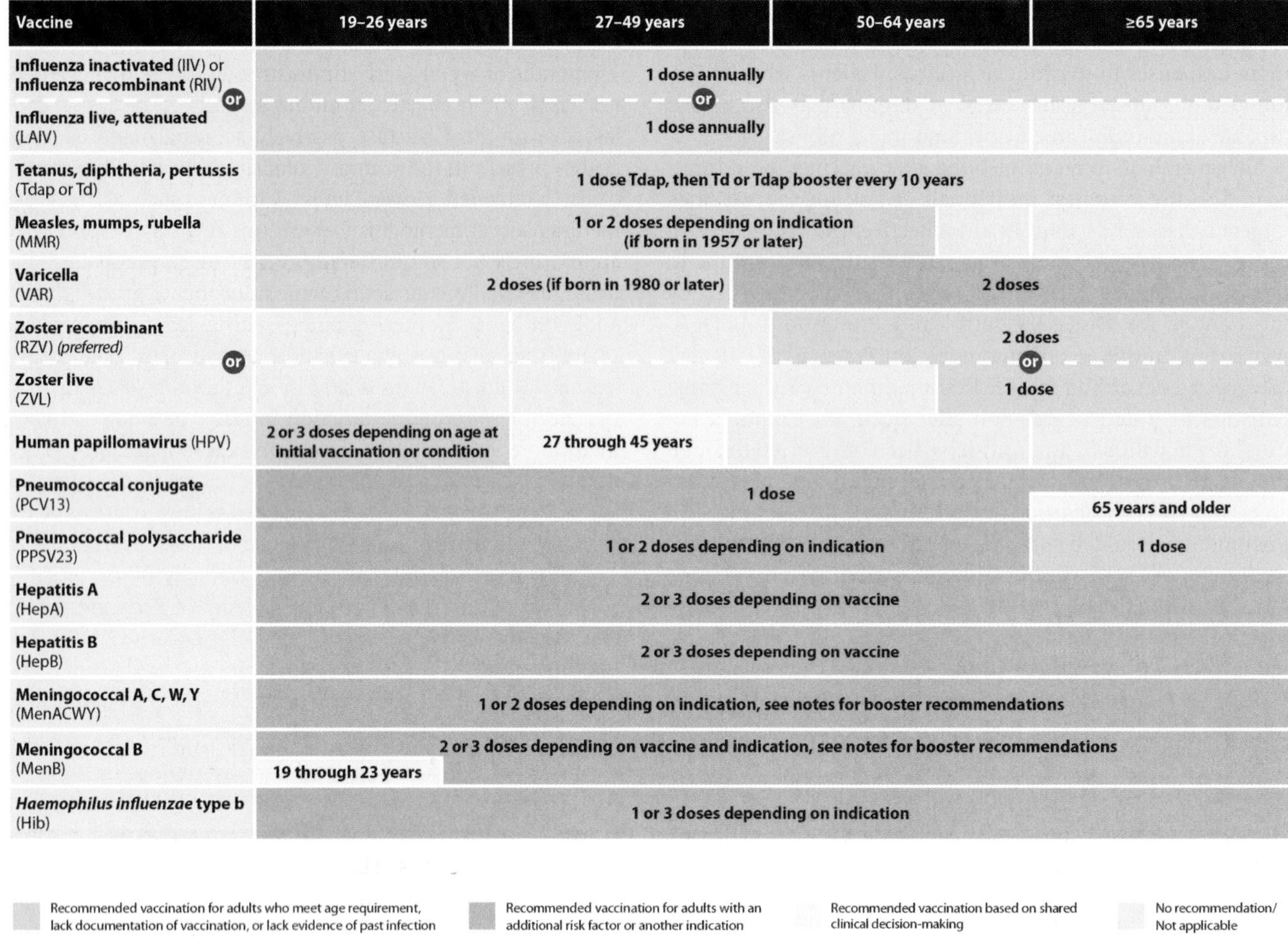

Vaccine	19–26 years	27–49 years	50–64 years	≥65 years
Influenza inactivated (IIV) or **Influenza recombinant** (RIV)	1 dose annually			
or	or			
Influenza live, attenuated (LAIV)	1 dose annually			
Tetanus, diphtheria, pertussis (Tdap or Td)	1 dose Tdap, then Td or Tdap booster every 10 years			
Measles, mumps, rubella (MMR)	1 or 2 doses depending on indication (if born in 1957 or later)			
Varicella (VAR)	2 doses (if born in 1980 or later)		2 doses	
Zoster recombinant (RZV) *(preferred)*			2 doses	
or			or	
Zoster live (ZVL)				1 dose
Human papillomavirus (HPV)	2 or 3 doses depending on age at initial vaccination or condition	27 through 45 years		
Pneumococcal conjugate (PCV13)	1 dose			65 years and older
Pneumococcal polysaccharide (PPSV23)	1 or 2 doses depending on indication			1 dose
Hepatitis A (HepA)	2 or 3 doses depending on vaccine			
Hepatitis B (HepB)	2 or 3 doses depending on vaccine			
Meningococcal A, C, W, Y (MenACWY)	1 or 2 doses depending on indication, see notes for booster recommendations			
Meningococcal B (MenB)	19 through 23 years; 2 or 3 doses depending on vaccine and indication, see notes for booster recommendations			
***Haemophilus influenzae* type b** (Hib)	1 or 3 doses depending on indication			

Recommended vaccination for adults who meet age requirement, lack documentation of vaccination, or lack evidence of past infection

Recommended vaccination for adults with an additional risk factor or another indication

Recommended vaccination based on shared clinical decision-making

No recommendation/ Not applicable

FIGURE 25–7 Recommended adult immunization schedule—United States, 2020. *(Courtesy of the Centers for Disease Control and Prevention.)*

Nature of Vaccine

The nature of the vaccine is another important factor influencing the quality of the immune response. In general, the most immunogenic vaccines consist of live, attenuated organisms that are able to replicate in the host, and the least immunogenic vaccines consist of purified components (subunits) derived from the pathogen. Vaccine antigens with a low level of immunogenicity require an adjuvant (see discussion that follows).

Connections

Principles of Immunologic Memory

Memory B and T lymphocytes are generated because of active immunity. These memory cells can be activated quickly if the individual is exposed to the same antigen at a later time, reducing the lag period before antibody production. Antibody titers rise quickly and reach higher levels than those produced after the first exposure to the antigen. Antibody concentrations remain high for a long period and provide long-lasting immunity. The protection provided by the memory response serves as the basis for repeated vaccine injections during routine immunization schedules. It also provides the host with lifelong immunity after recovery from a natural infection with a pathogen.

Adjuvants

An **adjuvant** is a substance that is administered together with a vaccine antigen to produce an enhanced immune response. The term *adjuvant,* coined by Ramon in 1926, is derived from the Latin word *adjuvare,* which means "to help."

A diverse group of molecules can function as vaccine adjuvants, including emulsions, mineral salts, microbial products, small molecules, microparticles, and liposomes. These molecules are thought to activate pathways of the innate immune system, inducing the release of cytokines that promote inflammation and stimulate cells of the adaptive immune system. Adjuvants can be broadly classified as *antigen delivery systems,* which enhance the uptake of antigens by antigen-presenting cells (APCs) or *immunopotentiators,* which activate dendritic cells to present antigens to T cells in humoral or cell-mediated immune responses. In some vaccine formulations, the two types of adjuvants have been combined together.

The ultimate purpose for using adjuvants in vaccines is to increase antibody titers and, for some vaccines, to induce cell-mediated immunity as well. Effective adjuvants can potentially reduce the dose of antigen needed in a vaccine, decrease the number of inoculations required, and increase the speed and duration of the immune response. They are capable of enhancing immunity in both young and elderly persons.

Three types of adjuvants that function as antigen delivery systems are aluminum salts, oil-in-water emulsions, and microparticles. Aluminum salts, such as aluminum hydroxide, aluminum phosphate, potassium aluminum sulfate ("alum"), or a mixture thereof, have been the most widely used type of adjuvant. They preferentially stimulate Th2 responses, which induce antibody production. The adjuvant activity of alum was discovered by Glenny in 1926 in his experimentation with diphtheria toxoid. Aluminum salts absorbed to antigens are used in several vaccine formulations today, including those against HAV, hepatitis B virus (HBV), HPV, diphtheria, tetanus, meningococcus, pneumococcal conjugates, and *H. influenza* type B.

Another type of adjuvant is an oil-in-water emulsion, composed of liquid dispersions of oil droplets stabilized with surfactants. Oil-in-water emulsions are mixed with vaccine antigens and are believed to stimulate the immune response by inducing release of chemokines and enhancing antigen uptake and migration of APCs. The first such adjuvant was discovered by Freund in the 1930s and is known as *Freund's complete adjuvant* (FCA). FCA is a powerful adjuvant containing killed mycobacteria. It has been used in animal studies but is not suitable for use in humans because it produces abscesses and scar formation at the site of inoculation. Freund's incomplete adjuvant (FIA), an oil-in-water emulsion without mycobacteria, has been used in some human vaccines but has strong side effects.

More recently developed oil-in-water emulsions include MF59 and the Adjuvant Systems AS01B and AS03. These adjuvants stimulate potent humoral and cell-mediated immune responses. MF59 contains the organic compound squalene and is used in a form of the seasonal influenza vaccine designed to stimulate immunity in adults aged 65 and older. AS01B is an adjuvant that is used in the recombinant vaccine for shingles; it is composed of monophosphoryl lipid A (MPL) and QS-21, a natural compound derived from the Chilean soapbark tree. AS03, a lipid emulsion containing D,L-α-tocopherol (vitamin E), squalene, and polysorbate 80, is approved for use in a vaccine to prevent avian (H5N1) influenza.

One type of microparticle that has been used in vaccines is called a *virosome*. Virosomes are spherical structures that consist of a phospholipid membrane that contains viral proteins but lacks viral nucleic acids. They can be used as a vaccine delivery system because they are capable of fusing with APCs to facilitate antigen presentation. Virosomes derived from influenza viruses have been incorporated in vaccines for influenza and hepatitis A.

Immunopotentiators function by targeting molecules that activate the cell-signaling pathways of the innate defense system. Novel adjuvants that bind to pattern-recognition receptors, such as the Toll-like receptors (TLRs), Rig-like receptors (RLRs), NOD-like receptors (NLRs), and C-type lectin receptors (see Chapter 2), have the ability to stimulate innate immunity and the release of cytokines that affect the adaptive immune responses. For example, a cytosine-phosphate-guanine (CpG) oligodeoxynucleotide that binds to TLR9 has been approved for use as an adjuvant in a hepatitis B vaccine for adults. MPL, which binds to TLR4, was used as an adjuvant component in a former vaccine for HPV and is being investigated in clinical trials for other vaccines.

Other immunopotentiators under investigation include poly-IC, a synthetic analog of double-stranded ribonucleic acid (RNA) that activates TLR3, and bacterial flagellin, which activates TLR5. Saponin-based adjuvants are also under study. These are plant-derived glycosides that are combined with antigen in nanoparticles called *immunostimulatory complexes* (ISCOMs). They are thought to stimulate strong antibody and cell-mediated responses by increasing antigen uptake and the activation of dendritic cells. Various cytokines, chemokines, and inactivated bacterial toxins are also being studied for their ability to act as immunopotentiators. Different combinations of adjuvants are also under investigation.

Challenges and Future Directions in Vaccine Development

Although conventional forms of vaccines have been highly effective in preventing numerous infections, there are still no vaccines for many diseases that cause major illnesses and death in the world. Several of these diseases are caused by viruses, bacteria, and parasites that have complex mechanisms of pathogenesis. They may display variability through genetic mutations or multistage life cycles or have developed other methods to escape attack by the immune system. For example, the ability of the immune system to eliminate HIV is hampered by the virus's capacity to infect and kill CD4+ T cells, integrate into the host genome, and rapidly mutate (see Chapter 24). *Plasmodium falciparum,* the cause of malaria, has posed a challenge for vaccine development through its ability to alter its surface antigens in the different stages of its complex life cycle. The vaccine for TB, BCG, is not optimally effective because mycobacteria can establish a carrier state and become reactivated during periods of immune suppression. Other infections that have posed a global challenge for effective vaccine development include hepatitis C, respiratory syncytial virus, Epstein-Barr virus (EBV), cytomegalovirus (CMV), herpes simplex, rhinovirus, and leishmaniasis.

New vaccine designs, adjuvants, and methods of vaccine administration are being studied in attempts to conquer these diseases. The potential for these to be successful will be aided by technical advances in multiple disciplines, including molecular genetics, structural biology, bioinformatics, nanotechnology, formulation, and techniques to monitor recipient immune response. Researchers will use these tools to identify antigens that can be formulated with potent adjuvants in producing vaccines that will stimulate a long-lasting, broad humoral response as well as effective T-cell responses. These advanced technologies will help accelerate the development of new, effective vaccines against major global diseases in the next generation.

Clinical Correlations

mRNA Vaccines

Vaccine technologies that incorporate messenger RNA (mRNA) molecules that code for vaccine antigens have been developed more recently. mRNA-based vaccines have sparked much interest among scientists because they show promise in generating immunity in a safe and effective manner and can be manufactured rapidly and inexpensively. At the time of this writing, several vaccine candidates for severe acute respiratory syndrome coronavirus-2 (SARS-CoV-2), the cause of the pandemic disease COVID-19, are in clinical trials.

Benefits and Adverse Effects of Vaccines

Vaccines are recognized as one of the 20th century's greatest medical achievements. Because of routine immunization, smallpox has been eradicated worldwide, and poliomyelitis has been eliminated from the Western world. Infectious diseases that were once leading causes of illness and death in the beginning of the 20th century, such as diphtheria and measles, have a greatly reduced incidence today, especially in developed nations. A study conducted by the CDC in 2007 found that the overall incidence of diseases for which vaccines had been developed before 1980 decreased by over 92%, and mortality from these diseases decreased by more than 99%. For example, the annual number of measles cases in the United States dropped from over 500,000 before implementation of the measles vaccine in 1963 to 120 cases in 2017. The estimated numbers of cases of selected vaccine-preventable diseases in the United States before and after implementation of their corresponding vaccines are shown in **Table 25–1**. The success of vaccination continues in the 21st century as immunization programs have expanded to countries throughout the world, preventing about 2.5 million deaths each year in children aged 5 and under.

An important feature of immunization is that it not only benefits the individuals receiving the vaccine but also reduces the risk of nearby persons, who have not been vaccinated, of contracting the infectious disease. When a sufficient proportion of individuals in a population have been immunized, unvaccinated individuals, such as newborns and immunocompromised patients, are offered some protection because there is little chance for the disease to spread in the community. This concept of extending protection to others in the population is known as **community immunity** or **herd immunity** and is of great importance to public health **(Fig. 25–8).**

Persons who have altered immunocompetence are at risk from certain immunizations and require special consideration.

Table 25–1 Estimated Number of Cases of Selected Vaccine-Preventable Diseases in the United States Annually***

DISEASE	ANNUAL NUMBER OF CASES IN PRE-VACCINE ERA	REPORTED ANNUAL CASES POST-VACCINE
Diphtheria	>21,000	0*
Haemophilus influenza	20,000	33*
Hepatitis A	>117,000	4,000**
Hepatitis B (acute)	>66,000	20,900**
Measles	>530,200	120*
Mumps	>162,300	6,109*
Pertussis	>200,700	18,975*
Pneumococcus	>63,000	30,400**
Polio	>16,300	0*
Rotavirus	>62,500	30,625**
Rubella	>47,700	7*
Smallpox	>29,000	0*
Tetanus	580	33*
Varicella	>4,000,000	102,128**

**Data from 2017.*

***Data from 2016.*

Table adapted from CDC Pinkbook *(https://www.cdc.gov/vaccines/pubs/pinkbook/downloads/appendices/e/impact.pdf; Accessed 12/29/2019) and Roush SW, Murphy TV. Historical comparisons of morbidity and mortality for vaccine-preventable diseases in the United States.* JAMA. *2007; 298:2155–2163.*

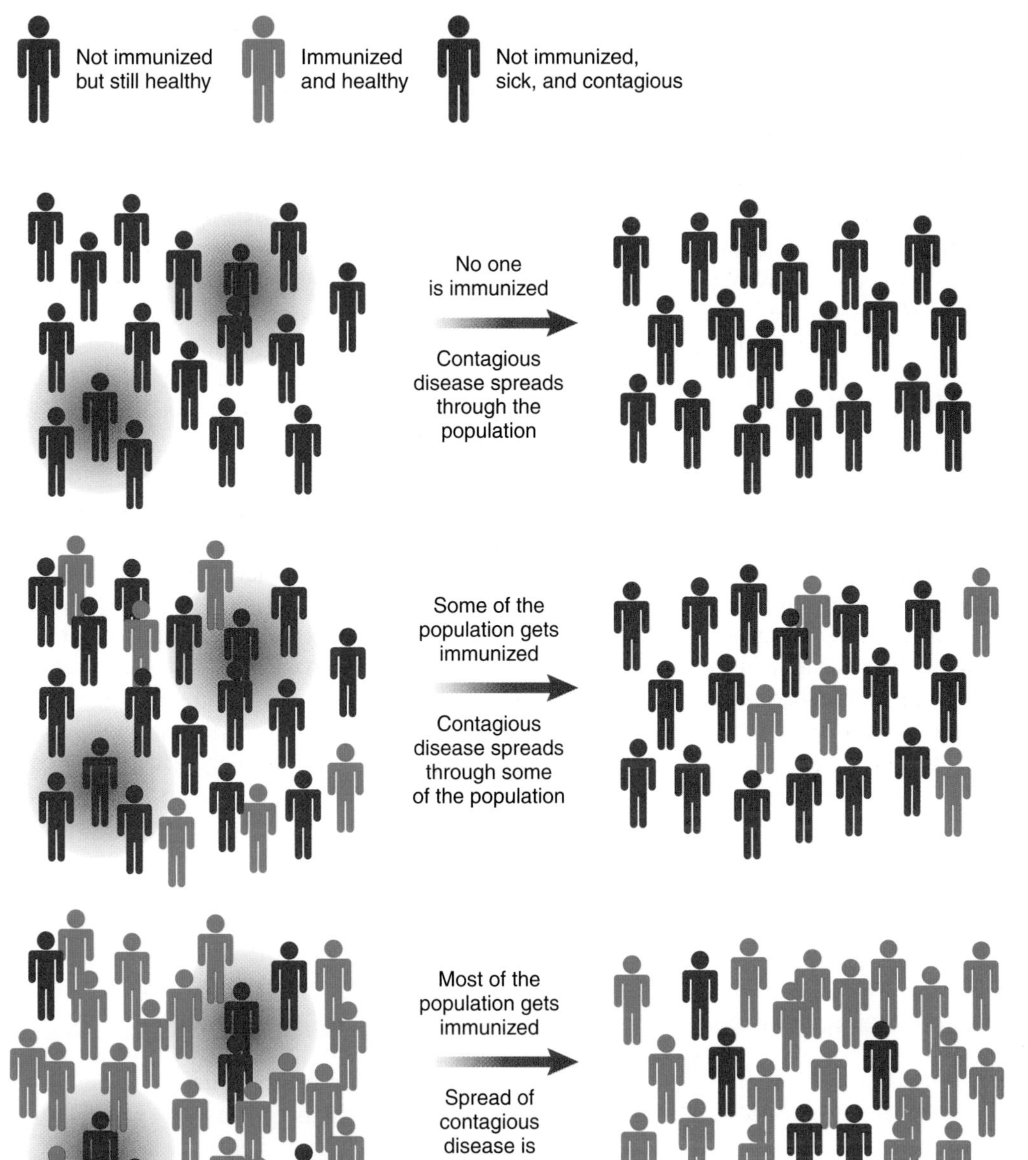
Not immunized
but still healthy
Immunized
and healthy
Not immunized,
sick, and contagious
No one
is immunized
Contagious
disease spreads
through the
population
Some of the
population gets
immunized
Contagious
disease spreads
through some
of the population
Most of the
population gets
immunized
Spread of
contagious
disease is
contained

FIGURE 25–8 Community immunity ("herd immunity"). *(Adapted from the National Institute of Allergy and Infectious Diseases. http://www.niaid.nih.gov/topics/pages/communityimmunity.aspx. Accessed November 30, 2015.)*

These individuals have decreased levels of humoral or cell-mediated immunity because of inherited primary immunodeficiency diseases or acquired deficiencies secondary to other conditions, such as HIV infection, hematologic malignancies, or treatment with immunosuppressive drugs or radiation (see Chapter 19).

The administration of live vaccines is contraindicated in immunodeficient individuals because they are highly susceptible to contracting infections; therefore, they should be immunized with inactivated or subunit vaccines. Although the organisms contained in live vaccines are attenuated and usually will not cause pathology in healthy individuals, they have the potential for uncontrolled replication and may cause disseminated disease in immunodeficient persons. For example, the vaccine for smallpox was known to cause a highly fatal condition in infants with severe combined immunodeficiency disease (SCID), involving progressive spread of necrotic lesions from the site of vaccine injection to adjacent areas of the skin, bone, and internal organs. Administration of the BCG vaccine for TB to infants with SCID or HIV infection has also resulted in disseminated, life-threatening infections. The CDC publishes specific recommendations for vaccination of persons with altered immunocompetence.

Vaccines can also produce adverse effects in previously healthy individuals, but fortunately, most of these are not severe. A local inflammatory response at the site of injection is frequently reported because of stimulation of TLRs by the vaccine antigen or adjuvant. Systemic inflammatory reactions are also common. These manifest with fever, irritability, nausea, vomiting, and myalgia 24 to 48 hours after injection of killed vaccines, or 14 to 21 days after receipt of a live vaccine, and generally resolve within 72 hours. Other adverse effects of vaccines include hypersensitivity reactions and effects related to the vaccine antigen or its administration.

Hypersensitivity reactions to vaccines may be local or systemic and can be immediate or delayed (see Connections box). immunoglobulin E (IgE)-mediated, type I (anaphylactic) hypersensitivity is usually triggered by vaccine additives such as gelatin (a stabilizer) or neomycin (an antibiotic used to prevent bacterial contamination). Anaphylactic reactions are rare, occurring in 0.65 cases per 1 million vaccine doses, on average. Development of an Arthus skin reaction because of local immune complex formation (type III hypersensitivity) has been reported in individuals who have received a booster shot of the tetanus vaccine and who possess residual antibodies from previous tetanus immunization (see Chapter 14). Contact dermatitis, a delayed (type IV) hypersensitivity reaction that appears 48 hours after vaccination, is considered harmless. It has been reported in some individuals in response to vaccine additives, including adjuvants such as alum, preservatives such as thimerosal and 2-phenoxyethanol, the toxin-inactivating agent formaldehyde, and antibiotics such as neomycin. Hypersensitivity develops infrequently in response to vaccines and human serum preparations and is more common when serum from animal sources is used for passive immunization.

Connections

Hypersensitivity Reactions

Reactions to vaccine components can be in the form of type I, III, or IV hypersensitivity. Recall the mechanisms of these reactions from Chapter 14. In sum:

Type I reactions: Individuals produce high levels of IgE antibody, which binds to mast cells and basophils. Binding of allergen to adjacent cell-bound IgE antibodies triggers the granules in these cells to release chemical mediators, which rapidly induce inflammatory reactions and smooth muscle contractions.

Type III reactions: Persons develop immunoglobulin G (IgG) and immunoglobulin M (IgM) antibodies that bind to vaccine or serum components. Complement binds to these complexes, activating the classical pathway and release of inflammatory mediators. Neutrophils are attracted to the areas of immune complex deposition, where they release lysosomal enzymes that destroy surrounding tissues.

Type IV reactions: Some individuals may develop a delayed response to a vaccine component. This is a cell-mediated reaction in which Th1 cells are stimulated to release cytokines that attract macrophages and cause inflammation.

Fortunately, other adverse effects associated with vaccines are rare. Interested readers can learn about effects associated with specific vaccines from vaccine information sheets and written inserts that accompany vaccine preparations and from the CDC website on vaccines and immunizations. The most dramatic example of such an effect was the development of paralytic poliomyelitis after use of the live, attenuated oral (Sabin) vaccine for polio. Occurring at a rate of approximately 1 case per 2.7 million doses of the vaccine, this event was caused by reversion of the Sabin polio virus type 3 to a neurovirulent strain. To avoid this tragic consequence, industrialized countries have stopped using the Sabin vaccine and replaced it with the injectable, killed Salk-type polio vaccine in their routine immunization schedules. Another example of a potentially serious vaccine consequence was the possible association of a vaccine for Lyme disease with the development of chronic arthritis that was resistant to treatment. This condition developed in individuals with the human leukocyte antigen (HLA) type DR-4, possibly because of a cross-reactive autoimmune response. Although the association of the vaccine with arthritis could not be definitively demonstrated, wide media coverage generated fear from the public, and the vaccine was withdrawn from the market in 2002, just 3 years after its licensure.

In 1998, public concern arose from a study conducted in England by Dr. Andrew Wakefield, who proposed a linkage between the MMR vaccine and development of a form of autism. Wakefield and his colleagues hypothesized that the vaccine caused intestinal inflammation and damage to the intestinal barrier, allowing pathogenic proteins to enter into the bloodstream and cause damage to the brain. It was not until 2010 that research studies using valid scientific designs proved Wakefield's findings to be unsubstantiated; his early papers were then retracted. Unfortunately, wide media coverage of Wakefield's claims had stirred up fears in the public, and many parents refused to get their children vaccinated.

Fears such as these, as well as religious or personal objections against immunization, have caused some individuals to delay or refuse vaccination for themselves or their children. Anti-vaccine public sentiments can result in lower-than-optimal vaccine coverage, leaving a significant number of individuals in the population unprotected against serious diseases. This situation, coupled with importation of diseases by unvaccinated individuals immigrating into a country, can lead to outbreaks of diseases that would normally be preventable. For example, in 2019, more than 1,270 cases of measles were reported in 31 states in the United States, mostly in people who had not been vaccinated against the disease or who had unknown vaccination status. Pertussis presents another challenge because immunity wanes 5 to 10 years after vaccination, requiring multiple boosters at various ages to maintain adequate protection. Failure to maintain immunity with up-to-date immunization has resulted in frequent outbreaks, with over 48,000 cases of pertussis reported in the United States in the year 2012. High vaccine coverage is essential to preventing such outbreaks and maintaining a healthy population.

Passive Immunization

As we previously discussed, passive immunity results from the transfer of preformed antibodies to an unimmunized host. Antibodies can be transferred naturally to a mother's fetus or infant in two ways: (1) A pregnant woman's IgG antibodies pass through the placenta to her unborn fetus, or (2) maternal immunoglobulin A (IgA) antibodies in breast milk and colostrum are ingested by the infant during the nursing process (see Chapter 5 and **Fig. 25–9**). These antibodies provide protection

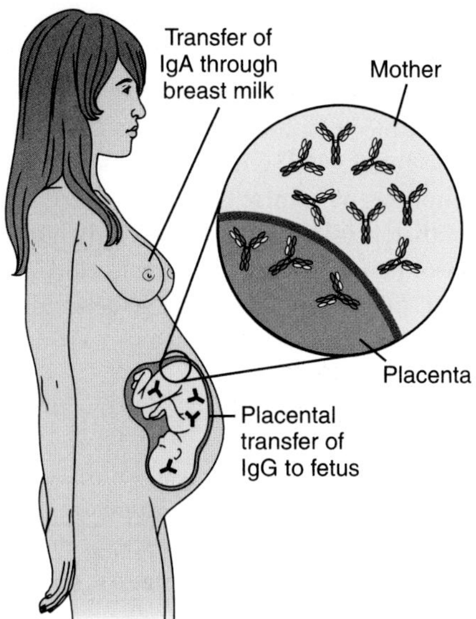

FIGURE 25–9 Passive immunity is transferred from a mother to her fetus or infant through the placenta (IgG) or breast milk (IgA).

to the newborn against pathogens to which the mother has developed immunity, either through natural infection or through vaccination. IgG antibodies protect the infant during its first few months of life, a time when the baby's own immune system is immature and has not yet encountered many antigens. IgA antibodies provide mucosal immunity, an important mechanism in attacking pathogens at their portals of entry into the body. Antibodies can also be passively transferred to a host as a means of immunoprophylaxis or immunotherapy.

Passive Immunization as Therapy for Infectious Diseases

The benefits of passive immunization were first discovered in the late 1800s by von Behring and Kitasto. The two scientists developed an antibody preparation against diphtheria and tetanus by injecting rabbits with small doses of the toxins responsible for these diseases. They went on to demonstrate that injection of serum from these rabbits into mice could protect the mice from infection with virulent forms of the bacteria that caused the two diseases. These historical experiments showed that protective substances (now known to be antibodies) could be generated in the blood and passively transfer their immune properties when injected into nonimmune individuals.

Today, human serum preparations are used to provide passive immunity to individuals who have been exposed to a pathogen but have not been vaccinated or developed immunity through natural infection. Two types of preparations are available: standard **human immune serum globulin** (also known as **HISG** or *gamma globulin*) and specific HISG. Standard HISG is a sterile preparation of concentrated antibodies made from pooled serum of several thousands of donors. In the United States, only donors who test negative for hepatitis B and HIV are used. The plasma from these individuals is enriched for immunoglobulins by a cold ethanol precipitation procedure, known as *Cohn's alcohol fractionation*. This is followed by depletion of blood coagulation factors, removal of IgG aggregates, and several virus inactivation steps to further ensure safety of the preparation. HISG consists predominantly of IgG; IgM and IgA are found in insignificant quantities because of their lower serum concentrations and rapid half-lives (see Chapter 5). HISG has been administered for more than 60 years as a prophylactic treatment to prevent infections in immunodeficient patients who are unable to produce sufficient amounts of antibodies (see Chapter 19). HISG contains antibodies specific for numerous antigens to provide generalized humoral protection against a variety of pathogens.

Antigen-specific immune globulins, also known as *hyperimmune globulins,* are prepared from pooled serum of human donors who have developed immunity against a particular pathogen through a recent natural infection or vaccination. These preparations contain a high concentration of antibody against the pathogen or its product and are used to treat individuals who have been potentially exposed to the pathogen but have not been immunized. The potency of the preparation is ensured by determining the antibody titer through laboratory testing. Specific HISGs have been developed for a variety of infectious diseases, including hepatitis A, hepatitis B (hepatitis B immune globulin; HBIG), varicella zoster, rabies, tetanus, and respiratory syncytial virus. Scientists have developed monoclonal antibody preparations that can be used as passive immunotherapy to provide protection to individuals infected with SARS-CoV-2, the virus that causes COVID-19. This work is based on observations that administration of convalescent plasma from patients recovering from infection with SARS-CoV-2 to hospitalized patients with COVID-19 improves clinical outcome and reduces mortality.

Specific immune globulins for some antigens have also been prepared from animal sera, usually horse serum. Examples of these include antitoxins for tetanus, diphtheria, and botulism, as well as antisera against snake venoms. **Antitoxins** are antibodies that specifically bind to epitopes on bacterial toxins. They protect against the harmful effects of these toxins by neutralizing their activity.

Advantages and Limitations of Passive Immunization

As we previously mentioned in this chapter, the main advantage of passive immunization is that it provides immediate immunity to the host. This is because the antibodies are already present in the serum that is being transferred and the host does not have to experience the lag period required for its own immune system to be activated by the antigen (see Chapter 5). This immediate protection can be especially beneficial in situations in which unimmunized individuals have been exposed to a harmful antigen; they would develop disease symptoms and possibly die if they had to wait for an immune response to occur. For example, disease could be avoided in an unvaccinated person who had contact with soil that was potentially contaminated with tetanus-causing bacteria or who had an accidental needlestick involving blood from a hepatitis B patient. Hepatitis A could be prevented in customers who dined at a restaurant in which a food handler was found to have the infection, and death could be prevented in people who have been bitten by a poisonous snake or an animal with rabies. When a mother naturally transfers antibodies to her infant through the placenta or breast milk, her child is provided with immediate protection to a variety of pathogens until the child's own immune system can mature.

However, passive immunity is not long-lasting. The length of the immunity is limited by the biological half-life of the immunoglobulins. Therefore, patients with immunodeficiency diseases require repeated, periodic injections or intravenous administration of HISG to be adequately protected. In addition, no memory lymphocytes are generated, so an individual will not be protected if exposure to the same antigen occurs at a later time in life. Another disadvantage of passive immunization is that hypersensitivity reactions, although rare with HISG, can occur frequently after therapy with animal serum. These reactions involve type I hypersensitivity (anaphylaxis) or type III hypersensitivity (serum sickness) (see Chapter 14).

Connections

Half-Life of Immunoglobulins

Recall from Chapter 5 that the half-life for IgG, the predominant immunoglobulin in human serum, is 23 days, whereas the half-life of the other immunoglobulin classes is 6 days or fewer. For this reason, the effects of passive immunization are temporary.

Immunosuppressive Effects of Passive Immunization

In addition to its protective effects, passive immunization of gamma globulins can also have immunosuppressive effects in certain situations. For example, in Chapter 14, we discussed how the administration of Rh-immune globulin can prevent hemolytic disease of the newborn. Rh-immune globulin inhibits the production of anti-Rh antibodies in an Rh-negative mother toward paternally derived Rh antigens on her fetus. In addition, it has been found that intravenous immunoglobulin therapy can modulate the proinflammatory activities of IgG antibodies in patients with autoimmune diseases. Over 30 years ago, it was discovered that intravenous infusion of HISG results in an immediate increase in platelet counts and improvement of symptoms in patients with immune thrombocytopenia (ITP). Similar results have been found in patients with other inflammatory disorders. Intravenous immunoglobulin therapy is approved by the Food and Drug Administration (FDA) for treatment of ITP, chronic inflammatory demyelinating polyneuropathy (CIDP), and Kawasaki's disease, and its effects are being studied in other chronic inflammatory disorders.

The way in which intravenous immunoglobulins inhibit the inflammatory response is unclear, but several mechanisms have been proposed. The antibodies in the HISG preparation contain many antigen specificities and may mediate killing of target cells by antibody-dependent cellular cytotoxicity (ADCC); prevent interactions of ligands with cell surface receptors; inhibit cytokines; neutralize autoantibodies; or bind to activated complement components, such as C3a and C5a, blocking their activity. HISG may also block engulfment of immune complexes by saturating the Fc receptors on phagocytic cells. Other possible mechanisms by which HISG may modulate immune activity include enhancement of T regulatory (Treg) cell function, modulation of dendritic cell activation, or inhibition of B cells.

Monoclonal Antibodies

Monoclonal antibodies, as we discussed in Chapter 5, are derived from a single clone of B cells; therefore, they have exquisite specificity for a particular epitope of an antigen. This specificity is being harnessed in the use of monoclonal antibodies as agents of passive immunization, most notably for the treatment of cancer and autoimmune diseases. Numerous monoclonal antibodies have been approved by the FDA and the European Medicines Agency (EMA) for the treatment of patients with hematologic malignancies, solid tumors, autoimmune disorders, and a variety of other conditions, including cardiovascular disease, transplant rejection, and allergic asthma. A list of approved monoclonal antibody therapies as well as those undergoing review is available from The Antibody Society. Examples of monoclonal antibodies that have been widely used as therapeutic agents include rituximab, directed against the CD20 antigen on B cells, for treatment of non-Hodgkin lymphoma; trastuzumab, directed against HER2/neu, for treatment of certain breast cancers; and adalimumab, directed against tumor necrosis factor-α (TNF-α), used for reduction of inflammation in patients with rheumatoid arthritis. These and other examples of monoclonal antibodies approved by the FDA for therapeutic use in patients are listed in **Table 25–2.**

As we previously discussed in Chapter 5, monoclonal antibodies were originally developed using mouse B cells to produce hybridomas that secreted antibody to the desired antigen. When these monoclonal antibodies were used as therapeutic agents in humans, immune responses were likely to occur to the foreign epitopes on the mouse immunoglobulins, resulting in the production of *human anti-mouse antibodies (HAMAs)*. HAMAs significantly limited the usefulness of the monoclonal antibody therapy because they caused type I (anaphylactic) or type III (immune complex) hypersensitivity reactions.

Connections

Monoclonal Antibodies and Mice

Monoclonal antibodies were originally produced from mice, by injecting the mice with the desired antigen, isolating B cells from spleens of the immunized animals, and fusing them with cultured mouse myeloma cells to produce immortal hybrid cell lines known as "hybridomas" (see Chapter 5). Cell culture techniques were used to isolate the hybridomas that produced the desired antibody. The monoclonal antibodies purified from these cultures consisted entirely of mouse protein.

Table 25–2 Examples of FDA-Approved Monoclonal Antibodies Used for Immunotherapy

NAME*	TYPE	SPECIFICITY	KEY DISEASE INDICATION(S)
Adalimumab (Humira)	Human	TNF-α	Rheumatoid arthritis, psoriatic arthritis, ankylosing spondylitis, Crohn's disease, plaque psoriasis, juvenile idiopathic arthritis
Alemtuzumab (Campath)	Humanized	CD52	Chronic lymphocytic leukemia Multiple sclerosis
Basiliximab (Simulect)	Chimeric	CD25	Kidney transplant rejection
Bevacizumab (Avastin)	Humanized	Vascular endothelial growth factor (VEGF)	Colorectal cancer, non–small-cell lung carcinoma, renal cell carcinomas, glioblastoma
Daratumumab (Darzalex)	Human	CD38	Multiple myeloma
Ipilimumab (Yervoy)	Human	CTLA-4	Melanoma
Omalizumab (Xolair)	Humanized	IgE	Allergic asthma
Pembrolizumab (Keytruda)	Humanized	PD-1	Melanoma, non–small-cell lung cancer, Hodgkin lymphoma, Merkel cell carcinoma
Rituximab (Rituxan)	Chimeric	CD20	Non-Hodgkin lymphoma, chronic lymphocytic leukemia, rheumatoid arthritis, granulomatosis with polyangiitis, microscopic polyangiitis
Trastuzumab (Herceptin)	Humanized	HER2/neu	Breast cancer, gastric adenocarcinoma, gastroesophageal junction adenocarcinoma

**Brand names are in parentheses.*

CD = cluster of differentiation; CTLA-4 = cytotoxic T-lymphocyte–associated protein 4; HER2 = human epidermal growth factor receptor 2; IgE = immunoglobulin E; PD-1 = programmed cell death protein 1; TNF = tumor necrosis factor.

Over the years, the development of recombinant DNA technology has allowed scientists to produce monoclonal antibodies that have an increasingly larger human component, making them less likely to trigger an adverse immune reaction. Initially, chimeric antibodies were developed, which consisted of a mouse-derived immunoglobulin variable region combined with a human-derived constant region **(Fig. 25–10)**. This was followed by the production of humanized antibodies, which contain all human sequences except for the antigen-binding complementarity-determining regions, which are mouse derived. Today, it is possible to produce fully human monoclonal antibodies by phage display, a technique in which genes coding for a specific antibody molecule are cloned in bacteriophages or by transgenic mouse technologies involving incorporation of the immunoglobulin genes of interest into genetically modified mice. These antibodies have a low potential for immunogenicity and are becoming more widely available for therapeutic use.

The World Health Organization (WHO) assigned a nomenclature that designates all monoclonal antibodies by the suffix "*-mab*" and includes a portion called an "infix" to indicate their mouse/human component (the infix has been dropped in monoclonal antibodies produced after mid-2017). Mouse monoclonal antibodies can be identified by the infix/suffix, "*-omab*." Chimeric antibodies include "*-ximab*" in their names. Humanized antibodies have been denoted by "*-zumab*," and fully human antibodies are indicated by "*-umab*." The WHO nomenclature also includes terminology to indicate the target antigen of the monoclonal antibody. For example, the infix "tu" designates a tumor antigen, such as in the antibody ri<u>tu</u>ximab.

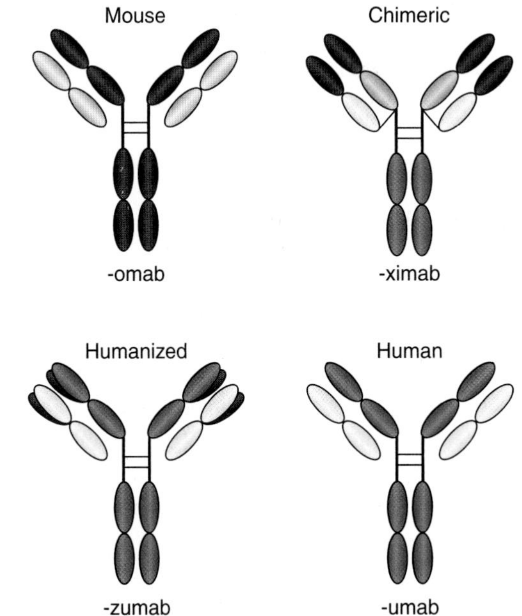

FIGURE 25–10 Monoclonal antibodies used as therapeutic agents can be made in mice, but humans may react to the foreign protein. The antigen-binding portion of the molecule can be grafted onto the constant regions of human antibodies to reduce such reactivity. It is also possible to humanize such antibodies so that only parts of the variable regions are incorporated into human antibody molecules.

The development of humanized and fully human antibodies has especially had an impact in the treatment of autoimmune diseases and cancer. Monoclonal antibodies targeting TNF-α bind to the cytokine to neutralize its activity and have been very beneficial in reducing the pathogenesis associated with rheumatoid arthritis and other autoimmune disorders (see Chapter 15). Monoclonal antibodies used in cancer therapy are able to mediate killing of tumor cells by a variety of mechanisms (see Chapter 17). They can directly kill tumor cells by binding to cell surface receptors or other membrane-bound proteins, causing apoptosis or inhibition of signaling and cell proliferation. They can also bind to the tumor cells and facilitate their destruction through opsonization and phagocytosis, ADCC, activation of the complement cascade, or activation of T cells. Because of their ability to specifically target a diverse range of molecules, monoclonal antibodies are considered to be one of the most successful cancer therapies in the last 20 years.

Clinical Correlations

Monoclonal Antibodies Directed Against Inhibitory Receptors

Cytotoxic T-lymphocyte–associated protein 4 (CTLA-4) and programmed cell death protein 1 (PD-1) are inhibitory receptors that become more numerous on T cells during a prolonged immune response. These receptors are also known as *immune checkpoints* because they are upregulated in order to prevent overactivation of the immune system, which could potentially lead to autoimmunity. Persistent high levels of tumor antigens can cause upregulation of these receptors, which, in turn, reduces the effectiveness of T-cell responses in destroying tumors. Monoclonal antibodies have been developed against CTLA-4 and PD-1, with the goal of blocking these inhibitory receptors and decreasing suppression of anti-tumor responses. Therapeutic use of these antibodies has been observed to increase life expectancy in patients with advanced cancers, including melanoma, renal cell carcinoma, and non–small-cell lung cancer.

Various modifications of monoclonal antibodies have also been developed for passive immunotherapy. Fragments of monoclonal antibodies, such as the Fab portion, have been used to enhance their effectiveness or ability to penetrate tissues in the body. For example, ranibizumab is a recombinant humanized monoclonal antibody Fab fragment that binds to human vascular endothelial growth factor A (VEGF-A) and prevents it from binding to its receptors. This antibody fragment has been used to suppress vascularization and delay vision loss in some forms of macular degeneration.

Some monoclonal antibodies have been conjugated to drugs or toxins, allowing these agents to be delivered to a specific site, such as tumor cells in the body. For example, Brentuximab vedotin, a monoclonal antibody targeting the CD30 antigen that has been linked to the anti-tubulin agent monomethyl auristatin E, has been used successfully to treat patients with systemic anaplastic large-cell lymphoma who have not responded to other treatments.

Another modification has been the development of bifunctional monoclonal antibodies, in which two immunoglobulin chains with different antigen specificities have been fused into a single molecule. This allows the two antigens to be brought close together when they are bound by the antibody. For example, the antibody blinatumomab, which is capable of binding to both CD3 on T cells and CD19 on B cells from acute lymphoblastic leukemia (ALL), has been used to recruit cytotoxic T cells to kill the malignant B cells in adult patients with relapsed B-cell ALL.

Adoptive Immunotherapy

While passive immunization is aimed at providing the humoral component of the immune response, adoptive immunotherapy involves transferring cells of the immune system to increase the cell-mediated immune response of the recipient. The cells transferred can be derived from a donor individual or from the recipients themselves. In the case of *autologous* transfers, the cells are removed from the patient, treated in vitro to become more immunologically reactive, and infused back into the same patient. The cells transferred in adoptive immunotherapy can be naturally derived or genetically engineered to target a particular antigen. Heterogeneous cell types can be transferred, although most applications have focused on the transfer of T-cell–mediated activity.

Adoptive Immunotherapy for Cancer

Human studies involving adoptive cell transfer have led to the development of innovative immunotherapies for cancer patients. Cancer immunotherapy with adoptively transferred cells is based on the observation of immune responses against tumor cells in animal studies. In the 1960s, researchers discovered that lymph node cells from mice immunized with chemically or virally induced tumors were able to protect against growth of the same tumor type when they were transferred to genetically identical recipients. They found that this immune response was enhanced in the presence of the cytokine interleukin 2 (IL-2). Scientists later began to look for the ability of lymphoid cells actually found within a tumor mass to mount an anti-tumor response. Through their work, they identified a heterogeneous population of T cells that can demonstrate cytotoxic effects against the tumor. These cells came to be known as **tumor-infiltrating lymphocytes (TILs).** TILs appear to be ineffective in eliminating the tumor at their natural site, possibly because they are not present in adequate numbers, they become anergic because of chronic activation, or they are surrounded by Treg cells and myeloid-derived suppressor cells. However, Rosenberg and his colleagues at the National Institutes of Health (NIH) found that they could enrich for and expand the TIL population in vitro by incubating cells from the tumor in the presence of IL-2.

In 1986, Rosenberg's group demonstrated protective effects of autologous TILs against metastases in mice. In 1988, the researchers applied a similar approach to humans. In their landmark publication, the scientists showed that TILs isolated from patients with metastatic melanoma and expanded in vitro could mediate tumor regression when given back to the same patients. In this adoptive immunotherapy procedure, which has been improved over the years, tumors are surgically removed, dissected into fragments, and incubated in culture in the presence of IL-2 for a few weeks. During the incubation period, the TILs proliferate and kill the residual tumor cells. T cells showing potent anti-tumor activity are isolated from the mixture and further expanded in the presence of IL-2, anti-CD3 antibody, and irradiated mononuclear cells derived from normal peripheral blood. These purified, potent TILs are then infused into the same patient from which the tumor fragments were derived. The expanded TILs migrate back to the tumor, where they mediate its destruction (see Fig 17–12).

Adoptive transfer of autologous TILs along with IL-2 into cancer patients has had the greatest impact in those with metastatic melanoma, resulting in tumor regression and increased disease-free survival in a significant percentage of treated individuals. The success of this treatment is thought to be the result of the high level of immunogenicity of melanoma tumors and pretreatment of patients with total body irradiation, which is thought to deplete regulatory and suppressor cells within the host that could inhibit the anti-tumor effects of the TILs. Adoptive TIL therapy is also being investigated in patients with other types of tumors who have exhausted other treatment options. Efforts are under way to improve techniques to reduce the cost of this expensive, personalized treatment so that it can be available to a larger number of patients.

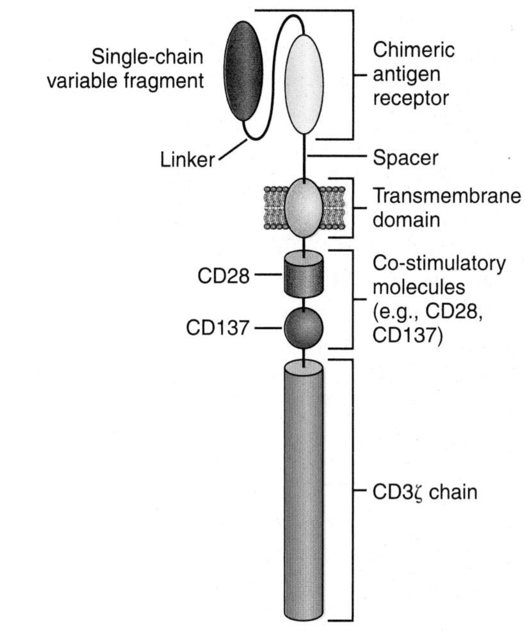

FIGURE 25–11 Structure of a CAR-T–cell receptor. Key components of the receptor include a single-chain variable fragment from a monoclonal antibody that will bind to the tumor antigen, a spacer region and transmembrane domain, costimulatory molecules, and part of the CD3 molecule.

CAR-T–Cell Therapy

An area of high interest to immunologists is the development of genetically engineered T cells that express high-affinity T-cell receptors (TCRs) for specific tumor antigens, known as **CAR-T cells** (chimeric antigen receptor T cells). Normally, T cells express receptors consisting of α and β chains complexed with CD3. These receptors recognize a specific antigen associated with a class I or class II major histocompatibility complex (MHC) molecule (see Chapter 4). In contrast, CAR-T cells possess receptors made from a tumor-specific single-chain variable fragment of a monoclonal antibody molecule linked to the CD3ζ chain of the TCR and a costimulatory molecule such as CD28 to enhance cytokine production and proliferation of the T cells **(Fig. 25–11).** These receptors are capable of strongly binding to the tumor antigen in the absence of an MHC molecule and thus are not MHC-restricted.

In CAR-T–cell therapy, a patient's white blood cells (WBCs) are collected by leukapheresis, and the T cells within the sample are stimulated to proliferate in vitro by incubation with IL-2 and anti-CD3. Then, the gene coding for the chimeric antigen receptor specific for the patient's tumor antigen is introduced into the expanded T cells using viral vectors or nonviral transfection methods. The genetically modified T cells are expanded in culture and infused back into the patient after he or she has received total body irradiation and lympho-depleting chemotherapy to enhance engraftment and potency of the infused cells. At the time of this writing, the following CAR-T–cell therapies have been approved by the FDA for patients in whom other treatments have not worked: tisagenlecleucel (Kymriah), a CAR-T–cell therapy directed against the CD-19 antigen for treatment of B-cell ALL in children and adults younger than 25 years, as well as adult patients with large B-cell lymphoma; and axicabtagene ciloleucel (Yescarta), another CD-19 directed therapy for adult patients with large B-cell lymphoma.

Other Applications of Adoptive Immunotherapy

Hematopoietic stem-cell transplantation is another area in which medical practitioners are using adoptive immunotherapy. These stem cells are routinely used as a treatment for certain immunodeficiency disorders (see Chapter 19). Autologous or allogeneic transplantation of hematopoietic stem cells can also be used to restore the immune system in patients who have been treated with chemotherapy and a high dose of total body irradiation. The treatment has been used most commonly in patients with multiple myeloma, non-Hodgkin lymphoma, or acute leukemias.

Clinical trials are also under way for other applications related to transplant immunology that may have a significant clinical impact. For example, clinical trials involving adoptive transfer of Treg cells to transplant patients are being conducted in an attempt to prevent graft rejection or graft-versus-host disease (GVHD). In addition, medical scientists are adoptively transferring cytotoxic T cells to transplant recipients to treat opportunistic infections with viruses such as CMV, EBV, and adenovirus and their associated complications, which can be life threatening in these immunosuppressed patients.

SUMMARY

- Immunity is the condition of resistance to a disease. Immunization is the process by which immunity is acquired. There are three types of immunization—active, passive, and adoptive.
- Active immunization involves stimulation of an individual's own immune system to mount an adaptive immune response to an antigen, because of either natural infection or receipt of a vaccine.
- Passive immunization involves the transfer of premade antibodies from an immune host to a nonimmune host. This type of immunity can occur naturally, by transfer of maternal IgG antibodies through the placenta to the fetus or by transfer of IgA antibodies from a mother to her infant through breast milk. Passive immunity can also be transferred artificially through commercial antibody preparations such as human immune serum globulin.
- Adoptive immunotherapy is achieved by transferring cells of the immune system to a nonimmune host. The cells can be derived either from a genetically different (allogeneic) host or they can be stimulated in vitro before re-introduction into the same (autologous) individual.
- Active immunity takes time to develop but provides long-lasting protection to the host because of the production of immunologic memory. Passive immunity provides immediate protection but is short-lived because antibody titers decline at a rate that is determined by the biological half-life of the immunoglobulins. Adoptive immunity provides long-lasting protection if the cells become established in the host.
- A traditional vaccine is a microbially derived antigen suspension that is administered to a healthy host in order to stimulate an immune response that will prevent the host from developing an infectious disease. Thus, vaccines are used for immunoprophylaxis.
- In 1796, Dr. Edward Jenner was the first to publicize the procedure of vaccination by using material from cowpox skin lesions to immunize against the deadly disease smallpox. In the 1800s, Louis Pasteur used the principle of attenuation, or weakened microorganisms, to produce vaccines against chicken cholera, anthrax, and rabies.
- In the 20th century, vaccine development grew exponentially because of new methods to attenuate microorganisms, production of toxoids, and technologies that allowed viruses to be grown in cell culture. In the latter part of the 20th century, the first recombinant vaccine, produced by genetic engineering, was developed.
- Conventional vaccines may be composed of live, attenuated (weakened, nonpathogenic) microorganisms; inactivated (killed) microorganisms; or antigenic subunits such as recombinant antigens or toxoids. Toxoids are bacterial toxins that have been inactivated so that they are no longer pathogenic but are still immunogenic.
- Adjuvants are substances that are often included in vaccines in order to increase the immune response to the target antigens. Examples of adjuvants include aluminum salts and oil-in-water emulsions. They are believed to enhance the immune response by promoting migration of APCs and increased antigen uptake and by inducing the release of proinflammatory cytokines and chemokines.
- The effectiveness of a vaccine is not only influenced by the nature of the vaccine but also by the age and immune status of the host. To obtain an optimal immune response, vaccines must be administered according to recommended schedules.
- Vaccines protect not only the individuals who have received the vaccines but also their contacts, a phenomenon known as "community immunity" or "herd immunity."
- Vaccines are considered to be one of the greatest achievements of medicine. The benefits of vaccines greatly outweigh their risks. Rarely, vaccines can cause side effects such as hypersensitivity reactions. Live vaccines should not be administered to patients with immunodeficiency disorders because they can replicate uncontrollably and cause disseminated disease.
- Passive immunization with preformed antibody preparations is administered in order to provide immediate humoral immunity to unimmunized persons.
- Patients with humoral immunodeficiencies are routinely treated with standard HISG, prepared from pooled serum of many donors, to provide protection against a variety of pathogens. Specific HISG containing antibody against a particular pathogen can be used to treat nonimmune, healthy individuals who have had contact with the pathogen to provide immediate protection.
- Antitoxins are antibodies directed against toxins from pathogenic bacteria. They can be isolated from the serum of laboratory animals that have been injected with the toxin and used to prevent diseases such as tetanus, diphtheria, and botulism by passive immunization.
- Passive immunization of immunoglobulins can also be used as immunosuppressive therapy for certain autoimmune and chronic inflammatory disorders, as well as to prevent hemolytic disease of the newborn.
- Monoclonal antibodies have specificity for a particular antigenic epitope. They are being used as therapeutic agents for cancers, autoimmune diseases, and various other conditions.
- Monoclonal antibodies were originally 100% mouse derived because they were produced by hybridoma technology. Advancement in genetic technologies has allowed scientists to make hybrid antibodies that consist partially of mouse protein and partially of human protein. These antibodies can be characterized as chimeric, humanized, or fully human, depending on the amount of the human component. Administration of these antibodies reduces the chance that the recipients will produce

human-anti-mouse antibodies (HAMAs) and develop hypersensitivity reactions.

- Adoptive immunotherapy involves the transfer of cells of the immune system to provide immunity. Examples include treatment of melanoma patients with autologous IL-2 activated tumor-infiltrating lymphocytes (TILs), CAR-T–cell therapy for selected B-cell malignancies, and administration of hematopoietic stem cells to patients with hematologic malignancies who have been treated with high doses of chemotherapy and irradiation.

Study Guide: Major Features of Active Immunity, Passive Immunity, and Adoptive Immunity

	MECHANISM	EXAMPLES	ADVANTAGES	LIMITATIONS
Active Immunity	Activation of humoral and cell-mediated responses in an individual's own immune system by exposure to an antigen	Natural infection with a pathogen Immunization with a vaccine	Long-term immunologic memory to the antigen is generated	Delay in initiation of immune response
Passive Immunity	Transfer of antibodies from immunized host(s) to nonimmune individuals	Passage of IgG through the placenta, from a pregnant woman to her fetus Passage of IgA through breast milk, from mother to infant Standard human immune serum globulin Specific human immune serum globulin Antitoxins Rh-immune globulin Monoclonal antibodies	Provides immediate protection to the recipient	Immunity is temporary, declining with the half-life of the antibodies Immunologic memory is not generated Hypersensitivity can develop, especially when sera of animal origin are used
Adoptive Immunity	Transfer of cells of the immune system to nonimmune individuals	Adoptive immunotherapy with activated TILs or CAR-T cells to cancer patients Hematopoietic stem cell transplantation	Can transfer cell-mediated immunity	Patient's own immune cells must be depleted to increase chance of successful therapy Allogeneic cells may be rejected

Study Guide: Characteristics of Conventional Vaccines

	COMPOSITION	EXAMPLES	ADVANTAGES	LIMITATIONS
Attenuated	Live pathogens that have been weakened by growth under modified culture conditions	BCG (Bacillus Calmette Guerin) Typhoid fever Oral polio (Sabin) Measles (rubeola) Mumps German measles (rubella) Chickenpox (varicella) Shingles (zoster) Influenza (nasal mist) Rotavirus	Induce both humoral and cell-mediated immunity Effective in inducing immunity after a single dose	Cannot be administered to immunocompromised individuals Rare potential to mutate to a pathogenic form Maternal antibodies can interfere with immune response to the vaccine in infants Require careful handling and storage
Inactivated	Killed microorganisms	Intramuscular polio (Salk) Influenza (intramuscular or intradermal) Hepatitis A	Can safely be given to immunocompromised individuals	Stimulates humoral immunity but little or no cell-mediated immunity May require two or more booster doses to produce protective immunity

(continued)

Study Guide: Characteristics of Conventional Vaccines—cont'd

	COMPOSITION	EXAMPLES	ADVANTAGES	LIMITATIONS
Subunit	One or more purified components of a pathogen	Toxoids Purified proteins Polysaccharides Recombinant antigens	Induces an immune response to the pathogenic component(s) of a microorganism Safer than administration of an intact organism	Requires two or more booster doses to produce protective immunity Requires an adjuvant to increase immunogenicity Must be multivalent if a broad immune response is desired
a. Toxoids	Bacterial toxins that have been chemically inactivated so that they are not pathogenic	Diphtheria Tetanus	See information for subunit vaccines in this table	Requires two or more booster doses to produce protective immunity Requires an adjuvant to increase immunogenicity
b. Purified Components	Biochemically purified components of a microorganism	Pertussis (whooping cough)	See information for subunit vaccines in this table Produces fewer side effects than whole bacteria	See information for subunit vaccines in this table
c. Polysaccharides	Biochemically purified polysaccharide from bacterial capsule	Streptococcal pneumonia *Haemophilus influenzae* type b Neisserial meningitis	See information for subunit vaccines in this table	See information for subunit vaccines in this table Requires conjugation to a carrier protein to induce IgG production and long-term immunity
d. Recombinant Antigen	Protein produced by genetically modified nonpathogenic bacteria, yeast, or mammalian cells	Hepatitis B Human papilloma virus (cervical, anal, genital cancers) Influenza Varicella zoster (shingles)	Highly purified protein that is safer than administration of intact organism	See information for subunit vaccines in this table Cannot be used to produce antigens other than proteins

CASE STUDIES

1. A 2-year-old boy has made numerous visits to his doctor because he has suffered from recurring respiratory and ear infections. An immunologic workup revealed that the child had a low number of B cells and decreased immunoglobulin concentrations. Based on these results, the boy was diagnosed with an antibody immunodeficiency disease.

Questions

a. What childhood vaccines could safely be administered to this child? What is the composition of these vaccines?
b. What childhood vaccines should not be administered to this child? Why?
c. How can the child be protected against the diseases for which he is unable to receive vaccination?

2. Suppose you ate lunch at a popular restaurant a few days ago. Your local health department puts out a notice that several of the customers who dined at the restaurant recently have confirmed cases of hepatitis A and that the source of infection was traced to a supply of green onions that had been used in the salads. Public health officials advise anyone who has eaten at the

restaurant in the last 2 weeks to visit the local county health department to receive passive immunization to prevent the infection.

Questions

a. What type of passive immunization should be administered, and what is the main benefit of this treatment?

b. If you received this treatment and did not develop hepatitis A, would you be immune to this virus 10 years from now? Why or why not?

REVIEW QUESTIONS

1. Suppose an individual develops antibodies in response to a streptococcal pharyngitis infection. This is an example of
   a. active immunity.
   b. passive immunity.
   c. adoptive immunity.
   d. immunoprophylaxis.

2. Which of the following illustrates passive immunity?
   a. Development of high antibody titers in a healthy person after receipt of the hepatitis B vaccine
   b. Recovery of a patient from a hepatitis A infection
   c. Passage of IgG antibodies through the placenta of a pregnant woman to her fetus
   d. Transfer of tumor-infiltrating lymphocytes to a cancer patient

3. Which of the following is *not* a characteristic of passive immunity?
   a. Transfer of antibodies
   b. Occurs naturally or because of therapy
   c. Provision of immediate protection
   d. Development of long-term memory

4. What was one of the major contributions of Louis Pasteur to vaccine development?
   a. Development of the smallpox vaccine
   b. Use of attenuated microorganisms in vaccines
   c. Inactivation of bacterial toxins for vaccines
   d. Discovery of recombinant vaccine antigens

5. The antigenic component of the hepatitis B vaccine differs from those of many of the conventional vaccines in that it consists of a
   a. live, attenuated virus.
   b. inactivated virus.
   c. cryptic antigen.
   d. recombinant antigen.

6. Which of the following describes the properties of a toxoid?
   a. Both pathogenic and immunogenic
   b. Pathogenic but not immunogenic
   c. Not pathogenic but immunogenic
   d. Neither pathogenic nor immunogenic

7. Suppose a vaccine was available in two forms: attenuated and inactivated. What is an advantage of the attenuated form?
   a. It can be used in immunocompromised patients.
   b. It induces both humoral and cell-mediated immunity.
   c. There is no interference of the immune response in infants by maternal antibodies.
   d. It does not require special handling and storage to maintain its effectiveness.

8. What factor(s) influence the effectiveness of a person's immune response to a vaccine?
   a. Age of the recipient
   b. The individual's immune status
   c. The nature of the vaccine
   d. All of the above

9. Chimeric antigen receptors in CAR-T cells are composed of which of the following components?
   a. α and β chains of the TCR in complex with CD3
   b. α and β chains of the TCR in complex with class I MHC
   c. Single-chain variable fragment of a monoclonal antibody complexed with class I MHC
   d. Single-chain variable fragment of a monoclonal antibody complexed with CD3 and a costimulatory molecule

10. When one individual becomes immunized by receiving a series of vaccine injections according to schedule, the resulting protection extends to that individual's nearby contacts. This concept is known as
    a. immunologic memory.
    b. neighborhood immunity.
    c. herd immunity.
    d. contagious immunity.

11. Which preparation would you recommend for treatment of a patient with an antibody deficiency?
    a. Monoclonal antibody
    b. Specific human immune serum globulin
    c. Standard human immune serum globulin
    d. Animal serum antitoxins

12. Immunoglobulins consisting of a mouse-derived variable region combined with a human-derived constant region are known as
    a. monoclonal antibodies.
    b. chimeric antibodies.
    c. humanized antibodies.
    d. fully human antibodies.

13. HAMAs are
    a. mouse-derived antibodies that have been used for therapy.
    b. monoclonal antibodies with therapeutic benefits.
    c. human antibodies that are produced against mouse proteins.
    d. antitoxins that can provide immediate immunity.

14. What is a major characteristic of adoptive immunotherapy?
    a. It involves the transfer of cells to deliver immunity.
    b. It involves the transfer of cytokines to deliver immunity.
    c. It can only occur in the presence of autologous cells.
    d. Its purpose is to increase the humoral immune response.

15. Infusion of TILs into a cancer patient is an example of
    a. active immunity.
    b. adoptive immunity.
    c. passive immunity.
    d. natural immunity.

Glossary

Accuracy: The ability of a test to actually measure what it claims to measure.

Acquired immunodeficiency syndrome (AIDS): A disease affecting the immune system caused by HIV.

Activation unit: The combination of complement components C1, C4b, and C2b that form the enzyme C3 convertase, whose substrate is C3.

Active immunity: Immunity resulting from natural exposure to an infectious agent or administration of a vaccine.

Acute-phase reactants: Normal serum proteins that increase rapidly because of infection, injury, or trauma to the tissues.

Acute rejection (AR): A type of rejection that occurs days to weeks after transplantation as a result of cellular mechanisms and antibody formation.

Acute rheumatic fever: A disease that develops as a sequel to Group A streptococcal pharyngitis, characterized by the presence of antibodies that cross-react with heart tissue.

Adaptive immunity: A type of resistance that is characterized by specificity for each individual pathogen, or microbial agent, and the ability to remember a prior exposure, which results in an increased response to that pathogen upon repeated exposure.

Adaptive T regulatory 1 (Tr1) cells: CD4+ T cells induced from antigen-activated naïve T cells under the influence of interleukin-10. These cells exert suppressive activities.

Adjuvant: A substance administered with an immunogen that enhances and potentiates the immune response.

Adoptive immunity: Immunity resulting from the transfer of cells of the immune system (usually lymphocytes) from an immunized host to a nonimmune individual.

Adoptive immunotherapy: Administration of immune cells to treat patients with conditions such as immunodeficiency diseases or cancer.

Affinity: The initial force of attraction that exists between a Fab site on an antibody and one epitope or a determinant site on the corresponding antigen.

Affinity maturation: Process during the immune response whereby somatic mutations in B cells result in immunoglobulin receptors that can bind the antigen more strongly.

Agammaglobulinemias: Immunodeficiency diseases in which antibody levels in the blood are significantly decreased.

Agglutination: The process by which particulate antigens such as cells aggregate to form large complexes when a specific antibody is present.

Agglutination inhibition: An agglutination reaction based on competition between antigen-coated particles and soluble patient antigens for a limited number of antibody-combining sites. Lack of agglutination is a positive test result.

Agglutinin: An antibody that causes clumping or agglutination of the cells that triggered its formation.

Allele: An alternate form of a gene that codes for a slightly different form of the same product.

Allelic exclusion: The selection of an allele on one chromosome only.

Allergen: An antigen that triggers a type I hypersensitivity response (i.e., an allergy).

Allergy immunotherapy (AIT): Therapy involving administration of increasing doses of an allergen with the goal of inducing immune tolerance to the allergen.

Alloantigen: An antigen that is found in another member of the host's species and that is capable of eliciting an immune response in the host.

Allograft: Tissue transferred from an individual of one species into another individual of the same species.

Allotype: A minor variation in amino acid sequence in a particular class of immunoglobulin molecules that is inherited in Mendelian fashion.

Alpha-fetoprotein (AFP): A tumor marker that is commonly elevated in patients with primary hepatocellular carcinoma and nonseminomatous testicular cancer.

Alpha$_1$-antitrypsin (AAT): An acute-phase protein that acts as an inhibitor of proteases released from white blood cells (WBCs).

Alternative pathway: A means of activating complement proteins without an antigen–antibody combination. This pathway is triggered by constituents of microorganisms.

Amplification: Copying of nucleic acids to increase the amount available for testing.

Analyte: The substance being measured in an immunoassay.

Analytic sensitivity: The lowest measurable amount of an analyte.

Analytic specificity: An assay's ability to generate a negative result when the analyte is not present.

Anamnestic response: The memory, or secondary, immune response.

Anaphylatoxin: A small peptide formed during complement activation that causes increased vascular permeability, contraction of smooth muscle, and release of histamine from basophils and mast cells.

Anaphylaxis: A life-threatening response to an allergen characterized by the systemic release of histamine.

Anergy: A state of immune unresponsiveness to a specific antigen.

Antagonism: Effect that occurs when the action of one cytokine counteracts the activity of another cytokine.

Antibodies: Glycoproteins produced by B lymphocytes and plasma cells in response to foreign substance exposure. Antibodies are also known as *immunoglobulins.*

Antibody array: A multiplex assay that uses antibody-coated beads to identify target antigens, such as tumor antigens.

Antibody-dependent cellular cytotoxicity (ADCC): The process of destroying antibody-coated target cells by natural killer cells, monocytes, macrophages, and neutrophils, all of which have specific receptors for an antibody.

Antibody–drug conjugates: Antibody that is attached to toxins or radioisotopes to help specifically destroy cancer cells.

Anti-centromere antibodies: Autoantibodies that bind to proteins in the centromere (the middle region of a chromosome where the sister chromatids are joined); associated with the CREST syndrome.

Anti-cyclic citrullinated peptide (anti-CCP or ACPA): Autoantibodies to proteins that contain an atypical amino acid called *citrulline* (a modified arginine), produced by granulocytes and monocytes. This antibody is highly specific for rheumatoid arthritis.

Anti-DNase B: An antibody directed against DNase B, which is secreted by Group A streptococci.

Antigen: Macromolecule that is capable of eliciting formation of immunoglobulins (antibodies) or sensitized lymphocytes in an immunocompetent host.

Antigen-dependent phase: The final phase of B-cell development, which occurs when a B cell is stimulated by an antigen and undergoes transformation to a blast stage, resulting in the formation of memory cells and antibody-secreting plasma cells.

Antigen-independent phase: The first phase of B-cell development in the bone marrow, which results in mature B cells that have not yet been exposed to antigen.

Antigen presentation: The process by which degraded peptides within cells are transported to the plasma membrane with major histocompatibility class (MHC) molecules so that T cells can then recognize them.

Antigen switching: A protective mechanism used by parasites that involves varying synthesis of surface antigens to evade an immune response by the host.

Antigenic concealment: Means by which parasites hide their antigens from the host by remaining inside of the host's cells without their antigens being displayed.

Antigenic mimicry: A mechanism by which parasites express epitopes that are similar or identical to host molecules, thus protecting the parasite from being recognized and eliminated by the immune system.

Antigenic shedding: A mechanism by which parasites can evade the immune system by shedding surface antigens that bind to the host's antibodies and cells.

Antigenic variation: A change in parasite antigens due to genetic modifications that allows them to escape the immune response.

Anti-glomerular basement membrane (anti-GBM) disease: An autoimmune disease characterized by production of antibodies to the basement membranes in the kidneys and lungs; formerly known as *Goodpasture's syndrome*.

Anti-HBe: Antibody to a hepatitis B capsid antigen.

Anti-HBs: Antibody to hepatitis B surface antigen.

Anti-histone antibodies: Autoantibodies to histones, which are nucleoproteins found in chromatin. Elevated levels are associated with drug-induced lupus.

Anti-neutrophil cytoplasmic antibody (ANCA): Autoantibodies produced against proteins in the neutrophil granules; these antibodies are strongly associated with vascular inflammatory syndromes.

Anti-nuclear antibody (ANA): Antibody produced to different components of the nucleus in several autoimmune diseases. Examples include anti-DNA, anti-deoxyribonucleoprotein, and anti-ribonuclear protein antibodies, all of which may be present in systemic lupus erythematosus.

Anti-phospholipid antibodies: A heterogeneous group of autoantibodies that bind to phospholipids or phospholipid–protein complexes.

Antiretroviral therapy (ART): Therapeutic drugs that suppress the replication of a retrovirus such as HIV.

Anti-RNP antibody: Autoantibodies directed against ribonucleoprotein (RNP), which consists of several nonhistone proteins complexed to a small nuclear RNA called *U1-nRNP.* These antibodies are found in some patients with autoimmune rheumatic diseases.

Antitoxin: Antibody used in passive immunization for the purpose of neutralizing a bacterial toxin.

Apoptosis: A normal process of programmed cell death.

Arthus reaction: A type III hypersensitivity skin reaction that occurs when an individual has a large amount of circulating antibody and is exposed to the antigen intradermally, resulting in localized deposition of immune complexes.

ASO titer: A test for the diagnosis of poststreptococcal sequelae, based on the neutralization of streptolysin O by antistreptolysin O found in patient serum.

Aspergillosis: An opportunistic fungal infection predominantly caused by *Aspergillus fumigatus.*

Ataxia-telangiectasia (AT): An autosomal recessive syndrome that results in a combined defect of cellular and humoral immunity. The defect is in a gene responsible for recombination of immunoglobulin superfamily genes.

Atopy: An inherited tendency to respond to naturally occurring allergens; it results in the continual production of immunoglobulin E (IgE).

Attenuation: A process of producing nonpathogenic bacteria or viruses for use in vaccines. These organisms have been weakened by treatment with a chemical, exposure to elevated or cold temperatures, or repeated passage in cell culture.

Atypical hemolytic uremic syndrome (aHUS): A rare genetic disorder associated with defects in complement regulation that cause microvascular thrombosis and affect the kidneys.

Autoantibody: An antibody produced against an antigen found in an individual's own cells, tissues, or organs.

Autoantigen: An antigen that belongs to the host and is not capable of eliciting an immune response under normal circumstances.

Autocrine: Effect produced by a cell that stimulates the same cell.

Autograft: Tissues removed from one location of an individual's body and reintroduced in another location in the same individual.

Autoimmune disease: A condition in which damage to body organs results from the presence of autoantibodies or autoreactive cells.

Autoimmune hemolytic anemia: An autoimmune disorder in which patients form antibodies that destroy their own red blood cells (RBCs).

Autoimmune hepatitis (AIH): Autoimmune disease in which patients produce antibodies that damage the liver; formerly known as autoimmune hepatitis.

Autoimmune liver disease: An autoimmune disease that mainly affects the liver, including autoimmune hepatitis (AIH), primary biliary cholangitis (PBC), and primary sclerosing cholangitis (PSC).

Autoimmune thyroid disease (AITD): An autoimmune disease that affects the function of the thyroid gland, caused by the formation of antibodies or sensitized cells; includes Hashimoto's disease and Graves' disease.

Automatic sampling: Automatic pipetting of a sample that is programmed into an instrument for testing of that sample.

Avidity: The strength with which a multivalent antibody binds a multivalent antigen.

B lymphocytes: Cells derived from the bone marrow which play a key role in the humoral immune response; they develop into plasma cells that produce specific antibodies.

Basophil: A type of white blood cell (WBC) found in peripheral blood, containing granules that release substances that are involved in allergic reactions.

Batch analyzer: An instrument that permits analysis of several different samples at the same time.

Bence Jones proteins: Monoclonal immunoglobulin light chains found in the urine of patients with multiple myeloma.

Benign: Tissue that is not malignant.

Biohazard: A biological substance that poses a threat to human health, for example, contaminated blood or body fluids.

Biohazardous material: Patient specimens that may contain potentially harmful infectious agents.

Bioinformatics: Field of study that combines biology, computer science, statistics, mathematics, and other information sciences to develop and use methods to analyze large sets of biological data.

Biomarker profiling: The use of proteomic methods to identify unique patterns of proteins that are associated with a disease, such as a specific type of cancer.

Biotin: A vitamin of the B-complex family that has an affinity for streptavidin; the complex is used for labeling in some types of immunoassays.

Bloodborne pathogens (BBPs): Pathogens such as HIV and hepatitis B virus (HBV) that can be transmitted by contact with contaminated blood or blood products.

Blowout pipette: A type of pipette in which the last drop of liquid must be forced out using a pipetting bulb or other device to deliver an accurate volume.

Bone marrow: The largest tissue in the body, located in the long bones, which functions in the generation of hematopoietic cells and B cell maturation.

Borrelia burgdorferi: A spirochete bacterium that is the causative agent of Lyme disease.

Branched-chain DNA (bDNA): A technique used to detect a small amount of DNA via several hybridization steps that create a branching effect with several nucleic acid probes.

Bruton's tyrosine kinase (Btk) deficiency: An X-linked recessive immunodeficiency disease that results in a lack of mature B lymphocytes and immunoglobulins of all classes.

Bystander lysis: A phenomenon that occurs in complement activation when C3b becomes deposited on host cells, making them a target for destruction by phagocytic cells.

C1 inhibitor (C1-INH): A glycoprotein that acts to dissociate C1r and C1s from C1q, thus inhibiting the first active enzyme formed in the classical complement cascade.

C3 glomerulopathies (C3G): Diseases involving the glomeruli of the kidneys.

C4-binding protein (C4BP): A protein in the complement system that serves as a cofactor for factor 1 in the inactivation of C4b.

Cancer: A disease characterized by the presence of a malignant tumor.

Cancer antigen 125 (CA 125): A glycosylated protein that is used clinically as a marker for ovarian cancer.

Cancer vaccines: Vaccines that have been developed for the purpose of preventing or treating cancer.

Candidiasis: An opportunistic fungal infection caused by *Candida albicans* and other *Candida* species.

Capture (sandwich) immunoassays: Immunoassays that detect an antigen by its ability to bind to an antibody attached to a solid phase as well as a detector antibody that contains a label, such as an enzyme.

Carcinoembryonic antigen (CEA): An oncofetal protein that may be elevated in patients with cancers of the breast, gastrointestinal tract, pancreas, or lung.

Carcinogenesis: The process by which a cell is transformed into a malignant tumor.

Carcinoma: Malignant tumor derived from the skin or epithelial linings of internal organs or glands.

CAR-T cells: Genetically modified T cells possessing a chimeric antigen receptor that binds to an antigen that can serve as a target for adoptive immunotherapy.

Cascade: A series of steps that occur in a progressive manner, for example, the classical pathway of complement or the secretion of a cytokine by a cell that activates target cells to produce additional cytokines.

CD4 T cell: Type of lymphocyte that provides help to B cells to initiate antibody production (T helper cell) or, less commonly, inhibits the immune response (T regulatory cell).

CD45: A leukocyte marker present on all white blood cells (WBCs); used to identify WBC populations in flow cytometry analyses.

Celiac disease: An autoimmune disease affecting the small intestine and other organs.

Cell cycle: The sequence of events that occurs between cell divisions and consists of the following phases: G1 (Gap 1), S (DNA synthesis), G2 (Gap 2), and M (Mitosis).

Cell-mediated immunity: A type of immunity in which T cells produce cytokines that help to regulate both the innate and adaptive immune response.

Central tolerance: Destruction of potentially self-reactive T and B cells as they mature in either the thymus or the bone marrow.

Ceruloplasmin: An acute-phase reactant that acts as the principal copper-transporting protein in human plasma.

Chain of infection: A continuous link between three elements—a source, a method of transmission, and a susceptible host.

Chain termination sequencing: A modification of the DNA replication process, which utilizes modified nucleotide bases called *dideoxynucleotide triphosphates* (ddNTPs). When these are incorporated into the growing DNA chain, synthesis stops.

Chancre: The initial lesion that develops on the external genitalia in syphilis.

Chemical Hygiene Plan: A plan that identifies appropriate work practices, standard operating procedures, and safety considerations in regard to the use of chemicals in the laboratory.

Chemiluminescence: The production of light energy by a chemical reaction.

Chemiluminescent immunoassay: A technique that employs a chemical attached to either an antigen or antibody. Light is emitted because of a chemical reaction and indicates that an antigen–antibody combination has taken place.

Chemiluminescent microparticle immunoassay (CMIA): A heterogeneous immunoassay that uses a chemiluminescent tag and antibody-coated microparticles as a reagent.

Chemokines: A large family of homologous cytokines that promote migration of white blood cells through chemotaxis.

Chemotaxin: A protein or other substance that acts as a chemical messenger to produce chemotaxis.

Chemotaxis: The migration of cells in the direction of a chemical messenger.

Chromosome: Structure in the nucleus that carries genetic information, consisting of DNA complexed with nuclear proteins.

Chronic granulomatous disease (CGD): An immunodeficiency inherited in either an X-linked or autosomal recessive fashion that results in an inability of the neutrophils to produce the reactive forms of oxygen necessary for normal bacterial killing.

Chronic rejection: Rejection of a graft that usually occurs after the first year of transplantation and results from progressive fibrosis of blood vessels in the grafted tissue.

Class I MHC (HLA) molecules: Proteins coded for by genes at three loci (A, B, C) in the major histocompatibility complex. They are expressed on all nucleated cells and are important to consider in the transplantation of tissues.

Class II MHC (HLA) molecules: Proteins coded for by the DR, DP, and DQ loci of the major histocompatibility complex. They are found on B cells, macrophages, activated T cells, monocytes, dendritic cells, and endothelium and are important to consider in the transplantation of tissues.

Class switching: The production of immunoglobulins other than immunoglobulin M (IgM) by daughter cells of antigen-exposed B lymphocytes.

Classical pathway: A series of steps involved in the activation of complement that begins with antigen–antibody binding.

Clinical and Laboratory Standards Institute (CLSI): An organization that develops clinical laboratory testing standards based on input from industry, government, and health-care professionals.

Clinical Laboratory Improvement Amendments (CLIA): Federal regulatory standards that apply to all clinical laboratory testing in the United States.

Clonal deletion: The process of eliminating clones of lymphocytes that would be capable of an autoimmune response.

Clonal expansion: Proliferation of lymphocytes during an immune response to create a population of identical cells, all capable of responding to the same antigen.

Clonal selection hypothesis: A theory postulated to explain the specificity of antibody formation, based on the premise that each lymphocyte is genetically programmed to produce a specific type of antibody and is selected by contact with an antigen.

Cloned-enzyme donor immunoassay (CEDIA): A homogeneous competitive immunoassay that uses a β-galactosidase enzyme that has been genetically engineered in two parts: acceptor and donor.

Clusters of differentiation (CD): Antigenic markers of leukocytes that are identified by groups of monoclonal antibodies expressing common or overlapping reactivity.

Coccidioidomycosis: A fungal disease caused by *Coccidioides immitis* that is endemic to the southwestern United States and may be characterized by primary pulmonary infection.

Coefficient of variation (CV): The average distance each data point in a normal distribution is from the mean. It is expressed as a percentage of the mean.

Cold agglutinins: Antibodies that react below 30°C, typically formed in response to diseases such as *Mycoplasma* pneumonia and certain viral infections.

Colony-stimulating factor (CSF): A family of cytokines in human serum that promote hematopoiesis and the differentiation of monocytes, granulocytes, and erythrocytes.

Commensalistic: A relationship between two species of organisms in which there is no benefit or harm to either organism.

Common variable immunodeficiency (CVI): A heterogeneous group of immunodeficiency disorders that usually appears in patients between the ages of 20 and 30 years. It is characterized by a deficiency of one or more classes of immunoglobulins.

Community immunity: Concept of extending protection to unvaccinated individuals by reducing spread of an infection when a significant proportion of individuals in the population have been immunized; also known as *herd immunity*.

Competitive immunoassay: An immunoassay in which unlabeled and labeled antigen compete for a limited number of binding sites on reagent antibody.

Complement: A series of proteins that are normally present in serum and whose overall functions are mediation of inflammation and destruction of foreign cells.

Complement-dependent cytotoxicity (CDC): Killing of cells that results from attachment of antibody with activation of complement.

Complement receptor type 1 (CR1): A cell-bound regulator of complement activation. It assists in degrading C3b and C4b and mediates transport of C3b-coated immune complexes to the liver and spleen.

Complementary or copy DNA (cDNA): A DNA sequence made from ribonucleic acid (RNA) using the enzyme reverse transcriptase and nucleotide base-pairing rules.

Conformational epitope: Key antigenic site that results from the folding of one chain or multiple chains, bringing certain amino acids from different segments of a linear sequence or sequences into close proximity with each other so that they can be recognized together.

Congenital syphilis: The transfer of syphilis from an infected mother to her fetus during pregnancy.

Conidia: Asexual reproductive structures produced by fungi at the tip of hyphae; also known as *spores*.

Constant region: The carboxy-terminal segment of antibody molecules (half of immunoglobulin light chains plus three-quarters of heavy chains) that consists of a polypeptide sequence found in all chains of that type.

Contact dermatitis: A delayed hypersensitivity reaction caused by T-cell sensitization to low-molecular-weight compounds, such as nickel and rubber, that come in contact with the skin.

Control mean: The average of all data points.

Coombs reagent: An anti-human immunoglobulin reagent used to enhance the detection of immunoglobulin G (IgG) antibodies in blood bank testing.

C-reactive protein (CRP): A trace constituent of serum that increases rapidly following infection or trauma to the body and acts as an opsonin to enhance phagocytosis.

CREST syndrome: A subset of scleroderma named after its five major features: calcinosis, Raynaud's phenomenon, esophageal dysmotility, sclerodactyly, and telangiectasia.

Crossmatch: Incubation of donor lymphocytes with recipient serum to determine the presence of antibodies, which would indicate rejection of a potential transplant.

Cross-reactivity: A phenomenon that occurs when an antibody reacts with an antigen that is structurally similar to the original antigen that induced antibody production.

Cryoglobulins: Immunoglobulins of the immunoglobulin M (IgM) or IgG class that precipitate at cold temperatures, causing occlusion of blood vessels in the extremities if a patient is exposed to the cold.

Cryptococcosis: A fungal disease caused by *Cryptococcus neoformans* and characterized as a pulmonary infection that may spread to the central nervous system and the brain.

C-type lectin receptors (CLRs): Plasma-membrane receptors found on white blood cells (WBCs) that bind to mannan and β-glucans in fungal cell walls.

Cyst: Inactive form of a parasite that can transmit infection.

Cytogenetics: The branch of genetics devoted to the study of chromosomes.

Cytokine: Small protein that acts as a chemical messenger to affect the function or activity of other cells, especially cells of the immune system.

Cytomegalovirus (CMV): A virus in the herpes family that is responsible for infection, ranging from a mononucleosis-like syndrome to a life-threatening illness in immunocompromised patients.

Cytotoxic T cell: T cells that bear the CD8 marker and function to kill virus-infected cells and tumor cells by triggering apoptosis.

Decay-accelerating factor (DAF): A glycoprotein found on peripheral red blood cells (RBCs), endothelial cells, fibroblasts, and epithelial cell surfaces that is capable of dissociating C3 convertases formed by both the classical and alternative pathways of complement.

Defensins: Small cationic proteins that, when released from lysosomal granules, can kill bacteria and many fungi by destroying their cell walls.

Delayed hypersensitivity: Type IV or T-cell–mediated hypersensitivity; so named because its manifestations are not seen until 24 to 48 hours after exposure to the inducing antigen.

Delta check: A QA procedure that compares a patient's test results with the previous results.

Dendritic cell: Tissue cells covered with long membranous extensions that make them resemble nerve cell dendrites.

Deoxyribonucleic acid (DNA): The nucleic acid whose sugar is deoxyribose. It is the primary genetic material of all cellular organisms and DNA viruses.

Dermatomyositis (DM): A systemic autoimmune rheumatic disease that involves the skin.

Diagnostic sensitivity: The proportion of people who have a specific disease or condition and who have a positive test result.

Diagnostic specificity: The proportion of people who do not have a disease or condition and who have a negative test result.

Diapedesis: The process by which cells are capable of moving from the circulating blood to the tissues by squeezing through the wall of a blood vessel.

DiGeorge syndrome: A congenital defect of the third and fourth pharyngeal pouches that affects thymic development, leading to a T-cell deficiency.

Diluent: One of two entities needed for making up a solution. It is the medium into which the solute is added.

Direct agglutination: A clumping of cells that occurs when antibodies react with antigens that are naturally found on the surface of the cells.

Direct allorecognition: Pathway in which recipient T cells recognize intact human leukocyte (HLA) molecules on donor cells.

Direct antiglobulin test (DAT): A technique to determine in vivo attachment of antibody or complement to red blood cells (RBCs), using anti-human globulin to cause a visible agglutination reaction.

Direct immunofluorescence assay: A technique to identify a specific antigen using an antibody that has a fluorescent tag attached.

Domain: Region of an antibody molecule that consists of approximately 110 amino acids.

Double-negative (DN) thymocyte: Stage in the development of T cells when neither CD4 nor CD8 is expressed.

Double-positive (DP) thymocyte: Stage in the development of T cells when both CD4 and CD8 antigens are expressed.

Double-stranded DNA (dsDNA) antibodies: Autoantibodies produced against double-stranded DNA that are diagnostic for systemic lupus erythematosus (SLE).

Dual-parameter dot plot: Grouping of cells based on two different characteristics, one of which is plotted on the *x*-axis and the other on the *y*-axis.

Ectoparasite: Multicelled parasitic organism that lives on the skin of the host.

Effector cells: Mature, functional T lymphocytes or B lymphocytes that carry out the functions of immune responses.

Electrochemiluminescence immunoassay (ECLIA): A modified chemiluminescence immunoassay in which an antibody reagent is labeled with ruthenium, which is oxidized at the surface of an electrode and releases light when it is returned to its reduced state.

Electrophoresis: The separation of molecules in an electrical field based on differences in charge and size.

ELISA: See *enzyme-linked immunosorbent assay.*

ELISpot: A modified ELISA technique that detects the frequency of cultured cells that secrete a particular cytokine.

Endocrine: Internal secretion of substances, such as hormones or cytokines, directly into the bloodstream that causes systemic effects.

Endogenous pyrogen: A substance produced by the body that causes fever. Interleukin-1 is an example.

Endotoxin: A component of the cell walls of gram-negative bacteria, which consists of the portion of lipopolysaccharide (LPS) called *lipid A*. Endotoxin is a potent stimulator of cytokine release that can lead to septic shock.

Endpoint method: A radial immunodiffusion technique in which antigen is allowed to diffuse out until the point of equivalence is reached.

Enzyme: A protein that acts as a catalyst for a specific biochemical reaction; commonly used as a label in immunoassays.

Enzyme immunoassay (EIA): An assay that uses an enzyme label to detect an antigen–antibody reaction; the enzyme acts on a substrate to produce a colored product, light, or fluorescence.

Enzyme-linked immunosorbent assay (ELISA): An immunoassay that employs an enzyme label on one of the reactants.

Enzyme-multiplied immunoassay technique (EMIT): A homogeneous immunoassay based on the principle of change in enzyme activity as a specific antigen–antibody interaction occurs in solution.

Eosinophil: A white blood cell (WBC) that contains reddish-orange granules on Wright-stained blood smears and is involved in allergic reactions.

Epigenetics: The study of modifications in gene expression that are not caused by changes in the nucleotide sequence of DNA.

Epitope: The key portion of the immunogen against which the immune response is directed; also known as the *determinant site.*

Epitope spreading: An expansion of an immune response to unrelated antigens, which may be involved in the development of autoimmunity.

Epstein-Barr virus (EBV): A DNA virus of the herpesvirus family.

Erythropoietin (EPO): A colony-stimulating factor that increases red blood cell (RBC) production in the bone marrow.

Examination variable: A variable that includes reagent and test performance, instrument calibration and maintenance, personnel requirements, and technical competence.

Exotoxin: Potent protein released from living bacteria (mostly gram-positive) that causes harm to the host by binding to a specific cellular receptor.

External defense system: Structural barriers that prevent most infectious agents from entering the body.

External quality assessment (EQA): The testing of unknown samples received from an outside agency.

Extractable nuclear antigen (ENA): A member of a family of small nuclear proteins associated with uridine-rich ribonucleic acid (RNA) that can stimulate the production of autoantibodies; examples are Sm and RNP.

Extrinsic parameter: In flow cytometry, properties of a cell such as a surface protein that require addition of a fluorescent-labeled antibody for their detection.

F(ab')$_2$: Fragment of an immunoglobulin molecule obtained by pepsin cleavage that consists of two light chains and two heavy-chain halves held together by disulfide bonding. This piece has two antigen-binding sites.

Fab fragment: Fragment of an immunoglobulin molecule obtained by papain cleavage that consists of a light chain and one-half of a heavy chain held together by disulfide bonding.

Factor H: A control protein in the complement system. It acts as a cofactor with factor I to break down C3b formed during complement activation.

Factor I: A serine protease that cleaves C3b and C4b formed during complement activation. A different cofactor is required for each of these reactions.

Fc fragment: Fragment of an immunoglobulin molecule obtained by papain cleavage that consists of the carboxy-terminal halves of two heavy chains. These two halves are held together by disulfide bonds. This fragment spontaneously crystallizes at 4°C.

Fibrinogen: An acute-phase reactant that changes to fibrin and forms clots in the bloodstream.

Flocculation: The formation of downy masses of precipitate that occurs over a narrow range of antigen concentration.

Flow cytometer: An automated system in which single cells in a fluid are analyzed in terms of intrinsic light-scattering characteristics as well as extrinsic properties.

Flow cytometry: An automated system for identifying cells based on the scattering of light as cells flow single file through a laser beam.

Fluorescence in situ hybridization (FISH): A technique used to identify a specific region of DNA in a chromosome through binding of fluorescent-tagged complementary DNA probes.

Fluorescence polarization immunoassay (FPIA): An immunoassay based on the change in polarization of fluorescent light emitted from a labeled molecule when it is bound by antibody.

Fluorescent anti-nuclear antibody (FANA) testing: Testing to identify the presence of antibody to nuclear antigens, using human epithelial cells and a fluorescent-labeled anti-human immunoglobulin.

Fluorescent treponemal antibody absorption (FTA-ABS) test: A confirmatory test for syphilis, which detects antibodies to *Treponema pallidum* by using anti-human immunoglobulin with a fluorescent label.

Fluorochrome: See *fluorophores*.

Fluorophores: Compounds that absorb energy from an incident light source and convert that energy into light of a longer wavelength and lower energy as the excited electrons return to the ground state.

Fomite: An inanimate object that can become contaminated with an infectious agent and transmit the agent to a new host.

Forward-angle light scatter (FSC): Light scattered at an angle of less than 90 degrees, which indicates the size of a cell.

Fungi: Organisms made up of eukaryotic cells with rigid walls composed of chitin, mannan, and sometimes cellulose.

Gate: A set of filters placed around a population of interest to analyze various parameters (extrinsic and intrinsic) of the cells contained within the selected region.

Gel electrophoresis: Method of separating either proteins or DNA based on their size and electrical charge. Samples are placed in wells on the gel and exposed to an electrical current.

Genes: Specific sequences of nucleotides in chromosomes that carry information for a protein or a noncoding RNA molecule.

Genetic code: A set of three nucleotides that code for one amino acid.

Genome: The entire set of genes in an organism.

Genomics: The study of all the genes in an organism.

Germinal center: The interior of a secondary follicle where blast transformation of B cells takes place.

Globally Harmonized System (GHS): An international system that standardizes the classification of hazardous chemicals and the symbols used for these hazards on labels and in safety data sheets.

Goodpasture's syndrome: An autoimmune disease characterized by the presence of an autoantibody to collagen in the glomerular (kidney) or alveolar (lung) basement membranes; also known as *anti-glomerular basement membrane disease*.

Graduated pipette: A pipette that has markings all along its length to allow for varying amounts of liquid to be measured.

Graft-versus-host disease (GVHD): A condition that results from transplantation of immunocompetent cells into an immunodeficient host. The transfused cells attack the tissues of the recipient within the first 100 days posttransplant.

Granulocyte colony-stimulating factor (G-CSF): A cytokine produced by fibroblasts and epithelial cells that enhances the production of neutrophils.

Granulocyte-macrophage colony-stimulating factor (GM-CSF): A cytokine produced by T cells and other cell lines that stimulates increased production of granulocytic cells and macrophages.

Granuloma: An organized cluster of inflammatory cells formed in some type IV hypersensitivity responses.

Granulomatosis with polyangiitis (PGA): An autoimmune disease involving inflammation of the small- to medium-sized blood vessels and the production of anti-neutrophil cytoplasmic antibody (ANCA); formerly known as *Wegener's granulomatosus*.

Graves' disease: An autoimmune disease characterized by hyperthyroidism caused by the presence of antibody to thyroid-stimulating hormone receptors. Antigen–antibody combination results in continual release of thyroid hormones.

Group A streptococcus (GAS): Gram-positive, catalase-negative cocci often found in pairs or chains that are responsible for diseases ranging from pharyngitis to necrotizing fasciitis.

Gummas: Localized areas of granulomatous inflammation on bones, skin, and subcutaneous tissue caused by tertiary syphilis.

Hairy-cell leukemia: Chronic leukemia characterized by the formation of large mononuclear cells with irregular cytoplasmic projections found in bone marrow.

Haplotype: A set of genes that are located close together on a chromosome and are usually inherited as a single unit.

Hapten: A simple chemical group that can bind to antibody once it is formed but that cannot stimulate antibody formation unless bound to a larger carrier molecule.

Haptoglobin: An acute-phase reactant that binds irreversibly to free hemoglobin released by intravascular hemolysis.

Hashimoto's thyroiditis: An autoimmune disease that results in hypothyroidism caused by the presence of antithyroglobulin and thyroid peroxidase antibodies, which progressively destroy the thyroid gland.

Heavy (H) chain: One of the polypeptide units that makes up an immunoglobulin molecule. Each immunoglobulin monomer consists of two heavy chains paired with two light chains.

Heavy-chain diseases: B-cell lymphomas characterized by the production of monoclonal immunoglobulin heavy chains that are not attached to light chains.

Helicobacter pylori: A gram-negative spiral bacterium that is a major cause of gastric and duodenal ulcers.

Helminth: Parasitic worm, such as a flatworm, tapeworms or roundworm.

Hemagglutination: An antigen–antibody reaction that results in the clumping of red blood cells (RBCs).

Hemagglutination inhibition: A test for detecting antibodies to certain viruses, based on lack of agglutination that results from antibody neutralizing the virus.

Hematopoiesis: The production of blood cells from multipotent hematopoietic stem cells in the bone marrow.

Hematopoietic growth factors: Cytokines or other factors in the blood that stimulate formation and differentiation of blood cells.

Hemolytic disease of the fetus and newborn (HDFN): A cytotoxic reaction that destroys an infant's red blood cells (RBCs) because of placental transfer of maternal antibodies to Rh antigens.

Hemolytic titration (CH_{50}) assay: An assay that measures complement-activating ability by determining the amount of patient serum required to lyse 50% of a standardized concentration of antibody-sensitized sheep erythrocytes.

Hemolytic uremic syndrome (HUS): A condition characterized by hemolytic anemia, low platelet count, and acute renal failure caused by either a Shiga toxin related to an infection or complement dysregulation.

Hepatitis: Inflammation of the liver that can be caused by several viruses as well as noninfectious factors, such as radiation, exposure to chemicals, or autoimmune diseases.

Hepatitis A virus (HAV): An RNA virus that can cause hepatitis; transmitted by the fecal–oral route, close person-to-person contact, or ingestion of contaminated food or water.

Hepatitis B surface antigen (HBsAg): The surface antigen of hepatitis B virus, the first marker to appear in hepatitis B infection.

Hepatitis B virus (HBV): A DNA virus that can cause hepatitis; it is transmitted by a parenteral route, through sexual contact, or acquired perinatally.

Hepatitis Be antigen (HBeAg): Antigen associated with the capsid of hepatitis B virus.

Hepatitis C virus (HCV): A ribonucleic acid (RNA) virus that can cause hepatitis; it is transmitted sexually or through contaminated blood or needles.

Hepatitis D virus (HDV): A ribonucleic acid (RNA) virus that can cause hepatitis; it requires the presence of hepatitis B virus (HBV) for its replication and expression.

Hepatitis E virus (HEV): A ribonucleic acid (RNA) virus that can cause hepatitis; it is transmitted by the fecal–oral route or ingestion of contaminated food or water.

Herd immunity: Concept of extending protection to unvaccinated individuals by reducing spread of an infection when a significant proportion of individuals in the population have been immunized; also known as *community immunity*.

Hereditary angioedema (HAE): A disease characterized by swelling of the extremities, the skin, the gastrointestinal tract, and other mucosal surfaces because of a deficiency in the complement inhibitor C1NH.

Heteroantigen: An antigen of a species different from that of the host, such as other animals, plants, or microorganisms.

Heterogeneous immunoassay: Immunoassay in which enzyme is used as a label and that requires a separation step to separate free from bound analyte.

Heterophile antibody: Antibody that is capable of reacting with similar antigens from two or more unrelated species; commonly found in patients with infectious mononucleosis.

Heterophile antigen: An antigen that exists in unrelated plants or animals but is either identical or closely related so that antibody to one will cross-react with antibody to the other.

High-dose hook effect: Limitation of antibody-based assays caused by massive amounts of tumor marker antigens present.

Hinge region: The flexible portion of the heavy chain of an immunoglobulin molecule that is located between the first and second constant regions. This allows the molecule to bend to let the two antigen-binding sites operate independently.

Histamine: A vasoactive amine released from mast cells and basophils during an allergic reaction.

Histoplasmosis: An infection caused by the fungus *Histoplasma. capsulatum*.

HLA antibody screen: Test for HLA antibodies in candidates and recipients of solid-organ transplants.

HLA genotype: Actual alleles, for human leukocyte antigen (HLA) antigens, that are inherited.

HLA matching: The pairing up of donor and recipient in a transplant on the basis of similar human leukocyte antigen (HLA) antigens.

HLA phenotype: The expression of human leukocyte antigen (HLA) genes that actually appear as proteins on cells.

HLA typing: Laboratory testing used to identify the human leukocyte antigen (HLA) antigens or genes in a transplant candidate or donor.

Hodgkin lymphoma (HL): A malignant disease that typically begins in one lymph node and is characterized by the presence of Reed-Sternberg cells, giant multinucleated cells that are usually transformed B lymphocytes.

Homogeneous immunoassay: An immunoassay in which no separation step is necessary. It is based on the principle of a decrease in enzyme activity when specific antigen–antibody combination occurs.

Human chorionic gonadotropin (hCG): A hormone that is synthesized by trophoblasts and used as a marker for tumors of the ovaries, testes, and trophoblast cells.

Human epidermal growth factor receptor 2 (HER2): A transmembrane receptor that binds human epidermal growth factor; it is overexpressed in a certain type of breast cancer.

Human immune serum globulin (HISG): A sterile preparation of concentrated antibodies made from pooled serum of thousands of donors; used as a prophylactic treatment in patients with antibody deficiencies.

Human immunodeficiency virus (HIV): A retrovirus that is the etiologic agent of AIDS.

Human leukocyte antigen (HLA): Protein coded for by the human major histocompatibility class (MHC) genes that has essential roles in the immune response and the rejection of foreign transplants.

Human T-cell lymphotropic virus type I (HTLV-I): A ribonucleic acid (RNA) retrovirus that causes adult T-cell leukemia or lymphoma and HTLV associated myelopathy/tropical spastic paraparesis.

Human T-cell lymphotropic virus type II (HTLV-II): A ribonucleic acid (RNA) retrovirus that is thought to be associated with neurological disease, certain hematologic and dermatological diseases, and an increased incidence of infections.

Humoral immunity: Protection from disease resulting from substances in the serum (e.g., antibodies).

Hybridization: Specific binding of two single-stranded DNA segments, as in binding of a probe with a known nucleic acid sequence to an unknown piece of DNA.

Hybridoma: A cell line resulting from the fusion of a myeloma cell and a B cell. These can be maintained in tissue culture indefinitely and can produce a very specific type of antibody known as a *monoclonal antibody*.

Hyperacute rejection: Rejection of tissue that occurs within minutes or hours following transplantation, because of antibodies to ABO and human leukocyte antigen (HLA) antigens that are already present in the graft recipient.

Hypercytokinemia: Dysregulation of cytokines, producing hyperstimulation of the immune response.

Hypersensitivity: A heightened state of immune responsiveness.

Hyphae: Filamentous tubular branching structures characteristic of some fungi.

Idiotype: The variable portion of light and heavy immunoglobulin chains that is unique to a particular immunoglobulin molecule. This region constitutes the antigen-binding site.

IgM anti-HBc: Antibody that is the first to appear in hepatitis B infection. It is of the immunoglobulin M (IgM) class and is directed against the core antigen on the virus particle.

Immature B cell: A phase in the growth of B cells characterized by the appearance of complete immunoglobulin M (IgM) antibody molecules on the cell surface.

Immediate hypersensitivity: Reaction to an allergen that occurs in minutes and can be life-threatening.

Immune adherence: The ability of phagocytic cells to bind complement-coated particles.

Immune checkpoint inhibitors: Monoclonal antibodies that enhance patients' T-cell responses to tumors by blocking inhibitory pathways that inactivate T cells; examples include antibodies to CTLA-4, PD-1, and PD-L1.

Immunity: The condition of being resistant to infection.

Immunization: The process by which immunity is acquired.

Immunoblotting: A technique used to identify antibodies to complex antigens. It consists of electrophoresis of the antigen mix followed by transfer of the pattern to nitrocellulose paper for reaction with patient serum.

Immunochromatography: A rapid technique in which the analyte is applied at one end of a strip and migrates toward the distal end, where the results can be visualized in minutes.

Immunodeficiencies: Inherited or acquired disorders in which a part of the body's immune system is missing or dysfunctional.

Immunoediting: The ability of tumor cells to escape immune surveillance through suppression of immunogenicity.

Immunofixation electrophoresis (IFE): A semiquantitative gel precipitation technique in which proteins are first separated by electrophoresis, then incubated with antibodies to individual proteins that are added directly to the gel surface; used commonly to identify monoclonal immunoglobulins.

Immunofluorescence assay (IFA): Test used to identify cellular antigens or antibodies to those antigens using an antibody with a fluorescent tag.

Immunogen: Any substance that is capable of inducing an immune response.

Immunogenicity: The ability of an immunogen to stimulate a host response.

Immunoglobulin (Ig): Glycoproteins in the serum portion of the blood that are a major component of humoral immunity.

Immunohistochemistry: The use of labeled antibodies to directly detect tumor markers in tissue.

Immunologic diversion: A mechanism by which parasites enhance their survival in the host by inducing the production of proteins that divert the attention of the immune system.

Immunologic subversion: A mechanism by which parasites can avoid the effector mechanisms of the immune response by producing proteins that act as homologues of various components of the immune system.

Immunologic tolerance: A state of immune unresponsiveness directed against a specific antigen.

Immunology: The study of the reactions of a host when foreign substances are introduced into the body.

Immunometric assay: An immunoassay in which antibody to the target antigen is bound to the solid phase; also known as a *capture* or *sandwich* immunoassay.

Immunophenotyping: Identifying cells according to their surface antigen expression.

Immunoprophylaxis: The use of immunization to prevent disease.

Immunosubtraction (immunotyping): A procedure that uses capillary electrophoresis to identify monoclonal immunoglobulin components.

Immunosuppressive agent: An agent used to suppress an antigraft immune response to transplanted tissue.

Immunosurveillance: The mechanisms by which the immune system patrols the body for the presence of cancerous or pre-cancerous cells and eliminates them before they become clinically evident.

Immunotherapy: Treatment that uses the ability of the immune system to destroy tumor cells.

Immunotoxins: Antibodies conjugated to toxins to help destroy cancer cells.

Immunoturbidimetry: A technique for determining the concentration of particles in a solution based on the change in absorbance, caused by a reduction in light intensity that occurs when an incident beam is passed through a solution in which antigen-antibody complexes are forming.

Impetigo: A skin infection caused by bacteria such as Group A streptococci.

In situ hybridization (ISH): Molecular assays that detect targets "in place" as they appear in tissues, cells, and subcellular structures.

Indigenous microbiota: Symbiotic microorganisms that reside on and colonize the surfaces of an individual, also known as *normal flora.*

Indirect allorecognition: Pathway by which the immune system recognizes foreign human leukocyte antigen (HLA) proteins on a donor graft; it involves the uptake, processing, and presentation of foreign HLA proteins by the recipient's antigen-presenting cells (APCs) to recipient T cells to produce antibodies and cell-mediated responses against the graft.

Indirect antiglobulin test (IAT): A laboratory method that detects in vitro binding of antibody to red blood cells (RBCs); it is used in the crossmatching of blood to prevent a transfusion reaction.

Indirect ELISAs: Enzyme immunoassays that detect an antibody in the test sample using a labeled antibody reagent.

Indirect immunofluorescence (IIF) assay: A technique to identify antigen by using two antibodies: one that is specific to the antigen and a second that is an anti-human immunoglobulin with a fluorescent tag.

Infection control: Procedures used to control and monitor infections occurring within health-care facilities.

Infectivity: An organism's ability to establish an infection; the proportion of individuals exposed to a pathogen through horizontal transmission (i.e., person-to-person contact) who will become infected.

Inflammasome: A protein oligomer that contains caspase enzymes and other proteins associated with apoptosis; it may be defective in some autoinflammatory disorders.

Inflammation: Cellular and humoral mechanisms involved in the overall reaction of the body to injury or invasion by an infectious agent.

Inflammatory myopathies (IMs): A group of systemic autoimmune diseases characterized by chronic inflammation of the skeletal muscles and progressive muscle weakness.

Innate lymphoid cell (ILC): Family of cells that contribute to innate immunity and tissue remodeling; ILCs develop from the common lymphoid progenitor and have lymphoid morphology but do not possess antigen-specific receptors.

Innate (natural) immunity: The ability of the individual to resist infection by means of normally present body functions.

Integrins: Molecules on certain leukocytes that cause adhesion to endothelial cells.

Interferons (IFNs): Cytokines produced by T cells and other cell lines that inhibit viral synthesis or act as immune regulators.

Interleukin (IL): A group of cytokines produced by leukocytes and other cells that regulate adaptive immune responses and the inflammatory process.

Internal defense system: Defense mechanism inside the body in which both cells and soluble factors play essential parts.

Intrinsic parameter: Light-scattering properties that are a part of the cell, such as size and granularity.

Invariant chain: A protein that associates with human leukocyte antigen (HLA) class II antigens shortly after they are synthesized to prevent interaction of their binding sites with any endogenous peptides in the endoplasmic reticulum.

Isograft (syngeneic graft): Graft that involves the transfer of tissue between two genetically identical members of the same species.

Isohemagglutinin: Antibody that agglutinates red blood cells (RBCs) of other individuals of the same species; in humans, they are directed against the A or B antigens on RBCs.

Isothermal: An amplification process using a reaction that proceeds at a single temperature.

Isotype: A unique amino acid sequence that is common to all immunoglobulin molecules of a given class in a given species.

Isotype switching: A genetically-driven process by which B cells change their antibody production from immunoglobulin M (IgM) to another immunoglobulin class.

Joining (J) chain: A glycoprotein with a molecular weight of 15,000 that serves to link immunoglobulin monomers together. J chains are found only in immunoglobulin M (IgM) and secretory immunoglobulin A (IgA) molecules.

Kappa (κ) chain: One of two types of immunoglobulin light chains that are present in approximately two-thirds of all immunoglobulin molecules.

Karyotype analysis: A test used to examine the chromosomes in a cell sample for numerical or structural abnormalities.

Lambda (λ) chain: One of two types of immunoglobulin light chains that are present in approximately one-third of all immunoglobulin molecules.

Lancefield group: A means of classifying streptococci on the basis of differences in the cell wall carbohydrate.

Lateral flow immunochromatographic assay (LFA): Immunochromatographic assay for rapid antigen detection.

Lattice: The combination of antibody and multivalent antigen to produce a stable complex that results in a visible reaction.

Law of mass action: A law used to mathematically describe the equilibrium relationship between soluble reactants and insoluble products. It can be applied to antigen–antibody relationships.

Lean system: A system used in the laboratory that focuses on the elimination of waste to allow a facility to do more with less and at the same time increase customer and employee satisfaction.

Lectin pathway: A pathway for the activation of complement based on binding of mannose-binding protein to constituents on bacterial cell walls.

***Leptospira* species:** Spirochete bacteria that cause leptospirosis.

Leptospirosis: Infection caused by tightly coiled spirochete bacteria called *leptospires.*

Leukemia: A progressive malignant disease of blood-forming organs, characterized by proliferation of leukocytes and their precursors in the bone marrow.

Leukocytes: White blood cells (WBCs).

Leukotrienes (LT): A class of secondary mediators released from mast cells and basophils during type I hypersensitivity reactions.

Light (L) chain: Small chain in an immunoglobulin molecule that is bound to the larger chain by disulfide bonds. The two types of light chains are called *kappa* and *lambda.*

Linear epitope: Amino acids following one another on a single polypeptide chain that act as a key antigenic site.

Leptospirosis: Infection caused by tightly coiled spirochetes called *leptospires.*

Lyme disease: A disease caused by infection with the spirochete bacteria *Borrelia burgdorferi.*

Lymph node: A secondary lymphoid organ that is located along a lymphatic duct and whose purpose is to filter lymphatic fluid from the tissues and act as a site for processing of foreign antigen.

Lymphocyte: The key white blood cell (WBC) involved in the adaptive immune response.

Lymphomas: Cancers of the lymphoid cells that tend to proliferate as solid tumors.

Macrophage: A white blood cell (WBC) that engulfs and kills microbes and presents antigen to T cells.

Macrophage colony-stimulating factor (M-CSF): A cytokine that induces growth of hematopoietic cells destined to become monocytes and macrophages.

Major histocompatibility complex (MHC): The genes that control expression of a large group of proteins originally identified on leukocytes but now known to be found on all nucleated cells in the body. These proteins regulate the immune response and play a role in graft rejection.

MALDI-TOF: Matrix-associated laser desorption ionization time-of-flight mass spectrometry, a technique used to analyze proteins to identify a substance or microorganism in a sample.

Malignant: A descriptive term for cancerous tumors that can circulate to other parts of the body and invade nearby organs.

Mannose-binding lectin (MBL): A protein present in the blood that binds to mannose on bacterial cells and initiates the lectin pathway for complement activation.

Mast cell: A tissue cell that plays a role in allergic reactions.

Membrane attack complex (MAC): The combination of complement components C5b, C6, C7, C8, and C9 that becomes inserted into the target-cell membrane, causing lysis.

Membrane cofactor protein (MCP): A protein found on all epithelial and endothelial cells that helps to control complement-mediated lysis by acting as a cofactor for Factor I–mediated cleavage of C3b.

Memory cell: Progeny of an antigen-activated B or T cell that is able to respond to antigen more quickly than the parent cell.

Metastasis: Process of malignant cells traveling through the body, thereby causing new foci of malignancy.

MHC restriction: The selection of thymocytes that will only interact with the major histocompatibility complex (MHC) antigens found on host cells.

MIA: see *Multiplex immunoassay.*

Microarray: A technology that enables simultaneous analysis of thousands of genes in a sample by hybridization with a panel of molecular probes that are complementary to portions of specific genes or chromosome regions; the probes are spotted onto separate locations on a small glass slide or nylon membrane.

Microbiome: The collection of microorganisms that exists on the body, including bacteria, viruses, yeast, and fungi.

Micropipette: Mechanical pipette that delivers volumes in the microliter (μL) range; used when very small volumes are needed.

Microscopic agglutination test (MAT): A technique that is the gold standard for diagnosing leptospirosis.

Minor histocompatibility antigens (mHAs): Non-human leukocyte antigen (HLA) proteins that can induce a weak graft rejection response when introduced into an individual possessing a different polymorphic variant.

Mitogen: A substance that stimulates mitosis in all T cells or all B cells, regardless of antigen specificity.

Mixed connective tissue disease (MCTD): An autoimmune disorder characterized by overlapping features of limited cutaneous systemic sclerosis (SSc), systemic lupus erythematosus (SLE), polymyositis, and rheumatoid arthritis.

Mixed lymphocyte reaction (MLR): An assay that measures the proliferation of responder T cells to non-self antigens in a potential transplant donor.

Molecular mimicry: The similarity between an infectious agent and a self-antigen that causes antibody formed in response to the former to cross-react with the latter.

Monoclonal: Derived from a single clone of identical cells.

Monoclonal antibody: Very specific antibody derived from a single antibody-producing cell that has been cloned or duplicated.

Monoclonal gammopathy: A disorder in which a clone of lymphoid cells causes overproduction of a single immunoglobulin component called a *paraprotein.*

Monoclonal gammopathy of undetermined significance (MGUS): A premalignant plasma cell disorder characterized by the presence of monoclonal immunoglobulin in the serum, a plasma bone marrow count of less than 10%, and absence of clinical features. Some cases may progress to multiple myeloma through time.

Monocyte: The largest white blood cell (WBC) in peripheral blood. It migrates to the tissues to become a macrophage.

Multiple myeloma: A malignancy of mature plasma cells that results in a monoclonal increase in an immunoglobulin component, most commonly IgG.

Multiple sclerosis (MS): An autoimmune disease in which the myelin sheath of axons becomes progressively destroyed by antibodies to myelin proteins.

Multiplex immunoassay (MIA): An automated immunoassay that uses a mixture of polystyrene beads conjugated with different antigens or antibodies as the solid phase and a fluorescent-tagged antibody to simultaneously detect multiple antibodies or antigens in a sample by flow cytometry.

Mumps virus: A single-stranded ribonucleic acid (RNA) virus that is the causative agent of mumps, a disease characterized by swelling of the parotid glands.

Mutation: A permanent change in the nucleotide sequence within a gene or chromosome.

Mutualistic: A relationship between a human host and microbial species in which both organisms benefit.

Myasthenia gravis (MG): An autoimmune disease characterized by progressive muscle weakness caused by formation of antibody to acetylcholine receptors.

Mycelial fungi: Multicellular fungi that are made up of intertwined hyphae and reproduce through the production of spores.

Mycoplasma pneumoniae: A small gram-negative bacterium that lacks a cell wall and is the cause of upper respiratory infections.

Mycoses: Infections or Diseases produced by fungi.

Natural killer (NK) cell: A type of lymphocyte that has the ability to kill target cells such as tumor cells and virus-infected cells without prior exposure to them.

Negative predictive value: The probability that a person with a negative screening test does not have the disease being tested for.

Negative selection: The process by which T cells that can respond to self-antigen are destroyed in the thymus.

Neoplasm: An abnormal cell mass; a tumor.

Nephelometry: A technique for determining the concentration of particles in a solution by measuring the light scattered at a particular angle from the incident beam as it passes through the solution.

Neutrophil: A white blood cell (WBC) with a multilobed nucleus and a large number of neutral staining granules on a blood smear treated with Wright stain. Its main function is phagocytosis.

Next-generation sequencing (NGS): A technique that is able to sequence large numbers of DNA templates simultaneously (massively parallel sequencing), yielding hundreds of thousands of short nucleotide sequences in a single run.

Noncompetitive immunoassay: An immunoassay in which patient antigen is captured by antibody bound to a solid phase and detected by subsequent addition of a labeled antibody. The amount of label measured is directly proportional to the amount of patient antigen present in the test sample.

Non-Hodgkin or lymphocytic lymphoma (NHL): A wide range of cancers of the lymphoid tissue, of which B-cell lymphomas represent the majority.

Nontreponemal tests: Serological tests for syphilis that detect antibody to cardiolipin and instead of specific antitreponemal antibody.

Nucleic acid: A sequence of nucleotides that carries the genetic information for a protein; DNA or RNA.

Nucleolus: A prominent structure within the nucleus where transcription and processing of ribosomal ribonucleic acid (rRNA) and assembly of the ribosomes takes place.

Nucleosome antibodies: Autoantibodies against DNA–histone complexes [also known as nucleosomes or deoxyribonucleoprotein (DNP)].

Nucleotide: A unit of DNA or ribonucleic acid (RNA) composed of a phosphorylated ribose or deoxyribose sugar and a nitrogen base.

Occupational Safety and Health Administration (OSHA): A federal agency that monitors and enforces safety regulations for workers.

Oncofetal antigens: Antigens that are expressed in the developing fetus and in rapidly dividing tissue, such as that associated with tumors, but that are absent in normal adult tissue.

Oncogene: Gene that encodes a protein capable of inducing cellular transformation.

Opportunistic illnesses: Infections or malignancies that primarily occur in individuals who are immunocompromised.

Opsonins: Serum proteins that attach to a foreign substance and enhance phagocytosis (from the Greek word meaning "to prepare for eating").

Opsonization: Coating of a foreign antigen with antibody or complement to enhance phagocytosis.

Ouchterlony double diffusion: A qualitative gel precipitation technique in which both antigen and antibody diffuse out from wells cut in the gel. The pattern obtained indicates whether or not antigens are identical.

Oxidative burst: An increase in oxygen consumption in phagocytic cells, which generate oxygen radicals used to kill engulfed microorganisms.

p24 antigen: A structural core antigen that is part of HIV.

Paracrine: Secretions such as cytokines that affect only target cells in close proximity.

Paraprotein (M protein): A single immunoglobulin component produced by a malignant clone of lymphoid cells in lymphoproliferative diseases.

Parasite: Microorganism that survives by living off of another organism.

Parasitic: Relationship in which an organism causes harm to its host.

Paratope: An antigen-binding site on an antibody molecule.

Parenteral: Mode of transmission other than through the intestinal tract, most notably bloodborne transmission.

Paroxysmal cold hemoglobinuria: A condition in which patients produce a biphasic autoantibody that binds to red blood cells (RBCs) at cold temperatures and activates complement at 37°C to produce an intermittent hemolysis.

Paroxysmal nocturnal hemoglobinuria (PNH): A disease characterized by complement-mediated hemolysis of erythrocytes resulting from a deficiency of decay-accelerating factor on the red blood cells (RBCs).

Particle agglutination (PA) test: Agglutination test that uses antigen-coated gel particles or red blood cells to detect antibody to *Treponema pallidum.*

Passive agglutination: A reaction in which particles coated with antigens not normally found on their surfaces clump together because of their combination with antibody.

Passive immunity: A type of immunity that results from the transfer of antibodies from immunized hosts to a nonimmune individual.

Passive immunodiffusion: A precipitation reaction in a gel in which antigen–antibody combination occurs by means of diffusion.

Passive immunotherapy: Passive immunization of an individual with commercial preparations of antibodies formed by other hosts to prevent or treat a disease.

Pathogen-associated molecular patterns (PAMPs): Structural patterns of carbohydrates, nucleic acids, or bacterial peptides on microorganisms that are recognized by pathogen recognition receptors (PRRs) on the cells of the innate immune system.

Pathogenicity: The inherent capacity of an organism to cause disease.

Pattern recognition receptors (PRRs): Receptors on cells of the innate immune system that bind to PAMPs on pathogenic microorganisms.

Percent panel reactive antibody (%PRA): Proportion of potential transplant donors in a donor pool possessing one or more human leukocyte antigen (HLA) antigens to which the recipient has antibodies; a calculation that determines the likelihood that a donor and recipient will be incompatible based on HLA frequencies in a large donor population

Periarteriolar lymphoid sheath (PALS): White pulp of splenic tissue, which is made up of lymphocytes, macrophages, plasma cells, and granulocytes. It surrounds the central arterioles.

Peripheral tolerance: Destruction or repression of lymphocytes in the peripheral lymphoid organs that could respond to self-antigens.

Personal protective equipment (PPE): Items such as gowns, masks, gloves, and face shields used to protect the body from infectious agents.

Phagocytosis: From the Greek word *phagein*, meaning "cell eating," the engulfment of cells or particulate matter by neutrophils, macrophages, or other cells.

Phagolysosome: The structure formed by the fusion of cytoplasmic granules and a phagosome during the process of phagocytosis.

Phagosome: A vacuole formed within a phagocytic cell as pseudopodia surround a particle during the process of phagocytosis.

Plasma cell: A differentiated B cell that actively secretes antibody.

Plasma cell dyscrasias: Immunoproliferative diseases characterized by overproduction of a single immunoglobulin component by a clone of lymphoid cells.

Plasmid: A self-replicating genetic element located in the cytoplasm of a bacterium, which has a limited number of genes that can be transferred between bacteria.

Pleiotropy: Many different actions of a single cytokine. The cytokine may affect the activities of more than one kind of cell and have more than one kind of effect on the same cell.

Polyclonal: Derived from many clones of cells. Polyclonal antibodies are derived from many clones of B cells or plasma cells, and are therefore diverse in terms of their antigen specificity.

Polymerase chain reaction (PCR): A means of amplifying tiny quantities of nucleic acid using a heat-stable polymerase enzyme and a primer pair that is specific for the DNA sequence desired.

Polymorphism: The presence of two or more different genetic compositions (e.g., human leukocyte antigen [HLA] genes) among individuals in a population.

Polymyositis (PM): A systemic rheumatic autoimmune disorder that involves inflammation of the skeletal muscles.

Positive predictive value: The percentage of all positives in a serological test that are true positives.

Positive selection: The process of selecting immature T lymphocytes for survival on the basis of expression of high levels of CD3 and the ability to respond to self-major histocompatibility complex (MHC) antigens.

Postexamination variable: A process that affects the reporting of results and correct interpretation of data.

Postexposure prophylaxis (PEP): Course of preventative treatment provided after exposure to potentially infectious organisms.

Poststreptococcal glomerulonephritis: A condition that damages the glomeruli of the kidney, caused by an initial immune response to a streptococcal infection.

Postzone: Lack of a visible reaction in an antigen–antibody combination, caused by an excess of antigen.

Pre-B cell: The stage of development of a B cell where the heavy-chain part of the antibody molecule is present.

Precipitation: The combination of soluble antigen with soluble antibody to produce visible insoluble complexes.

Precision: The ability to consistently reproduce the same result upon repeated testing of the same sample.

Preexamination variable: A variable that occurs before the actual testing of the specimen and includes test requests, patient preparation, timing, specimen collection, handling, and storage.

Primary antibody response: The initial response to a foreign antigen, characterized by a long lag phase and a slow rise in antibody and consisting of mostly immunoglobulin M (IgM).

Primary biliary cholangitis (PBC): An autoimmune disease that involves progressive destruction of the intrahepatic bile ducts; formerly known as primary biliary cirrhosis

Primary follicle: A cluster of B cells that have not yet been stimulated by antigen.

Primary immunodeficiency disease (PID): Inherited diseases in which part of the immune system is absent or dysfunctional.

Primary lymphoid organs: The organs in which lymphocytes mature: these are the bone marrow and the thymus.

Primer: Short sequences of DNA, usually 20 to 30 nucleotides long, used to hybridize specifically to a particular target DNA to help initiate replication of the DNA.

Pro-B cell: A stage in B-cell development in which rearrangement of the genes that code for the heavy-chain region of an antibody molecule occur.

Probe: A nucleic acid, several hundred to a few thousand bases in length, with a known sequence that is used to identify the presence of a complementary DNA or ribonucleic acid (RNA) sequence in an unknown sample.

Proficiency testing: The laboratory testing of unknown samples received from an outside agency.

Properdin: A protein that stabilizes the C3 convertase generated in the alternative complement pathway.

Prostate-specific antigen (PSA): A glycoprotein that is produced specifically by epithelial cells in the prostate gland; PSA is a widely used marker for prostate cancer.

Proteome: The total complement or set of proteins expressed by an organism or cell.

Proteomics: The field of study that involves identification and quantification of the array of proteins present in a sample.

Proto-oncogenes: Normal genes that stimulate cell proliferation and growth; mutations can convert these genes into cancer-promoting oncogenes.

Protozoa: A diverse group of single-celled organisms that can live and multiply inside of human hosts.

Prozone: Lack of a visible reaction in antigen–antibody combination caused by the presence of excess antibody. This may result in a false-negative reaction.

Purine-nucleoside phosphorylase (PNP) deficiency: A disease characterized by lack of the enzyme purine nucleoside phosphorylase, which leads to accumulation of a purine metabolite that is toxic to T cells and a defect in cell-mediated immunity.

Pyrosequencing: A DNA sequencing method that relies on the generation of light when nucleotides are added to a growing strand of DNA.

Quality assessment (QA): The overall process of guaranteeing quality patient care. It involves the continual monitoring of the entire test process from test ordering and specimen collection through reporting and interpreting results.

Quality control (QC): The materials, procedures, and techniques that monitor the accuracy, precision, and reliability of a laboratory test.

Quality indicator: Measurements developed by each laboratory to determine if the quality system essentials are being met.

Quality management (QM): The overall process of guaranteeing quality patient care.

Quality management system (QMS): A system that incorporates the objectives of total quality management and continuous quality improvement to ensure quality results, staff competence, and efficiency within an organization.

Quality system essentials (QSEs): Methods to meet the requirements of regulatory, accreditation, and standard-setting organizations.

Quantitative PCR (qPCR): A molecular test involving accumulation of a polymerase chain reaction (PCR) product in real time during amplification of a nucleic acid sequence.

Radial immunodiffusion (RID): A precipitation technique in which antibody is uniformly distributed in the support gel, and antigen is applied to a well cut into the gel. As the antigen diffuses out from the well, an antigen–antibody combination occurs until the zone of equivalence is reached.

Radioimmunoassay (RIA): A technique used to measure small concentrations of an analyte, using a radioactive label on one of the immunologic reactants.

Random access analyzer: An analyzer that can run multiple tests on multiple samples using multiple analytes.

Rapid antigen detection system (RDTS): See *lateral flow immunochromatographic assay.*

Rapid immunoassays: Membrane-based tests based on immunochromatography and commonly used as point-of-care assays.

Rapid plasma reagin (RPR) test: A slide flocculation test for syphilis that detects antibody to cardiolipin.

Rate nephelometry: A technique that measures the rate of light scattering after the reagent antibody is added to a sample containing patient antigen. The rate change is directly related to antigen concentration if the concentration of antibody is kept constant.

Reagin: An antibody formed during the course of syphilis that is directed against cardiolipin released from host tissues and not against *Treponema pallidum*.

Recognition unit: The complement component that consists of the C1qrs complex. This must bind to at least two Fc regions on antibody molecule(s) to initiate the classical complement cascade.

Recombinant protein vaccine: A vaccine produced by cloning the gene coding for the vaccine antigen into the genome of bacteria, yeast, or cultured cells.

Redundancy: A phenomenon that occurs when different cytokines have the same effect.

Reference interval: The range of values found in healthy individuals who do not have the condition detected by the assay.

Reliability: The ability to maintain both precision and accuracy in laboratory testing.

Reportable range: The range of values that will generate a positive result for the specimens assayed by the test procedure.

Restriction endonucleases: Enzymes that cleave DNA at specific recognition sites that are typically 4 to 6 base pairs long.

Restriction fragment length polymorphisms (RFLPs): Variations in nucleotides within DNA that change where restriction enzymes cleave the DNA. Where mutations occur, different-size pieces of DNA are obtained, resulting in an altered electrophoretic pattern.

Reverse passive agglutination: A reaction in which carrier particles coated with antibody clump together because of a combination with antigen.

Reverse transcriptase: An enzyme produced by certain ribonucleic acid (RNA) viruses to convert viral RNA into DNA.

Rheumatoid arthritis (RA): An autoimmune disease that affects the synovial membrane of multiple joints. It is characterized by the presence of the autoantibodies *anti-CCP* and *rheumatoid factor.*

Rheumatoid factor (RF): An antibody of the immunoglobulin M (IgM) class produced by patients with rheumatoid arthritis that is directed against immunoglobulin G (IgG).

Ribonucleic acid (RNA): The nucleic acid containing the sugar ribose. It is the primary genetic material of RNA viruses and plays a role in the transcribing of genetic information in cells.

Rickettsiae: Small gram-negative fastidious bacteria that are obligate intracellular parasites and are responsible for diseases such as Rocky Mountain spotted fever and typhus.

Rocky Mountain spotted fever (RMSF): A disease caused by infection with *R. rickettsii.*

Root cause analysis (RCA): A problem-solving protocol used to identify the causes of adverse events in a health-care setting.

Rubella virus: A ribonucleic acid (RNA) virus that causes German measles and congenital infection.

Rubeola virus: A single-stranded ribonucleic acid (RNA) virus that causes measles.

S protein: A control protein in the complement cascade that interferes with binding of the C5b67 complex to a cell membrane, thus preventing cell lysis.

Safety data sheet (SDS): A document that contains information on physical and chemical characteristics of a substance, fire, explosion reactivity, health hazards, primary routes of entry, exposure limits and carcinogenic potential, precautions for safe handling, spill clean-up, and emergency first aid information.

Sandwich immunoassay: An immunoassay in which antibody to the target antigen is bound to the solid phase; also known as a *capture* or *immunometric* immunoassay.

Sarcoma: A type of cancer derived from bone or soft tissues such as fat, muscles, tendons, cartilage, nerves, and blood vessels.

Scarlet fever: An illness with a characteristic rash and fever that is caused by the erythrogenic toxins released from Group A streptococcal bacteria.

Secondary antibody response: A second or memory response to an antigen, characterized by a shortened lag period, a more rapid rise in antibody, and higher serum levels for a longer period of time.

Secondary follicle: A cluster of B cells that are proliferating in response to a specific antigen.

Secondary immunodeficiency: An immunodeficiency that is acquired secondary to other conditions, such as certain infections, malignancies, autoimmune disorders, and immunosuppressive therapies.

Secondary lymphoid organs: Organs that include the spleen, lymph nodes, appendix, tonsils, and other mucosal-associated lymphoid tissue where the main contact with foreign antigens takes place.

Secretory component (SC): A protein that is synthesized in epithelial cells and added to immunoglobulin A (IgA) to facilitate transport of IgA to mucosal surfaces.

Self-tolerance: The ability of the immune system to accept self-antigens and not initiate a response against them.

Sensitization: (1) The combination of antibody with a single antigenic determinant on the surface of a cell without agglutination. (2) Induction of an immune response.

Serial dilution: A method of decreasing the strength of an antibody solution by using the same dilution factor for each step.

Seroconversion: Change of a serological test result from antibody negative to antibody positive from samples obtained during the course of an immune response.

Serological pipette: A graduated or measuring pipette that has marks all along its length all the way down to the tip.

Serology: The study of the noncellular portion of the blood known as *serum*.

Serotype: A group of related bacteria or viruses that share specific antigens that can be identified by serological testing.

Serum: The liquid portion of the blood minus the clotting factors.

Serum amyloid A (SAA): An acute-phase protein that acts as a chemical messenger to activate monocytes and macrophages in order to increase inflammation.

Serum sickness: A type III hypersensitivity reaction that results from the production of antibodies to animal serum used in passive immunization.

Severe combined immunodeficiency (SCID): An inherited deficiency of both cell-mediated and antibody-mediated immunity that results in overwhelming infections and death in infancy if not treated successfully.

Shift: An abrupt change in the mean that may be caused by a malfunction of an instrument or a new lot number of reagents.

Side (right angle) scatter (SSc): Light scattered at 90 degrees in a flow cytometer that indicates the complexity of a cell, determined by characteristics such as granularity.

Single-nucleotide polymorphisms (SNPs): Variants of a particular DNA sequence involving a single base pair; these variations are shared by at least 2% of a population and result in the generation of different alleles.

Single-parameter histogram: Plot of a chosen parameter or measurement on the *x*-axis against the number of events on the *y*-axis.

Single-positive (SP) stage: A stage in T-cell development characterized by the presence of surface CD4 or CD8 but not both markers.

Single step, competitive, immunochromatographic method: A rapid immunoassay in which antigen in a patient sample is added to a membrane containing detection antibody adsorbed onto colloidal gold particles.

Six Sigma: A method employed by health-care organizations to reduce variables and decrease errors.

Sjögren's syndrome: An autoimmune disorder characterized by the presence of dry eyes, dry mouth, and connective tissue disease.

Sm antigen: An extractable nuclear antigen; autoantibodies to Sm are specific for systemic lupus erythematosus.

Solute: The substance being diluted (e.g. serum) during preparation of a dilution.

Spirochetes: Long, slender, helically coiled bacteria containing flagella that wind around the bacterial cell wall and exhibit a characteristic corkscrew motility.

Spleen: The largest secondary lymphoid organ in the body, located in the upper left quadrant of the abdomen. Its function is to filter out aged cells and foreign antigens.

SS-A/Ro: An extractable nuclear antigen consisting of small, uridine-rich ribonucleic acid (RNA) complexed to cellular protein; found in a significant percentage of patients with Sjögren's syndrome.

SS-B/La: An extractable nuclear antigen consisting of small, uridine-rich ribonucleic acid (RNA) complexed to cellular protein; found in a significant percentage of patients with Sjögren syndrome.

Standard deviation (SD): A measurement statistic that describes the average distance of each data point in a normal distribution from the mean.

Standard of care: The attention, caution, and prudence that a reasonable person in the same circumstances would exercise in performing laboratory testing.

Standard Precautions (SPs): Guidelines describing personnel protection that should be used for the care of all patients, including hand washing, gloves, mask, eye protection, face shield, gown, patient-care equipment, environmental control, linens, taking care to prevent injuries, and patient placement.

Streptavidin (SAv): A bacterial protein that has a strong affinity for biotin; the complex is used for labeling in some types of immunoassays.

Streptococcus pyogenes: Group A streptococci; gram-positive cocci that have several clinical manifestations, including pharyngitis, impetigo, scarlet fever, acute rheumatic fever, and post-streptococcal glomerulonephritis.

Streptolysin O: A protein capable of lysing red blood cells (RBCs) and white blood cells (WBCs), which is produced by some groups of streptococci as they grow.

Streptozyme: A serological test for infection with Group A streptococci that detects five different antibodies to streptococcal products.

Superantigens: Microbial proteins that can act as potent T-cell mitogens because they bind to both class II major histocompatibility complex (MHC) molecules and T-cell receptors, regardless of antigen specificity.

Surrogate light chain: Two short polypeptide chains noncovalently associated with each other that appear before actual light chains are formed by a developing B cell.

Symbiotic: A relationship in which two species live together, often maintaining a long-term, but not necessarily a beneficial, interaction (e.g., a bacterium and a human).

Synergistic: Effect of cytokines that complement and enhance each other.

Syngeneic graft: The transfer of tissue or organs between genetically identical individuals such as identical twins.

Syphilis: A sexually transmitted disease caused by the spirochete bacterium *Treponema pallidum.*

Systemic lupus erythematosus (SLE): A chronic inflammatoryautoimmune disease characterized by the presence of antinuclear antibodies. Symptoms may include swelling of the joints, an erythematous rash, and deposition of immune complexes in the kidneys.

Systemic sclerosis (SSc): A systemic autoimmune disease characterized by excessive fibrosis and vascular abnormalities that affect the skin, joints, and internal organs; also known as *scleroderma*.

T-dependent antigen: An antigen that requires T-cell help in order for B cells to respond.

T follicular helper (Tfh) cell: A subpopulation of T helper cells that remain in the lymph nodes, where they interact with B cells and plasma cells.

T helper (Th) cells: Lymphocytes that express the CD4 antigen. Their function is to provide help to B cells in recognizing foreign antigen and producing antibody to it.

T helper 1 (Th1) cells: T cells that are developed through the expression of interleukin-12 (IL-12) by dendritic cells and that are primarily responsible for cell-mediated immunity.

T helper 2 (Th2) cells: T cells that are developmentally regulated by interleukin-4 (IL-4) and whose main function is to drive antibody-mediated immunity.

T helper 17 (Th17) cells: A subset of T cells that play an important role in host defense against bacterial and fungal infections at mucosal surfaces. They secrete interleukin-17 (IL-17), which attracts neutrophils to the site of infection.

T-independent antigens: Antigens that are able to elicit antibody formation in the absence of T cells.

T lymphocytes: Cells that mature in the thymus which play important roles in cell-mediated immunity and produce cytokines that assist the humoral immune response.

***T. pallidum* particle agglutination (TP-PA) test:** A particle agglutination test that detects antibodies to *Treponema pallidum* to aid in the diagnosis of syphilis.

T regulatory (Treg) cell: A subpopulation of T cells that play an important role in suppressing the immune response to self-antigens.

Tertiary syphilis: The last stage of syphilis that appears months to years after secondary infection. It is characterized by granulomatous inflammation, cardiovascular disease, and central nervous system involvement.

Tetrapeptide: The basic four-chain unit common to all immunoglobulin molecules, consisting of two large heavy chains and two smaller light chains.

The Joint Commission (TJC): An independent body that certifies and accredits health-care organizations in the United States,

Thymocyte: Immature lymphocyte, found in the thymus, that undergoes differentiation to become a mature T cell.

Thymus: A small, flat, bilobed organ found in the thorax of humans, which serves as the site for differentiation of T cells.

Thyroglobulin (Tg): A large iodinated glycoprotein from which the active thyroid hormone triiodothyronine (T3) and its precursor, thyroxine (T4), are synthesized.

Thyroid peroxidase (TPO): An enzyme that oxidizes iodine ions to form the iodine atoms that are incorporated into thyroglobulin to facilitate the synthesis of the thyroid hormones T3 and T4.

Thyroid-stimulating hormone (TSH): A hormone produced by the pituitary gland that binds to specific receptors, on the thyroid gland causing thyroglobulin to be broken down into secretable T3 and T4.

Thyroid-stimulating hormone receptor antibodies (TRAbs): Antibodies that are directed against the receptor for thyroid-stimulating hormone. Some of these antibodies are associated with Graves' disease and result in overstimulation of the thyroid gland, while others prevent thyroid-stimulating hormone (TSH) from binding to its receptor and cause decreased thyroid function.

Thyroid-stimulating immunoglobulins (TSIs): Autoantibodies directed against the thyroid-stimulating hormone (TSH) receptor, which are responsible for the hyperthyroidism seen in Graves' disease.

Thyrotoxicosis: A condition caused by overproduction of thyroid hormones, as seen in Graves' disease.

Thyrotropin-releasing hormone (TRH): A hormone secreted by the hypothalamus that acts on the pituitary gland to induce the release of thyroid-stimulating hormone (TSH).

Tissue transglutaminase (tTG): An intestinal enzyme that converts the glutamine residues in gliadin to glutamic acid; autoantibodies to tTG are commonly produced in patients with celiac disease.

Titer: A number that represents the relative concentration of an antibody. It is the reciprocal of the highest dilution in which a positive reaction occurs.

Toll-like receptors (TLRs): Receptors found on human leukocytes and other cell types that recognize microorganisms and aid in their destruction.

Toxoid: A chemically inactivated bacterial toxin used in some vaccines.

Toxoplasma gondii: The protozoal organism that causes toxoplasmosis, an infection that can have severe consequences in immunocompromised individuals and congenitally infected infants.

TP-PA test: See *T. pallidum particle agglutination (TP-PA) test.*

Transcription: The process of generating a messenger ribonucleic acid (RNA) strand from DNA. This is used to code for protein.

Transforming growth factor-β (TGF-β): A cytokine that induces antiproliferative activity in a variety of cell types and downregulation of the inflammatory response.

Transient hypogammaglobulinemia: A condition characterized by low immunoglobulin levels that occurs in infants around 2 to 3 months of age. It is believed to be caused by delayed maturation of one or more components of the immune system and usually corrects itself spontaneously.

Translation: The process by which messenger ribonucleic acid (RNA) is used to make functional proteins.

Transporters associated with antigen processing (TAP 1 and TAP 2): Proteins that are responsible for the adenosine triphosphate (ATP)-dependent transport of newly synthesized short peptides from the cytoplasm to the lumen of the endoplasmic reticulum for binding to class I human leukocyte antigen (HLA) antigens.

Trend: A gradual change in the mean in one direction that may be caused by a gradual deterioration of reagents or deterioration of instrument performance.

Treponema pallidum: A spirochete that is the causative agent of syphilis.

Treponemal tests: Serological tests for syphilis that detect antibodies directed against *Treponema pallidum*.

Tumor: An abnormal cell mass that can either be benign or malignant.

Tumor-infiltrating lymphocyte (TIL): Lymphocyte within a tumor mass that are able to react with antigens on tumor cells to help destroy them.

Tumor marker: Biological substances found in increased amounts in the blood, body fluids, or tissues of patients with a specific type of cancer.

Tumor necrosis factor (TNF): Family of cytokines that mediate the innate defense against gram-negative bacteria and effect adaptive immune responses.

Tumor suppressor genes: Genes that control the entry of cells into the cell cycle and prevent cells from completing the cycle if they contain damaged DNA or other abnormalities. Mutations in these genes can cause unregulated cell proliferation and contribute to tumor growth.

Turnaround time (TAT): The amount of time required between the point at which a test is ordered by the health-care provider and the results are reported to the health-care provider.

22q11.2 deletion syndrome: An autosomal dominant disorder caused by a deletion in chromosome 22, region q11, resulting in underdevelopment of the thymus and a T-cell deficiency.

Type 1 diabetes mellitus (T1D): A chronic autoimmune disease characterized by insufficient insulin production, caused by progressive destruction of the beta cells of the pancreas.

Type I hypersensitivity: An allergic reaction in which antigen-specific immunoglobulin E (IgE) antibody binds to mast cells and basophils, triggering degranulation and the release of chemical mediators; also known as *anaphylactic hypersensitivity.*

Type II hypersensitivity: An immune reaction in which immunoglobulin G (IgG) or immunoglobulin M (IgM) antibodies are produced to cell surface receptors, causing damage to the cells, dysfunction of the cells, or overstimulation of the function of the cells; also known as *antibody-mediated cytotoxic hypersensitivity.*

Type III hypersensitivity: An immune reaction in which immunoglobulin G (IgG) or immunoglobulin M (IgM) antibodies react with soluble antigens to form small complexes that deposit in the tissues and activate complement to induce inflammation; also known as *complex-mediated hypersensitivity.*

Type IV hypersensitivity: A cell-mediated response involving the release of cytokines that induce inflammation and tissue damage 24 to 72 hours after contact with an antigen.

Typhus: Diseases characterized by fever, rash, and a cough caused by *Rickettsiae* bacteria.

Urease: An enzyme that breaks down urea to form ammonia and bicarbonate. Presence of urease is used as an indicator of *Helicobacter pylori* infection.

Vaccine: An antigen preparation derived from a pathogen that is administered to healthy individuals in order to produce immunity to an infectious disease.

Variable: Anything that can be changed or altered in laboratory testing.

Variable region: The amino-terminal region of an immunoglobulin that has a unique amino acid sequence and is responsible for the antigen specificity of an antibody.

Variants: Changes in a nucleotide sequence.

Varicella-zoster virus (VZV): A herpes virus that causes chickenpox and zoster, or shingles.

Venereal Disease Research Laboratory (VDRL) test: A flocculation test for the cardiolipin antibody produced in syphilis patients; an example of a nontreponemal test.

Viral load tests: Quantitative tests for nucleic acid from viruses such as HIV. These tests are used to predict disease progression and to monitor the effects of antiretroviral therapy.

Viremia: The presence of a virus circulating in the blood.

Virulence: A quantitative trait of an organism that refers to the extent of pathology it can cause when it infects a host.

Virulence factors: Characteristics of a microorganism that can increase its pathogenicity by contributing to its ability to establish itself in the host, invade or damage host tissue, or evade the host immune response.

Virus-like particle: Particles (VLPs) formed when proteins from a viral capsid or envelope assemble to produce structures similar to the virus from which they were derived; VLPs are the major component of some viral vaccines.

Volumetric pipette: A pipette that is marked and calibrated to deliver only one volume of a specified liquid.

Waldenström macroglobulinemia: An immunoproliferative disease caused by a malignancy of lymphocytes that results in production of immunoglobulin M (IgM) paraproteins.

Wegener's granulomatosis (WG): See *granulomatosis with polyangiitis (PGA).*

Weil's disease: Severe systemic leptospirosis involving renal and hepatic failure.

Western blot test: A confirmatory test that has been used for some infections (e.g., HIV, Lyme disease) based on separation of antigens from the pathogen by electrophoresis followed by transfer or blotting of the antigen pattern to a supporting medium for reaction with test serum.

Wiskott-Aldrich syndrome (WAS): A rare X-linked recessive syndrome characterized by immunodeficiency, eczema, and thrombocytopenia.

Xenograft: The transfer of tissue from an individual of one species to an individual of another species, such as animal tissue transplanted to a human.

Yeast: A unicellular form of certain fungi that reproduces asexually by budding, in which the parent cell divides into two unequal parts.

Zone of equivalence: The point in an antigen–antibody reaction at which the number of multivalent sites of antigen and antibody are approximately equal, resulting in optimal antigen-antibody reaction (e.g., precipitation).

References

1. Introduction to Immunity and the Immune System

1. Abbas AK, Lichtman AH, Pillai S. *Cellular and Molecular Immunology*. 9th ed. Philadelphia: Elsevier; 2018:13–37.
2. Altfeld M, Fadda L, Frieta D, Bhardwaj N. DCs and NK cells: Critical effectors in the immune response to HIV-1. *Nat Rev Immunol*. 2011;11:176–186.
3. Bell A, Harmening DM, Hughes VC. Morphology of human blood and marrow. In: *Clinical Hematology and Fundamentals of Hemostasis*. 5th ed. Philadelphia: F.A. Davis; 2009:1–44.
4. Berche P. Louis Pasteur, from crystals of life to vaccination. *Clin Microbiol Infec*. 2012;18(suppl 5): 1–6. doi:10.1111/j.1469-0691.2012.03945.x
5. Blom B, Spits H. Development of human lymphoid cells. *Annu Rev Immunol*. 2006;24:287–320.
6. Bonilla FA, Oettgen HC. Adaptive immunity. *J Allergy Clin Immunol*. 2010;125:S33–S40.
7. Chapel H, Hacney M, Misbah S, Snowden N. *Essentials of Clinical Immunology*. 6th ed. Chichester, UK; 2014:2–33.
8. Ciesla B. Leukopoiesis, WBC differential, and lymphocyte function. In: Ciesla B, ed. *Hematology in Practice*. 3rd ed. Philadelphia: F.A. Davis; 2019.
9. Clark G, Stockinger H, Balderas R, van Zelm MC, et al. Nomenclature of CD molecules from the tenth human leukocyte differentiation antigen workshop. *Clin & Trans Immunol*. 2016;5, e57. doi:10.1038/cti.2015.38
10. Czader M. Mature lymphoid neoplasms. In: Keohane E, Smith LJ, Walenga JM, eds. *Rodak's Hematology: Clinical Principles and Applications*. 5th ed. St. Louis: Elsevier/Saunders; 2016:619–641.
11. Delves PJ, Martin SJ, Burton DR, Roitt IM. *Roitt's Essential Immunology*. 13th ed. Chichester, UK: John Wiley and Sons; 2017:3–51.
12. Engel P, Boumsell L, Balderas R, et al. CD nomenclature 2015: human leukocyte differentiation antigen workshops as a driving force in immunology. *J Immunol*. 2015;195(10):4555–4563.
13. Gordon S. Elie Metchnikoff: father of natural immunity. *Eur J Immunol*. 2008;38:3257–3264.
14. Greenberg S. History of immunology. In: Paul WE, ed. *Fundamental Immunology*. 7th ed. Philadelphia: Lippincott Williams & Wilkins; 2013:22–46.
15. Haynes BF, Soderberg KA, Fauci AS. Introduction to the immune system. In: Jameson J, Fauci AS, Kasper DL, Hauser SL, Longo DL, Loscalzo J, eds. *Harrison's Principles of Internal Medicine*. 20th ed. New York: McGraw-Hill. http://accessmedicine.mhmedical.com/content.aspx?bookid=2129§ionid=192284326. Accessed August 9, 2019.
16. History of immunology. http:// www.bioexplorer.net/history_of_biology/immunology/. Accessed November 9, 2018.
17. Human cell differentiation molecules. hcdm.org. Accessed November 7, 2018.
18. Johnson JK, Miller JS. Current strategies exploiting NK-cell therapy to treat haematologic malignancies. *Int J Immunogenet*. 2018;45:237–246.
19. Keratin.com. Silkworms and chickens—Louis Pasteur. *Immunology History III*. http://www.keratin.com/am/am003.shtml. Accessed August 9, 2019.
20. Lugli E, Hudspeth K, Roberto A, Mavilio D. Tissue-resident and memory properties of human T-cell and NK-cell subsets. *Eur J Immunol*. 2016.46:1809–1847.
21. Magher RC. Hematopoiesis. In: Keohane E, Smith LJ, Walenga JM, eds. *Rodak's Hematology: Clinical Principles and Applications*. 5th ed. St. Louis: Elsevier/Saunders; 2016:76–94.
22. Mandal A, Viswanathan C. Natural killer cells: in health and disease. *Hematol Oncol Stem Cell Ther*. 2015; 8(2):47–55.
23. Mathur S, Schexneider K, Hutchison RE, Mahi, G. Hematopoiesis. In: McPherson RA, Pincus MR, eds. *Henry's Clinical Diagnosis and Management by Laboratory Method*. 23rd ed. Philadelphia: Elsevier Saunders; 2016:540–558.
24. McPherson RA, Massey HD. Overview of the immune system and immunologic disorders. In: McPherson RA, Pincus MR, eds. *Henry's Clinical Diagnosis and Management by Laboratory Method*. 23rd ed. Philadelphia: Elsevier Saunders; 2016:856–861.
25. Meagher RC. Hematopoiesis. In: Keohane E, Smith LJ, Walenga JM, eds. *Rodak's Hematology: Clinical Principles and Applications*. 5th ed. St. Louis: Elsevier /Saunders; 2016:76–94.
26. Punt J, Stranford SA, Jones PP, Owen, JA. *Kuby Immunology*. 8th ed. New York: WH Freeman; 2019:31–68.
27. Roquiz W, Al Diffalha S, Kini AR. Leukocyte development, kinetics, and functions. In: Keohane E, Smith LJ, Walenga JM, eds. *Rodak's Hematology: Clinical Principles and Applications*. 5th ed. St. Louis: Elsevier/Saunders; 2016:149–166.
28. Sato K, Fujita S. Dendritic cells—nature and classification. *Allergol Int*. 2007;56:183–191.
29. Spits H, Artis D, Colonna M, Diefenbach A, Di Santo JP, Eberl G, et al. Innate lymphoid cells—a proposal for uniform nomenclature. *Nat Rev Immunol*. 2013;13(2):145–149.
30. Sun JC, Beilke JN, Lanier LL. Adaptive immune features of natural killer cells. *Nature*. 2009;457:557–561.
31. Sun JC, Lanier LL. NK cell development, homeostasis and function: parallels with CD8+ T cells. *Nat Rev Immunol*. 2011;11:645–657.
32. Vajpayee N, Graham SS, Bern S. Basic examination of blood and bone marrow. In: McPherson RA, Pincus MR, eds. *Henry's Clinical Diagnosis and Management by Laboratory Method*. 23rd ed. Philadelphia: Elsevier Saunders; 2016:510–553.
33. Vikhanski L. *Immunity: How Elie Metchnikoff Changed the Course of Modern Medicine*. Chicago, IL: Chicago Review Press; 2016.
34. Zielinski CE, Corti D, Mele F, et al. Dissecting the human immunological memory for pathogens. *Immunol Rev*. 2011;240:40–51.

2. Innate Immunity

1. Algarra M, Gomes D, Esteves da Silva JCG. Current analytical strategies for C-reactive protein quantification in blood. *Clinica Chimica Acta*. 2013;415:1–9.
2. Bergin DA, Reeves EP, Meleady P, et al. A-1 antitrypsin regulates human neutrophil chemotaxis induced by soluble immune complexes and IL-8. *J Clin Invest*. 2010 (December);120(12):4236–4250.
3. Bernink JH, Peters CP, Munneke M, et al. Human type 1 innate lymphoid cells accumulate in inflamed mucosal tissues. *Nat Immunol*. 2013;14(3):221–229. doi:10.1038/ni.2534
4. Boekholdt SM, Kastelein JJ. C-reactive protein and cardiovascular risk: more fuel to the fire. *Lancet*. 2010;375(9709):95–96. doi:10.1016/S0140-6736(09)62098-5
5. Braga F, Panteghini M. Biologic variability of C-reactive protein: is the available information reliable? *Clinica Chimica Acta*. 2012;413:1179–1183.

6. Buckley DI, Fu R., Freeman M, Rogers K, Helfand M. C-reactive protein as a risk factor for coronary heart disease: a systematic review and meta-analyses for the U.S. Preventive Services Task Force. *Ann Intern Med.* 2009;151(7):483–495.
7. Campbell KS, Hasegawa J. Natural killer cell biology: an update and future directions. *J Allergy Clin Immunol.* 2013;132(3):536–544.
8. Carty M, Bowie AG. Recent insights into the role of Toll-like receptors in viral infection. *Clin Exp Immunol.* 2010;161:397–406.
9. Carvalho FA, Koren O, Goodrich JK, et al. Transient inability to manage proteobacteria promotes chronic gut inflammation in TLR5-deficient mice. *Cell Host Microbe.* 2012;12(2):139–152. doi:10.1016/j.chom.2012.07.004
10. Das SK, Ray K. Wilson's disease: an update. *Nat Clin Pract Neurol.* 2006;2:482–493.
11. Davis BK, Wen H, Ting JP. The inflammasome NLRs in immunity, inflammation, and associated diseases. *Annu Rev Immunol.* 2011;29: 707–735. doi:10.1146/annurev-immunol-031210-101405
12. Deguine J, Bousso P. Dynamics of NK cell interactions in vivo. *Immunol Rev.* 2013;252:154–159.
13. Deobagkar-Lele M, Bhaskarla C, Dhanaraju R, et al. Innate immunity and the 2011 Nobel Prize. *Resonance.* 2012;17(10): 974–995.
14. Di Santo JP. Natural killer cell developmental pathways. A question of balance. *Ann Rev Immunol.* 2006;24:257–286.
15. Eberl G, Colonna M, Di Santo JP, McKenzie AN. Innate lymphoid cells. Innate lymphoid cells: a new paradigm in immunology. *Science.* 2015;348(6237):aaa6566. doi:10.1126/science .aaa6566
16. Faty A, Ferre P, Commans S. The acute phase protein serum amyloid A induces lipolysis and inflammation in human adipocytes through distinct pathways. *PLOS One.* 2012 (April);7(4):e34031. http://www.plosone.org. Accessed May 4, 2014.
17. Fritzma GA. Thrombolytic disorders and laboratory assessment. In: Smith LJ, Walenga, JM, Keohane EM, eds. *Hematology: Clinical Principles and Applications.* 5th ed. Philadelphia: Elsevier Saunders; 2016:667–712.
18. Fritzma MG, Fritzma GA. Normal hemostasis and coagulation. In: Smith LJ, Walenga JM, Keohane EM, eds. *Hematology: Clinical Principles and Applications.* 5th ed. Philadelphia: Elsevier Saunders; 2016:642–666.
19. Grad E, Danenberg HD. C-reactive protein and atherosclerosis: cause or effect? *Blood Rev.* 2013;27:23–29.
20. Greene DN, Elliott-Jelf MC, Straseki JA, Grenache DG. Facilitating the laboratory diagnosis of α1-antitrypsin deficiency. *Am J Clin Path.* 2013;139:184–191.
21. Harmening DM, Lawrence LW, Green R, Schaub CR. Hemolytic anemias. In: Harmening DM, ed. *Clinical Hematology and Fundamentals of Hemostasis.* 5th ed. Philadelphia: F.A. Davis; 2009:252–279.
22. Harmening DM, Marty J, Strauss RG. Cell biology, disorders of neutrophils, infectious mononucleosis, and related lymphocytosis. In: Harmening DM, ed. *Clinical Hematology and Fundamentals of Hemostasis.* 5th ed. Philadelphia: F.A. Davis; 2009:305–330.
23. Hutchinson WL, Koenig W, Frohlich M, et al. Immunoradiometric assay of circulating C-reactive protein: age-related values in the adult general population. *Clin Chem.* 2000;46:934–938.
24. Jacobson TA, Ito MK, Maki KC, et al. (2014). National Lipid Association recommendations for patient-centered management of dyslipidemia: part 1—executive summary. *J Clin Lipidol.* 2014;8(5):473–488. doi:10.1016/j.jacl.2014.07.007
25. Jeong E, Lee JY. Intrinsic and extrinsic regulation of innate immune receptors. *Yonsei Med J.* 2011;52(3):379–392.
26. Kumar H, Kawai T, Akira S. Pathogen recognition by the innate immune system. *Int Rev Immunol.* 2011;30:16–34.
27. Landis-Piwowar K. Granulocytes and monocytes. In: McKenzie S, Williams L, eds. *Clinical Laboratory Hematology.* 3rd ed. Upper Saddle River, NJ: Pearson; 2015:Chapter 7:97–121.
28. Liu G, Zhang L, Zhao Y. Modulation of immune responses through direct activation of Toll-like receptors to T cells. *Clin Exp Immunol.* 2010;160:168–175.
29. Mahajan RD, Mishra B, Singla P. Ceruloplasmin—an update. *Int J Pharm Sci Rev Res.* 2011(July-Aug);9(2):116–119.
30. Malle E, Sodin-Semrl S, Kovacevic A. Serum amyloid A: an acute-phase protein involved in tumour pathogenesis. *Cell Mol Life Sci.* 2009;66:9–26. doi:10.1007/s00018-008-8321-x
31. McPherson RA. Specific proteins. In: McPherson RA, Pincus MR, eds. *Henry's Clinical Diagnosis and Management by Laboratory Methods.* 23rd ed. St. Louis: Elsevier Saunders; 2017:253–266.
32. Means TK, Latz E, Hayashi F, Murali MR, Golenbock DT, Luster AD. Human lupus autoantibody-DNA complexes activate DCs through cooperation of CD32 and TLR9. *J Clin Invest.* 2005;115(2):407–417. doi:10.1172/JCI23025
33. Medzhitov R, Shevach EM, Trinchieri G, Mellor AL. Highlights of 10 years of immunology. *Nat Rev Immunol.* 2011;11:693–702.
34. Moro K, Yamada T, Tanabe M, et al. Innate production of T(H)2 cytokines by adipose tissue-associated c-Kit(+)Sca-1(+) lymphoid cells. *Nature.* 2010;463(7280):540–544. doi:10.1038/nature08636
35. Motta V, Soares F, Sun T, Philpott DJ. NOD-like receptors: versatile cytosolic sentinels. *Physiol Rev.* 2015;95(1):149–178. doi:10.1152/physrev.00009.2014
36. Nantasenamat C, Prachayasittikul V, Bulow L. Molecular modeling of the human hemoglobin-haptoglobin complex sheds light on the protective mechanisms of haptoglobin. *PLOS One.* 2013(April);8(4):e62996.
37. Nauseef WM. Assembly of the phagocyte NADPH oxidase. *Histochem Cell Biol.* 2004;122:277–291.
38. Neill DR, Wong SH, Bellosi A, et al. Nuocytes represent a new innate effector leukocyte that mediates type-2 immunity. *Nature.* 2010;464(7293):1367–1370. doi:10.1038/nature08900
39. Orange JS. Human natural killer cell deficiencies. *Curr Opin Allergy Clin Immunol.* 2006;6:399–409.
40. Pepys MB, Hirschfield GM. C-reactive protein: a critical update. *J Clin Invest.* 2003;111:1805–1812.
41. Rigottier-Gois L. Dysbiosis in inflammatory bowel diseases: the oxygen hypothesis. *ISME J.* 2013;7(7): 1256–1261. doi:10.1038/ismej.2013.80
42. Schroder K, Tschopp J. The inflammasomes. *Cell.* 2010;140(6): 821–832. doi:10.1016/j.cell.2010.01.040
43. Segal AW. How neutrophils kill microbes. *Annu Rev Immunol.* 2005;23:197–223.
44. Song C, Hsu K, Yamen E, et al. Serum amyloid A induction of cytokines in monocytes/macrophages and lymphocytes. *Atherosclerosis.* 2007;(2009):374–383. doi:10.1016/j.atherosclerosis.2009.05.007
45. Stoller JK, Aboussouan LS. α1 antitrypsin deficiency. *Lancet.* 2005;365:2225–2236.
46. Van Holten TC, Waanders LF, de Groot PG, et al. Circulating biomarkers for predicting cardiovascular disease risk; a systemic review and comprehensive overview of meta-analyses. *PLOS One.* 2013(April);8(4):e62080.
47. Vivier E, Raulet DH, Moretta A, et al. Innate or adaptive immunity? The example of natural killer cells. *Science.* 2011;33(6013):44–49.
48. Woodhouse S. C-reactive protein: from acute phase reactant to cardiovascular disease risk factor. *MLO.* 2002(March);34(3):12–20.

49. Yerbury JJ, Rybehyn MS, Esterbrook-Smith SB, et al. The acute phase protein haptoglobin is a mammalian extracellular chaperone with an action similar to clusterin. *Biochemistry.* 2005;44:10914–10925.

3. Nature of Antigens and the Major Histocompatibility Complex

1. Abbas AK, Lichtman AH, Pillai S. *Cellular and Molecular Immunology.* 9th ed. Philadelphia: Elsevier; 2018:117–144.
2. Berzofsky JA, Berkower IJ. Immunogenicity and antigen structure. In: Paul WE, ed. *Fundamental Immunology.* 7th ed. Philadelphia: Wolters Kluwer/Lippincott Williams & Wilkins; 2012:539–582.
3. Bolstad N, Warren DJ, Nustad K. Heterophilic antibody interference in immunometric assays. *Best Pract Res Clin Endocrinol Metab.* 2013;27(5):647–661.
4. Chen B, Li J, He C, et al. Role of HLA-B27 in the pathogenesis of ankylosing spondylitis. *Mol Med Rep.* 2017;15(4):1943–1951.
5. Cooling L, Downs T. Immunohematology. In: McPherson RA, Pincus MR, eds. *Henry's Clinical Diagnosis and Management by Laboratory Methods.* 23rd ed. St. Louis: Elsevier Inc; 2017:680–734.
6. Delves PJ, Martin SJ, Burton DR, Roitt IM. *Roitt's Essential Immunology.* 12th ed. Chichester, UK: Wiley-Blackwell; 2011:79–112.
7. Di Carluccio AR, Triffon CF, Chen W. Perpetual complexity: predicting human CD8(+) T-cell responses to pathogenic peptides. *Immunol Cell Biol.* 2018:96(4):358–369.
8. Fagoaga OR. Human leukocyte antigen: the major histocompatibility complex of man. In: McPherson RA, Pincus MR, eds. *Henry's Clinical Diagnosis and Management by Laboratory Methods.* 23rd ed. St. Louis: Elsevier Inc; 2017:955–972.
9. HLA Informatics Group, Anthony Nolan Research Institute. HLA allele numbers: assigned as of September 2018. http://hla.alleles.org/nomenclature/stats.html. Accessed December 12, 2018.
10. Karch CP, Burkhard P. Vaccine technologies: from whole organisms to rationally designed protein assemblies. *Biochem Pharmacol.* 2016 Nov 15;120:1–14.
11. Koch J, Tampe R. The macromolecular peptide-loading complex in MHC class I-dependent antigen presentation. *Cell Mol Life Sci.* 2006;63:653–662.
12. Lan X, Zhang MM, Pu CL, et al. Impact of human leukocyte antigen mismatching on outcomes of liver transplantation: a meta-analysis. *World J Gastroenterol.* 2010;16(27):3457–3464.
13. Murphy KP. *Janeway's Immunobiology.* 8th ed. New York: Garland Science, Taylor and Francis Group; 2011:201–234.
14. Owen JA, Punt J, Stranford SA, Jones PP. *Kuby Immunology.* 7th ed. New York: WH Freeman and Co.; 2013:261–298.
15. Parham P. *The Immune System.* 4th ed. New York: Garland Science, Taylor and Francis Group; 2015:120–144.

4. Adaptive Immunity

1. Abbas AK, Lichtman AH, Pillai S. *Cellular and Molecular Immunology.* 9th ed. Philadelphia: Saunders Elsevier; 2017.
2. Meng X, Yang B, Suen WC. Prospects for modulating the CD40/CD40L pathway in the therapy of the hyper-IgM syndrome. *Innate Immun.* 2018;24(1):4–10.
3. Murphy K. *Janeway's Immunobiology.* 9th ed. New York: Garland Science, Taylor and Francis Group; 2017.
4. Parham P. *The Immune System.* 4th ed. New York: Garland Science, Taylor and Francis Group; 2015:113–148.
5. Paul WE. *Fundamental Immunology.* 7th ed. Philadelphia: Lippincott, Williams and Wilkins; 2012.
6. Stevens CD. Adaptive immunity. In: Stevens CD and Miller L. *Clinical Immunology and Serology: A Laboratory Perspective.* 4th ed. Philadelphia: F.A. Davis Company; 2017:45–60.

5. Antibody Structure and Function

1. Brandtzaeg P, Johansen F. Mucosal B cells: phenotypic characteristics, transcriptional regulation, and homing properties. *Immunol Rev.* 2005;206:32–63.
2. Burnet FM. A modification of Jerne's theory of antibody production using the concept of clonal selection. *Aust J Sci.* 1957;20:67–69.
3. Chaplin DD. Overview of the immune system. *J Allergy Clin Immunol.* 2010;125:S3–S23.
4. Chaudhuri J, Basu U, Zarrin A, et al. Evolution of the immunoglobulin heavy chain class switch recombination mechanism. *Adv Immunol.* 2007;94:157–214.
5. Cobb RM, Oestreich KJ, Osipovich OA, Oltz EM. Accessibility control of V(D)J recombination. *Adv Immunol.* 2006;91:45–110.
6. Dreyer WJ, Bennett JC. The molecular basis of antibody formation: a paradox. *Proc Natl Acad Sci USA.* 1965;54:864.
7. Dudley DD, Chaudhuri J, Bassing CH, Alt FW. Mechanism and control of V(d)J recombination versus class switch recombination: similarities and differences. *Adv Immunol.* 2005;86:43–112.
8. Edelman GM. The structure and function of antibodies. *Sci Am.* 1970;223:34.
9. Jerne NK. The natural selection theory of antibody production. *Proc Natl Acad Sci USA.* 1955;41:849–857.
10. Johansson SGO. The history of IgE: from discovery to 2010. *Curr Allergy Asthm R.* 2011;11(2):173–177.
11. MacKay IR. History of immunology in Australia: events and identities. *Int Med J.* 2006;36:394–398.
12. Male D, Brostoff J, Roth DB, Roitt IM. *Immunology.* 8th ed. Philadelphia: Elsevier Saunders; 2013:51–70.
13. McPherson RA, Riley RS, Massey HD. Laboratory evaluation of immunoglobulin function and humoral immunity. In: McPherson RA, Pincus MR, eds. *Henry's Clinical Diagnosis and Management by Laboratory Methods.* 23rd ed. St. Louis: Elsevier Inc; 2017:913–928.
14. Monteiro RC. Role of IgA and IgA Fc receptors in inflammation. *J Clin Immunol.* 2010;30:1–9.
15. Nezlin R, Ghetie V. Interactions of immunoglobulins outside the antigen-combining site. *Adv Immunol.* 2004;82:155–215.
16. Owen JA, Punt J, Stranford SA. *Kuby Immunology.* 7th ed. New York: WH Freeman and Company; 2013:65–103, 225–259, 329–356, 415–450.
17. Porter RR. The structure of antibodies. *Sci Am.* 1967;217:81.
18. Schroeder HW Jr, Wald D, Greenspan NS. Immunoglobulins: structure and function. In: Paul WE, ed. *Fundamental Immunology.* 6th ed. Philadelphia: Lippincott Williams & Wilkins; 2013:129–149.
19. Schroeder HW, Cavacini L. Structure and function of immunoglobulins. *J Allergy Clin Immunol.* 2010;125(2S2):S41–S52.
20. Wines B, Hogarth P. IgA receptors in health and disease. *Tissue Antigens.* 2006;68:103–114.
21. Woof JM, Kerr MA. The function of immunoglobulin A in immunity. *J Path.* 2006;208:270–282.
22. Woof JM, Mestecky J. Mucosal immunoglobulins. *Immunol Rev.* 2005;206:64–82.

Monoclonal Antibodies

1. Bruggemann M, Osborn MJ, Ma B, Buelow R. Strategies to obtain divers and specific human monoclonal antibodies from transgenic animals. *Transplantation.* 2017;101(8):1770–1776.

2. Buss NAPS, Henderson SJ, McFarlane M, et al. Monoclonal antibody therapeutics: history and future. *Curr Opin Pharmacol.* 2012;12:615–622.
3. Delves PJ, Martin SJ, Burton DR, Roitt IM. *Roitt's Essential Immunology.* 12th ed. Chichester, UK: Wiley-Blackwell; 2011: 141–187.
4. Kohler G, Milstein C. Continuous cultures of fused cells secreting antibody of predefined specificity. *Nature.* 1975;256:495–497.
5. National Cancer Institute. Biological therapies for cancer. http://www:cancer.gov/cancertopics/factsheet/Therapy/biological. Accessed January 1, 2019.
6. Owen JA, Punt J, Stranford SA. *Kuby Immunology.* 7th ed. New York: WH Freeman; 2013:653–692.
7. Owens RJ., Young RJ. The genetic engineering of monoclonal antibodies. *J Immunol Methods.* 1994;168:149–165.
8. Sapra P, Shor B. Monoclonal antibody-based therapies in cancer: advances and challenges. *Pharmacol Therapeut.* 2013;138:452–469.
9. Stryjewska A, Kiepura K, Librowski T, Lochnyski S. Biotechnology and genetic engineering in the new drug development. Part II. Monoclonal antibodies, modern vaccines and gene therapy. *Pharmacological Reports.* 2013;65:1086–1101.
10. Watkins NA, Ouwehand WH. Introduction to antibody engineering and phage display. *Vox Sang.* 2000;78:72–79.
11. Yamada T. Therapeutic monoclonal antibodies. *Keio J Med.* 2011;60(2):37–46.

6. Cytokines

1. Abbas AK, Lichtman AH, Pillai S. *Cellular and Molecular Immunology.* 9th ed. Philadelphia: Saunders Elsevier; 2017:35–85.
2. Drutskaya MS, Efimov GA, Kruglov AA, Nedospasov SA. Can we design a better anti-cytokine therapy? *J Leukoc Biol.* 2017 Sep;102(3):783–790. doi:10.1189/jlb.3MA0117-025R. Epub 2017 May 25. Review. PubMed PMID: 28546502.
3. Eder K, Baffy N, Falus A, Fulop AK. The major inflammatory mediator interleukin-6 and obesity. *Inflamm Res.* 2009 Nov;58(11):727–736. doi:10.1007/s00011-009-0060-4. Epub 2009 Jun 19. Review. PubMed PMID: 19543691.
4. Heuertz RM, Ezekiel UR. Cytokines. In: Stevens CD, Miller L, eds. *Clinical Immunology and Serology: A Laboratory Perspective.* 4th ed. Philadelphia: F.A. Davis Company; 2017:77–90.
5. Jakimovski D, Kolb C, Ramanathan M, Zivadinov R, Weinstock-Guttman B. Interferon β for multiple sclerosis. *Cold Spring Harb Perspect Med.* 2018 Nov 1;8(11):pii:a032003. doi:10.1101/cshperspect.a032003. Review. PubMed PMID: 29311124.
6. Justiz Vaillant AA, Qurie A. Interleukin. [Updated 2019 Jun 12]. In: *StatPearls* [Internet]. Treasure Island, FL: StatPearls Publishing; 2019 Jan. https://www.ncbi.nlm.nih.gov/books/NBK499840/
7. Leonard WJ, Lin JX, O'Shea JJ. The γ(c) family of cytokines: basic biology to therapeutic ramifications. *Immunity.* 2019 Apr 16; 50(4):832–850. doi:10.1016/j.immuni.2019.03.028. Review. PubMed PMID: 30995502.
8. Madera S, Rapp M, Firth MA, Beilke JN, Lanier LL, Sun JC. Type I IFN promotes NK cell expansion during viral infection by protecting NK cells against fratricide. *J Exp Med.* 2016 Feb 8;213(2): 225–233. doi:10.1084/jem.20150712. Epub 2016 Jan 11. PubMed PMID: 26755706; PubMed Central PMCID: PMC4749923.
9. Murphy K. *Janeway's Immunobiology.* 9th ed. New York: Garland Science, Taylor and Francis Group; 2017.
10. Oxford JS, Gill D. Unanswered questions about the 1918 influenza pandemic: origin, pathology, and the virus itself. *Lancet Infect Dis.* 2018 Nov;18(11):e348–e354. doi:10.1016/S1473-3099(18)30359-1. Epub 2018 Jun 20. Review. PubMed PMID: 29935779.
11. Paul WE. *Fundamental Immunology.* 7th ed. Philadelphia: Lippincott, Williams and Wilkins; 2012:601–707.
12. Shevach EM. Foxp3(+) T regulatory cells: Still many unanswered questions—a perspective after 20 years of study. *Front Immunol.* 2018 May 15;9:1048. doi:10.3389/fimmu.2018.01048. eCollection 2018. Review. PubMed PMID: 29868011; PubMed Central PMCID: PMC5962663.
13. Zitvogel L, Galluzzi L, Kepp O, Smyth MJ, Kroemer G. Type I interferons in anticancer immunity. *Nat Rev Immunol.* 2015 Jul;15(7):405–414. doi:10.1038/nri3845. Epub 2015 Jun 1. Review. PubMed PMID: 26027717.

7. The Complement System

Pathways of the Complement System

1. Barnum S, Schein T. *The Complement Fact Book.* Oxford, UK: Elsevier Ltd.; 2018.
2. Carroll MC, Fischer MB. Complement and the immune response. *Curr Opin Immunol.* 1997;9(1):64–69.
3. Eisen DP, Minchinton RM. Impact of mannose-binding lectin on susceptibility to infectious diseases. *Clin Infect Dis.* 2003;37(11):1496–1505.
4. Fearon DT. Activation of the alternative complement pathway. *CRC Crit Rev Immunol.* 1979;1(1):1–32.
5. Flierman R, Daha MR. The clearance of apoptotic cells by complement. *Immunobiology.* 2007;212(4-5):363–370.
6. Frakking FN J, Brouwer, N, van Eijkelenburg NKA, et al. Low mannose-binding lectin (MBL) levels in neonates with pneumonia and sepsis. *Clin Exp Immunol.* 2007;150(2):255–262.
7. Garred P, Genster N, Pilely K, et al. A journey through the lectin pathway of complement-MBL and beyond. *Immunol Rev.* 2016;274(1):74–97.
8. Harrison RA. The properdin pathway: an "alternative activation pathway" or a "critical amplification loop" for C3 and C5 activation? *Semin Immunopathol.* 2018;40(1):15–35.
9. Janssen BJ, Christodoulidou A, McCarthy A, Lambris JD, Gros P.. Structure of C3b reveals conformational changes that underlie complement activity. *Nature.* 2006;444(7116):213–216.
10. Lachmann PJ. Looking back on the alternative complement pathway. *Immunobiology.* 2018;223(8–9):519–523.
11. Lewis MJ, Botto M. Complement deficiencies in humans and animals: links to autoimmunity. *Autoimmunity.* 2006;39(5): 367–378.
12. Matsushita M, Endo Y, Fujita T. Structural and functional overview of the lectin complement pathway: its molecular basis and physiological implication. *Arch Immunol Ther Exp (Warsz).* 2013;61(4):273–283.
13. Medzhitov R, Janeway Jr. C. Innate immunity. *N Engl J Med.* 2000;343(5):338–344.
14. Morgan P. Complement. In: Paul WE, ed. *Fundamental Immunology.* Philadelphia: Lippincott-Raven; 2013:863–890.
15. Nilsson B, Nilsson Ekdahl K. The tick-over theory revisited: is C3 a contact-activated protein? *Immunobiology.* 2012;217(11):1106–1110.
16. Pillemer L. The properdin system. *Trans N Y Acad Sci.* 1955;17(7):526–530.
17. Punt J, Stranford SA, Jones PP, Owen JA. *Kuby Immunology.* 8th ed. New York: WH Freeman and Co.; 2019:165–204.
18. Rawal N, Pangburn MK. Structure/function of C5 convertases of complement. *Int Immunopharmacol.* 2001;1(3):415–422.

19. Sörman A, Zhang L, Ding Z, Heyman B How antibodies use complement to regulate antibody responses. *Mol Immunol.* 2014;61(2):79–88.
20. Troldborg A, Hansen A, Hansen SW, et al. Lectin complement pathway proteins in healthy individuals. *Clin Exp Immunol.* 2017;188(1):138–147.
21. Ugurlar D, Howes SC, Jan de Kreuk B, et al. Structures of C1-IgG1 provide insights into how danger pattern recognition activates complement. *Science.* 2018;359(6377):794–797.
22. Vidarsson G, Dekkers G, Rispens T. IgG subclasses and allotypes: from structure to effector functions. *Front Immunol.* 2014;5:520.
23. Volanakis JE, Narayana SV. Complement factor D, a novel serine protease. *Protein Sci.* 1996;5(4):553–564.
24. Walport MJ. Complement. First of two parts. *N Engl J Med.* 2001;344(14):1058–1066.
25. Wang G, de Jong RN, van den Bremer ETJ, et al. Molecular basis of assembly and activation of complement component C1 in complex with immunoglobulin G1 and antigen. *Mol Cell.* 2016;63(1):135–145.
26. Wedgwood RJ, Pillemer L. The nature and interactions of the properdin system. *Acta Haematol.* 1958;20(1–4):253–259.
27. Xu Y, Narayana SV, Volanakis JE. Structural biology of the alternative pathway convertase. *Immunol Rev.* 2001;180:123–135.
28. Yaseen S, Demopulos G, Dudler T, et al. Lectin pathway effector enzyme mannan-binding lectin-associated serine protease-2 can activate native complement C3 in absence of C4 and/or C2. *FASEB J.* 2017;31(5):2210–2219.

Complement System Controls

1. Ahearn JM, Fearon DT. Structure and function of the complement receptors, CR1 (CD35) and CR2 (CD21). *Adv Immunol.* 1989;46:183–219.
2. Carroll MC. The complement system in B cell regulation. *Mol Immunol.* 2004;41(2–3):141–146.
3. Degn SE, Thiel S, Nielsen O, et al. MAp19, the alternative splice product of the MASP2 gene. J Immunol Methods. 2011;373(1–2):89–101.
4. DiScipio RG. Ultrastructures and interactions of complement factors H and I. *J Immunol.* 1992;149(8):2592–2599.
5. Holers VM. Complement and its receptors: new insights into human disease. *Annu Rev Immunol.* 2014;32:433–459.
6. Kerr FK, Thomas AR, Wijeyewickrema, LC, et al. Elucidation of the substrate specificity of the MASP-2 protease of the lectin complement pathway and identification of the enzyme as a major physiological target of the serpin, C1-inhibitor. *Mol Immunol.* 2008;45(3):670–677.
7. Killick J, Morisse G, Sieger D, Astier, AL. Complement as a regulator of adaptive immunity. *Semin Immunopathol.* 2018;40(1):37–48.
8. Naama JK, Niven IP, Zoma A, Mitchell WS, Whaley K. Complement, antigen-antibody complexes and immune complex disease. *J Clin Lab Immunol.* 1985;17(2):59–67.
9. Nilsson SC, Blom AM. Purification and functional characterization of factor I. *Methods Mol Biol.* 2014;1100:177–188.
10. Preissner KT. Structure and biological role of vitronectin. *Annu Rev Cell Biol.* 1991;7:275–310.
11. Smedbraten J, Mjøen G, Hartmann A, et al. Low level of MAp44, an inhibitor of the lectin complement pathway, and long-term graft and patient survival; a cohort study of 382 kidney recipients. *BMC Nephrol.* 2016;17(1):148.
12. Smith BO, Mallin RL, Krych-Goldberg M, et al. Structure of the C3b binding site of CR1 (CD35), the immune adherence receptor. *Cell.* 2002;108(6):769–780.
13. Zeerleder S. C1-inhibitor: more than a serine protease inhibitor. *Semin Thromb Hemost.* 2011;37(4):362–374.

Complement Receptors

1. Kishore U, Reid KB. C1q: structure, function, and receptors. *Immunopharmacology.* 2000;49(1–2):159–170.
2. Vorup-Jensen T, Jensen RK. Structural Immunology of Complement Receptors 3 and 4. *Front Immunol.* 2018;9:2716.

Biologic Manifestations of Complement Activation

1. Arbore G, Kemper C, Kolev M. Intracellular complement—the complosome—in immune cell regulation. *Mol Immunol.* 2017;89:2–9.
2. Carroll MC. The complement system in regulation of adaptive immunity. *Nat Immunol.* 2004;5(10):981–986.
3. Chenoweth DE. The properties of human C5a anaphylatoxin. The significance of C5a formation during hemodialysis. *Contrib Nephrol.* 1987;59:51–71.
4. Coulthard LG, Hawksworth OA, Woodruff TM. Complement: the emerging architect of the developing brain. *Trends Neurosci.* 2018;41(6):373–384.
5. Freeley S, Kemper C, Le Friec G. The "ins and outs" of complement-driven immune responses. *Immunol Rev.* 2016;274(1):16–32.
6. Hugli TE. Structure and function of the anaphylatoxins. *Springer Semin Immunopathol.* 1984;7(2–3):193–219.
7. Kemper C, Kohl J. Novel roles for complement receptors in T cell regulation and beyond. *Mol Immunol.* 2013;56(3):181–190.
8. Laursen NS, Magnani F, Gottfredsen RH, Petersen SV, Andersen GR. Structure, function and control of complement C5 and its proteolytic fragments. *Curr Mol Med.* 2012;12(8):1083–1097.
9. Luchena C, Zuazo-Ibarra J, Alberdi E, Matute C, Capetillo-Zarate E. Contribution of neurons and glial cells to complement-mediated synapse removal during development, aging and in Alzheimer's disease. *Mediators Inflamm.* 2018;2018:2530414.
10. Manthey HD, Woodruff TM, Taylor SM, Monk PN. Complement component 5a (C5a). *Int J Biochem Cell Biol.* 2009;41(11):2114–2117.
11. McPherson RA, Huber SA, Jenny NS. Mediators of inflammation: complement, cytokines and adhesion molecules. In: McPherson RA, Pincus MR, eds. *Henry's Clinical Diagnosis and Management by Laboratory Methods.* St. Louis: Elsevier; 2017:929–943.
12. Peng Q, Li K, Sacks SH, Zhou W.. The role of anaphylatoxins C3a and C5a in regulating innate and adaptive immune responses. *Inflamm Allergy Drug Targets.* 2009;8(3):236–246.

Complement and Disease States

1. Greve J, Strassen U, Gorczyza M, et al. Prophylaxis in hereditary angioedema (HAE) with C1 inhibitor deficiency. *J Dtsch Dermatol Ges.* 2016;14(3):266–275.
2. Grumach AS, Kirschfink M. Are complement deficiencies really rare? Overview on prevalence, clinical importance and modern diagnostic approach. *Mol Immunol.* 2014;61(2):110–117.
3. Heitzeneder S, Seidel M, Förster-Waldl E, Heitger A. Mannan-binding lectin deficiency—Good news, bad news, doesn't matter? *Clin Immunol.* 2012;143(1):22–38.
4. Hill A, DeZern AE, Kinoshita T, Brodsky RA. Paroxysmal nocturnal haemoglobinuria. *Nat Rev Dis Primers.* 2017;3:17028.
5. Nicolas C, Vuiblet V, Baudouin V, et al. C3 nephritic factor associated with C3 glomerulopathy in children. *Pediatr Nephrol.* 2014;29(1):85–94.
6. Sjoholm AG, Jönsson G, Braconier, JH, Sturfelt G, Truedsson L. Complement deficiency and disease: an update. *Mol Immunol.* 2006;43(1–2):78–85.

7. Skattum L, van Deuren M, van der Poll T, Truedsson L. Complement deficiency states and associated infections. *Mol Immunol.* 2011;48(14):1643–1655.
8. Zuraw BL, Christiansen SC. HAE pathophysiology and underlying mechanisms. *Clin Rev Allergy Immunol.* 2016;51(2):216–229.

Laboratory Detection of Complement and Therapeutic Drug Monitoring

1. Frazer-Abel A. The effect on the immunology laboratory of the expansion in complement therapeutics. *J Immunol Methods.* 2018;461:30–36.
2. Frazer-Abel A, Giclas PC. Update on laboratory tests for the diagnosis and differentiation of hereditary angioedema and acquired angioedema. *Allergy Asthma Proc.* 2011;32(suppl 1):17–21.
3. Frazer-Abel A, Sepiashvili L, Mbughuni MM, Willrich MAV. Overview of laboratory testing and clinical presentations of complement deficiencies and dysregulation. *Adv Clin Chem.* 2016;77:1–75.
4. Gatault P, Brachet G, Ternant D, et al. Therapeutic drug monitoring of eculizumab: rationale for an individualized dosing schedule. *mAbs.* 2015;7(6):1205–1211.
5. Giclas PC Analysis of complement in the clinical laboratory. In: Detrick HR, Folds J, eds. *Manual of Molecular and Clinical Laboratory Immunology.* Washington, DC: ASM Press; 2006:115–117.
6. Greenbaum LA, Fila M, Ardissino G, et al. Eculizumab is a safe and effective treatment in pediatric patients with atypical hemolytic uremic syndrome. *Kidney Int.* 2016;89(3):701–711.
7. Hillmen P, Young NS, Schubert J, et al. The complement inhibitor eculizumab in paroxysmal nocturnal hemoglobinuria. *N Engl J Med.* 2006;355(12):1233–1243.
8. Jager U, D'Sa S, Schörgenhofer C, et al. Inhibition of complement C1s improves severe hemolytic anemia in cold agglutinin disease: a first-in-human trial. *Blood.* 2018;133(9):893–901.
9. Jaskowski TD, Martins TB, Litwin CM, Hill, HR. Comparison of three different methods for measuring classical pathway complement activity. *Clin Diagn Lab Immunol.* 1999;6(1):137–139.
10. Jokiranta TS. HUS and atypical HUS. *Blood.* 2017;129(21):2847–2856.
11. Kabat EA, Mayer MM. *Experimental Immunochemistry.* 2nd ed. Springfield, IL: Thomas;1961:905
12. Legendre CM, Licht C, Loirat C. Eculizumab in atypical hemolytic-uremic syndrome. *N Engl J Med.* 2013;369(14):1379–1380.
13. Liu LL, Liu, N, Chen Y, et al. Glomerular mannose-binding lectin deposition is a useful prognostic predictor in immunoglobulin A nephropathy. *Clin Exp Immunol.* 2013;174(1):152–160.
14. Loirat C, et al. An international consensus approach to the management of atypical hemolytic uremic syndrome in children. *Pediatr Nephrol.* 2016;31(1):15–39.
15. Mollnes TE, Jokiranta TS, Truedsson L, et al. Complement analysis in the 21st century. *Mol Immunol.* 2007;44(16):3838–3849.
16. Prohaszka Z, Nilsson B, Frazer-Abel A, et al. Complement analysis 2016: Clinical indications, laboratory diagnostics and quality control. *Immunobiology.* 2016;221(11):1247–1258.
17. Ricklin D, Barratt-Due A, Mollnes TE. Complement in clinical medicine: Clinical trials, case reports and therapy monitoring. *Mol Immunol.* 2017;89:10–21.
18. Ricklin D, Mastellos DC, Reis ES, Lambris JD, et al. The renaissance of complement therapeutics. *Nat Rev Nephrol.* 2018;14(1):26–47.
19. Segarra A, Romero K, Agraz I, et al. Mesangial C4d deposits in early IgA nephropathy. *Clin J Am Soc Nephrol.* 2018;13(2):258–264.
20. Servais A, Noël LH, Frémeaux-Bacchi V, Lesavre P. C3 glomerulopathy. *Contrib Nephrol.* 2013;181:185–193.
21. Volokhina EB, Westra D, van der Velden TJAM, van de Kar NCAJ, Mollnes TE, van den, Heuvel LP. Complement activation patterns in atypical haemolytic uraemic syndrome during acute phase and in remission. *Clin Exp Immunol.* 2015;181(2):306–313.
22. Wehling C, Amon O, Bommer M, et al. Monitoring of complement activation biomarkers and eculizumab in complement-mediated renal disorders. *Clin Exp Immunol.* 2017;187(2):304–315.
23. Wen L, Atkinson JP, Giclas PC. Clinical and laboratory evaluation of complement deficiency. *J Allergy Clin Immunol.* 2004;113(4):585–593; quiz 594.
24. Willrich MAV, Andreguetto BD, Sridharan M, et al. The impact of eculizumab on routine complement assays. *J Immunol Methods.* 2018;460:63–71.

8. Safety and Quality Management

1. Baer DM. Standards for transporting specimens. *MLO.* 2005;37(11):38.
2. Bloodborne Pathogens standard 1910. 1030(d)(4)(ii)(A). https://www.osha.gov/pls/oshaweb/owadisp.show_document?p_id=10051&p_table=STANDARDS. Accessed October 29, 2018.
3. Centers for Disease Control and Prevention. Clinical Laboratory Improvement Amendments. Test complexities. June 11, 2018. https://www.cdc.gov/clia/index.html Accessed October 26, 2018.
4. Centers for Disease Control and Prevention. Guideline for handwashing hygiene in health-care settings. *MMWR.* 2002;51(rr16): 1–48. http://www.cdc.gov/handhygiene/. Accessed October 31, 2018.
5. Centers for Disease Control and Prevention. Updated U.S. public health service guidelines for the management of occupational exposures to HBV, HCV, and HIV and recommendations for postexposure prophylaxis. https://www.cdc.gov/mmwr/PDF/rr/rr5011.pdf. Accessed October 31, 2018.
6. Centers for Medicare and Medicaid Services, Department of Health and Human Services. Clinical Laboratory Iprovement Amendments, proficiency testing and PT referral booklet. https://www.cms.gov/Regulations-and-Guidance/Legislation/CLIA/Downloads/CLIAbrochure8.pdf. Accessed October 31, 2018.
7. Centers for Medicare and Medicaid Services, Department of Health and Human Services. Current Clinical Laboratory Improvement Amendments regulations and guidelines. http://www.cms.gov/Regulations-and-Guidance/CLIA. Accessed October 31, 2018.
8. CLIA Program and Medicare Laboratory Services. https://www.cms.gov/Outreach-and-Education/Medicare-Learning-Network-MLN/MLNProducts/Downloads/CLIABrochure.pdf. Accessed October 26, 2018.
9. Clinical and Laboratory Standards Institute. *Protection of Laboratory Workers From Occupationally Acquired Infections: Approved Guideline.* 4th ed. CLSI Document M29-A4. Clinical and Laboratory Standards Institute, Wayne, PA: Clinical and Laboratory Standards Institute; 2014.
10. Clinical and Laboratory Standards Institute. *Quality Management System: A Model for Laboratory Services: Approved Guideline.* 4th ed. CLSI document QM SO1-A4. Wayne, PA: Clinical and Laboratory Standards Institute; 2011.
11. Clinical and Laboratory Standards Institute. *Quality Practices in Noninstrumented Point of Care Testing: An Instructional Manual and Resources for Health Care Workers. Approved Guideline.* CLSI document POCT08-A. Wayne, PA: Clinical and Laboratory Standards Institute; 2010.
12. College of American Pathologists. *Commission on Laboratory Accreditation, Immunology Checklist.* Skokie, IL: College of American Pathologists; 2007.

13. Hazardous materials: infectious substances; harmonizing with the United Nations recommendations. http://www.federalregister.gov/articles/2005/05/19/05-9717/hazardous-materials-infectious-substances-harmonization-with-the-UN recommendations. Accessed October 31, 2018.
14. Hill E. The role of Six Sigma in a modern quality management strategy. *Medical Laboratory Observer (MLO)*. https://www.mlo-online.com/the-role-of-six-sigma-in-a-modern-quality-management-strategy. July 24, 2018. Accessed October 26, 2018.
15. International Air Transportation Association Regulations. Dangerous goods regulations (DGR). 58th ed. 2017. https://www.iata.org/whatwedo/cargo/dgr/Documents/infectious-substance-classification-DGR56-en.pdf. Accessed October 31, 2018.
16. NIOSH Alert. *Preventing Allergic Reactions to Natural Rubber Latex in the Workplace*. DHHS (NIOSH) Publication 97–135. Cincinnati, OH: National Institute for Occupational Safety and Health; 1997.
17. Occupational exposure to bloodborne pathogens, final rule. *Federal Register.* January 18, 2001. https://www.federalregister.gov/documents/2001/01/18/01-1207/occupational-exposure-to-bloodborne-pathogens-needlestick-and-other-sharps-injuries-final-rule. Accessed October 30, 2018.
18. Occupational exposure to hazardous chemicals in laboratories, final rule. *Federal Register.* https://www.federalregister.gov/documents/2013/01/22/2013-00788/occupational-exposure-to-hazardous-chemicals-in-laboratories-non-mandatory-appendix-technical. Accessed October 31, 2018.
19. Occupational Safety and Health Administration. *Enforcement Procedures for the Occupational Exposure to Bloodborne Pathogens Standard.* Directive CPL 02-02-069. Washington, DC: Occupational Safety and Health Administration; 2001. https://www.osha.gov/sites/default/files/enforcement/directives/CPL_02-02-069.pdf. Accessed October 30, 2018.
20. Occupational Safety and Health Administration. Laboratory safety chemical hygiene plan. OSHA occupational exposure to hazardous chemical in laboratories standard. (29 CFR 1910.1450.) January 22, 2013. Accessed October 31, 2018.
21. Scungio D. Keeping the laboratory environment clean and safe. *Medical Laboratory Observer (MLO)*. June 21, 2018. https://www.mlo-online.com/continuing-education/article/13017006/keeping-the-laboratory-environment-clean-and-safe. Accessed August 21, 2020.
22. Siegel JD, Rhinehart E, Jackson M, Chiarello L; Healthcare Infection Control Practices Advisory Committee. 2007 Guideline for isolation precautions: preventing transmission of infectious agents in healthcare settings. https://www.cdc.gov/infectioncontrol/guidelines/isolation/index.html. Accessed October 30, 2018.
23. Strasinger SK, DiLorenzo MS. *The Phlebotomy Textbook*. 4th ed. Philadelphia: F.A. Davis; 2018.
24. Strasinger SK, DiLorenzo MS. *Urinalysis and Body Fluids*. 6th ed. Philadelphia: F.A. Davis; 2014.
25. The Joint Commission. *National Patient Safety Goals Effective January 2019*. Laboratory Accreditation Program. https://www.jointcommission.org/assets/1/6/NPSG_Chapter_LAB_Jan2019.pdf. Accessed October 27, 2018.
26. Top laboratory deficiencies across accreditation agencies. *Clin Lab News (CLN), an AACC Publication*. 2018 July;44(6):38.
27. U.S. Department of Health and Human Services. Public Health Service, CDC, NIH. *Biosafety in Microbiological and Biomedical Laboratories (BMBL)*. 5th ed. Washington, DC: U.S. Department of Health and Human Services; 2011. https://www.cdc.gov/labs/BMBL.html. Accessed October 29, 2018.
28. U.S. Department of Labor, Occupational Safety and Health Administration. Bloodborne pathogens and needlestick prevention standards. https://www.osha.gov/SLTC/bloodbornepathogens/standards.html. Accessed October 31, 2018.
29. U.S. Department of Transportation. Transporting infectious substances safely. https://hazmatonline.phmsa.dot.gov/services/publication_documents/Transporting%20Infectious%20Substances%20Safely.pdf. Accessed October 31, 2018.

9. Principles of Serological Testing

1. Ashwood ER, Bruns DE. Clinical evaluation of methods. In: Burtis CA, Bruns DE, eds. *Tietz Fundamentals of Clinical Chemistry and Molecular Diagnostics.* 7th ed. St. Louis: Elsevier Saunders; 2015:32–39.
2. Estridge BH, Reynolds AP. *Basic Clinical Laboratory Techniques.* 5th ed. Clifton Park, NY: Thomson Delmar Learning; 2008:85–96.
3. Lo SF. Principles of basic techniques and laboratory safety. In: Burtis CA, Bruns DE, eds. *Tietz Fundamentals of Clinical Chemistry and Molecular Diagnostics.* 7th ed. St. Louis: Elsevier Saunders; 2015:107–128.

10. Precipitation and Agglutination Reactions

1. Alper CA, Johnson AM. Immunofixation electrophoresis: a technique for the study of protein polymorphism. *Vox Sang.* 1969;17:445.
2. Aoyagi K, Ashihara Y, Kasahara Y. Immunoassay and immunochemistry. In: McPherson RA, Pincus MR, eds. *Henry's Clinical Diagnosis and Management by Laboratory Methods.* 23rd ed. Philadelphia: Elsevier Saunders; 2017:862–889.
3. Blaney KD, Howard PR. *Basic and Applied Concepts of Blood Banking and Transfusion Practices.* 3rd ed. St. Louis: Elsevier Mosby; 2013:1–27.
4. Csako G. Immunofixation electrophoresis for identification of proteins and specific antibodies. *Methods Mol Biol.* 2012;869:147–171.
5. Delves PJ, Martin SJ, Burton DR, Roitt IM. *Roitt's Essential Immunology.* 12th ed. Oxford, UK: Wiley-Blackwell; 2011:113–140.
6. Fahey JL, McKelvey EM. Quantitative determination of serum immunoglobulins in antibody-agar plates. *J Immunol.* 1965;94:84.
7. Gaikwad UN, Rajurkar M. Diagnostic efficiency of Widal slide agglutination test against Widal tube agglutination test in enteric fever. *Int J Med Public Health.* 2014;4(3):227–230.
8. Kricka LJ, Park JY. Immunochemical techniques. In: Rifai N, Horvath AR, Wittwer CT, eds. *Tietz Fundamentals of Clinical Chemistry and Molecular Diagnostics.* 6th ed. St. Louis: Elsevier; 2018:348–367.
9. Kricka LJ, Park JY. Optical techniques. In: Rifai N, Horvath AR, Wittwer CT, eds. *Tietz Fundamentals of Clinical Chemistry and Molecular Diagnostics.* 6th ed. St. Louis: Elsevier; 2018:200–223.
10. Lapage G. Dr. HE Durham. *Nature.* 1945;156:742.
11. Levinson SS. Urine immunofixation electrophoresis remains important and is complementary to serum free light chain. *Clin Chem Lab Med.* 2011;49(11):1801–1804.
12. Lindsley MD. Serological and molecular diagnosis of fungal infections. In: Detrick B, Schmitz JL, Hamilton RG, eds. *Manual of Molecular and Clinical Laboratory Immunology.* 8th ed. Washington, DC: ASM Press; 2016:503–534.
13. Litwin CM, Litwin SE, Hill HR. Diagnostic methods for group A streptococcal infections. In: Detrick B, Schmitz JL, Hamilton RG, eds. *Manual of Molecular and Clinical Laboratory Immunology.* 8th ed. Washington, DC: ASM Press; 2016:394–403.

14. Male D, Brostoff J, Roth DB, Roitt IM. *Immunology.* 8th ed. Philadelphia: Elsevier Saunders; 2013:51–70.
15. Mancini G, Carbonara AO, Heremans JF. Immunochemical quantitation of antigens by single radial immunodiffusion. *Immunochem.* 1965;2:235.
16. Pincus MR, Lifshitz MS, Bock JA. Analysis: Principles of instrumentation. In: McPherson RA, Pincus MR, eds. *Henry's Clinical Diagnosis and Management by Laboratory Methods.* 23rd ed. Philadelphia: Elsevier Saunders; 2017:33–59.
17. Punt J, Stranford SA, Jones PP, Owen JA. *Kuby Immunology.* 8th ed. New York: WH Freeman. 2019:762–766.
18. Tille P. *Bailey and Scott's Diagnostic Microbiology.* 14th ed. St. Louis: Elsevier Mosby; 2017:144–160.

11. Labeled Immunoassays

1. CAP Today. Chemistry and immunoassay analyzers, mid- and high-volume labs. 2019. https://www.captodayonline.com/chemistry-immuno-mid-high/. Accessed February 21, 2020.
2. Cinquanta L, Fontana DE, Bizzaro N. Chemiluminescent immunoassay technology: what does it change in autoantibody detection? *Auto Immun Highlights.* 2017;8(1):9.
3. Engvall E, Perlmann P. Enzyme-linked immunosorbent assay, ELISA. 3. Quantitation of specific antibodies by enzyme-labeled anti-immunoglobulin in antigen-coated tubes. *J Immunol.* 1972;109(1):129–135.
4. Li J, Wagar EA, Meng QH. Comprehensive assessment of biotin interference in immunoassays. *Clin Chim Acta.* 2018;487:293–298.
5. MEDTOX Diagnostics. PROFILE®-V for MEDTOXScan. 2017. https://www.medtoxdiagnostics.com/medtoxscan/. Accessed February 21, 2020.
6. Miao D, Guyer KM, Dong F, et al. GAD65 autoantibodies detected by electrochemiluminescence assay identify high risk for type 1 diabetes. *Diabetes.* 2013;62(12):4174–4178.
7. Sanavio B, Krol S. On the slow diffusion of point-of-care systems in therapeutic drug monitoring. *Front Bioeng Biotechnol.* 2015; 3:20. doi:10.3389/fbioe.2015.00020
8. Skelley DS, Brown LP, Besch PK. Radioimmunoassay. *Clin Chem.* 1973;19(2):146–186.
9. Snyder MR. A basic guide to ANA testing. *Clinical Laboratory News.* 2019;45(3):15–18.
10. Straseski JA, Stolbach A, Clarke W. Opiate-positive immunoassay screen in a pediatric patient. *Clin Chem.* 2010;56(8):1220–1223.
11. Tacker DH, Robinson R, Perrotta PL. Abbott ARCHITECT iPhenytoin assay versus similar assays for measuring free phenytoin concentrations. *Lab Med.* 2014;45(2):176–181.
12. Yalow RS, Berson SA. Immunoassay of endogenous plasma insulin in man. *J Clin Invest.* 1960;39(7):1157–1175.

12. Molecular Diagnostic Techniques

1. Afshan N, Bashir M, Tipu HN, Hussain M. Optimization of an in-house PCR method for the detection of HLA-B*27 alleles. *Biomed Rep.*2018;8(4):385–390.
2. Antonov J, Goldstein DR, Oberli A, et al. Reliable gene expression measurements from degraded RNA by quantitative real-time PCR depend on short amplicons and a proper normalization. *Lab Invest.* 2005;85:1040–1050.
3. Barbazuk W, Schnable PS. SNP discovery by transcriptome pyrosequencing. *Meth Mole Biol.* 2011;729:225–246.
4. Buckingham L. *Molecular Diagnostics: Fundamentals, Methods and Clinical Applications.* 3rd ed. Philadelphia: F.A. Davis; 2019.
5. Cottrell C, Al-Kateb H, Bredemeyer AJ, et al. Validation of a next-generation sequencing assay for clinical molecular oncology. *J Mol Diagn.* 2013;16:89–105.
6. Dhama K, Karthik K, Chakraborty S, et al. Loop-mediated isothermal amplification of DNA (LAMP): a new diagnostic tool lights the world of diagnosis of animal and human pathogens: a review. *Pakistani Journal of Biological Science,* 2014;17(2):151–166.
7. Dunn P. Human leucocyte antigen typing: techniques and technology, a critical appraisal. *Int J Immunogenet.* 2011;38: 463–473.
8. Esposito S, Zampiero A, Terranova L, et al. Pneumococcal bacterial load colonization as a marker of mixed infection in children with alveolar community-acquired pneumonia and respiratory syncytial virus or rhinovirus infection. *Pediatr Infect Dis J.* 2013;32:1199–1204.
9. Gabriel C, Danzer M, Hackl C, et al. Rapid high-throughput human leukocyte antigen typing by massively parallel pyrosequencing for high-resolution allele identification. *Hum Immunol.* 2009;70:960–964.
10. Giachetti C, Linnen JM, Kolk DP, et al. Highly sensitive multiplex assay for detection of human immunodeficiency virus type 1 and hepatitis C virus RNA. *J Clinical Microbiol.* 2002;40:2408–2419.
11. Glenn G, Andreou LV. Analysis of DNA by Southern blotting. *Method Enzymol.* 2013;529:47–63.
12. Grossmann V, Roller A, Klein HU, et al. Robustness of amplicon deep sequencing underlines its utility in clinical applications. *J Mol Diagn.* 2013;15:473–484.
13. Harrington C, Lin EI, Olson MT, Eshleman JR. Fundamentals of pyrosequencing. *Arch Pathol Lab Med.* 2013;137: 1296–1303.
14. Higuchi R, Fockler C, Dollinger G, Watson R. Kinetic PCR analysis: real-time monitoring of DNA amplification reactions. *Biotechnol.* 1993;11:1026–1030.
15. Jennings LJ, Arcila ME, Corless C, et al. Guidelines for validation of next-generation sequencing-based oncology panels: a joint consensus recommendation of the Association for Molecular Pathology and College of American Pathologists. *J Mol Diagn.* 2017;19(3):341–365.
16. Jennings LJ, Kirschmann D. Genetic testing requires NGS and Sanger methodologies. *Ped Neurol Briefs.* 2016;30(9):36.
17. Keslar K, Lin M, Zmijewska AA, et al. Multicenter evaluation of a standardized protocol for noninvasive gene expression profiling. *Am J Transplant.* 2013;13:1891–1897.
18. Khan Z, Poetter K, Park DJ. Enhanced solid phase PCR: mechanisms to increase priming by solid support primers. *Analyt Biochem.* 2008;375:391–393.
19. Kircher M, Heyn P, Kelso J. Addressing challenges in the production and analysis of Illumina sequencing data. *BMC Genomics.* 2011;382:1–14.
20. Kurt K, Alderborn A, Nilsson M, et al. Multiplexed genotyping of methicillin-resistant *Staphylococcus aureus* isolates by use of padlock probes and tag microarrays. *J Clin Microbiol.* 2009;47(3):577–585.
21. Kwoh D, Davis GR, Whitfield KM, et al. Transcription-based amplification system and detection of amplified human immunodeficiency virus type 1 with a bead-based sandwich hybridization format. *P Natl Acad Sci.* 1989;86:1173–1777.
22. Lachmann N, Todorova K, Schulze H, Schönemann C. Luminex(®) and its applications for solid organ transplantation, hematopoietic stem cell transplantation, and transfusion. *Transfus Med Hemoth.* 2013;40:182–189.
23. Lank S, Wiseman RW, Dudley DM, O'Connor DH. A novel single cDNA amplicon pyrosequencing method for high-throughput, cost-effective sequence-based HLA class I genotyping. *Hum Immunol.* 2010;71:1011–1017.

24. Liu L, Li Y, Li S, et al. Comparison of next-generation sequencing systems. *J Biomed Biotech.* 2012;1–12. doi:10.1155/2012/251364. Accessed October 29, 2020.
25. Marsh S. Nomenclature for factors of the HLA system, updates. *HLA.* 2019;93(6):511–541.
26. Maxam A, Gilbert W. A new method for sequencing DNA. *P Natl Acad Sci.* 1977;74:560–564.
27. Nakano M, Komatsu J, Matsuura S, et al. Single-molecule PCR using water-in-oil emulsion. *J Biotech.* 2003;102:117–124.
28. Nelson N, Cheikh AB, Matsuda E, Becker MM. Simultaneous detection of multiple nucleic acid targets in a homogeneous format. *Biochem.* 1996;35:8429–8438.
29. Neumann F, Hernández-Neuta I, Grabbe M, et al. Padlock probe assay for detection and subtyping of seasonal influenza. *Clin Chem,* 2018;64(12):1704–1712.
30. Nyrén P. The history of pyrosequencing. *Meth Mol Biol.* 2007;373:1–14.
31. Oliver, M. The invader assay for SNP genotyping. *Mutat Res.* 2005;573:103–110.
32. Parameswaran P, Jalili R, Tao L, et al. A pyrosequencing-tailored nucleotide barcode design unveils opportunities for large-scale sample multiplexing. *Nucleic Acids Res.* 2007;35:e130.
33. Pas S, Molenkamp R, Schinkel J, et al. Performance evaluation of the new Roche cobas AmpliPrep/cobas TaqMan HCV test, version 2.0, for detection and quantification of hepatitis C virus RNA. *J Clinical Microbiol.* 2013;51:238–242.
34. Pearson WR, Lipman DJ. Improved tools for biological sequence comparison. *Proc Natl Acad Sci.* 1988;85(8):2444–2448.
35. Prosperi M, Prosperi L, Bruselles A, et al. Combinatorial analysis and algorithms for quasispecies reconstruction using next-generation sequencing. *BMC Bioinformatics,* 2011;12:1–13.
36. Rothberg JM, Hinz W, Rearick TM, et al. An integrated semiconductor device enabling non-optical genome sequencing. *Nature.* 2011;475(7356):348–352.
37. Sander JD, Joung JK. CRISPR-Cas systems for editing, regulating and targeting genomes. *Nat Biotechnol.* 2014;32(4):347–355.
38. Sanger F, Nicklen S, Coulson AR. DNA sequencing with chain-terminating inhibitors. *P Natl Acad Sci.* 1977;74:5463–5467.
39. Santamaria P, Lindstrom AL, Boyce-Jacino MT, et al. HLA class I sequence-based typing. *Hum Immunol.* 1993;37:39–50.
40. Singh DD, Hawkins RD, Lahesmaa R, Tripathi SK. CRISPR/Cas9 guided genome and epigenome engineering and its therapeutic applications in immune mediated diseases. *Sem Cell Develop Biol.* 2019;18:30111–30113.
41. Sykes P, Neoh SH, Brisco MJ, et al. Quantitation of targets for PCR by use of limiting dilution. *Biotechniques.* 1992;13:444–449.
42. Vermehren J, Yu ML, Monto A, et al. Multi-center evaluation of the Abbott RealTime HCV assay for monitoring patients undergoing antiviral therapy for chronic hepatitis C. *Clin Virol.* 2011;52:133–137.
43. Vogelstein K, Kinzler KW. Digital PCR. *P Natl Acad Sci.* 1999;96:9236–9241.
44. Wajid B, Serpedin E. Review of general algorithmic features for genome assemblers for next generation sequencers. *Genom Proteom Bioinform.* 2012;10:58–73.
45. Wirtz C, Sayer D. Data analysis of HLA sequencing using Assign-SBT v3.6+ from Conexio. *Meth Mol Biol.* 2012;882:87–121.
46. Worthey EA, Mayer AN, Syverson, GD, et al. Making a definitive diagnosis: successful clinical application of whole exome sequencing in a child with intractable inflammatory bowel disease. *Genet Med.* 2011;13(3):255–262.
47. Yan L, Zhou J, Zheng Y, et al. Isothermal amplified detection of DNA and RNA. *Mol Biosyst.* 2014;10(5):970–1003.

13. Flow Cytometry and Laboratory Automation

1. Alexiou GA, Vartholomatos E, Goussia A, et al. DNA content is associated with malignancy of intracranial neoplasms. *Clin Neurol Neurosurg.* 2013(Sep);115(9):1784–1787.
2. Appold K. Checklist for buying a chemistry analyzer. *Clin Lab Prod.* 2013(Nov);12–15.
3. Armbruster DA, Overcash DR, Reyes J. Clinical chemistry automation in the 21st century—Amat Victoria Curam. *Clin Biochem Rev.* 2014;35(3)143–153.
4. Association for Molecular Pathology. Association for Molecular Pathology statement: recommendations for in-house development and operation of molecular diagnostic tests. *Am J Clin Path.* 1999;111:449–463.
5. BD Biosciences. BD LSR Fortessa X-20 Flow Cytometer. http://www.bdbiosciences.com/us/instruments/research/cell-analyzers/bd-lsrfortessa-x-20/m/1519232/overview. Accessed May 16, 2019.
6. Bleesing JJH, Fleischer TA. Immunophenotyping. *Semin Hematol.* 2001;38(2):100.
7. Borowitz MJ, Craig FE, Digiuseppe JA, et al. Guidelines for the diagnosis and monitoring of paroxysmal nocturnal hemoglobinuria and related disorders by flow cytometry. *Cytometry B Clin Cytom.* 2010(Jul);78(4):211–230.
8. Carter PH, Resto-Ruiz S, Washington GC, et al. Flow cytometric analysis of whole blood lysis, three anticoagulants, and five cell preparations. *Cytometry.* 1992;13:68–74.
9. Centers for Disease Control and Prevention. Revised surveillance case definition for HIV infection—United States, 2014. https://www.cdc.gov/mmwr/preview/mmwrhtml/rr6303a1.htm. Accessed May 16, 2019.
10. Chen JC, Davis BH, Wood B, Warzynski MJ. Multicenter clinical experience with flow cytometric method for fetomaternal hemorrhage detection. *Cytometry.* 2002;50:285–290.
11. College of American Pathologists. Automated immunoassay analyzers. http://www.cap.org/apps/docs/cap_today/surveys/0608_ImmunoSurvey.pdf. Accessed May 6, 2019.
12. Cortelazzo S, Ponzoni M, Ferreri AJ, Hoelzer D. Lymphoblastic lymphoma. *Crit Rev Oncol Hematol.* 2011(Sep);79(3):330–343.
13. Degheidy H, Salem DAA, Yuan CM, Stetler-Stevenson M. Chronic lymphocytic leukemia, the prototypic chronic leukemia for flow cytometric analysis. In: Detrick B, Schmitz JL, Hamilton RG, eds. *Manual of Molecular and Clinical Laboratory Immunology.* 8th ed. Washington, DC: ASM Press; 2016:226–234.
14. DiGiuseppe JA. Acute lymphoblastic leukemia: diagnosis and minimal residual disease detection by flow cytometric immunophenotyping. In: Detrick B, Schmitz JL, Hamilton RG, eds. *Manual of Molecular and Clinical Laboratory Immunology.* 8th ed. Washington, DC: ASM Press; 2016:207–216.
15. Fernandes BJ, vonDadelszen P, Fazal I, et al. Flow cytometric assessment of feto-maternal hemorrhage; a comparison with Betke-Kleihauer. *Prenat Diagn.* 2007;27(7):641–643.
16. Giorgi JVA, Kesson M, Chou CC. Immunodeficiency and infectious diseases. In: Rose NL, deMacario CE, Fahey JL, Friedman H, Penn GM, eds. *Manual of Clinical Laboratory Immunology.* 4th ed. Washington, DC: ASM Press; 1992:174–181.
17. Golightly MG. Dihydrorhodamine (DHR) flow cytometry test for chronic granulomatous disease (CGD): a simple test for routine clinical flow cytometry. *Int Clin Cytom Soc.* 2011 (Winter);2(1).
18. Harris HL, Jaffe ES, Stein H, et al. A revised European-American classification of lymphoid neoplasms: a proposal from the International Lymphoma Study Group. *Blood.* 1994;84:1361–1392.
19. Kricka LJ, Park, JY. Optical techniques. In: Burtis CA, Burns DE, eds. *Tietz Fundamentals of Clinical Chemistry and Molecular Diagnostics.* 7th ed. St. Louis: Elsevier Saunders; 2015:129–150.

20. Margolick JB, Munoz A, Donnenberg A, et al. Failure of T-cell homeostasis preceding AIDS in HIV infection. *Nat Med.* 1995;1:674–680.
21. Moon TC, Legrys VA. Teaching method validation in the clinical laboratory science curriculum. *Clin Lab Sci.* 2008;21(1):19–24.
22. National Committee for Clinical Laboratory Standards. *Clinical Applications of Flow Cytometry Quality Assurance and Immunophenotyping of Peripheral Blood Lymphocytes.* H42-A. Wayne, PA: National Committee for Clinical Laboratory Standards; 1998.
23. Remaley AT, Hortin GL. Protein analysis for diagnostic applications. In: Detrick B, Hamilton RG, Folds JD, et al, eds. *Manual of Molecular and Clinical Laboratory Immunology.* 7th ed. Washington, DC: ASM Press; 2006:7–21.
24. Renzi P, Ginns LC. Analysis of T cell subsets in normal adults. Comparison of whole blood lysis technique to Ficoll-Hypaque separation by flow cytometry. *Immunol Meth.* 1987;98:53–56.
25. Srinivasula S, Lempicki RA, Adelsberger JW, et al. Differential effects of HIV viral load and CD4 count on proliferation of naive and memory CD4 and CD8 T lymphocytes. *Blood.* 2011 (Jul 14);118(2):262–270.
26. Sunheimer RL, Lifshitz MS, Threatte G. Analysis: clinical laboratory automation. In: McPherson RA, Pincus MR, eds. *Henry's Clinical Diagnosis and Management by Laboratory Methods.* 22nd ed. Philadelphia: Elsevier Saunders; 2011:64–72.
27. Turgeon ML. Automated procedures. In: *Immunology and Serology in Laboratory Medicine.* 5th ed. St. Louis: Mosby; 2014:170–182.
28. Van Dongen JJM, Lhermitte L, Bottcher S, et al. EuroFlow antibody panels for standardized n-dimensional flow cytometric immunophenotyping of normal, reactive, and malignant leukocytes. *Leukemia.* 2012;26:1908–1975.
29. Vardiman JW. The World Health Organization classification of neoplastic diseases of the hematopoietic and lymphoid tissues. An overview with emphasis on myeloid neoplasms. *Chem Biol Interact.* 2010(Mar 19);184(1–2):16–20.
30. Wood BL, Soma L. Acute myeloid leukemia: diagnosis and minimal residual disease detection by flow cytometric immunophenotyping. In: Detrick B, Schmitz JL, Hamilton RG, eds. *Manual of Molecular and Clinical Laboratory Immunology.* 8th ed. Washington, DC: ASM Press; 2016:217–225.

14. Hypersensitivity

Hypersensitivity—General

1. Owen JA, Punt J, Stranford SA. *Kuby Immunology.* 7th ed. New York: W.H. Freeman; 2013:485–516.

Type I Hypersensitivity—Mechanism

1. Boyce JA. The biology of the mast cell. *Allergy Asthma Proc.* 2004;25:27–30.
2. Brown JM, Wilson TM, Metcalfe DD. The mast cell and allergic diseases: role in pathogenesis and implications for therapy. *Clin Exp Allergy.* 2007;38:4–18.
3. Fishbein AB, Fuleihan RL. The hygiene hypothesis revisited: does exposure to infectious agents protect us from allergy? *Curr Opin Pediatr.* 2012;24(1):98–102.
4. Galli SJ, Tsai M. IgE and mast cells in allergic disease. *Nature Med.* 2012;18:693–704.
5. Gould HJ, Sutton BJ, Beavil AJ, et al. The biology of IgE and the basis of allergic disease. *Annu Rev Immunol.* 2003;21:579–628.
6. Granada M, Wilk JB, Tuzova M, et al. A genome-wide association study of plasma total IgE concentrations in the Framingham heart study. *J Allergy Clin Immun.* 2012;129(3):840–845.e21.
7. Holloway JA, Yang IA, Holgate ST. Genetics of allergic disease. *J Allergy Clin Immunol.* 2010;125:S81–S94.
8. Jatzlauk G, Bartel S, Heine H, Schloter M, Krauss-Etschmann S. Influences of environmental bacteria and their metabolites on allergies, asthma, and host microbiota. *Allergy.* 2017; Dec;72(12):1859–1867.
9. MacGalshan D. IgE receptor and signal transduction in mast cells and basophils. *Curr Opin Immunol.* 2008;20:717–723.
10. Parham P. IgE-mediated immunity and allergy. In: *The Immune System.* 4th ed. New York: Garland Science; 2015:401–431.
11. Stone KD, Prussin C, Metcalfe DD. IgE, mast cells, basophils, and eosinophils. *J Allergy Clin Immunol.* 2010;125:S73–S80.
12. Vercilli D. Discovering susceptibility genes for asthma and allergy. *Nat Rev Immunol.* 2008;8:169–182.
13. Vercelli D. Remembrance of things past: HLA genes come back on the allergy stage. *J Allergy Clin Immunol.* 2012;129:846–847.
14. Wlasiuk G, Vercelli D. The farm effect, or: when, what and how a farming environment protects from asthma and allergic disease. *Curr Opin Allergy CI.* 2012;12(5):461–466.

Type I Hypersensitivity—Clinical Conditions and Therapy

1. American Academy of Allergy, Asthma & Immunology. Allergy statistics. https://www.aaaai.org/about-aaaai/newsroom/allergy-statistics. Accessed July 16, 2018.
2. Asthma and Allergy Foundation of America. Allergy facts and figures. http://www.aafa.org/display.cfm?id=9&sub=30. Accessed July 16, 2018.
3. Berings M, Karaasian C, Altunbulakli C, et al. Advances and highlights in allergen immunotherapy: on the way to sustained clinical and immunologic tolerance. *J Allergy Clin Immunol.* 2017;140:1250–1267.
4. Burks AW, Calderon MA, Casale T, et al. Update on allergy immunotherapy: American Academy of Allergy, Asthma & Immunology/European Academy of Allergy and Clinical Immunology/PRACTALL consensus report. *J Allergy Clin Immunol.* 2013;131(5):1288–1296.e3.
5. Casale TB, Stokes JR. Future forms of immunotherapy. *J Allergy Clin Immunol.* 2011;127(1):8–15.
6. Centers for Disease Control and Prevention. Latex allergy. https://www.cdc.gov/healthcommunication/toolstemplates/entertainmented/tips/LatexAllergy.html. Accessed July 16, 2018.
7. European Academy of Allergy and Clinical Immunology. EAACI guidelines on allergen immunotherapy: executive statement. *Allergy.* 2018;73:739–743.
8. Fried AJ, Oettgen HC. Anti-IgE in the treatment of allergic disorders in pediatrics. *Curr Opin Pediatr.* 2010;22(6):758–764.
9. Gawchik DO. Latex allergy. *Mt Sinai J Med.* 2011;78:759–772.
10. Homberger H, Hamilton RG. Allergic diseases. In: Elkins M, Davenport R, Mintz PD, eds. *Henry's Clinical Diagnosis and Management by Laboratory Methods.* 23rd ed. St. Louis: Elsevier Inc; 2017:1057–1070.
11. Kuhl K, Hanania NA. Targeting IgE in asthma. *Curr Opin Pulm Med.* 2012;18(1):1–5.
12. LoVerde D, Iweala OI, Eginli A, Krishnaswamy G. Anaphylaxis. *Chest.* 2018;153(2):528–543.
13. Luccioli S, Escobar-Gutierrez A, Bellanti JA. Allergic diseases and asthma. In: Bellanti JA, Escobar-Gutierrez A, Tsokos GC, eds. *Immunology IV: Clinical Applications in Health and Disease.* Bethesda, MD: I Care Press; 2012:685–765.
14. Stokes JR, Casale TB. Allergic rhinitis and asthma: celebrating 100 years of immunotherapy. *Curr Opin Immunol.* 2011;23(6):808–813.

15. Taylor JS, Erkek E. Latex allergy: diagnosis and management. *Dermatol Ther.* 2004;17(4):289–301.
16. Wu M, Mcintosh J, Liu J. Current prevalence rate of latex allergy: why it remains a problem? *J Occup Health.* 2016;58:138–144.

Allergy Testing

1. Canonica GW, Ansotegui IJ, Pawankar R, et al. A WAO–ARIA–GA2 LEN consensus document on molecular-based allergy diagnostics. *World Allergy Org J.* 2013;6:1–17. doi:10.1186/1939-4551-6-17
2. Carr TF, Saltoun CA. Skin testing in allergy. *Allergy Asthma Proc.* 2012;33(suppl 1):S6–S8.
3. Cox L. Overview of serological-specific IgE antibody testing in children. *Curr Allergy Asthm R.* 2011;11(6):447–453.
4. Hamilton RG. Immunological methods in the diagnostic allergy clinical and research laboratory, In: Detrick B, Schmitz JL, Hamilton RG, eds. *Manual of Molecular and Clinical Laboratory Immunology.* 8th ed. Washington, DC: ASM Press; 2016:795–800.
5. Hamilton RG, Williams PB, Specific IgE Testing Task Force of the American Academy of Allergy, Asthma & Immunology. American College of Allergy, Asthma and Immunology. Human IgE antibody serology: a primer for the practicing North American allergist /immunologist. *J Allergy Clin Immunol.* 2010;126(1):33–38.
6. Heffler E, Puggioni F, Peveri S, Montagni M, Canonica GW. Extended IgE profile based on an allergen macroarray: a novel tool for precision medicine in allergy diagnosis. *World Allergy Org J.* 2018;11:7. doi:10.1186/s40413-018-0186-3.
7. Jensen-Jarolim E, Jensen AN, Canonica GW. Debates in allergy medicine: molecular allergy diagnosis with ISAC will replace screenings by skin prick test in the future. *World Allergy Org J.* 2017;10:33. doi:10.1186/s40413-017-0164-1
8. Kranke B, Aberer W. Skin testing for IgE-mediated drug allergy. *Immunol Allergy Clin.* 2009;29(3):503–516.
9. Larenas-Linnemann D, Luna-Pech JA, Mösges R. Debates in allergy medicine: allergy skin testing cannot be replaced by molecular diagnosis in the near future. *World Allergy Org J.* 2017;10:32. doi:10.1186/s40413-017-0164-1.
10. Pomes A, Davies JA, Gadermaier G, et al. WHO/IUIS allergen nomenclature: providing a common language. *Mol Immunol.* 2018; 100:3–13. doi:10.1016/j.molimm.2018.03.003
11. Thermo Scientific. ImmunoCAP lab tests. 2012. http://www.phadia.com/Products/Allergy-testing-products/ImmunoCAP-Assays/. Accessed July 14, 2018.
12. Tourlas K, Burman D. Allergy testing. *Prim Care Clin Office Prac.* 2016;43:363–374.
13. Volcheck GW. Which diagnostic tests for common allergies? Where to start when you face an allergy puzzle. *Postgrad Med.* 2001;109(5):71–72.
14. WHO/IUIS Allergen Nomenclature Sub-Committee. Allergen nomenclature. http://www.allergen.org/pubs.php. Accessed July 14, 2018.

Type II Hypersensitivity

1. Blaney KD, Howard PR. *Concepts of Immunohematology.* 2nd ed. St. Louis: Mosby, Elsevier; 2009:284–303.
2. Cooling L, Downs T. Immunohematology. In: Elkins M, Davenport R, Mintz PD, eds. *Henry's Clinical Diagnosis and Management by Laboratory Methods.* 23rd ed. St. Louis: Elsevier Inc; 2017:680–734.
3. D'Arena G, Taylor RP, Cascavilla N, Lindorfer MA. Monoclonal antibodies: new therapeutic agents for autoimmune hemolytic anemia? *Endocr Metab Immune Disord Drug Targets.* 2008;8(1):62–68.
4. Davenport RD, Mintz PD. Transfusion medicine. In: Elkins M, Davenport R, Mintz PD, eds. *Henry's Clinical Diagnosis and Management by Laboratory Methods.* 23rd ed. St. Louis: Elsevier Inc; 2017:735–750.
5. Delaney M, Wendel S, Bercovitz RS, et al. Transfusion reactions: prevention, diagnosis, and treatment. *Lancet.* 2016;388:2825–2836.
6. Dzieczkowski JS, Tiberghien P, Anderson KC. Transfusion biology and therapy. In: Jameson JL, Fauci A, Kasper D, Hauser S, Longo DL, Loscalzo J, eds. *Harrison's Principles of Internal Medicine.* 20th ed. New York: McGraw-Hill; 2018. http://accessmedicine.mhmedical.com.libproxy1.upstate.edu/content.aspx?bookid=2129§ionid=192280223. Accessed July 16, 2018.
7. Garratty G, Dzik W, Issitt PD, et al. Terminology for blood group antigens and genes—historical origins and guidelines in the new millennium. *Transfusion.* 2000;40(4):477–489.
8. Grotzke M. The thyroid gland. In: Bishop ML, Fody EP, Schoeff LE, eds. *Clinical Chemistry.* 8th ed. Philadelphia: Lippincott, Williams & Wilkins; 2018:476–487.
9. Harmening DM, Rodberg K, Green EB. Autoimmune hemolytic anemias. In: Harmening DM, ed. *Modern Blood Banking & Transfusion Practices.* 6th ed. Philadelphia: F.A. Davis; 2012:439–473.
10. Hendrickson JE, Delaney M. Hemolytic disease of the fetus and newborn: modern practice and future investigations. *Transfusion Med Rev.* 2016;30:159–164.
11. Kennedy MS. Hemolytic disease of the newborn (HDFN). In: Harmening DM, ed. *Modern Blood Banking & Transfusion Practices.* 6th ed. Philadelphia: F.A. Davis; 2012:427–438.
12. Luzzatto L. Hemolytic anemias. In: Jameson JL, Fauci A, Kasper D, Hauser S, Longo DL, Loscalzo J, eds. *Harrison's Principles of Internal Medicine.* 20th ed. New York: McGraw-Hill; 2018. http://accessmedicine.mhmedical.com.libproxy1.upstate.edu/content.aspx?bookid=2129§ionid=192017418. Accessed July 16, 2018.
13. McNicholl FP. Clinical syndromes associated with cold agglutinins. *Transfus Sci.* 2000;22:125–133.
14. Miller LE, Ludke HR, Peacock JE, Tomar RH. *Manual of Laboratory Immunology.* 2nd ed. Philadelphia: Lea & Febiger; 1991:360–364.
15. Murray NA, Roberts IA. Haemolytic disease of the newborn. *Arch Dis Child Fetal Neonatal Ed.* 2007;92(2):F83–F88.
16. Storry JR, Castilho L, Chen Q, Daniels G, Denomme G. International Society of Blood Transfusion Working Party on red cell immunogenetics and terminology: report of the Seoul and London meetings. *ISBT Sci Ser.* 2016 Aug;11(2):118–122. doi:10.1111/voxs.12280
17. Storry JR, Olsson ML. Genetic basis of blood group diversity. *Br J Haematol.* 2004;126(6):759–771.
18. Torres R, Kenney B, Tormey CA. Diagnosis, treatment, and reporting of adverse effects of transfusion. *Lab Medicine.* 2012;43(5):217–231.

Type III Hypersensitivity

1. Bellanti JA, Escobar-Gutierrez A. Mechanisms of immunologic injury. In: Bellanti JA, Escobar-Gutierrez A, Tsokos GC, eds. *Immunology IV: Clinical Applications in Health and Disease.* Bethesda, MD: I Care Press; 2012:661–683.
2. Bellanti JA, Escobar-Gutierrez A, Joost JJ. Cytokines, chemokines, and the immune system. In: Bellanti JA, Escobar-Gutierrez A, Tsokos GC, eds. *Immunology IV: Clinical Applications in Health and Disease.* Bethesda, MD: I Care Press; 2012:287–366.

Type IV Hypersensitivity

1. Akuthota P, Wechsler ME. Hypersensitivity pneumonitis and pulmonary infiltrates with eosinophilia. In: Jameson JL, Fauci

A, Kasper D, Hauser S, Longo DL, Loscalzo J, eds. *Harrison's Principles of Internal Medicine.* 20th ed. New York: McGraw-Hill; 2018. http://accessmedicine.mhmedical.com.libproxy1.upstate.edu/content.aspx?bookid=2129§ionid=186950464. Accessed July 16, 2018.

2. American Thoracic Society. Targeted tuberculin testing and treatment of latent tuberculosis infection. *MMWR Recommendations & Reports.* 2000;49(RR-6):1–51.
3. Belknap R, Daley CL. Interferon gamma release assays. *Clin Lab Med.* 2014;34:337–349.
4. Borkowska DI, Napiorkowska AM, Brzezinska SA, et al. From latent tuberculosis infection to tuberculosis. News in diagnostics (QuantiFERON-Plus). *Polish J Microbiol.* 2017;66(1): 5–8.
5. Centers for Disease Control and Prevention. Updated guidelines for using interferon gamma release assays to detect Mycobacterium tuberculosis infection—United States, 2010. *MMWR.* 2010;59(RR-5):1–26.
6. Gladman AC. Toxicodendron dermatitis: poison ivy, oak, and sumac. *Wilderness Environ Med.* 2006;17(2):120–128.
7. Jacob SE, Steele T. Allergic contact dermatitis: early recognition and diagnosis of important allergens. *Dermatol Nurs.* 2006;18(5):433–439, 446.
8. Jacob SE, Zapolanski T. Systemic contact dermatitis. *Dermatitis.* 2008;19(1):9–15.
9. Jensen PA, Lambert LA, Iademarco MF, Ridzon R, CDC. Guidelines for preventing the transmission of mycobacterium tuberculosis in health-care settings, 2005. *MMWR Rec Rep.* 2005;54(RR-17):1–141.
10. Karlberg AT, Bergstrom MA, Borje A, et al. Allergic contact dermatitis—formation, structural requirements, and reactivity of skin sensitizers. *Chem Res Toxicol.* 2008;21(1):53–69.
11. Lee PW, Elsaie ML, Jacob SE. Allergic contact dermatitis in children: common allergens and treatment: a review. *Curr Opin Pediatr.* 2009;21(4):491–498.
12. Litwin CM. Immunological tests in tuberculosis. In: Detrick B, Schmitz JL, Hamilton RG, eds. *Manual of Molecular and Clinical Laboratory Immunology.* 8th ed. Washington, DC: ASM Press; 2016:433–443.
13. McCormick T, Shearer W. Delayed-type hypersensitivity skin testing. In: Detrick B, Hamilton RG, Folds JD, eds. *Manual of Molecular and Clinical Laboratory Immunology.* 7th ed. Washington, DC: ASM Press; 2006:234–240.
14. Moesgaard F, Lykkegaard Nielsen M, Norgaard Larsen P, et al. Cell-mediated immunity assessed by skin testing (multitest). I. Normal values in healthy Danish adults. *Allergy.* 1987;42(8):591–596.
15. Patel AM, Ryu JH, Reed CE. Hypersensitivity pneumonitis: current concepts and future questions. *J Allergy Clin Immunol.* 2001;108:661–670.
16. Peiser M, Tralau T, Heidler J, et al. Allergic contact dermatitis: epidemiology, molecular mechanisms, in vitro methods and regulatory aspects. Current knowledge assembled at an international workshop at BfR, Germany. *Cell Mol Life Sci.* 2012;69(5): 763–781.
17. Qiagen, Inc. QuantiFERON-TB Gold Plus (QFT-Plus) Package Insert 08/2017.

15. Autoimmunity

Epidemiology and Etiology of Autoimmune Diseases

1. Abbas AK, Lichtman AH, Pillai S. Immunologic tolerance and autoimmunity. In: Abbas AK, Lichtman AH, Pillai S. *Cellular and Molecular Immunology.* 9th ed. Philadelphia: Elsevier; 2018:325–350.
2. American Autoimmune Diseases Related Association. Autoimmune disease list. https://www.aarda.org/diseaselist/. Accessed January 20, 2020.
3. Anaya JM, Ramirez-Santana C, Alzate MA, Molano-Gonzalez N, Rojas-Villarraga A. The autoimmune ecology. *Front Immunol.* 2016;7(Article 139): 1–31. doi:10.3389/fimmu.2016.00139
4. Autoimmune Registry. Estimates of prevalence for autoimmune disease. http://www.autoimmuneregistry.org/autoimmune-statistics. Accessed January 20, 2020.
5. Chervonsky AV. Microbiota and autoimmunity. *Cold Spring Harb Perspect Bio* 2013;5(3):a007294.
6. Cusick MF, Libbey JE, Fujinami RS. Molecular mimicry as a mechanism of autoimmune disease. *Clin Rev Allergy Immunol.* 2012;42(1):102–111.
7. Kyttaris V, Tsokos GC. Tolerance, autoimmunity, and autoinflammation. In: Bellanti JA, Escobar-Gutierrez A, Tsokos GC, eds. *Immunology IV: Clinical Applications in Health and Disease.* Bethesda, MD: I Care Press; 2012:767–798.
8. Lu Q. The critical importance of epigenetics in autoimmunity. *J Autoimmun.* 2013;41:1–5.
9. National Institute of Health. Medline Plus. Autoimmune diseases. https://medlineplus.gov/autoimmunediseases.html#cat_79. Accessed January 20, 2020.
10. Ngo ST, Steyen FJ, McCombe PA. Gender differences in autoimmune disease. *Front Neuroendocrin.* 2014;35:347–369.
11. Pillai S. Rethinking mechanisms of autoimmune pathogenesis. *J Autoimmun.* 2013;45:97–103.
12. Proft T, Fraser JD. Bacterial superantigens. *Clin Exp Immunol.* 2003;133(3):299–306.
13. Quintero OL, Amador-Patarroyo MJ, Montoya-Ortiz G, et al. Autoimmune disease and gender: plausible mechanisms for the female predominance of autoimmunity. *J Autoimmun.* 2012;38(2–3):J109–J119.
14. Selmi C, Leung PS, Sherr DH, et al. Mechanisms of environmental influence on human autoimmunity: A National Institute of Environmental Health Sciences expert panel workshop. *J Autoimmun.* 2012;39(4):272–284.
15. Sfriso P, Ghirardello A, Botsios C, et al. Infections and autoimmunity: the multifaceted relationship. *J Leukoc Biol.* 2010;87(3):385–395.
16. Vadasz Z, Toubi E. Frontier issues in autoimmunity: publications in 2009–2010. *IMAJ.* 2010;12(12):757–761.
17. Wahren-Herlenius M, Dorner T. Immunopathogenic mechanisms of systemic autoimmune disease. *Lancet.* 2013;382(9894): 819–831.

Systemic Lupus Erythematosus

1. Araujo-Fernandez S, Ahijon-Lana M, Isenberg DA. Drug-induced lupus: including anti-tumour necrosis factor and interferon induced. *Lupus.* 2014;23(6):545–553.
2. Aringer M, Costenbader K, Daikh D, et al. 2019 European League Against Rheumatism/American College of Rheumatology classification criteria for systemic lupus erythematosus. *Arthrit Rheumatol.* 2019;71(9):1400–1412. doi:10.1002/art.40930
3. Baer AN, Witter FR, Petri M. Lupus and pregnancy. *Obstet Gynecol Surv.* 2011;66(10):639–653.
4. Campbell R, Jr, Cooper GS, Gilkeson GS. Two aspects of the clinical and humanistic burden of systemic lupus erythematosus: mortality risk and quality of life early in the course of disease. *Arthritis Rheum.* 2008;59(4):458–464.

5. Cozzani E, Drosera M, Gasparini G, Parodi A. Serology of lupus erythematosus: correlation between immunopathological features and clinical aspects. *Autoimmune Dis.* 2014;2014:321–359.
6. Fanouriakis A, Kostopoulou M, Alunno A. I. 2019 update of the EULAR recommendations for the management of systemic lupus erythematosus. *Ann Rheum Dis.* 2019;78:736–745.
7. Gergely P, Jr, Isaak A, Szekeres Z, et al. Altered expression of Fc gamma and complement receptors on B cells in systemic lupus erythematosus. *Ann NY Acad Sci.* 2007;1108:183–192.
8. Gualtierotti R, Biggioggero M, Penatti AE, Meroni PL. Updating on the pathogenesis of systemic lupus erythematosus. *Autoimmun Rev.* 2010;10(1):3–7.
9. Hahn B. Systemic lupus erythematosus. In: Jameson J, Fauci AS, Kasper DL, Hauser SL, Longo DL, Loscalzo J, eds. *Harrison's Principles of Internal Medicine.* 20th ed. New York: McGraw-Hill; 2018. http://accessmedicine.mhmedical.com/content.aspx?bookid=2129§ionid=192284866. Accessed January 20, 2020.
10. Heinlen LD, McClain MT, Merrill J, et al. Clinical criteria for systemic lupus erythematosus precede diagnosis, and associated autoantibodies are present before clinical symptoms. *Arthrit Rheum.* 2007;56(7):2344–2351.
11. Kuhn A, Bonsmann G, Anders HJ, et al. The diagnosis and treatment of systemic lupus erythematosus. *Dtsch Arztebl Int.* 2015;112:423–432.
12. Marks SD, Tullus K. Autoantibodies in systemic lupus erythematosus. *Pediatr Nephrol.* 2012;27(10):1855–1868.
13. Mok CC. Systemic lupus erythematosus: what should family physicians know in 2018? *Hong Kong Med J.* 2018;24:501–511.
14. Nowling TK, Gilkeson GS. Mechanisms of tissue injury in lupus nephritis. *Arthritis Res Ther.* 2011;13(6):250.
15. O'Neill S, Cervera R. Systemic lupus erythematosus. *Best Pract Res Clin Rh.* 2010;24(6):841–855.
16. Petri M, Orbai AM, Alarcon GS, et al. Derivation and validation of the systemic lupus international collaborating clinics classification criteria for systemic lupus erythematosus. *Arthrit Rheum.* 2012;64(8):2677–2686.
17. Rahman A, Isenberg DA. Systemic lupus erythematosus. *N Engl J Med.* 2008;358(9):929–939.
18. Rodriguez-Garcia V, Dias SS, Isenberg D. Recent advances in the treatment of systemic lupus erythematosus. *Int J Clin Rheumatol.* 2014;9(1):89–100.
19. Smith PP, Gordon C. Systemic lupus erythematosus: clinical presentations. *Autoimmun Rev.* 2010;10(1):43–45.
20. Tsokos GC. Systemic lupus erythematosus. A disease with a complex pathogenesis. *Lancet.* 2001;358(suppl):S65.
21. von Muhlen A, Nakamura RM. Clinical and laboratory evaluation of systemic rheumatic diseases. In: McPherson RA, Pincus MR, eds. *Henry's Clinical Diagnosis and Management by Laboratory Methods.* 22nd ed. Philadelphia: Elsevier Saunders; 2011:973–990.

Antinuclear Antibodies

1. Aarden LA, de Groot ER, Feltkamp TE. Immunology of DNA. III. *Crithidia luciliae,* a simple substrate for the determination of anti-dsDNA with the immunofluorescence technique. *Ann NY Acad Sci.* 1975;254:505–515.
2. Al-Zougbi A. Antinuclear antibody. *Medscape.* https://emedicine.medscape.com/article/2086616-overview#a1. Updated 2014. Accessed February 29, 2020.
3. Chan EKL, Damoiseaux J, Carballo OG, et al. Report of the First International Consensus on Standardized Nomenclature of Antinuclear Antibody HEp-2 Cell Patterns (ICAP) 2014–2015. *Front Immunol.* 2015, Aug 20;6:412.
4. Chan EKL, Damoiseaux J, de Melo Cruvinel W, et al. Report on the Second International Consensus on ANA Pattern (ICAP) Workshop in Dresden 2015. *Lupus.* 2016;25:797–804.
5. Damoiseaux J, Andrade LEC, Carballo OG, et al. Clinical relevance of HEp-2 indirect immunofluorescent patterns: the International Consensus on ANA Patterns (ICAP) perspective. *Ann Rheum Dis.* 2019;78:879–889.
6. Dellavance A, de Melo Cruvinel W, Carvalho Francescanonio PL, Coelho Andrade LE. Antinuclear antibody tests. In: Detrick B, Schmitz JL, Hamilton RG, eds. *Manual of Molecular and Clinical Laboratory Immunology.* 8th ed. Washington, DC: ASM Press; 2016:843–858.
7. Ghillani P, Rouquette AM, Desgruelles C, et al. Evaluation of the LIAISON ANA screen assay for antinuclear antibody testing in autoimmune diseases. *Ann NY Acad Sci.* 2007;1109:407–413.
8. Hanly JG, Su L, Farewell V, Fritzler MJ. Comparison between multiplex assays for autoantibody detection in systemic lupus erythematosus. *J Immunol Methods.* 2010;358(1–2):75–80.
9. Hanly JG, Thompson K, McCurdy G, et al. Measurement of autoantibodies using multiplex methodology in patients with systemic lupus erythematosus. *J Immunol Methods.* 2010;352(1–2):147–152.
10. Hutchison KW, Wener MH, Gilliland BG, Astion ML. Medical training solutions. Antinuclear antibody online training course. University of Washington, Dept. of Laboratory Medicine Website. https://medtraining.org/labcontent.aspx. Updated 2013. Accessed February 29, 2020.
11. ICAP Consensus on ANA Patterns. Website. https://www.anapatterns.org/index.php. Updated 2019. Accessed February 29, 2020.
12. Jeong S, Yang D, Lee W, et al. Diagnostic value of screening enzyme immunoassays compared to indirect immunofluorescence for anti-nuclear antibodies in patients with systemic rheumatic diseases: a systematic review and meta-analysis. *Sem Arthrit Rheumat.* 2018;48:334–342.
13. Kim J, Lee W, Kim G-T, et al. Diagnostic utility of automated indirect immunofluorescence compared to manual indirect immunofluorescence for antinuclear antibodies in patients with systemic lupus erythematosus: a systematic review and meta-analysis. *Sem Arthrit Rheumat.* 2019;48:728–735.
14. Kumar Y, Bhatia A, Minz RW. Antinuclear antibodies and their detection methods in diagnosis of connective tissue diseases: a journey revisited. *Diagn Pathol.* 2009;4:1.
15. Li ZY, Han RL, Yan ZL, Li LJ, Feng ZR. Antinuclear antibodies detection: a comparative study between automated recognition and conventional visual interpretation. *J Clin Lab Anal.* 2019;33:e22619.
16. Meroni PL, Bizzaro N, Cavazzana I, et al. Automated tests of ANA immunofluorescence as throughput autoantibody detection technology: strengths and limitations. *BMC Med.* 2014;12:38.
17. Meroni PL, Chan EK, Damoiseaux J, et al. Unending story of the indirect immunofluorescence assay on HEp-2 cells: old problems and new solutions? *Ann Rheum Dis.* 2019;78:e46.
18. Meroni PL, Schur PH. ANA screening: an old test with new recommendations. *Ann Rheum Dis.* 2010;69(8):1420–1422.
19. Pisetsky DS. Antinuclear antibody testing—misunderstood or misbegotten? *Nature Rev.* 2017;13:495–502.
20. Reeves W, Han S, Massini J, Li Y. Immunodiagnosis and laboratory assessment of systemic lupus erythematosus. In: Detrick B, Schmitz JL, Hamilton RG, eds. *Manual of Molecular and Clinical Laboratory Immunology.* 8th ed. Washington, DC: ASM Press; 2016:868–877.

21. Reeves WH, Satoh M, Lyons R, et al. Detection of autoantibodies against proteins and ribonucleoproteins by double immunodiffusion and immunoprecipitation. In: Detrick B, Hamilton RG, Folds JD, eds. *Manual of Molecular and Clinical Laboratory Immunology.* 7th ed. Washington, DC: ASM Press; 2006:1007–1018.
22. Tiwary AK, Kumar P. Paradigm shift in antinuclear antibody negative lupus: current evidence. *Indian J Dermatol Venereol Leprol.* 2018;84:384–387.
23. Van Hoovels L, Schouwers S, Van den Bremt S, et al. Variation in antinuclear antibody detection by automated indirect immunofluorescence analysis. *Ann Rheum Dis.* 2019;78:e48.
24. Zeus Scientific IFA ANA HEp-2 pattern guide. Website. https://www.zeusscientific.com/pattern-guide. Updated 2020. Accessed February 29, 2020.

Phospholipid Antibodies

1. Marlar RA, Fink LM, Miller JL. Laboratory approach to thrombotic risk. In: McPherson RA, Pincus MR, eds. *Henry's Clinical Diagnosis and Management by Laboratory Methods.* 22nd ed. Philadelphia: Elsevier; 2011:823–830.
2. Murphy M, Harris N. In: Detrick B, Schmitz JL, Hamilton RG, eds. *Manual of Molecular and Clinical Laboratory Immunology.* 8th ed. Washington, DC: ASM Press; 2016:905–908.
3. Vlachoyiannopoulos PG, Samarkos M, Sikara M, Tsiligros P. Antiphospholipid antibodies: laboratory and pathogenetic aspects. *Crit Rev Clin Lab Sci.* 2007;44(3):271–338.

Rheumatoid Arthritis

1. Aletaha D, Neogi T, Silman AJ, et al. 2010 Rheumatoid arthritis classification criteria: an American College of Rheumatology/European League Against Rheumatism collaborative initiative. *Arthrit Rheum.* 2010;62(9):2569–2581.
2. Arnett FC, Edworthy SM, Bloch DA. The American Rheumatism Association 1987 criteria for the classification of rheumatoid arthritis. *Arthrit Rheum.* 1988;31(3):315–324.
3. Chauffe AD, Bubb MR. Antibody and biomarker testing in rheumatoid arthritis. In: Detrick B, Schmitz JL, Hamilton RG, eds. *Manual of Molecular and Clinical Laboratory Immunology.* 8th ed. Washington, DC: ASM Press; 2016: 897–904.
4. Chen S-J, Lin G-J, Chen J-W, et al. Immunopathogenic mechanisms and novel immune-modulated therapies in rheumatoid arthritis. *Int J Mol Sci.* 2019;20:1332. doi:10.3390/ijms20061332
5. Emery P, McInnes IB, van Vollerhoven R, Kraan MC. Clinical identification and treatment of a rapidly progressing disease state in patients with rheumatoid arthritis. *Rheumatology.* 2008;47:392–398.
6. Farid SS, Azizi G, Mirshafiey A. Anti-citrullinated protein antibodies and their clinical utility in rheumatoid arthritis. *Int J Rheum Dis.* 2013;16(4):379–386.
7. Hill J. The what, whys, and wherefores of rheumatoid arthritis. *Nurs Res Care.* 2008;10:123–126.
8. Holers VM. Autoimmunity to citrullinated proteins and the initiation of rheumatoid arthritis. *Curr Opin Immunol.* 2013;25(6):728–735.
9. Ingegnoli F, Castelli R, Gualtierotti R. Rheumatoid factors: clinical applications. *Dis Markers.* 2013;35(6):727–734.
10. Jung YO, Kim HA. Recent paradigm shifts in the diagnosis and treatment of rheumatoid arthritis. *Korean J Intern Med.* 2012;27(4):378–387.
11. Kay J, Upchurch KS. ACR/EULAR 2010 rheumatoid arthritis classification criteria. *Rheumatology.* 2012;51(suppl 6):5–9.
12. Klareskog L, Catrina AI, Paget S. Rheumatoid arthritis. *Lancet.* 2009;373(9664):659–672.
13. Lee AN, Beck CE, Hall M. Rheumatoid factor and anti-CCP autoantibodies in rheumatoid arthritis: a review. *Clin Lab Sci.* 2008;21(1):15–18.
14. Niewold TB, Harrison MJ, Paget SA. Anti-CCP antibody testing as a diagnostic and prognostic tool in rheumatoid arthritis. *QJM.* 2007;100(4):193–201.
15. Sanmarti R, Ruiz-Esquide V, Hernandez MV. Rheumatoid arthritis: a clinical overview of new diagnostic and treatment approaches. *Curr Top Med Chem.* 2013;13(6):698–704.
16. Scott DL. Biologics-based therapy for the treatment of rheumatoid arthritis. *Clin Pharmacol Ther.* 2012;91(1):30–43.
17. Scott DL, Wolfe F, Huizinga TW. Rheumatoid arthritis. *Lancet.* 2010;376(9746):1094–1108.
18. Shah A, St. Clair E. Rheumatoid arthritis. In: Jameson J, Fauci AS, Kasper DL, Hauser SL, Longo DL, Loscalzo J, eds. *Harrison's Principles of Internal Medicine.* 20th ed. New York: McGraw-Hill; 2018. http://accessmedicine.mhmedical.com/content.aspx?bookid=2129§ionid=192284979. Accessed March 1, 2020.
19. Smolen JS, Aletaha D, Barton A, et al. Rheumatoid arthritis. *Nature Rev Dis Primers.* 2018;4:1–23.

Other Systemic Autoimmune Rheumatic Diseases (SARDs)

1. Denton CP, Khanna D. Systemic sclerosis. *The Lancet.* 2017;390:1685–1699.
2. Findlay A, Goyal N, Mozaffar T. An overview of polymyositis and dermatomyositis. *Muscle & Nerve.* 2015;51(5):638–656.
3. Greenberg SA, Amato AA. Inflammatory myopathies. In: Jameson J, Fauci AS, Kasper DL, Hauser SL, Longo DL, Loscalzo J, eds. *Harrison's Principles of Internal Medicine.* 20th ed. New York: McGraw-Hill; 2018. http://accessmedicine.mhmedical.com/content.aspx?bookid=2129§ionid=19228568. Accessed May 14, 2020.
4. Kuwana M. Immunodiagnosis of scleroderma. In: Detrick B, Schmitz JL, Hamilton RG, eds. *Manual of Molecular and Clinical Laboratory Immunology.* 8th ed. Washington, DC: ASM Press; 2016:888–896.
5. Moutsopoulos HM. Sjögren's syndrome. In: Jameson J, Fauci AS, Kasper DL, Hauser SL, Longo DL, Loscalzo J, eds. *Harrison's Principles of Internal Medicine.* 20th ed. New York: McGraw-Hill; 2018. http://accessmedicine.mhmedical.com/content.aspx?bookid=2129§ionid=19228527. Accessed May 14, 2020.
6. Shiboski CH, Shiboski SC, Seror R, et al. 2016 American College of Rheumatology/European League Against Rheumatism classification criteria for primary Sjögren's syndrome. *Ann Rheum Dis.* 2017;76:9–16.
7. Stefanski A-L, Tomiak C, Pleyer U, et al. The diagnosis and treatment of Sjogren's syndrome. *Dtsch Arztebl Int,* 2017;114:354–361.
8. Varga J. Systemic sclerosis (scleroderma) and related disorders. In: Jameson J, Fauci AS, Kasper DL, Hauser SL, Longo DL, Loscalzo J, eds. *Harrison's Principles of Internal Medicine.* 20th ed. New York: McGraw-Hill; 2018. http://accessmedicine.mhmedical.com/content.aspx?bookid=2129§ionid=15921472. Accessed May 14, 2020.

Granulomatosis With Polyangiitis and ANCA

1. Alberici F, Martorana D, Bonatti F, et al. Genetics of ANCA-associated vasculitides: HLA and beyond. *Clin Exp Rheum.* 2014;32(2 suppl 82):S90–S97.

2. Bossuyt X, Cohen Tervaert J-W, Arimura Y. Revised 2017 international consensus on testing of ANCAs in granulomatosis with polyangiitis and microscopic polyangiitis. *Nature Rev Rheum.* 2017;13:684–692.
3. Burlingame RW, Buchner CE, Hanly JG, Walsh NM. Antineutrophil cytoplasmic antibodies (ANCA) and strategies for diagnosing ANCA-associated vasculitides. In: Detrick B, Schmitz JL, Hamilton RG, eds. *Manual of Molecular and Clinical Laboratory Immunology.* 8th ed. Washington, DC: ASM Press; 2016:909–916.
4. Cartin-Ceba R, Peikert T, Specks U. Pathogenesis of ANCA-associated vasculitis. *Curr Rheumatol Rep.* 2012;14(6): 481–493.
5. Csernok E. ANCA testing: the current stage and perspectives. *Clin Exp Nephrol.* 2013;17(5):615–618.
6. Flores-Suarez LF. Antineutrophil cytoplasm autoantibodies: usefulness in rheumatology. *Reumatologia Clinica.* 2012;8(6):351–357.
7. Holding S. Challenges and opportunities from the revised international consensus on ANCA testing. *Annals of Clinical Biochemistry.* 2019;56(1):4–6.
8. Hutchison KW, Wener MH, Gilliland BG, Astion ML. *Medical Training Solutions.* ANCA online training course. University of Washington, Dept. of Laboratory Medicine. Medical Training Solutions. Website. http://medtraining.org/labcontent.aspx. Updated 2013. Accessed September 22, 2014.
9. Langford CA, Fauci AS. The vasculitis syndromes. In: Jameson J, Fauci AS, Kasper DL, Hauser SL, Longo DL, Loscalzo J, eds. *Harrison's Principles of Internal Medicine.* 20th ed. New York: McGraw-Hill; 2018. http://accessmedicine.mhmedical.com/content.aspx?bookid=2129§ionid=192285458. Accessed May 16, 2020.
10. Moosig F, Lamprecht P, Gross WL. Wegener's granulomatosis: the current view. *Clin Rev Allergy Immunol.* 2008;35(1–2):19–21.
11. Radice A, Bianchi L, Sinico RA. Anti-neutrophil cytoplasmic autoantibodies: methodological aspects and clinical significance in systemic vasculitis. *Autoimmun Rev.* 2013;12(4):487–495.
12. Savige J, Gillis D, Benson E, et al. International consensus statement on testing and reporting of antineutrophil cytoplasmic antibodies (ANCA). *Am J Clin Pathol.* 1999;111(4):507–513.
13. Schilder AM. Wegener's granulomatosis vasculitis and granuloma. *Autoimmun Rev.* 2010;9(7):483–487.
14. Sinico RA, Radice A. Antineutrophil cytoplasmic antibodies (ANCA) testing: detection methods and clinical application. *Clin Exp Rheum.* 2014;32(2 suppl 82):S112–S117.
15. Tarabishy AB, Schulte M, Papaliodis GN, Hoffman GS. Wegener's granulomatosis: clinical manifestations, differential diagnosis, and management of ocular and systemic disease. *Surv Ophthalmol.* 2010;55(5):429–444.
16. Weeda LW, Jr, Coffey SA. Wegener's granulomatosis. *Oral & Maxillofac Surg Clinics N Am.* 2008;20(4):643–649.

Autoimmune Thyroid Diseases

1. Ahmed R, Al-Shaikh S, Akhtar M. Hashimoto thyroiditis: a century later. *Adv Anat Pathol.* 2012;19(3):181–186.
2. ARUP Consult. Autoimmune thyroiditis. https://arupconsult.com/content/thyroiditis-autoimmune. Accessed May 18, 2020.
3. Brown RS. Autoimmune thyroid disease: unlocking a complex puzzle. *Curr Opin Pediatr.* 2009;21(4):523–528.
4. Burel CL, Rose NR, Barbesino G, et al. Endocrinopathies: chronic thyroiditis, Addison disease, pernicious anemia, Graves disease, diabetes, hypophysitis. In: Detrick B, Schmitz JL, Hamilton RG, eds. *Manual of Molecular and Clinical Laboratory Immunology.* 8th ed. Washington, DC: ASM Press; 2016:930–953.
5. Caturegli P, De Remigis A, Rose NR. Hashimoto thyroiditis: clinical and diagnostic criteria. *Autoimmun Rev.* 2014;13(4–5):391–397.
6. Chuma-Bitcon V, Gruson D. The role of laboratory diagnostics in patient management for Graves' disease. *MLO.* 2016, June 22. https://www.mlo-online.com/home/article/13008698/the-role-of-laboratory-diagnostics-in-patient-management-for-graves-disease. Accessed May 18, 2020.
7. Gopinath B, Musselman R, Beard N, et al. Antibodies targeting the calcium binding skeletal muscle protein calsequestrin are specific markers of ophthalmopathy and sensitive indicators of ocular myopathy in patients with Graves' disease. *Clin Exp Immunol.* 2006;145(1):56–62.
8. Grotzke M. The thyroid gland. In: Bishop ML, Fody EP, Schoeff LE, eds. *Clinical Chemistry.* 8th ed. Philadelphia: Lippincott Williams and Wilkins; 2018:476–487; 489–501.
9. Jacobson EM, Huber A, Tomer Y. The HLA gene complex in thyroid autoimmunity: from epidemiology to etiology. *J Autoimmun.* 2008;30(1–2):58–62.
10. Jacobson EM, Tomer Y. The genetic basis of thyroid autoimmunity. *Thyroid.* 2007;17(10):949–961.
11. Jameson J, Mandel SJ, Weetman AP. Hyperthyroidism. In: Jameson J, Fauci AS, Kasper DL, Hauser SL, Longo DL, Loscalzo J, eds. *Harrison's Principles of Internal Medicine.* 20th ed. New York: McGraw-Hill; 2018. http://accessmedicine.mhmedical.com/content.aspx?bookid=2129§ionid=179924631. Accessed May 18, 2020.
12. Jameson J, Mandel SJ, Weetman AP. Hypothyroidism. In: Jameson J, Fauci AS, Kasper DL, Hauser SL, Longo DL, Loscalzo J. eds. Harrison's Principles of Internal Medicine, 20e New York, NY: McGraw-Hill;. http://accessmedicine.mhmedical.com/content.aspx?bookid=2129§ionid=179924583. Accessed May 18, 2020.
13. Lytton SD, Kahaly GJ. Bioassays for TSH-receptor autoantibodies: an update. *Autoimmun Rev.* 2010;10(2):116–122.
14. McKenna TJ. Graves' disease. *Lancet.* 2001;357(9270):1793–1796.
15. Menconi F, Marcocci C, Marino M. Diagnosis and classification of Graves' disease. *Autoimmun Rev.* 2014;13(4–5):398–402.
16. Rocchi R. Critical issues on Graves' ophthalmopathy. *MLO.* 2006, May 12;38(5):10.
17. Sinclair D. Clinical and laboratory aspects of thyroid autoantibodies. *Ann Clin Biochem.* 2006;43(Pt 3):173–183.
18. Weetman AP. Graves' disease. *N Engl J Med.* 2000;343(17): 1236–1248.

Type I Diabetes Mellitus

1. American Diabetes Association. Classification and diagnosis of diabetes: standards of medical care in diabetes 2020. *Diabetes Care.* 2020;43(suppl. 1):S14–S31. doi:10.2337/dc20-S002.
2. ARUP Consult. Diabetes-associated autoantibodies. https://arupconsult.com/ati/diabetes-associated-autoantibodies. Accessed May 19, 2020.
3. Burel CL, Rose NR, Barbesino G, et al. Endocrinopathies: chronic thyroiditis, Addison disease, pernicious anemia, Graves disease, diabetes, hypophysitis. In: Detrick B, Schmitz JL, Hamilton RG, eds. *Manual of Molecular and Clinical Laboratory Immunology.* 8th ed. Washington, DC: ASM Press; 2016:930–953.
4. Bylund DJ, Nakamura RM. Organ-specific autoimmune diseases. In: McPherson RA, Pincus MR, eds. *Henry's Clinical Diagnosis and Management by Laboratory Methods.* 22nd ed. Philadelphia: Elsevier Saunders; 2011:1003–1020.
5. Canivell S, Gomis R. Diagnosis and classification of autoimmune diabetes mellitus. *Autoimmun Rev.* 2014;13(4–5):403–407.

6. Cerna M. Genetics of autoimmune diabetes mellitus. *Wien Med Wochenschr.* 2008;158(1–2):2–12.
7. Imam K. Clinical features, diagnostic criteria and pathogenesis of diabetes mellitus. *Adv Exp Med Biol.* 2012;771:340–355.
8. Powers AC, Niswender KD, Evans-Molina C. Diabetes mellitus: diagnosis, classification, and pathophysiology. In: Jameson J, Fauci AS, Kasper DL, Hauser SL, Longo DL, Loscalzo J, eds. *Harrison's Principles of Internal Medicine.* 20th ed. New York: McGraw-Hill; 2018. https://accessmedicine.mhmedical.com/content.aspx?sectionid=192288322. Accessed May 19, 2020.
9. Powers AC, Niswender KD, Rickels MR. Diabetes mellitus: management and therapies. In: Jameson J, Fauci AS, Kasper DL, Hauser SL, Longo DL, Loscalzo J, eds. *Harrison's Principles of Internal Medicine.* 20th ed. New York: McGraw-Hill; 2018. http://accessmedicine.mhmedical.com/content.aspx?bookid=2129§ionid=192288412. Accessed May 19, 2020.
10. Taplin CE, Barker JM. Autoantibodies in type 1 diabetes. *Autoimmunity.* 2008;41(1):11–18.
11. von Herrath M, Peakman M, Roep B. Progress in immune-based therapies for type 1 diabetes. *Clin Exp Immunol.* 2013;172(2):186–202.
12. Wenzlau JM, Hutton JC. Novel diabetes autoantibodies and prediction of type 1 diabetes. *Curr Diabetes Rep.* 2013;13(5):608–615.
13. Zhang L, Nakayama M, Eisenbarth GS. Insulin as an autoantigen in NOD/human diabetes. *Curr Opin Immunol.* 2008;20(1):111–118.

Celiac Disease

1. Brown NK, Guandalini S, Semrad C, Kupfer SS. A clinician's guide to celiac disease HLA genetics. *Am J Gastroenterol.* 2019;114:1587–1592. doi:10.14309/ajg.0000000000000310
2. Fasano A, Catassi C. Clinical practice. Celiac disease. *N Engl J Med.* 2012;367(25):2419–2426.
3. Green PH, Cellier C. Celiac disease. *N Engl J Med.* 2007;357(17):1731–1743.
4. Guandalini S, Assiri A. Celiac disease: a review. *JAMA Pediatrics.* 2014;168(3):272–278.
5. Husby S, Murray JA, Katzka DA. AGA clinical practice update on diagnosis and monitoring of celiac disease—changing utility of serology and histologic measures: expert review. *Gastroenterology.* 2019;156:885–889.
6. Leffler DA, Schuppan D. Update on serologic testing in celiac disease. *Am J Gastroenterol.* 2010;105(12):2520–2524.
7. Lerner A, Ramesh A, Matthias T. Serologic diagnosis of celiac disease: new biomarkers. *Gastroenterol Clin N Am.* 2019;48:307–317. doi:10.1016/j.gtc.2019.02.009
8. Lindfors K, Ciacci C, Kurppa K, et al. Coeliac disease. *Nature Rev.* 2019; 5(3);1–18. doi:10.1038/s41572-018-0054-z
9. Lundin KE, Sollid LM. Advances in coeliac disease. *Curr Opin Gastroenterol.* 2014;30(2):154–162.
10. Ma MX, John M, Forbes GM. Diagnostic dilemmas in celiac disease. *Expert Rev Gastroenterol Hepatol.* 2013;7(7):643–655.

Autoimmune Liver Diseases

1. ARUP Laboratories. Mitochondrial M2 antibody, IgG (ELISA). https://ltd.aruplab.com/Tests/Pub/0050065. Accessed May 21, 2021.
2. Bogdanos DP, Komorowski L. Disease-specific autoantibodies in primary biliary cirrhosis. *Clinica Chimica Acta.* 2011;412(7–8):502–512.
3. Bowlus CL, Gershwin ME. The diagnosis of primary biliary cirrhosis. *Autoimmun Rev.* 2014;13(4–5):441–444.
4. Carbone M, Neuberger JM. Autoimmune liver disease, autoimmunity and liver transplantation. *J Hepatol.* 2014;60(1):210–223.
5. de Boer YS, van Gerven NM, Zwiers A, et al. Genome-wide association study identifies variants associated with autoimmune hepatitis type 1. *Gastroenterology.* 2014;147(2):443–452.
6. Grotzke M. The thyroid gland. In: Bishop ML, Fody EP, Schoeff LE, eds. *Clinical Chemistry.* 7th ed. Philadelphia: Lippincott Williams and Wilkins; 2013:489–501.
7. Heneghan MA, Yeoman AD, Verma S, Smith AD, Longhi MS. Autoimmune hepatitis. *Lancet.* 2013;382(9902):1433–1444.
8. Hennes EM, Zeniya M, Czaja AJ, Parés A, Dalekos GN, Krawitt EL: Simplified criteria for the diagnosis of autoimmune hepatitis. *Hepatology.* 2008;48:169–176.
9. Hirschfield GM. Diagnosis of primary biliary cirrhosis. *Best Pract Res Clin Ga.* 2011;25(6):701–712.
10. Leung PSC, Manns MP, Coppel RL, Gershwin ME. Detection of antimitochondrial autoantibodies in primary biliary cholangitis and liver kidney microsomal antibodies in autoimmune hepatitis. In: Detrick B, Schmitz JL, Hamilton RG, eds. *Manual of Molecular and Clinical Laboratory Immunology.* 8th ed. Washington, DC: ASM Press; 2016:966–974.
11. Liberal R, Grant CR, Longhi MS, Mieli-Vergani G, Vergani D. Diagnostic criteria of autoimmune hepatitis. *Autoimmun Rev.* 2014;13(4–5):435–440.
12. Liberal R, Grant CR, Mieli-Vergani G, Vergani D. Autoimmune hepatitis: a comprehensive review. *J Autoimmun.* 2013;41:126–139.
13. Lohse, AW, Wiegard C. Diagnostic criteria for autoimmune hepatitis. *Best Prac Res: Clin Gastroenterol; Kidlington.* 2011, Dec;25(6):665–671. doi:10.1016/j.bpg.2011.10.004
14. Mells GF, Kaser A, Karlsen TH. Novel insights into autoimmune liver diseases provided by genome-wide association studies. *J Autoimmun.* 2013;46:41–54.
15. Nguyen DL, Juran BD, Lazaridis KN. Primary biliary cirrhosis. *Best Pract Res Clin Ga.* 2010;24(5):647–654.

Multiple Sclerosis

1. Brownlee WJ, Hardy TA, Fazekas F, Miller DH. Diagnosis of multiple sclerosis: progress and challenges. *Lancet.* 2017;389:1336–1346.
2. Compston A, Coles A. Multiple sclerosis. *Lancet.* 2002;359(9313):1221–1231.
3. Cree BC, Hauser SL. Multiple sclerosis. In: Jameson J, Fauci AS, Kasper DL, Hauser SL, Longo DL, Loscalzo J, eds. *Harrison's Principles of Internal Medicine.* 20th ed. New York: McGraw-Hill; 2018. http://accessmedicine.mhmedical.com/content.aspx?bookid=2129§ionid=192533073. Accessed May 22, 2020.
4. Lo Sasso B, Agnello L, Bivona G, Bellia C, Ciaccio M. Cerebrospinal fluid analysis in multiple sclerosis diagnosis: an update. *Medicina.* 2019;55:245. doi:10.3390/medicina55060245
5. Milo R, Miller A. Revised diagnostic criteria of multiple sclerosis. *Autoimmun Rev.* 2014;13(4–5):518–524.
6. Sykes E, Posey Y. Immunochemical characteristics of immunoglobulins in serum, urine, and cerebrospinal fluid. In: Detrick B, Schmitz JL, Hamilton RG, eds. *Manual of Molecular and Clinical Laboratory Immunology.* 8th ed. Washington, DC: ASM Press; 2016:89–100.
7. Tavazzi E, Rovaris M, La Mantia L. Drug therapy for multiple sclerosis. *CMAJ.* 2014;186(11):833–840.
8. Thompson AJ, Banwell BL, Barkhof F, et al. Diagnosis of multiple sclerosis: 2017 revisions of the McDonald criteria. *Lancet Neurol.* 2018;17:162.

Myasthenia Gravis

1. Amato AA. Myasthenia gravis and other diseases of the neuromuscular junction. In: Jameson J, Fauci AS, Kasper DL, Hauser SL, Longo DL, Loscalzo J, eds. *Harrison's Principles of Internal Medicine.* 20th ed. New York: McGraw-Hill; 2018. http://accessmedicine.mhmedical.com/content.aspx?bookid=2129§ionid=192533554. Accessed May 22, 2020.
2. ARUP Laboratories. Myasthenia gravis testing. https://ltd.aruplab.com/api/ltd/pdf/127. Accessed May 24, 2020.
3. Berrih-Aknin S, Le Panse R. Myasthenia gravis: a comprehensive review of immune dysregulation and etiological mechanisms. *J Autoimmun.* 2014;52:90–100.
4. Cavalcante P, Bernasconi P, Mantegazza R. Autoimmune mechanisms in myasthenia gravis. *Curr Opin Neurol.* 2012;25(5):621–629.
5. Cromar A, Lozier BK, Haven TR, Hill HR. Detection of acetylcholine receptor blocking antibodies by flow cytometry. *Am J Clin Pathol.* January 2016;145:81–85.
6. Dalakas MC. Novel future therapeutic options in myasthenia gravis. *Autoimmun Rev.* 2013;12(9):936–941.
7. Gilhus NE. Myasthenia gravis. *N Engl J Med.* 2016;375:2570.
8. Levinson AI, Lisak RP. Myasthenia gravis. In: Detrick B, Schmitz JL, Hamilton RG, eds. *Manual of Molecular and Clinical Laboratory Immunology.* 8th ed. Washington, DC: ASM Press; 2016:954–960.
9. Spillane J, Higham E, Kullmann DM. Myasthenia gravis. *BMJ.* 2012;345:e8497.
10. Yan M, Xing GL, Xiong WC, Mei L. Agrin and LRP4 antibodies as new biomarkers of myasthenia gravis. *Ann N Y Acad Sci.* 2018 Feb;1413(1):126–135. doi:10.1111/nyas.13573
11. Zagoriti Z. Recent advances in genetic predisposition of myasthenia gravis. *Biomed Res Int.* 2013;2013:1–12.

Anti-Glomerular Basement Membrane Disease (Goodpasture's Syndrome)

1. Bergs L. Goodpasture syndrome. *Crit Care Nurse.* 2005;25(5):50–54.
2. Collins AB, Smith RN, Colvin RB. Western blot analysis for the detection of anti-glomerular basement membrane antibodies and anti-phospholipase A2 receptor antibodies. In: Detrick B, Schmitz JL, Hamilton RG, eds. *Manual of Molecular and Clinical Laboratory Immunology.* 8th ed. Washington, DC: ASM Press; 2016:385–390.
3. Dammacco F, Battaglia S, Gesualdo L, Racanelli V. Goodpasture's disease: a report of ten cases and a review of the literature. *Autoimmunity Reviews.* 2013;12(11):1101–1108.
4. Hellmark T, Segelmark M. Diagnosis and classification of Goodpasture's disease (anti-GBM). *J Autoimmun.* 2014;48–49:108–112.
5. Lahmer T, Heemann U. Anti-glomerular basement membrane antibody disease: a rare autoimmune disorder affecting the kidney and the lung. *Autoimmunity Reviews.* 2012;12(2):169–173.
6. McAdoo SP, Pusey CD. Anti-glomerular basement membrane disease. *Semin Respir Crit Care Med.* 2018;39:494–503.
7. Segelmark M, Hellmark T. Anti-glomerular basement membrane disease: an update on subgroups, pathogenesis and therapies. *Nephrol Dial Transplant.* 2019;34:1826–1832.

16. Transplantation Immunology

1. Abbas A, Lichtman A, Pillai S. *Cellular and Molecular Immunology.* 9th ed. Philadelphia: Elsevier; 2018:373–396.
2. Afzali B, Lechler RI, Hernandez-Fuentes MP. Allorecognition and the alloresponse: clinical implications. *Tissue Antigens.* 2007;69:545–556.
3. Angaswamy N, Tiriveedhi V, Sarma NJ, et al. Interplay between immune responses to HLA and non-HLA self-antigens in allograft rejection. *Hum Immunol.* 2013;74:1478–1485.
4. Baxter-Lowe L-A. Chimerism testing. In: Detrick B, Schmitz J, Hamilton R, eds. *Manual of Molecular and Clinical Laboratory Immunology.* 8th ed. Washington, DC: ASM Press; 2016:1161–1168.
5. Bray RA, Nickerson PW, Kerman RH, Gebel HM. Evolution of HLA antibody detection: technology emulating biology. *Immunol Res.* 2004;29:41–54.
6. Cardinal H, Dieude M, Hebert MJ. The emerging importance of non-HLA autoantibodies in kidney transplant complications. *J Am Soc Nephrol.* 2017;28:400–406.
7. Cechova H, Leontovycova M, Pavlatova L. Chimerism as an important marker in post-transplant monitoring. *HLA.* 2018;92(S2):60–63. doi:10.1111/tan.13407
8. Coleman B, Tsongalis GJ. *Molecular Diagnostics for the Clinical Laboratorian.* 2nd ed. New York: Humana Press; 2005.
9. Colombo MB, Haworth SE, Poli F, et al. Luminex technology for anti-HLA antibody screening: evaluation of performance and of impact on laboratory routine. *Cytometry B Clin Cytom.* 2007;72:465–471.
10. Colvin RB. Antibody-mediated renal allograft rejection: diagnosis and pathogenesis. *J Am Soc Nephrol.* 2007;18:1046–1056.
11. Colvin RB. Chronic allograft nephropathy. *N Engl J Med.* 2003;349:2288–2290.
12. D'Orsogna LJ, Roelen DL, Doxiadis II, Claas FH. Alloreactivity from human viral specific memory T-cells. *Transpl Immunol.* 2010;23:149–155.
13. Dickinson AM, Norden J, Li S, et al. Graft-versus-leukemia effect following hematopoietic stem cell transplantation for leukemia. *Front Immunol.* 2017;8:496.
14. Farag SS, Fehniger TA, Ruggeri L, Velardi A, Caligiuri MA. Natural killer cell receptors: new biology and insights into the graft-versus-leukemia effect. *Blood.* 2002;100:1935–1947.
15. Gebel HM, Bray RA, Nickerson P. Pre-transplant assessment of donor-reactive, HLA-specific antibodies in renal transplantation: contraindication vs. risk. *Am J Transplant.* 2003;3:1488–1500.
16. Goker H, Haznedaroglu IC, Chao NJ. Acute graft-vs-host disease: pathobiology and management. *Exp Hematol.* 2001;29:259–277.
17. Halloran P, Lui S. *Primer on Transplantation.* Yhorofare, NJ: American Society of Transplant Physicians; 1998.
18. Lee SJ, Klein J, Haagenson M, et al. High-resolution donor-recipient HLA matching contributes to the success of unrelated donor marrow transplantation. *Blood.* 2007;110:4576–4583.
19. Leichtman A. *Primer on Transplantation.* Thorofare, NJ: American Society of Transplant Physicians; 1998.
20. Ruggeri L, Capanni M, Urbani E, et al. Effectiveness of donor natural killer cell alloreactivity in mismatched hematopoietic transplants. *Science.* 2002;295:2097–2100.
21. Simpson E, Scott D, James E, et al. Minor H antigens: genes and peptides. *Transpl Immunol.* 2002;10:115–123.
22. Singh N, Samant H, Hawby A, Samaniego M. Biomarkers of rejection in kidney transplantation. *Current Opinion in Organ Transplantation.* 2018;23:1–8.
23. Siu JHY, Surendrakumar V, Richards JA, Pettigrew GJ. T cell allorecognition pathways in solid organ transplantation. *Front Immunol.* 2018;9:2548.

24. Taniguchi M, Rebellato LM, Cai J, et al. Higher risk of kidney graft failure in the presence of anti-angiotensin II type-1 receptor antibodies. *Am J Transplant.* 2013;13:2577–2589.
25. Thielke J, Kaplan B, Benedetti E. The role of ABO-incompatible living donors in kidney transplantation: state of the art. *Semin Nephrol.* 2007;27:408–413.
26. UNOS (United Network for Organ Sharing). Transplant trends. https://unos.org/data/transplant-trends/#transplants_by_organ_type+year. Accessed November 19, 2020.
27. Wiebe C, Gibson IW, Blydt-Hansen TD, et al. Evolution and clinical pathologic correlations of de novo donor-specific HLA antibody post kidney transplant. *Am J Transplant.* 2012;12:1157–1167.
28. World Health Organization. Haematopoietic stem cell transplantation HSCtx. http://www.who.int/transplantation/hsctx/en. Accessed November 19, 2020.
29. .Zou Y, Stastny P, Susal C, Dohler B, Opelz G. Antibodies against MICA antigens and kidney-transplant rejection. *N Engl J Med.* 2007;357:1293–1300.
30. Zwirner NW, Dole K, Stastny P. Differential surface expression of MICA by endothelial cells, fibroblasts, keratinocytes, and monocytes. *Hum Immunol.* 1999;60:323–330.

17. Tumor Immunology

Tumor Biology

1. American Cancer Society. Cancer facts & figures 2020. https://www.cancer.org/research/cancer-facts-statistics/all-cancer-facts-figures/cancer-facts-figures-2020.html. Updated 2020. Accessed May 29, 2020.
2. American Cancer Society. How is breast cancer staged? https://www.cancer.org/cancer/breast-cancer/understanding-a-breast-cancer-diagnosis/stages-of-breast-cancer.html. Updated 2019. Accessed May 29, 2020.
3. American Cancer Society. Known and probable human carcinogens. https://www.cancer.org/cancer/cancer-causes/general-info/known-and-probable-human-carcinogens.html. Updated 2020. Accessed May 29, 2020.
4. Benson JR, Liau SS. Cancer genetics: a primer for surgeons. *Surg Clin N Am.* 2008;88(4):681–704.
5. Environmental Working Group. Re-thinking carcinogens. https://www.ewg.org/research/rethinking-carcinogens/hallmarks-cancer-how-normal-cells-turn-cancer-cells. Accessed May 29. 2020.
6. Hanahan D, Coussens LM. Accessories to the crime: functions of cells recruited to the tumor microenvironment. *Cancer Cell.* 2012;21:309–322.
7. Hanahan D, Weinberg RA. The Hallmarks of Cancer. *Cell.* 2000;100(1):57–70.
8. Hanahan D, Weinberg RA. The hallmarks of cancer: the next generation. *Cell.* 2011;144(5):646–674.
9. Mak TW, Saunders ME. Tumor immunology. In: Mak TW, Saunders ME. *The Immune Response: Basic and Clinical Principles.* Boston, MA: Elsevier/Academic; 2006:826–871.
10. National Cancer Institute. Fact sheet: cancer staging. https://www.cancer.gov/about-cancer/diagnosis-staging/staging. Updated 2015. Accessed May 29, 2020.
11. National Cancer Institute. What is cancer? https://www.cancer.gov/about-cancer/understanding/what-is-cancer. Accessed May 29, 2020.
12. Owen JA, Punt J., Stranford SA. *Kuby Immunology.* 7th ed. New York: WH Freeman and Co.; 2013:627–651.
13. World Health Organization. Cancer. https://www.who.int/en/news-room/fact-sheets/detail/cancer. Updated 2018. Accessed May 29, 2020.

Tumor Antigens

1. Abbas AK, Lichtman AH, Pillai S. Immunity to tumors. In: Abbas AK, Lichtman AH, Pillai S. *Cellular and Molecular Immunology.* 8th ed. Philadelphia: Elsevier Saunders; 2018:397–416.
2. De Duve Institute. Cancer antigenic peptide database. https://caped.icp.ucl.ac.be/Peptide/list. Accessed May 30, 2020.
3. Finn OJ. Human tumor antigens: yesterday, today, and tomorrow. *Cancer Immunol Res.* 2017;5(5);347–354.
4. Finnigan JP, Rubinsteyn A, Hammerbacher J, Bhardwaj N. Mutation-derived tumor antigens: novel targets in cancer immunotherapy. *Oncology,* 2015;29(12):970–975.
5. Prestwich RJ, Errington F, Hatfield P, et al. The immune system—is it relevant to cancer development, progression and treatment? *Clin Oncol-UK (Royal College of Radiologists).* 2008;20(2):101–112.
6. Smith CC, Selitsky SR, Chai S, Armistead PM, Vincent BJ, Serody JS. Alternative tumour- specific antigens. *Nature Rev Cancer.* 2019;19:465–478.

Clinically Relevant Serum Tumor Markers

1. American Society of Clinical Oncology. Assays and predictive markers. https://www.asco.org/research-guidelines/quality-guidelines/guidelines/assays-and-predictive-markers. Accessed June 1, 2020.
2. American Urological Association. Early detection of prostate cancer (2018). https://www.auanet.org/guidelines/prostate-cancer-early-detection-guideline. Accessed June 3, 2020.
3. Andriole GL, Crawford ED, Grubb RL, et al. Prostate cancer screening in the randomized prostate, lung, colorectal, and ovarian cancer screening trial: mortality results after 13 years of follow-up. *J Natl Cancer Inst.* 2012;104(2):125–132.
4. ARUP Consult. Prostate cancer—PSA. https://arupconsult.com/content/prostate-cancer. Accessed June 3, 2020.
5. ARUP Laboratories. ARUP consult. https://www.arupconsult.com/. Accessed June 1, 2020.
6. Borza T, Konijeti R, Kibel AS. Early detection, PSA screening, and management of overdiagnosis. *Hematology—Oncology Clinics of North America.* 2013;27(6):1091–1110.
7. Brennan DJ, O'Connor DP, Rexhepaj E, Ponten F, Gallagher WM. Antibody-based proteomics: fast-tracking molecular diagnostics in oncology. *Nat Rev Cancer.* 2010;10(9):605–617.
8. Buys SS, Partridge E, Black A, et al. Effect of screening on ovarian cancer mortality: the prostate, lung, colorectal and ovarian (PLCO) cancer screening randomized controlled trial. *JAMA.* 2011;305(22):2295–2303.
9. Diamandis EP, Hoffman BR, Sturgeon CM. National Academy of Clinical Biochemistry laboratory medicine practice guidelines for the use of tumor markers. *Clin Chem.* 2008;54(11):1935–1939.
10. Duffy MJ. Carcinoembryonic antigen as a marker for colorectal cancer: is it clinically useful? *Clin Chem.* 2001;47(4):624–630.
11. El-Serag HB, Kanwal F, Davila JA, Kramer J, Richardson P. A new laboratory-based algorithm to predict development of hepatocellular carcinoma in patients with hepatitis C and cirrhosis. *Gastroenterology.* 2014;146(5):1249–1255.e1.
12. Emerson JF, Lai KKY. Endogenous antibody interferences in immunoassays. *Lab Med.* 2013;44(1):69–73.
13. Gentry-Maharaj A, Menon U. Screening for ovarian cancer in the general population. *Best Pract Res Clin Ob.* 2012;26(2):243–256.
14. Gupta S, Bent S, Kohlwes J. Test characteristics of alpha-fetoprotein for detecting hepatocellular carcinoma in patients with hepatitis C. A systematic review and critical analysis. *Ann Intern Med.* 2003;139(1):46–50.

15. Hayes JH, Barry MJ. Screening for prostate cancer with the prostate-specific antigen test: a review of current evidence. *JAMA.* 2014;311(11):1143–1149.
16. Henry NL, Hayes DF. Cancer biomarkers. *Mol Oncol.* 2012;6(2):140–146.
17. Jain S, Pincus MR, Bluth MH, et al. Diagnosis and management of cancer using serologic and other body fluid markers. In: McPherson RA, Pincus MR, eds. *Henry's Clinical Diagnosis and Management by Laboratory Methods.* 23rd ed. Philadelphia: Elsevier Saunders; 2017:1432–1450.
18. Loeb S, Catalona WJ. Prostate-specific antigen in clinical practice. *Cancer Lett.* 2007;249(1):30–39.
19. McCudden CR, Willis MS. Circulating tumor markers: basic concepts and clinical applications. In: Bishop ML, Fody EP, Schoeff LE, eds. *Clinical Chemistry: Principles, Techniques, and Correlations.* 8th ed. Philadelphia: Wolters Kluwer Health/Lippincott Williams & Wilkins; 2018:646–659.
20. Medeiros LR, Rosa DD, da Rosa MI, Bozzetti MC. Accuracy of CA 125 in the diagnosis of ovarian tumors: a quantitative systematic review. *Eur J Obstet Gyn R B.* 2009;142(2):99–105.
21. National Academy of Clinical Biochemistry. Guideline summaries. *Oncology.* https://www.guidelinecentral.com/summaries/specialties/oncology/. Accessed June 1, 2020.
22. National Comprehensive Cancer Network. NCCN guidelines. https://www.nccn.org/professionals/physician_gls/. Accessed June 1, 2020.
23. Ostrov BE, Amsterdam D. The interference of monoclonal antibodies with laboratory diagnosis: clinical and diagnostic implications. *Immunol Invest.* 2013;42(8):673–690.
24. Painter JT, Clayton NP, Herbert RA. Useful immunohistochemical markers of tumor differentiation. *Toxicol Pathol.* 2010;38(1):131–141.
25. Pritzker KP. Cancer biomarkers: easier said than done. *Clin Chem.* 2002;48(8):1147–1150.
26. Schroder FH, Hugosson J, Roobol MJ, et al. Prostate-cancer mortality at 11 years of follow-up. *N Engl J Med.* 2012;366(11):981–990.
27. Sokoll L, Chan D. Tumor markers. In: Clarke W, Dufour D, eds. *Contemporary Practice in Clinical Chemistry.* Washington, DC: AACC Press; 2006.
28. Sturgeon C. Practice guidelines for tumor marker use in the clinic. *Clin Chem.* 2002;48(8):1151–1159.
29. Sturgeon CM, Duffy MJ, Hofmann BR, et al. National Academy of Clinical Biochemistry laboratory medicine practice guidelines for use of tumor markers in liver, bladder, cervical, and gastric cancers. *Clin Chem.* 2010;56(6):e1–e48.
30. Sturgeon CM, Duffy MJ, Stenman UH, et al. National Academy of Clinical Biochemistry laboratory medicine practice guidelines for use of tumor markers in testicular, prostate, colorectal, breast, and ovarian cancers. *Clin Chem.* 2008;54(12):e11–e79.
31. Sturgeon CM, Lai LC, Duffy MJ. Serum tumour markers: how to order and interpret them. *BMJ.* 2009;339:b3527.
32. Tan E, Gouvas N, Nicholls RJ, et al. Diagnostic precision of carcinoembryonic antigen in the detection of recurrence of colorectal cancer. *Surg Oncol.* 2009;18(1):15–24.
33. U.S. Preventative Services Taskforce. Prostate cancer screening. https://www.uspreventiveservicestaskforce.org/uspstf/recommendation/prostate-cancer-screening. Accessed June 3, 2020.
34. U.S. Preventive Services Task Force. Screening for prostate cancer. U.S. Preventive Services Task Force recommendation statement. *JAMA.* 2018;319(18):1901–1913. doi:10.1001/jama.2018.3710
35. Wald NJ. Prenatal screening for open neural tube defects and Down syndrome: three decades of progress. *Prenat Diagn.* 2010;30(7):619–621.
36. Wolf AMD, Wender RC, Etzioni RB, et al. American Cancer Society guideline for the early detection of prostate cancer. *CA Cancer J Clin.* 2010;60:70–98.

Molecular Methods in Cancer Diagnosis

1. Aboud OA, Weiss RH. New opportunities from the cancer metabolome. *Clin Chem.* 2013;59(1):138–146.
2. Bedeir A, Krasinskas AM. Molecular diagnostics of colorectal cancer. *Arch Pathol Lab Med.* 2011;135(5):578–587.
3. Buckingham L. *Molecular Diagnostics: Fundamentals, Methods, and Clinical Applications.* 3rd ed. Philadelphia: F.A. Davis Co.; 2019.
4. Burnet FM. The concept of immunological surveillance. *Progress Exp Tumor Res.* 1970;13:1–27.
5. Cherkis KA, Schroeder BE. Molecular testing as a tool for the management of metastatic cancer patients. *MLO.* 2014;46(3):8–10.
6. Chow MT, Moller A, Smyth MJ. Inflammation and immune surveillance in cancer. *Semin Cancer Biol.* 2012;22(1):23–32.
7. De Abreu FB, Wells WA, Tsongalis GJ. The emerging role of the molecular diagnostics laboratory in breast cancer personalized medicine. *Am J Pathol.* 2013;183(4):1075–1083.
8. Dunn GP, Old LJ, Schreiber RD. The immunobiology of cancer immunosurveillance and immunoediting. *Immunity.* 2004;21(2):137–148.
9. Food and Drug Administration. Table of pharmacogenomic biomarkers in drug labeling. https://www.fda.gov/drugs/science-and-research-drugs/table-pharmacogenomic-biomarkers-drug-labeling. Updated 2020. Accessed June 5, 2020.
10. A comparison of antibody arrays and mass spectrometry in protein profiling and biomarker research. *Genetic Engineering and Biotechnology News.* 2019. https://www.genengnews.com/biomarker-discovery/a-comparison-of-antibody-arrays-and-mass-spectrometry-in-protein-profiling-and-biomarker-research/. Accessed June 5, 2020.
11. Klein G, Sjogren HO, Klein E, Hellstrom KE. Demonstration of resistance against methylcholanthrene-induced sarcomas in the primary autochthonous host. *Cancer Res.* 1960;20:1561–1572.
12. McVeigh TP, Kerin MJ. Clinical use of the Oncotype DX genomic test to guide treatment decisions for patients with invasive breast cancer. *Breast Cancer—Targets and Therapy.* 2017:9:393–400.
13. Melo JV, Barnes DJ. Chronic myeloid leukaemia as a model of disease evolution in human cancer. *Nat Rev Cancer.* 2007;7(6):441–453.
14. National Cancer Institute and National Human Genome Research Institute. The Cancer Genome Atlas Program. https://www.cancer.gov/about-nci/organization/ccg/research/structural-genomics/tcga. Accessed June 5, 2020.
15. Petrucelli N, Daly MB, Feldman GL. BRCA1 and BRCA2 hereditary breast and ovarian cancer. http://www.ncbi.nlm.nih.gov/books/NBK1247/. Updated 2016. Accessed June 5, 2020.
16. Portier BP, Gruver AM, Huba MA, et al. From morphologic to molecular: established and emerging molecular diagnostics for breast carcinoma. *New Biotechnol.* 2012;29(6):665–681.
17. Prehn RT, Main JM. Immunity to methylcholanthrene-induced sarcomas. *J Nat Cancer Inst.* 1957;18:769–778.
18. Pusztai L, Mazouni C, Anderson K, Wu Y, Symmans WF. Molecular classification of breast cancer: limitations and potential. *Oncologist.* 2006;11(8):868–877.
19. Schreiber H. Cancer immunology. In: Paul WE, ed. *Fundamental Immunology.* 7th ed. Philadelphia: Lippincott Williams & Wilkins; 2013:1200–1234.
20. Soliman H, Shah V, Srkalovic G, et al. MammaPrint guides treatment decisions in breast cancer: results of the IMPACt trial. *BMC Cancer.* 2020; 20:81. doi:10.1186/s12885-020-6534-z

21. Tan HT, Lee YH, Chung MC. Cancer proteomics. *Mass Spectrom Rev.* 2012;31(5):583–605.

Interactions Between the Immune System and Tumors

1. Abbas AK, Lichtman AH, Pillai S. Immunity to tumors. In: *Cellular and Molecular Immunology.* 8th ed. Philadelphia: Elsevier Saunders; 2018:397–416.
2. Adam JK, Odhav B, Bhoola KD. Immune responses in cancer. *Pharmacol Ther.* 2003;99(1):113–132.
3. Burnet FM. The concept of immunological surveillance. *Progress in Experimental Tumor Research.* 1970;13:1–27.
4. Chow MT, Moller A, Smyth MJ. Inflammation and immune surveillance in cancer. *Semin Cancer Biol.* 2012;22(1):23–32.
5. Dunn GP, Old LJ, Schreiber RD. The immunobiology of cancer immunosurveillance and immunoediting. *Immunity.* 2004;21(2): 137–148.
6. Finn OJ. Cancer immunology. *N Engl J Med.* 2008;358(25): 2704–2715.
7. Gonzalez H, Hagerling C, Werb Z. Roles of the immune system in cancer: from tumor initiation to metastatic progression. *Genes & Development.* 2018;32:1267–1284.
8. Klein G, Sjogren HO, Klein E, Hellstrom KE. Demonstration of resistance against methylcholanthrene-induced sarcomas in the primary autochthonous host. *Cancer Res.* 1960;20:1561–1572.
9. Prehn RT, Main JM. Immunity to methylcholanthrene-induced sarcomas. *J Nat Cancer Inst.* 1957;18:769–778.
10. Schreiber H. Cancer immunology. In: Paul WE, ed. *Fundamental Immunology.* 7th ed. Philadelphia: Lippincott Williams & Wilkins; 2013:1200–1234.
11. Swann JB, Smyth MJ. Immune surveillance of tumors. *J Clin Invest.* 2007;117(5):1137–1146.
12. Whiteside T. Immune responses to malignancies. *J Allergy Clin Immunol.* 2010 February; 125(202):S272–S283. doi:10.1016/j.jaci.2009.09.045
13. Whiteside TL. The tumor microenvironment and its role in promoting tumor growth. *Oncogene.* 2008;27(45):5904–5912.

Immunotherapy

1. Antignani A, Fitzgerald D. Immunotoxins: the role of the toxin. *Toxins.* 2013;5(8):1486–1502.
2. Bhutani D, Vaishampayan UN. Monoclonal antibodies in oncology therapeutics: present and future indications. *Expert Opin Biol Th.* 2013;13(2):269–282.
3. Cancer Research Institute. Cancer vaccines: preventive, therapeutic, personalized. https://www.cancerresearch.org/immunotherapy/treatment-types/cancer-vaccines. Accessed June 10, 2020.
4. Chen X, Cai HH. Monoclonal antibodies for cancer therapy approved by FDA. *MOJ Immunol.* 2016;4(2):00120. doi:10.15406/moji.2016.04.00120
5. Dezfouli S, Hatzinisiriou I, Ralph SJ. Use of cytokines in cancer vaccines/immunotherapy: recent developments improve survival rates for patients with metastatic malignancy. *Curr Pharm Des.* 2005;11(27):3511–3530.
6. Foltz IN, Karow M, Wasserman SM. Evolution and emergence of therapeutic monoclonal antibodies: what cardiologists need to know. *Circulation.* 2013;127(22):2222–2230.
7. Gajewski TF. Cancer immunotherapy. *Mol Oncol.* 2012;6(2): 242–250.
8. Goldman B, DeFrancesco L. The cancer vaccine roller coaster. *Nat Biotechnol.* 2009;27(2):129–139.
9. Guo Y, Lei K, Tang L. Neoantigen vaccine delivery for personalized anticancer immunotherapy. *Front Immunol.* 2018;2. doi:10.3389/fimmu.2018.01499.
10. He J, Hu Y, Hu M, Li B. Development of PD-1/PD-L1 pathway in tumor immune microenvironment and treatment for non-small cell lung cancer. *Nature.com Scientific Reports.* 2015;5:13110. doi:10.1038/srep13110
11. Kantoff PW, Higano CS, Shore ND, et al. Sipuleucel-T immunotherapy for castration-resistant prostate cancer. *N Engl J Med.* 2010;363(5):411–422.
12. Kawai K, Miyazaki J, Joraku A, Nishiyama H, Akaza H. Bacillus Calmette-Guerin (BCG) immunotherapy for bladder cancer: current understanding and perspectives on engineered BCG vaccine. *Cancer Sci.* 2013;104(1):22–27.
13. Krishnamurthy A, Jimeno A. Bispecific antibodies for cancer therapy: a review. *Pharm Ther.* 2018;185:122–134.
14. Lieschke GJ, Burgess AW. Granulocyte colony-stimulating factor and granulocyte-macrophage colony-stimulating factor (2). *N Engl J Med.* 1992;327(2):99–106.
15. McCarthy EF. The toxins of William B. Coley and the treatment of bone and soft-tissue sarcomas. *Iowa Orthopedic J.* 2006;26:154–158.
16. Mchayleh W, Bedi P, Sehgal R, Solh M. Chimeric antigen receptor T-cells: the future is now. *J Clin Med.* 2019;8:207. doi:10.3390/jcm8020207
17. National Cancer Institute. Fact sheet. https://www.cancer.gov/about-cancer/treatment/types/immunotherapy/bio-therapies-fact-sheet. Updated 2018. Accessed June 12, 2020.
18. National Cancer Institute. Immunotherapy to treat cancer. https://www.cancer.gov/about-cancer/treatment/types/immunotherapy. Updated 2019. Accessed June 10, 2020.
19. National Institutes of Health. ClinicalTrials.Gov. https://clinicaltrials.gov/ct2/home. Accessed June 10, 2020.
20. Saloustros E, Tryfonidis K, Georgoulias V. Prophylactic and therapeutic strategies in chemotherapy-induced neutropenia. *Expert Opin Pharmacother.* 2011;12(6):851–863.
21. Scott AM, Allison JP, Wolchok JD. Monoclonal antibodies in cancer therapy. *Cancer Imm.* 2012;12:14.
22. Sievers EL, Senter PD. Antibody-drug conjugates in cancer therapy. *Annu Rev Med.* 2013;64:15–29.
23. Snook AE, Waldman SA. Advances in cancer immunotherapy. *Disc Med.* 2013;15(81):120–125.
24. Tagawa M. Cytokine therapy for cancer. *Curr Pharm Des.* 2000;6(6):681–699.
25. Tarhini AA, Gogas H, Kirkwood JM. IFN-alpha in the treatment of melanoma. *J Immunol.* 2012;189(8):3789–3793.
26. Thomas A, Teicher BA, Hassan R. Antibody–drug conjugates for cancer therapy. *Lancet Oncol.* 2016;17:e254–262.
27. Tonia T, Mettler A, Robert N, et al. Erythropoietin or darbepoetin for patients with cancer. *Cochrane DB Syst Rev.* 2012;12:003407.
28. van den Boorn JG, Hartmann G. Turning tumors into vaccines: co-opting the innate immune system. *Immunity.* 2013;39(1):27–37.
29. Wu S, Zhang Y, Xu L, et al. Multicenter, randomized study of genetically modified recombinant human interleukin-11 to prevent chemotherapy-induced thrombocytopenia in cancer patients receiving chemotherapy. *Support Care Cancer.* 2012;20(8):1875–1884.
30. Zolot RS, Basu S, Million RP. Antibody-drug conjugates. *Nat Rev Drug Discov.* 2013;12(4):259–260.

18. Immunoproliferative Diseases

Classification of Hematologic Malignancies

1. Arber DA, Orazi A, Hasserjian R, et al. The 2016 revision to the World Health Organization classification of myeloid neoplasms and acute leukemia. *Blood.* 2016; 127(20):2391–2405.

2. Baiocchi RA. Classification of malignant lymphoid disorders. In: Kaushansky K, Lichtman MA, Prchal JT, Levi MM, Press OW, Burns LJ, et al, eds. *Williams Hematology.* 9th ed. New York: McGraw-Hill; 2016. https://accessmedicine.mhmedical.com/content.aspx?bookid=1581§ionid=108072816. Accessed June 15, 2020.
3. Bennett JM, Catovsky D, Daniel MT, et al. Proposals for the classification of the acute leukaemias: French-American-British Cooperative Group. *Br J Haematol.* 1976;33:451–458.
4. Bennett JM, Catovsky D, Daniel MT, et al. The French-American-British (FAB) Co-operative Group. Proposals for the classification of the myelodysplastic syndromes. *Br J Haematol.* 1982;51:189–199.
5. Harris ML, Jaffe ES, Diebold J, et al. The World Health Organization classification of hematological malignancies. Report of the Clinical Advisory Committee meeting, Airline House, Virginia, November 1997. *Mod Pathol.* 2000;13:193.
6. Keohane EM. Introduction to hematologic neoplasms. In: Keohane EM, Otto CN, Walenga JM. *Rodak's Hematology.* 6th ed. St. Louis: Elsevier Inc; 2020:466–476.
7. Swerdlow SH, Campo E, Harris NL, et al, eds. *WHO Classification of Tumours of Haematopoietic and Lymphoid Tissues.* 4th ed. Lyon, France: IARC Press; 2008:10–15, 171–175, 194–195.
8. Vardiman JV, Thiele J, Arber DA, et al. The 2008 revision of the World Health Organization (WHO) classification of myeloid neoplasms and acute leukemia: rationale and important changes. *Blood.* 2009;114:937–951.

Leukemias

1. American Society of Clinical Oncology. Cancer.Net. Leukemia—acute lymphocytic. https://www.cancer.net/cancer-types/leukemia-acute-lymphocytic-all. Accessed June 15, 2020.
2. Colby-Graham MF, Chordas C. The childhood leukemias. *J Pediatric Nursing.* 2003;18(2):87–95.
3. Hutchison RE, Schexneider KI. Leukocytic disorders. In: McPherson RA, Pincus MR. *Henry's Clinical Diagnosis and Management by Laboratory Methods.* 23rd ed. Philadelphia: Elsevier; 2017:606–658.
4. Kebriaei P, Anastasi J, Larson RA. Acute lymphoblastic leukemia: diagnosis and classification. *Best Practice Res Clinic Haematol.* 2001;15(4):597–621.
5. Larson RA. Acute lymphoblastic leukemia. In: Kaushansky K, Lichtman MA, Prchal JT, Levi MM, Press OW, Burns LJ, et al, eds. *Williams Hematology.* 9th ed. New York: McGraw-Hill; 2016. https://accessmedicine.mhmedical.com/content.aspx?bookid=1581§ionid=108072900. Accessed June 18, 2020.
6. Marionneaux S. Maslak P. Mature lymphoid neoplasms. In: Keohane EM, Otto CN, Walenga JM. *Rodak's Hematology.* 6th ed. St. Louis: Elsevier Inc; 2020:603–625.
7. Omman RA, Kini AR. Acute leukemias. In: Keohane EM, Otto CN, Walenga JM. *Rodak's Hematology.* 6th ed. St. Louis: Elsevier Inc; 2020:540–544.
8. Riley RS, Massey D, Jackson-Cook C, et al. Immunophenotypic analysis of acute lymphocytic leukemia. *Hematol Oncol Clin N Am.* 2002;16:245–299.
9. Tiacci E, Schiavoni G, Forconi F, et al. Simple genetic diagnosis of hairy cell leukemia by sensitive detection of the BRAF-V600E mutation. *Blood.* 2012;119(1):192–196.
10. Venkataraman G, Aguhar C, Kreitman RJ, et al. Characteristic CD103 and CD123 expression pattern defines hairy cell leukemia. *Am J Clin Path.* 2011;136:625–630.
11. Zenz T, Mertens D, Küppers R, et al. From pathogenesis to treatment of chronic lymphocytic leukaemia. *Nature Rev Cancer.* 2010;10:37–50.

Lymphomas

1. Dreyling M. Mantle cell lymphoma. In: Kaushansky K, Lichtman MA, Prchal JT, Levi MM, Press OW, Burns LJ, et al, eds. *Williams Hematology.* 9th ed. New York: McGraw-Hill; 2016. https://accessmedicine.mhmedical.com/content.aspx?bookid=1581§ionid=108075164. Accessed June 23, 2020.
2. Evans AG, Friedberg JW. Burkitt lymphoma. In: Kaushansky K, Lichtman MA, Prchal JT, Levi MM, Press OW, Burns LJ, et al, eds. *Williams Hematology.* 9th ed. New York: McGraw-Hill; 2016.https://accessmedicine.mhmedical.com/content.aspx?bookid=1581§ionid=108075470. Accessed June 23, 2020.
3. Kapatai G, Murray P. Contribution of the Epstein-Barr virus to the molecular pathogenesis of Hodgkin lymphoma. *J Clin Pathol.* 2007;60:1342–1349.
4. Karube K, Niino D, Kimura Y, Ohshima K. Classical Hodgkin lymphoma, lymphocyte depleted type: clinicopathological analysis and prognostic comparison with other types of classical Hodgkin lymphoma. *Path Res Prac.* 2013;209(4):201–207.
5. Küppers R, Engert A, Hansmann M-L. Hodgkin lymphoma. *J Clin Invest.* 2012;122(10):3429–3447.
6. Press OW. Hodgkin lymphoma. In: Kaushansky K, Lichtman MA, Prchal JT, Levi MM, Press OW, Burns LJ, et al, eds. *Williams Hematology.* 9th ed. New York: McGraw-Hill;.2016. https://accessmedicine.mhmedical.com/content.aspx?bookid=1581§ionid=108074485. Accessed June 21, 2020.
7. Shankland KR, Armitage JO, Hancock BW. Non-Hodgkin lymphoma. *Lancet.* 2012;380:848–857.

MGUS, SMM, and Multiple Myeloma

1. American Cancer Society. Drug therapy for multiple myeloma. https://www.cancer.org/cancer/multiple-myeloma/treating/chemotherapy.html. Accessed June 25, 2020.
2. American Cancer Society. Key statistics about multiple myeloma. https://www.cancer.org/cancer/multiple-myeloma/about/key-statistics.html. Accessed June 24, 2020.
3. Bianchi G, Ghobrial IM. Does my patient with a serum monoclonal spike have multiple myeloma? *Hematol Oncol Clin N Am.* 2012;26:383–393.
4. Bird JM, Owen RG, S'Da S, et al. Guidelines for the diagnosis and management of multiple myeloma 2011. *Br J Hematology.* 2011;154:32–75.
5. Caers J, Vekemans M-C, Bries G, et al. Diagnosis and follow-up of monoclonal gammopathies of undetermined significance; information for referring physicians. *Ann Med.* 2013;45:413–422.
6. Cancer.Net. Multiple myeloma. https://www.cancer.net/cancer-types/multiple-myeloma/view-all. Accessed June 25, 2020.
7. International Myeloma Foundation. International Myeloma Working Group (IMWG) criteria for the diagnosis of multiple myeloma. https://www.myeloma.org/international-myeloma-working-group-imwg-criteria-diagnosis-multiple-myeloma. Accessed June 24, 2020.
8. Kuehl WM, Bergsagel PL. Molecular pathogenesis of multiple myeloma and its premalignant precursor. *J Clin Invest.* 2012;122(10):3456–3463.
9. Kyle RA, Durie BG, Rajkumar SV, et al. Monoclonal gammopathy of undetermined significance (MGUS) and smoldering (asymptomatic) multiple myeloma: IMWG consensus perspectives risk factors for progression and guidelines for monitoring and management. *Leukemia.* 2010;24:1121–1127.
10. Niels WCJ, Palumbo A, Johnsen HE, et al. The clinical relevance and management of monoclonal gammopathy of undetermined

significance and related disorders: recommendations from the European Myeloma Network. *Haematologica.* 2014;99(6):984–996.
11. Rajkumar SV. Multiple myeloma: 2016 update on diagnosis, risk-stratification, and management. *Am J Hematol.* 2016 July;91(7):719–734. doi:10.1002/ajh.24402
12. Rajkumar SV. Updated diagnostic criteria and staging system for multiple myeloma. https://ascopubs.org/doi/10.1200/EDBK_159009. Accessed June 24, 2020.
13. Rajkumar SV, Dimopoulos MA, Palumbo A, et al. International Myeloma Working Group updated criteria for the diagnosis of multiple myeloma. *Lancet Oncol.* 2014;15(12):e538–e548. doi:10.1016/S1470-2045(14)70442-5
14. Rajkumar SV, Kyle RA, Therneau TM, et al. Serum free light chain ratio is an independent risk factor for progression in monoclonal gammopathy of undetermined significance. *Blood.* 2005;106(3):812–817.
15. Rajkumar SV, Landgren O, Mateos MV. Smoldering multiple myeloma. *Lancet Oncol.* 2014;15:e538–548.
16. Zingone A, Kuehl WM. Pathogenesis of monoclonal gammopathy of undetermined significance and progression to multiple myeloma. *Sem Hematol.* 2011;48(1):4–12.

Other Plasma Cell Dyscrasias

1. Bianchi G, Anderson KC, Harris NL, Sohani AR. The heavy chain diseases: clinical and pathologic features. *Oncology.* 2014;28(1):45.
2. Cancer.Net. Waldenström's macroglobulinemia. https://www.cancer.net/cancer-types/waldenstrom%E2%80%99s-macroglobulinemia/introduction. Accessed June 26, 2020.
3. Genetics Home Reference. Waldenström macroglobulinemia. https://ghr.nlm.nih.gov/condition/waldenstrom-macroglobulinemia#resources. Accessed June 26, 2020.
4. Gertz M. Waldenström macroglobulinemia. *Hematol.* 2012;17(S1):S112–S116.
5. Gertz MA. Waldenström macroglobulinemia: 2013 update on diagnosis, risk stratification, and management. *Am J Hematol.* 2013;88:703–711.
6. Saheen SP, Talwalker SS, Lin P, et al. Waldenström macroglobulinemia: a review of the entity and its differential diagnosis. *Adv Anat Pathol.* 2012;19(1):11–27.
7. Vital A. Paraproteinemic neuropathies. *Bran Pathol.* 2001;11:399–407.
8. Wahner-Roedler DL, Kyle RA. Heavy chain diseases. *Best Pract Res Clin Ha.* 2005;18(4):729–746.
9. Witzig TE, Wahner-Roedler DL. Heavy chain disease. *Curr Treat Option On.* 2002;3:247–254.

Laboratory Evaluation of Immunoproliferative Diseases

1. Buckingham L. *Molecular Diagnostics. Fundamentals, Methods, and Clinical Applications.* 3rd ed. Philadelphia: F.A. Davis Co.; 2019:369–416.
2. Craig FE, Foon KA. Flow cytometric immunophenotyping for hematologic neoplasms. *Blood.* 2008;11(8):3941–3967.
3. Dispenzieri A, Kyle R, Gertz M, et al. International Myeloma Working Group guidelines for serum-free light chain analysis in multiple myeloma and related disorders. *Leukemia.* 2009;23:215–224.
4. Jenner E. Serum free light chains in clinical laboratory diagnostics. *Clin Chim Acta.* 2014;427:15–20.
5. Katzmann J, Kyle RA, Benson J, et al. Screening panels for detection of monoclonal gammopathies. *Clin Chem.* 2009;55:1517–1522.
6. Korbet SM, Schwartz MM. Disease of the month. Multiple myeloma. *J Am Soc Nephrol.* 2006;17:2533–2545.
7. McPherson RA, Riley RS, Massey HD. Laboratory evaluation of immunoglobulin function and humoral immunity. In: McPherson RA, Pincus MR. *Henry's Clinical Diagnosis and Management by Laboratory Methods.* 23rd ed. Philadelphia: Elsevier; 2017:913–928.
8. Merker JD, Valouev A, Gotlib J. Next-generation sequencing in hematologic malignancies: what will be the dividends? *Ther Adv Hematol.* 2012;3(6):333–339.
9. Mullighan CG. Genome sequencing of lymphoid malignancies. *Blood.* 2013;122(24):3899–3907.
10. Simons A, Sikkema-Raddatz B, deLeeuw N, et al. Genome-wide arrays in routing diagnostics of hematologic malignancies. *Hum Mutat.* 2012;33(6):941–948.
11. The Binding Site. *Immunofixation (IFE) Kit. Product Insert.* Birmingham, UK: The Binding Site Group, Ltd.; 2010, July.
12. Viva Products application note. Urine protein concentration with vivaproducts concentrators. http://www.vivaproducts.com/downloads/urine-protein-concentration-w-concentrators.pdf. Accessed June 26, 2020.
13. Wood BL, Cherian S, Borowitz MJ. The flow cytometric evaluation of hematopoietic neoplasia. In: McPherson RA, Pincus MR. *Henry's Clinical Diagnosis and Management by Laboratory Methods.* 23rd ed. Philadelphia: Elsevier; 2017:659–680.

19. Immunodeficiency Diseases

1. Aiuti A, Roncarolo MG, Naldini L. Gene therapy for ADA-SCID, the first marketing approval of an ex vivo gene therapy in Europe: paving the road for the next generation of advanced therapy medicinal products. *EMBO Molecular Medicine.* 2017;737–740.
2. Anonymous. Primary immunodeficiency diseases. Report of an IUIS Scientific Committee. International Union of Immunological Societies. *Clin Exp Immunol.* 1999;118(suppl 1):1–28.
3. Barnidge DR, Dispenzieri A, Merlini M, Katzmann JA, Murray DL. Monitoring free light chains in serum using mass spectrometry. *Clin Chem Lab Med.* 2016;54:1073–1083.
4. Bousfiha A, Jeddane L, Ailal F, et al. A phenotypic approach for IUIS PID classification and diagnosis: guidelines for clinicians at the bedside. *J Clin Immunol.* 2013;33:1078–1087.
5. Bousfiha A, Jeddane L, Picard C, et al. The 2017 IUIS phenotypic classification for primary immunodeficiencies. *J Clin Immunol.* 2018;8(1):129–143.
6. Buckley R. Primary immunodeficiency diseases due to defects in lymphocytes. *N Engl J Med.* 2000;343:1313–1324.
7. Cavazzana M, Bushman FD, Miccio A, Andre-Schmutz I, Six E. Gene therapy targeting haematopoietic stem cells for inherited diseases: progress and challenges. *Nature Rev.* 2019;18:447–462.
8. Centers for Disease Control and Prevention. Newborn screening: severe combined immunodeficiency (SCID). https://www.cdc.gov/newbornscreening/scid.html. Accessed August 21, 2020.
9. Chinen J, Lawrence M, Dorsey M, Kobrynski LJ. Practical approach to genetic testing for primary immunodeficiencies. *Ann Allergy Asthma Immunol.* 2019 Aug 28;123(5):433–439.
10. Fischer A. Human primary immunodeficiency diseases. *Immunity.* 2007;27:835–845.
11. Fischer A. Primary immune deficiency diseases. In: Jameson J, Fauci AS, Kasper DL, Hauser SL, Longo DL, Loscalzo J, eds. *Harrison's Principles of Internal Medicine.* 20th ed. New York: McGraw-Hill; 2018. http://accessmedicine.mhmedical.com/content.aspx?bookid=2129§ionid=181950913. Accessed November 15, 2019.
12. Fischer A. Primary immunodeficiency diseases: an experimental model for molecular medicine. *Lancet.* 2001;357:1863–1869.
13. Fleisher TA. Back to basics: primary immune deficiencies: window into the immune system. *Pediatr Rev.* 2006;27(10):363–372.

14. Gennery AR, Cant AJ. Cord blood stem cell transplantation in primary immune deficiencies. *Curr Opin Allergy CI.* 2007;7:528–534.
15. Giclas PC. Hereditary and acquired complement deficiencies. In: Detrick B, Schmitz JL, Hamilton RG, eds. *Manual of Molecular and Clinical Laboratory Immunology.* 8th ed. Washington, DC: ASM Press; Washington, DC; 2016:749–765.
16. Gilmour KC, Chandra A, Kumararatne DS. Primary antibody deficiency diseases. In: Detrick B, Schmitz JL, Hamilton RG, Folds JD, eds. *Manual of Molecular and Clinical Laboratory Immunology.* 8th ed. Washington, DC: ASM Press; 2016:737–748.
17. Holland SM, Neutropenia and neutrophil defects. In: Detrick B, Schmitz JL, Hamilton RG, eds. *Manual of Molecular and Clinical Laboratory Immunology.* 8th ed. Washington, DC: ASM Press; 2016:765–774.
18. Immune Deficiency Foundation. Specific disease types. https://primaryimmune.org/about-primary-immunodeficiencies/specific-disease-types/ Accessed November 12, 2019.
19. Kelly BT, Tam JS, Verbsky JW, Routes JM. Screening for severe combined immunodeficiency. *Clin Epidemiol.* 2013;5:363–369.
20. Latz E, Xiao TS, Stutz A. Activation and regulation of the inflammasomes. *Nature Rev Immunol.* 2013;13:397–411.
21. Lederman HM. The primary immunodeficiency diseases. In: Detrick B, Schmitz JL, Hamilton RG, eds. *Manual of Molecular and Clinical Laboratory Immunology.* 8th ed. Washington, DC: ASM Press; 2016:713–714.
22. Maggina P, Gennary AR. Classification of primary immunodeficiencies: need for a revised approach? *J Allergy Clin Immunol.* 2012;131:292–294.
23. Mallott J, Kwan A, Church J, et al. Newborn screening for SCID identifies patients with ataxia telangiectasia. *J Clin Immunol.* 2013;33:540–549.
24. McCusker C, Upton J, Warrington R. Primary immunodeficiency. *Allergy Asthma Clin Immunol.* 2018;14(suppl 2):141–152. doi:10.1186/s13223-018-0290-5
25. Noël A-C, Pelluard F, Delezoide A-L, et al. Fetal phenotype associated with the 22q11 deletion. *Am J Med Genet Part A.* 2014;9999:1–8.
26. Pallav K, Xu H, Leffler DA, Kabbani T, Kelly CP. Immunoglobulin A deficiency in celiac disease in the United States. *J Gastroenterol Hepatol.* 2016 Jan;31(1):133–137.
27. Peacocke M, Siminovitch KA. Wiskott-Aldrich syndrome: new molecular and biochemical insights. *J Am Acad Dermatol.* 1992;27(4):507–519.
28. Peterson MM. Myeloperoxidase deficiency. *Medscape.* https://emedicine.medscape.com/article/887599-overview#a5. Updated October 19, 2016. Accessed November 14, 2019.
29. Picard C, Gasper HB, Al-Herz W, et al. International Union of Immunological Societies: 2017 Primary Immunodeficiency Diseases Committee report on inborn errors of immunity. *J Clin Immunol.* 2018;38:96–128.
30. PID App for Android. Google play. https://play.google.com/store/apps/details?id=com.horiyasoft.pidclassification. Accessed October 30, 2019.
31. PID Classification. Apple App Store. https://apps.apple.com/us/app/pid-phenotypical-diagnosis/id1160729399. Accessed October 30, 2019.
32. Puck J. Prenatal diagnosis and genetic analysis of X-linked immunodeficiency disorders. *Pediatr Res.* 1993;33(suppl):S29.
33. Puck JM. Primary immunodeficiency diseases. *JAMA.* 1997;278:1835–1841.
34. Roifman CM, Verbsky JW, Routes JM. Approach to the diagnosis of severe combined immunodeficiency: newborn screening. In: Detrick B, Schmitz JL, Hamilton RG, eds. *Manual of Molecular and Clinical Laboratory Immunology.* 8th ed. Washington, DC: ASM Press; Washington, DC; 2016:715–720.
35. Rosenzweig D, Fleisher TA. Laboratory evaluation for T cell function. *J Allergy Clin Immunol.* 2013;131(2):622–623e.4.
36. Stiehm RE. The four most common pediatric immunodeficiencies. *Adv Exp Med Biol.* 2007;601:15–26.
37. Taddei I, Morishima M, Huynh T, Lindsay EA. Genetic factors are major determinants of phenotypic variability in a mouse model of the DiGeorge/del22q11 syndromes. *PNAS.* 2001;98(20):11428–11431.
38. U.S. National Library of Medicine. Genetics home reference. https://ghr.nlm.nih.gov/condition/ Accessed November 12, 2019.
39. van de Vijver E1, van den Berg TK, Kuijpers TW. Leukocyte adhesion deficiencies. *Hematol Oncol Clin North Am.* 2013 Feb;27(1):101–116.
40. Verbsky JW, Grossman WJ. Cellular and genetic basis of primary immune deficiencies. *Pediatr Clin N Am.* 2006;53:649–684.

20. Serological and Molecular Detection of Bacterial Infections

Bacterial Infections, Immune Defenses, Laboratory Detection

1. Black JG. *Microbiology Principles and Explorations.* 6th ed. Hoboken, NJ: Wiley; 2005:446–469.
2. Centers for Disease Control and Prevention. Summary of notifiable infectious diseases and conditions—United States, 2015. https://www.cdc.gov/mmwr/volumes/64/wr/mm6453a1.htm. Accessed October 25, 2018.
3. Farley TA, Cohen DA, Elkins W. Asymptomatic sexually transmitted diseases: the case for screening. *Prev Med.* 2003;36:502–509.
4. Findley BB, McFadden G. Anti-immunology: evasion of the host immune system by bacterial and viral pathogens. *Cell.* 2006;124:767–782.
5. Gordon GI, Ley RE, Wilson R, et al. *Extending Our View of Self: The Human Gut Microbiome Initiative (HGMI)* [white paper]. Bethesda, MD: National Human Genome Research Institute; 2005.
6. He QY, Lau GK, Zhou Y, et al. Serum biomarkers of hepatitis B virus infected liver inflammation: a proteomic study. *Proteomics.* 2003;3(5):666–674.
7. Korenromp EL, Sudaryo MK, de Vlas SJ, et al. What proportion of episodes of gonorrhoea and chlamydia becomes symptomatic? *Int. J. STD AIDS.* 2002;13:91–101.
8. Kuakarn S, SomParn P, Tangkijvanich P, et al. Serum proteins in chronic hepatitis B patients treated with peginterferon alfa-2b. *World J Gastroenterol.* 2013;19(31):5067–5075.
9. Mahon CR, Lehman DC. *Textbook of Diagnostic Microbiology* 6th ed. St. Louis: W.B. Saunders Company; 2018.
10. Mak TW, Saunders M. *The Immune Response: Basic and Clinical Principles.* Burlington, MA: Elsevier Academic Press; 2006:641–694.
11. Ndao M, Rainczuk A, Rioux MC, et al. Is SELDITOF a valid tool for diagnostic biomarkers? *Trends Parasitol.* 2010;26(12):561–567.
12. Nettleman MD. Biological warfare and infection control. *Infect Control Hosp Epidemiol.* 1991;12:368–372.
13. Que Y, Morielloon P. *Staphylococcus aureus* (including staphylococcal toxic shock). In: Mandell GL, Bennett JE, Dolin R, eds. *Principles and Practice of Infectious Diseases.* 7th ed. Philadelphia: Churchill Livingstone Elsevier; 2009:2543–2578.
14. Sajid M, Kawde A-N, Daud M. Designs, formats and applications of lateral flow assay: a literature review. *Journal of Saudi Chemical*

Society. 2014;19(6):689–705. doi:10.1016/j.jscs.2014.09.001. Accessed October 25, 2018.

15. Tancrede C. Role of human microflora in health and disease. *Eur J Clin Microbiol Infect Dis.* 1992;11(11):1012–1015.
16. Tang N, Tornatore P, Weinberger SR. Current developments in SELDI affinity technology. *Mass Spectrom Rev.* 2004;23(1): 34–44.
17. The Body's Ecosystem. http://www.the-scientist.com/?articles.view/articleNo/40600/title/The-Body-s-Ecosystem. Accessed October 25, 2018.
18. Tille PM. *Bailey and Scott's Diagnostic Microbiology.* 14th ed. St. Louis: Mosby Elsevier; 2017.
19. Verweij JJ, Canales M, Polman K, et al. Molecular diagnosis of *Strongyloides stercoralis* in faecal samples using real-time PCR. *Trans R Soc Trop Med Hyg.* 2009;103(4):342–346.
20. Wright GL. SELDI protein chip MS: a platform for biomarker discovery and cancer diagnosis. *Exp Rev Mol Diagnos.* 2002;2(6): 549–563.
21. Yansouni CP, Merckx J, Libman MD, Ndao M. Recent advances in clinical parasitology diagnostics. *Curr Infect Dis Rep.* 2014;16:434.

Group A Streptococci

1. Active Bacterial Core Surveillance. Active bacterial core surveillance (ABCS) report, emerging infections program network: group A streptococcus 2016. http://www.cdc.gov/abcs/index.html. Accessed October 25, 2018.
2. Centers for Disease Control and Prevention, Biotechnology Core Branch Facility. Introduction to emm typing: M protein gene (emm) typing *Streptococcus pyogenes.* http://www.cdc.gov/streplab/M-ProteinGene-typing.html. Accessed May 31, 2019.
3. Davies HD, McGeer A, Schwartz B, et al. Invasive group A streptococcal infections in Ontario, Canada, Ontario Group A Streptococcal Study Group. *N Eng J Med.* 2001;335:547–554.
4. Fischetti VA. Streptococcal M protein. *Sci Am.* 1991;264:58.
5. Lang MM, Towers C. Identifying poststreptococcal glomerulonephritis. *Nurse Pract.* 2001;26:34.
6. Larson HS. Streptococcaceae. In: Mahan CR, Manuselis G, eds. *Textbook of Diagnostic Microbiology.* 2nd ed. Philadelphia: WB Saunders; 2000:345–371.
7. Lewis JB, Neilson EG. Glomerular diseases. In: Jameson J, Fauci AS, Kasper DL, Hauser SL, Longo DL, Loscalzo J, eds. *Harrison's Principles of Internal Medicine.* 20th ed. New York: McGraw-Hill; 2018. http://accessmedicine.mhmedical.com/content.aspx?bookid=2129§ionid=192281295. Accessed May 31, 2019.
8. Lewis LS. Impetigo work-up. *Medscape.* emedicine.medscape.com/article/965254-workup. Accessed May 31, 2019.
9. Litwin CM, Litwin SE, Hill HR. Diagnostic methods for group A streptococcal infections. In: Detrick B, Schmitz JL, Hamilton RG, eds. *Manual of Molecular and Clinical Laboratory Immunology.* 8th ed. Washington, DC: ASM Press; 2016:394–403.
10. Moses AE, Goldberg S, Korenman Z, et al. Invasive group A streptococcal infections. *Israel Emerg Infect Dis.* 2002;8:421–426.
11. Sauda M, Wu W, Conran P, et al. Streptococcal pyrogenic exotoxin B enhances tissue damage initiated by other *Streptococcus pyogenes* products. *J Infect Dis.* 2001;184:723–731.
12. Spellerberg B, Brandt C. Streptococcus. In: Jorgensen JH, Pfaller MA, eds. *Manual of Clinical Microbiology.* 11th ed. Washington, DC: ASM Press; 2015:383–402.
13. Stevens DL, Kaplan EL. *Streptococcal Infections—Clinical Aspects, Microbiology, and Molecular Pathogenesis.* New York: Oxford University Press; 2000.
14. Wessels MR. Streptococcal and enterococcal infections. In: Braunwald E, Fauci AS, Kasper EL, et al, eds. *Harrison's Principles of Internal Medicine.* 15th ed. New York: McGraw-Hill; 2001:901–909.

Helicobacter pylori

1. Allen LA, Schlesinger LS, Kang B. Virulent strains of *Helicobacter pylori* demonstrate delayed phagocytosis and stimulate homotypic phagosome fusion in macrophages. *J Exp Med.* 2000;191:115–128.
2. Atherton J, Cao P, Peek RM, et al. Mosaicism in vacuolating cytotoxin alleles of *Helicobacter pylori:* association of specific vacA types with cytotoxin production and peptic ulceration. *J Biol Chem.* 1995;270:1771–1777.
3. D'Elios MM, Manghetti M, De Carli M, et al. T helper 1 effector cells specific for *Helicobacter pylori* in the gastric antrum of patients with peptic ulcer disease. *J Immunol.* 1997;158:962–967.
4. Dunn BE, Phadnis SH. Diagnosis of *Helicobacter pylori* infection and assessment of eradication. In: Detrick B, Schmitz JL, Hamilton RG, eds. *Manual of Molecular and Clinical Laboratory Immunology.* 8th ed. Washington, DC: ASM Press; 2016:404–411.
5. Everhart JE, Kruszon-Moran D, Perez-Perez GI, et al. Seroprevalence and ethnic differences in *Helicobacter pylori* infection among adults in the United States. *J Infect Dis.* 2000;181:1359–1363.
6. Graham DY, Lew GM, Malaty HM, et al. Factors influencing the eradication of *Helicobacter pylori* with triple therapy. *Gastroenterology.* 1992;102:493–496.
7. Hazell SL, Lee A, Brady L, et al. *Campylobacter pylori* and gastritis: association with intracellular spaces and adaptation to an environment of mucus as important factors in colonization of the gastric epithelium. *J Infect Dis.* 1986;153:658–663.
8. Lawson AJ. *Helicobacter.* In: Jorgensen JH, Pfaller MA, eds. *Manual of Clinical Microbiology.* 11th ed. Washington, DC: ASM Press; 2015:1013–1027.
9. Letley DP, Rhead JL, Twells RJ, et al. Determinants of non-toxicity in the gastric pathogen *Helicobacter pylori. J Biol Chem.* 2003;278: 26734–26741.
10. Malfertheiner P, Megraud F, O'Moran C, and the European *Helicobacter pylori* Study Group (EHPSG). Current concepts in the management of *Helicobacter pylori* infection—the Maastricht 2-2000 Consensus Report. *Alim Pharmacol Ther.* 2002;16:167–180, 200.
11. Marshall BJ. History of the discovery of *Campylobacter pylori.* In: Blaser MJ. Campylobacter pylori *in Gastritis and Peptic Ulcer Disease.* New York: Igaku Shoin; 1989:7–23.
12. Megraud F. Impact of *Helicobacter pylori* virulence in the outcome of gastroduodenal disease: lessons from the microbiologist. *Digest Dis.* 2001;19:99–103.
13. Megraud F, Lehours P. *Helicobacter pylori* detection and antimicrobial susceptibility testing. *Clin Microbiol Rev.* 2007;20(2):280–322.
14. Mohammadi M, Nedrud J, Redline R, et al. Murine CD4 T-cell response to *Helicobacter* infection: TH1 cells enhance gastritis and TH2 cells reduce bacterial load. *Gastroenterology.* 1997;113:1848–1857.
15. National Institutes of Health Consensus Conference. *Helicobacter pylori* in peptic ulcers. *JAMA.* 1994;272:65–69.
16. Peek RM, Blaser MJ. *Helicobacter pylori* and gastrointestinal tract adenocarcinomas. *Nat Rev Cancer.* 2002;2:28–37.
17. Segal ED, Cha J, Lo J, et al. Altered states: involvement of phosphorylated CagA in the induction of host cellular growth changes by *Helicobacter pylori. Proc Natl Acad Sci USA.* 1999;96:14559–14564.

18. Sokic-Milutinovic T, Wex T, Todorovic V, et al. Anti-CagA and anti-VacA antibodies in *Helicobacter pylori*-infected patients with and without peptic ulcer disease in Serbia and Montenegro. *Scand J Gastroenterol.* 2004;3:222–226.
19. Suzuki M, Miura S, Suematsu M, et al. *Helicobacter pylori*-associated ammonia production enhances neutrophil-dependent gastric mucosal cell injury. *Am J Physiol.* 1992;263:G719–G725.
20. Wang J, Brooks EG, Bamford KB, et al. Negative selection of T cells by *Helicobacter pylori* as a model for bacterial strain selection by immune evasion. *J Immunol.* 2001;167:926–934.
21. Wotherspoon AC, Ortiz Hidalgo C, Falzon MR, et al. *Helicobacter pylori*-associated gastritis and primary B-cell gastric lymphoma. *Lancet.* 1991;338:1175–1176.

Mycoplasma pneumoniae

1. Baum SG. *Mycoplasma pneumoniae* and atypical pneumoniae. In: Mandell GL, Bennett JE, Dolin R, eds. *Principles and Practice of Infectious Diseases.* 7th ed. Philadelphia: Churchill Livingstone Elsevier; 2009:2486.
2. Beersma MFC, Dirven K, van Dam AP, et al. Evaluation of 12 commercial tests and the complement fixation test for *Mycoplasma pneumoniae*-specific immunoglobulin G (IgG) and IgM antibodies, with PCR used as the "gold standard." *J Clin Microbiol.* 2005;43:2277–2285.
3. Biofire Diagnostics. *FilmArray Respiratory Panel Information Sheet.* Salt Lake City, UT: Biofire Diagnostics; 2014.
4. Feizi T, Taylor-Robinson D. Cold agglutinin anti-I and *Mycoplasma pneumoniae. Immunology.* 1967;13:405.
5. Fink CG, Sillis M, Read SJ, et al. Neurologic disease associated with *Mycoplasma pneumoniae* infection: PCR evidence against a direct invasive mechanism. *Clin Mol Pathol.* 1995;48:51–54.
6. Foy HM. Infections caused by *Mycoplasma pneumoniae* and possible carrier state in different populations of patients. *Clin Infect Dis.* 1993;17(suppl. 1):S37–S46.
7. Lind K, Spencer ES, Anderson HK. Cold agglutinin production and cytomegalovirus infection. *Scand J Infect Dis.* 1974;6:109.
8. McCormack JG. Mycoplasma pneumoniae and the erythema multiforme–Stevens-Johnson syndrome. *J Infect.* 1981;3:32.
9. Nisar N, Guleria R, Kumar S, et al. Mycoplasma pneumoniae and its role in asthma. *Postgrad Med J.* 2007;83:100–104.
10. Razin S, Yogev D, Naot Y. Molecular biology and pathogenicity of mycoplasmas. *Microbiol Mol Biol Rev.* 1998;62:1094–1156.
11. Rosenfield RE, Schmidt PJ, Calvo RC, et al. Anti-i, a frequent cold agglutinin in infectious mononucleosis. *Vox Sang.* 1965;10:631.
12. Schalock PC, Dinulos JGH. *Mycoplasma pneumoniae*-induced Stevens-Johnson syndrome without skin lesions: fact or fiction? *J Am Acad Dermatol.* 2005;52:312–315.
13. Schubothe H. The cold hemagglutinin disease. *Semin Hematol.* 1966;3:27.
14. Shmuel R, David Y, Yehudith N. Molecular biology and pathogenicity of mycoplasmas. *Microbiol Mol Biol Rev.* 1998;62:1094–1156.
15. Waites KB. New concepts of *Mycoplasma pneumoniae* infections in children. *Pediatr Pulmonol.* 2003;36:267–278.
16. Waites KB, Brown MB, Simecka JW. Mycoplasma: immunologic and molecular diagnostic methods. In: Detrick B, Schmitz JL, Hamilton RG, eds. *Manual of Molecular and Clinical Laboratory Immunology.* 8th ed. Washington, DC: ASM Press; 2016:444–452.
17. Waites KB, Taylor-Robinson DT. Mycoplasma and ureoplasma. In: Murray PR, Baron EJ, Jorgensen JH, et al, eds. *Manual of Clinical Microbiology.* 9th ed. Washington, DC: ASM Press; 2007:1004–1020.
18. Yang J, Hooper W, Phillips D, et al. Cytokines in *Mycoplasma pneumoniae* infections. *Cytokine Growth Factor Rev.* 2004;15:157–168.

Rickettsial Infections

1. Anderson B, Friedman H, Bendinelli M. *Rickettsial Infection and Immunity.* New York: Plenum Press; 1997.
2. Blanton LS, Walker DH. The *Rickettsiaceae, Anaplasmataceae,* and *Coxiellaceae*. In: Detrick B, Schmitz JL, Hamilton RG, eds. *Manual of Molecular and Clinical Laboratory Immunology.* 8th ed. Washington, DC: ASM Press; 2016:461–472.
3. Centers for Disease Control and Prevention. *Rocky Mountain Spotted Fever Statistics and Epidemiology.* Atlanta, GA: Centers for Disease Control and Prevention; updated April 7, 2020. http://www.cdc.gov/rmsf/stats/. Accessed August 21, 2020.
4. Centers for Disease Control and Prevention. *Rocky Mountain Spotted Fever (RMSF)—Symptoms, Diagnosis, and Treatment.* Atlanta, GA: Centers for Disease Control and Prevention; 2019.
5. Elghetany TM, Walker DH. Hemostatic changes in Rocky Mountain spotted fever and Mediterranean spotted fever. *Am J Clin Pathol.* 1999;112:159–168.
6. Eremeeva ME, Dasch GA. *Rickettsial (Spotted & Typhus Fevers) & Related Infections (Anaplasmosis & Ehrlichiosis).* Atlanta, GA: Centers for Disease Control and Prevention; 2019. http://www.cdc.gov/travel/yellowbook/2014/chapter-3-infectious-diseases-related-to-travel/rickettsial-spotted-and-typhus-fevers-and-related-infections-anaplasmosis-and-ehrlichiosis. Accessed August 21, 2020.
7. Harrell GT, Aikawa JK. Pathogenesis of circulatory failure in Rocky Mountain spotted fever. Alteration in the blood volume and the thiocyanate space at various stages of the disease. *Arch Intern Med.* 1949;83:331–347.
8. Li H, Walker DH. rOmpA is a critical protein for the adhesion of *Rickettsia rickettsii* to host cells. *Microb Pathog.* 1998;24:289–298.
9. Perine PL, Chandler BP, Krause DK, et al. A clinico-epidemiological study of epidemic typhus in Africa. *Infect Dis.* 1992;14:1149–1158.
10. Uchiyama T, Kawano H, Kusuhara Y. The major outer membrane protein rOmpB of spotted fever group rickettsiae functions in the rickettsial adherence to and invasion of Vero cells. *Microb Infect.* 2006:801–809.
11. Walker DH. *Rickettsia rickettsii* and other spotted fever group *Rickettsiae* (Rocky Mountain spotted fever and other spotted fevers). In: Mandell GL, Bennett JE, Dolin R, eds. *Principles and Practice of Infectious Diseases.* 7th ed. Philadelphia: Churchill Livingstone Elsevier; 2009:2499–2507.
12. Walker DH, Bouyer DH. Rickettsia and orientia. In: Murray PR, Baron EJ, Jorgensen JH, et al, eds. *Manual of Clinical Microbiology.* 9th ed. Washington, DC: ASM Press; 2007:1036–1045.
13. Walker DH, Ismail N. Emerging and re-emerging rickettsioses: endothelial cell infection and early disease events. *Nat Rev Microbiol.* 2008;6:375–386.

21. Spirochete Diseases

Syphilis

1. American Red Cross. Blood donation eligibility criteria. http://www.redcrossblood.org/donating-blood/eligibility-requirements/eligibility-criteria-topic. Accessed June 10, 2019.
2. Binnicker MJ. Which algorithm should be used to screen for syphilis? *Curr Opin Infect Dis.* 2012;25(1):79–85.
3. Binnicker MJ, Jespersen DJ, Rollins LO. Treponema-specific tests for serodiagnosis of syphilis: comparative evaluation of seven assays. *J Clin Microbiol.* 2011;49:1313.

4. Blanco DR, Miller JN, Lovett MA. Surface antigens of the syphilis spirochete and their potential as virulence determinants. *Emerg Infect Dis.* 1997;3:11–20.
5. Centers for Disease Control and Prevention. http://www.cdc.gov/std/syphilis/DCL-Syphilis-MMWR-2-10-2011.pdf. Accessed June 10, 2019.
6. Centers for Disease Control and Prevention. Discordant results from reverse sequence syphilis screening: five laboratories, United States, 2006–2010. *MMWR.* 2011;60(05):133–137.
7. Centers for Disease Control and Prevention. Newborn syphilis cases more than double in four years, reaching 20-year high: press release; September 25, 2018. https://www.cdc.gov/nchhstp/newsroom/2018/std-surveillance-report-2017-press-release.html. Accessed June 10, 2019.
8. Centers for Disease Control and Prevention. Outbreak of syphilis among men who have sex with men—Southern California, 2000. *MMWR.* 2001;50(38):117–120.
9. Centers for Disease Control and Prevention. Primary and secondary syphilis among men who have sex with men—New York City, 2001. *MMWR.* 2002;51(38):853–856.
10. Centers for Disease Control and Prevention. Primary and secondary syphilis—United States, 2005–2013. *MMWR.* 2014;63(18):402–406.
11. Centers for Disease Control and Prevention. Sexually transmitted disease (STD) surveillance 2017: data and statistics (2013–2017). http//www.cdc.gov/std/stats/. Accessed June 10, 2019.
12. Chhabra RS, Brion LP, Castro M, Freundlich L, Glaser JH. Comparison of maternal sera, cord blood, and neonatal sera for detecting presumptive congenital syphilis: relationship with maternal treatment. *Pediatrics.* 1993;91:88–91.
13. Cole MJ, Perry KR, Parry JV. Comparative evaluation of 15 serological assays for the detection of syphilis infection. *Eur J Clin Microbiol.* 2007;26(10):705–713.
14. Doherty L, Fenton KA, Jones J, et al. Syphilis: old problem, new strategy. *BMJ.* 2002;325:153–165.
15. Dunseth CD, Ford BA, Krasowski MD. Traditional versus reverse syphilis algorithms: a comparison at a large academic medical center. *Pract Lab Med.* 2017;8:52–59.
16. Gayet-Ageron A, Lautenschlager S, Ninet B, et al. Sensitivity, specificity and likelihood ratios of PCR in the diagnosis of syphilis: a systematic review and meta-analysis. *Sex Transmitted Dis.* 2013;89(3):251–256.
17. Goldmeier D, Hay P. A review and update on adult syphilis, with particular reference to its treatment. *Int J STD AIDS.* 1993;4:70–82.
18. Gomez E, Jespersen DJ, Harring JA, Binnicker MJ. Evaluation of the Bio-Rad BioPlex 2200 syphilis multiplex flow immunoassay for the detection of IgM- and IgG-class antitreponemal antibodies. *Clin Vaccine Immunol.* 2010;17:966.
19. Heymans R, vander Helm JJ, deVries HJC, et al. Clinical value of *Treponema pallidum* real time PCR for diagnosis of syphilis. *J Clin Microbiol.* 2010;48(2):497–502.
20. Larsen SA, Pope V, Johnson RE, Kennedy RJ, eds. *A Manual of Tests for Syphilis.* Washington, DC: American Public Health Association; 1998.
21. LaSala PR, Smith MB. Spirochete infections. In: McPherson RA, Pincus MR, eds. *Henry's Clinical Diagnosis and Management by Laboratory Methods.* 22nd ed. Philadelphia: WB Saunders; 2011:1129–1144.
22. Lukehart SA. Syphilis. In: Jameson J, Fauci AS, Kasper DL, Hauser SL, Longo DL, Loscalzo J, eds. ***Harrison's Principles of Internal Medicine.*** 20th ed. New York: McGraw-Hill; 2018. http://accessmedicine.mhmedical.com/content.aspx?bookid=2129§ionid=192023811. Accessed June 10, 2019.
23. McKenna C, Schroeter A, Kierland R, et al. The fluorescent treponemal antibody absorbed (FTA-ABS) test beading phenomenon in connective tissue diseases. *Mayo Clin Proc.* 1973;48:545–548.
24. Michelow IC, Wendel GD Jr, Norgard MV, et al. Central nervous system infection in congenital syphilis. *N Engl J Med.* 2002;346:1792–1798.
25. Morshed MG, Singh AE. Recent trends in the serologic diagnosis of syphilis. *Clin Vaccine Immunol.* 2015; 22:137–147.
26. Noordhoek G, Wolters EC, De Jonge MEJ, Van Embden JDA. Detection by polymerase chain reaction of *Treponema pallidum* DNA in cerebrospinal fluid from neurosyphilis patients before and after antibiotic treatment. *J Clin Microbiol.* 1991;29:1976–1984.
27. Orton S, Liu H, Dodd R, Williams A. Prevalence of circulating *Treponema pallidum* DNA and RNA in blood donors with confirmed-positive syphilis tests. *Transfusion.* 2002;42:94–99.
28. Patel JA, Chonmaitree T. Syphilis screen at delivery: a need for uniform guidelines. *Am J Dis Child.* 1993;147:256–258.
29. Peeling RW, Mabey D, Kamb ML, et al. Syphilis. *Nat Rev Dis Primers.* 2017 Oct 12;3:17073. Published online. doi:10.1038/nrdp.2017.73
30. Pope V. Use of treponemal test to screen for syphilis. *Infect Med.* 2004;21:399–404.
31. Pope V, Fears MB, Morrill WE, et al. Comparison of the Serodia *Treponema pallidum* particle agglutination, Captia Syphilis-G, and SpiroTek Reagin II tests with standard test techniques for diagnosis of syphilis. *J Clin Microbiol.* 2000;38:2543–2545.
32. Ropper AH. Neurosyphilis. *New Engl J Med.* 2019;381:1358–1363.
33. Sánchez PJ, Wendel GD, Grimprel E, et al. Evaluation of molecular methodologies and rabbit infectivity testing for the diagnosis of congenital syphilis and neonatal central nervous system invasion by *Treponema pallidum. J Infect Dis.* 1993;167:148–157.
34. Schiff E, Lindberg M. Neurosyphilis. *South Med J.* 2002;95:1083–1087.
35. Schmitz JL. Laboratory diagnosis of syphilis. In: Detrick B, Schmitz JL, Hamilton RG. *Manual of Clinical Laboratory Immunology.* 8th ed. Washington, DC: ASM Press; 2016:412–417.
36. Sena AC, White BL, Sparling PF. Novel *Treponema pallidum serologic* tests: a paradigm shift in syphilis screening for the 21st century. *Clin Infect Dis.* 2010;51(6):700–708.
37. Symptomatic early neurosyphilis among HIV-positive men who have sex with men—four cities, United States, January 2002–June 2004. *MMWR.* 2007;56(25):625–628.
38. Tsimis ME, Sheffield JS. Update on syphilis and pregnancy. *Birth Defects Res.* 2017 Mar 15; 109(5):347–352.
39. World Health Organization. *Global Incidence and Prevalence of Selected Curable Sexually Transmitted Infections–2008.* Geneva: World Health Organization; 2018. http://www.who.int/reproductive-health/publications/rtis/stisestimates/en/. Accessed January 15, 2019.
40. Woznicova V, Votava M, Flasarova M. Clinical specimens for PCR detection of syphilis. *Epidemiol Mikrobiol Immunol.* 2007;56:66–71.

Lyme Disease

1. Aguero-Rosenfeld ME, Wang G, Schwartz I, Wormser GP. Diagnosis of *Lyme borreliosis. Clin Micro Rev.* 2005;18:484–509.
2. Branda JA, Strle K, Nigrovic LE, et al. Evaluation of modified 2-tiered serodiagnostic testing algorithms for early Lyme disease. *Clin Infec Dis.* 2017;64:1074–1080.

3. Brown SL, Hansen SL, Langone JJ. Role of serology in diagnosis of Lyme disease. *JAMA.* 1999;282:62–66.
4. Burgdorfer W, Barbour AG, Hayes SF, et al. Lyme disease—A tick-borne spirochetosis? *Science.* 1982;216:1317.
5. Centers for Disease Control and Prevention. Lyme disease diagnosis and testing. http://www.cdc.gov/lyme/diagnosistesting/index.html. Accessed June 10, 2019.
6. Centers for Disease Control and Prevention. Lyme disease vaccination. http://www.cdc.gov/lyme/prev/vaccine.html. Accessed June 10, 2019.
7. Centers for Disease Control and Prevention. Notice to readers: caution regarding testing for Lyme disease. *MMWR.* 2005;54:125–126.
8. Centers for Disease Control and Prevention. Recommendations for test performance and interpretation from the Second National Conference on Serological Diagnosis of Lyme Disease. *MMWR.* 1995;44:590–591.
9. Centers for Disease Control and Prevention. Summary of notifiable diseases—United States, 2008–2015. *MMWR.* 2017;66(22):1–12.
10. Dressler F, Whalen JA, Reinhardt BN, Steere AC. Western blotting in the serodiagnosis of Lyme disease. *J Infect Dis.* 1993;167: 392–400.
11. Engstrom SM, Shoop E, Johnson RC. Immunoblot interpretation criteria for serodiagnosis of early Lyme disease. *J Clin Microbiol.* 1995;33:419–427.
12. Feder HM, Johnson BJ, O'Connell S, et al. A critical appraisal of "chronic Lyme disease." *N Engl J Med.* 2007;357:1422–1430.
13. Golightly MG. Laboratory considerations in the diagnosis and management of Lyme borreliosis. *Am J Clin Path.* 1993;99:168–174.
14. Golightly MG, Benach J. Tick-borne diseases. *Rev Clin Micro.* 1999;10(1):1–10.
15. Grodzicki RL, Steere AC. Comparison of immunoblotting and indirect enzyme-linked immunosorbent assay using different antigen preparations for diagnosing early Lyme disease. *J Infect Dis.* 1988;157(4):790–797.
16. Hercogova J. Review: Lyme borreliosis. *Int J Dermatol.* 2001;40:547–550.
17. Kalish RA, Kaplan RF, Taylor E, et al. Evaluation of study patients with Lyme disease, 10–20 year follow-up. *J Infect Dis.* 2001;183:453–460.
18. Lyme Info.Net. Lyme disease vaccine. http://www.lymeinfo.net/vaccine.html. Accessed June 10, 2019.
19. Magnarelli LA, Miller JN, Anderson JF, Riviere GR. Cross-reactivity of nonspecific Treponemal antibodies in serologic tests for Lyme disease. *J Clin Micro.* 1990;28:1276–1279.
20. Mahon CR, Lehman DC. The spirochetes. In: *Textbook of Diagnostic Microbiology.* 6th ed. St. Louis: Elsevier Saunders;2019: 524–525.
21. Marques AR. Revisiting the Lyme disease serodiagnostic algorithm: the momentum gathers. *J Clin Microbiol.* 2018;56(8):1–7.
22. Mead P, Petersen J, Hinckley A. Updated CDC recommendation for serologic diagnosis of Lyme disease. *MMWR Morb Mortal Wkly Rep.* 2019;68:703. doi:10.15585/mmwr.mm6832a4
23. Nadelman RB, Nowakowski J, Fish D, et al. Prophylaxis with single-dose doxycycline for the prevention of Lyme disease after an *Ixodes scapularis* tick bite. *N Engl J Med.* 2001;345:79–84.
24. Pfister HW, Wilske B, Weber K. *Lyme borreliosis:* basic science and clinical aspects. *Lancet.* 1994;343:1013–1016.
25. Rosa PA, Schwan TG. A specific and sensitive assay for the Lyme disease spirochete *Borrelia burgdorferi* using the polymerase chain reaction. *J Infect Dis.* 1989;160:1018–1029.
26. Schriefer ME. Borrelia. In: Jorgensen JH, Pfaller MA, eds. *Manual of Clinical Microbiology.* 11th ed., vol. 1. Washington, DC: ASM Press; 2015:1037–1054.
27. Smith RP, Schoen RT, Rahn DW, et al. Clinical characteristics and treatment outcome of early Lyme disease in patients with microbiologically confirmed erythema migrans. *Ann Intern Med.* 2002;136:421–428.
28. Steere AC. *Lyme borreliosis.* In: Jameson J, Fauci AS, Kasper DL, Hauser SL, Longo DL, Loscalzo J, eds. *Harrison's Principles of Internal Medicine.* 20th ed. New York: McGraw-Hill; 2018. http://accessmedicine.mhmedical.com/content.aspx?bookid=2129§ionid=192024028. Accessed June 10, 2019.
29. Steere AC. Lyme disease. *N Engl J Med.* 2001;345:115–124.
30. Steere AC, Malawista SE, Snydman DR, et al. Lyme arthritis: an epidemic of oligoarticular arthritis in children and adults in three Connecticut communities. *Arthritis Rheum.* 1977;20:7–17.
31. Wang G, Aguero-Rosenfeld ME. Lyme disease, relapsing fever, and leptospirosis In: Detrick B, Schmitz JL, Hamilton RG. *Manual of Clinical Laboratory Immunology.* 8th ed. Washington, DC: ASM Press; 2016:419–432.
32. Wormser GP, Dattwyler RJ, Shapiro ED, et al. The clinical assessment, treatment, and prevention of Lyme disease, human granulocytic anaplasmosis, and babesiosis: clinical practice guidelines by the Infectious Diseases Society of America. *Clin Inf Dis.* 2006;43:1089–1134.

Leptospirosis

1. Ahmed A, Grobusch MP, Klatser PR, Hartskeerl RA. Molecular approaches in the detection and characterization of *Leptospira. J Bacteriol Parasitol.* 2012;3:133.
2. Centers for Disease Control and Prevention. Leptospirosis: healthcare workers. 2018. https://www.cdc.gov/leptospirosis/health_care_workers/index.html. Updated August 4, 2020. Accessed August 21, 2020.
3. Chappel RJ, Goris MG, Palmer MF, Hartskeerl RA. Impact of proficiency testing on results of the microscopic agglutination test for diagnosis of leptospirosis. *J Clin Microbiol.* 2004;42:5484–5488.
4. Edwards CN, Levett PN. Prevention and treatment of leptospirosis. *Expert Rev Anti Infect Ther.* 2004;2:293–298.
5. Levitt PN. Leptospira. In: Jorgensen JH, Pfaller MA, eds. *Manual of Clinical Microbiology.* 11th ed., vol. 1. Washington, DC: ASM Press; 2015:1028–1036.
6. Monahan AM, Miller IS, Nally JE. Leptospirosis: risk during recreational activities. *J Appl Microbiol.* 2009;107:707–716.
7. Thaipadunpanit J, Chierakul W, Wuthiekanun V, et al. Diagnostic accuracy of real-time PCR assays targeting 16S rRNA and LipL32 genes for human leptospirosis in Thailand: a case control study. *PLoS One.* 2011;6:e16236.
8. Tile PM. The spirochetes. Chapter 45. In: Tile PM. *Bailey and Scott's Diagnostic Microbiology.* 14th ed. St. Louis: Mosby; 2018.

22. Serological and Molecular Diagnosis of Parasitic and Fungal Infections

Parasitic Infections—General

1. Abu-Shakra M, Buskila D, Yehuda Shoenfeld Y. Molecular mimicry between host and pathogen: examples from parasites and implication. *Immunol Lett.* 1999;67(2):147–152.
2. Abu-Shakra M, Shoenfeld Y. Parasitic infection and autoimmunity. *Autoimmunity.* 1991;9(4):337–344.
3. Akira S, Uematsu S, Takeuchi O. Pathogen recognition and innate immunity. *Cell.* 2006;124:783–801.

4. Araujo FG. Diagnosis of parasitic diseases. *Mem Inst Oswaldo Cruz Rio J.* 1988;83(suppl 1):464–465.
5. Barry JD. The relative significance of mechanisms of antigenic variation in African Trypanosomes. *Parasitol Today.* 1997;13:212–218.
6. Bhattacharyya MK, Norris DE, Kumar N. Molecular players of homologous recombination in protozoan parasites: implications for generating antigenic variation. *Infect Genet Evol.* 2004;4(2): 91–98.
7. Centers for Disease Control and Prevention. Malaria diagnosis (United States). https://www.cdc.gov/malaria/diagnosis_treatment/diagnosis.html. Accessed July 9, 2019.
8. Centers for Disease Control and Prevention. Serum/plasma specimens—detection of antibodies—general information. https://www.cdc.gov/dpdx/diagnosticprocedures/serum/antibodydetection.html. Accessed July 9, 2019.
9. Chandra RK. Immune responses in parasitic diseases. Part B: mechanisms. *Rev Infect Dis.* 1982;4(4):756–762.
10. Collier L, Balows A, Sussman M, eds. *Topley and Wilson's Microbiology and Microbial Infections.* 9th ed. New York: Oxford University Press;1998:69–70.
11. Donati D, Mok B, Chêne A, et al. Increased B cell survival and preferential activation of the memory compartment by a malaria polyclonal B cell activator. *J Immunol.* 2006;177:3035–3044.
12. Dunne DW, Butterworth AE, Fulford AJH, et al. Immunity after treatment of human schistosomiasis: association between IgE antibodies to adult worm antigens and resistance to reinfection. *Eur J Immunol.* 1992;22:1483–1494.
13. Falella FJ, Delaney KM, Moorman AC, et al. Declining morbidity and mortality among patients with advanced human immunodeficiency virus infection. *N Engl J Med.* 1998;338(13):853–860.
14. FilmArray gastrointestinal panels. https://www.biomerieux-diagnostics.com/filmarrayr-gi-panel. Accessed July 9, 2019.
15. Franchi L, Eigenbrod T, Munoz-Planillo R, Nunez G. The inflammasome: a caspase-1-activation platform that regulates immune responses and disease pathogenesis. *Nat Immunol.* 2009;10:241–247.
16. Garcia LS. *Diagnostic Medical Parasitology.* 5th ed. Washington, DC: ASM Press; 2007:567–591.
17. Garcia LS, Paltridge GP, Shimizu RY. General approaches for detection and identification of parasites. In: Jorgensen JH, Pfaller MA, eds. *Manual of Clinical Laboratory Immunology.* 11th ed. Washington, DC: ASM Press; 2015:2317–2337.
18. Garcia ME, Blanco JL. Principales enfermedades fu´ngicas que afectan a los animales dome´sticos. *Rev Iberoam Micol.* 2000;17:S2–S7.
19. Hagan P, Blumenthal UJ, Dunn D, Simpson AJ, Wilkins HA. Human IgE, IgG4 and resistance to reinfection with *Schistosoma haematobium. Nature.* 1991;349:243–245.
20. Hotez PJ. *Forgotten People, Forgotten Diseases: The Neglected Tropical Diseases and Their Impact on Global Health and Development.* Washington, DC: ASM Press; 2013.
21. Jenkins SJ, Hewitson JP, Jenkins GR, et al. Modulation of the host's immune response by schistosome larvae. *Parasite Immunol.* 2005;27:385–393.
22. John DT, Petri WA. *Markell and Voge's Medical Parasitology.* 9th ed. Philadelphia: Elsevier Saunders; 2006:112.
23. Khouri R, Bafica A, Silva Mda P, et al. IFN-beta impairs superoxide-dependent parasite killing in human macrophages: evidence for a deleterious role of SOD1 in cutaneous leishmaniasis. *J Immunol.* 2009;182(4):2525–2531.
24. Maddison SE. Serodiagnosis of parasitic diseases. *Clin Microbiol Rev.* 1991;4(4):457–469.
25. Male D, Brostoff J, Roth D, Roitt I. *Immunology.* 7th ed. Philadelphia: Mosby Elsevier; 2006:277–298.
26. Montoya JG, Remington JS. Management of *Toxoplasma gondii* infection during pregnancy. *Clin Infect Dis.* 2008;47(4):554–566.
27. Moody A. Rapid diagnostic tests for malaria parasites. *Clin Microbiol Rev.* 2002;15(1):66–78.
28. Murray CJ, Rosenfeld LC, Lim SS, et al. Global malaria mortality between 1980 and 2010: a systematic analysis. *Lancet.* 2012;379:413–431.
29. Pappas MG. Recent applications of the Dot-ELISA in immunoparasitology, *Vet Parasitol.* 1988;29(2):105–129.
30. Persing D, Mathiesen D, Marshall WF, et al. Detection of *Babesia microti* by polymerase chain reaction. *J Clin Microbiol.* 1992;30(8):2097–2103.
31. Playfair JHL. Effective and ineffective immune responses to parasites: evidence from experimental models. *Curr Top Microbiol Immunol.* 1978;80:37–64.
32. Sadick MD, Raff HV. Differences in expression and exposure of promastigote and amastigote membrane molecules in *Leishmania tropica. Infect Immun.* 1985;47(2):395–400.
33. Salzet M, Capron A, Stefano GB. Molecular crosstalk in host–parasite relationships: schistosome- and leech–host interactions. *Parasitol Today.* 2000;16(12):536–540.
34. Shimizu RY, Garcia LS. Specimen collection, transport, and processing. In: Jorgensen JH, Pfaller MA, eds. *Manual of Clinical Laboratory Immunology.* 11th ed. Washington, DC: ASM Press; 2015:2293–2309.
35. State and Local Health Departments, CDC. Update: trends in AIDS incidence, deaths, and prevalence—United States, 1996. *MMWR.* 1997;46:165–173.
36. Swan H, Sloan L, Muyombwe A, et al. Evaluation of a real-time polymerase chain reaction assay for the diagnosis of malaria in patients from Thailand. *Am J Trop Med Hyg.* 2005;73(5):850–854.
37. World Health Organization. Revised Global Burden of Disease (GBD) 2002 estimates: Mortality, incidence, prevalence, YLL, YLD and DALYs by sex, cause and region, estimates for 2002 as reported in the World Health Report 2004. Accessed August 21, 2020.
38. Zandman-Goddard G, Shoenfeld Y. Parasitic infection and autoimmunity, *Lupus.* 2009;18:1144–1148.

Toxoplasmosis

1. Bjerkås I. Neuropathology and host–parasite relationship of acute experimental toxoplasmosis of the blue fox *(Alopex lagopus). Vet Pathol.* 1990;27(6):381–390.
2. Centers for Disease Control and Prevention. Toxoplasmosis: Laboratory Diagnosis. https://www.cdc.gov/dpdx/toxoplasmosis/index.html. Accessed November 19, 2020.
3. Dunn D, Wallon M, Peyron F, et al. Mother-to-child transmission of toxoplasmosis: risk estimates for clinical counselling. *Lancet.* 1999;353(9167):1829–1833.
4. Hedman K, Lappalainen M, Seppala I, Makela O. Recent primary *Toxoplasma* infection indicated by a low avidity of specific IgG. *J Infect Dis.* 1989;159:736–739.
5. Jones JL, Kruszon-Moran D, Elder S, et al. *Toxoplasma gondii* infection in the United States, 2011–2014. *Am J Trop Med Hyg.* 2018;98(2):551–557.
6. Lappalainen M, Koskela P, Koskiniemi M, et al. Toxoplasmosis acquired during pregnancy: improved serodiagnosis based on avidity of IgG. *J Infect Dis.* 1993;167(3):691–697.
7. Lappalainen M, Koskiniemi M, Hiilesmaa V, et al. Outcome of children after maternal primary *Toxoplasma* infection during pregnancy with emphasis on avidity of specific IgG. *Pediatr Infect Dis J.* 1995;14:354–356.

8. Liesenfeld O, Montoya JG, Kinney S, et al. Effect of testing for IgG avidity in the diagnosis of *Toxoplasma gondii* infection in pregnant women: experience in a US reference laboratory. *J Infect Dis.* 2001;183(8):1248–1253.
9. Lin MH, Chen TC, Kuo TT, et al. Real-time PCR for quantitative detection of *Toxoplasma gondii. J Clin Microbiol.* 2000;38(11):4121–4125.
10. Luft BJ, Remington JS. Toxoplasmic encephalitis in AIDS. *Clin Infect Dis.* 1992;15(2):211–222.
11. Pelloux H, Brun E, Vernet G, et al. Determination of anti-*Toxoplasma gondii* immunoglobulin G avidity: adaptation to the Vidas system (bioMe´rieux). *Diagn Microbiol Infect Dis.* 1998;32:69–73.
12. Remington JS, McLeod R, Thulliez P, Desmonts G. Toxoplasmosis. In: Remington JS, Klein JO, eds. *Infectious Diseases of the Fetus and Newborn Infant.* 5th ed. Philadelphia: Saunders; 2001:205–346.
13. Ruskin J, Remington JS. Toxoplasmosis in the compromised host. *Ann Intern Med.* 1976;84(2):193–199.
14. Wong SY, Remington JS. Biology of *Toxoplasma gondii. AIDS.* 1993;7(3):299–316.

Fungal Infections—General

1. Baddley JW, Stroud TP, Salzman D, Pappas PG. Invasive mold infections in allogeneic bone marrow transplant recipients. *Clin Infect Dis.* 2001;32:1319–1324.
2. Beutler BA. TLRs and innate immunity. *Blood.* 2009;113: 1399–1407.
3. Brooks GF. *Jawetz, Melnick & Adelberg's Medical Mycology.* 24th ed. London: McGraw-Hill Medical; 2007.
4. Casadevall A, Feldmesser M, Pirofski L. Induced humoral immunity and vaccination against major human fungal pathogens. *Curr Opin Microbiol.* 2002;5:386–391.
5. De Pauw B, Walsh TJ, Donnelly JP, et al. Revised definitions of invasive fungal disease from the European Organization for Research and Treatment of Cancer/Invasive Fungal Infections Cooperative Group and the National Institute of Allergy and Infectious Diseases Mycoses Study Group (EORTC/MSG) Consensus Group. *Clin Infect Dis.* 2008;46(12):1813–1821.
6. Ferwerda B, Ferwerda G, Plantinga TS, et al. Human dectin-1 deficiency and mucocutaneous fungal infections. *N Engl J Med.* 2009;361:1760–1767.
7. Hawksworth DL, Lücking R. 2017. Fungal diversity revisited: 2.2to3.8millionspecies.*MicrobiolSpectrum.*5(4):FUNK-0052-2016. doi:10.1128/microbiolspec.FUNK-0052-2016.
8. Janeway CA, Medzhitov R. Innate immune recognition. *Annu Rev Immunol.* 2002;20:197–216.
9. Karageorgopoulos DE, Evridiki, K. Vouloumanou K, et al. b-D-glucan assay for the diagnosis of invasive fungal infections: a meta-analysis. *Clin Infect Dis.* 2011;52(6):750–770.
10. Kirk PM, Cannon PF, Minter DW, Stalpers JA. *Dictionary of the Fungi.* 10th ed. Wallingford, UK: CABI; 2008.
11. Levitz SM. Overview of host defenses in fungal infections. *Clin Infect Dis.* 1992;14:S37–S42.
12. Marr KA, Carter RA, Crippa F, et al. Epidemiology and outcome of mould infections in hematopoietic stem cell transplant recipients. *Clin Infect Dis.* 2002;34:909–917.
13. Martinon F, Mayor A, Tschopp J. The inflammasomes: guardians of the body. *Annu Rev Immunol.* 2009;27:229–265.
14. Medzhitov R. Recognition of microorganisms and activation of the immune response. *Nature.* 2007;449:819–826.
15. Medzhitov R. Toll-like receptors and innate immunity. *Nat Rev Immunol.* 2001;1(2):135–145.
16. Pfaller MA, Diekema DJ. Rare and emerging opportunistic fungal pathogens: concern for resistance beyond *Candida albicans* and *Aspergillus fumigatus. J Clin Microbiol.* 2004;42:4419–4431.
17. Polonelli L, Casadevall A, Han Y, et al. The efficacy of acquired humoral and cellular immunity in the prevention and therapy of experimental fungal infections. *Med Mycol.* 2000;38(suppl. 1): 281–292.
18. Rippon JW. *Medical Mycology: The Pathogenic Fungi and Pathogenic Actinomycetes.* 3rd ed. Philadelphia: WE Saunders; 1988.
19. Romani L. Cell mediated immunity to fungi: a reassessment. *Med Mycol.* 2008;46:515–529.
20. Romani L. Immunity to fungal infections. *Nat Rev Immunol.* 2004;4(1):1–23.
21. Shinobu S, Yoichiro I. Dectin-1 and dectin-2 in innate immunity against fungi. *Int Immunol.* 2011;23(8):467–472.
22. Stringer J, Beard C, Miller R, Wakefield A. A new name *(Pneumocystis jiroveci)* for pneumocystis from humans. *Emerging Infectious Diseases* [serial online]. 2002, September;8(9):891–896. Ipswich, MA: MEDLINE with Full Text. Accessed January 4, 2019.
23. Takeuchi O, Akira S. Pattern recognition receptors and inflammation. *Cell.* 2010;140(6):805–820.
24. Taylor PR, Tsoni SV, Willment JA, et al. Dectin-1 is required for b-glucan recognition and control of fungal infection. *Nat Immunol.* 2007;8:31–38.
25. Vautier S, Sousa Mda G, Brown GD. C-type lectins, fungi and Th17 responses. *Cytokine Growth Factor Rev.* 2010;21:405–412.
26. Wisplinghoff H, Bischoff T, Tallent SM, et al. Nosocomial bloodstream infections in US hospitals: analysis of 24,179 cases from a prospective nationwide surveillance study. *Clin Infect Dis.* 2004;39:309–317.
27. Zelante T, Iannitti R, De Luca A, Romani L. IL-22 in antifungal immunity. *Eur J Immunol.* 2011;41:270–275.
28. Zhang SX. Enhancing molecular approaches for diagnosis of fungal infections. *Future Microbiol.* 2013;8:1599–1611.

Aspergillus *Species*

1. Donnelly JP. Polymerase chain reaction for diagnosing invasive aspergillosis: getting closer but still a ways to go. *Clin Infect Dis.* 2006;42:487–489.
2. Greenberger PA. Allergic bronchopulmonary aspergillosis. *J Allergy Clin Immunol.* 2002;110(5):685–692.
3. Hebart H, Loffler J, Meisner C, et al. Early detection of *Aspergillus* infection after allogeneic stem cell transplantation by polymerase chain reaction screening. *J Infect Dis.* 2000;181:1713–1719.
4. Loeffler J, Hebart H, Cox P, et al. Nucleic acid sequence-based amplification of Aspergillus RNA in blood samples. *J Clin Microbiol.* 2001;39:1626–1629.
5. Mennink-Kersten MA, Donnelly JP, Verweij PE. Detection of circulating galactomannan for the diagnosis and management of invasive aspergillosis. *Lancet Infect Dis.* 2004;4:349–357.
6. Stevens DA, Moss RB, Kurup VP, et al. Allergic bronchopulmonary aspergillosis in cystic fibrosis—state of the art: Cystic Fibrosis Foundation Consensus Conference. *Clin Infect Dis.* 2003;37(suppl 3):S225–S264.
7. Summerbell R. Ascomycetes, aspergillus, fusarium, sporothrix, piedraia, and their relatives. In: Howard DH. *Pathogenic Fungi in Humans and Animals.* 2nd ed. New York: Marcel Dekker; 2003:237–498.
8. Wald A, Leisenring W, van Burik J-A, et al. Epidemiology of *Aspergillus* infections in a large cohort of patients undergoing bone marrow transplantation. *J Infect Dis.* 1997;175(6): 1459–1466.

9. White PL, Linton CJ, Perry MD, et al. The evolution and evaluation of a whole blood polymerase chain reaction assay for the detection of invasive aspergillosis in hematology patients in a routine clinical setting. *Clin Infect Dis.* 2006;42:479–486.
10. Young RC, Bennett JE. Invasive aspergillosis. Absence of detectable antibody response. *Am Rev Resp Dis.* 1971;104:710–716.
11. Zmeili OS, Soubani AO. Pulmonary aspergillosis: a clinical update. *QJM.* 2007;100(6):317–334.

Candida *Species*

1. Avni T, Leibovici L, Mical PM. PCR diagnosis of invasive candidiasis: systematic review and metanalysis. *J Clin Microbiol.* 2011;49(2):665.
2. Costa C, Costa JM, Desterke C, et al. Real-time PCR coupled with automated DNA extraction and detection of galactomannan antigen in serum by enzyme-linked immunosorbent assay for diagnosis of invasive aspergillosis. *J Clin Microbiol.* 2002;40:2224–2227.
3. Cuenca-Estrella M, Verweij PE, Arendrup MC. ESCMID guideline for the diagnosis and management of *Candida* diseases 2012: diagnostic procedures. *Clin Microbiol Infect.* 2012;18 (suppl 7):9–18.
4. Gudlaugsson O, Gillespie S, Lee K, et al. Attributable mortality of nosocomial candidemia, revisited. *Clin Infect Dis.* 2003;37: 1172–1177.
5. Mikulska M, Calandra T, Sanguinetti M, Poulain D, Viscoli C. The Third European Conference on Infections in Leukemia Group. The use of mannan antigen and anti-mannan antibodies in the diagnosis of invasive candidiasis: recommendations from the Third European Conference on Infections in Leukemia. *Crit Care.* 2010;14:R222.
6. Pappas PG. Invasive candidiasis. *Infect Dis Clin N Am.* 2006;20: 485–506.
7. Reddy GR, Georgy SA, Pillai MG, Sudevan R. Antifungal susceptibility in blood stream infections with *Candida:* an experience from a tertiary care hospital in Kerala, India. *Res Rev: J Pharm Toxicol Stud.* 2018;6(1):43-46.
8. Saijo S, Fujikado N, Furuta T, et al. Dectin-1 is required for host defense against *Pneumocystis carinii* but not against *Candida albicans. Nat Immunol.* 2007:8:39–46.
9. Trick WE, Fridkin SK, Edwards JR, et al. Secular trend of hospital-acquired candidemia among intensive care unit patients in the United States during 1989–1999. *Clin Infect Dis.* 2002;35:627–630.
10. Zilberberg MD, Shorr AF, Kollef MH. Secular trends in Candidemia-related hospitalization in the United States, 2000–2005. *Infect Control Hosp Epidemiol.* 2008;29(10):978–980.

Cryptococcus neoformans

1. Bennett, JE, Bailey JW. Control for rheumatoid factor in the latex test for cryptococcosis. *Am J Clin Pathol.* 1971;56:360–365.
2. Binnicker MJ, Jespersen DJ, Bestrom JE, Rollins LO. Comparison of four assays for the detection of cryptococcal antigen. *Clin Vaccine Immunol.* 2012;19(12):1988–1990.
3. Boulware DR, Rolfes MA, Rajasingham R, et al. Multisite validation of cryptococcal antigen lateral flow assay and quantification by laser thermal contrast. *Emerg Infect Dis.* 2014;20(1):45–53.
4. Casadevall A, Perfect JR. *Cryptococcus neoformans.* Washington, DC: ASM Press; 1988.
5. Dolan CT. Specificity of the latex-cryptococcal antigen test. *Am J Clin Pathol.* 1972;58:358–364.
6. Emmons CW. Isolation of *Cryptococcus neoformans* from soil. *J Bacteriol.* 1951;62(6):685–690.
7. Emmons CW. Saprophytic sources of *Cryptococcus neoformans* associated with the pigeon. *Am J Hyg.* 1955;62(3):227–232.
8. Eng RHK, Person A. Serum cryptococcal antigen determination in the presence of rheumatoid factor. *J Clin Microbiol.* 1981;14:700–702.
9. Gordon MA, Lapa EW. Elimination of rheumatoid factor in the latex test for cryptococcosis. *Am J Clin Pathol.* 1974;61:488–494.
10. Hay RJ, Mackenzie DWR. False positive latex test for cryptococcal antigen in cerebrospinal fluid. *J Clin Pathol.* 1982;35:244–245.
11. Henson DJ, Hill AR. Cryptococcal pneumonia: a fulminate presentation. *Am J Med.* 1984;288(5):221–222.
12. Huffnagle GB. Role of cytokines in T cell immunity to a pulmonary *Cryptococcus neoformans* infection. *Biol Signals.* 1996;5:215–222.
13. Kauffman CA, Bergman AG, Severance PJ, et al. Detection of cryptococcal antigen. Comparison of two latex agglutination tests. *Am J Clin Pathol.* 1981;75(1):106–109.
14. Levitz SM. The ecology of *Cryptococcus neoformans* and the epidemiology of cryptococcosis. *Rev Infect Dis.* 1991;13:1163–1169.
15. McNeil JI, Kan VL. Decline in the incidence of cryptococcosis among HIV-related patients. *J Acquir Immune Defic Syndr Hum Retrovirol.* 1995;9(2):206–208.
16. Murphy JW. Cryptococcal immunity and immunostimulation. *Adv Exp Med Biol.* 1992;319:225–230.
17. Perfect JR. Cryptococcosis. *Infect Dis Clin N Am.* 1989;3(1):77–102.
18. Snow RM, Dismukes WE. Cryptococcal meningitis: diagnostic value of cryptococcal antigen in cerebrospinal fluid. *Arch Intern Med.* 1975;135(9):1155–1157.
19. van Elden LJ, Walenkamp AM, Lipovsky MM. Declining number of patients with cryptococcosis in the Netherlands in the era of highly active antiretroviral therapy. *AIDS.* 2000;14(7): 2787–2788.

Histoplasma capsulatum

1. Allendoerfer R, Deepe GS, Jr. Intrapulmonary response to *Histoplasma capsulatum* in alpha interferon knockout mice. *Infect Immun.* 1997;65:2564–2569.
2. DiSalvo AF, Ajello L, Palmer JW, et al. Isolation of *Histoplasma capsulatum* from Arizona bats. *Am J Epidemiol.* 1969;89(5): 606–614.
3. Kauffman CA. Histoplasmosis: a clinical and laboratory update. *Clin Micro Rev.* 2007;20(1):115–132.
4. Wheat, LJ. Laboratory diagnosis of histoplasmosis: update. *Semin Respir Infect.* 2000;16:131–140.
5. Wheat LJ, Kauffman CA. Histoplasmosis. *Infect Dis Clin N Am.* 2003;17:1–19.
6. Wheat LJ, Kohler RB, Tewari RP. Diagnosis of disseminated histoplasmosis by detection of *Histoplasma capsulatum* antigen in serum and urine specimens. *N Engl J Med.* 1986;314(2):83–88.
7. Williams BM, Fojtasek P, Connolly-Stringfield P, Wheat JL. Diagnosis of histoplasmosis by antigen detection during an outbreak in Indianapolis, Ind. *Arch Pathol Lab Med.* 1994;118:1205–1208.
8. Zhou P, Sieve MC, Bennett J, et al. IL-12 prevents mortality in mice infected with *Histoplasma capsulatum* through induction of IFN-alpha. *J Immunol.* 1995;155:785–795.

Coccidiodes immitis

1. Blair JE, Currier JT. Significance of isolated positive IgM serologic results by enzyme immunoassay for coccidioidomycosis. *Mycopathologia.* 2008;166(2):77–82.
2. Galgiani JN. Coccidioidomycosis: a regional disease of national importance: rethinking approaches for control. *Ann Intern Med.* 1999;130:293–300.
3. Gifford MA. San Joaquin fever. In: *Annual Report Kern County Health Department for Fiscal Year July 1, 1935 to June 30, 1936*, pp. 22–23.

4. Shubitz L, Peng T, Perrill R, et al. Protection of mice against *Coccidioides immitis* intranasal infection by vaccination with recombinant antigen 2/PRA. *Infect Immun.* 2002;70:3287–3289.
5. Smith CE, Beard RR, Whiting EG, et al. Varieties of coccidioidal infection in relation to the epidemiology and control of the disease. *Am J Public Health.* 1946;36(12):1394–1402.
6. Smith CE, Whiting EG, Baker EE, et al. The use of coccidioidin. *Am Rev Tuberc Pulm Dis.* 1948;57(4):330–360.
7. Sunenshine RH, Anderson S, Erhart L, et al. Public health surveillance for coccidioidomycosis in Arizona. *Ann NY Acad Sci.* 2007;1111:96–102.
8. Valdivia L, Nix D, Wright M, et al. Coccidioidomycosis as a common cause of community-acquired pneumonia. *Emerg Infect Dis.* 2006;12(6):958–962.
9. Wieden MA, Lundergan LL, Blum J, et al. Detection of coccidioidal antibodies by 33-kDa spherule antigen, *Coccidioides* EIA, and standard serologic tests in sera from patients evaluated for coccidioidomycosis. *J Infect Dis.* 1996;173(5):1273–1277.

23. Serological and Molecular Detection of Viral Infections

Viruses: Immune Defenses and Escape Mechanisms

1. Abbas AK, Lichtman AH, Pillai S. Immunity to microbes. In: *Cellular and Molecular Immunology.* 9th ed. Philadelphia: Elsevier Saunders; 2018:351–372.
2. Mak TW, Saunders ME. *The Immune Response: Basic and Clinical Principles.* Burlington, MA: Elsevier Academic Press; 2006:664–680.
3. McNabb, KM. Clinical virology. In: Mahon CR, Lehman DC, Manuselis G, eds. *Textbook of Diagnostic Microbiology.* 5th ed. Maryland Heights, MO: Elsevier Saunders; 2015:688–726.
4. Punt J, Stranford SA, Jones PP, Owen JA, *Kuby Immunology.* 8th ed. New York: WH Freeman and Co.; 2019:644–651.
5. Williams MA, Bevan MJ. Effector and memory CTL differentiation. *Annu Rev Immunol.* 2007;25:171–192.

Hepatitis—General

1. Dienstag JL. Acute viral hepatitis. In: Jameson J, Fauci AS, Kasper DL, Hauser SL, Longo DL, Loscalzo J, eds. *Harrison's Principles of Internal Medicine.* 20th ed. New York: McGraw-Hill; 2018. http://accessmedicine.mhmedical.com/content.aspx?bookid=2129§ionid=159214492. Accessed July 17, 2019.
2. Niesters HG, Riezebos-Brilman A, Van Leer-Buter CC. Viral hepatitis. In: Detrick B, Schmitz JL, Hamilton RG, eds. *Manual of Molecular and Clinical Laboratory Immunology.* 8th ed. Washington, DC: ASM Press; 2016:620–638.

Hepatitis A and Hepatitis E

1. Anderson DA, Counihan NA. Hepatitis A and E viruses. In: Jorgensen JH, Pfaller MA, Carroll KC, Veralovic J, Carroll KC, Funke G, et al, eds. *Manual of Clinical Microbiology.* Vol. 2. 11th ed. Washington, DC: ASM Press; 2015:1584–1598.
2. Centers for Disease Control and Prevention. Hepatitis A questions and answers for health professionals. https://www.cdc.gov/hepatitis/hav/havfaq.htm#vaccine. Updated November 9, 2018. Accessed January 15, 2019.
3. Centers for Disease Control and Prevention. Hepatitis E questions and answers for health professionals: overview and statistics. https://www.cdc.gov/hepatitis/hev/hevfaq.htm#section2. Updated May 9, 2018. Accessed January 15, 2019.
4. Dalton HR, Hunter JG, Bendall RP. Hepatitis E. *Curr Opin Infect Dis.* 2013;26(5):471–478.
5. Fiore AE, Wasley A, Bell BP. Prevention of hepatitis A through active or passive immunization. *MMWR.* 2006;55(RR07):1–23.
6. Fujiwara S, Yokokawa Y, Morino K, et al. Chronic hepatitis E: a review of the literature. *J Viral Hepat.* 2014;21(2):78–89.
7. Heo NY, Lim YS, An J, et al. Multiplex polymerase chain reaction test for the diagnosis of acute viral hepatitis A. *Clin Mol Hepatol.* 2012;18(4):397–403.
8. Jeong SH, Lee HS. Hepatitis A: clinical manifestations and management. *Intervirology.* 2010;53(1):15–19.
9. Kamar N, Dalton HR, Abravanel F, Izopet J. Hepatitis E virus infection. *Clin Microbiol Rev.* 2014;27(1):116–138.
10. Matheny SC, Kingery JE. Hepatitis A. *Am Fam Physician.* 2012;86(11):1027–1034.
11. Nainan OV, Xia G, Vaughan G, Margolis HS. Diagnosis of hepatitis A virus infection: a molecular approach. *Clin Microbiol Rev.* 2006;19(1):63–79.
12. Perez-Gracia MT, Mateos Lindemann ML, Caridad Montalvo Villalba M. Hepatitis E: current status. *Rev Med Virol.* 2013;23(6): 384–398.
13. Qiu F, Cao J, Su Q, Bi S. Multiplex hydrolysis probe real-time PCR for simultaneous detection of hepatitis A virus and hepatitis E virus. *Int J Mol Sci.* 2014;15:9780–9788.
14. World Health Organization. Hepatitis A. https://www.who.int/immunization/diseases/hepatitisA/en/. Updated October 19, 2015. Accessed January 15, 2019.
15. World Health Organization. Hepatitis E. https://www.who.int/en/news-room/fact-sheets/detail/hepatitis-e. Updated September 19, 2018. Accessed January 15, 2019.
16. World Health Organization. Hepatitis E fact sheet. https://www.who.int/news-room/fact-sheets/detail/hepatitis-e. Accessed August 21, 2020.
17. Zhu FC, Zhang J, Zhang XF, et al. Efficacy and safety of a recombinant hepatitis E vaccine in healthy adults: a large-scale, randomised, double-blind placebo-controlled, phase 3 trial. *Lancet.* 2010;376(9744):895–902.

Hepatitis B and Hepatitis D

1. Alvarado-Mora MV, Locarnini S, Rizzetto M, Pinho JR. An update on HDV: virology, pathogenesis and treatment. *Antivir Ther (Lond).* 2013;18(3 Pt B):541–548.
2. Centers for Disease Control and Prevention. Viral hepatitis statistics and surveillance. https://www.cdc.gov/hepatitis/statistics/index.htm . Accessed August 21, 2020.
3. Dienstag JL. Hepatitis B virus infection. *N Eng J Med.* 2008;359(14):1486–1500.
4. Farci P. Delta hepatitis: an update. *J Hepatol.* 2003;39(suppl 1): S212–S219.
5. Ganem D, Prince AM. Hepatitis B virus infection—natural history and clinical consequences. *N Eng J Med.* 2004;350(11): 1118–1129.
6. Horvat RT, Tegtmeier GE Taylor R. Hepatitis B and D viruses. In: Veralovic J, Carroll KC, Funke G, Jorgensen JH, Pfaller MA, Carroll KC, et al, eds. *Manual of Clinical Microbiology.* Vol. 2. 11th ed. Washington, DC: ASM Press; 2015: 1841–1858.
7. Hughes SA, Wedemeyer H, Harrison PM. Hepatitis delta virus. *Lancet.* 2011;378(9785):73–85.
8. Kao J. Diagnosis of hepatitis B virus infection through serological and virological markers. *Exp Rev Gas Hep.* 2008;2(4): 553–562.
9. Le Gal F, Gordien E, Affolabi D, et al. Quantification of hepatitis delta virus RNA in serum by consensus real-time PCR indicates different patterns of virological response to interferon therapy in chronically infected patients. *J Clin Microbiol.* 2005;43(5):2363–2369.

10. Mast EE, Margolis HS, Fiore AE, et al. A comprehensive immunization strategy to eliminate transmission of hepatitis B virus infection in the United States. *MMWR.* 2005;54(RR16):1–23.
11. Nebbia G, Peppa D, Maini MK. Hepatitis B infection: current concepts and future challenges. *Q J Med.* 2012;105:109–113.
12. Noureddin M, Gish R. Hepatitis delta: epidemiology, diagnosis and management 36 years after discovery. *Curr Gastroenterol Rep.* 2014;16(1):365.
13. Servoss JC, Friedman LS. Serologic and molecular diagnosis of hepatitis B infection. *Infect Dis Clin N Am.* 2006;20:47–61.
14. Shepard CW, Simard EP, Finelli L, et al. Hepatitis B virus infection: epidemiology and vaccination. *Epidemiol Rev.* 2006;28:112–125.
15. Wilkins T, Zimmerman D, Schade RR. Hepatitis B: diagnosis and treatment. *Am Fam Physician.* 2010;81(8):965–972.
16. World Health Organization. Hepatitis B fact sheet. https://www.who.int/news-room/fact-sheets/detail/hepatitis-b. Accessed August 21, 2020.

Hepatitis C

1. Amjad M, Moudgal V, Faisal M. Laboratory methods for diagnosis and management of hepatitis C virus infection. *Lab Medicine.* 2013;44(4):292–299.
2. Centers for Disease Control and Prevention. Hepatitis C questions and answers for health professionals: overview and statistics. https://www.cdc.gov/hepatitis/hcv/hcvfaq.htm#section1. Updated July 2, 2019. Accessed July 18, 2019.
3. Centers for Disease Control and Prevention. 1999 USPHS/IDSA guidelines for the prevention of opportunistic infections in persons infected with the human immunodeficiency virus. *MMWR.* 1999;48(RR-10):1–59.
4. Centers for Disease Control and Prevention. Recommendations for prevention and control of hepatitis C virus (HCV) infection and HCV-related chronic disease. *MMWR.* 1998;47 (RR-19):1–40.
5. Centers for Disease Control and Prevention. Testing for HCV infection: an update of guidance for clinicians and laboratorians. *MMWR.* 2013;62(18):362–365.
6. Chan J. Hepatitis C. *Disease-A-Month.* 2014;60(5):201–212.
7. Cheney CP, Chopra S, Graham C. Hepatitis C. *Infect Dis Clin N Am.* 2000;14(3):633–665.
8. DeLemos AS, Chung RT. Hepatitis C treatment: an incipient therapeutic revolution. *Trends Mol Med.* 2014;20(6):315–321.
9. Duddempudi AT, Bernstein DE. Hepatitis B and C. *Clin Geriatr Med.* 2014;30(1):149–167.
10. Forman MS, Valsamakis A. Hepatitis C virus. In: Jorgensen JH, Pfaller MA, Carroll KC, et al, eds. *Manual of Clinical Microbiology.* Vol. 2. 11th ed. Washington, DC: ASM Press; 2015:1599–1616.
11. Ghany MG, Strader DB, Thomas DL, Seeff LB. American Association for the Study of Liver Diseases. Diagnosis, management, and treatment of hepatitis C: an update. *Hepatology.* 2009;49(4):1335–1374.
12. Gower E, Estes C, Blach S, et al. Global epidemiology and genotype distribution of the hepatitis C virus infection. *J Hepatol.* 2014;61(1 suppl):S45–S57.
13. Moyer VA. U.S. Preventive Services Task Force. Screening for hepatitis C virus infection in adults: U.S. preventive services task force recommendation statement. *Ann Intern Med.* 2013;159(5):349–357.
14. Parisi MR, Soldini L, Vidoni G, et al. Point-of-care testing for HCV infection: recent advances and implications for alternative screening. *New Microbiologica.* 2014;37(4):449–457.
15. Scheel TK, Rice CM. Understanding the hepatitis C virus life cycle paves the way for highly effective therapies. *Nat Med.* 2013;19(7):837–849.
16. Scott JD, Gretch DR. Molecular diagnostics of hepatitis C infection. *JAMA.* 2007;297:724–732.
17. Smith BD, Morgan RL, Beckett GA, et al. Recommendations for the identification of chronic hepatitis C virus infection among persons born during 1945–1965. *MMWR Rec Rep.* 2012;61(RR-4):1–32.
18. Vermeersch P, Van Ranst M, Lagrou K. Validation of a strategy for HCV antibody testing with two enzyme immunoassays in a routine clinical laboratory. *J Clin Virol.* 2008;42(4):394–398.
19. Villar LM, Cruz HD, Barbosa JR, et al. Update on hepatitis B and C virus diagnosis. *World J of Virol.* 2015, Nov 12; 4(4):323–342.
20. World Health Organization. Hepatitis C. https://www.who.int/en/news-room/fact-sheets/detail/hepatitis-c. Updated July 18, 2018. Accessed January 16, 2019.

Epstein-Barr Virus

1. Balfour Jr HH, Hogquist KA, Verghese PS. Epstein-Barr virus and cytomegalovirus. In: Detrick B, Schmitz JL, Hamilton RG, eds. *Manual of Molecular and Clinical Laboratory Immunology.* 8th ed. Washington, DC: ASM Press; 2016:563–577.
2. Cohen JI. Epstein-Barr virus infections, including infectious mononucleosis. In: Jameson J, Fauci AS, Kasper DL, Hauser SL, Longo DL, Loscalzo J, eds. *Harrison's Principles of Internal Medicine.* 20th ed. New York: McGraw-Hill; 2018. http://accessmedicine.mhmedical.com/content.aspx?bookid=2129§ionid=192024765. Accessed July 17, 2019.
3. Dunmire SK, Verghese PS, Balfouur HH. Review: primary Epstein-Barr virus infection. *J Clin Virol.* 2018;102:84–92.
4. Ebell MH. Epstein-Barr virus infectious mononucleosis. *Am Fam Physician.* 2004;70(7):1279–1290.
5. Feng Z, Li Z, Sui B, Xu G, Xia T. Serologic diagnosis of infectious mononucleosis by chemiluminescent immunoassay using capsid antigen p18 of Epstein-Barr virus. *Clin Chim Acta.* 2005;354:77–82.
6. Gartner BC, Preiksaitis J. Epstein-Barr virus. In: Versalovic J, Carroll KC, Funke G, Jorgensen JH, Pfaller MA, Carroll KC, et al, eds. *Manual of Clinical Microbiology.* Vol. 2. 11th ed. Washington, DC: ASM Press; 2015:1738–1753.
7. Gottschalk S, Rooney CM, Heslop HE. Post-transplant lymphproliferative disorders. *Annu Rev Med.* 2005;56:29–44.
8. Jenson HB. Epstein-Barr virus. *Pediatr Rev.* 2011;32:375–383.
9. Junker AK. Epstein-Barr virus. *Pediatr Rev.* 2005;26(3):79–85.
10. Odumade OA, Hogquist KA, Balfour HH. Progress and problems in understanding and managing primary Epstein-Barr virus infections. *Clin Microbiol Rev.* 2011;24(1):193–209.
11. Robinson BJ, Pierson SL McNabb KM. Clinical virology. In: Mahon CR, Lehman DC, Manuselis G, eds. *Textbook of Diagnostic Microbiology.* 5th ed. Maryland Heights, MO: Elsevier Saunders; 2015:688–726.
12. Williams H, Crawford DH. Epstein-Barr virus: the impact of scientific advances on clinical practice. *Blood.* 2006;107(3):862–869.

Cytomegalovirus

1. Adler SP, Marshall B. Cytomegalovirus infections. *Pediatr Rev.* 2007;28(3):92–100.
2. Ariza-Heredia EJ, Nesher L, Chemaly RF. Cytomegalovirus diseases after hematopoietic stem cell transplantation: a mini-review. *Cancer Lett.* 2014;342(1):1–8.

3. Bale JF. Congenital cytomegalovirus infection. In: Tselis AC, Booss J, eds. *Handbook of Clinical Neurology.* Amsterdam, The Netherlands: Elsevier BV; 2014:319–326.
4. Centers for Disease Control and Prevention. Cytomegalovirus and congenital CMV infection: interpretation of laboratory tests. https://www.cdc.gov/cmv/clinical/lab-tests.html. Accessed July 17, 2019.
5. Fowler KB, Boppana SB. Congenital cytomegalovirus (CMV) infection and hearing deficit. *J Clin Virol.* 2006:35;226–231.
6. Fowler KB, Boppana SR. Congenital cytomegalovirus infection. *Sem Perinatol.* 2018(42);149–154.
7. Fu TM, An Z, Wang D. Progress on pursuit of human cytomegalovirus vaccines for prevention of congenital infection and disease. *Vaccine.* 2014;32(22):2525–2533.
8. Hodinka RL. Human cytomegalovirus. In: Jorgensen JH, Pfaller MA, Carroll KC, et al, eds. *Manual of Clinical Microbiology.* Vol. 2. 11th ed. Washington, DC: ASM Press; 2015:1718–1737.
9. Kotton C, Hirsch MS. Cytomegalovirus and human herpesvirus types 6, 7, and 8. In: Jameson J, Fauci AS, Kasper DL, Hauser SL, Longo DL, Loscalzo J, eds. *Harrison's Principles of Internal Medicine.* 20th ed. New York: McGraw-Hill; 2018. http://accessmedicine.mhmedical.com/content.aspx?bookid=2129§ionid=192024819. Accessed July 17, 2019.
10. Lancini D, Faddy HM, Flower R, Hogan C. Cytomegalovirus disease in immunocompetent adults. *Med J Aust.* 2014;201(10): 578–580.
11. Landry ML, Ferguson D. 2-hour cytomegalovirus pp65 antigenemia assay for rapid quantitation of cytomegalovirus in blood samples. *J Clin Microbiol.* 2000;38(1):427–428.
12. Lazzarotto T, Guerra B, Gabrielli L, et al. Update on the prevention, diagnosis and management of cytomegalovirus infection during pregnancy. *Clin Microbiol Infect.* 2011;17(9):1285–1293.
13. Mendelson E, Aboudy Y, Smetana Z, et al. Laboratory assessment and diagnosis of congenital viral infections: rubella, cytomegalovirus (CMV), varicella-zoster virus (VZV), herpes simplex virus (HSV), parvovirus B19 and human immunodeficiency virus (HIV). *Reprod Toxicol.* 2006;21:350–382.
14. Pillet S, Roblin X, Cornillon J, et al. Quantification of cytomegalovirus viral load. *Exp Rev Anti Infe.* 2014;12(2):193–210.
15. Ross SA, Boppana SB. Congenital cytomegalovirus infection: outcome and diagnosis. *Semin Pediatr Infect Dis.* 2005;16(1):44–49.
16. Walker SP, Palma-Dias R, Wood EM, et al. Cytomegalovirus in pregnancy: to screen or not to screen. *BMC Pregnancy and Childbirth.* 2013;13:96–103.
17. Wang D, Fu TM. Progress on human cytomegalovirus vaccines for prevention of congenital infection and disease. *Curr Opin Virol.* 2014;6:13–23.

Varicella Zoster Virus

1. Bader MS. Herpes zoster: diagnostic, therapeutic, and preventive approaches. *Postgrad Med.* 2013;125(5):78–91.
2. Breuer J, Harper DR, Kangro HO. Varicella zoster. In: Zuckerman AJ, Banatvala JE, Pattison JR, eds. *Principles and Practice of Clinical Virology.* 4th ed. Chichester, England: John Wiley & Sons; 2000:47–77.
3. Centers for Disease Control and Prevention. Shingles (herpes zoster) vaccination. https://www.cdc.gov/shingles/vaccination.html. Updated October 25, 2019. Accessed January 29, 2019.
4. Gershon AA, Gershon MD. Pathogenesis and current approaches to control of varicella-zoster virus infections. *Clin Microbiol Rev.* 2013;26(4):728–743.
5. Kimberlin DW, Whitley RJ. Varicella-zoster vaccine for the prevention of herpes zoster. *N Engl J Med.* 2007;356:1338–1343.
6. Marin M, Gurtis D, Chaves SS, et al. Prevention of varicella: recommendations of the advisory committee on immunization practices (ACIP). *MMWR.* 2007;56(RR-4):1–40.
7. McCrary ML, Severson J, Trying SK. Varicella zoster virus. *J Am Acad Dermatol.* 1999;41:1–14.
8. Oxman MN, Levin MJ, Johnson GR, et al. A vaccine to prevent herpes zoster and postherpetic neuralgia in older adults. *N Engl J Med.* 2000;343:222.
9. Puchhammer-Stockl E, Aberle S. Varicella-zoster virus. In: Jorgensen JH, Pfaller MA, Carroll KC, et al, eds. *Manual of Clinical Microbiology.* Vol. 2. 11th ed. Washington, DC: ASM Press; 2015:1704–1717.
10. Sauerbrei A, Wutzler P. Serological detection of varicella-zoster virus-specific immunoglobulin G by an enzyme-linked immunosorbent assay using glycoprotein antigen. *J Clin Microbiol.* 2006;44(9):3094–3097.
11. Schmid DS, Loparev V. Varicella virus. In: Detrick B, Schmitz JL, Hamilton RG, eds. *Manual of Molecular and Clinical Laboratory Immunology.* 8th ed. Washington, DC: ASM Press; 2016:556–562.
12. Stover BH, Bratcher DF. Varicella-zoster virus: infection, control, and prevention. *Am J Infect Control.* 1998;26(3):369–381.
13. Whitley RJ. Varicella-zoster virus infections. In: Jameson J, Fauci AS, Kasper DL, Hauser SL, Longo DL, Loscalzo J, eds. *Harrison's Principles of Internal Medicine.* 20th ed. New York: McGraw-Hill; 2018. http://accessmedicine.mhmedical.com/content.aspx?bookid=2129§ionid=192024718. Accessed July 17, 2019.
14. Zhou F, Harpaz R, Jumaan AO, et al. Impact of varicella vaccination on health care utilization. *JAMA.* 2005;294(7): 797–802.

Rubella, Rubeola, and Mumps Viruses

1. Bellini WJ, Icenogle JP. Measles and rubella viruses. In: Jorgensen JH, Pfaller MA, Carroll KC, et al, eds. *Manual of Clinical Microbiology.* Vol. 2. 11th ed. Washington, DC: ASM Press; 2015:1519–1535.
2. Bellini WJ, Rota JS, Lowe LE, et al. Subacute sclerosing panencephalitis: more cases of this fatal disease are prevented by measles immunization than was previously recognized. *J Infec Dis.* 2005;192:1686–1693.
3. Binnicker MJ, Jespersen DJ, Rollins LO. Evaluation of the Bio-Rad bioplex measles, mumps, rubella, and varicella-zoster virus IgG multiplex bead immunoassay. *Clin Vaccine Immunol.* 2011:1524–1526.
4. Centers for Disease Control and Prevention. Epidemiology of vaccine-preventable diseases. *The Pinkbook Website.* http://www.cdc.gov/vaccines/pubs/pinkbook/index.html. Published May 2012. Updated June 29, 2018. Accessed July 17, 2019.
5. Centers for Disease Control and Prevention. Measles (rubeola). Clinical features. https://www.cdc.gov/measles/hcp/index.html. Updated February 5, 2018. Accessed July 18, 2019.
6. Centers for Disease Control and Prevention. Measles (rubeola). Measles cases and outbreaks. https://www.cdc.gov/measles/cases-outbreaks.html. Updated January 10, 2019. Accessed January 29, 2019.
7. Centers for Disease Control and Prevention. Mumps cases and outbreaks. https://www.cdc.gov/mumps/outbreaks.html. Updated January 10, 2019. Accessed January 29, 2019.

8. Centers for Disease Control and Prevention. Mumps: questions and answers about lab testing. http://www.cdc.gov/mumps/lab/qa-lab-test-infect.html#realtime-pcr. Updated 2017. Accessed July 17, 2019.
9. Centers for Disease Control and Prevention. Pregnancy and rubella. https://www.cdc.gov/rubella/pregnancy.html Updated September 15, 2017. Accessed July 18, 2019.
10. Centers for Disease Control and Prevention. Rubella (German measles, three day measles) overview. https://www.cdc.gov/rubella/about/symptoms.html. Updated September 15, 2017. Accessed July 18, 2019.
11. Centers for Disease Control and Prevention. Serology: IgG avidity detection. https://www.cdc.gov/rubella/lab/serology.html. Updated September 28, 2017. Accessed July 18, 2019.
12. DeSantis M, Cavaliere AF, Straface G, et al. Rubella infection in pregnancy. *Reprod Toxicol.* 2006;21:390–398.
13. DiPaola F, Michael A, Mandel ED. A casualty of the immunization wars: the reemergence of measles. *JAAPA.* 2012;25(6):50–54.
14. Hamkar R, Javilvand S, Mokhtari-Azad T, et al. Assessment of IgM enzyme immunoassay and IgG avidity assay for distinguishing between primary and secondary immune response to rubella vaccine. *J Virol Meth.* 2005;130:59–65.
15. Hodinka RL, Moshal KL. Childhood infections. In: Storch GA, ed. *Essentials of Diagnostic Virology.* New York: Churchill Livingstone; 2000:167–186.
16. Hummel KB, Lowe L, Bellini WJ, Rota PA. Development of quantitative gene-specific real-time RT-PCR assays for detection of measles virus in clinical specimens. *J Virol Meth.* 2006;132:166–173.
17. Leland DS. Parainfluenza and mumps viruses. In: Jorgensen JH, Pfaller MA, Carroll KC, et al, eds. *Manual of Clinical Microbiology.* Vol. 2. 11th ed. Washington, DC: ASM Press; 2015:1487–1497.
18. Leland DS, Relich RF. Measles, mumps, and rubella viruses. In: Detrick B, Schmitz JL, Hamilton RG, eds. *Manual of Molecular and Clinical Laboratory Immunology.* 8th ed. Washington, DC: ASM Press; 2016:610–619.
19. Mace M, Cointe D, Six C, et al. Diagnostic value of reverse transcription-PCR of amniotic fluid for prenatal diagnosis of congenital rubella infection in pregnant women with confirmed primary rubella infection. *J Clin Microbiol.* 2004;42(10):4818–4820.
20. McLean HQ, Fiebelkorn AP, Tempte JL, Wallace GS. Prevention of measles, rubella, congenital rubella syndrome, and mumps, 2013. Summary recommendations of the Advisory Committee on Immunization Practices (ACIP). *MMWR.* 2013;62(4):1–34.
21. Michel Y, Saloum K, Tournier C, et al. Rapid molecular diagnosis of measles virus infection in an epidemic setting. *J Med Virol.* 2013;85:723–730.
22. Mubareka S, Richards H, Gray M, Tipples GA. Evaluation of commercial rubella immunoglobulin G avidity assays. *J Clin Microbiol.* 2007;45(1):231–233.
23. Portella G, Galli C. Multicentric evaluation of two chemiluminescent immunoassays for IgG and IgM antibodies towards rubella virus. *J Clin Virol.* 2010;49:105–110.
24. Public Health Agency of Canada. Archived guidelines for the prevention and control of mumps outbreaks in Canada. Appendix 4. Laboratory guidelines for the diagnosis of mumps. http://www.phac-aspc.gc.ca/publicat/ccdr-rmtc/10vol36/36s1/appendix-annexe-4-eng.php. Updated June 17, 2009. Accessed April 29, 2015.
25. Rainwater-Lovett K, Moss WJ. Measles (Rubeola). In: Jameson J, Fauci AS, Kasper DL, Hauser SL, Longo DL, Loscalzo J, eds. *Harrison's Principles of Internal Medicine.* 20th ed. New York: McGraw-Hill; 2018. http://accessmedicine.mhmedical.com/content.aspx?bookid=2129§ionid=192025856. Accessed July 17, 2019.
26. Rubin SA. Mumps. In: Jameson J, Fauci AS, Kasper DL, Hauser SL, Longo DL, Loscalzo J, eds. *Harrison's Principles of Internal Medicine.* 20th ed. New York: McGraw-Hill; 2018. http://accessmedicine.mhmedical.com/content.aspx?bookid=2129§ionid=192025962. Accessed July 17, 2019.
27. Shanley JD. The resurgence of mumps in young adults and adolescents. *Cleveland Clinic J Med.* 2007;74(1):42–48.
28. Tipples G, Hiebert J. Detection of measles, mumps, and rubella viruses. In: Stephenson JR, Warnes A, eds. *Methods in Molecular Biology. Diagnostic Virology Protocols.* Vol. 665. New York, Springer Science and Business Media; 2011:183–193.
29. Zimmerman LA, Reef SE. Rubella (German measles). In: Jameson J, Fauci AS, Kasper DL, Hauser SL, Longo DL, Loscalzo J, eds. *Harrison's Principles of Internal Medicine.* 20th ed. New York: McGraw-Hill; 2018. http://accessmedicine.mhmedical.com/content.aspx?bookid=2129§ionid=192025918. Accessed July 17, 2019.

Human T-Cell Lymphotropic Viruses

1. Abrams A, Akahata Y, Jacobson S. The prevalence and significance of HTLV-I/II seroindeterminate Western blot patterns. *Viruses.* 2011;3(8):1320–1331.
2. Araujo A, Hall WW. Human T-lymphotropic virus type II and neurological disease. *Ann Neurol.* 2004;56(1):10–19.
3. Biswas HH, Kaidarova Z, Garrity G, et al. HTLV outcomes study: increased all-cause and cancer mortality in HTLV-II infection. *J Acquir Immune Defic Syndr.* 2010;54:290–296.
4. Chang YB, Kaidarova Z, Hindes D, et al. Seroprevalence and demographic determinants of human T-lymphotropic virus type 1 and 2 infections among first-time blood donors—United States, 2000–2009. *J Infect Dis.* 2014;209(4):523–531.
5. Ishitsuka K, Tamura K. Human T-cell leukaemia virus type I and adult T-cell leukaemia-lymphoma. *Lancet Oncol.* 2014;15(11):e517–e526.
6. Longo DL, Fauci AS. The human retroviruses. In: Jameson J, Fauci AS, Kasper DL, Hauser SL, Longo DL, Loscalzo J, eds. *Harrison's Principles of Internal Medicine.* 20th ed. New York: McGraw-Hill; 2018. http://accessmedicine.mhmedical.com/content.aspx?bookid=2129§ionid=192025194. Accessed July 17, 2019.
7. Martin-Davila P, Fortun J, Lopez-Velez R, et al. Transmission of tropical and geographically restricted infections during solid-organ transplantation. *Clin Microbiol Rev.* 2008;21(1):60–96.
8. Qayyum S, Choi JK. Adult T-cell leukemia/lymphoma. *Arch Pathol Lab Med.* 2014;138(2):282–286.
9. Satou Y, Matsuoka M. Virological and immunological mechanisms in the pathogenesis of human T-cell leukemia virus type 1. *Rev Med Virol.* 2013;23(5):269–280.
10. Switzer WM, Heneine W, Owen SM. Human T-cell lymphotropic viruses. In: Jorgensen JH, Pfaller MA, Carroll KC, et al, eds. *Manual of Clinical Microbiology.* Vol. 2. 11th ed. Washington, DC: ASM Press; 2015:1458–1469.
11. Verdonck K, Gonzalez E, Van Dooren S, et al. Human T-lymphotropic virus 1: recent knowledge about an ancient infection. *Lancet Infect Dis.* 2007;7(4):266–281.
12. Waters A, Oliveira AL, Coughlan S, et al. Multiplex real-time PCR for the detection and quantitation of HTLV-1 and HTLV-2 proviral load: addressing the issue of indeterminate HTLV results. *J Clin Virol.* 2011;52(1):38–44.

24. Laboratory Diagnosis of HIV Infection

General

1. Abbas AK, Lichtman AH, Pillai S. Congenital and acquired immunodeficiencies. In: *Cellular and Molecular Immunology.* 9th ed. Philadelphia: Elsevier; 2018:459–487.
2. Centers for Disease Control and Prevention. HIV basic statistics. https://www.cdc.gov/hiv/basics/statistics.html. Accessed October 26, 2019.
3. Centers for Disease Control and Prevention. HIV in the United States and dependent areas. Website. https://www.cdc.gov/hiv/statistics/overview/ataglance.html?CDC_AA_refVal=https%3A%2F%2Fwww.cdc.gov%2Fhiv%2Fstatistics%2Fbasics%2Fataglance.html. Updated October 30, 2019. Accessed November 21, 2019.
4. Collier L, Oxford J. *Human Virology.* 3rd ed. New York: Oxford University Press; 2006:179–188.
5. Fauci AS, Folkers GK, Lane H. Human immunodeficiency virus disease: AIDS and related disorders. In: Jameson J, Fauci AS, Kasper DL, Hauser SL, Longo DL, Loscalzo J, eds. *Harrison's Principles of Internal Medicine.* 20th ed. New York: McGraw-Hill; 2018. http://accessmedicine.mhmedical.com/content.aspx?bookid=2129§ionid=192025263. Accessed October 27, 2019.
6. Johnston MI, Fauci AS. An HIV vaccine—evolving concepts. *N Engl J Med.* 2007;356(20):2073–2081.
7. Kandathil AJ, Ramalingam S, Kannangai R, David S, Sridharan G. Molecular epidemiology of HIV. *Indian J Med Res.* 2005;121:333–344.
8. Karim SS, Karim QA, Gouws E, Baxter C. Global epidemiology of HIV-AIDS. *Infect Dis Clin N Am.* 2007;21:1–17.
9. Kwon DS, Walker BD. Ch. 42. Immunology of human immunodeficiency virus infection. In: Paul WE, ed. *Fundamental Immunology.* 7th ed. Philadelphia: Wolters Kluwer Health/Lippincott Williams & Wilkins; 2013:1016–1031.
10. Maartens G, Celum C, Lewin SR. HIV infection: epidemiology, pathogenesis, treatment, and prevention. *Lancet.* 2014;384:258–271.
11. Punt J, Stranford SA, Jones PP, Owen JA. Chapter 18 Immunodeficiency disorders. In: *Kuby Immunology.* 8th ed. New York: WH Freeman and Co; 2013:681–717.
12. World Health Organization. HIV/AIDS fact sheet. Website. https://www.who.int/news-room/fact-sheets/detail/hiv-aids. Updated November 15, 2019. Accessed December 5, 2019.

HIV Characteristics

1. Barre-Sinoussi F, Chermann, JC, Rey F, et al. Isolation of a T-lymphotropic retrovirus from a patient at risk for acquired immunodeficiency syndrome (AIDS). *Science.* 1983;220:868–870.
2. Clavel F, Guétard D, Brun-Vézinet F, et al. Isolation of a new human retrovirus from West African patients. *Science.* 1986;223:343–346.
3. Coffin J, Swanstrom R. HIV pathogenesis: dynamics and genetics of viral populations and infected cells. *Cold Spring Harb Perspect Med.* 2013;3:1–16.
4. Gallo RC, Salahuddin SZ, Popovic M, et al. Human T-lymphotropic retrovirus, HTLV-III isolated from AIDS patients and donors at risk for AIDS. *Science.* 1984;224:500–503.
5. Levy JA, Hoffman AD, Kramer SM, Landis JA, Shimabukuro JM, Oshiro LS.. Isolation of lymphocytopathic retroviruses from San Francisco patients with AIDS. *Science.* 1984;225:840–842.
6. Liu R, Paxton WA, Choe S, et al. Homozygous defect in HIV-1 co-receptor accounts for resistance of some multiply-exposed individuals to HIV-1 infection. *Cell.* 86:367–377.
7. Samson M, Libert F, Doranz BJ, et al. Resistance to HIV-1 infection in Caucasian individuals bearing mutant alleles of the CCR-5 chemokine receptor gene. *Nature.* 1996;382:722–725.

Transmission and Precautions

1. Centers for Disease Control and Prevention. Achievements in public health: reduction in perinatal transmission of HIV infection—United States, 1985–2005. *MMWR.* 2006;55(21):592–597.
2. Centers for Disease Control and Prevention. HIV and occupational exposure. https://www.cdc.gov/hiv/workplace/healthcareworkers.html. Updated September 5, 2019. Accessed November 21, 2019.
3. Centers for Disease Control and Prevention. Public health service guidelines for the management of health-care worker exposures to HIV and recommendations for postexposure prophylaxis. *MMWR.* 1998;47:211–215.
4. Centers for Disease Control and Prevention. Recommendations for prevention of HIV transmission in health-care settings. *MMWR.* 1987;36 (suppl no. 2S):1S–17S.
5. Centers for Disease Control and Prevention. Updated U.S. Public Health Service guidelines for the management of occupational exposures to HBV, HCV, and HIV and recommendations for postexposure prophylaxis. *MMWR.* 2001;50(RR11):1–42.
6. Centers for Disease Control and Prevention. Updated U.S. Public Health Service guidelines for the management of occupational exposures to HIV and recommendations for postexposure prophylaxis. September 25, 2013. https://stacks.cdc.gov/view/cdc/20711. Updated May 23, 2018. Accessed November 21, 2019.
7. Dodd RY, Notari EP, Stramer SL. Current prevalence and incidence of infectious disease markers and estimated window period risk in the American Red Cross blood donor population. *Transfusion.* 2002;42:975–979.
8. Kuhar D, Henderson D, Struble K, et al. Updated U.S. public health service guidelines for the management of occupational exposures to human immunodeficiency virus and recommendations for postexposure prophylaxis. *Infect Control Hosp Epidemiol.* 2013;34(9):875–892. doi:10.1086/672271
9. Occupational Safety & Health Administration. Bloodborne pathogens standard 29 CFR 1910.1030. https://www.osha.gov/laws-regs/regulations/standardnumber/1910/1910.1030. Accessed November 21, 2019.
10. Panlilio AL, Cardo DM, Grohskopf LA, Heneine W, Ross CS. Updated U.S. public health service guidelines for the management of occupational exposures to HIV and recommendations for postexposure prophylaxis. *MMWR.* 2005;54(RR09):1–17.

Immunologic Manifestations of HIV

1. Carrington M, Alter G. Innate control of HIV. *Cold Spring Harb Perspect Med.* 2012;2:a007070.
2. Collins KL. Resistance of HIV-infected cells to cytotoxic T lymphocytes. *Microbes Infect.* 2004;6:494–500.
3. Frost SDW, Trkola A, Gunthard HF, Richman DD. Antibody responses in primary HIV infection. *Curr Opin HIVAIDS.* 2008;3(1):45–51.
4. Lackner AA, Lederman MM, Rodriguez B. HIV pathogenesis: the host. *Cold Spring Harb Perspect Med.* 2012; 2(9):a007005.
5. Lane HC, Fauci AS. Immunologic abnormalities in the acquired immunodeficiency syndrome. *Annu Rev Immunol.* 1985;3: 477–500.
6. Paranjape RS. Immunopathogenesis of HIV infection. *Indian J Med Res.* 2005;121(4):240–255.

7. Swanstrom R, Coffin J. HIV pathogenesis: the virus. *Cold Spring Harb Perspect Med.* 2012;2:a007443.

Clinical Symptoms of HIV Infection

1. Centers for Disease Control and Prevention. 1993 revised classification system for HIV infection and expanded surveillance case definition for AIDS among adolescents and adults. *MMWR.* 1992;41(No. RR-17):961–962.
2. Centers for Disease Control and Prevention. 1994 revised classification system for human immunodeficiency virus infection in children less than 13 years of age. *MMWR.* 1994;43 (No. RR-12):1–10.
3. Centers for Disease Control and Prevention. Revised surveillance case definitions for HIV infection among adults, adolescents, and children aged <18 months and for HIV infection and AIDS among children aged 18 months to <13 years. *MMWR.* 2008;57(No. RR-10):1–8.
4. Centers for Disease Control and Prevention. Revised surveillance case definition for HIV infection—United States, 2014. *MMWR.* 2014;63(3):1–10.
5. Centers for Disease Control and Prevention. Revision of the case definition of acquired immunodeficiency syndrome for national reporting—United States. *MMWR.* 1985;34:373–375.
6. Centers for Disease Control and Prevention. Revision of the CDC surveillance case definition for acquired immunodeficiency syndrome. *MMWR.* 1987;36(1):1S–15S.
7. Centers for Disease Control and Prevention. Update on acquired immunodeficiency syndrome (AIDS)—United States. *MMWR.* 1982;31:507–514.
8. European Collaborative Study. Children born to women with HIV infection: natural history and risk of transmission. *Lancet.* 1991;337:253–260.
9. Peckham C, Gibb D. Mother-to-child transmission of the human immunodeficiency virus (HIV). *N Engl J Med.* 1995;333(5):298–302.
10. Price RW, Brew B, Sidtis J, Rosenblum M, Scheck AC, Cleary P. The brain in AIDS: central nervous system HIV-1 infection and AIDS dementia complex. *Science.* 1988;239:586–592.
11. Rodes B, Toro C, Paxinos E, et al. Differences in disease progression in a cohort of long-term non-progressors after more than 16 years of HIV-1 infection. *AIDS.* 2004;18(8):1109–1116.
12. Zetola NM, Pilcher CD. Diagnosis and management of acute HIV infection. *Infect Dis Clin N Am.* 2007;21:19–48.

Treatment and Vaccine Development

1. Chen LF, Hoy J, Lewin SR. Ten years of highly active antiretroviral therapy for HIV infection. *MJA.* 2007;186(3):146–151.
2. Connor EM, Sperling RS, Gelber R, et. al. Reduction of maternal-infant transmission of human immunodeficiency virus type 1 with zidovudine treatment. *N Engl J Med.* 1994;331:1173–1180.
3. Dept. of Health and Human Services. AIDS info. http://aidsinfo.nih.gov/guidelines. Updated November 2019. Accessed November 21, 2019.
4. Haynes BF, McElrath MJ. Progress in HIV-1 vaccine development. *Curr Opin HIV AIDS.* 2013;8:326–332.
5. Marsden MD, Zack JA. HIV/AIDS eradication. *Bioorganic & Med Chem Lett.* 2013;23:4003–4010.
6. Robinson HL. HIV/AIDS vaccines: 2018. *Clin Pharmacol & Therapeutics.* 2018;104(6):1062–1073.
7. Shapiro SZ. Clinical development of candidate HIV vaccines: different problems for different vaccines. *AIDS Res Human Retroviruses.* 2014;30(4):325–329.
8. Stephenson KE. Therapeutic vaccination for HIV: hopes and challenges. *Curr Opin HIV AIDS.* 2018;13(5):408–415.
9. U.S. Public Health Service. Preexposure prophylaxis for the prevention of HIV infection in the United States—2014. A clinical practice guideline. *CDC Stacks.* 2014:1–67.
10. World Health Organization. Update of recommendations on first and second-line antiretroviral regimens. https://apps.who.int/iris/bitstream/handle/10665/325892/WHO-CDS-HIV-19.15-eng.pdf?ua=1. Updated July 2019. Accessed November 21, 2019.
11. Younai FS. Thirty years of the human immunodeficiency virus epidemic and beyond. *Int J Oral Science.* 2013;5:191–199.

Laboratory Testing for HIV Infection

1. Association of Public Health Laboratories. Suggested reporting language for the HIV laboratory diagnostic testing algorithm 2018. https://www.aphl.org/aboutAPHL/publications/Documents/ID-2019Jan-HIV-Lab-Test-Suggested-Reporting-Language.pdf. Accessed December 6, 2019.
2. Barnett D, Denny TN. Ch. 13 Lymphocyte immunophenotyping in human immunodeficiency virus infection: for richer, for poorer. In: Carey JL, McCoy Jr JP, Keren DF, eds. *Flow Cytometry in Clinical Diagnosis.* 4th ed. Chicago, IL: American Society for Clinical Pathology Press; 2007:259–274.
3. Baum P, Heilek G. Viral load monitoring: shifting paradigms in clinical practice. *MLO.* 2013;45(11):8.
4. Bentsen C, McLaughlin L, Mitchell E, et al. Performance evaluation of the Bio-Rad laboratories GS HIV combo ag/ab EIA, a 4th generation HIV assay for the simultaneous detection of HIV p24 antigen and antibodies to HIV-1 (groups M and O) and HIV-2 in human serum or plasma. *Journal of Clinical Virology.* 2011;52(suppl 1):S57–S61.
5. Boyle DS, Hawkins KR, Steele MS, Singhal M, Cheng X. Emerging technologies for point-of-care CD4 T-lymphocyte counting. *Trends Biotechnol.* 2012;30(1):45–54.
6. Branson BM, Handsfield HH, Lampe MA, et al. Centers for Disease Control and Prevention (CDC). Revised recommendations for HIV testing of adults, adolescents, and pregnant women in health-care settings. *MMWR.* 2006;55(RR-14):1–17.
7. Branson BM, Owen SM. Ch. 82 Human immunodeficiency viruses. In: Jorgensen J, Pfaller M, Carroll K. *Manual of Clinical Microbiology.* 11th ed. Washington, DC: ASM Press; 2015:1436–1457.
8. Branson BM, Owen SM, Wesolowski LG, et al. Laboratory testing for the diagnosis of HIV infection: updated recommendations. *CDC Stacks Website.* http://stacks.cdc.gov/view/cdc/23447. Updated June 27, 2014. Accessed December 18, 2014.
9. Centers for Disease Control and Prevention. Guidelines for performing single-platform absolute CD4+ T cell determinations with CD45 gating for persons infected with human immunodeficiency virus. *MMWR.* 2003;52(RR-2):1–13.
10. Centers for Disease Control and Prevention. Interpretation and use of the Western blot assay for serodiagnosis of human immunodeficiency virus type I infections. *MMWR.* 1989;38(S-7):1–7.
11. Centers for Disease Control and Prevention. 1997 revised guidelines for performing CD4+ T-cell determinations in persons infected with human immunodeficiency virus. *MMWR.* 1997;46(RR-2):1–29.
12. Centers for Disease Control and Prevention. Protocols for confirmation of rapid HIV tests. *MMWR.* 2004;53(10):221–222.
13. Centers for Disease Control and Prevention. Revised recommendations for HIV testing of adults, adolescents, and pregnant women in health care settings. *MMWR.* 2006;55(RR-14):1–17.

14. Consortium for retrovirus serology standardizations. Serologic diagnosis of human immunodeficiency virus infection by Western blot testing. *JAMA*. 1988;260:674–679.
15. Constantine NT, Zink H. HIV testing technologies after two decades of evolution. *Indian J Med Res*. 2005;121(4):519–538.
16. Curtis KA, Johnson JA, Owen SM. Principles and procedures of human immunodeficiency virus diagnosis. In: Detrick B, Schmitz JL, Hamilton RG, eds. *Manual of Molecular and Clinical Laboratory Immunology*. 8th ed. Washington, DC: ASM Press; 2016:696–710.
17. Delaney KP, Branson BM, Uniyal A, et al. Performance of an oral fluid rapid HIV-1/2 test: experience from four CDC studies. *AIDS*. 2006;20:1655–1660.
18. Donovan M, Palumbo P. Diagnosis of HIV: challenges and strategies for HIV prevention and detection among pregnant women and their infants. *Clin Perinatol*. 2010;37(4):751–763.
19. Durant J, Clevenbergh P, Halfon P, et al. Drug-resistance genotyping in HIV-1 therapy. *Lancet*. 1999;353:2195–2199.
20. Food and Drug Administration. Complete list of donor screening assays for infectious agents and HIV diagnostic assays. Website. https://www.fda.gov/vaccines-blood-biologics/complete-list-donor-screening-assays-infectious-agents-and-hiv-diagnostic-assays. Updated September 2019. Accessed November 22, 2019.
21. Greenwald JL, Burstein GR, Pincus J, Branson B. A rapid review of rapid HIV antibody tests. *Curr Infect Dis Reports*. 2006;8:125–131.
22. Health Resources and Services Administration. National HIV curriculum 2019. https://www.hiv.uw.edu/go/screening-diagnosis. Accessed December 6, 2019.
23. Hirsch M, Brun-Vézinet F, D'Aquila RT, et al. Antiretroviral drug resistance testing in adult HIV-1 infection. Recommendations of an international AIDS Society—USA panel. *JAMA*. 2000;28:2417–2426.
24. Hurt CB, Nelson JAE, Hightow-Weidman LB, Miller WC. Selecting an HIV test: a narrative review for clinicians and researchers. *Sex Trans Dis*. 2017;44(12):739–746.
25. Kapler R. Understanding the CDC's updated HIV test protocol. *MLO Med Lab Obs*. 2016 Feb;48(2):8–14.
26. Mellors JW, Munoz A, Giorgi JV, et al. Plasma viral load and CD4+ lymphocytes as prognostic markers of HIV-1 infection. *Ann Intern Med*. 1997;126(12):946–954.
27. Moyer VA. U.S. Preventive Services Task Force. Screening for HIV: U.S. preventive services task force recommendation statement. *Ann Intern Med*. 2013;159(1):51–60.
28. Myers JE, El-Sadr WM, Zerbe A, Branson BM. Rapid HIV self-testing: long in coming but opportunities beckon. *AIDS*. 2013;27(11):1687–1695.
29. Nasrullah M, Wesolowski LG, Meyer WA, 3rd, et al. Performance of a fourth-generation HIV screening assay and an alternative HIV diagnostic testing algorithm. *AIDS*. 2013;27(5):731–737.
30. Nolte FS, Caliendo AM. Molecular microbiology. In: Jorgensen J, Pfaller M, Carroll K. *Manual of Clinical Microbiology*. 11th ed. Washington, DC: ASM Press; 2015:54–90.
31. Obermeier M, Symons J, Wensing AMJ. HIV population genotypic tropism testing and its clinical significance. *Curr Opin HIV AIDS*. 2012;7(5):470–477.
32. O'Brien TR, George JR, Epstein JS, Holmberg SD, Schochetman G. Testing for antibodies to human immunodeficiency virus type 2 in the United States. *MMWR*. 1992;41(RR-12):1–9.
33. Owen SM. Testing for acute HIV infection: implications for treatment as prevention. *Curr Opin HIV AIDS*. 2012;7(2):125–130.
34. Quest diagnostics. HIV-1 infection: laboratory tests for selecting antiretroviral therapy. *Quest Diagnostics Website*. https://testdirectory.questdiagnostics.com/test/test-guides/TG_HIV_Antiretroviral_Therapy/hiv-1-infection-laboratory-tests-for-selecting-antiretroviral-therapy. Updated 2016. Accessed November 22, 2019.
35. Read JS, the Committee on Pediatric AIDS. Diagnosis of HIV-1 infection in children younger than 18 months in the United States. *Pediatrics*. 2007;120:e1547–e1562.
36. Rowley CF. Developments in CD4 and viral load monitoring in resource-limited settings. *Clin Infect Dis*. 2014;58(3):407–412.
37. Schappert J, Wians Jr FH, Schiff E, et al. Multicenter evaluation of the Bayer ADVIA centaur HIV 1/O/2 enhanced (EHIV) assay. *Clinica Chimica Acta*. 2006;372(1–2):158–166.
38. Sherin K, Klekamp BG, Beal J, Martin M. What is new in HIV infection? *Am Fam Med*. 2014;89(4):265–272.
39. Wade D, Daneau G, Aboud S, Vercauteren GH, Urassa WS, Kestens L. WHO multicenter evaluation of FACSCount CD4 and pima CD4 T-cell count systems: instrument performance and misclassification of HIV-infected patients. *JAIDS*. 2014;66(5):e98–107.

25. Immunization and Vaccines

Vaccines

1. Briere EC, Rubin L, Moro PL, et al. Prevention and control of *Haemophilus influenzae* type b disease: recommendations of the Advisory Committee on Immunization Practices (ACIP). *MMWR*. 2014;63(1):1–14.
2. Centers for Disease Control and Prevention. About pertussis outbreaks. *Pertussis (Whooping Cough) Website*. http://www.cdc.gov/pertussis/outbreaks/about.html. Updated November 18, 2019. Accessed August 21, 2020.
3. Centers for Disease Control and Prevention. Historical perspectives: a centennial celebration: Pasteur and the modern era of immunization. *MMWR*. 1985;34(26):389–390.
4. Centers for Disease Control and Prevention. History of smallpox. https://www.cdc.gov/smallpox/history/history.html. Accessed December 29, 2019.
5. Centers for Disease Control and Prevention. Immunization schedules. http://www.cdc.gov/vaccines/schedules/index.html. Updated February 3, 2020. Accessed August 21, 2020.
6. Centers for Disease Control and Prevention. Impact of vaccines in the 20th and 21st centuries. https://www.cdc.gov/vaccines/pubs/pinkbook/downloads/appendices/e/impact.pdf. Accessed December 29, 2019.
7. Centers for Disease Control and Prevention. Measles cases and outbreaks. https://www.cdc.gov/measles/cases-outbreaks.html. Accessed December 29, 2019.
8. Centers for Disease Control and Prevention. Reported cases and deaths from vaccine preventable diseases, United States. https://www.cdc.gov/vaccines/pubs/pinkbook/downloads/appendices/e/reported-cases.pdf. Accessed December 29, 2019.
9. Centers for Disease Control and Prevention. The Pink Book. General recommendations on immunization. https://www.cdc.gov/vaccines/pubs/pinkbook/genrec.html. Accessed December 29, 2019.
10. Centers for Disease Control and Prevention. Update: vaccine side effects, adverse reactions, contraindications, and precautions. Recommendations of the Advisory Committee on Immunization Practices (ACIP). *MMWR Rec Reports*. 1996;45(RR-12):1–35.
11. Coffman RL, Sher A, Seder RA. Vaccine adjuvants: putting innate immunity to work. *Immunity*. 2010;33(4):492–503.
12. DeGregorio E, D'Oro U, Bertholet S, Rappuoli R. Vaccines. In: Paul WE, ed. *Fundamental Immunology*. 7th ed. Philadelphia: Lippincott Williams & Wilkins; 2013:1032–1068.

13. De Gregorio E, Rappuoli R. Vaccines for the future: learning from human immunology. *Microb Biotechnol.* 2012;5(2):149–155.
14. de Souza Apostólico J, Alves Santos Lunardelli V, Coirada FC, Boscardin SB, Rosa DS. Adjuvants: classification, modus operandi, and licensing. *J Imm Res.* 2016. doi:10.1155/2016/1459394. Accessed January 2, 2020.
15. Di Pasquale A, Preiss S, Da Silva FT, Garçon N. Vaccine adjuvants: from 1920 to 2015 and beyond. *Vaccines.* 2015;3: 320–343; doi:10.3390/vaccines3020320
16. Ezeanolue E, Harriman K, Hunter P, Kroger A, Pellegrini C. General best practice guidelines for immunization. Best practices guidance of the Advisory Committee on Immunization Practices (ACIP). https://www.cdc.gov/vaccines/hcp/acip-recs/general-recs/index.html. Updated April 20, 2017. Accessed on January 1, 2020.
17. Fiore AE, Wasley A, Bell BP. Prevention of hepatitis A through active or passive immunization: recommendations of the Advisory Committee on Immunization Practices (ACIP). *MMWR Rec Rep.* 2006;55(RR-7):1–23.
18. Glenny A, Pope C, Waddington H, Wallace V. The antigenic value of toxoid precipitated by potassium-alum. *J Path Bacteriol.* 1926;29:38–45.
19. Grohskopf LA, Alyanak E, Broder KR, Walter EB, Fry AM, Jernigan DB, Atmar RL. Prevention and control of seasonal influenza with vaccines: recommendations of the Advisory Committee on Immunization Practices—United States, 2019–2020 season. *MMWR.* 2019:68(3):1–21.
20. Hebert CJ, Hall CM, Odoms LN. Lessons learned and applied: what the 20th century vaccine experience can teach us about vaccines in the 21st century. *Hum Vaccines Immunother.* 2012;8(5):560–568.
21. Heidary N, Cohen DE. Hypersensitivity reactions to vaccine components. *Dermatitis.* 2005;16(3):115–120.
22. Hilleman MR. Vaccines in historic evolution and perspective: a narrative of vaccine discoveries. *J Hum Virol.* 2000;3(2):63–76.
23. Jackson BR, Iqbal S, Mahon B. Updated recommendations for the use of typhoid vaccine *MMWR.* 2015;64(11):305–308.
24. Karch CP, Burkhard P. Vaccine technologies: from whole organisms to rationally designed protein assemblies. *Biochem Pharmacol.* 2016;120:1–14. doi:10.1016/j.bcp.2016.05.001
25. Koff WC, Burton DR, Johnson PR, et al. Accelerating next-generation vaccine development for global disease prevention. *Science.* 340(2013). doi:10.1126/science.1232910
26. Kroger AT, Sumaya CV, Pickering LK, Atkinson WL. General recommendations on immunization. Recommendations of the Advisory Committee on Immunization Practices. *MMWR.* 2011;60(2):1–61.
27. Lambert LC, Fauci AS. Influenza vaccines for the future. *N Engl J Med.* 2010;363(21):2036–2044.
28. Lattanzi M, Rappuoli R, Stadler K. The use of vaccines and antibody preparations. In: Bellanti JA, Escobar-Gutierrez A, Joost JJ, eds. *Immunology IV: Clinical Applications in Health and Disease.* Bethesda, MD: I Care Press;2012:891–937.
29. Liang JL, Tiwari T, Moro P, et al. Prevention of pertussis, tetanus, and diphtheria with vaccines in the United States: recommendations of the Advisory Committee on Immunization Practices (ACIP). *MMWR Rec Rep.* 2018;67(2):1–44.
30. MacNeil JR, Rubin L, Folaranmi T, Ortega-Sanchez IR, Patel M, Martin SW. Prevention and control of meningococcal disease: recommendations of the Advisory Committee on Immunization Practices (ACIP). *MMWR Rec Rep.* 2015;64(41):1171–1176.
31. Makela PH. Vaccines: coming of age after 200 years. *FEMS Microbiol Rev.* 2000;24(1):9–20.
32. Marin M, Guris D, Chaves SS, et al. Prevention of varicella: recommendations of the Advisory Committee on Immunization Practices (ACIP). *MMWR Rec Rep.* 2007;56(RR-4):1–40.
33. Mascola JR, Fauci AS. Novel vaccine technologies for the 21st century. *Nature Rev Immunol.* doi:10.1038/s41577-019-0243-3. Accessed January 2, 2020.
34. Matanock A, Lee G, Gierke R, Kobayashi M, Leidner A, Pilishvili T. Use of 13-valent pneumococcal conjugate vaccine and 23-valent pneumococcal polysaccharide vaccine among adults aged ≥65 years: updated recommendations of the Advisory Committee on Immunization Practices. *MMWR.* 2019;68(46);1069–1075.
35. McClure CC, Cataldi JR, O'Leary ST. Vaccine hesitancy: where we are and where we are going. *Clin Ther.* 2017; 39(8):1550–1562.
36. McLean HQ, Fiebelkorn HP, Tempte JL, Wallace GS. Prevention of measles, rubella, congenital rubella syndrome, and mumps, 2013: recommendations of the Advisory Committee on Immunization Practices (ACIP). *MMWR.* 2013;62(4):1–34.
37. National Institute of Allergy and Infectious Diseases. Community immunity ("herd" immunity). http://www.niaid.nih.gov/topics/pages/communityimmunity.aspx. Updated 2010. Accessed November 15, 2013.
38. Nelson NP, Link-Gelles R, Romero JR, et al. Update: recommendations of the Advisory Committee on Immunization Practices for use of hepatitis A vaccine for postexposure prophylaxis and for preexposure prophylaxis for international travel. *MMWR.* 2018;67(43);1216–1220.
39. Nigrovic LE, Thompson KM. The Lyme vaccine: a cautionary tale. *Epidemiol Infect.* 2007;135(1):1–8.
40. Owen JA, Punt J, Stranford SA. *Kuby Immunology.* 7th ed. New York: WH Freeman and Co.; 2013:574–591.
41. Pallansch MA. Ending use of oral poliovirus vaccine—a difficult move in the polio endgame. *N Eng J Med.* 2018;379(9):801–802.
42. Pardi N, Hogan MJ, Porter FW, Weissman D. mRNA vaccines—a new era in vaccinology. *Nature Reviews Drug Discovery* 2018; 17:261–279.
43. Petrosky E, Bocchini JA, Hariri S, et al. Use of 9-valent human papillomavirus (HPV) vaccine: updated HPV vaccination recommendations of the Advisory Committee on Immunization Practices (ACIP). *MMWR.* 2015;64(11):300–304.
44. Plotkin SA. Six revolutions in vaccinology. *Pediatr Infect Dis J.* 2005;24(1):1–9.
45. Plotkin SA. Vaccines: past, present and future. *Nat Med.* 2005;11(4 suppl):S5–11.
46. Plotkin SA, Plotkin SL. The development of vaccines: how the past led to the future. *Nat Rev Microbiol.* 2011;9(12):889–893.
47. Prevots DR, Burr RK, Sutter RW, Murphy TV. Poliomyelitis prevention in the United States. Updated recommendations of the Advisory Committee on Immunization Practices (ACIP). *MMWR Rec Rep.* 2000;49(RR-5):1–22.
48. Rao TSS, Andrade C. The MMR vaccine and autism: sensation, refutation, retraction, and fraud. *Indian J Psychiatry.* 2011;53(2):95–96.
49. Riedel S. Edward Jenner and the history of smallpox and vaccination. *BUMC Proceedings.* 2005;18(1):21–25.
50. Roush SW, Murphy TV. Historical comparisons of morbidity and mortality for vaccine-preventable diseases in the United States. *JAMA.* 2007;298(18):2155–2163.
51. Rueckert C, Guzman CA. Vaccines: from empirical development to rational design. *PLOS Pathog.* 2012;8(11):1–7.
52. Schillie S, Vellozzi C, Reingold A, et al. Prevention of hepatitis B virus infection in the United States: recommendations of the Advisory Committee on Immunization Practices. *MMWR.* 2018;67(1):1–31.

53. Siegrist CA. Mechanisms underlying adverse reactions to vaccines. *J Comp Pathol.* 2007;137(suppl 1):S46–S50.
54. Succi RC. Vaccine refusal—what we need to know. *J Pediatr (Rio J).* 2018;94:574–581.
55. U.S. Food and Drug Administration. Common ingredients in US licensed vaccines. https://www.fda.gov/vaccines-blood-biologics/safety-availability-biologics/common-ingredients-us-licensed-vaccines. Accessed December 29, 2019.
56. Vaccine. *Taber's Medical Dictionary Website.* http://www.tabers.com/tabersonline/view/Tabers-Dictionary/739755/all/vaccine?q=vaccine#23. Accessed December 29, 2019.
57. World Health Organization. Immunization, vaccines, and biologicals. https://www.who.int/immunization/global_vaccine_action_plan/en/. Accessed December 29, 2019.

Passive Immunotherapy and Monoclonal Antibodies

1. Foltz IN, Karow M, Wasserman SM. Evolution and emergence of therapeutic monoclonal antibodies: what cardiologists need to know. *Circulation.* 2013;127(22):2222–2230.
2. Grundmann K. Emil von Behring: the founder of serum therapy. Nobel prizes and laureates. *Website.* http://www.nobelprize.org/nobel_prizes/medicine/laureates/1901/behring-article.html. Accessed January 2, 2020.
3. Kantha SS. A centennial review: the 1890 tetanus antitoxin paper of von Behring and Kitasato and the related developments. *Keio J Med.* 1991;40(1):35–39.
4. Keller MA, Stiehm ER. Passive immunity in prevention and treatment of infectious diseases. *Clin Microbiol Rev.* 2000;13(4):602–614.
5. Schwab I, Nimmerjahn F. Intravenous immunoglobulin therapy: how does IgG modulate the immune system? *Nat Rev Immunol.* 2013;13(3):176–189.
6. Scott AM, Allison JP, Wolchok JD. Monoclonal antibodies in cancer therapy. *Cancer Immun.* 2012;12:14.
7. Seidel JA, Otsuka A, Kabashima K. Anti-PD-1 and Anti-CTLA-4 therapies in cancer: mechanisms of action, efficacy, and limitations. *Front Oncol.* 2018, March 28. doi:10.3389/fonc.2018.00086
8. Singh S, Kumar NK, Dwiwedi P, et al. Monoclonal antibodies: a review. *Curr Clin Pharmacol.* 2018;13(2):85–99.
9. Stiehm ER. Standard and special human immune serum globulins as therapeutic agents. *Pediatrics.* 1979;63(2):301–319.
10. The Antibody Society. *Antibody Therapeutics Approved or in Regulatory Review in the EU or US.* https://www.antibodysociety.org/resources/approved-antibodies/. Accessed January 2, 2020.
11. Yuvienco C, Schwartz S. Monoclonal antibodies in rheumatic diseases. *Med Health, Rhode Island.* 2011;94(11):320–324.

Adoptive Immunotherapy

1. Copelan EA. Hematopoietic stem-cell transplantation. *N Engl J Med.* 2006;354(17):1813–1826.
2. Klein E, Sjogren HO. Humoral and cellular factors in homograft and isograft immunity against sarcoma cells. *Cancer Res.* 1960;20:452–461.
3. Lee S, Margolin K. Tumor-infiltrating lymphocytes in melanoma. *Curr Oncol Rep.* 2012;14(5):468–474.
4. Mchayleh M, Bedi P, Sehgal R, Solh M. Chimeric antigen receptor T-cells: the future is now. *J Clin Med.* 2019;8:207. doi:10.3390/jcm8020207
5. Pagliara D, Savoldo B. Cytotoxic T lymphocytes for the treatment of viral infections and posttransplant lymphoproliferative disorders in transplant recipients. *Curr Opin Infect Dis.* 2012;25(4):431–437.
6. Percia K, Varela JC, Oelke M, Schneck J. Adoptive T cell immunotherapy for cancer. *Rambam Maimonides Med J.* 2015;6(1):e0004:1–9.
7. Restifo NP, Dudley ME, Rosenberg SA. Adoptive immunotherapy for cancer: harnessing the T cell response. *Nat Rev Immunol.* 2012;12(4):269–281.
8. Rosenberg SA, Packard BS, Aebersold PM, et al. Use of tumor-infiltrating lymphocytes and interleukin-2 in the immunotherapy of patients with metastatic melanoma. A preliminary report. *N Engl J Med.* 1988;319(25):1676–1680.
9. Schliesser U, Streitz M, Sawitzki B. Tregs: application for solid-organ transplantation. *Curr Opin Organ Tran.* 2012;17(1):34–41.
10. Slettenmark B, Klein E. Cytotoxic and neutralization tests with serum and lymph node cells of isologous mice with induced resistance against gross lymphomas. *Cancer Res.* 1962;22:947–954.

Answer Key

Chapter 1 Introduction to Immunity and the Immune System

Answers to Case Studies

1. **a.** Because the swelling has occurred within 2 days, it is most likely caused by an innate immune response. The adaptive immune response takes longer to develop because it depends on lymphocytes recognizing a specific antigen. Swelling and redness in the tissue is caused by neutrophils leaving the bloodstream by means of diapedesis in response to the presence of bacteria. **b.** In addition to neutrophils, there may also be macrophages and dendritic cells present.

2. **a.** The adaptive immune system is characterized by specificity and memory. When exposed to the same foreign substance numerous times, the response is increased each time. Thus, with a serious disease such as tetanus, getting a booster shot of a similar but harmless substance will stimulate the immune system each time a booster is given. Restimulating the adaptive immune response provides greater protection than the innate immune system on its own, which could possibly be overwhelmed by pathogens such as the bacteria that cause tetanus. **b.** The most important cells involved in a response to a vaccine are the cells involved in acquired immunity, namely, T cells and B cells. T cells help B cells to stimulate the development of plasma cells, which actively produce antibody, and memory cells, which can be transformed to become active plasma cells in a very short time if the individual was re-exposed to tetanus in the future.

Answers to Review Questions

1. c	2. d	3. a	4. a	5. d	6. b	7. a
8. d	9. c	10. a	11. b	12. a	13. b	14. c
15. a	16. b	17. c	18. d	19. c	20. b	

Chapter 2 Innate Immunity

Answers to Case Studies

1. **a.** Although Rick's cholesterol levels were within normal limits for both HDL and total cholesterol, an increase in CRP has been associated with a greater risk of a future heart attack. Higher fibrinogen levels are also associated with an increased risk for a future cardiovascular event, although increased fibrinogen is not as great a risk factor as increased CRP. A rise in both of these acute-phase reactants indicates an underlying inflammatory process. Such a process is associated with atherosclerosis, a condition that damages coronary blood vessels. Rick's wife should encourage him to follow a healthy diet and to lose weight through exercise.

2. **a.** CRP is one of the first indicators of a possible infection. Levels also rise in the case of a malignancy, heart attack, or trauma to the body. If the infection was bacterial, an increase in the white blood cell (WBC) count should have been seen. This increase would mainly be because of recruitment of neutrophils to help fight the invading organism. However, if an infection is caused by a virus, there is typically no increase in the WBC count. As an acute-phase reactant, CRP levels increase dramatically within 24 hours, long before specific antibody can be detected. **b.** An increase in CRP would likely be seen if the student had infectious mononucleosis, a viral infection. However, CRP doesn't specifically indicate which type of viral infection may be present. The symptoms are consistent with the possibility of mononucleosis, but other conditions can't be ruled out. Repeating the mono test in a few days will allow enough time for a detectable level of antibody to form, and the diagnosis could be confirmed.

Answers to Review Questions

1. a	2. c	3. c	4. a	5. d	6. b	7. c
8. b	9. d	10. c	11. a	12. d	13. a	14. b
15. b	16. d					

Chapter 3 Nature of Antigens and the Major Histocompatibility Complex

Answers to Case Studies

1. **a.** Because every child inherits one haplotype (set of genes) from the mother and one from the father, 50% of the HLA antigens would match the mother, and 50% would match the father. It would never be more than that, unless the mother and father have at least one antigen in common. **b.** According to the law of independent assortment, there would be a 1:4 chance that the sister would be an exact match, a 1:2 chance that a sister would share half of the same alleles, and a 1:4 chance that a sister would share no alleles, having received the opposite haplotype from each parent. **c.** It is possible that a cadaver kidney may actually be a better match if neither sister is an exact match. The most important alleles to match are HLA A, B, and DR. If a cadaver match has more than one allele in common with the recipient at each of these loci, then it would be a closer match.

2. **a.** Of all the different antigens that have been purified by the other scientists working on the project, proteins generally make the best immunogens. This is because of all the biomolecules listed, only protein antigens can be processed and presented to T cells. B cells can respond to essentially all of the listed biomolecules—but an effective antibody response requires cooperation between T cells and B cells. **b.** Antigen alone is often insufficient to stimulate an immune response. For this reason, the zombie plague vaccine should be formulated with an adjuvant. Incorporating an adjuvant into the inoculum will function to stimulate an innate response and

may also keep the antigen concentrated at the site of vaccination—both of these adjuvant properties will help potentiate the response against the zombie virus antigen.

Answers to Review Questions

1. d 2. b 3. a 4. c 5. d 6. a 7. b
8. a 9. a 10. c 11. b 12. c 13. a 14. b
15. c 16. b 17. a

Chapter 4 Adaptive Immunity

Answers to Case Studies

1. a. The normal CD19+ cell count indicates that there is not a lack of B cells, which are presumably capable of responding to antigen and producing antibodies. The low CD4+ T-cell count indicates that there is a decrease in T helper (Th) cells. Th cells are necessary for a response to T-dependent antigens. The decreased CD4+ count means that B cells are not activated by The cells, and class switching to IgG does not occur. Memory B cells are not produced either. **b.** A lack of Th cells severely limits the B-cell response, resulting in increased bacterial infections.

2. a. CD8+ T cells are responsible for the destruction of cancer cells as well as any intracellular pathogens, such as viruses. Although antibodies may be produced, they are not very effective against cancerous cells or virally infected cells. Thus, an important arm of the adaptive immune system would not be working, and an individual would be more susceptible to certain kinds of infections or to cancer.

Answers to Review Questions

1. b 2. d 3. a 4. a 5. c 6. b 7. d
8. c 9. a 10. b 11. a 12. c 13. d 14. c
15. b 16. a 17. d

Chapter 5 Antibody Structure and Function

Answers to Case Studies

1. a. The presence of IgM only is an indicator of an early acute infection. IgM is the first antibody to appear, followed by IgG. In a reactivated case of mono, a small amount of IgM might be present, but IgG would also be present. Thus, the patient is encountering the virus for the first time. **b.** The memory cells triggered by the first exposure to the virus would cause production of IgG in a much shorter time, and there would be a greater increase in IgG compared with the amount of IgM present.

2. a. The increase in IgE is an indicator that the cold symptoms may actually be caused by an allergy. This is especially evident in the springtime, when pollen levels are high. The child should be tested for specific allergies to determine the cause of the symptoms. Treatment with antihistamine and avoidance of the allergen will help to relieve the symptoms. **b.** Chronic respiratory infections may be caused by a decrease or lack of IgA, but this is not the case here. Normal levels of IgG, IgM, and IgA indicate that this child is not immunocompromised.

Answers to Review Questions

1. a 2. a 3. b 4. d 5. c 6. a 7. d
8. a 9. a 10. c 11. b 12. a 13. c 14. d
15. b 16. b 17. c 18. b 19. d 20. a 21. c

Chapter 6 Cytokines

Answers to Case Study

a. G-CSF, **b.** IFN-γ and IL-2. **c.** IL-4 and IL-10.

Answers to Review Questions

1. b 2. a 3. d 4. d 5. c 6. a 7. d
8. b 9. c 10. d 11. b 12. b 13. a 14. c
15. b 16. d

Chapter 7 The Complement System

Answers to Case Studies

1. a. A decreased CH50 indicates a problem with the classical pathway. The decreased AH50 indicates a problem with the alternative pathway as well. Having both assays low strongly suggests a deficiency in the shared terminal pathway rather than two individual pathway deficiencies. **b.** Levels of C3 and C4 are normal, indicating that a deficiency is downstream of these components. This is consistent with the likelihood of a terminal pathway deficiency. Because the defense against encapsulated bacteria such as meningococci is reduced if there is a decrease in C5 through C9, the patient's symptoms are in accord with this conclusion. **c.** To confirm the actual deficiency, testing for the individual components C5 through C9 should be performed. Because this type of deficiency reduces the overall functioning of the complement system, patients should receive prompt therapy when signs of infection are noted.

2. a. Although the abdominal pain and vomiting could be caused by several infectious agents, the normal white blood cell count decreases the likelihood of a bacterial infection. The accompanying swelling of the hands and legs may be an indicator of a possible inflammatory problem associated with continuous activation of the complement system. Because this has been a recurring problem, the likelihood of an immune problem is increased. Because total serum protein is within the normal range, it is unlikely that the deficiency is from a lack of antibody production. A decrease of one complement component would not be apparent on a total protein determination. **b.** Reduced levels of both C4 and C2 could be from inheritance of defective genes for both components. However, the possibility of that is extremely rare. A more plausible explanation is that the deficiency of both C2 and C4 is caused by overconsumption rather than a lack of production. The normal level of C1q indicates it is likely not an acquired complement deficiency. **c.** A lack of C1-INH would result in overconsumption of C4 and C2. As this is the most common hereditary deficiency of the complement system, this represents a likely explanation for the symptoms. This can be verified by testing for this particular component.

Answers to Review Questions

1. b 2. a 3. d 4. e 5. c 6. a 7. d
8. a 9. e 10. d 11. a 12. b 13. e 14. a
15. a 16. d 17. d 18. d 19. c 20. a

Chapter 8 Safety and Quality Management

Answer to Case Studies

1. a. Gloves should never be removed when working with patient specimens. When they are, hands should be sanitized immediately using the correct procedure. Any contamination of the laboratory bench should be treated with sodium hypochlorite, and the paper towels should be disposed of in the regulated medical waste container. Because the supervisor's laboratory coat was disposable and became contaminated, it should be discarded in the regulated medical waste container and replaced with a new coat. Pipetting should have been done behind a Plexiglass shield because this would have prevented the spill onto the laboratory coat. **b.** Reservoir. The hands and contaminated fomites (laboratory coat and laboratory bench) that contain blood are ideal reservoirs for infectious agents. **c.** To break the chain, disinfect the work area with 1:10 sodium hypochlorite solution and sanitize hands to kill the infectious agent and eliminate the reservoir.

2. a. Take corrective action. All proficiency survey specimens are tested in the same manner as patient specimens by the laboratory personnel. **b.** Take corrective action. QC is performed at scheduled times, such as at the beginning of each shift or before testing patient samples, in the same manner as a patient specimen to evaluate the daily performance of instruments. **c.** Accept. **d.** Take corrective action. Documentation of QC includes dating and initialing the material when it is first opened and recording the manufacturer's lot number and the expiration date each time a control is run and the test result is obtained.

3. a. Report critical test results to the appropriate health-care staff on a timely basis. Document the name of the person receiving the results. **b.** The Joint Commission National Patient Safety Goals.

Answers to Review Questions

1. c 2. a 3. a 4. c 5. c 6. c 7. b
8. d 9. a 10. c 11. b 12. b 13. d 14. b
15. d 16. d 17. d 18. d 19. c 20. b
21. 2, 1, 2, 3, 2, 2 22. b 23. d 24. d 25. c

Chapter 9 Principles of Serological Testing

Answers to Case Study

a. The serological pipette must be emptied completely to obtain the correct volume because it is marked to contain (TC) rather than to deliver (TD). Therefore, it should have been blown out to expel the last drop of liquid, or the measurement should have been made from point to point, for example, by filling the pipette up to the 0.8-mL mark and then letting it drain to the 0.9-mL mark.

b. The 1.9 diluent was not correct. In order to make a 1:40 dilution with 0.1 mL of serum, the calculations are as follows:

$$1/40 = 0.1/x$$

$x = 4.0$ mL (This represents the total volume.)

$4.0 - 0.1 = 3.9$ mL of diluent to make a 1:40 dilution.

Answers to Review Questions

1. b 2. a 3. c 4. a 5. c 6. d 7. b
8. a 9. b 10. a 11. d 12. c 13. b 14. a
15. d 16. c 17. b 18. c 19. d 20. a

Chapter 10 Precipitation and Agglutination Reactions

Answers to Case Studies

1. a. The results indicate normal levels of IgG and IgM, but there is a decreased level of IgA. This most likely indicates a selective IgA deficiency, the most common genetic immunodeficiency. **b.** A decrease in serum IgA most likely indicates a decrease in secretory IgA, the immunoglobulin that is found on mucosal surfaces. Individuals with a selective IgA deficiency are more prone to respiratory tract and gastrointestinal tract infections because IgA represents the first line of defense against pathogens that invade mucosal surfaces. **c.** Nephelometry is a more sensitive method for measuring immunoglobulin levels. It is able to detect small quantities of immunoglobulin present. Results are obtained faster in comparison with RID; because the process is automated, it is not subject to human error in reading the results. Other errors that may occur with RID include overfilling or underfilling of wells, nicking of wells, and inaccurate incubation time or temperature. Therefore, nephelometry has largely replaced RID for the measurement of immunoglobulin levels.

2. a. The TP-PA test is a particle agglutination test used to look for the presence of antibodies to *T. pallidum*, the bacterium that causes syphilis. In this test, dilutions of patient serum are incubated with gel particles that have been sensitized with *T. pallidum* antigen, and the wells are examined for agglutination. A smooth mat of particles covering the well indicates that a lattice has been formed and thus represents a positive result. **b.** If the 1:40 result was negative, whereas the 1:80 result was positive, this is an example of a prozone phenomenon, in which there was an excess of antibody molecules in the 1:40 dilution that inhibited lattice formation, but equivalence was reached when the antibody was diluted to 1:80. **c.** The positive result indicates that the patient has been exposed to *T. pallidum* but cannot differentiate between a current infection and a past exposure. This would have to be determined by performing additional laboratory tests and taking a through medical history.

Answers to Review Questions

1. c 2. d 3. b 4. d 5. b 6. a 7. b
8. a 9. d 10. a 11. c 12. a 13. c 14. b
15. c 16. b 17. d 18. a

Chapter 11 Labeled Immunoassays

Answers to Case Study

a. This is an example of the high-dose hook effect (also called *antigen excess* or *postzone effect*). It occurs commonly in immunoassay measurements of tumor markers. The tumor marker concentration generally reflects the tumor burden, such that large tumors tend to generate very high concentrations of the test marker in blood. This causes the value to fall outside of the reportable range of the test method, which leads to loss of the linear relationship between detected signal and analyte concentration.

b. Dilute the patient sample. In this case, the technologist prepared a 1:10 dilution of the sample, based on the patient's first reported value (1,250 U/mL) and the test assay reportable range. This is illustrated in the two test results performed on Instrument B at the patient's 3-month follow-up. The initial test result run on Instrument B before dilution was 110 U/mL. After making a 1:10 dilution, the instrument result is 95 U/mL. Accounting for dilution factor, the final reported result is 950 U/mL, indicating that the original, undiluted sample result of 110 U/mL performed on Instrument B was falsely low because of antigen excess. If the diluted test result had instead been 11 U/mL for a final value of 110 U/mL, this could be reflective of successful treatment of the patient.

c. Immunoassay manufacturers often develop capture and detection antibodies using slightly different epitopes, meaning the reagent antibodies detect different parts of the test marker molecule. As such, the lack of standardization across different manufacturer methods means that test results may not be equivalent in the same person simply because the methods are different. For this reason, it is essential to have reference interval (normal range) cutoffs determined for each method. In the case study, the cutoff value for Instrument A is 38 U/mL, whereas for Instrument B, a cutoff of 55 U/mL is appropriate. Ideally, the same instrument/method should be used to measure the patient's tumor marker concentration for serial (repeat) testing to ensure the results are correctly interpreted.

d. In the event the original laboratory (test method) could not be used for follow-up, interpretation of the test result should be based on the manufacturer-specific cutoff value.

Answers to Review Questions

1. c	2. a	3. d	4. a	5. c	6. b	7. a
8. b	9. d	10. d	11. b	12. c	13. b	14. b
15. a						

Chapter 12 Molecular Diagnostic Techniques

Answers to Case Studies

1. a. Normal tissue that expresses PD-L1, such as tonsil, is a control for recognition of the epitope by the primary antibody. Cultured cells from cell lines expressing PD-L1 are provided with reagent sets and should also be included with each run as a standard for the reagents provided. An adjacent section cut from the test tissue run without addition of the primary antibody is a negative control for reagent quality and specificity. Tumor tissues that do not express PD-L1 are used to assess staining quality. Tissue that gives no staining on tumor cells but contains tumor-associated macrophages/immune cells that may express PD-L1 provides an internal positive control.

b. PD-L1 is the ligand for the PD-1 transmembrane protein, a member of the immunoglobulin superfamily. PD-1 is expressed in pro-B cells and is thought to play a role in their differentiation and is also important in T-cell function, contributing to the prevention of autoimmune diseases. PD-L1 is an immune inhibitory receptor ligand that is expressed by T cells and B cells and various types of tumor cells. It is also a transmembrane protein, and the interaction of this ligand with its receptor (PD-1) inhibits T-cell activation and cytokine production. This interaction prevents the autoimmune response; however, expression of PD-L1 on tumor cells provides an escape from the immune response by inactivating recognition of cytotoxic T cells. Clinical intervention using immunotherapeutic antibodies to PD-1 or PD-L1 (immune checkpoint inhibitors) reestablishes the immune response to tumor cells expressing PD-L1.

c. Clinical trials have shown that patients with tumors showing greater than 50% PD-L1 expression will respond well to immunotherapy with antibodies to PD-L1 or its receptor, PD-1. With PD-L1 expression of 60%, this patient will likely receive immunotherapy. Tumor cells that do not express PD-L1 will be less likely to respond to these agents; therefore, testing for its expression can guide treatment strategy. If expression is lower than 50%, alternate treatment strategies may be considered. Because of variations in test methods, treatment guidelines are continually updated.

2. a. The second option is correct. The amplification control should always be present to demonstrate that the PCR is working and to avoid false negatives. A reagent blank (no template) control is included to detect contamination. In a true negative, the amplification control would be positive, whereas the test target is negative. The previous test results do not necessarily predict that the current test results should be positive. Because the amplification control did not work, the current results are not interpretable.

b. The first option is correct. Because the amplification control is positive, the PCR is working, and the result is a true negative. The reagent blank (no template) control, not the amplification control, is used to detect contamination. In a true negative, the amplification control would be positive, whereas the test target is negative. The previous results may be reviewed for clinical interpretation of the result but do not predict a positive result in the current sample.

c. No. The test sensitivity goes to 50 copies/mL, meaning that there may be fewer than 50 copies/mL present that will not be detected by the test method. Although the previous results do not predict a positive result, because there is a history of the presence of virus, a residual low level of viral copies could be present. The results should be reported as "less than 50 copies/mL" to indicate the limited capacity of the test to detect the presence of HIV below 50 copies/mL.

Answers to Review Questions

1. a 2. d 3. b 4. b 5. a 6. b 7. a 8. d 9. a 10. d 11. b 12. b 13. a 14. c 15. c

Chapter 13 Flow Cytometry and Laboratory Automation

Answers to Case Studies

1. a. The result may represent an error of specificity, given that the newer instrument is getting positive results on specimens that were negative by the older method. However, the newer instrument could be more sensitive than the older one, so these could actually be positive samples. **b.** To resolve this discrepancy, known positive and negative controls should be run. The positive controls need to include those at the lower limit of detection, as well as more highly positive samples. This would help to determine if the new instrument is actually more sensitive rather than lacking in specificity.

2. a. The flow cytometry pattern in A indicates that the majority of lymphocytes are B cells because they are CD19+. The population most affected appears to be CD3+, which are T cells. Pattern B suggests that of the CD3+ lymphocytes, the majority are CD8+, or cytotoxic T cells. The CD4+ count is very low. **b.** T helper cells are necessary to provide help to B cells so that they can respond by making antibody. Thus, the child is unable to make IgG in response to potential pathogens she might encounter in the environment. **c.** This child should be tested for HIV. That would explain the decrease in CD4+ T cells. Tests for leukemia/lymphoma should also be ordered to rule out hematopoietic disorders affecting the CD4+ T-cells.

Answers to Review Questions

1. d 2. c 3. b 4. c 5. a 6. b 7. c 8. c 9. a 10. d 11. c 12. c 13. c 14. d 15. d 16. b 17. d 18. b 19. d 20. d

Chapter 14 Hypersensitivity

Answers to Case Studies

1. a. An increase in eosinophils is typically found in allergic individuals. Interleukins released by stimulated Th1 cells are involved in the recruitment of eosinophils from the bone marrow. Although there are other causes of eosinophilia, such as a parasitic infection, an increased number most often indicates an allergic reaction. **b.** The patient can have a skin-prick test performed to determine which allergens he is sensitized to. The patient would know his results immediately because a positive test would be indicated by formation of wheal-and-flare reactions within 20 minutes at the site(s) of injection. If he is unable to discontinue any antihistamines he might be taking, or if a clear area of skin in his forearm or back could not be found, a solid-phase immunoassay for allergen-specific IgE could be performed. **c.** A solid-phase immunoassay for total IgE could be performed to monitor the patient's response to allergen immunotherapy. If the therapy is successful, the IgE concentration in the patient's serum should decrease to a level within the reference range for patients his age.

2. a. A positive DAT indicates that the red blood cells (RBCs) are coated with either antibody or complement components. The destruction of some RBCs is the reason for the man's symptoms. **b.** The most likely cause of the positive DAT is the presence of an antibody of the IgM class. It might be an anti-I, triggered by *Mycoplasma pneumonia*. This is a cold-reacting antibody. **c.** A DAT that is only positive with anti-C3d indicates that only complement products are present on the RBCs. This is a further indication that the antibody is an IgM antibody because it does not remain on the cells at 37°C but does trigger complement activation, which can cause the cell destruction.

Answers to Review Questions

1. c 2. b 3. d 4. b 5. a 6. b 7. d 8. b 9. c 10. c 11. a 12. b 13. d 14. d 15. c 16. d

Chapter 15 Autoimmunity

Answers to Case Studies

1. a. In systemic lupus erythematosus, a low titer of rheumatoid factor is often present. Conversely, a low titer of anti-nuclear antibodies can be associated with rheumatoid arthritis. Thus, these two conditions cannot be differentiated on the basis of the rapid RF and ANA test results alone. **b.** The decreased RBC count may be caused by the presence of a low-level autoantibody directed against red blood cells, often associated with lupus. **c.** A fluorescent anti-nuclear antibody (FANA) test is a good screening tool to help distinguish between these two conditions. A homogeneous pattern would be indicative of lupus, whereas a speckled pattern can sometimes be found in rheumatoid arthritis or lupus. Therefore, if a speckled pattern is obtained, more specific testing for ENA antibodies should be done.The presence of anti-Sm antibody would be diagnostic for lupus. This is what was found in this case.

2. a. The low T4 level, enlarged thyroid gland, and presence of anti-thyroglobulin antibody are all indicators of Hashimoto's thyroiditis. **b.** Anti-thyroglobulin antibodies progressively destroy thyroglobulin produced by the thyroid. Thyroglobulin is normally cleaved in the thyroid to produce the secretable hormones triiodothyronine (T3) and thyroxine (T4). The presence of anti-thyroglobulin antibodies causes enlargement of the thyroid because of the immune response, and hypothyroidism results, characterized by fatigue and weight gain. **c.** Graves' disease is also an autoimmune illness that affects the thyroid, but it is characterized by hyperthyroidism. In this disease, antibodies to thyroid-stimulating hormone receptors are produced, sending a signal to the thyroid to constantly produce T3 and T4. Symptoms include nervousness, insomnia, restlessness, and weight loss, exactly opposite of the characteristics of Hashimoto's thyroiditis.

Answers to Review Questions

1. a	2. d	3. d	4. a	5. d	6. b	7. a
8. c	9. d	10. c	11. a	12. b	13. d	14. a
15. c						

Chapter 16 Transplantation Immunology

Answers to Case Studies

1. a. The most compatible donor for this patient would be Friend 2. Sibling 1 has the B35 antigen for which the patient possesses HLA antibody. Sibling 2 also has the B35 antigen and is also ABO incompatible. Friend 1 is ABO incompatible. Friend 2 is ABO identical and does not express the HLA-B35 antigen and is thus the most appropriate donor.

2. a. Maybe; for an unrelated donor, one can't be sure that they have the same alleles at each locus even if they have the same low-resolution type. **b.** The physician requested high-resolution HLA in order to determine if the donor and recipient had the same alleles at each locus. Serological typing (phenotyping) provides low-resolution results, as indicated. The best outcomes for a transplant occur if the recipient and donor are matched at the HLA allele level. High-resolution typing of the donor was performed. The donor's B locus typing indicated he or she had the alleles HLA-A*02:05 and HLA-B*44:03. Thus, they were actually mismatched for two alleles. Based on this finding, this donor was declined, and an additional search was conducted.

3. a. 34%. **b.** A cPRA value of 34% means that 34% of the people in the likely donor pool possess one or more of the antigens corresponding to the antibodies identified in this patient serum (HLA-A, B8, DR17).

Answers to Review Questions

1. b	2. c	3. d	4. d	5. b	6. b	7. a
8. d	9. a	10. b	11. b	12. d	13. a	14. c
15. b						

Chapter 17 Tumor Immunology

Answers to Case Studies

1. a. If no further CA 15-3 is being produced by tumor tissue, levels will decrease at the rate of the biological half-life for the molecule. Because CA 15-3 levels are not decreasing at this rate, a residual tumor is suspected. **b.** HER2 overexpression indicates that therapy with the monoclonal antibody Herceptin may be successful. **c.** Because the tumor lacks estrogen and progesterone receptors, hormone-suppressing therapy is unlikely to improve the prognosis.

2. a. No other tissues in men are known to produce PSA, so another source is extremely unlikely. **b.** PSA velocity is the rate of PSA increase between determinations. Because PSA increases with age and prostatic enlargement, examining PSA velocity is an attempt to separate benign and malignant conditions, as velocity is higher in malignancy. Most experts agree that PSA velocities that exceed 0.35 ng/mL per year indicate consideration for biopsy in men with low PSA levels and that PSA velocity should not be used alone but, rather, in conjunction with other laboratory tests when making the decision. **c.** The proportion of free PSA is within the interval associated with a low risk of prostate cancer. Furthermore, the patient's PSA velocity did not exceed 0.35 ng/mL per year, and the digital rectal examination did not detect any obvious sign of malignancy. Given the man's age, benign prostatic hypertrophy is likely, and further PSA testing after a waiting period may be warranted in lieu of a biopsy.

Answers to Review Questions

1. d	2. b	3. a	4. c	5. d	6. d	7. a
8. c	9. d	10. d	11. a	12. a	13. b	14. a
15. c						

Chapter 18 Immunoproliferative Diseases

Answers to Case Studies

1. a. The patient has evidence of anemia and pneumonia. The elevated erythrocytic sedimentation rate (ESR) is a nonspecific indicator of inflammation or elevated serum proteins. Based upon these findings, the physician requested the measurement of serum immunoglobulins. Elevated serum immunoglobulins can produce an elevated ESR. The extremely high IgG levels indicate that a monoclonal gammopathy is probably present. The patient is most likely suffering from multiple myeloma. Infiltration of cancerous myeloma cells into the bone marrow is likely to be responsible for the patient's anemia; despite having pneumonia, the white blood cell count is only slightly elevated. The back pain could also be caused by infiltration of myeloma cells into the vertebrae. The age of the patient is appropriate for the diagnosis of multiple myeloma. **b.** The diagnosis could be confirmed by performing a bone marrow biopsy because having more than 10% plasma cells in the bone marrow is one of the diagnostic criteria for multiple myeloma. Radiographs could reveal the presence of lytic bone lesions responsible for the patient's back pain. In addition, serum protein electrophoresis (SPE) could be used to detect a monoclonal band, and immunofixation electrophoresis (IFE) would be used to identify the suspected monoclonal IgG and possibly detect Bence Jones proteins in the patient's urine. Free light-chain assays can be used to determine the concentration of monoclonal light chains in the serum and the k/λ ratio.

2. a. Although hairy-cell leukemia (HCL) cells are not generally seen in the bone marrow, the hematologic bone marrow studies describe malignant cells characteristic of HCL. Splenomegaly is often seen in patients with HCL. **b.** Malignant HCL cells often express CD20 and CD25, the markers found in this patient. In addition, CD103 is a sensitive and specific marker for this disease. Although not tested for in this patient, CD123 is also a specific marker for HCL.

Answers to Review Questions

1. c 2. c 3. a 4. c 5. d 6. a 7. d
8. b 9. a 10. d 11. b 12. a 13. c 14. d
15. a

Chapter 19 Immunodeficiency Diseases

Answers to Case Studies

1. **a.** The constant bacterial infections coupled with laboratory results indicate an immunodeficiency disease, likely Bruton's tyrosine kinase deficiency or severe combined immunodeficiency syndrome (SCID). **b.** In both conditions, an X-linked recessive gene can be inherited, which affects males almost exclusively. **c.** To differentiate between the two immunodeficiency states, several types of testing are recommended. Measurement of serum IgA, IgM, and IgG levels should be performed to determine if, in fact, all classes of antibody are absent. Enumeration of classes of lymphocytes should also be determined by flow cytometry. In SCID, both T- and B-cell development is affected, and both lymphocyte populations would be deficient, whereas in Bruton's tyrosine kinase deficiency, only B-cell development is affected. Because the differential indicates that some lymphocytes are present, this would point to Bruton's tyrosine kinase deficiency. Flow cytometry findings confirming the presence of T cells can validate this diagnosis.

2. **a.** The patient's specimen is seen in region 4. Note the faint, diffuse IgG and light-chain bands. IgA or IgM bands are barely visible. Specimen 1 is a normal control. Specimen 2 contains a monoclonal IgG kappa protein. Specimen 3 is a concentrated 24-hour urine specimen that contains albumin. **b.** Her history and the SPE results indicate that she is immunocompromised and producing very little antibody. The faint immunoglobulin bands confirm the other laboratory findings.

Answers to Review Questions

1. c 2. c 3. d 4. a 5. b 6. a 7. d
8. d 9. a 10. b 11. d 12. a 13. c 14. d
15. b

Chapter 20 Serological and Molecular Detection of Bacterial Infections

Answers to Case Studies

1. **a.** Poststreptococcal glomerulonephritis. **b.** *Streptococcus pyogenes* (group A streptococci). **c.** Streptococcal antigen–antibody complexes may deposit in the glomeruli of the kidneys, or antibody formed against the organisms may cross-react with antigens in the glomeruli. These immune responses stimulate an inflammatory response that causes damage to the glomeruli, leading to renal impairment and function. The rapid GAS test was negative because the organism is no longer present in the throat and the patient did not present with pharyngitis. **d.** A urinalysis is helpful because microscopic hematuria is typically present in children with acute poststreptococcal glomerulonephritis. The proteinuria rarely exceeds 3+ by dipstick; however, massive proteinuria and a nephrotic picture may be observed in a small percentage of patients. **e.** The streptozyme test measures antibodies against five extracellular streptococcal antigens: anti-streptolysin (ASO), anti-hyaluronidase (AHase), anti-streptokinase (ASKase), anti-nicotinamide-adenine dinucleotidase (anti-NAD), and anti-DNAse B. The streptozyme test is positive in 95% of patients with acute post-streptococcal glomerulonephritis caused by GAS pharyngitis.

2. **a.** *Mycoplasma pneumoniae.* **b.** The patient has only been ill for several days and has not had time to mount a serological response to the causative agent. IgG levels suggest that the patient had a previous exposure to the organism, and the level may represent residual IgG from an earlier exposure. **c.** Definitive diagnosis of *M. pneumoniae* requires documented seroconversion by paired specimens obtained 2 to 4 weeks apart, measuring both IgM and IgG. A four-fold rise in IgG levels is considered diagnostic. **d.** Cold agglutinin titers used for the diagnosis of *M. pneumoniae* infections are not very specific or very sensitive. Testing for cold agglutinins is no longer recommended for the detection of *M. pneumoniae* infections because the development of cold agglutinins occurs in other conditions, including some viral infections and collagen vascular diseases. Although not specific for of *M. pneumoniae* infection, a high cold agglutinin titer in a patient with community-acquired pneumonia symptoms (>1:64) is likely to be caused by *M. pneumoniae.*

Answers to Review Questions

1. d 2. c 3. b 4. b 5. d 6. a 7. b
8. d 9. c 10. c 11. a 12. b 13. c 14. c
15. b

Chapter 21 Spirochete Diseases

Answers to Case Studies

1. **a.** Almost 25% of individuals with Lyme disease do not exhibit the characteristic rash; therefore, its absence does not rule out the possibility of the disease. **b.** There are several conditions that can cause false-positive results in EIA testing, including syphilis, other treponemal diseases, infectious mononucleosis, and autoimmune diseases such as rheumatoid arthritis. Thus, low levels of antibody might indicate one of these other diseases. However, false-negative results in Lyme disease are also possible because of a low level of antibody production. Therefore, an indeterminate test neither rules out nor confirms the presence of Lyme disease. **c.** If there is a history of tick bite and patient symptoms are consistent with Lyme disease, then a confirmatory test such as a different EIA or a Western blot should be performed. The Western blot is fairly specific for Lyme disease. If 5 of 10 protein bands specific for *Borrelia burgdorferi* IgG antibodies are positive, this confirms the presence of Lyme disease.

2. **a.** Although it is possible that the mother's positive RPR test could be a false positive, it is also likely that the mother is in the latent stage of syphilis, with no obvious signs of the disease. Although syphilis is not sexually transmitted during this stage, it can be transmitted from a mother to her unborn

child. Many infants do not exhibit clinical signs of the disease at birth; however, if infected and untreated, a large percentage of babies develop later symptoms, including neurological deficits such as blindness and mental retardation. **b.** A positive RPR on cord blood could be from transplacental passage of the mother's IgG antibodies. A titer should be performed on the cord blood and a serum sample obtained from the infant in several weeks. If infection is present in the infant, the titer will remain the same or increase. An IgM capture assay could also be performed on the infant's serum. The presence of specific anti-treponemal IgM would indicate that the infant had been exposed to *Treponema pallidum* because IgM antibodies do not cross the placenta. **c.** Because there is a good chance that the infant is at risk for congenital syphilis, immediate treatment with penicillin can prevent any further neurological consequences. **d.** A positive RPR test indicates the presence of nonspecific reagin antibodies produced against host-cell cardiolipin, cholesterol, and lecithin. As these antibodies are generally produced during pregnancy and certain malignancies, syphilis diagnosis should be confirmed by doing a treponemal-specific test such as the TP-PA or FTA-ABS.

Answers to Review Questions

1. d 2. c 3. b 4. d 5. b 6. c 7. c
8. d 9. b 10. d 11. d 12. b 13. c 14. c
15. c 16. c 17. d 18. c

Chapter 22 Serological and Molecular Diagnosis of Parasitic and Fungal Infections

Answers to Case Studies

1. a. It cannot be determined by the test results available whether the baby has congenital toxoplasmosis. The IgG antibodies in the newborn may reflect maternal antibodies that crossed the placenta. The presence of IgG antibodies in the newborn may reflect either past or recent infection in the mother. IgM antibodies may persist for up to 18 months after infection with *T. gondii*. Thus, the greatest value of testing for IgM antibodies is in determining whether a woman has had a recent infection. If no IgM antibodies are detected and only IgG is detected, this excludes a recent infection before pregnancy. The presence of IgG and IgM in the mother may indicate a recent infection. **b.** Tests for IgA and IgM antibodies are commonly used for the diagnosis of infection in the newborn. If IgG, IgM, and IgA are detected, a diagnosis of congenital toxoplasmosis is established. If IgG antibodies are detected but serological test results for IgM and IgA antibodies are negative, follow-up serological testing in suspected cases is indicated. Maternally transferred antibodies usually decrease and disappear within 6 to 12 months. Established infection in the mother can also be indicated by the presence of high-avidity IgG antibodies.

2. a. The majority of patients with symptomatic cryptococcosis have an identified underlying immunocompromised condition. These include AIDS, prolonged treatment with corticosteroids, organ transplantation, advanced malignancy, diabetes, and sarcoidosis. The clinical symptoms and outcome of cryptococcal meningitis vary, in part because of the related underlying medical conditions and the immune status of the host. The most common symptoms are headache, altered mental status, personality changes, confusion, lethargy, and coma. Nausea and vomiting are also common and are caused by increased intracranial pressure. Onset of the disease is often subacute and worsens over several weeks. The patient in this case was immunosuppressed because of his long-term steroid use and presented with severe headaches, gait instability, and weakness upon standing. **b.** The simplest diagnostic test is an India ink test on the patient's CSF. Because of the large polysaccharide capsule produced by the organism, the India ink is displaced, allowing for visualization of the yeast. The serological tests for cryptococcal antigen in serum and CSF are highly sensitive and specific for the diagnosis of invasive disease. These newer methods include latex agglutination and immunochromatographic assays for the detection of the capsular antigen in serum and CSF.

Answers to Review Questions

1. d 2. d 3. d 4. a 5. b 6. b 7. a
8. a 9. d 10. b 11. d 12. a 13. b 14. d
15. c 16. c

Chapter 23 Serological and Molecular Detection of Viral Infections

Answers to Case Studies

1. a. The patient's clinical symptoms and increase in liver function enzymes indicate inflammation of the liver. In order to determine whether this inflammation is because of viral hepatitis and to identify the cause, the following tests should be ordered: (1) IgM anti-HAV to screen for hepatitis A, (2) HBsAg to screen for hepatitis B, (3) IgM anti-HBc to screen for hepatitis B in the core window period when HBsAg is absent, and (4) anti-HCV to screen for hepatitis C. **b.** In order to monitor hepatitis B infection, testing for HBsAg and HBeAg should be performed periodically to determine how long the infection is persisting and the relative infectivity of the patient. Tests for anti-HBe and anti-HBs are performed to indicate whether the infection has resolved and whether immunity has been established, respectively. **c.** In chronic hepatitis B, HBsAg persists in the serum for more than 6 months. Total anti-HBc is also present, and HBeAg may or may not be present, depending on the degree of disease progression. Anti-HBe and anti-HBs are usually not present but may have a delayed appearance in those individuals who eventually recover.

2. a. Many viruses can produce congenital abnormalities in an infant born to a mother infected during pregnancy. These include cytomegalovirus, rubella virus, and varicella zoster virus. The infant's symptoms and mother's history suggest infection with rubella virus. **b.** Ideally, the mother would have been tested at the time of her illness during her pregnancy for rubella antibodies. Demonstration of rubella-specific IgM antibody, seroconversion from negative to positive for rubella antibody, or a four-fold rise in antibody titer would have indicated an active rubella infection. However, because this was not done, the mother could be tested for rubella-specific IgG antibody, which would indicate rubella exposure in the past but would not provide information as to when the exposure occurred. **c.** The infant's serum should be tested for rubella-specific IgM antibody, preferably with an IgM antibody capture enzyme immunoassay. IgM antibodies, which cannot pass through the placenta, would have been produced by the fetus because of active rubella infection. IgG antibodies, on the other hand, are derived mainly from the mother's serum because of passive transfer through the placenta.

Answers to Review Questions

1. c 2. d 3. b 4. a 5. d 6. b 7. a
8. d 9. b 10. c 11. c 12. c 13. d 14. a
15. c

Chapter 24 Laboratory Diagnosis of HIV Infection

1. a. The physician should order an FDA-approved immunoassay that simultaneously detects antibodies to HIV-1, antibodies to HIV-2, and p24 antigen. **b.** If the combination immunoassay was positive, a rapid test for HIV-1 and HIV-2 antibodies should be performed to confirm the results and distinguish between infection by the two viruses. **c.** If it was determined that the woman truly has HIV infection, her CD4 T-cell counts should be monitored periodically to assess the effects of the virus on her immune system. In addition, she should be placed on antiretroviral therapy, and the effectiveness of the therapy should be evaluated by periodically performing viral load assays to monitor the amount of HIV RNA in her plasma.

2. a. HIV infection is transmitted from mother to infant by three ways: (1) passage through the placenta during pregnancy, (2) exposure to maternal blood during the delivery process, or (3) through breast milk. In order to reduce the risk of transmission, antiretroviral therapy should be administered to the mother during her pregnancy and to the infant after birth. In addition, the mother should be advised not to breastfeed her baby. **b.** Testing the infant's serum for HIV antibody would yield confusing results. This is because the IgG HIV antibodies in the mother's serum pass through the placenta during the pregnancy and would be detectable in the infant's serum. The result would be a false positive if the infant was not HIV-infected. **c.** Because of the problems associated with antibody testing, molecular methods are preferred to make a diagnosis of HIV infection in infants younger than 18 months of age. The preferred molecular test is a PCR that detects the presence of proviral HIV DNA in the infant's peripheral blood mononuclear cells. Alternately, a quantitative HIV RNA test could be performed on the infant's plasma.

Answers to Review Questions

1. c 2. c 3. d 4. a 5. d 6. b 7. a
8. b 9. c 10. d 11. d 12. a 13. a 14. b
15. d

Chapter 25 Immunization and Vaccines

Answers to Case Studies

1. a. The child could safely receive vaccines that do not contain a live component. These include the vaccines for hepatitis B (a recombinant antigen); diphtheria and tetanus (toxoids); pertussis, *Haemophilus* influenza b, and pneumococcus (subunit vaccines); and polio, hepatitis A, and influenza (the preparations containing inactivated virus). **b.** The child could not receive any live, attenuated vaccines because the organisms in these vaccines, although weakened, may not be controlled by the child's immune system and could cause serious, disseminated infections. Such vaccines include those against the viral diseases: measles, mumps, rubella, varicella, and rotavirus. The nasal mist form of the influenza vaccine should also not be administered because it contains live, attenuated virus. **c.** The child could be protected against these infections by receiving regular injections of human immune serum globulin (gamma globulin), a preparation that has been pooled from the serum of other individuals and that contains numerous premade antibodies. In addition, family members and close friends of the child should make sure that they are up to date on their own immunizations. By preventing the development of these diseases in themselves, they are ensuring that they cannot pass the pathogen along to the child. This concept, whereby protection against infectious diseases is extended to others in a population, is known as "community immunity" or "herd immunity."

2. a. Hepatitis A–specific human immune serum globulin, consisting of a high concentration of antibody to the hepatitis A virus, should be used to prevent the infection in anyone who has dined at the restaurant recently. Because this preparation is derived from individuals who have previously been exposed to hepatitis A, the antibodies are premade and provide immediate protection when they are administered within 2 weeks after exposure to the pathogen. **b.** Although human immune serum globulin provides immediate protection, that protection is only temporary because the antibody titers decline over time, according to the half-life of the immunoglobulin molecules. The half-life for IgG, which comprises the majority of the preparation, is 23 days. To achieve long-term immunity without actually acquiring the infection, you would need to be immunized with the hepatitis A vaccine. The vaccine, consisting of inactivated hepatitis A virus, would stimulate an immune response against the viral antigens and the generation of memory lymphocytes that could quickly be reactivated in case of a later exposure.

Answers to Review Questions

1. a 2. c 3. d 4. b 5. d 6. c 7. b
8. d 9. d 10. c 11. c 12. b 13. c 14. a
15. b

Index

References followed by the letter "f" are for figures, "t" are for tables.